PDR FOR NUTRITIONAL SUPPLEMENTS

FIRST EDITION

PDR®

for Nutritional Supplements™

MEDICAL ECONOMICS™

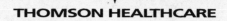

THOMSON HEALTHCARE

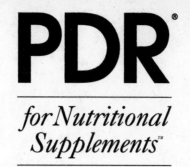

PDR® for Nutritional Supplements™

CHIEF EDITORS
Sheldon Saul Hendler, PhD, MD
David Rorvik, MS

PHARMACEUTICAL EDITOR
Thomas Fleming, RPh

ASSISTANT EDITORS
Maria Deutsch, MS, PharmD, CDE
Christine Wyble, PharmD

PRODUCTION MANAGER
Lydia F. Biagioli

SENIOR DATA MANAGER
Jeffrey D. Schaefer

INDEX SUPERVISOR
Johanna M. Mazur

INDEX EDITORS
Noel Deloughery
Shannon Reilly

PRODUCTION MANAGER, PRODUCT IDENTIFICATION GUIDE
Amy Brooks

ELECTRONIC PUBLISHING DESIGNER
Livio Udina

MANAGER, APPLICATION DEVELOPMENT
Thomas V. Dougherty

SENIOR TECHNOLOGY SPECIALIST
Stephen Crovatto

PROGRAMMER ANALYSTS
Kent Hudson
Chris McCabe

DESIGN DIRECTOR
Robert Hartman

PUBLISHING STAFF
Executive Vice President, Directory Services:
Paul Walsh

Vice President, Sales and Marketing:
Dikran N. Barsamian

National Sales Manager, Medical Economics Trade Sales: Bill Gaffney

Associate Product Manager: Jason Springer

Senior Business Manager: Mark S. Ritchin

Director of Direct Marketing: Michael Bennett

Direct Mail Manager: Lorraine M. Loening

Senior Marketing Analyst: Dina A. Maeder

Associate Promotion Manager: Linda Levine

Vice President, Clinical Communications and New Business Development:
Mukesh Mehta, RPh

New Business Development Manager:
Jeffrey D. Dubin

Editor, Directory Services: David W. Sifton

Project Manager: Edward P. Connor

Senior Associate Editor: Lori Murray

Assistant Editor: Gwynned L. Kelly

Director of Production: Brian Holland

Production Coordinators: Gianna Caradonna, Dee Ann DeRuvo, Melissa Katz, Christina Klinger

Format Editor: Stu W. Lehrer

Art Associate: Joan K. Akerlind

Digital Imaging Supervisor: Shawn W. Cahill

Digital Imaging Coordinator:
Frank J. McElroy, III

Fulfillment Managers: Stephanie DeNardi, Louis Bolcik

OFFICERS OF THOMSON HEALTHCARE:
Chief Executive Officer: Michael Tansey; *Chief Operating Officer:* Richard Noble; *Chief Financial Officer and Executive Vice President, Finance:* Paul Hilger; *Executive Vice President, Directory Services:* Paul Walsh; *Senior Vice President, Planning and Business Development:* William Gole; *Vice President, Human Resources:* Pamela M. Bilash

ISBN: 1-56363-364-7

Contents

Foreword

With three out of four Americans now using nutritional supplements on a regular basis, the need for an objective source of information on this contentious and confusing field has never been greater. Although the specific benefits of many familiar nutrients are widely known and thoroughly documented, the claims for many others remain highly speculative—and until now, there has been no single, comprehensive compendium to which to turn for an authoritative evaluation.

It's clear that a new kind of reference work has been urgently needed—a reference that weighs the available scientific evidence, makes the appropriate conclusions, and presents the pertinent facts in a clear, accessible manner. Drawing on over half a century's experience in the dissemination of pharmaceutical information, *Physicians' Desk Reference* is proud to present precisely such a reference: the new *PDR for Nutritional Supplements*.

This unique new handbook affords you the guidance of one of the nation's most respected authorities on clinical nutrition, Sheldon S. Hendler. With a PhD in biochemistry and molecular biology from Columbia University, postdoctoral training at the Salk Institute, and an MD from the University of California, San Diego, Dr. Hendler is superbly equipped to weigh the merits of therapeutic claims and present the evidence pro and con. As the editor of the *Journal of Medicinal Food* and the author of more than 50 peer-reviewed papers, he brings unmatched insight to this often controversial field.

With the assistance of co-author David Rorvik, science and medicine reporter for *Time Magazine* and contributor to a host of national publications, Dr. Hendler has forged a concise, yet comprehensive overview of the entire spectrum of current nutritional products, from the most widely used vitamins and minerals to exotica like shark cartilage and royal jelly. In all, you'll find over 200 monographs covering nearly 1,000 nutritional products. Included are an extensive array of amino acids and oligopeptides, fatty acids and other lipids, metabolites and cofactors, nucleic acids, proteins, glycosupplements, phytosupplements, hormonal products, and probiotics. Indeed, whatever a patient's concern may be, you're likely to find an answer here.

The monographs on these products are designed to arm you with all the information you need to forge rational recommendations and protect your patients' health. In addition to providing a penetrating summary of significant clinical research, they address all the practical issues encountered during routine use, from proper dosage to crucial precautions. Each monograph includes up to eleven standard sections. Here's a closer look at what they contain.

■ **Trade Names:** Listed here are the most widely distributed brands of the various formulations of the nutrient.

■ **Description:** This section provides a detailed discussion of the nature of the substance and its place in human biochemistry, along with its precise chemical structure.

■ **Actions and Pharmacology:** Here you'll find an overview of the nutrient's better documented actions, the proposed or verified mechanisms through which it exerts its effects, and its pharmacokinetics, including absorption, metabolism, and excretion.

■ **Indications and Usage:** Described here are the specific therapeutic uses proposed for the supplement, ranging from the accepted indications to the more speculative possibilities.

■ **Research Summary:** This section enumerates the leading claims made for the substance and evaluates the merits of each. Included are the most significant findings, both pro and con, drawn from retrospective reviews, meta-analyses, and controlled clinical trials.

■ **Contraindications, Precautions, Adverse Reactions:** Here you'll find the important safety considerations to remember when recommending the supplement and while monitoring the patient's progress.

■ **Interactions:** Listed here are the drugs, herbs, foods, and supplements with which the substance may interact. The effect of each combination is summarized, along with the appropriate action to take as a result.

■ **Overdosage:** This section presents the warning signs of overdose (if any are known) and summarized emergency treatment measures.

■ **Dosage and Administration:** Described here are typical dosage recommendations for each formulation of the substance, together with any special measures to be taken during administration.

■ **How Supplied:** This section lists available dosage forms and strengths of each formulation and salt.

■ **Literature:** Here you'll find relevant citations from the clinical literature.

To help you quickly locate the information you require, the monographs have been indexed by supplement name, trade names, nutritional category, indications, side effects, adjunctive uses, and manufacturers. You'll also find all the interactions cited in the text listed by both the agents in each combination. Here's an overview of what each index provides.

■ **Supplement Name Index:** This index lists nutrients by all the names most frequently employed in literature. Names that serve as monograph titles are highlighted by bold type. Alternative names and associated forms are cross-referenced to the appropriate monograph.

■ **Brand Name Index:** A guide to all the trade names cited in the monographs and combination-product tables. Items pictured in the book's Product Identification Guide are marked with a ◆ symbol.

■ **Category Index:** In this index, the monographs are listed by type, such as glycosupplements, hormones, and probiotics.

■ **Indications Index:** This index directs you to the nutrients customarily used for a particular therapeutic or preventive purpose. For ease of comparison with prescription and over-the-counter medications, the index employs the same headings found in the Indications Index of the *PDR Companion Guide.*

■ **Side Effects Index:** Here the monographs are grouped by potential adverse reactions cited in the text. Like the Indications Index, this index employs nomenclature used in the *PDR Companion Guide.*

■ **Interactions Guide:** This section lists problem combinations by both the name of the nutrient and the name of the interacting agent. Drug, herb, and food interactions are included. A description of the interaction's potential effect appears in each entry.

■ **Companion Drug Index:** This handy section suggests nutritional supplements that may be used, in conjunction with prescription drug therapy, to reverse drug-induced side effects, relieve symptoms of the illness itself, or treat sequelae of the initial disease. Supplements, together with their associated brands, are listed alphabetically under each condition. Brands pictured in the Product Identification Guide are marked with a ◆ symbol.

■ **Manufacturers Index:** Turn to this index for contact information on each supplier with products cited in the book. Listed products follow the company's contact information. Brands pictured in the Product Identification Guide are marked with a ◆ symbol.

Following the indices there's an extensive full-color Product Identification Guide that presents photos of some of the more popular commercial formulations. And at the end of the book, you'll find five tables designed to permit quick comparisons of combination products. Included are:

■ Calcium Combination Products
■ Iron Combination Products
■ Multivitamin Products
■ Multivitamin and Mineral Products
■ Vitamin B Complex Products

PDR for Nutritional Supplements is the product of one of the most thorough and inclusive examinations of the literature ever undertaken. Nevertheless, it's important to remember that it merely summarizes and synthesizes key data from the underlying reports, and of necessity includes neither every published report nor every recorded fact.

As in all scientific investigation, conclusions regarding the effectiveness of the supplements discussed in this compendium are based on the preponderance of current evidence and cannot be considered firm or final. The publisher does not warrant that any substance will unfailingly and uniformly exhibit the properties ascribed to it by researchers in the field.

Also, please remember that the products discussed in this book are marketed under the provisions of the Dietary Supplement and Health Education Act of 1994, which prohibits their sale for the diagnosis, treatment, cure, or prevention of any disease. The monographs in this compendium discuss scientific findings regarding the substance itself, and should not be construed as recommending any specific commercial preparation. Enumeration of specific products within a monograph implies no claim or warranty of their efficacy for any purpose, by either the manufacturer or the publisher. Furthermore, it should be understood that, just as omission of a product does not signify rejection, inclusion of a product does not imply endorsement, and that the publisher is not advocating the use of any product or substance described herein.

Please remember, too, that the potency and the purity of nutritional supplements are subject to substantial variation. Dosage ranges set forth in the monographs must therefore be employed only as general guidelines. Likewise, safety information found in the monographs applies only to the substance itself, and does not account for the effects of adulterants and variations in the manufacturing process.

In addition, the publisher does not guarantee that every possible hazard, adverse effect, contraindication, precaution, or consequence of overdose is included in the summaries presented here. The publisher has performed no independent verification of the data reported herein, and expressly disclaims responsibility for any error, whether inherent in the underlying literature or resulting from erroneous translation, transcription, or typography.

When patients approach you—as they surely will—for advice on the latest nutritional "discovery" to hit the nightly news, we hope that *PDR for Nutritional Supplements* will provide you with all the facts you need to offer sound, rational guidance firmly grounded in fact. Certainly such counseling is the aim of every dedicated health care professional. And at *PDR*, we fully share that goal.

Supplement Name Index

This index lists nutrients by the names most frequently employed in the literature. Names that serve as monograph titles appear in bold type. Alternative names and associated forms are cross-referenced to the appropriate monograph.

Brand Name Index

This index lists the trade names cited in the monographs and combination-product tables. Items pictured in the Product Identification Guide are marked with a [♦] symbol. A page number prefixed by "G" refers to the location of the product's photo. An italic page number denotes a listing in the combination-product tables.

Category Index

In this index, monographs are organized by type of nutrient. United States Adopted Names (USAN) and commonly used acronyms follow the supplement names when applicable. To locate supplements advocated for a specific medical problem or purpose, please consult the Indications Index.

Indications Index

Entries in this index are organized by specific complaint, enabling you to quickly review the nutritional measures appropriate to a given situation. United States Adopted Names (USAN) and commonly used acronyms follow the supplement names when applicable. For ease of comparison with prescription and over-the-counter medications, the index employs the same headings found in the Indications Index of the PDR Companion Guide.

Side Effects Index

Presented here is an alphabetical list of every potential side effect cited in the book. Under each side effect is a list of the monographs in which it appears. United States Adopted Names (USAN) and commonly used acronyms follow the supplement names when applicable. For ease of comparison with prescription and over-the-counter medications, the index employs the same headings found in the Side Effects Index of the PDR Companion Guide.

Interactions Guide

This section catalogs potentially adverse interactions between nutritional supplements and drugs, herbs, alcohol, food, tobacco, and other nutrients. Under each bold-face entry, you'll find a list of potentially interactive substances. A description of the interaction's effect follows each item in the list. All interactions are indexed under each element in the combination.

5-HT1 RECEPTOR AGONISTS
5-Hydroxytryptophan
(5-HTP may increase risk of side effects)
Myo-Inositol
(May have additive effects with Myo-Inositol)

5-HYDROXYTRYPTOPHAN
5-HT1 Receptor Agonists
(5-HTP may increase risk of side effects)
Carbidopa
(Increases 5-HTP levels in the brain)
Cyproheptadine Hydrochloride
(5-HTP may decrease effects)
Hypericum
(5-HTP may potentiate antidepressant effects and increase risk of side effects)
Methyldopa
(Inhibits 5-HTP metabolism to serotonin)
Methysergide Maleate
(5-HTP may decrease effects)
Monoamine Oxidase Inhibitors
(5-HTP may increase risk of side effects)
Phenoxybenzamine Hydrochloride
(Inhibits 5-HTP metabolism to serotonin)
Serotoninergic Agents
(5-HTP may potentiate antidepressant effects and increase risk of side effects)

Vitamin B6
(May enhance 5-HTP conversion to serotonin)

ACE INHIBITORS
Potassium
(Increased serum Potassium due to inhibition of aldosterone production)

ABCIXIMAB
Alpha-Tocopheryl Polyethylene
Glycol Succinate
(Enhanced antiplatelet effects of abciximab)
Gamma-Tocopherol
(Increased effects of abciximab)
Vitamin E
(Increased effects of abciximab)

ACARBOSE
Inositol Nicotinate
(High dose nicotinic acid may antagonize effects)
Niacin
(High dose nicotinic acid may antagonize effects)
Supplemental Enzymes
(Decreased efficacy of acarbose with amylase, pancreatin, and pancrelipase)

ACETAMINOPHEN
L-Methionine
(L-Methionine may decrease hepatic toxicity with overdosage)

Molybdenum
(High dose molybdate may inhibit acetaminophen metabolism)

ACETYL-L-CARNITINE
Didanosine
(May lead to decreased Acetyl-L-Carnitine levels)
Stavudine
(May lead to decreased Acetyl-L-Carnitine levels)
Valproic Acid
(May lead to L-Carnitine deficiencies)
Zalcitabine
(May lead to decreased Acetyl-L-Carnitine levels)

ACETYLCYSTEINE
Carbamazepine
(Reduced serum levels with NAC)
Nitrates and Nitrites
(May cause headaches with NAC)

ACITRETIN
Vitamin A
(May produce additive toxicity effects)

ACTIVATED CHARCOAL
Drugs, unspecified
(Avoid using Activated Charcoal within two hours of taking these products)
Food, unspecified
(Avoid using Activated Charcoal within two hours of taking these products)

Herbal Medicines, unspecified
(Avoid using Activated Charcoal within two hours of taking these products)

Nutritional Supplement
(Avoid using Activated Charcoal within two hours of taking these products)

ALCOHOL

Gamma-Hydroxybutyrate (GHB)
(May be life threatening with GHB)

Vitamin B6
(Chronic and excessive use may cause Vitamin B6 deficiency)

ALL-TRANS-RETINOIC ACID

Vitamin A
(May produce additive toxicity effects)

ALLIUM SATIVUM

Alpha-Tocopheryl Polyethylene Glycol Succinate
(Enhanced antithrombotic activity of garlic)

Borage Oil
(Interactions may occur with Borage Oil)

Eicosapentaenoic Acid (EPA)
(May interact with EPA)

Evening Primrose Oil
(EPO may increase bleeding tendencies)

Fish Oil
(May interact with Fish Oil)

Flaxseed Oil
(May interact with Flaxseed Oil)

Gamma-Tocopherol
(Enhanced antithrombotic activity of garlic)

Perilla Oil
(Increased antithrombotic effects with Perilla Oil)

Tocotrienols
(May enhance antithrombotic activity)

Vitamin E
(Enhanced antithrombotic activity of garlic)

ALPHA ADRENERGIC BLOCKERS

Inositol Nicotinate
(High dose nicotinic acid may potentiate hypotensive effects)

Niacin
(High dose nicotinic acid may potentiate hypotensive effects)

ALPHA-CAROTENE

Phytosterols
(Low serum levels due to Phytosterols)

ALPHA GALACTOSIDASE ENZYME

Prebiotics
(Decreased effectiveness of the soy oligosaccharides)

ALPHA TOCOPHERAL ACETATE

Gamma-Tocopherol
(Decreased plasma Gamma-Tocopherol levels)

ALPHA-LIPOIC ACID

Antidiabetic Drugs, unspecified
(Increased effect with Alpha-Lipoic Acid)

ALPHA-TOCOPHERYL POLYETHYLENE GLYCOL SUCCINATE

Abciximab
(Enhanced antiplatelet effects of abciximab)

Allium sativum
(Enhanced antithrombotic activity of garlic)

Antiplatelet Drugs
(Enhanced effects of antiplatelet drugs)

Aspirin
(Enhanced antiplatelet effects of aspirin)

Clopidogrel Bisulfate
(Enhanced antiplatelet effects of clopidogrel)

Coenzyme Q10
(Increased absorption of Coenzyme Q10)

Cyclosporine
(Increased absorption of cyclosporine)

Dipyridamole
(Enhanced antiplatelet effects of dipyridamole)

Eptifibatide
(Enhanced antiplatelet effects of eptifibatide)

Flavonoids
(Increased absorption of flavonoids)

Gamma-tocopherol
(Increased absorption when taken with TPGS; Decreased plasma levels with high doses of TPGS)

Ginkgo biloba
(Enhanced antithrombotic activity of gingko biloba)

Lipophilic drugs, unspecified
(Increased absorption of lipophilic drugs)

Polyphenols
(Increased absorption of polyphenols)

Selenium
(May function synergistically with Alpha-Tocopherol)

Ticlopidine Hydrochloride
(Enhanced antiplatelet effects of ticlopidine)

Tirofiban Hydrochloride
(Enhanced antiplatelet effects of tirofiban)

Tocotrienols
(Increased absorption when taken with TPGS; Decreased plasma levels with high doses of TPGS)

Vitamin A
(Increased absorption of Vitamin A)

Vitamin C
(May help maintain Alpha-Tocopherol in its reduced (antioxidant) form)

Vitamin D
(Increased absorption of Vitamin D)

Vitamin E
(Increased absorption with TPGS)

Vitamin K
(Increased absorption of Vitamin K)

Warfarin Sodium
(Enhanced anticoagulant response of warfarin)

ALPRAZOLAM
DHEA
  (May increase DHEA levels)

ALUMINUM HYDROXIDE
Vanadium
  (May decrease absorption of
  Vanadium)

**ALUMINUM-CONTAINING COMPOUNDS,
UNSPECIFIED**
Ascorbyl Palmitate
  (Large dose Vitamin C may
  increase urinary Aluminum
  excretion)
Silicon
  (Prevention of absorption due to
  Silicon)
Vitamin C
  (Large dose Vitamin C may
  increase urinary aluminum
  excretion)

AMILORIDE HYDROCHLORIDE
Potassium
  (Concomitant potassium-sparing
  diuretic and Potassium
  supplements can produce severe
  hyperkalemia)

AMINOBENZOIC ACID
(*See under* Para-Aminobenzoic Acid)

AMINOGLUTETHIMIDE
Chrysin
  (Chrysin may have additive
  effects)

AMIODARONE HYDROCHLORIDE
Arnica
  (Increased risk of prolonged QT
  interval when given with Arnica)
Vitamin B6
  (Concomitant Vitamin B6 may
  enhance amiodarone-induced
  photosensitivity)
Vitamin E
  (Alpha-tocopherol may ameliorate
  some adverse side effects of
  amiodarone)

AMITRIPTYLINE HYDROCHLORIDE
Arnica
  (Increased risk of prolonged QT
  interval when given with Arnica)

AMOXICILLIN
Bromelain
  (Bromelain may increase
  amoxicillin levels)

ANASTROZOLE
Chrysin
  (Chrysin may have additive
  effects)

ANDROSTENEDIOL
DHEA
  (May increase adverse effects of
  DHEA)

ANDROSTENEDIONE
DHEA
  (May increase adverse effects of
  DHEA)

ANTACIDS, ALUMINUM-CONTAINING
Fluoride
  (Decreased absorption of Fluoride)
Iron
  (Decreased absorption of Iron)
Phosphorus
  (Decreased absorption of
  Phosphorus)

ANTACIDS, MAGNESIUM-CONTAINING
Manganese
  (Decreased absorption of
  Manganese)

ANTACIDS, NON-ABSORBABLE
Lactulose
  (May increase Lactulose effects)

ANTACIDS, UNSPECIFIED
Indole-3-Carbinol
  (Block the conversion of Indole-3-
  Carbinol to DIM and ICZ)

**ANTIBIOTICS, BROAD SPECTRUM,
UNSPECIFIED**
Vitamin K
  (May decrease Vitamin K
  availability)

ANTIBIOTICS, UNSPECIFIED
Biotin
  (May decrease Biotin absorption)
Vitamin B12
  (May alter intestinal microflora to
  decrease Vitamin B12 absorption)

ANTICHOLINESTERASE DRUGS
Huperzine A
  (Additive effects and increased
  adverse effects with Huperzine A)

ANTICOAGULANT DRUGS, UNSPECIFIED
Borage Oil
  (Increased anticoagulant and
  antiplatelet effects with Borage
  Oil)
Bromelain
  (Bromelain may enhance
  anticoagulant effects)
Tiratricol (TRIAC)
  (Increased hypoprothrombinemic
  effect)

ANTICONVULSANTS
Gamma-Hydroxybutyrate (GHB)
  (May be life threatening with
  GHB)

**ANTIDEPRESSANT MEDICATIONS,
UNSPECIFIED**
Melatonin
  (May increase sedation and
  adverse effects with Melatonin)

ANTIDIABETIC DRUGS, UNSPECIFIED
Alpha-Lipoic Acid
  (Increased effect with Alpha-
  Lipoic Acid)
Coenzyme Q10 (CoQ10)
  (May need dosing adjustments)
D-Ribose
  (D-Ribose may cause
  hypoglycemia)
Glucosamine
  (Glucosamine may increase insulin
  resistance)

ANTIHISTAMINES
Gamma-Hydroxybutyrate (GHB)
  (May be life threatening with
  GHB)
L-Histidine
  (L-Histidine might decrease the
  efficacy of antihistamines)
Melatonin
  (May increase sedation and
  adverse effects with Melatonin)

ANTIPLATELET DRUGS

Alpha-Tocopheryl Polyethylene
Glycol Succinate
  (Enhanced effects of antiplatelet
  drugs)
Borage Oil
  (Increased anticoagulant and
  antiplatelet effects with Borage
  Oil)
Curcuminoids
  (Curcuminoids may enhance the
  antiplatelet effect)
Gamma-Tocopherol
  (Increased effects of antiplatelet
  drugs)
Green Tea Catechins
  (Enhanced effect with Green Tea
  Catechins)
Myco-Polysaccharides
  (Ganoderma may enhance
  antiplatelet effects)
Tocotrienols
  (Tocotrienol may potentiate
  antiplatelet effects)
Vitamin E
  (Increased effects of antiplatelet
  drugs)

ANTITHROMBOTIC AGENTS

Bromelain
  (Bromelain may enhance
  antithrombotic effects)

ANTITHYROID AGENTS

Iodine
  (May potentiate the hypothyroid
  effect of iodides)

ARGININE

(*See under* L-Arginine)

ARNICA

Amiodarone Hydrochloride
  (Increased risk of prolonged QT
  interval with Arnica)
Amitriptyline Hydrochloride
  (Increased risk of prolonged QT
  interval with Arnica)
Chlorpromazine
  (Increased risk of prolonged QT
  interval with Arnica)
Desipramine Hydrochloride
  (Increased risk of prolonged QT
  interval with Arnica)

Disopyramide
  (Increased risk of prolonged QT
  interval with Arnica)
Doxepin Hydrochloride
  (Increased risk of prolonged QT
  interval with Arnica)
Doxorubicin Hydrochloride
  (Increased cardiotoxicity with
  Arnica)
Haloperidol
  (Increased risk of prolonged QT
  interval with Arnica)
Pentamidine Isethionate
  (Increased risk of prolonged QT
  interval with Arnica)
Procainamide
  (Increased risk of prolonged QT
  interval with Arnica)
Prochlorperazine
  (Increased risk of prolonged QT
  interval with Arnica)
Quinidine
  (Increased risk of prolonged QT
  interval with Arnica)
Sotalol Hydrochloride
  (Increased risk of prolonged QT
  interval with Arnica)

AROMATASE INHIBITORS

Chrysin
  (Chrysin may have additive
  effects)

ASCORBATE

Chromium
  (Increased absorption of
  Chromium)

ASCORBIC ACID

(*See under* Vitamin C)

ASCORBYL PALMITATE

Aluminum-containing Compounds,
unspecified
  (Large dose Vitamin C may
  increase urinary Aluminum
  excretion)
Aspirin
  (May decrease Vitamin C
  absorption and large aspirin doses
  may cause Vitamin C deficiency)

Carbamazepine
  (Grapefruit flavonoids may
  increase bioavailability due to
  cytochrome P-450 3A4 inhibition)
Cisplatin
  (Vitamin C may potentiate
  antineoplastic activity)
Copper
  (High dose Vitamin C may
  decrease absorption)
Cyclosporine
  (Grapefruit flavonoids may
  increase bioavailability due to
  cytochrome P-450 3A4 inhibition)
Doxorubicin Hydrochloride
  (Vitamin C may potentiate
  antineoplastic activity)
Estrogen
  (Vitamin C may enhance
  inhibition of LDL formation)
Felodipine
  (Grapefruit flavonoids may
  increase bioavailability due to
  cytochrome P-450 3A4 inhibition)
Flavonoids
  (Vitamin C may have synergistic
  effects)
Glutathione
  (Vitamin C may maintain reduced
  Glutathione levels)
Iron Supplements
  (Vitamin C may cause iron
  overload)
Lovastatin
  (Grapefruit flavonoids may
  increase bioavailability due to
  cytochrome P-450 3A4 inhibition)
Nisoldipine
  (Grapefruit flavonoids may
  increase bioavailability due to
  cytochrome P-450 3A4 inhibition)
Paclitaxel
  (Vitamin C may potentiate
  antineoplastic activity)
Saquinavir
  (Grapefruit flavonoids may
  increase bioavailability due to
  cytochrome P-450 3A4 inhibition)
Simvastatin
  (Grapefruit flavonoids may
  increase bioavailability due to
  cytochrome P-450 3A4 inhibition)

ASPIRIN
Alpha-Tocopheryl Polyethylene
Glycol Succinate
  (Enhanced antiplatelet effects of
  aspirin)
Ascorbyl Palmitate
  (May decrease Vitamin C
  absorption and large aspirin doses
  may cause Vitamin C deficiency)
Borage Oil
  (Increased anticoagulant and
  antiplatelet effects with Borage
  Oil)
Eicosapentaenoic Acid (EPA)
  (May interact with EPA)
Evening Primrose Oil
  (EPO may increase bleeding
  tendencies)
Fish Oil
  (May interact with Fish Oil)
Flaxseed Oil
  (May interact with Flaxseed Oil)
Gamma-Tocopherol
  (Increased effects of aspirin)
Hemp Seed Oil
  (Increased bleeding and
  susceptibility to bruising)
Inositol Nicotinate
  (May decrease high dose nicotinic
  acid-induced flushing)
Melatonin
  (May decrease Melatonin levels)
Niacin
  (May decrease high dose nicotinic
  acid-induced flushing)
Perilla Oil
  (Increased antithrombotic effects
  with Perilla Oil)
Policosanol
  (Antithrombotic synergistic effect)
Vitamin C
  (May decrease Vitamin C
  absorption and large aspirin doses
  may cause Vitamin C deficiency)
Vitamin E
  (Increased effects of aspirin)

AZOLE ANTIFUNGALS
Red Yeast Rice
  (Increased risk of myopathy)

BACLOFEN
Glycine
  (Glycine may increase effect of
  baclofen)

BENTONITE
Drugs, unspecified
  (Bentonite may adsorb certain
  drugs)
Food, unspecified
  (Bentonite may adsorb certain
  food components)
Herbal Medicines, unspecified
  (Bentonite may adsorb certain
  herb components)
Nutritional Supplement
  (Bentonite may adsorb certain
  nutritional supplements)

BENZODIAZEPINES
Gamma-Hydroxybutyrate (GHB)
  (May be life threatening with
  GHB)
Melatonin
  (May increase sedation and
  adverse effects with Melatonin)

BETA BLOCKERS
Chromium
  (Elevated HDL cholesterol levels
  after two months of Chromium
  use)
Melatonin
  (May lead to decreased Melatonin
  levels)

BETA-CAROTENE
Cholestyramine
  (May decrease the absorption of
  Beta-Carotene)
Colestipol
  (May decrease the absorption of
  Beta-Carotene)
Fat Substitute
  (May decrease the absorption of
  Beta-Carotene)
Iron
  (Enhanced absorption of Iron)
Lutein
  (May decrease the absorption of
  Beta-Carotene)
Lutein and Zeaxanthin
  (Decreased absorption of Lutein
  and Zeaxanthin)

Lycopene
  (Increased absorption of
  Lycopene)
Mineral Oil
  (May decrease the absorption of
  Beta-Carotene)
Orlistat
  (May decrease the absorption of
  Beta-Carotene)
Pectin
  (Decreased absorption of Beta-
  Carotene)
Phytosterols
  (Low serum levels due to
  Phytosterols)
Piperine
  (Piperine may enhance the
  absorption)
Sodium Alginates and other Phyco-
Polysaccharides
  (Decreased absorption of Beta-
  Carotene)

BETAINE AND BETAINE HYDROCHLORIDE
Folic Acid
  (May be synergistic in lowering
  serum homocysteine levels)

BETHANECHOL CHLORIDE
Huperzine A
  (Additive effects and increased
  adverse effects with Huperzine A)

BEVERAGES, CAFFEINE-CONTAINING
Creatine
  (May interfere with effects of
  Creatine)

BEVERAGES, HOT
Inositol Nicotinate
  (May increase nicotinic acid-
  induced flushing)
Niacin
  (May increase nicotinic acid-
  induced flushing)

BEVERAGES, SULFITES
Thiamin
  (May inactivate Thiamin)

BEXAROTENE
Vitamin A
  (May produce additive toxicity
  effects)

BIOTIN

Antibiotics, unspecified
  (May decrease Biotin absorption)
Carbamazepine
  (May decrease Biotin levels)
Pantothenic Acid
  (May decrease Biotin absorption)
Phenobarbital
  (May decrease Biotin levels)
Phenytoin
  (May decrease Biotin levels)
Primidone
  (May decrease Biotin levels)

BISPHOSPHONATES

Bone Meal
  (Decreased absorption of the
  bisphosphonate)
Calcium
  (Decreased absorption of the
  bisphosphonate)
Ipriflavone
  (Additive effects with Ipriflavone)
Iron
  (Decreased absorption of the
  bisphosphonate)
Magnesium
  (Decreased absorption of the
  bisphosphonate)

BONE MEAL

Bisphosphonates
  (Decreased absorption of the
  bisphosphonate)
Calcitriol
  (Increased absorption of Calcium)
Dietary Fiber
  (Decreased absorption of Calcium)
Fructo-oligosaccharides
  (Increased absorption of Calcium)
Histamine H₂-receptor antagonists
  (Decreased absorption of Calcium)
Inositol
  (Decreased absorption of Calcium)
Inulin
  (Increased absorption of Calcium)
Levothyroxine Sodium
  (Decreased levothyroxine
  absorption and increased serum
  thyrotropin levels)
Oxalic Acid
  (Decreased absorption of Calcium)

Proton Pump Inhibitor
  (Decreased absorption of Calcium)
Quinolones
  (Decreased absorption of
  quinolones)
Sodium Alginate
  (Decreased absorption of Calcium)
Tetracyclines, unspecified
  (Decreased absorption of
  tetracyclines)
Vitamin D
  (Increased absorption of Calcium)

BORAGE OIL

Allium sativum
  (Interactions may occur with
  Borage Oil)
Anticoagulant drugs, unspecified
  (Increased anticoagulant and
  antiplatelet effects with Borage
  Oil)
Antiplatelet Drugs
  (Increased anticoagulant and
  antiplatelet effects with Borage
  Oil)
Aspirin
  (Increased anticoagulant and
  antiplatelet effects with Borage
  Oil)
Chlorpromazine
  (May cause seizures with Borage
  Oil)
Fish Oils
  (Increased antithrombotic activity
  with Borage Oil)
Ginkgo biloba
  (Interactions may occur with
  Borage Oil)
Nonsteroidal Anti-Inflammatory
Drugs
  (Increased anticoagulant and
  antiplatelet effects with Borage
  Oil)
Phenothiazines
  (May cause seizures with Borage
  Oil)
Warfarin Sodium
  (Increased anticoagulant and
  antiplatelet effects with Borage
  Oil)

BORON

Ipriflavone
  (Additive effects with Ipriflavone)
Magnesium
  (Increased Magnesium levels)

BREWER'S YEAST

Monoamine Oxidase Inhibitors
  (May cause hypertension with
  Brewer's Yeast)
Pargyline Hydrochloride
  (May cause hypertension with
  Brewer's Yeast)
Phenelzine Sulfate
  (May cause hypertension with
  Brewer's Yeast)
Tranylcypromine Sulfate
  (May cause hypertension with
  Brewer's Yeast)

BROMELAIN

Amoxicillin
  (Bromelain may increase
  amoxicillin levels)
Anticoagulant drugs, unspecified
  (Bromelain may enhance
  anticoagulant effects)
Antithrombotic Agents
  (Bromelain may enhance
  antithrombotic effects)
Curcuminoids
  (Bromelain may enhance the
  absorption of Curcuminoids)
Quercetin
  (Increased absorption of
  Quercetin)
Tetracyclines, unspecified
  (Bromelain may increase
  tetracycline levels)

BUMETANIDE

Thiamin
  (Chronic use may cause Thiamin
  deficiency)

C-GLUOSYLFLAVONES

Iodine
  (Inhibit thyroid peroxidase
  activity)

CAFFEINE

Green Tea Catechins
  (Synergistic effect with Green Tea
  Catechins in enhancing
  thermogenesis)

Zinc
(Decreased absorption of Zinc)

CALCITONIN, UNSPECIFIED
Gelatin Hydrolysates
(Gelatin Hydrosylates may enhance the osteoporosis treatment effects)
Hydrolyzed Collagen
(Enhanced effect in the treatment of osteoporosis with Hydrolyzed Collagen)
Ipriflavone
(Additive effects with Ipriflavone)

CALCITRIOL
Bone Meal
(Increased absorption of Calcium)
Calcium
(Increased absorption of Calcium)

CALCIUM
Bisphosphonates
(Decreased absorption of the bisphosphonate)
Calcitriol
(Increased absorption of Calcium)
Dietary Fiber
(Decreased absorption of Calcium)
Fluoride
(Decreased absorption of Fluoride)
Fructo-oligosaccharides
(Increased absorption of Calcium)
Histamine H₂-receptor antagonists
(Decreased absorption of Calcium)
Inositol
(Decreased absorption of Calcium)
Inositol Hexaphosphate
(May form chelates with Inositol Hexaphosphate)
Inulins
(Inulins may enhance absorption of dietary and supplemental Calcium)
Ipriflavone
(Additive effects with Ipriflavone)
Iron
(Decreased absorption of Iron)
L-Lysine
(L-Lysine may increase Calcium absorption)

Lactulose
(Lactulose may enhance absorption of dietary and supplemental Calcium)
Levothyroxine Sodium
(Decreased levothyroxine absorption and increased serum thyrotropin levels)
Magnesium
(Decreased absorption of Magnesium)
Manganese
(Decreased absorption of Manganese)
Medium-Chain Triglycerides
(MCT may facilitate the absorption of Calcium)
Oxalic Acid
(Decreased absorption of Calcium)
Pectin
(Decreased absorption of Calcium)
Phytic Acid
(Decreased absorption of Calcium)
Prebiotics
(Enhanced absorption of Calcium)
Proton Pump Inhibitor
(Decreased absorption of Calcium)
Psyllium
(Decreased absorption of Calcium)
Quinolones
(Decreased absorption of quinolones)
Sodium Alginate
(Decreased absorption of Calcium)
Sodium Alginates and other Phyco-Polysaccharides
(Decreased absorption of Calcium)
Soy Protein
(Reduced availability of Calcium)
Synbiotics
(Enhanced absorption of Calcium)
Tetracyclines, unspecified
(Decreased absorption of tetracyclines)
Thyroxine
(Decreased thyroxine absorption)
Transgalacto-Oligosaccharides
(Enhanced absorption of Calcium)
Vitamin B12
(May reverse metformin-induced decrease of Vitamin B12 absorption)

Vitamin D
(Concomitant Vitamin D is synergistic for corticosteroid-induced osteoporosis; increased absorption of Calcium)
Zinc
(Decreased Zinc absorption in postmenopausal women)

CALCIUM CHANNEL BLOCKERS, UNSPECIFIED
Inositol Nicotinate
(High dose nicotinic acid may potentiate hypotensive effects)
Niacin
(High dose nicotinic acid may potentiate hypotensive effects)

CALCIUM PANTOTHENATE
(*See under* Pantothenic Acid)

CARBAMAZEPINE
Acetylcysteine
(Reduced serum levels with NAC)
Ascorbyl Palmitate
(Grapefruit flavonoids may increase bioavailability due to cytochrome P-450 3A4 inhibition)
Biotin
(May decrease Biotin levels)
Folate
(May decrease Folate levels and increase homocysteine levels; High dose folic acid may decrease serum levels)
Nicotinamide
(Nicotinamide may decrease clearance)
Psyllium
(Reduced absorption of carbamazepine)
Vitamin B6
(Chronic use may decrease plasma pyridoxal 5'-phosphate)
Vitamin C
(Grapefruit flavonoids may increase bioavailability due to cytochrome P-450 3A4 inhibition)

CARBIDOPA
5-Hydroxytryptophan
(Increases 5-HTP levels in the brain)

Octacosanol
(Worsened dyskinesias in Parkinson's disease)

CAROTENOIDS
Chitosan
(Might bind to Chitosan)
Medium-Chain Triglycerides
(MCT may facilitate the absorption of carotenoids)

CEFAMANDOLE NAFATE
Vitamin K
(Can cause Vitamin K deficiency and hypoprothrombinemia)

CEFAZOLIN SODIUM
Vitamin K
(Can cause Vitamin K deficiency and hypoprothrombinemia)

CEFMENOXIME
Vitamin K
(Can cause Vitamin K deficiency and hypoprothrombinemia)

CEFOPERAZONE SODIUM
Vitamin K
(Can cause Vitamin K deficiency and hypoprothrombinemia)

CEFOTETAN
Vitamin K
(Can cause Vitamin K deficiency and hypoprothrombinemia)

CHITOSAN
Carotenoids
(Might bind to Chitosan)
Chondroitin Sulfate
(May decrease absorption of Chondroitin Sulfate)
Diet, lipid
(Might bind to Chitosan)
Flavonoids
(Might bind to Chitosan)
Lipophilic drugs, unspecified
(Might bind to Chitosan)
Vitamin A
(Might bind to Chitosan)
Vitamin C
(May enhance the benefits of Chitosan)
Vitamin D
(Might bind to Chitosan)

Vitamin E
(Might bind to Chitosan)
Vitamin K
(Might bind to Chitosan)
Zinc
(Might bind to Chitosan)

CHLORELLA
Warfarin Sodium
(Chlorella may interfere with effects)

CHLORIDE
Vanadium
(May decrease absorption of Vanadium)

CHLORPROMAZINE
Arnica
(Increased risk of prolonged QT interval when given with Arnica)
Borage Oil
(May cause seizures with Borage Oil)
Riboflavin (Vitamin B2)
(Inhibition of Riboflavin conversion to FMN and FAD)

CHOLECALCIFEROL
(*See under* Vitamin D)

CHOLESTYRAMINE
Beta-Carotene
(May decrease the absorption of Beta-Carotene)
Folate
(May decrease folic acid absorption)
Gamma-Tocopherol
(Decreased Gamma-Tocopherol absorption)
Inositol Nicotinate
(May reduce nicotinic acid absorption and may have synergistic antihyperlipidemic effects)
Lutein and Zeaxanthin
(Decreased absorption of Lutein and Zeaxanthin)
Lycopene
(Decreased absorption of Lycopene)

Niacin
(May reduce nicotinic acid absorption and may have synergistic antihyperlipidemic effects)
Psyllium
(Enhanced cholesterol-lowering action)
Riboflavin (Vitamin B2)
(Decreased absorption of Riboflavin)
Tocotrienols
(May decrease Tocotrienol absorption)
Vitamin A
(May decrease Vitamin A absorption)
Vitamin B12
(May decrease enterohepatic reabsorption of Vitamin B12)
Vitamin D
(May reduce Vitamin D absorption)
Vitamin E
(Decreased Vitamin E absorption)
Vitamin K
(May reduce Vitamin K absorption)

CHOLINE
Homocysteine
(Increased metabolism with Choline)
Huperzine A
(Additive effects and increased adverse effects with Huperzine A)
L-Carnitine
(May lead to increased L-Carnitine retention)
Methotrexate Sodium
(May decrease Choline metabolites)

CHOLINERGIC AGENTS
Huperzine A
(Additive effects and increased adverse effects with Huperzine A)

CHONDROITIN SULFATE
Chitosan
(May decrease absorption of Chondroitin Sulfate)

CHROMIUM

Ascorbate
(Increased absorption of
Chromium)
Beta Blockers
(Elevated HDL cholesterol levels
after two months of Chromium
use)
Phytic Acid
(Decreased absorption of
Chromium)
Sodium Alginates and other Phyco-
Polysaccharides
(Decreased absorption of
Chromium)
Vanadium
(May decrease absorption of
Vanadium)

CHRYSIN

Aminoglutethimide
(Chrysin may have additive
effects)
Anastrozole
(Chrysin may have additive
effects)
Aromatase Inhibitors
(Chrysin may have additive
effects)

CISPLATIN

Ascorbyl Palmitate
(Vitamin C may potentiate
antineoplastic activity)
Quercetin
(May cause genotoxicity in normal
tissues with Quercetin)
Vitamin C
(Vitamin C may potentiate
antineoplastic activity)

CLINDAMYCIN HYDROCHLORIDE

Pectin
(Decreased absorption of
clindamycin)

CLOPIDOGREL BISULFATE

Alpha-Tocopheryl Polyethylene
Glycol Succinate
(Enhanced antiplatelet effects of
clopidogrel)
Gamma-Tocopherol
(Increased effects of clopidogrel)

Vitamin E
(Increased effects of clopidogrel)

COENZYME Q10 (COQ10)

Alpha-Tocopheryl Polyethylene
Glycol Succinate
(Increased absorption of
Coenzyme Q10)
Antidiabetic Drugs, unspecified
(May need dosing adjustments)
Lovastatin
(Decreases CoQ10 levels)
Piperine
(Piperine may enhance the
absorption)
Pravastatin Sodium
(Decreases CoQ10 levels)
Propranolol Hydrochloride
(May inhibit some CoQ10-
dependent enzymes)
Simvastatin
(Decreases CoQ10 levels)
Warfarin Sodium
(May decrease the effectiveness of
warfarin)

COLCHICINE

Folate
(May decrease Folate levels)
Vitamin B12
(May decrease absorption of
Vitamin B12)

COLESTIPOL

Beta-Carotene
(May decrease the absorption of
Beta-Carotene)
Folate
(May decrease folic acid
absorption)
Gamma-Tocopherol
(Decreased Gamma-Tocopherol
absorption)
Inositol Nicotinate
(May reduce nicotinic acid
absorption and may have
synergistic antihyperlipidemic
effects)
Lutein and Zeaxanthin
(Decreased absorption of Lutein
and Zeaxanthin)
Lycopene
(Decreased absorption of
Lycopene)

Niacin
(May reduce nicotinic acid
absorption and may have
synergistic antihyperlipidemic
effects)
Riboflavin (Vitamin B2)
(Decreased absorption of
Riboflavin)
Tocotrienols
(May decrease Tocotrienol
absorption)
Vitamin A
(May decrease Vitamin A
absorption)
Vitamin B12
(May decrease enterohepatic
reabsorption of Vitamin B12)
Vitamin D
(May reduce Vitamin D
absorption)
Vitamin E
(Decreased Vitamin E absorption)
Vitamin K
(May reduce Vitamin K
absorption)

COPPER

Ascorbyl Palmitate
(High dose Vitamin C may
decrease absorption)
Diet high in fructose
(Decreased Copper levels)
Inositol Hexaphosphate
(May form chelates with Inositol
Hexaphosphate)
Iron
(Decreased Copper levels)
Molybdenum
(High dose of Molybdenum may
antagonize dietary Copper
absorption and high dose Copper
may antagonize Molybdenum
absorption)
Pectin
(Decreased absorption of Copper)
Penicillamine
(Decreased absorption of Copper
and penicillamine)
Phytic Acid
(Decreased absorption of Copper)
Psyllium
(Decreased absorption of Copper)

Soy Protein
  (Reduced availability of Copper)
Vitamin C
  (High dose Vitamin C may
  decrease absorption)
Zinc
  (Decreased absorption of Copper)

CREATINE
Beverages, caffeine-containing
  (May interfere with effects of
  Creatine)

CURCUMINOIDS
Antiplatelet Drugs
  (Curcuminoids may enhance the
  antiplatelet effect)
Bromelain
  (Bromelain may enhance the
  absorption of Curcuminoids)
Piperine
  (Piperine may enhance the
  absorption of Curcuminoids)
Warfarin Sodium
  (Curcuminoids may enhance the
  anticoagulant effect)

CYANOCOBALAMIN
(See under Vitamin B12)

CYCLOSERINE
Vitamin B6
  (May result in Vitamin B6
  deficiency)

CYCLOSPORINE
Alpha-Tocopheryl Polyethylene
Glycol Succinate
  (Increased absorption of
  cyclosporine)
Ascorbyl Palmitate
  (Grapefruit flavonoids may
  increase bioavailability due to
  cytochrome P-450 3A4 inhibition)
L-Arginine
  (L-Arginine may counteract
  antinaturetic effects)
Red Yeast Rice
  (Increased risk of myopathy)
Vitamin C
  (Grapefruit flavonoids may
  increase bioavailability due to
  cytochrome P-450 3A4 inhibition)

Vitamin E
  (Alpha-tocopherol may help to
  ameliorate renal side effects of
  cyclosporine)

CYPROHEPTADINE HYDROCHLORIDE
5-Hydroxytryptophan
  (5-HTP may decrease effects)

CYSTEINE
Iron
  (Increased absorption of Iron)

CYSTEINE-CONTAINING PROTIENS
Zinc
  (Increased absorption of Zinc)

D-GLUCARATE
Fluorouracil
  (Synergistic antitumor activity)
Retinoids
  (Synergistic chemopreventive
  effects)

D-RIBOSE
Antidiabetic Drugs, unspecified
  (D-Ribose may cause
  hypoglycemia)

DHEA
Alprazolam
  (May increase DHEA levels)
Androstenediol
  (May increase adverse effects of
  DHEA)
Androstenedione
  (May increase adverse effects of
  DHEA)
Danazol
  (May decrease DHEA levels)
Dexamethasone
  (May decrease DHEA levels)
Diltiazem Hydrochloride
  (May increase DHEA levels)
Insulin
  (May decrease DHEA levels)
Morphine Sulfate
  (May decrease DHEA levels)
Testosterone
  (May increase adverse effects of
  DHEA)

DL-PHENYLALANINE
(See under L-Phenylalanine)

DAIDZEIN
Ethanol
  (Daidzein/daidzin may increase the
  bioavailability of ingested ethanol)

DAIRY PRODUCTS
Fluoride
  (Decreased absorption of Fluoride)

DANAZOL
DHEA
  (May decrease DHEA levels)

DANTROLENE SODIUM
Glycine
  (Glycine may increase effects of
  dantrolene)

DAPSONE
Piperine
  (Piperine may inhibit metabolism)

DEGLYCYRRHIZINATED LICORICE (DGL)
Nitrofurantoin
  (Increased excretion rate of
  nitrofurantoin)

DESIPRAMINE HYDROCHLORIDE
Arnica
  (Increased risk of prolonged QT
  interval when given with Arnica)

DEXAMETHASONE
DHEA
  (May decrease DHEA levels)

DEXTROAMPHETAMINE
Pycnogenol
  (May be synergistic with
  Pycnogenol for attention deficit-
  hyperactivity disorder
  management)

DIAZEPAM
Glycine
  (Glycine may increase effects)

DIDANOSINE
Acetyl-L-Carnitine
  (May lead to decreased Acetyl-L-
  Carnitine levels)
L-Carnitine
  (May produce L-Carnitine
  deficiencies)

Riboflavin (Vitamin B2)
(Riboflavin may reverse nucleoside analogue-induced lactic acidosis in mild Riboflavin deficiencies)

DIET HIGH IN FRUCTOSE
Copper
(Decreased Copper levels)

DIET HIGH IN PROTEIN
Inositol Hexaphosphate
(May form chelates with Inositol Hexaphosphate)

DIET, LIPID
Chitosan
(Might bind to Chitosan)

DIETARY FIBER
Bone Meal
(Decreased absorption of Calcium)
Calcium
(Decreased absorption of Calcium)
Vitamin E
(May decrease the antioxidative effect of Alpha-Tocopherol and carotenoids)

DIGOXIN
Pectin
(Decreased absorption of digoxin)
Psyllium
(Reduced absorption of digoxin)

DILTIAZEM HYDROCHLORIDE
DHEA
(May increase DHEA levels)

DIMETHYL SULFOXIDE (DMSO)
Sulindac
(May decrease the effects of DMSO and increase side effects)

DIPYRIDAMOLE
Alpha-Tocopheryl Polyethylene Glycol Succinate
(Enhanced antiplatelet effects of dipyridamole)
Gamma-Tocopherol
(Increased effects of dipyridamole)
Vitamin E
(Increased effects of dipyridamole)

DISOPYRAMIDE
Arnica
(Increased risk of prolonged QT interval when given with Arnica)

DONEPEZIL HYDROCHLORIDE
Huperzine A
(Additive effects and increased adverse effects with Huperzine A)

DOXEPIN HYDROCHLORIDE
Arnica
(Increased risk of prolonged QT interval when given with Arnica)

DOXORUBICIN HYDROCHLORIDE
Arnica
(Increased cardiotoxicity with Arnica)
Ascorbyl Palmitate
(Vitamin C may potentiate antineoplastic activity)
L-Theanine
(L-Theanine may enhance antitumor effects and decrease adverse effects)
Riboflavin (Vitamin B2)
(Inhibition of Riboflavin conversion to FMN and FAD)
Vitamin C
(Vitamin C may potentiate antineoplastic activity)

DRUGS, UNSPECIFIED
Activated Charcoal
(Avoid using Activated Charcoal within two hours of taking these products)
Bentonite
(Bentonite may adsorb certain drugs)
Piperine
(Piperine may inhibit metabolism)

EICOSAPENTAENOIC ACID (EPA)
Allium sativum
(May interact with EPA)
Aspirin
(May interact with EPA)
Ginkgo biloba
(May interact with EPA)
Nonsteroidal Anti-Inflammatory Drugs
(May interact with EPA)

EPTIFIBATIDE
Alpha-Tocopheryl Polyethylene Glycol Succinate
(Enhanced antiplatelet effects of eptifibatide)
Gamma-Tocopherol
(Increased effects of eptifibatide)
Vitamin E
(Increased effects of eptifibatide)

ESTROGEN
Ascorbyl Palmitate
(Vitamin C may enhance inhibition of LDL formation)
Ipriflavone
(Additive effects with Ipriflavone)
Vitamin C
(Vitamin C may enhance inhibition of LDL formation)

ETHACRYNIC ACID
Thiamin
(Chronic use may cause Thiamin deficiency)

ETHAMBUTOL HYDROCHLORIDE
Piperine
(Piperine may inhibit metabolism)

ETHANOL
Daidzein
(Daidzein/daidzin may increase the bioavailability of ingested ethanol)
Inositol Nicotinate
(May increase nicotinic acid-induced flushing)
Niacin
(May increase nicotinic acid-induced flushing)

ETHIONAMIDE
Vitamin B6
(May increase Vitamin B6 requirements)

ETHYLENEDIAMINETETRAACETIC ACID
Vanadium
(May decrease absorption of Vanadium)

ETRETINATE
Vitamin A
(May produce additive toxicity effects)

EVENING PRIMROSE OIL

Allium sativum
  (EPO may increase bleeding
  tendencies)
Aspirin
  (EPO may increase bleeding
  tendencies)
Fish Oils
  (EPO may increase bleeding
  tendencies)
Ginkgo biloba
  (EPO may increase bleeding
  tendencies)
Nonsteroidal Anti-Inflammatory
Drugs
  (EPO may increase bleeding
  tendencies)
Phenothiazines
  (EPO lowers seizure threshold)
Warfarin Sodium
  (EPO may increase bleeding
  tendencies)

FAT SUBSTITUTE

Beta-Carotene
  (May decrease the absorption of
  Beta-Carotene)
Gamma-Tocopherol
  (Inhibits absorption of Gamma-
  Tocopherol)
Lutein and Zeaxanthin
  (Decreased absorption of Lutein
  and Zeaxanthin)
Lycopene
  (Reduced absorption of Lycopene)
Tocotrienols
  (May inhibit Tocotrienol
  absorption)
Vitamin A
  (May inhibit Vitamin A
  absorption)
Vitamin D
  (Inhibits Vitamin D absorption)
Vitamin E
  (Inhibits absorption of Vitamin E)
Vitamin K
  (May reduce Vitamin K
  absorption)

FATTY ACIDS

Medium-Chain Triglycerides
  (MCT may facilitate the
  absorption of fatty acids)

FATTY ACIDS, POLYUNSATURATED

Vitamin E
  (May increase Vitamin E
  requirements)

FELODIPINE

Ascorbyl Palmitate
  (Grapefruit flavonoids may
  increase bioavailability due to
  cytochrome P-450 3A4 inhibition)
Vitamin C
  (Grapefruit flavonoids may
  increase bioavailability due to
  cytochrome P-450 3A4 inhibition)

FIBER

(See under Dietary Fiber)

FIBRATES

Red Yeast Rice
  (Increased risk of myopathy)

FISH OIL

Allium sativum
  (May interact with Fish Oil)
Aspirin
  (May interact with Fish Oil)
Borage Oil
  (Increased antithrombotic activity
  with Borage Oil)
Evening Primrose Oil
  (EPO may increase bleeding
  tendencies)
Flaxseed Oil
  (May interact with Flaxseed Oil)
Ginkgo biloba
  (May interact with Fish Oil)
Nonsteroidal Anti-Inflammatory
Drugs
  (May interact with Fish Oil)

FLAVONOIDS

Alpha-Tocopheryl Polyethylene
Glycol Succinate
  (Increased absorption of
  flavonoids)
Ascorbyl Palmitate
  (Vitamin C may have synergistic
  effects)
Chitosan
  (Might bind to Chitosan)
Gamma-Tocopherol
  (Helps to maintain levels of
  reduced Gamma-Tocopherol)

Medium-Chain Triglycerides
  (MCT may facilitate the
  absorption of flavonoids)
Vitamin C
  (Vitamin C may have synergistic
  effects)
Vitamin E
  (Help to maintain levels of
  Vitamin E)

FLAXSEED OIL

Allium sativum
  (May interact with Flaxseed Oil)
Aspirin
  (May interact with Flaxseed Oil)
Fish Oils
  (May interact with Flaxseed Oil)
Ginkgo biloba
  (May interact with Flaxseed Oil)
Nonsteroidal Anti-Inflammatory
Drugs
  (May interact with Flaxseed Oil)
Warfarin Sodium
  (May interact with Flaxseed Oil)

FLUORIDE

Antacids, aluminum-containing
  (Decreased absorption of Fluoride)
Calcium
  (Decreased absorption of Fluoride)
Dairy products
  (Decreased absorption of Fluoride)

FLUORINE & FLUORIDE PREPARATIONS

Ipriflavone
  (Additive effects with Ipriflavone)

FLUOROURACIL

D-Glucarate
  (Synergistic antitumor activity)

FLUOXETINE HYDROCHLORIDE

Folate
  (Folic acid may enhance
  antidepressant effects)
Melatonin
  (Psychotic episode reported with
  Melatonin)

FLUVOXAMINE MALEATE

Melatonin
  (Increases the bioavailability of
  oral Melatonin)

FOLATE

Betaine and Betaine Hydrochloride
  (May be synergistic in lowering
  serum homocysteine levels)
Carbamazepine
  (May decrease Folate levels and
  increase homocysteine levels;
  High dose folic acid may decrease
  serum levels)
Cholestyramine
  (May decrease folic acid
  absorption)
Colchicine
  (May decrease Folate levels)
Colestipol
  (May decrease folic acid
  absorption)
Fluoxetine Hydrochloride
  (Folic acid may enhance
  antidepressant effects)
Food, unspecified
  (Decrease in folic acid
  availability)
Fosphenytoin
  (May decrease Folate levels and
  increase homocysteine levels;
  High dose folic acid may decrease
  serum levels)
Homocysteine
  (Increased metabolism with folic
  acid)
Lithium
  (Folic acid may increase efficacy)
Lometrexol
  (Folic acid may be synergistic and
  decrease adverse effects)
Metformin
  (Folic acid may reduce metformin-
  associated homocysteinemia)
Methotrexate
  (Folic acid may reduce toxic side
  effects)
Nonsteroidal Anti-Inflammatory
Drugs
  (Large doses may exert antifolate
  activity)
Phenobarbital
  (May decrease Folate levels and
  increase homocysteine levels;
  High dose folic acid may decrease
  serum levels)

Phenytoin
  (May decrease Folate levels and
  increase homocysteine levels;
  High dose folic acid may decrease
  serum levels)
Primidone
  (May decrease Folate levels and
  increase homocysteine levels;
  High dose folic acid may decrease
  serum levels)
Pyrimethamine
  (Folic acid may decrease
  antiparasitic effects)
Sulfasalazine
  (May decrease folic acid
  absorption)
Valproic Acid
  (May decrease Folate levels and
  increase homocysteine; High dose
  folic acid may decrease serum
  levels)
Vitamin B6
  (May be synergistic in lowering
  serum homocysteine levels)
Vitamin B12
  (Synergistic with Vitamin B12 to
  lower homocysteine levels)
Zinc
  (Folic acid may decrease Zinc
  absorption)

FOLIC ACID

(See under Folate)

FOOD, HOT

Inositol Nicotinate
  (May increase nicotinic acid-
  induced flushing)
Niacin
  (May increase nicotinic acid-
  induced flushing)

FOOD, SULFITES

Thiamin
  (May inactivate Thiamin)

FOOD, UNSPECIFIED

Activated Charcoal
  (Avoid using Activated Charcoal
  within two hours of taking these
  products)
Bentonite
  (Bentonite may adsorb certain
  food components)

Folate
  (Decrease in folic acid
  availability)
Thiamin
  (Antithiamin factors in food
  inactivate Thiamin)

FOSPHENYTOIN

Folate
  (May decrease Folate levels and
  increase homocysteine levels;
  High dose folic acid may decrease
  serum levels)
Vitamin B6
  (Vitamin B6 may lower plasma
  phenytoin levels)

FRUCTO-OLIGOSACCHARIDES

Bone Meal
  (Increased absorption of Calcium)
Calcium
  (Increased absorption of Calcium)
Magnesium
  (Increased absorption of
  Magnesium)

FRUCTOSE

(See under Diet high in fructose)

FUROSEMIDE

Thiamin
  (Chronic use may cause Thiamin
  deficiency)

GAMMA-HYDROXYBUTYRATE (GHB)

Alcohol
  (May be life threatening with
  GHB)
Anticonvulsants
  (May be life threatening with
  GHB)
Antihistamines
  (May be life threatening with
  GHB)
Benzodiazepines
  (May be life threatening with
  GHB)
Opiates
  (May be life threatening with
  GHB)
Protease Inhibitors
  (May be life threatening with
  GHB)

Skeletal Muscle Relaxants
(May be life threatening with GHB)
Tranquilizers
(May be life threatening with GHB)

GAMMA-TOCOPHEROL

Abciximab
(Increased effects of abciximab)
Allium sativum
(Enhanced antithrombotic activity of garlic)
Alpha Tocopheral Acetate
(Decreased plasma Gamma-Tocopherol levels)
Antiplatelet Drugs
(Increased effects of antiplatelet drugs)
Aspirin
(Increased effects of aspirin)
Cholestyramine
(Decreased Gamma-Tocopherol absorption)
Clopidogrel Bisulfate
(Increased effects of clopidogrel)
Colestipol
(Decreased Gamma-Tocopherol absorption)
Dipyridamole
(Increased effects of dipyridamole)
Eptifibatide
(Increased effects of eptifibatide)
Fat Substitute
(Inhibits absorption of Gamma-Tocopherol)
Flavonoids
(Helps to maintain levels of reduced Gamma-Tocopherol)
Ginkgo biloba
(Enhanced antithrombotic activity of gingko biloba)
Iron
(The ferrous form of iron can oxidize Gamma-Tocopherol to its pro-oxidant form)
Isoniazid
(Decreased Gamma-Tocopherol absorption)
Medium-Chain Triglycerides
(Enhanced Gamma-Tocopherol absorption)

Mineral Oil
(Decreased Gamma-Tocopherol absorption)
Neomycin
(Impaired utilization of Gamma-Tocopherol)
Ox Bile, Desiccated
(Increased Gamma-Tocopherol absorption)
Phytostanols
(Decreased plasma Gamma-Tocopherol levels)
Phytosterols
(Decreased plasma Gamma-Tocopherol levels)
Plant Phenolic Compounds
(Helps to maintain levels of reduced Gamma-Tocopherol)
Selenium
(Synergistic effect with Gamma-Tocopherol)
Sucralfate
(Interferes with Gamma-Tocopherol absorption)
Ticlopidine Hydrochloride
(Increased effects of ticlopidine)
Tirofiban Hydrochloride
(Increased effects of tirofiban)
Vitamin C
(Helps to maintain Gamma-Tocopherol in its reduced (antioxidant) form)
Warfarin Sodium
(Enhanced anticoagulant response of warfarin)

GAMMA-TOCOPHEROL

Alpha-Tocopheryl Polyethylene
Glycol Succinate
(Increased absorption when taken with TPGS; Decreased plasma levels with high doses of TPGS)

GANGLIONIC BLOCKING AGENTS

Inositol Nicotinate
(Nicotinic acid may potentiate effects)
Niacin
(Nicotinic acid may potentiate effects)

GARLIC

(*See under* Allium sativum)

GELATIN

(*See under* Gelatin Hydrolysates)

GELATIN HYDROLYSATES

Calcitonin, unspecified
(Gelatin Hydrosylates may enhance the osteoporosis treatment effects)

GEMFIBROZIL

Inositol Nicotinate
(High dose nicotinic acid may have synergistic antihyperlipidemic effects)
Niacin
(High dose nicotinic acid may have synergistic antihyperlipidemic effects)
Red Yeast Rice
(Increased risk of myopathy)

GENTAMICIN

L-Methionine
(Methionine may protect against ototoxicity)

GINKGO BILOBA

Alpha-Tocopheryl Polyethylene
Glycol Succinate
(Enhanced antithrombotic activity of gingko biloba)
Borage Oil
(Interactions may occur with Borage Oil)
Eicosapentaenoic Acid (EPA)
(May interact with EPA)
Evening Primrose Oil
(EPO may increase bleeding tendencies)
Fish Oil
(May interact with Fish Oil)
Flaxseed Oil
(May interact with Flaxseed Oil)
Gamma-Tocopherol
(Enhanced antithrombotic activity of gingko biloba)
Perilla Oil
(Increased antithrombotic effects with Perilla Oil)
Tocotrienols
(May enhance antithrombotic activity)

Vitamin E
(Enhanced antithrombotic activity
of ginkgo biloba)

GLUCOMANNAN

Vitamin A
(Decreased absorption of fat-
soluble vitamins)

Vitamin D
(Decreased absorption of fat-
soluble vitamins)

Vitamin E
(Decreased absorption of fat-
soluble vitamins)

Vitamin K
(Decreased absorption of fat-
soluble vitamins)

GLUCOSAMINE

Antidiabetic Drugs, unspecified
(Glucosamine may increase insulin
resistance)

GLUTAMINE PEPTIDES

Human Growth Hormone
(L-Glutamine may enhance
nutrient absorption with short
bowel syndrome)

Indomethacin
(L-Glutamine may inhibit
intestinal permeability caused by
indomethacin)

Methotrexate Sodium
(May decrease L-Glutamine
effects)

Paclitaxel
(L-Glutamine may prevent
paclitaxel adverse reactions)

GLUTATHIONE

Ascorbyl Palmitate
(Vitamin C may maintain reduced
Glutathione levels)

Vitamin C
(Vitamin C may maintain reduced
Glutathione levels)

GLYCINE

Baclofen
(Glycine may increase effects)

Dantrolene Sodium
(Glycine may increase effects)

Diazepam
(Glycine may increase effects)

L-Methionine
(L-Methionine may decrease
Glycine levels with low-protein
diet)

Tizanidine Hydrochloride
(Glycine may increase effects)

GOITROGENS

Iodine
(May compete with iodide and
cause hypothyroidism)

GRAPEFRUIT JUICE

Red Yeast Rice
(Increased risk of myopathy)

GREEN TEA CATECHINS

Antiplatelet Drugs
(Enhanced effect with Green Tea
Catechins)

Caffeine
(Synergistic effect with Green Tea
Catechins in enhancing
thermogenesis)

GUAIAC TEST

Iron
(High false positive occult blood
with Iron supplements)

HMG-COA REDUCTASE INHIBITORS

Inositol Nicotinate
(May produce rhabdomyolysis and
may have synergistic
antihyperlipidemic effects)

Niacin
(May produce rhabdomyolysis and
may have synergistic
antihyperlipidemic effects)

Pantethine
(May have additive lipid-
modulatory effects)

Red Yeast Rice
(Increased risk of adverse
reactions)

Tocotrienols
(Tocotrienols may have synergistic
cholesterol-lowering effects)

HALOPERIDOL

Arnica
(Increased risk of prolonged QT
interval when given with Arnica)

HEMP SEED OIL

Aspirin
(Increased bleeding and
susceptibility to bruising)

Nonsteroidal Anti-Inflammatory
Drugs
(Increased bleeding and
susceptibility to bruising)

Warfarin Sodium
(Increased bleeding and
susceptibility to bruising)

HERBAL MEDICINES, UNSPECIFIED

Activated Charcoal
(Avoid using Activated Charcoal
within two hours of taking these
products)

Bentonite
(Bentonite may adsorb certain
herb components)

HISTAMINE H₂-RECEPTOR ANTAGONISTS

Bone Meal
(Decreased absorption of Calcium)

Calcium
(Decreased absorption of Calcium)

Indole-3-Carbinol
(Block the conversion of Indole-3-
Carbinol to DIM and ICZ)

Iron
(Decreased absorption of carbonyl
iron)

L-Histidine
(L-Histidine might decrease the
efficacy of histamine H₂-receptor
antagonists)

Vitamin B12
(May decrease absorption of
dietary Vitamin B12, not
supplemental)

HOMOCYSTEINE

Choline
(Increased metabolism with
Choline)

Folic Acid
(Increased metabolism with folic
acid)

Vitamin B6
(Increased metabolism with
Vitamin B6)

Vitamin B12
(Increased metabolism with
Vitamin B12)

HUMAN GROWTH HORMONE

Glutamine Peptides
(L-Glutamine may enhance nutrient absorption with short bowel syndrome)

L-Glutamine
(L-Glutamine may enhance nutrient absorption with short bowel syndrome)

HUPERZINE A

Anticholinesterase drugs
(Additive effects and increased adverse effects with Huperzine A)

Bethanechol Chloride
(Additive effects and increased adverse effects with Huperzine A)

Choline
(Additive effects and increased adverse effects with Huperzine A)

Cholinergic Agents
(Additive effects and increased adverse effects with Huperzine A)

Donepezil Hydrochloride
(Additive effects and increased adverse effects with Huperzine A)

Phosphatidylcholine
(Additive effects and increased adverse effects with Huperzine A)

Physostigmine Salicylate
(Additive effects and increased adverse effects with Huperzine A)

Tacrine Hydrochloride
(Additive effects and increased adverse effects with Huperzine A)

HYDRALAZINE

Vitamin B6
(May increase Vitamin B6 requirements)

HYDROLYZED COLLAGEN

Calcitonin, unspecified
(Enhanced effect in the treatment of osteoporosis with Hydrolyzed Collagen)

HYPERICUM

5-Hydroxytryptophan
(5-HTP may potentiate antidepressant effects and increase risk of side effects)

Myo-Inositol
(May have additive effects with Myo-Inositol)

IBUPROFEN

L-Arginine
(L-Arginine may increase absorption)

IDARUBICIN HYDROCHLORIDE

L-Theanine
(L-Theanine may enhance antitumor effects and decrease adverse effects)

INDOLE-3-CARBINOL

Antacids, unspecified
(Block the conversion of Indole-3-Carbinol to DIM and ICZ)

Histamine H2-receptor antagonists
(Block the conversion of Indole-3-Carbinol to DIM and ICZ)

Proton Pump Inhibitor
(Block the conversion of Indole-3 Carbinol to DIM and ICZ)

Tamoxifen Citrate
(May be synergistic with Indole-3-Carbinol in protecting against breast cancer)

INDOMETHACIN

Glutamine Peptides
(L-Glutamine may inhibit intestinal permeability caused by indomethacin)

L-Glutamine
(L-Glutamine may inhibit intestinal permeability caused by indomethacin)

INOSITOL

Bone Meal
(Decreased absorption of Calcium)

Calcium
(Decreased absorption of Calcium)

Iron
(Decreased absorption of Iron)

Magnesium
(Decreased absorption of Magnesium)

Zinc
(Decreased absorption of Zinc)

INOSITOL HEXAPHOSPHATE

Calcium
(May form chelates with Inositol Hexaphosphate)

Copper
(May form chelates with Inositol Hexaphosphate)

Diet high in protein
(May form chelates with Inositol Hexaphosphate)

Iron
(May form chelates with Inositol Hexaphosphate)

Magnesium
(May form chelates with Inositol Hexaphosphate)

Manganese
(May form chelates with Inositol Hexaphosphate)

Zinc
(May form chelates with Inositol Hexaphosphate)

INOSITOL NIACINATE

(*See under* Inositol Nicotinate)

INOSITOL NICOTINATE

Acarbose
(High dose nicotinic acid may antagonize effects)

Alpha Adrenergic Blockers
(High dose nicotinic acid may potentiate hypotensive effects)

Aspirin
(May decrease high dose nicotinic acid-induced flushing)

Beverages, hot
(May increase nicotinic acid-induced flushing)

Calcium Channel Blockers, Unspecified
(High dose nicotinic acid may potentiate hypotensive effects)

Cholestyramine
(May reduce nicotinic acid absorption and may have synergistic antihyperlipidemic effects)

Colestipol
(May reduce nicotinic acid absorption and may have synergistic antihyperlipidemic effects)

Ethanol
(May increase nicotinic acid-
induced flushing)
Food, hot
(May increase nicotinic acid-
induced flushing)
Ganglionic Blocking Agents
(Nicotinic acid may potentiate
effects)
Gemfibrozil
(High dose nicotinic acid may
have synergistic antihyperlipidemic
effects)
HMG-CoA Reductase Inhibitors
(May produce rhabdomyolysis and
may have synergistic
antihyperlipidemic effects)
Metformin
(High dose nicotinic acid may
antagonize effects)
Miglitol
(High dose nicotinic acid may
antagonize effects)
Nicotine
(Transdermal nicotine may
enhance nicotinic acid-induced
flushing)
Nitrates and Nitrites
(High dose nicotinic acid may
potentiate hypotensive effects)
Nonsteroidal Anti-Inflammatory
Drugs
(May decrease high dose nicotinic
acid-induced flushing)
Pioglitazone Hydrochloride
(High dose nicotinic acid may
antagonize effects)
Repaglinide
(High dose nicotinic acid may
antagonize effects)
Rosiglitazone Maleate
(High dose nicotinic acid may
antagonize effects)
Sulfonylureas
(High dose nicotinic acid may
antagonize effects)
Warfarin Sodium
(Nicotinic acid may enhance
anticoagulant effects)

INSULIN
DHEA
(May decrease DHEA levels)

INTERLEUKEN-2
Melatonin
(Possible augmentation of the
antitumor effect by Melatonin)

INULIN
(*See under* Inulins)

INULINS
Bone Meal
(Increased absorption of Calcium)
Calcium
(Inulins may enhance absorption
of dietary and supplemental
Calcium)
Magnesium
(Inulins may enhance absorption
of dietary and supplemental
Magnesium)
Probiotics
(Inulins may increase beneficial
effects of Probiotics)

IODINE
Antithyroid Agents
(May potentiate the hypothyroid
effect of iodides)
C-Gluosylflavones
(Inhibit thyroid peroxidase
activity)
Goitrogens
(May compete with iodide and
cause hypothyroidism)
Lithium
(Potassium iodide and lithium may
result in hypothyroidism)
Selenium
(Synergistic activity in the
treatment of Kashin-Beck disease
and osteoarthropathy)
Soybean Preparations
(Inhibit thyroid peroxidase)
Warfarin Sodium
(Potassium iodide may decrease
the anticoagulant effectiveness of
warfarin)

IPRIFLAVONE
Bisphosphonates
(Additive effects with Ipriflavone)
Boron
(Additive effects with Ipriflavone)
Calcitonin, unspecified
(Additive effects with Ipriflavone)

Calcium
(Additive effects with Ipriflavone)
Estrogen
(Additive effects with Ipriflavone)
Fluorine & Fluoride Preparations
(Additive effects with Ipriflavone)
Nifedipine
(Increased serum levels with
Ipriflavone)
Selective Estrogen Receptor
Modulators
(Additive effects with Ipriflavone)
Theophylline
(Metabolism and elimination may
be inhibited by Ipriflavone)
Tolbutamide
(Increased serum levels with
Ipriflavone)
Vitamin D
(Additive effects with Ipriflavone)
Vitamin K
(Additive effects with Ipriflavone)

IRON
Antacids, aluminum-containing
(Decreased absorption of Iron)
Beta-Carotene
(Enhanced absorption of Iron)
Bisphosphonates
(Decreased absorption of the
bisphosphonate)
Calcium
(Decreased absorption of Iron)
Copper
(Decreased Copper levels)
Cysteine
(Increased absorption of Iron)
Gamma-Tocopherol
(The ferrous form of iron can
oxidize Gamma-Tocopherol to its
pro-oxidant form)
Guaiac
(High false positive occult blood
with Iron supplements)
Histamine H₂-receptor antagonists
(Decreased absorption of carbonyl
iron)
Inositol
(Decreased absorption of Iron)
Inositol Hexaphosphate
(May form chelates with Inositol
Hexaphosphate)

L-Cysteine
(Increased absorption of Iron)
Levodopa
(Decreased absorption of
levodopa)
Levothyroxine Sodium
(Decreased absorption of
levothyroxine)
Magnesium
(Decreased absorption of Iron)
N-Acetyl-L-Cysteine (NAC)
(Increased absorption of Iron)
Oxalic Acid
(Decreased absorption of Iron)
Pectin
(Decreased absorption of Iron)
Penicillamine
(Decreased absorption of
penicillamine)
Phytic Acid
(Decreased absorption of Iron)
Proton Pump Inhibitor
(Decreased absorption of carbonyl
iron)
Psyllium
(Decreased absorption of Iron)
Quinolones
(Decreased absorption of both the
quinolone and Iron)
Soy Protein
(Reduced availability of Iron)
Tannins
(Decreased absorption of Iron)
Tetracyclines, unspecified
(Decreased absorption of both the
tetracycline and Iron)
Tocotrienols
(Iron may cause oxidation of
tocotrienols)
Vanadium
(Decreased absorption of Iron)
Vitamin C
(Enhanced absorption of Iron)
Vitamin E
(Iron may cause oxidation of the
Tocopherols)
Zinc
(Decreased absorption of both Iron
and Zinc)

IRON SUPPLEMENTS
Ascorbyl Palmitate
(Vitamin C may cause iron
overload)
Liver Hydrolysate/Desiccated Liver
(Liver Hydrolysate and Desiccated
Liver may have additive effects)
Vitamin C
(Vitamin C may cause iron
overload)

ISONIAZID
Gamma-Tocopherol
(Decreased Gamma-Tocopherol
absorption)
Melatonin
(Possible enhanced effect with
Melatonin)
Piperine
(Piperine may inhibit metabolism)
Tocotrienols
(May decrease Tocotrienol
absorption)
Vitamin B6
(May result in Vitamin B6
deficiency)
Vitamin E
(Decreased Vitamin E absorption)

ISOTRETINOIN
Vitamin A
(May produce additive toxicity
effects)

KETOCONAZOLE
Vitamin D
(May decrease serum 1, 25-
dihydroxyvitamin D levels)

L-ARGININE
Cyclosporine
(L-Arginine may counteract
antinaturetic effects)
Ibuprofen
(L-Arginine may increase
absorption)
Nitrates, organic
(L-Arginine may potentiate
effects)
Sildenafil Citrate
(L-Arginine may potentiate
effects)

Yohimbine Hydrochloride
(L-Arginine may potentiate
effects)

L-CARNITINE
Choline
(May lead to increased
L-Carnitine retention)
Didanosine
(May produce L-Carnitine
deficiencies)
Stavudine
(May produce L-Carnitine
deficiencies)
Valproic Acid
(May produce L-Carnitine
deficiencies)
Zalcitabine
(May produce L-Carnitine
deficiencies)

L-CYSTEINE
Ascorbic Acid
(May inhibit the oxidation of
L-Cysteine)
Iron
(Increased absorption of Iron)
Zinc
(Increased absorption of Zinc)

L-GLUTAMINE
Human Growth Hormone
(L-Glutamine may enhance
nutrient absorption with short
bowel syndrome)
Indomethacin
(L-Glutamine may inhibit
intestinal permeability caused by
indomethacin)
Methotrexate Sodium
(May decrease L-Glutamine
effects)
Paclitaxel
(L-Glutamine may prevent
paclitaxel adverse reactions)

L-HISTIDINE
Antihistamines
(L-Histidine might decrease the
efficacy)
Histamine H2-receptor antagonists
(L-Histidine might decrease the
efficacy)

Medroxyprogesterone Acetate
(L-Histidine may enhance the
antineoplastic effect)
Zinc
(Enhanced absorption of Zinc)

L-LYSINE
Calcium
(L-Lysine may increase Calcium
absorption)

L-METHIONINE
Acetaminophen
(L-Methionine may decrease
hepatic toxicity with overdosage)
Gentamicin
(Methionine may protect against
ototoxicity)
Glycine
(L-Methionine may decrease
Glycine levels with low-protein
diet)
Methotrexate
(L-Methionine may decrease
hepatic toxicity with overdosage)
Zinc
(Increased absorption of Zinc)

L-PHENYLALANINE
Neuroleptics
(L-Phenylalanine may potentiate
tardive dyskinesia adverse effects)
Pargyline Hydrochloride
(L-Phenylalanine may cause
hypertension)
Phenelzine Sulfate
(L-Phenylalanine may cause
hypertension)
Selegiline Hydrochloride
(L-Phenylalanine may have
synergistic antidepressant effects)
Tranylcypromine Sulfate
(L-Phenylalanine may cause
hypertension)

L-THEANINE
Doxorubicin Hydrochloride
(L-Theanine may enhance
antitumor effects and decrease
adverse effects)
Idarubicin Hydrochloride
(L-Theanine may enhance
antitumor effects and decrease
adverse effects)

L-TYROSINE
Pargyline Hydrochloride
(L-Tyrosine may cause
hypertension)
Phenelzine Sulfate
(L-Tyrosine may cause
hypertension)
Tranylcypromine Sulfate
(L-Tyrosine may cause
hypertension)

LACTULOSE
Antacids, non-absorbable
(May increase Lactulose effects)
Calcium
(Lactulose may enhance
absorption of dietary and
supplemental Calcium)
Magnesium
(Lactulose may enhance
absorption of dietary and
supplemental Magnesium)
Probiotics
(Probiotics may increase Lactulose
beneficial effects)

LAMIVUDINE
Riboflavin (Vitamin B2)
(Riboflavin may reverse
nucleoside analogue-induced lactic
acidosis in mild Riboflavin
deficiencies)

LATAMOXEF
Vitamin K
(Can cause Vitamin K deficiency
and hypothrombinemia)

LAXATIVES, MAGNESIUM-CONTAINING
Manganese
(Decreased absorption of
Manganese)

LEVODOPA
Iron
(Decreased absorption of
levodopa)
Octacosanol
(Worsened dyskinesias in
Parkinson's disease)
Vitamin B6
(Vitamin B6 may reverse
therapeutic effects if not given
with carbidopa)

LEVOTHYROXINE SODIUM
Bone Meal
(Decreased levothyroxine
absorption and increased serum
thyrotropin levels)
Calcium
(Decreased levothyroxine
absorption and increased serum
thyrotropin levels)
Iron
(Decreased absorption of
levothyroxine)

LIPID
(*See under* Diet, lipid)

LIPOPHILIC DRUGS, UNSPECIFIED
Alpha-Tocopheryl Polyethylene
Glycol Succinate
(Increased absorption of lipophilic
drugs)
Chitosan
(Might bind to Chitosan)
Medium-Chain Triglycerides
(MCT may facilitate the
absorption of lipophilic drugs)

LITHIUM
Folate
(Folic acid may increase efficacy)
Iodine
(Potassium iodide and lithium may
result in hypothyroidism)
Potassium
(May increase Lithium toxicity)
Psyllium
(Reduced absorption of Lithium)

LIVER HYDROLYSATE/DESICCATED LIVER
Iron Supplements
(Liver Hydrolysate and Desiccated
Liver may have additive effects)

LOMETREXOL
Folate
(Folic acid may be synergistic and
decrease adverse effects)

LOVASTATIN
Ascorbyl Palmitate
(Grapefruit flavonoids may
increase bioavailability due to
cytochrome P-450 3A4 inhibition)
Coenzyme Q10 (CoQ10)
(Decreases CoQ10 levels)

Pectin
(Decreased absorption of
lovastatin)
Vitamin C
(Grapefruit flavonoids may
increase bioavailability due to
cytochrome P-450 3A4 inhibition)

LUTEIN
Beta-Carotene
(May decrease the absorption of
Beta-Carotene)
Pectin
(Decreased absorption of Lutein)
Sodium Alginates and other Phyco-
Polysaccharides
(Decreased absorption of Lutein)

LUTEIN AND ZEAXANTHIN
Beta-Carotene
(Decreased absorption of Lutein
and Zeaxanthin)
Cholestyramine
(Decreased absorption of Lutein
and Zeaxanthin)
Colestipol
(Decreased absorption of Lutein
and Zeaxanthin)
Fat Substitute
(Decreased absorption of Lutein
and Zeaxanthin)
Medium-Chain Triglycerides
(Enhanced absorption of Lutein
and Zeaxanthin)
Mineral Oil
(Decreased absorption of Lutein
and Zeaxanthin)
Oils, dietary
(Increased absorption of Lutein
and Zeaxanthin)
Pectin
(Decreased absorption of Lutein
and Zeaxanthin)

LYCOPENE
Beta-Carotene
(Increased absorption of
Lycopene)
Cholestyramine
(Decreased absorption of
Lycopene)
Colestipol Hydrochloride
(Decreased absorption of
Lycopene)

Fat Substitute
(Reduced absorption of Lycopene)
Medium-Chain Triglycerides
(Enhanced absorption of
Lycopene)
Mineral Oil
(Reduced absorption of Lycopene)
Oils, dietary
(Enhanced absorption of
Lycopene)
Pectin
(Decreased absorption of
Lycopene)
Phytosterols
(Low serum levels due to
Phytosterols)
Sodium Alginates and other Phyco-
Polysaccharides
(Decreased absorption of
Lycopene)

LYSINE
(See under L-Lysine)

MACROLIDE ANTIBIOTICS
Red Yeast Rice
(Increased risk of myopathy)

MAGNESIUM
Bisphosphonates
(Decreased absorption of the
bisphosphonate)
Boron
(Increased Magnesium levels)
Calcium
(Decreased absorption of
Magnesium)
Fructo-oligosaccharides
(Increased absorption of
Magnesium)
Inositol
(Decreased absorption of
Magnesium)
Inositol Hexaphosphate
(May form chelates with Inositol
Hexaphosphate)
Inulins
(Inulins may enhance absorption
of dietary and supplemental
Magnesium)
Iron
(Decreased absorption of Iron)

Lactulose
(Lactulose may enhance
absorption of dietary and
supplemental Magnesium)
Manganese
(Decreased absorption of
Manganese)
Medium-Chain Triglycerides
(MCT may facilitate the
absorption of Magnesium)
Oxalic Acid
(Decreased absorption of
Magnesium)
Pectin
(Decreased absorption of
Magnesium)
Phosphate Salts
(Decreased absorption of
Phosphate and Magnesium)
Phytic Acid
(Decreased absorption of
Magnesium)
Prebiotics
(Enhanced absorption of
Magnesium)
Psyllium
(Decreased absorption of
Magnesium)
Quinolones
(Decreased absorption of
quinolones)
Sodium Alginate
(Decreased absorption of
Magnesium)
Sodium Alginates and other Phyco-
Polysaccharides
(Decreased absorption of
Magnesium)
Soy Protein
(Reduced availability of
Magnesium)
Synbiotics
(Enhanced absorption of
Magnesium)
Tetracyclines, unspecified
(Decreased absorption of
tetracyclines)
Transgalacto-Oligosaccharides
(Enhanced absorption of
Magnesium)

MANGANESE

Antacids, magnesium-containing
(Decreased absorption of
Manganese)

Calcium
(Decreased absorption of
Manganese)

Inositol Hexaphosphate
(May form chelates with Inositol
Hexaphosphate)

Laxatives, magnesium-containing
(Decreased absorption of
Manganese)

Magnesium
(Decreased absorption of
Manganese)

Oxalic Acid
(Decreased absorption of
Manganese)

Phytic Acid
(Decreased absorption of
Manganese)

Sodium Alginates and other Phyco-
Polysaccharides
(Decreased absorption of
Manganese)

Soy Protein
(Reduced availability of
Manganese)

Tetracyclines, unspecified
(Reduced absorption of
Manganese)

MEDIUM-CHAIN TRIGLYCERIDES

Calcium
(MCT may facilitate the
absorption of Calcium)

Carotenoids
(MCT may facilitate the
absorption of carotenoids)

Fatty Acids
(MCT may facilitate the
absorption of fatty acids)

Flavonoids
(MCT may facilitate the
absorption of flavonoids)

Gamma-Tocopherol
(Enhanced Gamma-Tocopherol
absorption)

Lipophilic drugs, unspecified
(MCT may facilitate the
absorption of lipophilic drugs)

Lutein and Zeaxanthin
(Enhanced absorption of Lutein
and Zeaxanthin)

Lycopene
(Enhanced absorption of
Lycopene)

Magnesium
(MCT may facilitate the
absorption of Magnesium)

Tocotrienols
(May increase Tocotrienol
absorption)

Vitamin A
(MCT may facilitate the
absorption of Vitamin A)

Vitamin D
(MCT may facilitate the
absorption of Vitamin D)

Vitamin E
(MCT may facilitate the
absorption of Vitamin E)

Vitamin K
(MCT may facilitate the
absorption of Vitamin K)

MEDROXYPROGESTERONE ACETATE

L-Histidine
(L-Histidine may enhance the
antineoplastic effect)

MELATONIN

Antidepressant Medications,
unspecified
(May increase sedation and
adverse effects with Melatonin)

Antihistamines
(May increase sedation and
adverse effects with Melatonin)

Aspirin
(May decrease Melatonin levels)

Benzodiazepines
(May increase sedation and
adverse effects with Melatonin)

Beta Blockers
(May lead to decreased Melatonin
levels)

Fluoxetine Hydrochloride
(Psychotic episode reported with
Melatonin)

Fluvoxamine Maleate
(Increases the bioavailability of
oral Melatonin)

Interleuken-2
(Possible augmentation of the
antitumor effect by Melatonin)

Isoniazid
(Possible enhanced effect with
Melatonin)

Nonsteroidal Anti-Inflammatory
Drugs
(May decrease Melatonin levels)

Progestins
(Concomitant Melatonin may
cause additive effect in inhibiting
ovarian function)

METFORMIN

Folate
(Folic acid may reduce metformin-
associated homocysteinemia)

Inositol Nicotinate
(High dose nicotinic acid may
antagonize effects)

Niacin
(High dose nicotinic acid may
antagonize effects)

Vitamin B12
(May decrease absorption of
Vitamin B12)

METHIONINE

(See under L-Methionine)

METHOTREXATE

Folate
(Folic acid may reduce toxic side
effects)

L-Methionine
(L-Methionine may decrease
hepatic toxicity with overdosage)

METHOTREXATE SODIUM

Choline
(May decrease Choline
metabolites)

Glutamine Peptides
(May decrease L-Glutamine
effects)

L-Glutamine
(May decrease L-Glutamine
effects)

METHYLDOPA

5-Hydroxytryptophan
(Inhibits 5-HTP metabolism to
serotonin)

METHYSERGIDE MALEATE

5-Hydroxytryptophan
(5-HTP may decrease effects)

METOCLOPRAMIDE HYDROCHLORIDE

Riboflavin (Vitamin B2)
(Decreased absorption of
Riboflavin)

MIGLITOL

Inositol Nicotinate
(High dose nicotinic acid may
antagonize effects)

Niacin
(High dose nicotinic acid may
antagonize effects)

MINERAL OIL

Beta-Carotene
(May decrease the absorption of
Beta-Carotene)

Gamma-Tocopherol
(Decreased Gamma-Tocopherol
absorption)

Lutein and Zeaxanthin
(Decreased absorption of Lutein
and Zeaxanthin)

Lycopene
(Reduced absorption of Lycopene)

Tocotrienols
(May decrease Tocotrienol
absorption)

Vitamin A
(May decrease Vitamin A
absorption)

Vitamin D
(May reduce Vitamin D
absorption)

Vitamin E
(Decreased Vitamin E absorption)

Vitamin K
(May reduce Vitamin K
absorption)

MOLYBDENUM

Acetaminophen
(High dose molybdate may inhibit
acetaminophen metabolism)

Copper
(High dose of Molybdenum may
antagonize dietary Copper
absorption and high dose Copper
may antagonize Molybdenum
absorption)

MONOAMINE OXIDASE INHIBITORS

5-Hydroxytryptophan
(5-HTP may increase risk of side
effects)

Brewer's Yeast
(May cause hypertension with
Brewer's Yeast)

L-Phenylalanine
(L-Phenylalanine may cause
hypertension)

MORPHINE SULFATE

DHEA
(May decrease DHEA levels)

MYCO-POLYSACCHARIDES

Antiplatelet Drugs
(Ganoderma may enhance
antiplatelet effects)

MYO-INOSITOL

5-HT1 Receptor Agonists
(May have additive effects with
Myo-Inositol)

Hypericum
(May have additive effects with
Myo-Inositol)

Selective Serotonin Reuptake
Inhibitors
(May have additive effects with
Myo-Inositol)

N-ACETYL-L-CYSTEINE (NAC)

Iron
(Increased absorption of Iron)

Zinc
(Increased absorption of Zinc)

NEFAZODONE HYDROCHLORIDE

Red Yeast Rice
(Increased risk of myopathy)

NEOMYCIN

Gamma-Tocopherol
(Impaired utilization of Gamma-
Tocopherol)

Tocotrienols
(May decrease Tocotrienol effects)

Vitamin E
(Impaired utilization of
Vitamin E)

NEUROLEPTICS

L-Phenylalanine
(L-Phenylalanine may potentiate
tardive dyskinesia adverse effects)

NIACIN

Acarbose
(High dose nicotinic acid may
antagonize effects)

Alpha Adrenergic Blockers
(High dose nicotinic acid may
potentiate hypotensive effects)

Aspirin
(May decrease high dose nicotinic
acid-induced flushing)

Beverages, hot
(May increase nicotinic acid-
induced flushing)

Calcium Channel Blockers,
Unspecified
(High dose nicotinic acid may
potentiate hypotensive effects)

Cholestyramine
(May reduce nicotinic acid
absorption and may have
synergistic antihyperlipidemic
effects)

Colestipol
(May reduce nicotinic acid
absorption and may have
synergistic antihyperlipidemic
effects)

Ethanol
(May increase nicotinic acid-
induced flushing)

Food, hot
(May increase nicotinic acid-
induced flushing)

Ganglionic Blocking Agents
(Nicotinic acid may potentiate
effects)

Gemfibrozil
(High dose nicotinic acid may
have synergistic antihyperlipidemic
effects)

HMG-CoA Reductase Inhibitors
(May produce rhabdomyolysis and
may have synergistic
antihyperlipidemic effects)

Metformin
(High dose nicotinic acid may
antagonize effects)

Miglitol
(High dose nicotinic acid may
antagonize effects)

Nicotine
(Transdermal nicotine may enhance nicotinic acid-induced flushing)
Nitrates and Nitrites
(High dose nicotinic acid may potentiate hypotensive effects)
Nonsteroidal Anti-Inflammatory Drugs
(May decrease high dose nicotinic acid-induced flushing)
Pioglitazone Hydrochloride
(High dose nicotinic acid may antagonize effects)
Repaglinide
(High dose nicotinic acid may antagonize effects)
Rosiglitazone Maleate
(High dose nicotinic acid may antagonize effects)
Sulfonylureas
(High dose nicotinic acid may antagonize effects)
Warfarin Sodium
(Nicotinic acid may enhance anticoagulant effects)

NIACINAMIDE
(*See under* Nicotinamide)

NICOTINAMIDE
Carbamazepine
(Nicotinamide may decrease clearance)

NICOTINE
Inositol Nicotinate
(Transdermal nicotine may enhance nicotinic acid-induced flushing)
Niacin
(Transdermal nicotine may enhance nicotinic acid-induced flushing)

NICOTINIC ACID
Pantethine
(May have additive lipid-modulatory effects)
Red Yeast Rice
(Increased risk of myopathy)

NIFEDIPINE
Ipriflavone
(Increased serum levels with Ipriflavone)

NISOLDIPINE
Ascorbyl Palmitate
(Grapefruit flavonoids may increase bioavailability due to cytochrome P-450 3A4 inhibition)
Vitamin C
(Grapefruit flavonoids may increase bioavailability due to cytochrome P-450 3A4 inhibition)

NITRATES AND NITRITES
Acetylcysteine
(May cause headaches with NAC)
Inositol Nicotinate
(High dose nicotinic acid may potentiate hypotensive effects)
Niacin
(High dose nicotinic acid may potentiate hypotensive effects)

NITRATES, ORGANIC
L-Arginine
(L-Arginine may potentiate effects)

NITROFURANTOIN
Deglycyrrhizinated Licorice (DGL)
(Increased excretion rate of nitrofurantoin)

NONSTEROIDAL ANTI-INFLAMMATORY DRUGS
Borage Oil
(Increased anticoagulant and antiplatelet effects with Borage Oil)
Eicosapentaenoic Acid (EPA)
(May interact with EPA)
Evening Primrose Oil
(EPO may increase bleeding tendencies)
Fish Oil
(May interact with Fish Oil)
Flaxseed Oil
(May interact with Flaxseed Oil)
Folate
(Large doses may exert antifolate activity)

Hemp Seed Oil
(Increased bleeding and susceptibility to bruising)
Inositol Nicotinate
(May decrease high dose nicotinic acid-induced flushing)
Melatonin
(May decrease Melatonin levels)
Niacin
(May decrease high dose nicotinic acid-induced flushing)
Perilla Oil
(Increased antithrombotic effects with Perilla Oil)

NUTRITIONAL SUPPLEMENT
Activated Charcoal
(Avoid using Activated Charcoal within two hours of taking these products)
Bentonite
(Bentonite may adsorb certain nutritional supplements)
Curcuminoids
(Bromelain and Piperine may enhance the absorption of Curcuminoids)

OCTACOSANOL
Carbidopa
(Worsened dyskinesias in Parkinson's disease)
Levodopa
(Worsened dyskinesias in Parkinson's disease)

OILS, DIETARY
Lutein and Zeaxanthin
(Increased absorption of Lutein and Zeaxanthin)
Lycopene
(Enhanced absorption of Lycopene)

OPIATES
Gamma-Hydroxybutyrate (GHB)
(May be life threatening with GHB)

ORAL CONTRACEPTIVES
Riboflavin (Vitamin B2)
(Decreased serum levels of Riboflavin)
Vitamin A
(May increase serum retinol)

Vitamin B6
(May increase Vitamin B6 requirements)

ORLISTAT
Beta-Carotene
(May decrease the absorption of Beta-Carotene)
Tocotrienols
(May inhibit Tocotrienol absorption)
Vitamin A
(May decrease Vitamin A absorption)
Vitamin D
(May reduce Vitamin D absorption)
Vitamin K
(May reduce Vitamin K absorption)

OX BILE, DESICCATED
Gamma-Tocopherol
(Increased Gamma-Tocopherol absorption)
Tocotrienols
(May increase Tocotrienol absorption)
Vitamin E
(Increased absorption of Vitamin E)

OXALIC ACID
Bone Meal
(Decreased absorption of Calcium)
Calcium
(Decreased absorption of Calcium)
Iron
(Decreased absorption of Iron)
Magnesium
(Decreased absorption of Magnesium)
Manganese
(Decreased absorption of Manganese)
Zinc
(Decreased absorption of Zinc)

PACLITAXEL
Ascorbyl Palmitate
(Vitamin C may potentiate antineoplastic activity)

Glutamine Peptides
(L-Glutamine may prevent paclitaxel adverse reactions)
L-Glutamine
(L-Glutamine may prevent paclitaxel adverse reactions)
Vitamin C
(Vitamin C may potentiate antineoplastic activity)

PANTETHINE
HMG-CoA Reductase Inhibitors
(May have additive lipid-modulatory effects)
Nicotinic Acid
(May have additive lipid-modulatory effects)

PANTOTHENIC ACID
Biotin
(May decrease Biotin absorption)

PAPAIN
Quercetin
(Increased absorption of Quercetin)

PARA-AMINOBENZOIC ACID (PABA)
Sulfonamides
(Decreased effectiveness)

PARA-AMINOSALICYLIC ACID
Vitamin B12
(May decrease the absorption of Vitamin B12)

PARGYLINE HYDROCHLORIDE
Brewer's Yeast
(May cause hypertension with Brewer's Yeast)
L-Phenylalanine
(L-Phenylalanine may cause hypertension)
L-Tyrosine
(L-Tyrosine may cause hypertension)

PECTIN
Beta-Carotene
(Decreased absorption of Beta-Carotene)
Calcium
(Decreased absorption of Calcium)
Clindamycin Hydrochloride
(Decreased absorption of clindamycin)

Copper
(Decreased absorption of Copper)
Digoxin
(Decreased absorption of digoxin)
Iron
(Decreased absorption of Iron)
Lovastatin
(Decreased absorption of lovastatin)
Lutein
(Decreased absorption of Lutein)
Lutein and Zeaxanthin
(Decreased absorption of Lutein and Zeaxanthin)
Lycopene
(Decreased absorption of Lycopene)
Magnesium
(Decreased absorption of Magnesium)
Tetracycline Hydrochloride
(Decreased absorption of tetracycline)
Zinc
(Decreased absorption of Zinc)

PENICILLAMINE
Copper
(Decreased absorption of Copper and penicillamine)
Iron
(Decreased absorption of penicillamine)
Vitamin B6
(May result in Vitamin B6 deficiency)

PENTAMIDINE ISETHIONATE
Arnica
(Increased risk of prolonged QT interval when given with Arnica)

PERILLA OIL
Allium sativum
(Increased antithrombotic effects with Perilla Oil)
Aspirin
(Increased antithrombotic effects with Perilla Oil)
Ginkgo biloba
(Increased antithrombotic effects with Perilla Oil)

Nonsteroidal Anti-Inflammatory
Drugs
   (Increased antithrombotic effects
   with Perilla Oil)

PHENELZINE SULFATE
Brewer's Yeast
   (May cause hypertension with
   Brewer's Yeast)
L-Phenylalanine
   (L-Phenylalanine may cause
   hypertension)
L-Tyrosine
   (L-Tyrosine may cause
   hypertension)
Vitamin B6
   (May result in Vitamin B6
   deficiency)

PHENOBARBITAL
Biotin
   (May decrease Biotin levels)
Folate
   (May decrease Folate levels and
   increase homocysteine levels;
   High dose folic acid may decrease
   serum levels)
Vitamin B6
   (Vitamin B6 may lower
   phenobarbital plasma levels)
Vitamin D
   (May decrease serum 25-
   hydroxyvitamin D levels)

PHENOTHIAZINES
Borage Oil
   (May cause seizures with Borage
   Oil)
Evening Primrose Oil
   (EPO lowers seizure threshold)

PHENOXYBENZAMINE HYDROCHLORIDE
5-Hydroxytryptophan
   (Inhibits 5-HTP metabolism to
   serotonin)

PHENYLALANINE
(*See under* L-Phenylalanine)

PHENYTOIN
Biotin
   (May decrease Biotin levels)

Folate
   (May decrease Folate levels and
   increase homocysteine levels;
   High dose folic acid may decrease
   serum levels)
Piperine
   (Piperine may inhibit metabolism)
Vitamin B6
   (Vitamin B6 may lower phenytoin
   plasma levels)
Vitamin D
   (May decrease serum 25-
   hydroxyvitamin D levels)

PHOSPHATE SALTS
Magnesium
   (Decreased absorption of
   Phosphate and Magnesium)
Zinc
   (Decreased absorption of Zinc)

PHOSPHATIDYLCHOLINE
Huperzine A
   (Additive effects and increased
   adverse effects with Huperzine A)

PHOSPHORUS
Antacids, aluminum-containing
   (Decreased absorption of
   Phosphorus)
Zinc
   (Decreased absorption of Zinc)

PHYSOSTIGMINE SALICYLATE
Huperzine A
   (Additive effects and increased
   adverse effects with Huperzine A)

PHYTIC ACID
Calcium
   (Decreased absorption of Calcium)
Chromium
   (Decreased absorption of
   Chromium)
Copper
   (Decreased absorption of Copper)
Iron
   (Decreased absorption of Iron)
Magnesium
   (Decreased absorption of
   Magnesium)
Manganese
   (Decreased absorption of
   Manganese)

Zinc
   (Decreased absorption of Zinc)

PHYTONADIONE
(*See under* Vitamin K)

PHYTOSTANOLS
Gamma-Tocopherol
   (Decreased plasma Gamma-
   Tocopherol levels)
Tocotrienols
   (May decrease Tocotrienol levels)
Vitamin E
   (Decreased plasma Vitamin E
   levels)

PHYTOSTEROLS
Alpha-Carotene
   (Low serum levels due to
   Phytosterols)
Beta-Carotene
   (Low serum levels due to
   Phytosterols)
Gamma-Tocopherol
   (Decreased plasma Gamma-
   Tocopherol levels)
Lycopene
   (Low serum levels due to
   Phytosterols)
Tocotrienols
   (May decrease Tocotrienol levels)
Vitamin E
   (Low serum levels due to
   Phytosterols)

PIOGLITAZONE HYDROCHLORIDE
Inositol Nicotinate
   (High dose nicotinic acid may
   antagonize effects)
Niacin
   (High dose nicotinic acid may
   antagonize effects)

PIPERINE
Beta-Carotene
   (Piperine may enhance the
   absorption)
Coenzyme Q10
   (Piperine may enhance the
   absorption)
Curcuminoids
   (Piperine may enhance the
   absorption of Curcuminoids)
Dapsone
   (Piperine may inhibit metabolism)

Drugs, unspecified
(Piperine may inhibit metabolism)
Ethambutol Hydrochloride
(Piperine may inhibit metabolism)
Isoniazid
(Piperine may inhibit metabolism)
Phenytoin
(Piperine may inhibit metabolism)
Propanolol
(Piperine may inhibit metabolism)
Pyrazinamide
(Piperine may inhibit metbolism)
Rifampicin
(Piperine may inhibit metabolism)
Selenium
(Piperine may enhance the absorption)
Sulfadiazine
(Piperine may inhibit metabolism)
Theophylline
(Piperine may inhibit metabolism)
Vitamin B6
(Piperine may enhance the absorption)
Vitamin C
(Piperine may enhance the absorption)

PLANT PHENOLIC COMPOUNDS
Gamma-Tocopherol
(Helps to maintain levels of reduced Gamma-Tocopherol)
Vitamin E
(Help to maintain levels of Vitamin E)

POLICOSANOL
Aspirin
(Antithrombotic synergistic effect)

POLYPHENOLS
Alpha-Tocopheryl Polyethylene Glycol Succinate
(Increased absorption of polyphenols)

POTASSIUM
ACE Inhibitors
(Increased serum Potassium due to inhibition of aldosterone production)

Amiloride Hydrochloride
(Concomitant potassium-sparing diuretic and Potassium supplements can produce severe hyperkalemia)
Lithium
(May increase Lithium toxicity)
Spironolactone
(Concomitant potassium-sparing diuretic and Potassium supplements can produce severe hyperkalemia)
Triamterene
(Concomitant potassium-sparing diuretic and Potassium supplements can produce severe hyperkalemia)

POTASSIUM CHLORIDE
Vitamin B12
(May decrease absorption of dietary Vitamin B12)

PRAVASTATIN SODIUM
Coenzyme Q10 (CoQ10)
(Decreases CoQ10 levels)

PREBIOTICS
Alpha Galactosidase Enzyme
(Decreased effectiveness of the soy oligosaccharides)
Calcium
(Enhanced absorption of Calcium)
Magnesium
(Enhanced absorption of Magnesium)
Probiotics
(Synergistic effects with Prebiotics)

PRIMIDONE
Biotin
(May decrease Biotin levels)
Folate
(May decrease Folate levels and increase homocysteine levels; High dose folic acid may decrease serum levels)

PROBENECID
Riboflavin (Vitamin B2)
(Inhibit absorption of Riboflavin)

PROBIOTICS
Inulins
(Inulins may increase beneficial effects of Probiotics)
Lactulose
(Probiotics may increase Lactulose beneficial effects)
Prebiotics
(Enhanced effectiveness of the Probiotics)
Transgalacto-Oligosaccharides
(Enhanced beneficial effects of TOS)

PROCAINAMIDE
Arnica
(Increased risk of prolonged QT interval when given with Arnica)

PROCHLORPERAZINE
Arnica
(Increased risk of prolonged QT interval when given with Arnica)

PROGESTINS
Melatonin
(Concomitant Melatonin may cause additive effect in inhibiting ovarian function)

PROPANOLOL
Piperine
(Piperine may inhibit metabolism)

PROPANTHELINE BROMIDE
Riboflavin (Vitamin B2)
(Enhanced absorption of Riboflavin)

PROPRANOLOL HYDROCHLORIDE
Coenzyme Q10 (CoQ10)
(May inhibit some CoQ10-dependent enzymes)

PROTEASE INHIBITORS
Gamma-Hydroxybutyrate (GHB)
(May be life threatening with GHB)
Red Yeast Rice
(Increased risk of myopathy)

PROTEIN
(*See under* Diet high in Protein)

PROTON PUMP INHIBITOR
Bone Meal
(Decreased absorption of Calcium)

Calcium
(Decreased absorption of Calcium)
Indole-3-Carbinol
(Block the conversion of Indole-3 Carbinol to DIM and ICZ)
Iron
(Decreased absorption of carbonyl iron)
Vitamin B12
(May decrease absorption of dietary Vitamin B12, not supplemental)

PSYLLIUM
Calcium
(Decreased absorption of Calcium)
Carbamazepine
(Reduced absorption of carbamazepine)
Cholestyramine
(Enhanced cholesterol-lowering action)
Copper
(Decreased absorption of Copper)
Digoxin
(Reduced absorption of digoxin)
Iron
(Decreased absorption of Iron)
Lithium
(Reduced absorption of Lithium)
Magnesium
(Decreased absorption of Magnesium)
Warfarin Sodium
(Reduced absorption of warfarin sodium)
Zinc
(Decreased absorption of Zinc)

PSYLLIUM HUSK
(*See under* Psyllium)

PYCNOGENOL
Dextroamphetamine
(May be synergistic with Pycnogenol for attention deficit-hyperactivity disorder management)

PYRAZINAMIDE
Piperine
(Piperine may inhibit metbolism)

PYRIDOXINE HYDROCHLORIDE
(*See under* Vitamin B6)

PYRIMETHAMINE
Folate
(Folic acid may decrease antiparasitic effects)

QUERCETIN
Bromelains
(Increased absorption of Quercetin)
Cisplatin
(May cause genotoxicity in normal tissues when taken with Quercetin)
Papain
(Increased absorption of Quercetin)
Quinolones
(Competitively inhibited by Quercetin)

QUINACRINE HYDROCHLORIDE
Riboflavin (Vitamin B2)
(Inhibition of Riboflavin conversion to FMN and FAD)

QUINIDINE
Arnica
(Increased risk of prolonged QT interval when given with Arnica)

QUINOLONES
Bone Meal
(Decreased absorption of quinolones)
Calcium
(Decreased absorption of quinolones)
Iron
(Decreased absorption of both the quinolone and Iron)
Magnesium
(Decreased absorption of quinolones)
Quercetin
(Competitively inhibited by Quercetin)
Rutin
(Inhibition of activity due to Rutin)

RED YEAST RICE
Azole Antifungals
(Increased risk of myopathy)
Cyclosporine
(Increased risk of myopathy)

Fibrates
(Increased risk of myopathy)
Gemfibrozil
(Increased risk of myopathy)
Grapefruit Juice
(Increased risk of myopathy)
HMG-CoA Reductase Inhibitors
(Increased risk of adverse reactions)
Macrolide Antibiotics
(Increased risk of myopathy)
Nefazodone Hydrochloride
(Increased risk of myopathy)
Nicotinic Acid
(Increased risk of myopathy)
Protease Inhibitors
(Increased risk of myopathy)
Warfarin Sodium
(Increase in the INR as well as bleeding)

REPAGLINIDE
Inositol Nicotinate
(High dose nicotinic acid may antagonize effects)
Niacin
(High dose nicotinic acid may antagonize effects)

RETINOIDS
D-Glucarate
(Synergistic chemopreventive effects)

RIBOFLAVIN (VITAMIN B2)
Chlorpromazine
(Inhibition of Riboflavin conversion to FMN and FAD)
Cholestyramine
(Decreased absorption of Riboflavin)
Colestipol Hydrochloride
(Decreased absorption of Riboflavin)
Didanosine
(Riboflavin may reverse nucleoside analogue-induced lactic acidosis in mild Riboflavin deficiencies)
Doxorubicin Hydrochloride
(Inhibition of Riboflavin conversion to FMN and FAD)

Lamivudine
(Riboflavin may reverse nucleoside analogue-induced lactic acidosis in mild Riboflavin deficiencies)
Metoclopramide Hydrochloride
(Decreased absorption of Riboflavin)
Oral Contraceptives
(Decreased serum levels of Riboflavin)
Probenecid
(Inhibit absorption of Riboflavin)
Propantheline Bromide
(Enhanced absorption of Riboflavin)
Quinacrine Hydrochloride
(Inhibition of Riboflavin conversion to FMN and FAD)
Stavudine
(Riboflavin may reverse nucleoside analogue-induced lactic acidosis in mild Riboflavin deficiencies)
Tricyclic Antidepressants
(Inhibition of Riboflavin conversion to FMN and FAD)
Zidovudine
(Riboflavin may reverse nucleoside analogue-induced lactic acidosis in mild Riboflavin deficiencies)

RIFAMPICIN
Piperine
(Piperine may inhibit metabolism)

ROSIGLITAZONE MALEATE
Inositol Nicotinate
(High dose nicotinic acid may antagonize effects)
Niacin
(High dose nicotinic acid may antagonize effects)

RUTIN
Quinolones
(Inhibition of activity due to Rutin)
Vitamin C
(Prevention of Vitamin C oxidation, enhanced and/or inhibition of absorption with flavonoids)

SALICYLATES
Vitamin K
(Large doses may cause Vitamin K deficiency)

SAQUINAVIR
Ascorbyl Palmitate
(Grapefruit flavonoids may increase bioavailability due to cytochrome P-450 3A4 inhibition)
Vitamin C
(Grapefruit flavonoids may increase bioavailability due to cytochrome P-450 3A4 inhibition)

SELECTIVE ESTROGEN RECEPTOR MODULATORS
Ipriflavone
(Additive effects with Ipriflavone)

SELECTIVE SEROTONIN REUPTAKE INHIBITORS
Myo-Inositol
(May have additive effects with Myo-Inositol)

SELEGILINE HYDROCHLORIDE
L-Phenylalanine
(May have synergistic antidepressant effects)

SELENIUM
Alpha-Tocopheryl Polyethylene Glycol Succinate
(May function synergistically with Alpha-Tocopherol)
Gamma-Tocopherol
(Synergistic effect with Gamma-Tocopherol)
Iodine
(Synergistic activity in the treatment of Kashin-Beck disease, and osteoarthropathy)
Piperine
(Piperine may enhance the absorption)
Vitamin C
(Decreased absorption of Selenium)
Vitamin E
(Synergistic beneficial effects)

SEROTONINERGIC AGENTS
5-Hydroxytryptophan
(5-HTP may potentiate antidepressant effects and increase risk of side effects)

SILDENAFIL CITRATE
L-Arginine
(L-Arginine may potentiate effects)

SILICON
Aluminum-containing Compounds, unspecified
(Prevention of absorption due to Silicon)

SIMVASTATIN
Ascorbyl Palmitate
(Grapefruit flavonoids may increase bioavailability due to cytochrome P-450 3A4 inhibition)
Coenzyme Q10 (CoQ10)
(Decreases CoQ10 levels)
Vitamin C
(Grapefruit flavonoids may increase bioavailability due to cytochrome P-450 3A4 inhibition)

SKELETAL MUSCLE RELAXANTS
Gamma-Hydroxybutyrate (GHB)
(May be life threatening with GHB)

SODIUM ALGINATE
Bone Meal
(Decreased absorption of Calcium)
Calcium
(Decreased absorption of Calcium)
Magnesium
(Decreased absorption of Magnesium)

SODIUM ALGINATES AND OTHER PHYCO-POLYSACCHARIDES
Beta-Carotene
(Decreased absorption of Beta-Carotene)
Calcium
(Decreased absorption of Calcium)
Chromium
(Decreased absorption of Chromium)
Lutein
(Decreased absorption of Lutein)

Lycopene
(Decreased absorption of
Lycopene)
Magnesium
(Decreased absorption of
Magnesium)
Manganese
(Decreased absorption of
Manganese)
Zinc
(Decreased absorption of Zinc)

SOTALOL HYDROCHLORIDE
Arnica
(Increased risk of prolonged QT
interval when given with Arnica)

SOY PROTEIN
Calcium
(Reduced availability of Calcium)
Copper
(Reduced availability of Copper)
Iron
(Reduced availability of Iron)
Magnesium
(Reduced availability of
Magnesium)
Manganese
(Reduced availability of
Manganese)
Zinc
(Reduced availability of Zinc)

**SOY-CONTAINING DIETARY
SUPPLEMENTS**
Supplemental Enzymes
(Decreased prebiotic activity of
Soy products when taken with
alpha-galactosidase)

SOYBEAN PREPARATIONS
Iodine
(Inhibit thyroid peroxidase)

SPIRONOLACTONE
Potassium
(Concomitant potassium-sparing
diuretic and Potassium
supplements can produce severe
hyperkalemia)

SQUALENE
Vitamin K
(May reduce Vitamin K
absorption)

ST. JOHN'S WORT
(*See under* Hypericum)

STAVUDINE
Acetyl-L-Carnitine
(May lead to decreased Acetyl-L-
Carnitine levels)
L-Carnitine
(May produce L-Carnitine
deficiencies)
Riboflavin (Vitamin B2)
(Riboflavin may reverse
nucleoside analogue-induced lactic
acidosis in mild Riboflavin
deficiencies)

SUCRALFATE
Gamma-Tocopherol
(Interferes with Gamma-
Tocopherol absorption)
Tocotrienols
(May inhibit Tocotrienol
absorption)
Vitamin E
(Interferes with Vitamin E
absorption)

SULFADIAZINE
Piperine
(Piperine may inhibit metabolism)

SULFASALAZINE
Folate
(May decrease folic acid
absorption)

SULFITES
(*See under* Food, sulfites)

SULFONAMIDES
Para-Aminobenzoic Acid (PABA)
(Decreased effectiveness)

SULFONYLUREAS
Inositol Nicotinate
(High dose nicotinic acid may
antagonize effects)
Niacin
(High dose nicotinic acid may
antagonize effects)

SULINDAC
Dimethyl Sulfoxide (DMSO)
(May decrease the effects of
DMSO and increase side effects)

SUPPLEMENTAL ENZYMES
Acarbose
(Decreased efficacy of acarbose
when taken with amylase,
pancreatin, and pancrelipase)
Anticoagulant drugs, unspecified
(Enhanced anticoagulant activity
when taken with Bromelain)
Antithrombotic Agents
(Enhanced antithrombotic activity
when taken with Bromelain)
Soy-containing dietary supplements
(Decreased prebiotic activity of
Soy products when taken with
alpha-galactosidase)

SYMPATHOMIMETIC AGENTS
Tiratricol (TRIAC)
(Increased risk of coronary
insufficiency in patients with
coronary artery disease)

SYNBIOTICS
Calcium
(Enhanced absorption of Calcium)
Magnesium
(Enhanced absorption of
Magnesium)

TACRINE HYDROCHLORIDE
Huperzine A
(Additive effects and increased
adverse effects with Huperzine A)

TAMOXIFEN CITRATE
Indole-3-Carbinol
(May be synergistic with Indole-3-
Carbinol in protecting against
breast cancer)

TANNINS
Iron
(Decreased absorption of Iron)
Thiamin
(May inactivate Thiamin)
Zinc
(Decreased absorption of Zinc)

TESTOSTERONE
DHEA
(May increase adverse effects of
DHEA)

TETRACYCLINE HYDROCHLORIDE
Pectin
  (Decreased absorption of
  tetracycline)

TETRACYCLINES, UNSPECIFIED
Bone Meal
  (Decreased absorption of
  tetracyclines)
Bromelain
  (Bromelain may increase
  tetracycline levels)
Calcium
  (Decreased absorption of
  tetracyclines)
Iron
  (Decreased absorption of both the
  tetracycline and Iron)
Magnesium
  (Decreased absorption of
  tetracyclines)
Manganese
  (Reduced absorption of
  Manganese)

THEOPHYLLINE
Ipriflavone
  (Metabolism and elimination may
  be inhibited by Ipriflavone)
Piperine
  (Piperine may inhibit metabolism)
Vitamin B6
  (Vitamin B6 may increase risk of
  theophylline-induced seizures)

THIAMIN
Beverages, sulfites
  (May inactivate Thiamin)
Bumetanide
  (Chronic use may cause Thiamin
  deficiency)
Ethacrynic Acid
  (Chronic use may cause Thiamin
  deficiency)
Food, sulfites
  (May inactivate Thiamin)
Food, unspecified
  (Antithiamin factors in food
  inactivate Thiamin)
Furosemide
  (Chronic use may cause Thiamin
  deficiency)
Tannins
  (May inactivate Thiamin)

THYROID PREPARATIONS
Tiratricol (TRIAC)
  (Additive effects with Tiratricol)

THYROXINE
Calcium
  (Decreased thyroxine absorption)

TICLOPIDINE HYDROCHLORIDE
Alpha-Tocopheryl Polyethylene
Glycol Succinate
  (Enhanced antiplatelet effects of
  ticlopidine)
Gamma-Tocopherol
  (Increased effects of ticlopidine)
Vitamin E
  (Increased effects of ticlopidine)

TIRATRICOL (TRIAC)
Anticoagulant drugs, unspecified
  (Increased hypoprothrombinemic
  effect)
Sympathomimetic Agents
  (Increased risk of coronary
  insufficiency in patients with
  coronary artery disease)
Thyroid Preparations
  (Additive effects with Tiratricol)
Warfarin Sodium
  (Increased hypoprothrombinemic
  effect)

TIROFIBAN HYDROCHLORIDE
Alpha-Tocopheryl Polyethylene
Glycol Succinate
  (Enhanced antiplatelet effects of
  tirofiban)
Gamma-Tocopherol
  (Increased effects of tirofiban)
Vitamin E
  (Increased effects of tirofiban)

TIZANIDINE HYDROCHLORIDE
Glycine
  (Glycine may increase effects)

TOCOTRIENOLS
Allium sativum
  (May enhance antithrombotic
  activity)
Alpha-Tocopheryl Polyethylene
Glycol Succinate
  (Increased absorption when taken
  with TPGS; Decreased plasma
  levels with high doses of TPGS)

Antiplatelet Drugs
  (Tocotrienol may potentiate
  antiplatelet effects)
Cholestyramine
  (May decrease Tocotrienol
  absorption)
Colestipol
  (May decrease Tocotrienol
  absorption)
Fat Substitute
  (May inhibit Tocotrienol
  absorption)
Ginkgo biloba
  (May enhance antithrombotic
  activity)
HMG-CoA Reductase Inhibitors
  (Tocotrienols may have synergistic
  cholesterol-lowering effects)
Iron
  (May decrease Tocotrienol
  absorption)
Isoniazid
  (May decrease Tocotrienol
  absorption)
Medium-Chain Triglycerides
  (May increase Tocotrienol
  absorption)
Mineral Oil
  (May decrease Tocotrienol
  absorption)
Neomycin
  (May decrease Tocotrienol effects)
Orlistat
  (May inhibit Tocotrienol
  absorption)
Ox Bile, Desiccated
  (May increase Tocotrienol
  absorption)
Phytostanols
  (May decrease Tocotrienol levels)
Phytosterols
  (May decrease Tocotrienol levels)
Sucralfate
  (May inhibit Tocotrienol
  absorption)
Warfarin Sodium
  (Large dose Tocotrienols may
  enhance anticoagulant effects)

TOLBUTAMIDE
Ipriflavone
  (Increased serum levels with
  Ipriflavone)

TRANQUILIZERS

Gamma-Hydroxybutyrate (GHB)
  (May be life threatening with
  GHB)

TRANSGALACTO-OLIGOSACCHARIDES

Calcium
  (Enhanced absorption of Calcium)
Magnesium
  (Enhanced absorption of
  Magnesium)
Probiotics
  (Enhanced beneficial effects of
  TOS)

TRANYLCYPROMINE SULFATE

Brewer's Yeast
  (May cause hypertension with
  Brewer's Yeast)
L-Phenylalanine
  (L-Phenylalanine may cause
  hypertension)
L-Tyrosine
  (L-Tyrosine may cause
  hypertension)

TRIAMTERENE

Potassium
  (Concomitant potassium-sparing
  diuretic and Potassium
  supplements can produce severe
  hyperkalemia)

TRICYCLIC ANTIDEPRESSANTS

Riboflavin (Vitamin B2)
  (Inhibition of Riboflavin
  conversion to FMN and FAD)

TYROSINE

(*See under* L-Tyrosine)

VALPROIC ACID

Acetyl-L-Carnitine
  (May lead to L-Carnitine
  deficiencies)
Folate
  (May decrease Folate levels and
  increase homocysteine; High dose
  folic acid may decrease serum
  levels)
L-Carnitine
  (May produce L-Carnitine
  deficiencies)
Vitamin B6
  (Chronic use may decrease plasma
  pyridoxal 5'-phosphate)

VANADIUM

Aluminum Hydroxide
  (May decrease absorption of
  Vanadium)
Chloride
  (May decrease absorption of
  Vanadium)
Chromium
  (May decrease absorption of
  Vanadium)
Ethylenediaminetetraacetic Acid
  (May decrease absorption of
  Vanadium)
Iron
  (Decreased absorption of Iron)

VINPOCETINE

Warfarin Sodium
  (Changes in prothrombin time
  when used concomitantly)

VITAMIN A

Acitretin
  (May produce additive toxicity
  effects)
All-trans-retinoic Acid
  (May produce additive toxicity
  effects)
Alpha-Tocopheryl Polyethylene
Glycol Succinate
  (Increased absorption of
  Vitamin A)
Bexarotene
  (May produce additive toxicity
  effects)
Chitosan
  (Might bind to Chitosan)
Cholestyramine
  (May decrease Vitamin A
  absorption)
Colestipol
  (May decrease Vitamin A
  absorption)
Etretinate
  (May produce additive toxicity
  effects)
Fat Substitute
  (May inhibit Vitamin A
  absorption)
Glucomannan
  (Decreased absorption of fat-
  soluble vitamins)

Isotretinoin
  (May produce additive toxicity
  effects)
Medium-Chain Triglycerides
  (MCT may facilitate the
  absorption of Vitamin A)
Mineral Oil
  (May decrease Vitamin A
  absorption)
Oral Contraceptives
  (May increase serum retinol)
Orlistat
  (May decrease Vitamin A
  absorption)
Vitamin K
  (Large doses may decrease
  Vitamin A absorption)

VITAMIN B6

5-Hydroxytryptophan
  (May enhance 5-HTP conversion
  to serotonin)
Alcohol
  (Chronic and excessive use may
  cause Vitamin B6 deficiency)
Amiodarone Hydrochloride
  (Concomitant Vitamin B6 may
  enhance amiodarone-induced
  photosensitivity)
Carbamazepine
  (Chronic use may decrease plasma
  pyridoxal 5'-phosphate)
Cycloserine
  (May result in Vitamin B6
  deficiency)
Ethionamide
  (May increase Vitamin B6
  requirements)
Folate
  (May be synergistic in lowering
  serum homocysteine levels)
Fosphenytoin
  (Vitamin B6 may lower plasma
  phenytoin levels)
Homocysteine
  (Increased metabolism of
  Vitamin B6)
Hydralazine
  (May increase Vitamin B6
  requirements)
Isoniazid
  (May result in Vitamin B6
  deficiency)

Levodopa
(Vitamin B6 may reverse therapeutic effects if not given with carbidopa)

Oral Contraceptives
(May increase Vitamin B6 requirements)

Penicillamine
(May result in Vitamin B6 deficiency)

Phenelzine Sulfate
(May result in Vitamin B6 deficiency)

Phenobarbital
(Vitamin B6 may lower phenobarbital plasma levels)

Phenytoin
(Vitamin B6 may lower phenytoin plasma levels)

Piperine
(Piperine may enhance the absorption)

Theophylline
(Vitamin B6 may increase risk of theophylline-induced seizures)

Valproic Acid
(Chronic use may decrease plasma pyridoxal 5'-phosphate)

Vitamin B12
(Synergistic with Vitamin B12 to lower homocysteine levels)

VITAMIN B12

Antibiotics, unspecified
(May alter intestinal microflora to decrease Vitamin B12 absorption)

Calcium
(May reverse metformin-induced decrease of Vitamin B12 absorption)

Cholestyramine
(May decrease enterohepatic reabsorption of Vitamin B12)

Colchicine
(May decrease absorption of Vitamin B12)

Colestipol
(May decrease enterohepatic reabsorption of Vitamin B12)

Folate
(May be synergistic in lowering serum homocysteine levels)

Folic Acid
(Synergistic with Vitamin B12 to lower homocysteine levels)

Histamine H2-receptor antagonists
(May decrease absorption of dietary Vitamin B12, not supplemental)

Homocysteine
(Increased metabolism with Vitamin B12)

Metformin
(May decrease absorption of Vitamin B12)

Para-Aminosalicylic Acid
(May decrease the absorption of Vitamin B12)

Potassium Chloride
(May decrease absorption of dietary Vitamin B12)

Proton Pump Inhibitor
(May decrease absorption of dietary Vitamin B12, not supplemental)

Vitamin B6
(Synergistic with Vitamin B12 to lower homocysteine levels)

VITAMIN C

Alpha-Tocopheryl Polyethylene Glycol Succinate
(May help maintain Alpha-Tocopherol in its reduced (antioxidant) form)

Aluminum-containing Compounds, unspecified
(Large dose Vitamin C may increase urinary aluminum excretion)

Aspirin
(May decrease Vitamin C absorption and large aspirin doses may cause Vitamin C deficiency)

Carbamazepine
(Grapefruit flavonoids may increase bioavailability due to cytochrome P-450 3A4 inhibition)

Chitosan
(May enhance the benefits of Chitosan)

Cisplatin
(Vitamin C may potentiate antineoplastic activity)

Copper
(High dose Vitamin C may decrease absorption)

Cyclosporine
(Grapefruit flavonoids may increase bioavailability due to cytochrome P-450 3A4 inhibition)

Doxorubicin Hydrochloride
(Vitamin C may potentiate antineoplastic activity)

Estrogen
(Vitamin C may enhance inhibition of LDL formation)

Felodipine
(Grapefruit flavonoids may increase bioavailability due to cytochrome P-450 3A4 inhibition)

Flavonoids
(Vitamin C may have synergistic effects)

Gamma-Tocopherol
(Helps to maintain Gamma-Tocopherol in its reduced (antioxidant) form)

Glutathione
(Vitamin C may maintain reduced Glutathione levels)

Iron
(Enhanced absorption of Iron)

Iron Supplements
(Vitamin C may cause iron overload)

L-Cysteine
(May inhibit the oxidation of L-Cysteine)

Lovastatin
(Grapefruit flavonoids may increase bioavailability due to cytochrome P-450 3A4 inhibition)

Nisoldipine
(Grapefruit flavonoids may increase bioavailability due to cytochrome P-450 3A4 inhibition)

Paclitaxel
(Vitamin C may potentiate antineoplastic activity)

Piperine
(Piperine may enhance the absorption)

Rutin
  (Prevention of Vitamin C
  oxidation, enhanced and/or
  inhibition of absorption with
  flavonoids)
Saquinavir
  (Grapefruit flavonoids may
  increase bioavailability due to
  cytochrome P-450 3A4 inhibition)
Selenium
  (Decreased absorption of
  Selenium)
Simvastatin
  (Grapefruit flavonoids may
  increase bioavailability due to
  cytochrome P-450 3A4 inhibition)

VITAMIN D
Alpha-Tocopheryl Polyethylene
Glycol Succinate
  (Increased absorption of
  Vitamin D)
Bone Meal
  (Increased absorption of Calcium)
Calcium
  (Concomitant Vitamin D is
  synergistic for corticosteroid-
  induced osteoporosis; increased
  absorption of Calcium)
Chitosan
  (Might bind to Chitosan)
Cholestyramine
  (May reduce Vitamin D
  absorption)
Colestipol
  (May reduce Vitamin D
  absorption)
Fat Substitute
  (Inhibits Vitamin D absorption)
Glucomannan
  (Decreased absorption of fat-
  soluble vitamins)
Ipriflavone
  (Additive effects with Ipriflavone)
Ketoconazole
  (May decrease serum 1, 25-
  dihydroxyvitamin D levels)
Medium-Chain Triglycerides
  (MCT may facilitate the
  absorption of Vitamin D)
Mineral Oil
  (May reduce Vitamin D
  absorption)

Orlistat
  (May reduce Vitamin D
  absorption)
Phenobarbital
  (May decrease serum 25-
  hydroxyvitamin D levels)
Phenytoin
  (May decrease serum 25-
  hydroxyvitamin D levels)

VITAMIN E
Abciximab
  (Increased effects of abciximab)
Allium sativum
  (Enhanced antithrombotic activity
  of garlic)
Alpha-Tocopheryl Polyethylene
Glycol Succinate
  (Increased absorption when taken
  with TPGS)
Amiodarone Hydrochloride
  (Alpha-tocopherol may ameliorate
  some adverse side effects of this
  drug)
Antiplatelet Drugs
  (Increased effects of antiplatelet
  drugs)
Aspirin
  (Increased effects of aspirin)
Chitosan
  (Might bind to Chitosan)
Cholestyramine
  (Decreased Vitamin E absorption)
Clopidogrel Bisulfate
  (Increased effects of clopidogrel)
Colestipol
  (Decreased Vitamin E absorption)
Cyclosporine
  (Alpha-tocopherol may help to
  ameliorate renal side effects of
  cyclosporine)
Dietary Fiber
  (May decrease the antioxidative
  effect of Alpha-Tocopherol and
  carotenoids)
Dipyridamole
  (Increased effects of dipyridamole)
Eptifibatide
  (Increased effects of eptifibatide)
Fat Substitute
  (Inhibits absorption of Vitamin E)

Fatty Acids, polyunsaturated
  (May increase Vitamin E
  requirements)
Flavonoids
  (Help to maintain levels of
  Vitamin E)
Ginkgo biloba
  (Enhanced antithrombotic activity
  of ginkgo biloba)
Glucomannan
  (Decreased absorption of fat-
  soluble vitamins)
Iron
  (Ferrous form of Iron can oxidize
  unesterified Vitamin E to its pro-
  oxidant form)
Isoniazid
  (Decreased Vitamin E absorption)
Medium-Chain Triglycerides
  (Enhanced absorption of
  Vitamin E)
Mineral Oil
  (Decreased Vitamin E absorption)
Neomycin
  (Impaired utilization of
  Vitamin E)
Ox Bile, Desiccated
  (Increased absorption of
  Vitamin E)
Phytostanols
  (Decreased plasma Vitamin E
  levels)
Phytosterols
  (Low serum levels due to
  Phytosterols)
Plant Phenolic Compounds
  (Help to maintain levels of
  Vitamin E)
Selenium
  (Synergistic effect with
  Vitamin E)
Sucralfate
  (Interferes with Vitamin E
  absorption)
Ticlopidine Hydrochloride
  (Increased effects of ticlopidine)
Tirofiban Hydrochloride
  (Increased effects of tirofiban)
Vitamin K
  (May reduce Vitamin K
  absorption)

Warfarin Sodium
  (Enhanced anticoagulant response
  of warfarin)
Zidovudine
  (Vitamin E may ameliorate
  myelosuppressive side effects of
  zidovudine)

VITAMIN K

Alpha-Tocopheryl Polyethylene
Glycol Succinate
  (Increased absorption of
  Vitamin K)
Antibiotics, broad spectrum,
unspecified
  (May decrease Vitamin K
  availability)
Cefamandole Nafate
  (Can cause Vitamin K deficiency
  and hypoprothrombinemia)
Cefazolin Sodium
  (Can cause Vitamin K deficiency
  and hypoprothrombinemia)
Cefmenoxime
  (Can cause Vitamin K deficiency
  and hypoprothrombinemia)
Cefoperazone Sodium
  (Can cause Vitamin K deficiency
  and hypoprothrombinemia)
Cefotetan
  (Can cause Vitamin K deficiency
  and hypoprothrombinemia)
Chitosan
  (Might bind to Chitosan)
Cholestyramine
  (May reduce Vitamin K
  absorption)
Colestipol
  (May reduce Vitamin K
  absorption)
Fat Substitute
  (May reduce Vitamin K
  absorption)
Glucomannan
  (Decreased absorption of fat-
  soluble vitamins)
Ipriflavone
  (Additive effects with Ipriflavone)
Latamoxef
  (Can cause Vitamin K deficiency
  and hypothrombinemia)

Medium-Chain Triglycerides
  (May enhance Vitamin K
  absorption)
Mineral Oil
  (May reduce Vitamin K
  absorption)
Orlistat
  (May reduce Vitamin K
  absorption)
Salicylates
  (Large doses may cause Vitamin
  K deficiency)
Squalene
  (May reduce Vitamin K
  absorption)
Vitamin A
  (Large doses may decrease
  Vitamin A absorption)
Vitamin E
  (May reduce Vitamin K
  absorption)
Warfarin Sodium
  (Vitamin K can antagonize
  effects)

WARFARIN SODIUM

Alpha-Tocopheryl Polyethylene
Glycol Succinate
  (Enhanced anticoagulant response
  of warfarin)
Borage Oil
  (Increased anticoagulant and
  antiplatelet effects with Borage
  Oil)
Chlorella
  (Chlorella may interfere with
  effects)
Coenzyme Q10 (CoQ10)
  (May decrease the effectiveness of
  warfarin)
Curcuminoids
  (Curcuminoids may enhance the
  anticoagulant effect)
Evening Primrose Oil
  (EPO may increase bleeding
  tendencies)
Flaxseed Oil
  (May interact with Flaxseed Oil)
Gamma-Tocopherol
  (Enhanced anticoagulant response
  of warfarin)

Hemp Seed Oil
  (Increased bleeding and
  susceptibility to bruising)
Inositol Nicotinate
  (Nicotinic acid may enhance
  anticoagulant effects)
Iodine
  (Potassium iodide may decrease
  the anticoagulant effectiveness of
  warfarin)
Niacin
  (Nicotinic acid may enhance
  anticoagulant effects)
Psyllium
  (Reduced absorption of warfarin
  sodium)
Red Yeast Rice
  (Increase in the INR as well as
  bleeding)
Tiratricol (TRIAC)
  (Increased hypoprothrombinemic
  effect)
Tocotrienols
  (Large dose Tocotrienols may
  enhance anticoagulant effects)
Vinpocetine
  (Changes in prothrombin time
  when used concomitantly)
Vitamin E
  (Enhanced anticoagulant response
  of warfarin)
Vitamin K
  (Vitamin K can antagonize
  effects)
Wheat Grass/Barley Grass
  (Wheat Grass supplements may
  affect the INR)

WHEAT GRASS/BARLEY GRASS

Warfarin Sodium
  (Wheat Grass supplements may
  affect the INR)

YOHIMBINE HYDROCHLORIDE

L-Arginine
  (L-Arginine may potentiate
  effects)

ZALCITABINE

Acetyl-L-Carnitine
  (May lead to decreased Acetyl-L-
  Carnitine levels)

L-Carnitine
(May produce L-Carnitine deficiencies)

ZIDOVUDINE

Riboflavin (Vitamin B2)
(Riboflavin may reverse nucleoside analogue-induced lactic acidosis in mild Riboflavin deficiencies)

Vitamin E
(Vitamin E may ameliorate myelosuppressive side effects of zidovudine)

ZINC

Caffeine
(Decreased absorption of Zinc)

Calcium
(Decreased Zinc absorption in postmenopausal women)

Chitosan
(Might bind to Chitosan)

Copper
(Decreased absorption of Copper)

Cysteine-Containing Protiens
(Increased absorption of Zinc)

Folate
(Folic acid may decrease Zinc absorption)

Inositol
(Decreased absorption of Zinc)

Inositol Hexaphosphate
(May form chelates with Inositol Hexaphosphate)

Iron
(Decreased absorption of both Iron and Zinc)

L-Cysteine
(Enhanced absorption of Zinc)

L-Histidine
(Enhanced absorption of Zinc)

L-Methionine
(Increased absorption of Zinc)

N-Acetyl-L-Cysteine (NAC)
(Increased absorption of Zinc)

Oxalic Acid
(Decreased absorption of Zinc)

Pectin
(Decreased absorption of Zinc)

Phosphate Salts
(Decreased absorption of Zinc)

Phosphorus
(Decreased absorption of Zinc)

Phytic Acid
(Decreased absorption of Zinc)

Psyllium
(Decreased absorption of Zinc)

Sodium Alginates and other Phyco-Polysaccharides
(Decreased absorption of Zinc)

Soy Protein
(Reduced availability of Zinc)

Tannins
(Decreased absorption of Zinc)

Companion Drug Index

This index suggests nutritional supplements that may be used, in conjunction with prescription drug therapy, to reverse drug-induced side effects, relieve symptoms of the illness itself, or treat sequelae of the initial disease. Supplements, together with their associated brands, are listed alphabetically under each condition. Brands pictured in the Product Identification Guide are marked with a [♦] symbol and a page number giving the location of the photo. Italic page numbers refer to combination-product tables.

ALCOHOLISM, HYPOCALCEMIA SECONDARY TO

Alcoholism may be treated with disulfiram or naltrexone hydrochloride. The following products may be recommended for relief of hypocalcemia:

CALCIUM **74**

Alcalak Chewable Tablets (Textilease)

♦ Alka-Mints Chewable Tablets (Bayer) **G-3**

Antacid Chewable Tablets (Zenith Goldline)

Antacid Extra Strength Chewable Tablets (Cardinal)

Antacid Extra Strength Chewable Tablets (Zenith Goldline)

Antacid Extra Strength Tablets (McKesson)

Antacid Ultra Strength Chewable Tablets (Bergen Brunswig)

Ascocid Tablets (Key Company)

Cal-600 Tablets (PDK)

Cal-C-Caps Capsules (Key Company)

Cal-Carb Forte Tablets (Vitaline)

Cal-Carb Forte Wafers (Vitaline)

Cal-Cee Tablets (Key Company)

Cal-Citrate Capsules (Bio-Tech)

Cal-Citrate Tablets (Bio-Tech)

Cal-G Capsules (Key Company)

Cal-Gest Chewable Tablets (Rugby)

Cal-Glu Capsule (Bio-Tech)

Cal-Lac Capsules (Key Company)

Cal-Lac Tablets (Bio-Tech)

Cal-Mint Tablets (Freeda)

Calbon Tablets (Economed)

Calcarb 600 Tablets (Zenith Goldline)

Calci-Chew Tablets (R&D)

Calci-Mix Capsules (R&D)

Calcimin-300 Tablets (Key Company)

Calcio Del Mar Tablets (Marlop)

Calcionate Syrup (Hi-Tech)

Calcionate Syrup (Rugby)

Calciquid Syrup (Breckenridge)

Calciquid Syrup (Econolab)

Calcium 500 Chewable Tablets (Mason)

Calcium 500 Chewable Tablets (National Vitamin)

Calcium 500 Supplement Chewable Tablets (Bergen Brunswig)

Calcium 600 Capsules (McKesson)

Calcium 600 Tablets (Basic Vitamins)

Calcium 600 Tablets (Nature's Bounty)

Calcium 600 Tablets (Prime Marketing)

Calcium 600 Tablets (Rugby)

Calcium Antacid Chewable Tablets (Mason)

Calcium Antacid Chewable Tablets (Perrigo)

Calcium Antacid Extra Strength Chewable Tablets (Major Pharmaceuticals)

Calcium Antacid Extra Strength Chewable Tablets (Medicine Shoppe)

Calcium Antacid Extra Strength Tablets (Perrigo)

Calcium Antacid Ultra Strength Chewable Tablets (Major Pharmaceuticals)

Calcium Antacid Ultra Strength Chewable Tablets (Perrigo)

Calcium Citrate 950 Tablets (Basic Vitamins)

Calcium-600 Tablets (Key Company)

Calfort Tablets (Ampharco)

Calphron Powder (Nephro-Tech)

Caltrate 600 Tablets (Lederle)

Chooz Tablets (Heritage Consumer)

Citracal Economy Tablets (Mission)

Citracal Tablets (Mission)

Desempacho Tablets (D'Franssia)

Krebs Ionized Calcium Tablets (PhytoPharmica)

Life-Line Co-Co Bear Chewable Tablets (National Vitamin)

Liqui-Cal Chewable Tablets (Advanced Nutritional)

M2 Calcium Tablets (Miller Pharmacal)

Mallamint Chewable Tablets (Textilease)

Mylanta Calci Tabs Extra Strength (J&J • Merck)

Mylanta Calci Tabs Ultra Chewable Tablets (J&J • Merck)

Mylanta Children's Chewable Tablets (J&J • Merck)

Neo-Calglucon Syrup (Novartis Pharmaceuticals)

Nephro-Calci Tablets (R&D)

Nutralox Chewable Tablets (Hart Health)

♦ Os-Cal 500 Chewable Tablets (SmithKline Beecham) G-5

♦ Os-Cal 500 Tablets (SmithKline Beecham) G-5

Oysco 500 Tablets (Rugby)

Oyst-Cal 500 Tablets (Zenith Goldline)

Oyster Shell Calcium 500 Tablets (Medicine Shoppe)

Oyster Shell Calcium Natural Tablets (Cardinal)

Phoslo Tablets (Braintree)

Prelief Granules (AK Pharma)

Prelief Tablets (AK Pharma)

Revelation Powder (Alvin Last)

Ridactate Tablets (R.I.D.)

Rolaids Chewable Tablets (American Chicle)

Super Calcium Extra Strength Chewable Tablets (Mason)

Super Calcium Tablets (Mason)

Titralac Chewable Tablets (3M)

Titralac Extra Strength Chewable Tablets (3M)

Tums 500 Chewable Tablets (SmithKline Beecham)

♦ Tums Chewable Tablets (SmithKline Beecham) G-5

♦ Tums E-X Chewable Tablets (SmithKline Beecham) G-5

♦ Tums Ultra Chewable Tablets (SmithKline Beecham) G-5

Vitamin C Buffered Tablets (Nature's Bounty)

CALCIUM COMBINATION PRODUCTS *543t*

♦ AdvaCal Capsules (Lane Labs) G-4

Cal-600 w/Vitamin D Tablets (PDK)

Cal-Co3Y Capsules (Bio-Tech)

Cal/Mag Chelated Tablets (Freeda)

Cal/Mag Chewable Tablets (Freeda)

Calcarb 600 w/Vitamin D Tablets (Zenith Goldline)

Calcet Tablets (Mission)

Calcium & Magnesium Chelate Capsules (Key Company)

Calcium 500 w/Vitamin D Tablets (Basic Vitamins)

Calcium 500 w/Vitamin D Tablets (Mason)

Calcium 500 w/Vitamin D Tablets (Rexall Consumer)

Calcium 600 + Vitamin D Tablets (Perrigo)

Calcium 600 Plus Vitamin D Tablets (Nature's Bounty)

Calcium 600-D Tablets (Rugby)

Calcium 600/Vitamin D Tablets (Basic Vitamins)

Calcium 600/Vitamin D Tablets (Bergen Brunswig)

Calcium 600/Vitamin D Tablets (Cardinal)

Calcium 900 w/Vitamin D Capsules (Rexall Consumer)

Calcium 1200 w/Vitamin D Capsules (Rexall Consumer)

Calcium Carbonate/Vitamin D Tablets (Compumed)

Calcium Carbonate/Vitamin D Tablets (Heartland)

Calcium Carbonate/Vitamin D Tablets (Major Pharmaceuticals)

Calcium Carbonate/Vitamin D Tablets (National Vitamin)

Calcium Carbonate/Vitamin D Tablets (PD-Rx)

Calcium Carbonate/Vitamin D Tablets (Sky)

Calcium Citrate + D Tablets (Cardinal)

Calcium Citrate w/Vitamin D Tablets (Mason)

Calcium Citrate/Vitamin D Tablets (Bergen Brunswig)

Calcium-600 w/D Tablets (American Pharmacal)

Calcium/Magnesium/Zinc Tablets (Cardinal)

Calcium/Magnesium/Zinc Tablets (Rexall Consumer)

Calcium/Vitamin D Tablets (McKesson)

Calcium/Vitamin D Tablets (PD-Rx)

Calcium/Vitamin D Tablets (Vanguard)

Caltrate 600 + D Tablets (Lederle)

Citracal + D Tablets (Mission)

Citrus Calcium + D Tablets (Rugby)

Daily Calcium + Vitamin D Tablets (Nature's Bounty)

Ferosul Tablets (Major Pharmaceuticals)

Florical Capsules (Mericon)

Florical Tablets (Mericon)

Healthy Woman Bone Health Supplement Tablets (Personal Products Company)

Liqua-Cal Capsules (Key Company)

Liquid Calcium Capsules (Major Pharmaceuticals)

Liquid Calcium Plus Vitamin D Capsules (Mason)

Magnebind 200 Tablets (Nephro-Tech)

Magnebind 300 Tablets (Nephro-Tech)

Magnebind 400 Rx Tablets (Nephro-Tech)

Marblen Suspension (Fleming)

Marblen Tablets (Fleming)

Monocal Tablets (Mericon)

One-A-Day Bone Strength Tablets (Bayer)

♦ One-A-Day Calcium Plus Chewable Tablets (Bayer) .. **G-3**

♦ Os-Cal 250 + D Tablets (SmithKline Beecham) **G-5**

♦ Os-Cal 500 + D Tablets (SmithKline Beecham) **G-5**

Oysco 500 + D Tablets (Rugby)

Oysco D Tablets (Rugby)

Oyst-Cal-D 500 Tablets (Zenith Goldline)

Oyst-Cal-D Tablets (Zenith Goldline)

Oyster Shell Calcium 500 w/D Tablets (Medicine Shoppe)

Oyster Shell Calcium 1000/ Vitamin D Tablets (Mason)

Oyster Shell Calcium 1000/ Vitamin D Tablets (Rexall Consumer)

Oyster Shell Calcium Natural/Vit D Tablets (Cardinal)

Oyster Shell Calcium/ Vitamin D Tablets (American Pharmacal)

Oyster Shell Calcium/ Vitamin D Tablets (Basic Vitamins)

Oyster Shell Calcium/ Vitamin D Tablets (Bergen Brunswig)

Oyster Shell Calcium/ Vitamin D Tablets (Dixon-Shane)

Oyster Shell Calcium/ Vitamin D Tablets (Major Pharmaceuticals)

Oyster Shell Calcium/ Vitamin D Tablets (Mason)

Oyster Shell Calcium/ Vitamin D Tablets (McKesson)

Oyster Shell Calcium/ Vitamin D Tablets (National Vitamin)

Oyster Shell Calcium/ Vitamin D Tablets (Perrigo)

Oyster Shell Calcium/ Vitamin D Tablets (Reese)

Oyster Shell Calcium/ Vitamin D Tablets (Rexall Consumer)

Oyster Shell Calcium/ Vitamin D Tablets (Vanguard)

Oystercal-D 250 Tablets (Nature's Bounty)

Oystercal-D 500 Tablets (Nature's Bounty)

Parva-Cal 250 Tablets (Freeda)

Super Calcium w/Vitamin D Tablets (Mason)

Viactiv Chewable Tablets (Mead Johnson)

Vita-Calcium Wafers (Vitaline)

ALCOHOLISM, HYPOMAGNESEMIA SECONDARY TO

Alcoholism may be treated with disulfiram or naltrexone hydrochloride. The following products may be recommended for relief of hypomagnesemia:

MAGNESIUM **288**

Almora Tablets (Forest)

Chloromag Injection (Merit)

Dewee's Carminative Liquid (Humco)

Elite Magnesium Capsules (Miller Pharmacal)

M2 Magnesium Capsules (Miller Pharmacal)

Mag Delay Tablets (Major Pharmaceuticals)

Mag-200 Tablets (Optimox)

Mag-Carb Capsules (R&D)

Mag-Gel 600 Capsules (Cypress)

Mag-Ox 400 Tablets (Blaine)

Mag-SR Tablets (Cypress)

Mag-Tab Sr Tablets
(Niche)

Magimin Tablets (Key
Company)

Magimin-Forte Tablets
(Key Company)

Maglex Tablets (Lex)

Magnacaps Capsules (Key
Company)

Magnesium Carbonate
Powder (Freeda)

Magnesium Elemental
Tablets (National
Vitamin)

Magnesium Oxide Tablets
(Cypress)

Magonate Liquid (Fleming)

Magonate Natal Liquid
(Fleming)

Magonate Tablets
(Fleming)

Magtrate Tablets (Mission)

Slow-Mag Tablets (Quality
Care)

Slow-Mag Tablets (Shire
U.S.)

Sulfa-Mag Injection (Merit)

Uro-Mag Capsules (Blaine)

ALCOHOLISM, VITAMINS AND MINERALS DEFICIENCY SECONDARY TO

Alcoholism may be treated with disulfiram or naltrexone hydrochloride. The following products may be recommended for relief of vitamins and minerals deficiency:

MULTIVITAMIN PRODUCTS *550t*

BEC w/Zinc Tablets
(Bergen Brunswig)

♦ Bugs Bunny Plus Extra C
Chewable Tablets (Bayer) .. **G-3**

♦ Bugs Bunny Plus Iron
Chewable Tablets (Bayer) .. **G-3**

Cardiotek Tablets (Stewart-Jackson)

Cefol Tablets (Abbott
Hospital)

Circus Chews Children's
Chewable Tablets (Rexall
Consumer)

Daily Multiple Vitamins
Tablets (Marlex)

Daily Multiple Vitamins
Tablets (Rexall
Consumer)

Daily Multiple Vitamins w/
Iron Tablets (Rexall
Consumer)

Daily Multivitamins Tablets
(Sky)

♦ Flintstones Original
Children's Chewable
Tablets (Bayer) **G-3**

♦ Flintstones Plus Calcium
Chewable Tablets (Bayer) .. **G-3**

♦ Flintstones Plus Extra C
Chewable Tablets (Bayer) .. **G-3**

♦ Flintstones Plus Iron
Chewable Tablets (Bayer) .. **G-3**

Key-Plex Injection (Hyrex)

M.V.I. Pediatric Powder for
Injection (AstraZeneca LP)

M.V.I.-12 Injection
(AstraZeneca LP)

Multi-Vitamins Tablets
(Rugby)

Multivitamin Capsules
(Numark)

Once Daily Tablets (Prime
Marketing)

♦ One-A-Day Essential
Tablets (Bayer) **G-3**

Poly Vitamin Chewable
Tablets (Rugby)

Stress Formula Plus Zinc
Tablets (Rexall
Consumer)

Stress Formula Tablets
(Cardinal)

Stress Formula Tablets
(Rexall Consumer)

Therapeutic Multivitamin
Tablets (Bergen
Brunswig)

Ultra Tabs Tablets (Major
Pharmaceuticals)

Vitamins Children's
Chewable Tablets (Prime
Marketing)

**MULTIVITAMIN AND MINERAL
PRODUCTS** *553t*

♦ Alpha Betic Tablets
(Abkit) **G-3**

B-C w/Folic Acid Plus
Tablet (Geneva)

B-Complex Plus Tablets
(United Research)

B-Complex Vitamins Plus
Tablets (Teva)

B-Plex Plus Tablets (Zenith
Goldline)

Bacmin Tablets (Marnel)

Becomax RX Tablets
(Ampharco)

Berocca Plus Tablets
(Roche)

♦ Bugs Bunny Complete
Children's Chewable
Tablets (Bayer) **G-3**

Cerovite Senior Tablets
(Rugby)

Circavite T Tablets (Circle)

Clusinex Syrup
(Pharmakon)

Daily Multiple Vitamins/
Minerals Tablets
(Vanguard)

Dr. Art Ulene's Vitamin
Formula Packets (Feeling
Fine)

Equi-Roca Plus Tablets
(Equipharm)

Ferrex PC Tablets
(Breckenridge)

♦ Flintstones Complete
Children's Chewable
Tablets (Bayer) **G-3**

Formula B Plus Tablets
(Major Pharmaceuticals)

Glutofac-ZX Capsules
(Kenwood)

Hematin Plus Tablets
(Cypress)

Iromin-G Tablets (Mission)

Manly Machovites Tablets
(Neurovites)

Mega-Multi Capsules
(Innovative Health)

Niferex-PN Tablets
(Schwarz)

O-Cal FA Tablets
(Pharmics)

◆ One-A-Day 50 Plus Tablets
(Bayer) G-3
◆ One-A-Day Antioxidant
Capsules (Bayer) G-3
◆ One-A-Day Kids Complete
Chewable Tablets (Bayer) . . G-3
◆ One-A-Day Maximum
Tablets (Bayer) G-3
◆ One-A-Day Men's Tablets
(Bayer) G-3
◆ One-A-Day Women's
Tablets (Bayer) G-3
PMS Formula Tablets
(Neurovites)
Poly Vitamin w/Iron
Chewable Tablets
(Rugby)
Protect Plus Capsules (Gil)
Protect Plus Liquid (Gil)
Strovite Forte Tablets
(Everett)
Sunvite Platinum Tablets
(Rexall Consumer)
Sunvite Tablets (Rexall
Consumer)
Super Plenamins Extra
Strength Tablets (Rexall
Consumer)
Super Plenamins Tablets
(Rexall Consumer)
Support 500 Capsules
(Marin)
Support Liquid (Marin)
Thera Vite M Tablets
(PDK)
Thera-M w/Minerals
Tablets (Prime
Marketing)
◆ Theragran-M Tablets
(Bristol-Myers Products) G-3
Therapeutic Plus Vitamin
Tablets (Rugby)
Therobec Plus Tablets
(Qualitest)
Total Formula Original
Tablets (Vitaline)
V-C Forte Capsules
(Breckenridge)
Vicap Forte Tablets (Major
Pharmaceuticals)
Vicon Forte Tablets (UCB)

Vita-Min Rx Tablets (Bio-
Tech)
Vitacon Forte Tablets
(Amide)
Vitaplex Plus Tablets
(Amide)
Vitelle Nesentials Tablets
(Fielding)
THIAMIN **445**
VITAMIN B COMPLEX PRODUCTS . . **558t**
B-50 Complex Tablets
(Rexall Consumer)
B-100 Complex Tablets
(Rexall Consumer)
B-Ject-100 Injection
(Hyrex)
B-Plex Tablets (Contract
Pharmacal)
B-Plex Tablets (Zenith
Goldline)
Berocca Tablets (Roche)
Dialyvite Tablets
(Hillestad)
Formula B Tablets (Major
Pharmaceuticals)
Marlbee w/C Capsules
(Marlex)
Nephplex Rx Tablets
(Nephro-Tech)
Nephro-Vite Rx Tablets
(R&D)
Nephrocaps Capsules
(Fleming)
Primaplex Injection
(Primedics)
Stress B Complex with
Vitamin C Tablets
(Mission)
Strovite Tablets (Everett)
Therobec Tablets
(Qualitest)
Thex Forte Tablets (Lee)
Vicam Injection (Keene)
Vita-Bee w/C Tablets
(Rugby)
Vitamin B Complex 100
Injection (Hyrex)
Vitamin B Complex 100
Injection (McGuff)
Vitamin B Complex 100
Injection (Torrance)

Vitamin B Complex 100
Injection (Truxton)
Vitamin B Complex
Capsules (Rugby)
Vitamin B Complex w/
Vitamin C & B12
Injection (McGuff)
Vitamin B-100 Natural
Tablets (Cardinal)
Vitaplex Tablets (Amide)
Vitaplex Tablets (Medirex)

ANCYLOSTOMIASIS, IRON-DEFICIENCY ANEMIA SECONDARY TO

Ancylostomiasis may be treated with mebendazole or thiabendazole. The following products may be recommended for relief of iron-deficiency anemia:

IRON **234**
Dexferrum Injection
(American Regent)
Ed-In-Sol Elixir (Edwards)
Fe-40 Tablets (Bio-Tech)
◆ Feosol Caplets (SmithKline
Beecham) G-5
◆ Feosol Elixir (SmithKline
Beecham) G-5
◆ Feosol Tablets (SmithKline
Beecham) G-5
Feostat Chewable Tablets
(Forest)
Feostat Suspension (Forest)
Fer-Gen-Sol Liquid (Zenith
Goldline)
Fer-In-Sol Liquid (Mead
Johnson)
Fer-Iron Liquid (Rugby)
Feratab Tablets (Upsher-
Smith)
◆ Fergon Tablets (Bayer) G-3
Feronate Tablets (Prime
Marketing)
Ferosul Tablets (Major
Pharmaceuticals)
Ferretts Tablets (Pharmics)
Ferro-Caps Capsules
(Nature's Bounty)
Ferro-Time Capsules
(Time-Cap)

Ferrous Sulfate T.D.
Capsules (American
Pharmacal)

Ferrousal Tablets (Prime
Marketing)

Gentle Iron Capsules
(Solgar)

Infed Injection (Schein)

Ircon Tablets (Kenwood)

Iron Sol Elixir (Halsey)

Mol-Iron Tablets (Schering-
Plough)

Nephro-Fer Tablets (R&D)

Ridosol Tablets (R.I.D.)

Siderol Pediatric Tablets
(Marin)

♦ Slow Fe Tablets (Novartis

Slow Release Iron Tablets
(Cardinal)

Vitedyn-Slo Capsules
(Edyn)

Yieronia Elixir (R.I.D.)

Yierro-Gota Liquid (R.I.D.)

IRON COMBINATION PRODUCTS

Anemagen Capsules
(Ethex)

Anemagen FA Capsules
(Ethex)

Chromagen Capsules
(Savage)

Chromagen FA Tablets
(Savage)

Chromagen Forte Capsules
(Savage)

Conison Capsules (Ethex)

Contrin Capsules (Geneva)

DSS w/Iron Extended
Release Capsules
(American Pharmacal)

Daily Multiple Vitamins/
Iron Tablets (Vanguard)

Ed Cyte F Tablets
(Edwards)

Equi-Cyte F Tablets
(Equipharm)

Fe-Tinic 150 Forte
Capsules (Ethex)

Fero-Folic 500 Extended
Release Tablets (Abbott)

Fero-Grad-500 Extended
Release Tablets (Abbott)

Ferocon Capsules
(Breckenridge)

Ferotrinsic Capsules
(Contract Pharmacal)

Ferragen Capsules (Pecos)

Ferrex 150 Forte Capsules
(Breckenridge)

Ferro-Sequels Extended
Release Tablets
(Inverness)

Ferrous Fumarate DS
Extended Release
Capsules (Vita-Rx)

Fetrin Extended Release
Capsules (Lunsco)

Foltrin Capsules (Eon)

Fumatinic Extended
Release Capsules (Laser)

Hematin-F Tablets
(Cypress)

Hemocyte-F Tablets (U.S.
Pharmaceutical)

Iberet-Folic-500 Extended
Release Tablets (Abbott)

Icar-C Plus Tablets
(Hawthorn)

Icar-C Tablets (Hawthorn)

Infed Injection (Schein)

Ircon-FA Tablets
(Kenwood)

Irofol Tablets (Dayton)

Iron Advanced Tablets
(Rexall Consumer)

Iron w/Docusate Sodium
Extended Release Tablets
(Nature's Bounty)

Iron-Folic 500 Tablets
(Major Pharmaceuticals)

Martinic Capsules (Marlop)

Multi-Ferrous Folic
Extended Release Tablets
(United Research)

Multi-Vitamin w/Iron
Children's Liquid (Tri-
Med)

Multiret Folic-500
Extended Release Tablets
(Amide)

Multivitamins w/Iron
Children's Chewable
Tablets (Cardinal)

Myferon 150 Forte
Capsules (Me
Pharmaceuticals)

Nephro-Fer Rx Tablets
(R&D)

Nephro-Vite + FE Tablets
(R&D)

Nephron FA Tablets
(Nephro-Tech)

Niferex-150 Forte Capsules
(Schwarz)

Nu-Iron Plus Elixir (Merz)

Nutrinate Chewable Tablets
(Ethex)

One Tablet Daily w/Iron
Tablets (Zenith Goldline)

Prenafort Tablets (Cypress)

Promar Capsules (Marlop)

♦ Slow Fe w/Folic Acid
Extended Release Tablets

Stress Formula + Iron
Tablets (Cardinal)

Thera Hematinic Tablets
(Dixon-Shane)

Theragran Hematinic
Tablets (Apothecon)

Tolfrinic Tablets (Ascher)

Trinsicon Capsules
(Marlex)

Vitamins w/Iron Children's
Chewable Tablets
(Marlex)

Vitelle Irospan Extended
Release Tablets and
Extended Release
Capsules (Fielding)

Vitron-C Plus Tablets
(Novartis Consumer)

Vitron-C Tablets (Novartis
Consumer)

ANEMIA, IRON-DEFICIENCY

May result from the use of chronic
salicylate therapy or nonsteroidal
anti-inflammatory drugs. The
following products may be
recommended:

IRON

Dexferrum Injection
(American Regent)

Ed-In-Sol Elixir (Edwards)

Fe-40 Tablets (Bio-Tech)

♦ Feosol Caplets (SmithKline
Beecham) G-5
♦ Feosol Elixir (SmithKline
Beecham) G-5
♦ Feosol Tablets (SmithKline
Beecham) G-5
Feostat Chewable Tablets
(Forest)
Feostat Suspension (Forest)
Fer-Gen-Sol Liquid (Zenith
Goldline)
Fer-In-Sol Liquid (Mead
Johnson)
Fer-Iron Liquid (Rugby)
Feratab Tablets (Upsher-
Smith)
♦ Fergon Tablets (Bayer) G-3
Feronate Tablets (Prime
Marketing)
Ferosul Tablets (Major
Pharmaceuticals)
Ferretts Tablets (Pharmics)
Ferro-Caps Capsules
(Nature's Bounty)
Ferro-Time Capsules
(Time-Cap)
Ferrous Sulfate T.D.
Capsules (American
Pharmacal)
Ferrousal Tablets (Prime
Marketing)
Gentle Iron Capsules
(Solgar)
Infed Injection (Schein)
Ircon Tablets (Kenwood)
Iron Sol Elixir (Halsey)
Mol-Iron Tablets (Schering-
Plough)
Nephro-Fer Tablets (R&D)
Ridosol Tablets (R.I.D.)
Siderol Pediatric Tablets
(Marin)
♦ Slow Fe Tablets (Novartis
Consumer) G-5
Slow Release Iron Tablets
(Cardinal)
Vitedyn-Slo Capsules
(Edyn)
Yieronia Elixir (R.I.D.)
Yierro-Gota Liquid (R.I.D.)

IRON COMBINATION PRODUCTS ... *546t*
Anemagen Capsules
(Ethex)
Anemagen FA Capsules
(Ethex)
Chromagen Capsules
(Savage)
Chromagen FA Tablets
(Savage)
Chromagen Forte Capsules
(Savage)
Conison Capsules (Ethex)
Contrin Capsules (Geneva)
DSS w/Iron Extended
Release Capsules
(American Pharmacal)
Daily Multiple Vitamins/
Iron Tablets (Vanguard)
Ed Cyte F Tablets
(Edwards)
Equi-Cyte F Tablets
(Equipharm)
Fe-Tinic 150 Forte
Capsules (Ethex)
Fero-Folic 500 Extended
Release Tablets (Abbott)
Fero-Grad-500 Extended
Release Tablets (Abbott)
Ferocon Capsules
(Breckenridge)
Ferotrinsic Capsules
(Contract Pharmacal)
Ferragen Capsules (Pecos)
Ferrex 150 Forte Capsules
(Breckenridge)
Ferro-Sequels Extended
Release Tablets
(Inverness)
Ferrous Fumarate DS
Extended Release
Capsules (Vita-Rx)
Fetrin Extended Release
Capsules (Lunsco)
Foltrin Capsules (Eon)
Fumatinic Extended
Release Capsules (Laser)
Hematin-F Tablets
(Cypress)
Hemocyte-F Tablets (U.S.
Pharmaceutical)
Iberet-Folic-500 Extended
Release Tablets (Abbott)

Icar-C Plus Tablets
(Hawthorn)
Icar-C Tablets (Hawthorn)
Infed Injection (Schein)
Ircon-FA Tablets
(Kenwood)
Irofol Tablets (Dayton)
Iron Advanced Tablets
(Rexall Consumer)
Iron w/Docusate Sodium
Extended Release Tablets
(Nature's Bounty)
Iron-Folic 500 Tablets
(Major Pharmaceuticals)
Martinic Capsules (Marlop)
Multi-Ferrous Folic
Extended Release Tablets
(United Research)
Multi-Vitamin w/Iron
Children's Liquid (Tri-
Med)
Multiret Folic-500
Extended Release Tablets
(Amide)
Multivitamins w/Iron
Children's Chewable
Tablets (Cardinal)
Myferon 150 Forte
Capsules (Me
Pharmaceuticals)
Nephro-Fer Rx Tablets
(R&D)
Nephro-Vite + FE Tablets
(R&D)
Nephron FA Tablets
(Nephro-Tech)
Niferex-150 Forte Capsules
(Schwarz)
Nu-Iron Plus Elixir (Merz)
Nutrinate Chewable Tablets
(Ethex)
One Tablet Daily w/Iron
Tablets (Zenith Goldline)
Prenafort Tablets (Cypress)
Promar Capsules (Marlop)
♦ Slow Fe w/Folic Acid
Extended Release Tablets
(Novartis Consumer) G-3
Stress Formula + Iron
Tablets (Cardinal)
Thera Hematinic Tablets
(Dixon-Shane)

Theragran Hematinic
Tablets (Apothecon)
Tolfrinic Tablets (Ascher)
Trinsicon Capsules
(Marlex)
Vitamins w/Iron Children's
Chewable Tablets
(Marlex)
Vitelle Irospan Extended
Release Tablets and
Extended Release
Capsules (Fielding)
Vitron-C Plus Tablets
(Novartis Consumer)
Vitron-C Tablets (Novartis
Consumer)

ARTHRITIS

May be treated with corticosteroids
or nonsteroidal anti-inflammatory
drugs. The following products may
be recommended for relief of
symptoms:

BLACKCURRANT SEED OIL 55
BORAGE OIL 58
Borage Liquid Gold Liquid
(Health from the Sun)
Borage Oil Gla 240
Capsules (Health from
the Sun)
Borage Oil Omega-6
Capsules (Nature's Way)
Borage Power Capsules
(Nature's Herbs)
My Favorite Borage Oil
Capsules (Natrol)
Veg Borage Oil Capsules
(Twinlab)
CHICKEN COLLAGEN II 83
Arthred Hydrolyzed
Collagen Liquid (Source)
Bio-Cell Collagen Tablets
(Natrol)
Collagen II Tablets (Natrol)
Maxilife Chicken Collagen
Type II Capsules
(Twinlab)
COPPER 112
Coppermin Tablets (Key
Company)
Cu-5 Capsules (Bio-Tech)
Ocuvite Lutein Capsules
(Bausch & Lomb)

CURCUMINOIDS 117
Curcumin-Power Capsules
(Nature's Herbs)
DIMETHYL SULFOXIDE (DMSO) 132
Catalytic Formula Tablets
(Vitaline)
Rimso-50 Tablets
(Edwards)
EVENING PRIMROSE OIL 143
Evening Primrose De
Luxe-Hexan Capsules
(Health from the Sun)
Golden Primrose Capsules
(Carlson)
Mega Primrose Oil
Capsules (Twinlab)
My Favorite Evening
Primrose Oil Capsules
(Natrol)
Original Primrose For
Women Capsules
(Naturalife)
Primosa Capsules (Solaray)
Primrose Power Capsules
(Nature's Herbs)
Royal Brittany Evening
Primrose Oil Capsules
(Nature's Bounty)
Ultra EPO 1500 Capsules
(Nature's Plus)
Ultra EPO 1500 Capsules
(Source)
Veg Evening Primrose Oil
Capsules (Health from
the Sun)
FISH OIL 145
♦ Coromega Packets
(E.R.B.L.) G-4
FLOWER POLLEN 152
GAMMA-LINOLENIC ACID (GLA) 171
Mega GLA Capsules
(Source)
Super GLA Capsules
(Solgar)
GLUCOSAMINE 186
HEMP SEED OIL 206
L-CYSTEINE 259
L-HISTIDINE 265
NICOTINAMIDE 327
PANTOTHENIC ACID 341
Cal-Mincol Capsules (Bio-
Tech)

Panto-250 Tablets (Bio-
Tech)
Posture Tablets (Inverness)
S-ADENOSYL-L-METHIONE (SAME) . . . 410
SELENIUM 416

BURN INFECTIONS, SEVERE, NUTRIENTS DEFICIENCY SECONDARY TO

Severe burn infections may be
treated with anti-infectives. The
following products may be
recommended for relief of nutrients
deficiency:

ASCORBYL PALMITATE 33
MULTIVITAMIN PRODUCTS 550t
BEC w/Zinc Tablets
(Bergen Brunswig)
♦ Bugs Bunny Plus Extra C
Chewable Tablets (Bayer) . . G-3
♦ Bugs Bunny Plus Iron
Chewable Tablets (Bayer) . . G-3
Cardiotek Tablets (Stewart-
Jackson)
Cefol Tablets (Abbott
Hospital)
Circus Chews Children's
Chewable Tablets (Rexall
Consumer)
Daily Multiple Vitamins
Tablets (Marlex)
Daily Multiple Vitamins
Tablets (Rexall
Consumer)
Daily Multiple Vitamins w/
Iron Tablets (Rexall
Consumer)
Daily Multivitamins Tablets
(Sky)
♦ Flintstones Original
Children's Chewable
Tablets (Bayer) G-3
♦ Flintstones Plus Calcium
Chewable Tablets (Bayer) . . G-3
♦ Flintstones Plus Extra C
Chewable Tablets (Bayer) . . G-3
♦ Flintstones Plus Iron
Chewable Tablets (Bayer) . . G-3
Key-Plex Injection (Hyrex)
M.V.I. Pediatric Powder for
Injection (AstraZeneca LP)

M.V.I.-12 Injection
(AstraZeneca LP)

Multi-Vitamins Tablets
(Rugby)

Multivitamin Capsules
(Numark)

Once Daily Tablets (Prime
Marketing)

♦ One-A-Day Essential
Tablets (Bayer) G-3

Poly Vitamin Chewable
Tablets (Rugby)

Stress Formula Plus Zinc
Tablets (Rexall
Consumer)

Stress Formula Tablets
(Cardinal)

Stress Formula Tablets
(Rexall Consumer)

Therapeutic Multivitamin
Tablets (Bergen
Brunswig)

Ultra Tabs Tablets (Major
Pharmaceuticals)

Vitamins Children's
Chewable Tablets (Prime
Marketing)

**MULTIVITAMIN AND MINERAL
PRODUCTS** *553t*

♦ Alpha Betic Tablets
(Abkit) G-3

B-C w/Folic Acid Plus
Tablet (Geneva)

B-Complex Plus Tablets
(United Research)

B-Complex Vitamins Plus
Tablets (Teva)

B-Plex Plus Tablets (Zenith
Goldline)

Bacmin Tablets (Marnel)

Becomax RX Tablets
(Ampharco)

Berocca Plus Tablets
(Roche)

♦ Bugs Bunny Complete
Children's Chewable
Tablets (Bayer) G-3

Cerovite Senior Tablets
(Rugby)

Circavite T Tablets (Circle)

Clusinex Syrup
(Pharmakon)

Daily Multiple Vitamins/
Minerals Tablets
(Vanguard)

Dr. Art Ulene's Vitamin
Formula Packets (Feeling
Fine)

Equi-Roca Plus Tablets
(Equipharm)

Ferrex PC Tablets
(Breckenridge)

♦ Flintstones Complete
Children's Chewable
Tablets (Bayer) G-3

Formula B Plus Tablets
(Major Pharmaceuticals)

Glutofac-ZX Capsules
(Kenwood)

Hematin Plus Tablets
(Cypress)

Iromin-G Tablets (Mission)

Manly Machovites Tablets
(Neurovites)

Mega-Multi Capsules
(Innovative Health)

Niferex-PN Tablets
(Schwarz)

O-Cal FA Tablets
(Pharmics)

♦ One-A-Day 50 Plus Tablets
(Bayer) G-3

♦ One-A-Day Antioxidant
Capsules (Bayer) G-3

♦ One-A-Day Kids Complete
Chewable Tablets (Bayer) .. G-3

♦ One-A-Day Maximum
Tablets (Bayer) G-3

♦ One-A-Day Men's Tablets
(Bayer) G-3

♦ One-A-Day Women's
Tablets (Bayer) G-3

PMS Formula Tablets
(Neurovites)

Poly Vitamin w/Iron
Chewable Tablets
(Rugby)

Protect Plus Capsules (Gil)

Protect Plus Liquid (Gil)

Strovite Forte Tablets
(Everett)

Sunvite Platinum Tablets
(Rexall Consumer)

Sunvite Tablets (Rexall
Consumer)

Super Plenamins Extra
Strength Tablets (Rexall
Consumer)

Super Plenamins Tablets
(Rexall Consumer)

Support 500 Capsules
(Marin)

Support Liquid (Marin)

Thera Vite M Tablets
(PDK)

Thera-M w/Minerals
Tablets (Prime
Marketing)

♦ Theragran-M Tablets
(Bristol-Myers Products) G-3

Therapeutic Plus Vitamin
Tablets (Rugby)

Therobec Plus Tablets
(Qualitest)

Total Formula Original
Tablets (Vitaline)

V-C Forte Capsules
(Breckenridge)

Vicap Forte Tablets (Major
Pharmaceuticals)

Vicon Forte Tablets (UCB)

Vita-Min Rx Tablets (Bio-
Tech)

Vitacon Forte Tablets
(Amide)

Vitaplex Plus Tablets
(Amide)

Vitelle Nesentials Tablets
(Fielding)

**ORNITHINE ALPHA-
KETOGLUTARATE** 337

VITAMIN B COMPLEX PRODUCTS .. *558t*

B-50 Complex Tablets
(Rexall Consumer)

B-100 Complex Tablets
(Rexall Consumer)

B-Ject-100 Injection
(Hyrex)

B-Plex Tablets (Contract
Pharmacal)

B-Plex Tablets (Zenith
Goldline)

Berocca Tablets (Roche)

Dialyvite Tablets
(Hillestad)

Formula B Tablets (Major
Pharmaceuticals)
Marlbee w/C Capsules
(Marlex)
Nephplex Rx Tablets
(Nephro-Tech)
Nephro-Vite Rx Tablets
(R&D)
Nephrocaps Capsules
(Fleming)
Primaplex Injection
(Primedics)
Stress B Complex with
Vitamin C Tablets
(Mission)
Strovite Tablets (Everett)
Therobec Tablets
(Qualitest)
Thex Forte Tablets (Lee)
Vicam Injection (Keene)
Vita-Bee w/C Tablets
(Rugby)
Vitamin B Complex 100
Injection (Hyrex)
Vitamin B Complex 100
Injection (McGuff)
Vitamin B Complex 100
Injection (Torrance)
Vitamin B Complex 100
Injection (Truxton)
Vitamin B Complex
Capsules (Rugby)
Vitamin B Complex w/
Vitamin C & B12
Injection (McGuff)
Vitamin B-100 Natural
Tablets (Cardinal)
Vitaplex Tablets (Amide)
Vitaplex Tablets (Medirex)

VITAMIN C **486**
Asco-Caps Capsules (Key
Company)
Asco-Tabs-1000 Tablets
(Key Company)
Ascocid Powder (Key
Company)
Ascocid-500-D Tablets
(Key Company)
C Complex Tablets
(National Vitamin)
C-500-GR Tablets (Bio-
Tech)

C-Gram Tablets (Freeda)
C-Max Tablets (Bio-Tech)
C-Time Capsules (Time-
Cap)
C-Tym Capsules
(Economed)
C250 Chewable Tablets
(Nature's Bounty)
C250 w/Rose Hips Tablets
(Nature's Bounty)
C500 Capsules (Mason)
C500 Capsules (Nature's
Bounty)
C500 Plus Rose Hips/
Bioflavonoids Tablets
(Mason)
C500 Tablets (Rexall
Consumer)
C500 w/Rose Hips
Chewable Tablets (Rexall
Consumer)
C500 w/Rose Hips Tablets
(Nature's Bounty)
C500 w/Rose Hips Tablets
(Rexall Consumer)
C1000 Ascorbic Acid
Tablets (Mason)
C1000 Plus Rose Hips
Tablets (Rexall
Consumer)
C1000 Plus Rose Hips/
Bioflavonoids Tablets
(Mason)
C1000 Tablets (Mason)
C1000 Tablets (Nature's
Bounty)
C1000 Tablets (Rexall
Consumer)
C1000 w/Rose Hips
Tablets (Rexall
Consumer)
C1500 Plus Rose Hips/
Bioflavonoids Tablets
(Mason)
C1500 Tablets (Nature's
Bounty)
Cecon Liquid (Abbott)
Cemill 500 Tablets (Miller
Pharmacal)
Cemill 1000 Tablets
(Miller Pharmacal)

Cenolate Injection (Abbott
Hospital)
Cevi-Bid Tablets (Lee)
Chew-C Chewable Tablets
(Key Company)
Dull-C Powder (Freeda)
Ester C Tablets (Source)
Ester-C Capsules
(Swanson)
Ester-C Tablets (Swanson)
Fruit C Chewable Tablets
(Freeda)
♦ Halls Defense Lozenges
(Warner-Lambert) **G-6**
Mega-C Tablets (Merit)
Mega-C/A Plus Injection
(Merit)
Ortho/CS Injection (Merit)
Pellets C Capsules (Lemax)
Pure Vitamin C-Crystals
Powder (Nature's
Bounty)
Sunkist Vitamin C
Chewable Tablets
(Novartis Consumer)
Vicks Vitamin C Lozenge
(Procter & Gamble)
Vita-C Powder (Freeda)
Vitamin C Natural
Chewable Tablets
(Bergen Brunswig)
Vitamin C w/Rose Hips
Natural Tablets (Bergen
Brunswig)
Vitamin C w/Rose Hips
Natural Tablets
(Cardinal)
Vitamin C500 Plus Tablets
(Mason)

CANCER, NUTRIENTS DEFICIENCY SECONDARY TO

Cancer may be treated with
chemotherapeutic agents. The
following products may be
recommended for relief of nutrients
deficiency:

ASCORBYL PALMITATE **33**
MULTIVITAMIN PRODUCTS **550t**
BEC w/Zinc Tablets
(Bergen Brunswig)
♦ Bugs Bunny Plus Extra C
Chewable Tablets (Bayer) . . **G-3**

♦ Bugs Bunny Plus Iron
Chewable Tablets (Bayer) .. **G-3**
Cardiotek Tablets (Stewart-
Jackson)
Cefol Tablets (Abbott
Hospital)
Circus Chews Children's
Chewable Tablets (Rexall
Consumer)
Daily Multiple Vitamins
Tablets (Marlex)
Daily Multiple Vitamins
Tablets (Rexall
Consumer)
Daily Multiple Vitamins w/
Iron Tablets (Rexall
Consumer)
Daily Multivitamins Tablets
(Sky)
♦ Flintstones Original
Children's Chewable
Tablets (Bayer) **G-3**
♦ Flintstones Plus Calcium
Chewable Tablets (Bayer) .. **G-3**
♦ Flintstones Plus Extra C
Chewable Tablets (Bayer) .. **G-3**
♦ Flintstones Plus Iron
Chewable Tablets (Bayer) .. **G-3**
Key-Plex Injection (Hyrex)
M.V.I. Pediatric Powder for
Injection (AstraZeneca LP)
M.V.I.-12 Injection
(AstraZeneca LP)
Multi-Vitamins Tablets
(Rugby)
Multivitamin Capsules
(Numark)
Once Daily Tablets (Prime
Marketing)
♦ One-A-Day Essential
Tablets (Bayer) **G-3**
Poly Vitamin Chewable
Tablets (Rugby)
Stress Formula Plus Zinc
Tablets (Rexall
Consumer)
Stress Formula Tablets
(Cardinal)
Stress Formula Tablets
(Rexall Consumer)

Therapeutic Multivitamin
Tablets (Bergen
Brunswig)
Ultra Tabs Tablets (Major
Pharmaceuticals)
Vitamins Children's
Chewable Tablets (Prime
Marketing)

**MULTIVITAMIN AND MINERAL
PRODUCTS** *553t*
♦ Alpha Betic Tablets
(Abkit) **G-3**
B-C w/Folic Acid Plus
Tablet (Geneva)
B-Complex Plus Tablets
(United Research)
B-Complex Vitamins Plus
Tablets (Teva)
B-Plex Plus Tablets (Zenith
Goldline)
Bacmin Tablets (Marnel)
Becomax RX Tablets
(Ampharco)
Berocca Plus Tablets
(Roche)
♦ Bugs Bunny Complete
Children's Chewable
Tablets (Bayer) **G-3**
Cerovite Senior Tablets
(Rugby)
Circavite T Tablets (Circle)
Clusinex Syrup
(Pharmakon)
Daily Multiple Vitamins/
Minerals Tablets
(Vanguard)
Dr. Art Ulene's Vitamin
Formula Packets (Feeling
Fine)
Equi-Roca Plus Tablets
(Equipharm)
Ferrex PC Tablets
(Breckenridge)
♦ Flintstones Complete
Children's Chewable
Tablets (Bayer) **G-3**
Formula B Plus Tablets
(Major Pharmaceuticals)
Glutofac-ZX Capsules
(Kenwood)
Hematin Plus Tablets
(Cypress)
Iromin-G Tablets (Mission)

Manly Machovites Tablets
(Neurovites)
Mega-Multi Capsules
(Innovative Health)
Niferex-PN Tablets
(Schwarz)
O-Cal FA Tablets
(Pharmics)
♦ One-A-Day 50 Plus Tablets
(Bayer) **G-3**
♦ One-A-Day Antioxidant
Capsules (Bayer) **G-3**
♦ One-A-Day Kids Complete
Chewable Tablets (Bayer) .. **G-3**
♦ One-A-Day Maximum
Tablets (Bayer) **G-3**
♦ One-A-Day Men's Tablets
(Bayer) **G-3**
♦ One-A-Day Women's
Tablets (Bayer) **G-3**
PMS Formula Tablets
(Neurovites)
Poly Vitamin w/Iron
Chewable Tablets
(Rugby)
Protect Plus Capsules (Gil)
Protect Plus Liquid (Gil)
Strovite Forte Tablets
(Everett)
Sunvite Platinum Tablets
(Rexall Consumer)
Sunvite Tablets (Rexall
Consumer)
Super Plenamins Extra
Strength Tablets (Rexall
Consumer)
Super Plenamins Tablets
(Rexall Consumer)
Support 500 Capsules
(Marin)
Support Liquid (Marin)
Thera Vite M Tablets
(PDK)
Thera-M w/Minerals
Tablets (Prime
Marketing)
♦ Theragran-M Tablets
(Bristol-Myers Products) **G-3**
Therapeutic Plus Vitamin
Tablets (Rugby)
Therobec Plus Tablets
(Qualitest)

Total Formula Original
Tablets (Vitaline)
V-C Forte Capsules
(Breckenridge)
Vicap Forte Tablets (Major
Pharmaceuticals)
Vicon Forte Tablets (UCB)
Vita-Min Rx Tablets (Bio-
Tech)
Vitacon Forte Tablets
(Amide)
Vitaplex Plus Tablets
(Amide)
Vitelle Nesentials Tablets
(Fielding)

Easysoy Gold Super
Isoflavone Concentrate
Tablets (Twinlab)
Genistein Soy Isoflavones
(Source)
♦ Healthy Woman Soy
Menopause Tablets
(Personal Products
Company) **G-5**
Maxilife Mega Soy
Capsules (Health from
the Sun)
PC Soy Isoflavones
(Natrol)
Soy Essentials Tablets
(Enzymatic Therapy)
♦ Soy & Red Clover
Isoflavones Liquid
(Nature's Answer) **G-4**

Tocotrienol Antioxidant
Complex Capsules
(Source)
Tototrien-All Capsules
(Natrol)

B-50 Complex Tablets
(Rexall Consumer)
B-100 Complex Tablets
(Rexall Consumer)
B-Ject-100 Injection
(Hyrex)
B-Plex Tablets (Contract
Pharmacal)

B-Plex Tablets (Zenith
Goldline)
Berocca Tablets (Roche)
Dialyvite Tablets
(Hillestad)
Formula B Tablets (Major
Pharmaceuticals)
Marlbee w/C Capsules
(Marlex)
Nephplex Rx Tablets
(Nephro-Tech)
Nephro-Vite Rx Tablets
(R&D)
Nephrocaps Capsules
(Fleming)
Primaplex Injection
(Primedics)
Stress B Complex with
Vitamin C Tablets
(Mission)
Strovite Tablets (Everett)
Therobec Tablets
(Qualitest)
Thex Forte Tablets (Lee)
Vicam Injection (Keene)
Vita-Bee w/C Tablets
(Rugby)
Vitamin B Complex 100
Injection (Hyrex)
Vitamin B Complex 100
Injection (McGuff)
Vitamin B Complex 100
Injection (Torrance)
Vitamin B Complex 100
Injection (Truxton)
Vitamin B Complex
Capsules (Rugby)
Vitamin B Complex w/
Vitamin C & B12
Injection (McGuff)
Vitamin B-100 Natural
Tablets (Cardinal)
Vitaplex Tablets (Amide)
Vitaplex Tablets (Medirex)

Asco-Caps Capsules (Key
Company)
Asco-Tabs-1000 Tablets
(Key Company)
Ascocid Powder (Key
Company)

Ascocid-500-D Tablets
(Key Company)
C Complex Tablets
(National Vitamin)
C-500-GR Tablets (Bio-
Tech)
C-Gram Tablets (Freeda)
C-Max Tablets (Bio-Tech)
C-Time Capsules (Time-
Cap)
C-Tym Capsules
(Economed)
C250 Chewable Tablets
(Nature's Bounty)
C250 w/Rose Hips Tablets
(Nature's Bounty)
C500 Capsules (Mason)
C500 Capsules (Nature's
Bounty)
C500 Plus Rose Hips/
Bioflavonoids Tablets
(Mason)
C500 Tablets (Rexall
Consumer)
C500 w/Rose Hips
Chewable Tablets (Rexall
Consumer)
C500 w/Rose Hips Tablets
(Nature's Bounty)
C500 w/Rose Hips Tablets
(Rexall Consumer)
C1000 Ascorbic Acid
Tablets (Mason)
C1000 Plus Rose Hips
Tablets (Rexall
Consumer)
C1000 Plus Rose Hips/
Bioflavonoids Tablets
(Mason)
C1000 Tablets (Mason)
C1000 Tablets (Nature's
Bounty)
C1000 Tablets (Rexall
Consumer)
C1000 w/Rose Hips
Tablets (Rexall
Consumer)
C1500 Plus Rose Hips/
Bioflavonoids Tablets
(Mason)
C1500 Tablets (Nature's
Bounty)

Cecon Liquid (Abbott)

Cemill 500 Tablets (Miller Pharmacal)

Cemill 1000 Tablets (Miller Pharmacal)

Cenolate Injection (Abbott Hospital)

Cevi-Bid Tablets (Lee)

Chew-C Chewable Tablets (Key Company)

Dull-C Powder (Freeda)

Ester C Tablets (Source)

Ester-C Capsules (Swanson)

Ester-C Tablets (Swanson)

Fruit C Chewable Tablets (Freeda)

♦ Halls Defense Lozenges (Warner-Lambert) **G-6**

Mega-C Tablets (Merit)

Mega-C/A Plus Injection (Merit)

Ortho/CS Injection (Merit)

Pellets C Capsules (Lemax)

Pure Vitamin C-Crystals Powder (Nature's Bounty)

Sunkist Vitamin C Chewable Tablets (Novartis Consumer)

Vicks Vitamin C Lozenge (Procter & Gamble)

Vita-C Powder (Freeda)

Vitamin C Natural Chewable Tablets (Bergen Brunswig)

Vitamin C w/Rose Hips Natural Tablets (Bergen Brunswig)

Vitamin C w/Rose Hips Natural Tablets (Cardinal)

Vitamin C500 Plus Tablets (Mason)

VITAMIN E **505**

Alph-E Capsules (Key Company)

Alph-E-Mixed Capsules (Key Company)

Alpha-E Capsules (Advanced Nutritional)

Aquasol E Liquid (AstraZeneca LP)

Aquavit-E Liquid (Cypress)

Born Again Vitamin E Oil (Alvin Last)

DL-Alpha Tocopheryl E400 Capsules (Mason)

E-400-Mixed Capsules (Bio-Tech)

E-Max-1000 Capsules (Bio-Tech)

E-Pherol Tablets (Vitaline)

E100 Capsules (Nature's Bounty)

E200 Capsules (Nature's Bounty)

E200 Mixed Capsules (Rexall Consumer)

E400 Capsules (Nature's Bounty)

E400 Mixed Capsules (Rexall Consumer)

E400 Natural Capsules (Rexall Consumer)

E1000 Capsules (Nature's Bounty)

E1000 D-Alpha Capsules (Mason)

E1000 Mixed Capsules (Rexall Consumer)

Formula E 400 Capsules (Miller Pharmacal)

Liquid E Liquid (Freeda)

Nutr-E-Sol Capsules (Advanced Nutritional)

Nutr-E-Sol Liquid (Advanced Nutritional)

Total E-400 Capsules (Westlake)

Vitamin E Aqueous Liquid (Boca Pharmacal)

Vitamin E Aqueous Liquid (Silarx)

Vitamin E D-Alpha Capsules (Mason)

Vitamin E DL Alpha Capsules (Health Products)

Vitamin E DL-Alpha Capsules (Mason)

Vitamin E MTC Capsules (National Vitamin)

Vitamin E Mixed Capsules (Mason)

Vitamin E Mixed Tablets (Freeda)

Vitamin E Mixed Tocopherols Capsules (Swanson)

Vitamin E Natural Blend Capsules (Medicine Shoppe)

Vitamin E Natural Blend Capsules (Perrigo)

Vitamin E Natural Capsules (Basic Vitamins)

Vitamin E Natural Capsules (Bergen Brunswig)

Vitamin E Natural Capsules (Cardinal)

Vitamin E Natural Capsules (Dixon-Shane)

Vitamin E Natural Capsules (McKesson)

Vitamin E Natural Liquid (Geritrex)

Vitamin E Water Soluble Capsules (National Vitamin)

Vitamin E400 D Alpha Capsules (National Vitamin)

Vitamin E400 D-Alpha Capsules (Perrigo)

Vitamin E800 D-Alpha Capsules (Pharmavite)

WHEY PROTEINS **528**

Super Whey Pro Powder (Wallace)

Whey Ahead Powder (Twinlab)

Whey Protein Powder (Prolab)

CONGESTIVE HEART FAILURE, NUTRIENTS DEFICIENCY SECONDARY TO

Congestive heart failure may be treated with ACE inhibitors, cardiac glycosides or diuretics. The following products may be recommended for relief of nutrients deficiency:

MULTIVITAMIN PRODUCTS *550t*

BEC w/Zinc Tablets
(Bergen Brunswig)

♦ Bugs Bunny Plus Extra C
Chewable Tablets (Bayer) .. **G-3**

♦ Bugs Bunny Plus Iron
Chewable Tablets (Bayer) .. **G-3**

Cardiotek Tablets (Stewart-
Jackson)

Cefol Tablets (Abbott
Hospital)

Circus Chews Children's
Chewable Tablets (Rexall
Consumer)

Daily Multiple Vitamins
Tablets (Marlex)

Daily Multiple Vitamins
Tablets (Rexall
Consumer)

Daily Multiple Vitamins w/
Iron Tablets (Rexall
Consumer)

Daily Multivitamins Tablets
(Sky)

♦ Flintstones Original
Children's Chewable
Tablets (Bayer) **G-3**

♦ Flintstones Plus Calcium
Chewable Tablets (Bayer) .. **G-3**

♦ Flintstones Plus Extra C
Chewable Tablets (Bayer) .. **G-3**

♦ Flintstones Plus Iron
Chewable Tablets (Bayer) .. **G-3**

Key-Plex Injection (Hyrex)

M.V.I. Pediatric Powder for
Injection (AstraZeneca LP)

M.V.I.-12 Injection
(AstraZeneca LP)

Multi-Vitamins Tablets
(Rugby)

Multivitamin Capsules
(Numark)

Once Daily Tablets (Prime
Marketing)

♦ One-A-Day Essential
Tablets (Bayer) **G-3**

Poly Vitamin Chewable
Tablets (Rugby)

Stress Formula Plus Zinc
Tablets (Rexall
Consumer)

Stress Formula Tablets
(Cardinal)

Stress Formula Tablets
(Rexall Consumer)

Therapeutic Multivitamin
Tablets (Bergen
Brunswig)

Ultra Tabs Tablets (Major
Pharmaceuticals)

Vitamins Children's
Chewable Tablets (Prime
Marketing)

**MULTIVITAMIN AND MINERAL
PRODUCTS** *553t*

♦ Alpha Betic Tablets
(Abkit) **G-3**

B-C w/Folic Acid Plus
Tablet (Geneva)

B-Complex Plus Tablets
(United Research)

B-Complex Vitamins Plus
Tablets (Teva)

B-Plex Plus Tablets (Zenith
Goldline)

Bacmin Tablets (Marnel)

Becomax RX Tablets
(Ampharco)

Berocca Plus Tablets
(Roche)

♦ Bugs Bunny Complete
Children's Chewable
Tablets (Bayer) **G-3**

Cerovite Senior Tablets
(Rugby)

Circavite T Tablets (Circle)

Clusinex Syrup
(Pharmakon)

Daily Multiple Vitamins/
Minerals Tablets
(Vanguard)

Dr. Art Ulene's Vitamin
Formula Packets (Feeling
Fine)

Equi-Roca Plus Tablets
(Equipharm)

Ferrex PC Tablets
(Breckenridge)

♦ Flintstones Complete
Children's Chewable
Tablets (Bayer) **G-3**

Formula B Plus Tablets
(Major Pharmaceuticals)

Glutofac-ZX Capsules
(Kenwood)

Hematin Plus Tablets
(Cypress)

Iromin-G Tablets (Mission)

Manly Machovites Tablets
(Neurovites)

Mega-Multi Capsules
(Innovative Health)

Niferex-PN Tablets
(Schwarz)

O-Cal FA Tablets
(Pharmics)

♦ One-A-Day 50 Plus Tablets
(Bayer) **G-3**

♦ One-A-Day Antioxidant
Capsules (Bayer) **G-3**

♦ One-A-Day Kids Complete
Chewable Tablets (Bayer) .. **G-3**

♦ One-A-Day Maximum
Tablets (Bayer) **G-3**

♦ One-A-Day Men's Tablets
(Bayer) **G-3**

♦ One-A-Day Women's
Tablets (Bayer) **G-3**

PMS Formula Tablets
(Neurovites)

Poly Vitamin w/Iron
Chewable Tablets
(Rugby)

Protect Plus Capsules (Gil)

Protect Plus Liquid (Gil)

Strovite Forte Tablets
(Everett)

Sunvite Platinum Tablets
(Rexall Consumer)

Sunvite Tablets (Rexall
Consumer)

Super Plenamins Extra
Strength Tablets (Rexall
Consumer)

Super Plenamins Tablets
(Rexall Consumer)

Support 500 Capsules
(Marin)

Support Liquid (Marin)

Thera Vite M Tablets
(PDK)

Thera-M w/Minerals
Tablets (Prime
Marketing)

CONSTIPATION

May result from the use of ACE inhibitors, anticholinergics, anticonvulsants, antidepressants, beta blockers, bile acid sequestrants, butyrophenones, calcium and aluminum-containing antacids, calcium channel blockers, ganglionic blockers, hematinics, HMG-CoA reductase inhibitors, monoamine oxidase inhibitors, narcotic analgesics, nonsteroidal anti-inflammatory drugs or phenothiazines. The following products may be recommended:

CYSTIC FIBROSIS, NUTRIENTS DEFICIENCY SECONDARY TO

Cystic fibrosis may be treated with dornase alfa. The following products may be recommended for relief of nutrients deficiency:

Circus Chews Children's Chewable Tablets (Rexall Consumer)

Daily Multiple Vitamins Tablets (Marlex)

Daily Multiple Vitamins Tablets (Rexall Consumer)

Daily Multiple Vitamins w/ Iron Tablets (Rexall Consumer)

Daily Multivitamins Tablets (Sky)

♦ Flintstones Original Children's Chewable Tablets (Bayer) G-3

♦ Flintstones Plus Calcium Chewable Tablets (Bayer) .. G-3

♦ Flintstones Plus Extra C Chewable Tablets (Bayer) .. G-3

♦ Flintstones Plus Iron Chewable Tablets (Bayer) .. G-3

Key-Plex Injection (Hyrex)

M.V.I. Pediatric Powder for Injection (AstraZeneca LP)

M.V.I.-12 Injection (AstraZeneca LP)

Multi-Vitamins Tablets (Rugby)

Multivitamin Capsules (Numark)

Once Daily Tablets (Prime Marketing)

♦ One-A-Day Essential Tablets (Bayer) G-3

Poly Vitamin Chewable Tablets (Rugby)

Stress Formula Plus Zinc Tablets (Rexall Consumer)

Stress Formula Tablets (Cardinal)

Stress Formula Tablets (Rexall Consumer)

Therapeutic Multivitamin Tablets (Bergen Brunswig)

Ultra Tabs Tablets (Major Pharmaceuticals)

Vitamins Children's Chewable Tablets (Prime Marketing)

MULTIVITAMIN AND MINERAL PRODUCTS *553t*

♦ Alpha Betic Tablets (Abkit) G-3

B-C w/Folic Acid Plus Tablet (Geneva)

B-Complex Plus Tablets (United Research)

B-Complex Vitamins Plus Tablets (Teva)

B-Plex Plus Tablets (Zenith Goldline)

Bacmin Tablets (Marnel)

Becomax RX Tablets (Ampharco)

Berocca Plus Tablets (Roche)

♦ Bugs Bunny Complete Children's Chewable Tablets (Bayer) G-3

Cerovite Senior Tablets (Rugby)

Circavite T Tablets (Circle)

Clusinex Syrup (Pharmakon)

Daily Multiple Vitamins/ Minerals Tablets (Vanguard)

Dr. Art Ulene's Vitamin Formula Packets (Feeling Fine)

Equi-Roca Plus Tablets (Equipharm)

Ferrex PC Tablets (Breckenridge)

♦ Flintstones Complete Children's Chewable Tablets (Bayer) G-3

Formula B Plus Tablets (Major Pharmaceuticals)

Glutofac-ZX Capsules (Kenwood)

Hematin Plus Tablets (Cypress)

Iromin-G Tablets (Mission)

Manly Machovites Tablets (Neurovites)

Mega-Multi Capsules (Innovative Health)

Niferex-PN Tablets (Schwarz)

O-Cal FA Tablets (Pharmics)

♦ One-A-Day 50 Plus Tablets (Bayer) G-3

♦ One-A-Day Antioxidant Capsules (Bayer) G-3

♦ One-A-Day Kids Complete Chewable Tablets (Bayer) .. G-3

♦ One-A-Day Maximum Tablets (Bayer) G-3

♦ One-A-Day Men's Tablets (Bayer) G-3

♦ One-A-Day Women's Tablets (Bayer) G-3

PMS Formula Tablets (Neurovites)

Poly Vitamin w/Iron Chewable Tablets (Rugby)

Protect Plus Capsules (Gil)

Protect Plus Liquid (Gil)

Strovite Forte Tablets (Everett)

Sunvite Platinum Tablets (Rexall Consumer)

Sunvite Tablets (Rexall Consumer)

Super Plenamins Extra Strength Tablets (Rexall Consumer)

Super Plenamins Tablets (Rexall Consumer)

Support 500 Capsules (Marin)

Support Liquid (Marin)

Thera Vite M Tablets (PDK)

Thera-M w/Minerals Tablets (Prime Marketing)

♦ Theragran-M Tablets (Bristol-Myers Products) G-3

Therapeutic Plus Vitamin Tablets (Rugby)

Therobec Plus Tablets (Qualitest)

Total Formula Original Tablets (Vitaline)

V-C Forte Capsules (Breckenridge)

Vicap Forte Tablets (Major
Pharmaceuticals)
Vicon Forte Tablets (UCB)
Vita-Min Rx Tablets (Bio-
Tech)
Vitacon Forte Tablets
(Amide)
Vitaplex Plus Tablets
(Amide)
Vitelle Nesentials Tablets
(Fielding)

TAURINE **442**
Mega Taurine Capsules
(Twinlab)

VITAMIN A **462**
Active A Tablets (Source)

VITAMIN B COMPLEX PRODUCTS . . **558t**
B-50 Complex Tablets
(Rexall Consumer)
B-100 Complex Tablets
(Rexall Consumer)
B-Ject-100 Injection
(Hyrex)
B-Plex Tablets (Contract
Pharmacal)
B-Plex Tablets (Zenith
Goldline)
Berocca Tablets (Roche)
Dialyvite Tablets
(Hillestad)
Formula B Tablets (Major
Pharmaceuticals)
Marlbee w/C Capsules
(Marlex)
Nephplex Rx Tablets
(Nephro-Tech)
Nephro-Vite Rx Tablets
(R&D)
Nephrocaps Capsules
(Fleming)
Primaplex Injection
(Primedics)
Stress B Complex with
Vitamin C Tablets
(Mission)
Strovite Tablets (Everett)
Therobec Tablets
(Qualitest)
Thex Forte Tablets (Lee)
Vicam Injection (Keene)
Vita-Bee w/C Tablets
(Rugby)

Vitamin B Complex 100
Injection (Hyrex)
Vitamin B Complex 100
Injection (McGuff)
Vitamin B Complex 100
Injection (Torrance)
Vitamin B Complex 100
Injection (Truxton)
Vitamin B Complex
Capsules (Rugby)
Vitamin B Complex w/
Vitamin C & B12
Injection (McGuff)
Vitamin B-100 Natural
Tablets (Cardinal)
Vitaplex Tablets (Amide)
Vitaplex Tablets (Medirex)

VITAMIN D **498**
VITAMIN E **505**
Alph-E Capsules (Key
Company)
Alph-E-Mixed Capsules
(Key Company)
Alpha-E Capsules
(Advanced Nutritional)
Aquasol E Liquid
(AstraZeneca LP)
Aquavit-E Liquid (Cypress)
Born Again Vitamin E Oil
(Alvin Last)
DL-Alpha Tocopheryl E400
Capsules (Mason)
E-400-Mixed Capsules
(Bio-Tech)
E-Max-1000 Capsules (Bio-
Tech)
E-Pherol Tablets (Vitaline)
E100 Capsules (Nature's
Bounty)
E200 Capsules (Nature's
Bounty)
E200 Mixed Capsules
(Rexall Consumer)
E400 Capsules (Nature's
Bounty)
E400 Mixed Capsules
(Rexall Consumer)
E400 Natural Capsules
(Rexall Consumer)
E1000 Capsules (Nature's
Bounty)

E1000 D-Alpha Capsules
(Mason)
E1000 Mixed Capsules
(Rexall Consumer)
Formula E 400 Capsules
(Miller Pharmacal)
Liquid E Liquid (Freeda)
Nutr-E-Sol Capsules
(Advanced Nutritional)
Nutr-E-Sol Liquid
(Advanced Nutritional)
Total E-400 Capsules
(Westlake)
Vitamin E Aqueous Liquid
(Boca Pharmacal)
Vitamin E Aqueous Liquid
(Silarx)
Vitamin E D-Alpha
Capsules (Mason)
Vitamin E DL Alpha
Capsules (Health
Products)
Vitamin E DL-Alpha
Capsules (Mason)
Vitamin E MTC Capsules
(National Vitamin)
Vitamin E Mixed Capsules
(Mason)
Vitamin E Mixed Tablets
(Freeda)
Vitamin E Mixed
Tocopherols Capsules
(Swanson)
Vitamin E Natural Blend
Capsules (Medicine
Shoppe)
Vitamin E Natural Blend
Capsules (Perrigo)
Vitamin E Natural
Capsules (Basic
Vitamins)
Vitamin E Natural
Capsules (Bergen
Brunswig)
Vitamin E Natural
Capsules (Cardinal)
Vitamin E Natural
Capsules (Dixon-Shane)
Vitamin E Natural
Capsules (McKesson)
Vitamin E Natural Liquid
(Geritrex)

Vitamin E Water Soluble
Capsules (National
Vitamin)

Vitamin E400 D Alpha
Capsules (National
Vitamin)

Vitamin E400 D-Alpha
Capsules (Perrigo)

Vitamin E800 D-Alpha
Capsules (Pharmavite)

VITAMIN K **523**

DENTAL CARIES

May be treated with fluoride
preparations or vitamin and fluoride
supplements. The following products
may be recommended for relief of
symptoms:

FLUORIDE **154**

Flouritab Chewable Tablets
(Fluoritab)

Flouritab Liquid (Fluoritab)

Fluor-A-Day Chewable
Tablets (Pharmascience)

Fluor-A-Day Liquid
(Pharmascience)

Fluor-A-Day Lozenges
(Pharmascience)

Fluorabon Chewable
Tablets (Perry)

Fluorabon Solution (Perry)

Fluorinse Liquid (Oral B)

Flura-Loz Chewable
Tablets (Kirkman)

Lozengesi-Flur Lozenge
(Dreir)

Luride Chewable Tablets
(Colgate Oral)

Luride Liquid (Colgate
Oral)

Nafrinse Chewable Tablets
(Orachem)

Nafrinse Solution
(Orachem)

Neutracare Gel (Oral B)

Neutragard Fluoride Rinse
Solution (Pascal)

Pediaflor Drops (Ross)

Pharmaflur Chewable
Tablets (Pharmics)

Phos-Flur Gel (Colgate
Oral)

Phos-Flur Solution (Colgate
Oral)

Prevident 5000 Plus Cream
(Colgate Oral)

Prevident Cream (Colgate
Oral)

Prevident Solution (Colgate
Oral)

Thera-Flur-N Gel (Colgate
Oral)

DIABETES MELLITUS, CONSTIPATION SECONDARY TO

Diabetes mellitus may be treated
with insulins or oral hypoglycemic
agents. The following products may
be recommended for relief of
constipation:

GLUCOMANNAN **184**

LACTULOSE **243**

Cephulac Syrup (Aventis)

Cholac Syrup (Alra)

Chronulac Syrup (Aventis)

Constilac Syrup (Alra)

Constulose Solution
(Alpharma)

Duphalac Syrup (Solvay)

Enulose Solution
(Alpharma)

PECTIN **348**

Modified Citrus Pectin
Power Capsules (Nature's
Herbs)

PREBIOTICS **372**

PSYLLIUM **384**

Colon Care Formula
Psyllium Seed Capsules
(Yerba Prima)

Fiberall Powder (Novartis
Consumer)

Fiberall Wafers (Novartis
Consumer)

Fibro-XI Capsules (Key
Company)

Genfiber Powder (Zenith
Goldline)

Hydrocil Powder (Numark)

Konsyl Powder (Konsyl)

Konsyl-D Powder (Konsyl)

♦ Metamucil Powder and
Wafers (Procter &
Gamble) **G-5**

Modane Bulk Powder
(Savage)

♦ Perdiem Granules (Novartis
Consumer) **G-5**

Psyllium Husks 100% Pure
Powder (Yerba Prima)

Reguloid Powder (Carlson)

Reguloid Powder (Rugby)

Serutan Granules (Twinlab)

DIABETES MELLITUS, POORLY CONTROLLED, VITAMINS AND MINERALS DEFICIENCY SECONDARY TO

Diabetes mellitus may be treated
with insulins or oral hypoglycemic
agents. The following products may
be recommended for relief of
vitamins and minerals deficiency:

CHROMIUM **96**

MULTIVITAMIN PRODUCTS **550t**

BEC w/Zinc Tablets
(Bergen Brunswig)

♦ Bugs Bunny Plus Extra C
Chewable Tablets (Bayer) . . **G-3**

♦ Bugs Bunny Plus Iron
Chewable Tablets (Bayer) . . **G-3**

Cardiotek Tablets (Stewart-
Jackson)

Cefol Tablets (Abbott
Hospital)

Circus Chews Children's
Chewable Tablets (Rexall
Consumer)

Daily Multiple Vitamins
Tablets (Marlex)

Daily Multiple Vitamins
Tablets (Rexall
Consumer)

Daily Multiple Vitamins w/
Iron Tablets (Rexall
Consumer)

Daily Multivitamins Tablets
(Sky)

♦ Flintstones Original
Children's Chewable
Tablets (Bayer) **G-3**

♦ Flintstones Plus Calcium
Chewable Tablets (Bayer) . . **G-3**

♦ Flintstones Plus Extra C
Chewable Tablets (Bayer) . . **G-3**

♦ Flintstones Plus Iron
Chewable Tablets (Bayer) . . **G-3**

Key-Plex Injection (Hyrex)

M.V.I. Pediatric Powder for Injection (AstraZeneca LP)

M.V.I.-12 Injection (AstraZeneca LP)

Multi-Vitamins Tablets (Rugby)

Multivitamin Capsules (Numark)

Once Daily Tablets (Prime Marketing)

♦ One-A-Day Essential Tablets (Bayer) G-3

Poly Vitamin Chewable Tablets (Rugby)

Stress Formula Plus Zinc Tablets (Rexall Consumer)

Stress Formula Tablets (Cardinal)

Stress Formula Tablets (Rexall Consumer)

Therapeutic Multivitamin Tablets (Bergen Brunswig)

Ultra Tabs Tablets (Major Pharmaceuticals)

Vitamins Children's Chewable Tablets (Prime Marketing)

MULTIVITAMIN AND MINERAL PRODUCTS *553t*

♦ Alpha Betic Tablets (Abkit) G-3

B-C w/Folic Acid Plus Tablet (Geneva)

B-Complex Plus Tablets (United Research)

B-Complex Vitamins Plus Tablets (Teva)

B-Plex Plus Tablets (Zenith Goldline)

Bacmin Tablets (Marnel)

Becomax RX Tablets (Ampharco)

Berocca Plus Tablets (Roche)

♦ Bugs Bunny Complete Children's Chewable Tablets (Bayer) G-3

Cerovite Senior Tablets (Rugby)

Circavite T Tablets (Circle)

Clusinex Syrup (Pharmakon)

Daily Multiple Vitamins/ Minerals Tablets (Vanguard)

Dr. Art Ulene's Vitamin Formula Packets (Feeling Fine)

Equi-Roca Plus Tablets (Equipharm)

Ferrex PC Tablets (Breckenridge)

♦ Flintstones Complete Children's Chewable Tablets (Bayer) G-3

Formula B Plus Tablets (Major Pharmaceuticals)

Glutofac-ZX Capsules (Kenwood)

Hematin Plus Tablets (Cypress)

Iromin-G Tablets (Mission)

Manly Machovites Tablets (Neurovites)

Mega-Multi Capsules (Innovative Health)

Niferex-PN Tablets (Schwarz)

O-Cal FA Tablets (Pharmics)

♦ One-A-Day 50 Plus Tablets (Bayer) G-3

♦ One-A-Day Antioxidant Capsules (Bayer) G-3

♦ One-A-Day Kids Complete Chewable Tablets (Bayer) . . G-3

♦ One-A-Day Maximum Tablets (Bayer) G-3

♦ One-A-Day Men's Tablets (Bayer) G-3

♦ One-A-Day Women's Tablets (Bayer) G-3

PMS Formula Tablets (Neurovites)

Poly Vitamin w/Iron Chewable Tablets (Rugby)

Protect Plus Capsules (Gil)

Protect Plus Liquid (Gil)

Strovite Forte Tablets (Everett)

Sunvite Platinum Tablets (Rexall Consumer)

Sunvite Tablets (Rexall Consumer)

Super Plenamins Extra Strength Tablets (Rexall Consumer)

Super Plenamins Tablets (Rexall Consumer)

Support 500 Capsules (Marin)

Support Liquid (Marin)

Thera Vite M Tablets (PDK)

Thera-M w/Minerals Tablets (Prime Marketing)

♦ Theragran-M Tablets (Bristol-Myers Products) G-3

Therapeutic Plus Vitamin Tablets (Rugby)

Therobec Plus Tablets (Qualitest)

Total Formula Original Tablets (Vitaline)

V-C Forte Capsules (Breckenridge)

Vicap Forte Tablets (Major Pharmaceuticals)

Vicon Forte Tablets (UCB)

Vita-Min Rx Tablets (Bio-Tech)

Vitacon Forte Tablets (Amide)

Vitaplex Plus Tablets (Amide)

Vitelle Nesentials Tablets (Fielding)

TOCOTRIENOLS 453

Tocotrienol Antioxidant Complex Capsules (Source)

Tototrien-All Capsules (Natrol)

VANADIUM 459

VITAMIN B COMPLEX PRODUCTS . . *558t*

B-50 Complex Tablets (Rexall Consumer)

B-100 Complex Tablets (Rexall Consumer)

B-Ject-100 Injection (Hyrex)

B-Plex Tablets (Contract Pharmacal)

B-Plex Tablets (Zenith Goldline)

Berocca Tablets (Roche)

Dialyvite Tablets (Hillestad)

Formula B Tablets (Major Pharmaceuticals)

Marlbee w/C Capsules (Marlex)

Nephplex Rx Tablets (Nephro-Tech)

Nephro-Vite Rx Tablets (R&D)

Nephrocaps Capsules (Fleming)

Primaplex Injection (Primedics)

Stress B Complex with Vitamin C Tablets (Mission)

Strovite Tablets (Everett)

Therobec Tablets (Qualitest)

Thex Forte Tablets (Lee)

Vicam Injection (Keene)

Vita-Bee w/C Tablets (Rugby)

Vitamin B Complex 100 Injection (Hyrex)

Vitamin B Complex 100 Injection (McGuff)

Vitamin B Complex 100 Injection (Torrance)

Vitamin B Complex 100 Injection (Truxton)

Vitamin B Complex Capsules (Rugby)

Vitamin B Complex w/ Vitamin C & B12 Injection (McGuff)

Vitamin B-100 Natural Tablets (Cardinal)

Vitaplex Tablets (Amide)

Vitaplex Tablets (Medirex)

VITAMIN E **505**

Alph-E Capsules (Key Company)

Alph-E-Mixed Capsules (Key Company)

Alpha-E Capsules (Advanced Nutritional)

Aquasol E Liquid (AstraZeneca LP)

Aquavit-E Liquid (Cypress)

Born Again Vitamin E Oil (Alvin Last)

DL-Alpha Tocopheryl E400 Capsules (Mason)

E-400-Mixed Capsules (Bio-Tech)

E-Max-1000 Capsules (Bio-Tech)

E-Pherol Tablets (Vitaline)

E100 Capsules (Nature's Bounty)

E200 Capsules (Nature's Bounty)

E200 Mixed Capsules (Rexall Consumer)

E400 Capsules (Nature's Bounty)

E400 Mixed Capsules (Rexall Consumer)

E400 Natural Capsules (Rexall Consumer)

E1000 Capsules (Nature's Bounty)

E1000 D-Alpha Capsules (Mason)

E1000 Mixed Capsules (Rexall Consumer)

Formula E 400 Capsules (Miller Pharmacal)

Liquid E Liquid (Freeda)

Nutr-E-Sol Capsules (Advanced Nutritional)

Nutr-E-Sol Liquid (Advanced Nutritional)

Total E-400 Capsules (Westlake)

Vitamin E Aqueous Liquid (Boca Pharmacal)

Vitamin E Aqueous Liquid (Silarx)

Vitamin E D-Alpha Capsules (Mason)

Vitamin E DL Alpha Capsules (Health Products)

Vitamin E DL-Alpha Capsules (Mason)

Vitamin E MTC Capsules (National Vitamin)

Vitamin E Mixed Capsules (Mason)

Vitamin E Mixed Tablets (Freeda)

Vitamin E Mixed Tocopherols Capsules (Swanson)

Vitamin E Natural Blend Capsules (Medicine Shoppe)

Vitamin E Natural Blend Capsules (Perrigo)

Vitamin E Natural Capsules (Basic Vitamins)

Vitamin E Natural Capsules (Bergen Brunswig)

Vitamin E Natural Capsules (Cardinal)

Vitamin E Natural Capsules (Dixon-Shane)

Vitamin E Natural Capsules (McKesson)

Vitamin E Natural Liquid (Geritrex)

Vitamin E Water Soluble Capsules (National Vitamin)

Vitamin E400 D Alpha Capsules (National Vitamin)

Vitamin E400 D-Alpha Capsules (Perrigo)

Vitamin E800 D-Alpha Capsules (Pharmavite)

DIARRHEA

May result from the use of acarbose, ACE inhibitors, alprazolam, beta blockers, cardiac glycosides, chemotherapeutic agents, colchicine, diuretics, divalproex sodium, ethosuximide, fluoxetine hydrochloride, guanethidine monosulfate, hydralazine hydrochloride, levodopa, lithium carbonate, lithium citrate, magnesium-containing antacids, mesna, metformin hydrochloride, misoprostol, nonsteroidal anti-inflammatory drugs, olsalazine sodium, pancrelipase, potassium supplements, procainamide hydrochloride, reserpine, succimer, ticlopidine hydrochloride or valproic acid. The following products may be recommended:

PECTIN **348**

Modified Citrus Pectin Power Capsules (Nature's Herbs)

PROBIOTICS **377**

Acidophilus Lactocacilli w/ Pectin Capsules (Source)

Lacto Brev Capsules (Source)

Life Flora Capsules (Source)

Longest Living Acidophilus Capsules (Freelife)

NutraFlora Tablets (Source)

♦ Probiata Tablets (Wakunaga) **G-6**

PSYLLIUM **384**

Colon Care Formula Psyllium Seed Capsules (Yerba Prima)

Fiberall Powder (Novartis Consumer)

Fiberall Wafers (Novartis Consumer)

Fibro-XI Capsules (Key Company)

Genfiber Powder (Zenith Goldline)

Hydrocil Powder (Numark)

Konsyl Powder (Konsyl)

Konsyl-D Powder (Konsyl)

♦ Metamucil Powder and Wafers (Procter & Gamble) **G-5**

Modane Bulk Powder (Savage)

♦ Perdiem Granules (Novartis Consumer) **G-5**

Psyllium Husks 100% Pure Powder (Yerba Prima)

Reguloid Powder (Carlson)

Reguloid Powder (Rugby)

Serutan Granules (Twinlab)

SYNBIOTICS **441**

ZINC **534**

Cold-Eeze Lozenges (Quigley)

Ken-Zinc Lozenges (Kenyon Drug)

Krebs Ionized Zinc Tablets (PhytoPharmica)

M2 Zinc 50 Capsules (Miller Pharmacal)

Thera-Zinc Lozenges (Natrol)

Zinc Natural Tablets (Cardinal)

Zinc Preferred Capsules (Reese)

Zinc-15 Tablets (Key Company)

Zinc-50 Tablets (Key Company)

Zinc-Ease Lozenges (Republic)

Zincolate Capsules (Bio-Tech)

Zinimin Tablets (Key Company)

Zn Plus Protein Tablets (Miller Pharmacal)

Zn-50 Tablets (Bio-Tech)

DIARRHEA, INFECTIOUS

May be treated with ciprofloxacin, furazolidone or sulfamethoxazole-trimethoprim. The following products may be recommended for relief of symptoms:

PROBIOTICS **377**

Acidophilus Lactocacilli w/ Pectin Capsules (Source)

Lacto Brev Capsules (Source)

Life Flora Capsules (Source)

Longest Living Acidophilus Capsules (Freelife)

NutraFlora Tablets (Source)

♦ Probiata Tablets (Wakunaga) **G-6**

SYNBIOTICS **441**

YOGURT **532**

GASTRITIS, IRON-DEFICIENCY SECONDARY TO

Gastritis may be treated with histamine H_2 receptor antagonists, proton pump inhibitors or sucralfate. The following products may be recommended for relief of iron deficiency:

IRON **234**

Dexferrum Injection (American Regent)

Ed-In-Sol Elixir (Edwards)

Fe-40 Tablets (Bio-Tech)

♦ Feosol Caplets (SmithKline Beecham) **G-5**

♦ Feosol Elixir (SmithKline Beecham) **G-5**

♦ Feosol Tablets (SmithKline Beecham) **G-5**

Feostat Chewable Tablets (Forest)

Feostat Suspension (Forest)

Fer-Gen-Sol Liquid (Zenith Goldline)

Fer-In-Sol Liquid (Mead Johnson)

Fer-Iron Liquid (Rugby)

Feratab Tablets (Upsher-Smith)

♦ Fergon Tablets (Bayer) **G-3**

Feronate Tablets (Prime Marketing)

Ferosul Tablets (Major Pharmaceuticals)

Ferretts Tablets (Pharmics)

Ferro-Caps Capsules (Nature's Bounty)

Ferro-Time Capsules (Time-Cap)

Ferrous Sulfate T.D. Capsules (American Pharmacal)

Ferrousal Tablets (Prime
Marketing)

Gentle Iron Capsules
(Solgar)

Infed Injection (Schein)

Ircon Tablets (Kenwood)

Iron Sol Elixir (Halsey)

Mol-Iron Tablets (Schering-
Plough)

Nephro-Fer Tablets (R&D)

Ridosol Tablets (R.I.D.)

Siderol Pediatric Tablets
(Marin)

♦ Slow Fe Tablets (Novartis
Consumer) G-5

Slow Release Iron Tablets
(Cardinal)

Vitedyn-Slo Capsules
(Edyn)

Yieronia Elixir (R.I.D.)

Yierro-Gota Liquid (R.I.D.)

IRON COMBINATION PRODUCTS ... *546t*

Anemagen Capsules
(Ethex)

Anemagen FA Capsules
(Ethex)

Chromagen Capsules
(Savage)

Chromagen FA Tablets
(Savage)

Chromagen Forte Capsules
(Savage)

Conison Capsules (Ethex)

Contrin Capsules (Geneva)

DSS w/Iron Extended
Release Capsules
(American Pharmacal)

Daily Multiple Vitamins/
Iron Tablets (Vanguard)

Ed Cyte F Tablets
(Edwards)

Equi-Cyte F Tablets
(Equipharm)

Fe-Tinic 150 Forte
Capsules (Ethex)

Fero-Folic 500 Extended
Release Tablets (Abbott)

Fero-Grad-500 Extended
Release Tablets (Abbott)

Ferocon Capsules
(Breckenridge)

Ferotrinsic Capsules
(Contract Pharmacal)

Ferragen Capsules (Pecos)

Ferrex 150 Forte Capsules
(Breckenridge)

Ferro-Sequels Extended
Release Tablets
(Inverness)

Ferrous Fumarate DS
Extended Release
Capsules (Vita-Rx)

Fetrin Extended Release
Capsules (Lunsco)

Foltrin Capsules (Eon)

Fumatinic Extended
Release Capsules (Laser)

Hematin-F Tablets
(Cypress)

Hemocyte-F Tablets (U.S.
Pharmaceutical)

Iberet-Folic-500 Extended
Release Tablets (Abbott)

Icar-C Plus Tablets
(Hawthorn)

Icar-C Tablets (Hawthorn)

Infed Injection (Schein)

Ircon-FA Tablets
(Kenwood)

Irofol Tablets (Dayton)

Iron Advanced Tablets
(Rexall Consumer)

Iron w/Docusate Sodium
Extended Release Tablets
(Nature's Bounty)

Iron-Folic 500 Tablets
(Major Pharmaceuticals)

Martinic Capsules (Marlop)

Multi-Ferrous Folic
Extended Release Tablets
(United Research)

Multi-Vitamin w/Iron
Children's Liquid (Tri-
Med)

Multiret Folic-500
Extended Release Tablets
(Amide)

Multivitamins w/Iron
Children's Chewable
Tablets (Cardinal)

Myferon 150 Forte
Capsules (Me
Pharmaceuticals)

Nephro-Fer Rx Tablets
(R&D)

Nephro-Vite + FE Tablets
(R&D)

Nephron FA Tablets
(Nephro-Tech)

Niferex-150 Forte Capsules
(Schwarz)

Nu-Iron Plus Elixir (Merz)

Nutrinate Chewable Tablets
(Ethex)

One Tablet Daily w/Iron
Tablets (Zenith Goldline)

Prenafort Tablets (Cypress)

Promar Capsules (Marlop)

♦ Slow Fe w/Folic Acid
Extended Release Tablets
(Novartis Consumer) G-3

Stress Formula + Iron
Tablets (Cardinal)

Thera Hematinic Tablets
(Dixon-Shane)

Theragran Hematinic
Tablets (Apothecon)

Tolfrinic Tablets (Ascher)

Trinsicon Capsules
(Marlex)

Vitamins w/Iron Children's
Chewable Tablets
(Marlex)

Vitelle Irospan Extended
Release Tablets and
Extended Release
Capsules (Fielding)

Vitron-C Plus Tablets
(Novartis Consumer)

Vitron-C Tablets (Novartis
Consumer)

GASTROESOPHAGEAL REFLUX DISEASE

May be treated with histamine H_2
receptor antagonists, proton pump
inhibitors or sucralfate. The
following products may be
recommended for relief of
symptoms:

**SODIUM ALGINATES AND OTHER PHYCO-
POLYSACCHARIDES** **425**

HUMAN IMMUNODEFICIENCY VIRUS (HIV) INFECTIONS, NUTRIENTS DEFICIENCY SECONDARY TO

HIV infections may be treated with non-nucleoside reverse transcriptase inhibitors, nucleoside reverse transcriptase inhibitors or protease inhibitors. The following products may be recommended for relief of nutrients deficiency:

GLUTATHIONE **191**

MULTIVITAMIN PRODUCTS **550t**

BEC w/Zinc Tablets (Bergen Brunswig)

◆ Bugs Bunny Plus Extra C Chewable Tablets (Bayer) . . **G-3**

◆ Bugs Bunny Plus Iron Chewable Tablets (Bayer) . . **G-3**

Cardiotek Tablets (Stewart-Jackson)

Cefol Tablets (Abbott Hospital)

Circus Chews Children's Chewable Tablets (Rexall Consumer)

Daily Multiple Vitamins Tablets (Marlex)

Daily Multiple Vitamins Tablets (Rexall Consumer)

Daily Multiple Vitamins w/ Iron Tablets (Rexall Consumer)

Daily Multivitamins Tablets (Sky)

◆ Flintstones Original Children's Chewable Tablets (Bayer) **G-3**

◆ Flintstones Plus Calcium Chewable Tablets (Bayer) . . **G-3**

◆ Flintstones Plus Extra C Chewable Tablets (Bayer) . . **G-3**

◆ Flintstones Plus Iron Chewable Tablets (Bayer) . . **G-3**

Key-Plex Injection (Hyrex)

M.V.I. Pediatric Powder for Injection (AstraZeneca LP)

M.V.I.-12 Injection (AstraZeneca LP)

Multi-Vitamins Tablets (Rugby)

Multivitamin Capsules (Numark)

Once Daily Tablets (Prime Marketing)

◆ One-A-Day Essential Tablets (Bayer) **G-3**

Poly Vitamin Chewable Tablets (Rugby)

Stress Formula Plus Zinc Tablets (Rexall Consumer)

Stress Formula Tablets (Cardinal)

Stress Formula Tablets (Rexall Consumer)

Therapeutic Multivitamin Tablets (Bergen Brunswig)

Ultra Tabs Tablets (Major Pharmaceuticals)

Vitamins Children's Chewable Tablets (Prime Marketing)

MULTIVITAMIN AND MINERAL PRODUCTS **553t**

◆ Alpha Betic Tablets (Abkit) **G-3**

B-C w/Folic Acid Plus Tablet (Geneva)

B-Complex Plus Tablets (United Research)

B-Complex Vitamins Plus Tablets (Teva)

B-Plex Plus Tablets (Zenith Goldline)

Bacmin Tablets (Marnel)

Becomax RX Tablets (Ampharco)

Berocca Plus Tablets (Roche)

◆ Bugs Bunny Complete Children's Chewable Tablets (Bayer) **G-3**

Cerovite Senior Tablets (Rugby)

Circavite T Tablets (Circle)

Clusinex Syrup (Pharmakon)

Daily Multiple Vitamins/ Minerals Tablets (Vanguard)

Dr. Art Ulene's Vitamin Formula Packets (Feeling Fine)

Equi-Roca Plus Tablets (Equipharm)

Ferrex PC Tablets (Breckenridge)

◆ Flintstones Complete Children's Chewable Tablets (Bayer) **G-3**

Formula B Plus Tablets (Major Pharmaceuticals)

Glutofac-ZX Capsules (Kenwood)

Hematin Plus Tablets (Cypress)

Iromin-G Tablets (Mission)

Manly Machovites Tablets (Neurovites)

Mega-Multi Capsules (Innovative Health)

Niferex-PN Tablets (Schwarz)

O-Cal FA Tablets (Pharmics)

◆ One-A-Day 50 Plus Tablets (Bayer) **G-3**

◆ One-A-Day Antioxidant Capsules (Bayer) **G-3**

◆ One-A-Day Kids Complete Chewable Tablets (Bayer) . . **G-3**

◆ One-A-Day Maximum Tablets (Bayer) **G-3**

◆ One-A-Day Men's Tablets (Bayer) **G-3**

◆ One-A-Day Women's Tablets (Bayer) **G-3**

PMS Formula Tablets (Neurovites)

Poly Vitamin w/Iron Chewable Tablets (Rugby)

Protect Plus Capsules (Gil)

Protect Plus Liquid (Gil)

Strovite Forte Tablets (Everett)

Sunvite Platinum Tablets (Rexall Consumer)

Sunvite Tablets (Rexall Consumer)

Super Plenamins Extra
 Strength Tablets (Rexall
 Consumer)
Super Plenamins Tablets
 (Rexall Consumer)
Support 500 Capsules
 (Marin)
Support Liquid (Marin)
Thera Vite M Tablets
 (PDK)
Thera-M w/Minerals
 Tablets (Prime
 Marketing)
♦ Theragran-M Tablets
 (Bristol-Myers Products) **G-3**
Therapeutic Plus Vitamin
 Tablets (Rugby)
Therobec Plus Tablets
 (Qualitest)
Total Formula Original
 Tablets (Vitaline)
V-C Forte Capsules
 (Breckenridge)
Vicap Forte Tablets (Major
 Pharmaceuticals)
Vicon Forte Tablets (UCB)
Vita-Min Rx Tablets (Bio-
 Tech)
Vitacon Forte Tablets
 (Amide)
Vitaplex Plus Tablets
 (Amide)
Vitelle Nesentials Tablets
 (Fielding)

THIAMIN **445**
VITAMIN B COMPLEX PRODUCTS .. **558t**
B-50 Complex Tablets
 (Rexall Consumer)
B-100 Complex Tablets
 (Rexall Consumer)
B-Ject-100 Injection
 (Hyrex)
B-Plex Tablets (Contract
 Pharmacal)
B-Plex Tablets (Zenith
 Goldline)
Berocca Tablets (Roche)
Dialyvite Tablets
 (Hillestad)
Formula B Tablets (Major
 Pharmaceuticals)

Marlbee w/C Capsules
 (Marlex)
Nephplex Rx Tablets
 (Nephro-Tech)
Nephro-Vite Rx Tablets
 (R&D)
Nephrocaps Capsules
 (Fleming)
Primaplex Injection
 (Primedics)
Stress B Complex with
 Vitamin C Tablets
 (Mission)
Strovite Tablets (Everett)
Therobec Tablets
 (Qualitest)
Thex Forte Tablets (Lee)
Vicam Injection (Keene)
Vita-Bee w/C Tablets
 (Rugby)
Vitamin B Complex 100
 Injection (Hyrex)
Vitamin B Complex 100
 Injection (McGuff)
Vitamin B Complex 100
 Injection (Torrance)
Vitamin B Complex 100
 Injection (Truxton)
Vitamin B Complex
 Capsules (Rugby)
Vitamin B Complex w/
 Vitamin C & B12
 Injection (McGuff)
Vitamin B-100 Natural
 Tablets (Cardinal)
Vitaplex Tablets (Amide)
Vitaplex Tablets (Medirex)

HYPERTHYROIDISM, NUTRIENTS DEFICIENCY SECONDARY TO

Hyperthyroidism may be treated
with methimazole. The following
products may be recommended for
relief of nutrients deficiency:

IODINE **228**
Kelp Natural Iodine Tablets
 (Apothecary)
Kelp-Tabs (Key Company)
MULTIVITAMIN PRODUCTS **550t**
BEC w/Zinc Tablets
 (Bergen Brunswig)
♦ Bugs Bunny Plus Extra C
 Chewable Tablets (Bayer) .. **G-3**

♦ Bugs Bunny Plus Iron
 Chewable Tablets (Bayer) .. **G-3**
Cardiotek Tablets (Stewart-
 Jackson)
Cefol Tablets (Abbott
 Hospital)
Circus Chews Children's
 Chewable Tablets (Rexall
 Consumer)
Daily Multiple Vitamins
 Tablets (Marlex)
Daily Multiple Vitamins
 Tablets (Rexall
 Consumer)
Daily Multiple Vitamins w/
 Iron Tablets (Rexall
 Consumer)
Daily Multivitamins Tablets
 (Sky)
♦ Flintstones Original
 Children's Chewable
 Tablets (Bayer) **G-3**
♦ Flintstones Plus Calcium
 Chewable Tablets (Bayer) .. **G-3**
♦ Flintstones Plus Extra C
 Chewable Tablets (Bayer) .. **G-3**
♦ Flintstones Plus Iron
 Chewable Tablets (Bayer) .. **G-3**
Key-Plex Injection (Hyrex)
M.V.I. Pediatric Powder for
 Injection (AstraZeneca LP)
M.V.I.-12 Injection
 (AstraZeneca LP)
Multi-Vitamins Tablets
 (Rugby)
Multivitamin Capsules
 (Numark)
Once Daily Tablets (Prime
 Marketing)
♦ One-A-Day Essential
 Tablets (Bayer) **G-3**
Poly Vitamin Chewable
 Tablets (Rugby)
Stress Formula Plus Zinc
 Tablets (Rexall
 Consumer)
Stress Formula Tablets
 (Cardinal)
Stress Formula Tablets
 (Rexall Consumer)

Therapeutic Multivitamin
  Tablets (Bergen
  Brunswig)
Ultra Tabs Tablets (Major
  Pharmaceuticals)
Vitamins Children's
  Chewable Tablets (Prime
  Marketing)

**MULTIVITAMIN AND MINERAL
PRODUCTS** *553t*

♦ Alpha Betic Tablets
  (Abkit) **G-3**
B-C w/Folic Acid Plus
  Tablet (Geneva)
B-Complex Plus Tablets
  (United Research)
B-Complex Vitamins Plus
  Tablets (Teva)
B-Plex Plus Tablets (Zenith
  Goldline)
Bacmin Tablets (Marnel)
Becomax RX Tablets
  (Ampharco)
Berocca Plus Tablets
  (Roche)
♦ Bugs Bunny Complete
  Children's Chewable
  Tablets (Bayer) **G-3**
Cerovite Senior Tablets
  (Rugby)
Circavite T Tablets (Circle)
Clusinex Syrup
  (Pharmakon)
Daily Multiple Vitamins/
  Minerals Tablets
  (Vanguard)
Dr. Art Ulene's Vitamin
  Formula Packets (Feeling
  Fine)
Equi-Roca Plus Tablets
  (Equipharm)
Ferrex PC Tablets
  (Breckenridge)
♦ Flintstones Complete
  Children's Chewable
  Tablets (Bayer) **G-3**
Formula B Plus Tablets
  (Major Pharmaceuticals)
Glutofac-ZX Capsules
  (Kenwood)
Hematin Plus Tablets
  (Cypress)
Iromin-G Tablets (Mission)

Manly Machovites Tablets
  (Neurovites)
Mega-Multi Capsules
  (Innovative Health)
Niferex-PN Tablets
  (Schwarz)
O-Cal FA Tablets
  (Pharmics)
♦ One-A-Day 50 Plus Tablets
  (Bayer) **G-3**
♦ One-A-Day Antioxidant
  Capsules (Bayer) **G-3**
♦ One-A-Day Kids Complete
  Chewable Tablets (Bayer) .. **G-3**
♦ One-A-Day Maximum
  Tablets (Bayer) **G-3**
♦ One-A-Day Men's Tablets
  (Bayer) **G-3**
♦ One-A-Day Women's
  Tablets (Bayer) **G-3**
PMS Formula Tablets
  (Neurovites)
Poly Vitamin w/Iron
  Chewable Tablets
  (Rugby)
Protect Plus Capsules (Gil)
Protect Plus Liquid (Gil)
Strovite Forte Tablets
  (Everett)
Sunvite Platinum Tablets
  (Rexall Consumer)
Sunvite Tablets (Rexall
  Consumer)
Super Plenamins Extra
  Strength Tablets (Rexall
  Consumer)
Super Plenamins Tablets
  (Rexall Consumer)
Support 500 Capsules
  (Marin)
Support Liquid (Marin)
Thera Vite M Tablets
  (PDK)
Thera-M w/Minerals
  Tablets (Prime
  Marketing)
♦ Theragran-M Tablets
  (Bristol-Myers Products) **G-3**
Therapeutic Plus Vitamin
  Tablets (Rugby)
Therobec Plus Tablets
  (Qualitest)

Total Formula Original
  Tablets (Vitaline)
V-C Forte Capsules
  (Breckenridge)
Vicap Forte Tablets (Major
  Pharmaceuticals)
Vicon Forte Tablets (UCB)
Vita-Min Rx Tablets (Bio-
  Tech)
Vitacon Forte Tablets
  (Amide)
Vitaplex Plus Tablets
  (Amide)
Vitelle Nesentials Tablets
  (Fielding)

VITAMIN B COMPLEX PRODUCTS ... *558t*

B-50 Complex Tablets
  (Rexall Consumer)
B-100 Complex Tablets
  (Rexall Consumer)
B-Ject-100 Injection
  (Hyrex)
B-Plex Tablets (Contract
  Pharmacal)
B-Plex Tablets (Zenith
  Goldline)
Berocca Tablets (Roche)
Dialyvite Tablets
  (Hillestad)
Formula B Tablets (Major
  Pharmaceuticals)
Marlbee w/C Capsules
  (Marlex)
Nephplex Rx Tablets
  (Nephro-Tech)
Nephro-Vite Rx Tablets
  (R&D)
Nephrocaps Capsules
  (Fleming)
Primaplex Injection
  (Primedics)
Stress B Complex with
  Vitamin C Tablets
  (Mission)
Strovite Tablets (Everett)
Therobec Tablets
  (Qualitest)
Thex Forte Tablets (Lee)
Vicam Injection (Keene)
Vita-Bee w/C Tablets
  (Rugby)

Vitamin B Complex 100
Injection (Hyrex)

Vitamin B Complex 100
Injection (McGuff)

Vitamin B Complex 100
Injection (Torrance)

Vitamin B Complex 100
Injection (Truxton)

Vitamin B Complex
Capsules (Rugby)

Vitamin B Complex w/
Vitamin C & B12
Injection (McGuff)

Vitamin B-100 Natural
Tablets (Cardinal)

Vitaplex Tablets (Amide)

Vitaplex Tablets (Medirex)

HYPOKALEMIA

May result from the use of
aldesleukin, amphotericin B,
carboplatin, corticosteroids, diuretics,
etretinate, foscarnet sodium,
mycophenolate mofetil, pamidronate
disodium, tacrolimus, or thiazides.
The following products may be
recommended:

POTASSIUM **368**

HYPOMAGNESEMIA

May result from the use of
aldesleukin, aminoglycosides,
amphotericin B, caroboplatin,
cisplatin, cyclosporine, diuretics,
foscarnet, pamidronate, sargramostim
or tacrolimus. The following
products may be recommended:

MAGNESIUM **288**

Almora Tablets (Forest)

Chloromag Injection
(Merit)

Dewee's Carminative
Liquid (Humco)

Elite Magnesium Capsules
(Miller Pharmacal)

M2 Magnesium Capsules
(Miller Pharmacal)

Mag Delay Tablets (Major
Pharmaceuticals)

Mag-200 Tablets (Optimox)

Mag-Carb Capsules (R&D)

Mag-Gel 600 Capsules
(Cypress)

Mag-Ox 400 Tablets
(Blaine)

Mag-SR Tablets (Cypress)

Mag-Tab Sr Tablets
(Niche)

Magimin Tablets (Key
Company)

Magimin-Forte Tablets
(Key Company)

Maglex Tablets (Lex)

Magnacaps Capsules (Key
Company)

Magnesium Carbonate
Powder (Freeda)

Magnesium Elemental
Tablets (National
Vitamin)

Magnesium Oxide Tablets
(Cypress)

Magonate Liquid (Fleming)

Magonate Natal Liquid
(Fleming)

Magonate Tablets
(Fleming)

Magtrate Tablets (Mission)

Slow-Mag Tablets (Quality
Care)

Slow-Mag Tablets (Shire
U.S.)

Sulfa-Mag Injection (Merit)

Uro-Mag Capsules (Blaine)

HYPOPARATHYROIDISM

May be treated with vitamin D
sterols. The following products may
be recommended for relief of
symptoms:

CALCIUM **74**

Alcalak Chewable Tablets
(Textilease)

♦ Alka-Mints Chewable
Tablets (Bayer) **G-3**

Antacid Chewable Tablets
(Zenith Goldline)

Antacid Extra Strength
Chewable Tablets
(Cardinal)

Antacid Extra Strength
Chewable Tablets (Zenith
Goldline)

Antacid Extra Strength
Tablets (McKesson)

Antacid Ultra Strength
Chewable Tablets
(Bergen Brunswig)

Ascocid Tablets (Key
Company)

Cal-600 Tablets (PDK)

Cal-C-Caps Capsules (Key
Company)

Cal-Carb Forte Tablets
(Vitaline)

Cal-Carb Forte Wafers
(Vitaline)

Cal-Cee Tablets (Key
Company)

Cal-Citrate Capsules (Bio-
Tech)

Cal-Citrate Tablets (Bio-
Tech)

Cal-G Capsules (Key
Company)

Cal-Gest Chewable Tablets
(Rugby)

Cal-Glu Capsule (Bio-Tech)

Cal-Lac Capsules (Key
Company)

Cal-Lac Tablets (Bio-Tech)

Cal-Mint Tablets (Freeda)

Calbon Tablets (Economed)

Calcarb 600 Tablets
(Zenith Goldline)

Calci-Chew Tablets (R&D)

Calci-Mix Capsules (R&D)

Calcimin-300 Tablets (Key
Company)

Calcio Del Mar Tablets
(Marlop)

Calcionate Syrup (Hi-Tech)

Calcionate Syrup (Rugby)

Calciquid Syrup
(Breckenridge)

Calciquid Syrup (Econolab)

Calcium 500 Chewable
Tablets (Mason)

Calcium 500 Chewable
Tablets (National
Vitamin)

Calcium 500 Supplement
Chewable Tablets
(Bergen Brunswig)

Calcium 600 Capsules
(McKesson)

Calcium 600 Tablets (Basic
 Vitamins)
Calcium 600 Tablets
 (Nature's Bounty)
Calcium 600 Tablets
 (Prime Marketing)
Calcium 600 Tablets
 (Rugby)
Calcium Antacid Chewable
 Tablets (Mason)
Calcium Antacid Chewable
 Tablets (Perrigo)
Calcium Antacid Extra
 Strength Chewable
 Tablets (Major
 Pharmaceuticals)
Calcium Antacid Extra
 Strength Chewable
 Tablets (Medicine
 Shoppe)
Calcium Antacid Extra
 Strength Tablets (Perrigo)
Calcium Antacid Ultra
 Strength Chewable
 Tablets (Major
 Pharmaceuticals)
Calcium Antacid Ultra
 Strength Chewable
 Tablets (Perrigo)
Calcium Citrate 950
 Tablets (Basic Vitamins)
Calcium-600 Tablets (Key
 Company)
Calfort Tablets (Ampharco)
Calphron Powder (Nephro-
 Tech)
Caltrate 600 Tablets
 (Lederle)
Chooz Tablets (Heritage
 Consumer)
Citracal Economy Tablets
 (Mission)
Citracal Tablets (Mission)
Desempacho Tablets
 (D'Franssia)
Krebs Ionized Calcium
 Tablets (PhytoPharmica)
Life-Line Co-Co Bear
 Chewable Tablets
 (National Vitamin)
Liqui-Cal Chewable Tablets
 (Advanced Nutritional)

M2 Calcium Tablets
 (Miller Pharmacal)
Mallamint Chewable
 Tablets (Textilease)
Mylanta Calci Tabs Extra
 Strength (J&J • Merck)
Mylanta Calci Tabs Ultra
 Chewable Tablets (J&J •
 Merck)
Mylanta Children's
 Chewable Tablets (J&J •
 Merck)
Neo-Calglucon Syrup
 (Novartis
 Pharmaceuticals)
Nephro-Calci Tablets
 (R&D)
Nutralox Chewable Tablets
 (Hart Health)
♦ Os-Cal 500 Chewable
 Tablets (SmithKline
 Beecham) G-5
♦ Os-Cal 500 Tablets
 (SmithKline Beecham) G-5
Oysco 500 Tablets (Rugby)
Oyst-Cal 500 Tablets
 (Zenith Goldline)
Oyster Shell Calcium 500
 Tablets (Medicine
 Shoppe)
Oyster Shell Calcium
 Natural Tablets
 (Cardinal)
Phoslo Tablets (Braintree)
Prelief Granules (AK
 Pharma)
Prelief Tablets (AK
 Pharma)
Revelation Powder (Alvin
 Last)
Ridactate Tablets (R.I.D.)
Rolaids Chewable Tablets
 (American Chicle)
Super Calcium Extra
 Strength Chewable
 Tablets (Mason)
Super Calcium Tablets
 (Mason)
Titralac Chewable Tablets
 (3M)
Titralac Extra Strength
 Chewable Tablets (3M)

Tums 500 Chewable
 Tablets (SmithKline
 Beecham)
♦ Tums Chewable Tablets
 (SmithKline Beecham) G-5
♦ Tums E-X Chewable
 Tablets (SmithKline
 Beecham) G-5
♦ Tums Ultra Chewable
 Tablets (SmithKline
 Beecham) G-5
Vitamin C Buffered Tablets
 (Nature's Bounty)

**CALCIUM COMBINATION
PRODUCTS** *543t*
♦ AdvaCal Capsules (Lane
 Labs) G-4
Cal-600 w/Vitamin D
 Tablets (PDK)
Cal-Co3Y Capsules (Bio-
 Tech)
Cal/Mag Chelated Tablets
 (Freeda)
Cal/Mag Chewable Tablets
 (Freeda)
Calcarb 600 w/Vitamin D
 Tablets (Zenith Goldline)
Calcet Tablets (Mission)
Calcium & Magnesium
 Chelate Capsules (Key
 Company)
Calcium 500 w/Vitamin D
 Tablets (Basic Vitamins)
Calcium 500 w/Vitamin D
 Tablets (Mason)
Calcium 500 w/Vitamin D
 Tablets (Rexall
 Consumer)
Calcium 600 + Vitamin D
 Tablets (Perrigo)
Calcium 600 Plus Vitamin
 D Tablets (Nature's
 Bounty)
Calcium 600-D Tablets
 (Rugby)
Calcium 600/Vitamin D
 Tablets (Basic Vitamins)
Calcium 600/Vitamin D
 Tablets (Bergen
 Brunswig)
Calcium 600/Vitamin D
 Tablets (Cardinal)

Calcium 900 w/Vitamin D Capsules (Rexall Consumer)

Calcium 1200 w/Vitamin D Capsules (Rexall Consumer)

Calcium Carbonate/Vitamin D Tablets (Compumed)

Calcium Carbonate/Vitamin D Tablets (Heartland)

Calcium Carbonate/Vitamin D Tablets (Major Pharmaceuticals)

Calcium Carbonate/Vitamin D Tablets (National Vitamin)

Calcium Carbonate/Vitamin D Tablets (PD-Rx)

Calcium Carbonate/Vitamin D Tablets (Sky)

Calcium Citrate + D Tablets (Cardinal)

Calcium Citrate w/Vitamin D Tablets (Mason)

Calcium Citrate/Vitamin D Tablets (Bergen Brunswig)

Calcium-600 w/D Tablets (American Pharmacal)

Calcium/Magnesium/Zinc Tablets (Cardinal)

Calcium/Magnesium/Zinc Tablets (Rexall Consumer)

Calcium/Vitamin D Tablets (McKesson)

Calcium/Vitamin D Tablets (PD-Rx)

Calcium/Vitamin D Tablets (Vanguard)

Caltrate 600 + D Tablets (Lederle)

Citracal + D Tablets (Mission)

Citrus Calcium + D Tablets (Rugby)

Daily Calcium + Vitamin D Tablets (Nature's Bounty)

Ferosul Tablets (Major Pharmaceuticals)

Florical Capsules (Mericon)

Florical Tablets (Mericon)

Healthy Woman Bone Health Supplement Tablets (Personal Products Company)

Liqua-Cal Capsules (Key Company)

Liquid Calcium Capsules (Major Pharmaceuticals)

Liquid Calcium Plus Vitamin D Capsules (Mason)

Magnebind 200 Tablets (Nephro-Tech)

Magnebind 300 Tablets (Nephro-Tech)

Magnebind 400 Rx Tablets (Nephro-Tech)

Marblen Suspension (Fleming)

Marblen Tablets (Fleming)

Monocal Tablets (Mericon)

One-A-Day Bone Strength Tablets (Bayer)

♦ One-A-Day Calcium Plus Chewable Tablets (Bayer) .. G-3

♦ Os-Cal 250 + D Tablets (SmithKline Beecham) G-5

♦ Os-Cal 500 + D Tablets (SmithKline Beecham) G-5

Oysco 500 + D Tablets (Rugby)

Oysco D Tablets (Rugby)

Oyst-Cal-D 500 Tablets (Zenith Goldline)

Oyst-Cal-D Tablets (Zenith Goldline)

Oyster Shell Calcium 500 w/D Tablets (Medicine Shoppe)

Oyster Shell Calcium 1000/ Vitamin D Tablets (Mason)

Oyster Shell Calcium 1000/ Vitamin D Tablets (Rexall Consumer)

Oyster Shell Calcium Natural/Vit D Tablets (Cardinal)

Oyster Shell Calcium/ Vitamin D Tablets (American Pharmacal)

Oyster Shell Calcium/ Vitamin D Tablets (Basic Vitamins)

Oyster Shell Calcium/ Vitamin D Tablets (Bergen Brunswig)

Oyster Shell Calcium/ Vitamin D Tablets (Dixon-Shane)

Oyster Shell Calcium/ Vitamin D Tablets (Major Pharmaceuticals)

Oyster Shell Calcium/ Vitamin D Tablets (Mason)

Oyster Shell Calcium/ Vitamin D Tablets (McKesson)

Oyster Shell Calcium/ Vitamin D Tablets (National Vitamin)

Oyster Shell Calcium/ Vitamin D Tablets (Perrigo)

Oyster Shell Calcium/ Vitamin D Tablets (Reese)

Oyster Shell Calcium/ Vitamin D Tablets (Rexall Consumer)

Oyster Shell Calcium/ Vitamin D Tablets (Vanguard)

Oystercal-D 250 Tablets (Nature's Bounty)

Oystercal-D 500 Tablets (Nature's Bounty)

Parva-Cal 250 Tablets (Freeda)

Super Calcium w/Vitamin D Tablets (Mason)

Viactiv Chewable Tablets (Mead Johnson)

Vita-Calcium Wafers (Vitaline)

VITAMIN D 498

HYPOTHYROIDISM, CONSTIPATION SECONDARY TO

Hypothyroidism may be treated with thyroid hormones. The following products may be recommended for relief of constipation:

LACTULOSE **243**
Cephulac Syrup (Aventis)
Cholac Syrup (Alra)
Chronulac Syrup (Aventis)
Constilac Syrup (Alra)
Constulose Solution
(Alpharma)
Duphalac Syrup (Solvay)
Enulose Solution
(Alpharma)
PECTIN **348**
Modified Citrus Pectin
Power Capsules (Nature's
Herbs)
PREBIOTICS **372**
PSYLLIUM **384**
Colon Care Formula
Psyllium Seed Capsules
(Yerba Prima)
Fiberall Powder (Novartis
Consumer)
Fiberall Wafers (Novartis
Consumer)
Fibro-XI Capsules (Key
Company)
Genfiber Powder (Zenith
Goldline)
Hydrocil Powder (Numark)
Konsyl Powder (Konsyl)
Konsyl-D Powder (Konsyl)
♦ Metamucil Powder and
Wafers (Procter &
Gamble) **G-5**
Modane Bulk Powder
(Savage)
♦ Perdiem Granules (Novartis
Consumer) **G-5**
Psyllium Husks 100% Pure
Powder (Yerba Prima)
Reguloid Powder (Carlson)
Reguloid Powder (Rugby)
Serutan Granules (Twinlab)

INFECTIONS, BACTERIAL, UPPER RESPIRATORY TRACT

May be treated with amoxicillin
trihydrate, amoxicillin-clavulanate,
cephalosporins, doxycycline,
erythromycin, macrolide antibiotics,
minocycline hydrochloride or
penicillins. The following products
may be recommended for relief of
symptoms:

BROMELAIN **70**
Bromanase Tablets
(Kramer-Novis)
Bromelain 2400 Maximum
Strength Tablets
(Vitaline)

IRRITABLE BOWEL SYNDROME

May be treated with anticholinergic
combinations, dicyclomine
hydrochloride or hyoscyamine
sulfate. The following products may
be recommended for relief of
symptoms:

PSYLLIUM **384**
Colon Care Formula
Psyllium Seed Capsules
(Yerba Prima)
Fiberall Powder (Novartis
Consumer)
Fiberall Wafers (Novartis
Consumer)
Fibro-XI Capsules (Key
Company)
Genfiber Powder (Zenith
Goldline)
Hydrocil Powder (Numark)
Konsyl Powder (Konsyl)
Konsyl-D Powder (Konsyl)
♦ Metamucil Powder and
Wafers (Procter &
Gamble) **G-5**
Modane Bulk Powder
(Savage)
♦ Perdiem Granules (Novartis
Consumer) **G-5**
Psyllium Husks 100% Pure
Powder (Yerba Prima)
Reguloid Powder (Carlson)
Reguloid Powder (Rugby)
Serutan Granules (Twinlab)

ISCHEMIC HEART DISEASE

May be treated with beta blockers,
calcium channel blockers, isosorbide
dinitrate, isosorbide mononitrate or
nitroglycerin. The following
products may be recommended for
relief of symptoms:

L-CARNITINE **255**
♦ ProXeed Packets (Sigma-
Tau) **G-5**

NECATORIASIS, IRON-DEFICIENCY ANEMIA SECONDARY TO

Necatoriasis may be treated with
mebendazole or thiabendazole. The
following products may be
recommended for relief of iron-
deficiency anemia:

IRON **234**
Dexferrum Injection
(American Regent)
Ed-In-Sol Elixir (Edwards)
Fe-40 Tablets (Bio-Tech)
♦ Feosol Caplets (SmithKline
Beecham) **G-5**
♦ Feosol Elixir (SmithKline
Beecham) **G-5**
♦ Feosol Tablets (SmithKline
Beecham) **G-5**
Feostat Chewable Tablets
(Forest)
Feostat Suspension (Forest)
Fer-Gen-Sol Liquid (Zenith
Goldline)
Fer-In-Sol Liquid (Mead
Johnson)
Fer-Iron Liquid (Rugby)
Feratab Tablets (Upsher-
Smith)
♦ Fergon Tablets (Bayer) **G-3**
Feronate Tablets (Prime
Marketing)
Ferosul Tablets (Major
Pharmaceuticals)
Ferretts Tablets (Pharmics)
Ferro-Caps Capsules
(Nature's Bounty)
Ferro-Time Capsules
(Time-Cap)
Ferrous Sulfate T.D.
Capsules (American
Pharmacal)
Ferrousal Tablets (Prime
Marketing)
Gentle Iron Capsules
(Solgar)
Infed Injection (Schein)
Ircon Tablets (Kenwood)
Iron Sol Elixir (Halsey)
Mol-Iron Tablets (Schering-
Plough)
Nephro-Fer Tablets (R&D)
Ridosol Tablets (R.I.D.)

Siderol Pediatric Tablets
(Marin)
♦ Slow Fe Tablets (Novartis
Consumer) **G-5**
Slow Release Iron Tablets
(Cardinal)
Vitedyn-Slo Capsules
(Edyn)
Yieronia Elixir (R.I.D.)
Yierro-Gota Liquid (R.I.D.)

OSTEOPOROSIS

May be treated with bisphosphonates,
calcitonin or estrogens. The following
products may be recommended:

CALCIUM **74**

Alcalak Chewable Tablets
(Textilease)
♦ Alka-Mints Chewable
Tablets (Bayer) **G-3**
Antacid Chewable Tablets
(Zenith Goldline)
Antacid Extra Strength
Chewable Tablets
(Cardinal)
Antacid Extra Strength
Chewable Tablets (Zenith
Goldline)
Antacid Extra Strength
Tablets (McKesson)
Antacid Ultra Strength
Chewable Tablets
(Bergen Brunswig)
Ascocid Tablets (Key
Company)
Cal-600 Tablets (PDK)
Cal-C-Caps Capsules (Key
Company)
Cal-Carb Forte Tablets
(Vitaline)
Cal-Carb Forte Wafers
(Vitaline)
Cal-Cee Tablets (Key
Company)
Cal-Citrate Capsules (Bio-
Tech)
Cal-Citrate Tablets (Bio-
Tech)
Cal-G Capsules (Key
Company)
Cal-Gest Chewable Tablets
(Rugby)
Cal-Glu Capsule (Bio-Tech)

Cal-Lac Capsules (Key
Company)
Cal-Lac Tablets (Bio-Tech)
Cal-Mint Tablets (Freeda)
Calbon Tablets (Economed)
Calcarb 600 Tablets
(Zenith Goldline)
Calci-Chew Tablets (R&D)
Calci-Mix Capsules (R&D)
Calcimin-300 Tablets (Key
Company)
Calcio Del Mar Tablets
(Marlop)
Calcionate Syrup (Hi-Tech)
Calcionate Syrup (Rugby)
Calciquid Syrup
(Breckenridge)
Calciquid Syrup (Econolab)
Calcium 500 Chewable
Tablets (Mason)
Calcium 500 Chewable
Tablets (National
Vitamin)
Calcium 500 Supplement
Chewable Tablets
(Bergen Brunswig)
Calcium 600 Capsules
(McKesson)
Calcium 600 Tablets (Basic
Vitamins)
Calcium 600 Tablets
(Nature's Bounty)
Calcium 600 Tablets
(Prime Marketing)
Calcium 600 Tablets
(Rugby)
Calcium Antacid Chewable
Tablets (Mason)
Calcium Antacid Chewable
Tablets (Perrigo)
Calcium Antacid Extra
Strength Chewable
Tablets (Major
Pharmaceuticals)
Calcium Antacid Extra
Strength Chewable
Tablets (Medicine
Shoppe)
Calcium Antacid Extra
Strength Tablets (Perrigo)

Calcium Antacid Ultra
Strength Chewable
Tablets (Major
Pharmaceuticals)
Calcium Antacid Ultra
Strength Chewable
Tablets (Perrigo)
Calcium Citrate 950
Tablets (Basic Vitamins)
Calcium-600 Tablets (Key
Company)
Calfort Tablets (Ampharco)
Calphron Powder (Nephro-
Tech)
Caltrate 600 Tablets
(Lederle)
Chooz Tablets (Heritage
Consumer)
Citracal Economy Tablets
(Mission)
Citracal Tablets (Mission)
Desempacho Tablets
(D'Franssia)
Krebs Ionized Calcium
Tablets (PhytoPharmica)
Life-Line Co-Co Bear
Chewable Tablets
(National Vitamin)
Liqui-Cal Chewable Tablets
(Advanced Nutritional)
M2 Calcium Tablets
(Miller Pharmacal)
Mallamint Chewable
Tablets (Textilease)
Mylanta Calci Tabs Extra
Strength (J&J • Merck)
Mylanta Calci Tabs Ultra
Chewable Tablets (J&J •
Merck)
Mylanta Children's
Chewable Tablets (J&J •
Merck)
Neo-Calglucon Syrup
(Novartis
Pharmaceuticals)
Nephro-Calci Tablets
(R&D)
Nutralox Chewable Tablets
(Hart Health)
♦ Os-Cal 500 Chewable
Tablets (SmithKline
Beecham) **G-5**

♦ Os-Cal 500 Tablets
(SmithKline Beecham) **G-5**
Oysco 500 Tablets (Rugby)
Oyst-Cal 500 Tablets
(Zenith Goldline)
Oyster Shell Calcium 500
Tablets (Medicine
Shoppe)
Oyster Shell Calcium
Natural Tablets
(Cardinal)
Phoslo Tablets (Braintree)
Prelief Granules (AK
Pharma)
Prelief Tablets (AK
Pharma)
Revelation Powder (Alvin
Last)
Ridactate Tablets (R.I.D.)
Rolaids Chewable Tablets
(American Chicle)
Super Calcium Extra
Strength Chewable
Tablets (Mason)
Super Calcium Tablets
(Mason)
Titralac Chewable Tablets
(3M)
Titralac Extra Strength
Chewable Tablets (3M)
Tums 500 Chewable
Tablets (SmithKline
Beecham)
♦ Tums Chewable Tablets
(SmithKline Beecham) **G-5**
♦ Tums E-X Chewable
Tablets (SmithKline
Beecham) **G-5**
♦ Tums Ultra Chewable
Tablets (SmithKline
Beecham) **G-5**
Vitamin C Buffered Tablets
(Nature's Bounty)

**CALCIUM COMBINATION
PRODUCTS** **543t**
♦ AdvaCal Capsules (Lane
Labs) **G-4**
Cal-600 w/Vitamin D
Tablets (PDK)
Cal-Co3Y Capsules (Bio-
Tech)
Cal/Mag Chelated Tablets
(Freeda)

Cal/Mag Chewable Tablets
(Freeda)
Calcarb 600 w/Vitamin D
Tablets (Zenith Goldline)
Calcet Tablets (Mission)
Calcium & Magnesium
Chelate Capsules (Key
Company)
Calcium 500 w/Vitamin D
Tablets (Basic Vitamins)
Calcium 500 w/Vitamin D
Tablets (Mason)
Calcium 500 w/Vitamin D
Tablets (Rexall
Consumer)
Calcium 600 + Vitamin D
Tablets (Perrigo)
Calcium 600 Plus Vitamin
D Tablets (Nature's
Bounty)
Calcium 600-D Tablets
(Rugby)
Calcium 600/Vitamin D
Tablets (Basic Vitamins)
Calcium 600/Vitamin D
Tablets (Bergen
Brunswig)
Calcium 600/Vitamin D
Tablets (Cardinal)
Calcium 900 w/Vitamin D
Capsules (Rexall
Consumer)
Calcium 1200 w/Vitamin D
Capsules (Rexall
Consumer)
Calcium Carbonate/Vitamin
D Tablets (Compumed)
Calcium Carbonate/Vitamin
D Tablets (Heartland)
Calcium Carbonate/Vitamin
D Tablets (Major
Pharmaceuticals)
Calcium Carbonate/Vitamin
D Tablets (National
Vitamin)
Calcium Carbonate/Vitamin
D Tablets (PD-Rx)
Calcium Carbonate/Vitamin
D Tablets (Sky)
Calcium Citrate + D
Tablets (Cardinal)

Calcium Citrate w/Vitamin
D Tablets (Mason)
Calcium Citrate/Vitamin D
Tablets (Bergen
Brunswig)
Calcium-600 w/D Tablets
(American Pharmacal)
Calcium/Magnesium/Zinc
Tablets (Cardinal)
Calcium/Magnesium/Zinc
Tablets (Rexall
Consumer)
Calcium/Vitamin D Tablets
(McKesson)
Calcium/Vitamin D Tablets
(PD-Rx)
Calcium/Vitamin D Tablets
(Vanguard)
Caltrate 600 + D Tablets
(Lederle)
Citracal + D Tablets
(Mission)
Citrus Calcium + D
Tablets (Rugby)
Daily Calcium + Vitamin
D Tablets (Nature's
Bounty)
Ferosul Tablets (Major
Pharmaceuticals)
Florical Capsules (Mericon)
Florical Tablets (Mericon)
Healthy Woman Bone
Health Supplement
Tablets (Personal
Products Company)
Liqua-Cal Capsules (Key
Company)
Liquid Calcium Capsules
(Major Pharmaceuticals)
Liquid Calcium Plus
Vitamin D Capsules
(Mason)
Magnebind 200 Tablets
(Nephro-Tech)
Magnebind 300 Tablets
(Nephro-Tech)
Magnebind 400 Rx Tablets
(Nephro-Tech)
Marblen Suspension
(Fleming)
Marblen Tablets (Fleming)
Monocal Tablets (Mericon)

Chloromag Injection
(Merit)

Dewee's Carminative
Liquid (Humco)

Elite Magnesium Capsules
(Miller Pharmacal)

M2 Magnesium Capsules
(Miller Pharmacal)

Mag Delay Tablets (Major
Pharmaceuticals)

Mag-200 Tablets (Optimox)

Mag-Carb Capsules (R&D)

Mag-Gel 600 Capsules
(Cypress)

Mag-Ox 400 Tablets
(Blaine)

Mag-SR Tablets (Cypress)

Mag-Tab Sr Tablets
(Niche)

Magimin Tablets (Key
Company)

Magimin-Forte Tablets
(Key Company)

Maglex Tablets (Lex)

Magnacaps Capsules (Key
Company)

Magnesium Carbonate
Powder (Freeda)

Magnesium Elemental
Tablets (National
Vitamin)

Magnesium Oxide Tablets
(Cypress)

Magonate Liquid (Fleming)

Magonate Natal Liquid
(Fleming)

Magonate Tablets
(Fleming)

Magtrate Tablets (Mission)

Slow-Mag Tablets (Quality
Care)

Slow-Mag Tablets (Shire
U.S.)

Sulfa-Mag Injection (Merit)

Uro-Mag Capsules (Blaine)

Easysoy Gold Super
Isoflavone Concentrate
Tablets (Twinlab)

Genistein Soy Isoflavones
(Source)

♦ Healthy Woman Soy
Menopause Tablets
(Personal Products
Company) **G-5**

Maxilife Mega Soy
Capsules (Health from
the Sun)

PC Soy Isoflavones
(Natrol)

Soy Essentials Tablets
(Enzymatic Therapy)

♦ Soy & Red Clover
Isoflavones Liquid
(Nature's Answer) **G-4**

OSTEOPOROSIS, SECONDARY

May result from the use of
carbamazepine, chemotherapeutic
agents, methotrexate sodium,
phenytoin, prolonged glucocorticoid
therapy or thyroid hormones. The
following products may be
recommended:

Alcalak Chewable Tablets
(Textilease)

♦ Alka-Mints Chewable
Tablets (Bayer) **G-3**

Antacid Chewable Tablets
(Zenith Goldline)

Antacid Extra Strength
Chewable Tablets
(Cardinal)

Antacid Extra Strength
Chewable Tablets (Zenith
Goldline)

Antacid Extra Strength
Tablets (McKesson)

Antacid Ultra Strength
Chewable Tablets
(Bergen Brunswig)

Ascocid Tablets (Key
Company)

Cal-600 Tablets (PDK)

Cal-C-Caps Capsules (Key
Company)

Cal-Carb Forte Tablets
(Vitaline)

Cal-Carb Forte Wafers
(Vitaline)

Cal-Cee Tablets (Key
Company)

Cal-Citrate Capsules (Bio-
Tech)

Cal-Citrate Tablets (Bio-
Tech)

Cal-G Capsules (Key
Company)

Cal-Gest Chewable Tablets
(Rugby)

Cal-Glu Capsule (Bio-Tech)

Cal-Lac Capsules (Key
Company)

Cal-Lac Tablets (Bio-Tech)

Cal-Mint Tablets (Freeda)

Calbon Tablets (Economed)

Calcarb 600 Tablets
(Zenith Goldline)

Calci-Chew Tablets (R&D)

Calci-Mix Capsules (R&D)

Calcimin-300 Tablets (Key
Company)

Calcio Del Mar Tablets
(Marlop)

Calcionate Syrup (Hi-Tech)

Calcionate Syrup (Rugby)

Calciquid Syrup
(Breckenridge)

Calciquid Syrup (Econolab)

Calcium 500 Chewable
Tablets (Mason)

Calcium 500 Chewable
Tablets (National
Vitamin)

Calcium 500 Supplement
Chewable Tablets
(Bergen Brunswig)

Calcium 600 Capsules
(McKesson)

Calcium 600 Tablets (Basic
Vitamins)

Calcium 600 Tablets
(Nature's Bounty)

Calcium 600 Tablets
(Prime Marketing)

Calcium 600 Tablets
(Rugby)

Calcium Antacid Chewable
Tablets (Mason)

Calcium Antacid Chewable Tablets (Perrigo)

Calcium Antacid Extra Strength Chewable Tablets (Major Pharmaceuticals)

Calcium Antacid Extra Strength Chewable Tablets (Medicine Shoppe)

Calcium Antacid Extra Strength Tablets (Perrigo)

Calcium Antacid Ultra Strength Chewable Tablets (Major Pharmaceuticals)

Calcium Antacid Ultra Strength Chewable Tablets (Perrigo)

Calcium Citrate 950 Tablets (Basic Vitamins)

Calcium-600 Tablets (Key Company)

Calfort Tablets (Ampharco)

Calphron Powder (Nephro-Tech)

Caltrate 600 Tablets (Lederle)

Chooz Tablets (Heritage Consumer)

Citracal Economy Tablets (Mission)

Citracal Tablets (Mission)

Desempacho Tablets (D'Franssia)

Krebs Ionized Calcium Tablets (PhytoPharmica)

Life-Line Co-Co Bear Chewable Tablets (National Vitamin)

Liqui-Cal Chewable Tablets (Advanced Nutritional)

M2 Calcium Tablets (Miller Pharmacal)

Mallamint Chewable Tablets (Textilease)

Mylanta Calci Tabs Extra Strength (J&J • Merck)

Mylanta Calci Tabs Ultra Chewable Tablets (J&J • Merck)

Mylanta Children's Chewable Tablets (J&J • Merck)

Neo-Calglucon Syrup (Novartis Pharmaceuticals)

Nephro-Calci Tablets (R&D)

Nutralox Chewable Tablets (Hart Health)

♦ Os-Cal 500 Chewable Tablets (SmithKline Beecham) G-5

♦ Os-Cal 500 Tablets (SmithKline Beecham) G-5

Oysco 500 Tablets (Rugby)

Oyst-Cal 500 Tablets (Zenith Goldline)

Oyster Shell Calcium 500 Tablets (Medicine Shoppe)

Oyster Shell Calcium Natural Tablets (Cardinal)

Phoslo Tablets (Braintree)

Prelief Granules (AK Pharma)

Prelief Tablets (AK Pharma)

Revelation Powder (Alvin Last)

Ridactate Tablets (R.I.D.)

Rolaids Chewable Tablets (American Chicle)

Super Calcium Extra Strength Chewable Tablets (Mason)

Super Calcium Tablets (Mason)

Titralac Chewable Tablets (3M)

Titralac Extra Strength Chewable Tablets (3M)

Tums 500 Chewable Tablets (SmithKline Beecham)

♦ Tums Chewable Tablets (SmithKline Beecham) G-5

♦ Tums E-X Chewable Tablets (SmithKline Beecham) G-5

♦ Tums Ultra Chewable Tablets (SmithKline Beecham) G-5

Vitamin C Buffered Tablets (Nature's Bounty)

CALCIUM COMBINATION PRODUCTS *543t*

♦ AdvaCal Capsules (Lane Labs) G-4

Cal-600 w/Vitamin D Tablets (PDK)

Cal-Co3Y Capsules (Bio-Tech)

Cal/Mag Chelated Tablets (Freeda)

Cal/Mag Chewable Tablets (Freeda)

Calcarb 600 w/Vitamin D Tablets (Zenith Goldline)

Calcet Tablets (Mission)

Calcium & Magnesium Chelate Capsules (Key Company)

Calcium 500 w/Vitamin D Tablets (Basic Vitamins)

Calcium 500 w/Vitamin D Tablets (Mason)

Calcium 500 w/Vitamin D Tablets (Rexall Consumer)

Calcium 600 + Vitamin D Tablets (Perrigo)

Calcium 600 Plus Vitamin D Tablets (Nature's Bounty)

Calcium 600-D Tablets (Rugby)

Calcium 600/Vitamin D Tablets (Basic Vitamins)

Calcium 600/Vitamin D Tablets (Bergen Brunswig)

Calcium 600/Vitamin D Tablets (Cardinal)

Calcium 900 w/Vitamin D Capsules (Rexall Consumer)

Calcium 1200 w/Vitamin D Capsules (Rexall Consumer)

Calcium Carbonate/Vitamin D Tablets (Compumed)

Calcium Carbonate/Vitamin D Tablets (Heartland)

Calcium Carbonate/Vitamin D Tablets (Major Pharmaceuticals)

Calcium Carbonate/Vitamin D Tablets (National Vitamin)

Calcium Carbonate/Vitamin D Tablets (PD-Rx)

Calcium Carbonate/Vitamin D Tablets (Sky)

Calcium Citrate + D Tablets (Cardinal)

Calcium Citrate w/Vitamin D Tablets (Mason)

Calcium Citrate/Vitamin D Tablets (Bergen Brunswig)

Calcium-600 w/D Tablets (American Pharmacal)

Calcium/Magnesium/Zinc Tablets (Cardinal)

Calcium/Magnesium/Zinc Tablets (Rexall Consumer)

Calcium/Vitamin D Tablets (McKesson)

Calcium/Vitamin D Tablets (PD-Rx)

Calcium/Vitamin D Tablets (Vanguard)

Caltrate 600 + D Tablets (Lederle)

Citracal + D Tablets (Mission)

Citrus Calcium + D Tablets (Rugby)

Daily Calcium + Vitamin D Tablets (Nature's Bounty)

Ferosul Tablets (Major Pharmaceuticals)

Florical Capsules (Mericon)

Florical Tablets (Mericon)

Healthy Woman Bone Health Supplement Tablets (Personal Products Company)

Liqua-Cal Capsules (Key Company)

Liquid Calcium Capsules (Major Pharmaceuticals)

Liquid Calcium Plus Vitamin D Capsules (Mason)

Magnebind 200 Tablets (Nephro-Tech)

Magnebind 300 Tablets (Nephro-Tech)

Magnebind 400 Rx Tablets (Nephro-Tech)

Marblen Suspension (Fleming)

Marblen Tablets (Fleming)

Monocal Tablets (Mericon)

One-A-Day Bone Strength Tablets (Bayer)

♦ One-A-Day Calcium Plus Chewable Tablets (Bayer) .. G-3

♦ Os-Cal 250 + D Tablets (SmithKline Beecham) G-5

♦ Os-Cal 500 + D Tablets (SmithKline Beecham) G-5

Oysco 500 + D Tablets (Rugby)

Oysco D Tablets (Rugby)

Oyst-Cal-D 500 Tablets (Zenith Goldline)

Oyst-Cal-D Tablets (Zenith Goldline)

Oyster Shell Calcium 500 w/D Tablets (Medicine Shoppe)

Oyster Shell Calcium 1000/ Vitamin D Tablets (Mason)

Oyster Shell Calcium 1000/ Vitamin D Tablets (Rexall Consumer)

Oyster Shell Calcium Natural/Vit D Tablets (Cardinal)

Oyster Shell Calcium/ Vitamin D Tablets (American Pharmacal)

Oyster Shell Calcium/ Vitamin D Tablets (Basic Vitamins)

Oyster Shell Calcium/ Vitamin D Tablets (Bergen Brunswig)

Oyster Shell Calcium/ Vitamin D Tablets (Dixon-Shane)

Oyster Shell Calcium/ Vitamin D Tablets (Major Pharmaceuticals)

Oyster Shell Calcium/ Vitamin D Tablets (Mason)

Oyster Shell Calcium/ Vitamin D Tablets (McKesson)

Oyster Shell Calcium/ Vitamin D Tablets (National Vitamin)

Oyster Shell Calcium/ Vitamin D Tablets (Perrigo)

Oyster Shell Calcium/ Vitamin D Tablets (Reese)

Oyster Shell Calcium/ Vitamin D Tablets (Rexall Consumer)

Oyster Shell Calcium/ Vitamin D Tablets (Vanguard)

Oystercal-D 250 Tablets (Nature's Bounty)

Oystercal-D 500 Tablets (Nature's Bounty)

Parva-Cal 250 Tablets (Freeda)

Super Calcium w/Vitamin D Tablets (Mason)

Viactiv Chewable Tablets (Mead Johnson)

Vita-Calcium Wafers (Vitaline)

FLUORIDE **154**

Flouritab Chewable Tablets (Fluoritab)

Flouritab Liquid (Fluoritab)

Fluor-A-Day Chewable Tablets (Pharmascience)

Fluor-A-Day Liquid (Pharmascience)

Fluor-A-Day Lozenges (Pharmascience)

Fluorabon Chewable Tablets (Perry)

Fluorabon Solution (Perry)

Fluorinse Liquid (Oral B)

Flura-Loz Chewable
Tablets (Kirkman)

Lozengesi-Flur Lozenge
(Dreir)

Luride Chewable Tablets
(Colgate Oral)

Luride Liquid (Colgate
Oral)

Nafrinse Chewable Tablets
(Orachem)

Nafrinse Solution
(Orachem)

Neutracare Gel (Oral B)

Neutragard Fluoride Rinse
Solution (Pascal)

Pediaflor Drops (Ross)

Pharmaflur Chewable
Tablets (Pharmics)

Phos-Flur Gel (Colgate
Oral)

Phos-Flur Solution (Colgate
Oral)

Prevident 5000 Plus Cream
(Colgate Oral)

Prevident Cream (Colgate
Oral)

Prevident Solution (Colgate
Oral)

Thera-Flur-N Gel (Colgate
Oral)

IPRIFLAVONE **232**

Ostivone Capsules
(PhytoPharmica)

L-LYSINE **270**

L-Lysine Premium
Capsules (Ultimate)

MAGNESIUM **288**

Almora Tablets (Forest)

Chloromag Injection
(Merit)

Dewee's Carminative
Liquid (Humco)

Elite Magnesium Capsules
(Miller Pharmacal)

M2 Magnesium Capsules
(Miller Pharmacal)

Mag Delay Tablets (Major
Pharmaceuticals)

Mag-200 Tablets (Optimox)

Mag-Carb Capsules (R&D)

Mag-Gel 600 Capsules
(Cypress)

Mag-Ox 400 Tablets
(Blaine)

Mag-SR Tablets (Cypress)

Mag-Tab Sr Tablets
(Niche)

Magimin Tablets (Key
Company)

Magimin-Forte Tablets
(Key Company)

Maglex Tablets (Lex)

Magnacaps Capsules (Key
Company)

Magnesium Carbonate
Powder (Freeda)

Magnesium Elemental
Tablets (National
Vitamin)

Magnesium Oxide Tablets
(Cypress)

Magonate Liquid (Fleming)

Magonate Natal Liquid
(Fleming)

Magonate Tablets
(Fleming)

Magtrate Tablets (Mission)

Slow-Mag Tablets (Quality
Care)

Slow-Mag Tablets (Shire
U.S.)

Sulfa-Mag Injection (Merit)

Uro-Mag Capsules (Blaine)

MANGANESE **296**

NICOTINAMIDE **327**

PREBIOTICS **372**

SOY ISOFLAVONES **428**

Easysoy Gold Super
Isoflavone Concentrate
Tablets (Twinlab)

Genistein Soy Isoflavones
(Source)

♦ Healthy Woman Soy
Menopause Tablets
(Personal Products
Company) **G-5**

Maxilife Mega Soy
Capsules (Health from
the Sun)

PC Soy Isoflavones
(Natrol)

Soy Essentials Tablets
(Enzymatic Therapy)

♦ Soy & Red Clover
Isoflavones Liquid
(Nature's Answer) **G-4**

VITAMIN D **498**

VITAMIN K **523**

PANCREATIC INSUFFICIENCY, NUTRIENTS DEFICIENCY SECONDARY TO

Pancreatic insufficiency may be
treated with pancrelipase. The
following products may be
recommended for relief of nutrients
deficiency:

BROMELAIN **70**

Bromanase Tablets
(Kramer-Novis)

Bromelain 2400 Maximum
Strength Tablets
(Vitaline)

MULTIVITAMIN PRODUCTS **550t**

BEC w/Zinc Tablets
(Bergen Brunswig)

♦ Bugs Bunny Plus Extra C
Chewable Tablets (Bayer) . . **G-3**

♦ Bugs Bunny Plus Iron
Chewable Tablets (Bayer) . . **G-3**

Cardiotek Tablets (Stewart-
Jackson)

Cefol Tablets (Abbott
Hospital)

Circus Chews Children's
Chewable Tablets (Rexall
Consumer)

Daily Multiple Vitamins
Tablets (Marlex)

Daily Multiple Vitamins
Tablets (Rexall
Consumer)

Daily Multiple Vitamins w/
Iron Tablets (Rexall
Consumer)

Daily Multivitamins Tablets
(Sky)

♦ Flintstones Original
Children's Chewable
Tablets (Bayer) **G-3**

♦ Flintstones Plus Calcium
Chewable Tablets (Bayer) . . **G-3**

♦ Flintstones Plus Extra C
Chewable Tablets (Bayer) . . **G-3**

◆ Flintstones Plus Iron
   Chewable Tablets (Bayer) .. **G-3**
   Key-Plex Injection (Hyrex)
   M.V.I. Pediatric Powder for
   Injection (AstraZeneca LP)
   M.V.I.-12 Injection
   (AstraZeneca LP)
   Multi-Vitamins Tablets
   (Rugby)
   Multivitamin Capsules
   (Numark)
   Once Daily Tablets (Prime
   Marketing)
◆ One-A-Day Essential
   Tablets (Bayer) **G-3**
   Poly Vitamin Chewable
   Tablets (Rugby)
   Stress Formula Plus Zinc
   Tablets (Rexall
   Consumer)
   Stress Formula Tablets
   (Cardinal)
   Stress Formula Tablets
   (Rexall Consumer)
   Therapeutic Multivitamin
   Tablets (Bergen
   Brunswig)
   Ultra Tabs Tablets (Major
   Pharmaceuticals)
   Vitamins Children's
   Chewable Tablets (Prime
   Marketing)

**MULTIVITAMIN AND MINERAL
PRODUCTS** **553t**
◆ Alpha Betic Tablets
   (Abkit) **G-3**
   B-C w/Folic Acid Plus
   Tablet (Geneva)
   B-Complex Plus Tablets
   (United Research)
   B-Complex Vitamins Plus
   Tablets (Teva)
   B-Plex Plus Tablets (Zenith
   Goldline)
   Bacmin Tablets (Marnel)
   Becomax RX Tablets
   (Ampharco)
   Berocca Plus Tablets
   (Roche)
◆ Bugs Bunny Complete
   Children's Chewable
   Tablets (Bayer) **G-3**

Cerovite Senior Tablets
   (Rugby)
Circavite T Tablets (Circle)
Clusinex Syrup
   (Pharmakon)
Daily Multiple Vitamins/
   Minerals Tablets
   (Vanguard)
Dr. Art Ulene's Vitamin
   Formula Packets (Feeling
   Fine)
Equi-Roca Plus Tablets
   (Equipharm)
Ferrex PC Tablets
   (Breckenridge)
◆ Flintstones Complete
   Children's Chewable
   Tablets (Bayer) **G-3**
   Formula B Plus Tablets
   (Major Pharmaceuticals)
   Glutofac-ZX Capsules
   (Kenwood)
   Hematin Plus Tablets
   (Cypress)
   Iromin-G Tablets (Mission)
   Manly Machovites Tablets
   (Neurovites)
   Mega-Multi Capsules
   (Innovative Health)
   Niferex-PN Tablets
   (Schwarz)
   O-Cal FA Tablets
   (Pharmics)
◆ One-A-Day 50 Plus Tablets
   (Bayer) **G-3**
◆ One-A-Day Antioxidant
   Capsules (Bayer) **G-3**
◆ One-A-Day Kids Complete
   Chewable Tablets (Bayer) .. **G-3**
◆ One-A-Day Maximum
   Tablets (Bayer) **G-3**
◆ One-A-Day Men's Tablets
   (Bayer) **G-3**
◆ One-A-Day Women's
   Tablets (Bayer) **G-3**
   PMS Formula Tablets
   (Neurovites)
   Poly Vitamin w/Iron
   Chewable Tablets
   (Rugby)
   Protect Plus Capsules (Gil)
   Protect Plus Liquid (Gil)

Strovite Forte Tablets
   (Everett)
Sunvite Platinum Tablets
   (Rexall Consumer)
Sunvite Tablets (Rexall
   Consumer)
Super Plenamins Extra
   Strength Tablets (Rexall
   Consumer)
Super Plenamins Tablets
   (Rexall Consumer)
Support 500 Capsules
   (Marin)
Support Liquid (Marin)
Thera Vite M Tablets
   (PDK)
Thera-M w/Minerals
   Tablets (Prime
   Marketing)
◆ Theragran-M Tablets
   (Bristol-Myers Products) **G-3**
   Therapeutic Plus Vitamin
   Tablets (Rugby)
   Therobec Plus Tablets
   (Qualitest)
   Total Formula Original
   Tablets (Vitaline)
   V-C Forte Capsules
   (Breckenridge)
   Vicap Forte Tablets (Major
   Pharmaceuticals)
   Vicon Forte Tablets (UCB)
   Vita-Min Rx Tablets (Bio-
   Tech)
   Vitacon Forte Tablets
   (Amide)
   Vitaplex Plus Tablets
   (Amide)
   Vitelle Nesentials Tablets
   (Fielding)

VITAMIN A **462**
   Active A Tablets (Source)

VITAMIN B COMPLEX PRODUCTS .. **558t**
   B-50 Complex Tablets
   (Rexall Consumer)
   B-100 Complex Tablets
   (Rexall Consumer)
   B-Ject-100 Injection
   (Hyrex)
   B-Plex Tablets (Contract
   Pharmacal)

B-Plex Tablets (Zenith
   Goldline)
Berocca Tablets (Roche)
Dialyvite Tablets
   (Hillestad)
Formula B Tablets (Major
   Pharmaceuticals)
Marlbee w/C Capsules
   (Marlex)
Nephplex Rx Tablets
   (Nephro-Tech)
Nephro-Vite Rx Tablets
   (R&D)
Nephrocaps Capsules
   (Fleming)
Primaplex Injection
   (Primedics)
Stress B Complex with
   Vitamin C Tablets
   (Mission)
Strovite Tablets (Everett)
Therobec Tablets
   (Qualitest)
Thex Forte Tablets (Lee)
Vicam Injection (Keene)
Vita-Bee w/C Tablets
   (Rugby)
Vitamin B Complex 100
   Injection (Hyrex)
Vitamin B Complex 100
   Injection (McGuff)
Vitamin B Complex 100
   Injection (Torrance)
Vitamin B Complex 100
   Injection (Truxton)
Vitamin B Complex
   Capsules (Rugby)
Vitamin B Complex w/
   Vitamin C & B12
   Injection (McGuff)
Vitamin B-100 Natural
   Tablets (Cardinal)
Vitaplex Tablets (Amide)
Vitaplex Tablets (Medirex)

Alph-E Capsules (Key
   Company)
Alph-E-Mixed Capsules
   (Key Company)
Alpha-E Capsules
   (Advanced Nutritional)

Aquasol E Liquid
   (AstraZeneca LP)
Aquavit-E Liquid (Cypress)
Born Again Vitamin E Oil
   (Alvin Last)
DL-Alpha Tocopheryl E400
   Capsules (Mason)
E-400-Mixed Capsules
   (Bio-Tech)
E-Max-1000 Capsules (Bio-
   Tech)
E-Pherol Tablets (Vitaline)
E100 Capsules (Nature's
   Bounty)
E200 Capsules (Nature's
   Bounty)
E200 Mixed Capsules
   (Rexall Consumer)
E400 Capsules (Nature's
   Bounty)
E400 Mixed Capsules
   (Rexall Consumer)
E400 Natural Capsules
   (Rexall Consumer)
E1000 Capsules (Nature's
   Bounty)
E1000 D-Alpha Capsules
   (Mason)
E1000 Mixed Capsules
   (Rexall Consumer)
Formula E 400 Capsules
   (Miller Pharmacal)
Liquid E Liquid (Freeda)
Nutr-E-Sol Capsules
   (Advanced Nutritional)
Nutr-E-Sol Liquid
   (Advanced Nutritional)
Total E-400 Capsules
   (Westlake)
Vitamin E Aqueous Liquid
   (Boca Pharmacal)
Vitamin E Aqueous Liquid
   (Silarx)
Vitamin E D-Alpha
   Capsules (Mason)
Vitamin E DL Alpha
   Capsules (Health
   Products)
Vitamin E DL-Alpha
   Capsules (Mason)
Vitamin E MTC Capsules
   (National Vitamin)

Vitamin E Mixed Capsules
   (Mason)
Vitamin E Mixed Tablets
   (Freeda)
Vitamin E Mixed
   Tocopherols Capsules
   (Swanson)
Vitamin E Natural Blend
   Capsules (Medicine
   Shoppe)
Vitamin E Natural Blend
   Capsules (Perrigo)
Vitamin E Natural
   Capsules (Basic
   Vitamins)
Vitamin E Natural
   Capsules (Bergen
   Brunswig)
Vitamin E Natural
   Capsules (Cardinal)
Vitamin E Natural
   Capsules (Dixon-Shane)
Vitamin E Natural
   Capsules (McKesson)
Vitamin E Natural Liquid
   (Geritrex)
Vitamin E Water Soluble
   Capsules (National
   Vitamin)
Vitamin E400 D Alpha
   Capsules (National
   Vitamin)
Vitamin E400 D-Alpha
   Capsules (Perrigo)
Vitamin E800 D-Alpha
   Capsules (Pharmavite)

PARKINSON'S DISEASE, CONSTIPATION SECONDARY TO

Parkinson's disease may be treated
with centrally active anticholinergic
agents, dopaminergic agents or
selective inhibitor of MAO type B.
The following products may be
recommended for relief of
constipation:

Cephulac Syrup (Aventis)
Cholac Syrup (Alra)
Chronulac Syrup (Aventis)
Constilac Syrup (Alra)

Constulose Solution
(Alpharma)
Duphalac Syrup (Solvay)
Enulose Solution
(Alpharma)
PECTIN **348**
Modified Citrus Pectin
Power Capsules (Nature's
Herbs)
PREBIOTICS **372**
PSYLLIUM **384**
Colon Care Formula
Psyllium Seed Capsules
(Yerba Prima)
Fiberall Powder (Novartis
Consumer)
Fiberall Wafers (Novartis
Consumer)
Fibro-XI Capsules (Key
Company)
Genfiber Powder (Zenith
Goldline)
Hydrocil Powder (Numark)
Konsyl Powder (Konsyl)
Konsyl-D Powder (Konsyl)
♦ Metamucil Powder and
Wafers (Procter &
Gamble) **G-5**
Modane Bulk Powder
(Savage)
♦ Perdiem Granules (Novartis
Consumer) **G-5**
Psyllium Husks 100% Pure
Powder (Yerba Prima)
Reguloid Powder (Carlson)
Reguloid Powder (Rugby)
Serutan Granules (Twinlab)

PEPTIC ULCER DISEASE, IRON DEFICIENCY SECONDARY TO

Peptic ulcer disease may be treated with histamine H$_2$ receptor antagonists, proton pump inhibitors or sucralfate. The following products may be recommended for relief of iron deficiency:
IRON **234**
Dexferrum Injection
(American Regent)
Ed-In-Sol Elixir (Edwards)
Fe-40 Tablets (Bio-Tech)
♦ Feosol Caplets (SmithKline
Beecham) **G-5**

♦ Feosol Elixir (SmithKline
Beecham) **G-5**
♦ Feosol Tablets (SmithKline
Beecham) **G-5**
Feostat Chewable Tablets
(Forest)
Feostat Suspension (Forest)
Fer-Gen-Sol Liquid (Zenith
Goldline)
Fer-In-Sol Liquid (Mead
Johnson)
Fer-Iron Liquid (Rugby)
Feratab Tablets (Upsher-
Smith)
♦ Fergon Tablets (Bayer) **G-3**
Feronate Tablets (Prime
Marketing)
Ferosul Tablets (Major
Pharmaceuticals)
Ferretts Tablets (Pharmics)
Ferro-Caps Capsules
(Nature's Bounty)
Ferro-Time Capsules
(Time-Cap)
Ferrous Sulfate T.D.
Capsules (American
Pharmacal)
Ferrousal Tablets (Prime
Marketing)
Gentle Iron Capsules
(Solgar)
Infed Injection (Schein)
Ircon Tablets (Kenwood)
Iron Sol Elixir (Halsey)
Mol-Iron Tablets (Schering-
Plough)
Nephro-Fer Tablets (R&D)
Ridosol Tablets (R.I.D.)
Siderol Pediatric Tablets
(Marin)
♦ Slow Fe Tablets (Novartis
Consumer) **G-5**
Slow Release Iron Tablets
(Cardinal)
Vitedyn-Slo Capsules
(Edyn)
Yieronia Elixir (R.I.D.)
Yierro-Gota Liquid (R.I.D.)
IRON COMBINATION PRODUCTS . . . **546t**
Anemagen Capsules
(Ethex)

Anemagen FA Capsules
(Ethex)
Chromagen Capsules
(Savage)
Chromagen FA Tablets
(Savage)
Chromagen Forte Capsules
(Savage)
Conison Capsules (Ethex)
Contrin Capsules (Geneva)
DSS w/Iron Extended
Release Capsules
(American Pharmacal)
Daily Multiple Vitamins/
Iron Tablets (Vanguard)
Ed Cyte F Tablets
(Edwards)
Equi-Cyte F Tablets
(Equipharm)
Fe-Tinic 150 Forte
Capsules (Ethex)
Fero-Folic 500 Extended
Release Tablets (Abbott)
Fero-Grad-500 Extended
Release Tablets (Abbott)
Ferocon Capsules
(Breckenridge)
Ferotrinsic Capsules
(Contract Pharmacal)
Ferragen Capsules (Pecos)
Ferrex 150 Forte Capsules
(Breckenridge)
Ferro-Sequels Extended
Release Tablets
(Inverness)
Ferrous Fumarate DS
Extended Release
Capsules (Vita-Rx)
Fetrin Extended Release
Capsules (Lunsco)
Foltrin Capsules (Eon)
Fumatinic Extended
Release Capsules (Laser)
Hematin-F Tablets
(Cypress)
Hemocyte-F Tablets (U.S.
Pharmaceutical)
Iberet-Folic-500 Extended
Release Tablets (Abbott)
Icar-C Plus Tablets
(Hawthorn)
Icar-C Tablets (Hawthorn)

Infed Injection (Schein)

Ircon-FA Tablets
(Kenwood)

Irofol Tablets (Dayton)

Iron Advanced Tablets
(Rexall Consumer)

Iron w/Docusate Sodium
Extended Release Tablets
(Nature's Bounty)

Iron-Folic 500 Tablets
(Major Pharmaceuticals)

Martinic Capsules (Marlop)

Multi-Ferrous Folic
Extended Release Tablets
(United Research)

Multi-Vitamin w/Iron
Children's Liquid (Tri-
Med)

Multiret Folic-500
Extended Release Tablets
(Amide)

Multivitamins w/Iron
Children's Chewable
Tablets (Cardinal)

Myferon 150 Forte
Capsules (Me
Pharmaceuticals)

Nephro-Fer Rx Tablets
(R&D)

Nephro-Vite + FE Tablets
(R&D)

Nephron FA Tablets
(Nephro-Tech)

Niferex-150 Forte Capsules
(Schwarz)

Nu-Iron Plus Elixir (Merz)

Nutrinate Chewable Tablets
(Ethex)

One Tablet Daily w/Iron
Tablets (Zenith Goldline)

Prenafort Tablets (Cypress)

Promar Capsules (Marlop)

♦ Slow Fe w/Folic Acid
Extended Release Tablets
(Novartis Consumer) G-3

Stress Formula + Iron
Tablets (Cardinal)

Thera Hematinic Tablets
(Dixon-Shane)

Theragran Hematinic
Tablets (Apothecon)

Tolfrinic Tablets (Ascher)

Trinsicon Capsules
(Marlex)

Vitamins w/Iron Children's
Chewable Tablets
(Marlex)

Vitelle Irospan Extended
Release Tablets and
Extended Release
Capsules (Fielding)

Vitron-C Plus Tablets
(Novartis Consumer)

Vitron-C Tablets (Novartis
Consumer)

RENAL OSTEODYSTROPHY, HYPOCALCEMIA SECONDARY TO

Renal osteodystrophy may be treated with vitamin D sterols. The following products may be recommended for relief of hypocalcemia:

CALCIUM **74**

Alcalak Chewable Tablets
(Textilease)

♦ Alka-Mints Chewable
Tablets (Bayer) **G-3**

Antacid Chewable Tablets
(Zenith Goldline)

Antacid Extra Strength
Chewable Tablets
(Cardinal)

Antacid Extra Strength
Chewable Tablets (Zenith
Goldline)

Antacid Extra Strength
Tablets (McKesson)

Antacid Ultra Strength
Chewable Tablets
(Bergen Brunswig)

Ascocid Tablets (Key
Company)

Cal-600 Tablets (PDK)

Cal-C-Caps Capsules (Key
Company)

Cal-Carb Forte Tablets
(Vitaline)

Cal-Carb Forte Wafers
(Vitaline)

Cal-Cee Tablets (Key
Company)

Cal-Citrate Capsules (Bio-
Tech)

Cal-Citrate Tablets (Bio-
Tech)

Cal-G Capsules (Key
Company)

Cal-Gest Chewable Tablets
(Rugby)

Cal-Glu Capsule (Bio-Tech)

Cal-Lac Capsules (Key
Company)

Cal-Lac Tablets (Bio-Tech)

Cal-Mint Tablets (Freeda)

Calbon Tablets (Economed)

Calcarb 600 Tablets
(Zenith Goldline)

Calci-Chew Tablets (R&D)

Calci-Mix Capsules (R&D)

Calcimin-300 Tablets (Key
Company)

Calcio Del Mar Tablets
(Marlop)

Calcionate Syrup (Hi-Tech)

Calcionate Syrup (Rugby)

Calciquid Syrup
(Breckenridge)

Calciquid Syrup (Econolab)

Calcium 500 Chewable
Tablets (Mason)

Calcium 500 Chewable
Tablets (National
Vitamin)

Calcium 500 Supplement
Chewable Tablets
(Bergen Brunswig)

Calcium 600 Capsules
(McKesson)

Calcium 600 Tablets (Basic
Vitamins)

Calcium 600 Tablets
(Nature's Bounty)

Calcium 600 Tablets
(Prime Marketing)

Calcium 600 Tablets
(Rugby)

Calcium Antacid Chewable
Tablets (Mason)

Calcium Antacid Chewable
Tablets (Perrigo)

Calcium Antacid Extra
Strength Chewable
Tablets (Major
Pharmaceuticals)

Calcium Antacid Extra Strength Chewable Tablets (Medicine Shoppe)

Calcium Antacid Extra Strength Tablets (Perrigo)

Calcium Antacid Ultra Strength Chewable Tablets (Major Pharmaceuticals)

Calcium Antacid Ultra Strength Chewable Tablets (Perrigo)

Calcium Citrate 950 Tablets (Basic Vitamins)

Calcium-600 Tablets (Key Company)

Calfort Tablets (Ampharco)

Calphron Powder (Nephro-Tech)

Caltrate 600 Tablets (Lederle)

Chooz Tablets (Heritage Consumer)

Citracal Economy Tablets (Mission)

Citracal Tablets (Mission)

Desempacho Tablets (D'Franssia)

Krebs Ionized Calcium Tablets (PhytoPharmica)

Life-Line Co-Co Bear Chewable Tablets (National Vitamin)

Liqui-Cal Chewable Tablets (Advanced Nutritional)

M2 Calcium Tablets (Miller Pharmacal)

Mallamint Chewable Tablets (Textilease)

Mylanta Calci Tabs Extra Strength (J&J • Merck)

Mylanta Calci Tabs Ultra Chewable Tablets (J&J • Merck)

Mylanta Children's Chewable Tablets (J&J • Merck)

Neo-Calglucon Syrup (Novartis Pharmaceuticals)

Nephro-Calci Tablets (R&D)

Nutralox Chewable Tablets (Hart Health)

♦ Os-Cal 500 Chewable Tablets (SmithKline Beecham) G-5

♦ Os-Cal 500 Tablets (SmithKline Beecham) G-5

Oysco 500 Tablets (Rugby)

Oyst-Cal 500 Tablets (Zenith Goldline)

Oyster Shell Calcium 500 Tablets (Medicine Shoppe)

Oyster Shell Calcium Natural Tablets (Cardinal)

Phoslo Tablets (Braintree)

Prelief Granules (AK Pharma)

Prelief Tablets (AK Pharma)

Revelation Powder (Alvin Last)

Ridactate Tablets (R.I.D.)

Rolaids Chewable Tablets (American Chicle)

Super Calcium Extra Strength Chewable Tablets (Mason)

Super Calcium Tablets (Mason)

Titralac Chewable Tablets (3M)

Titralac Extra Strength Chewable Tablets (3M)

Tums 500 Chewable Tablets (SmithKline Beecham)

♦ Tums Chewable Tablets (SmithKline Beecham) G-5

♦ Tums E-X Chewable Tablets (SmithKline Beecham) G-5

♦ Tums Ultra Chewable Tablets (SmithKline Beecham) G-5

Vitamin C Buffered Tablets (Nature's Bounty)

CALCIUM COMBINATION PRODUCTS *543t*

♦ AdvaCal Capsules (Lane Labs) G-4

Cal-600 w/Vitamin D Tablets (PDK)

Cal-Co3Y Capsules (Bio-Tech)

Cal/Mag Chelated Tablets (Freeda)

Cal/Mag Chewable Tablets (Freeda)

Calcarb 600 w/Vitamin D Tablets (Zenith Goldline)

Calcet Tablets (Mission)

Calcium & Magnesium Chelate Capsules (Key Company)

Calcium 500 w/Vitamin D Tablets (Basic Vitamins)

Calcium 500 w/Vitamin D Tablets (Mason)

Calcium 500 w/Vitamin D Tablets (Rexall Consumer)

Calcium 600 + Vitamin D Tablets (Perrigo)

Calcium 600 Plus Vitamin D Tablets (Nature's Bounty)

Calcium 600-D Tablets (Rugby)

Calcium 600/Vitamin D Tablets (Basic Vitamins)

Calcium 600/Vitamin D Tablets (Bergen Brunswig)

Calcium 600/Vitamin D Tablets (Cardinal)

Calcium 900 w/Vitamin D Capsules (Rexall Consumer)

Calcium 1200 w/Vitamin D Capsules (Rexall Consumer)

Calcium Carbonate/Vitamin D Tablets (Compumed)

Calcium Carbonate/Vitamin D Tablets (Heartland)

Calcium Carbonate/Vitamin D Tablets (Major Pharmaceuticals)

Calcium Carbonate/Vitamin D Tablets (National Vitamin)

Calcium Carbonate/Vitamin D Tablets (PD-Rx)

Calcium Carbonate/Vitamin D Tablets (Sky)

Calcium Citrate + D Tablets (Cardinal)

Calcium Citrate w/Vitamin D Tablets (Mason)

Calcium Citrate/Vitamin D Tablets (Bergen Brunswig)

Calcium-600 w/D Tablets (American Pharmacal)

Calcium/Magnesium/Zinc Tablets (Cardinal)

Calcium/Magnesium/Zinc Tablets (Rexall Consumer)

Calcium/Vitamin D Tablets (McKesson)

Calcium/Vitamin D Tablets (PD-Rx)

Calcium/Vitamin D Tablets (Vanguard)

Caltrate 600 + D Tablets (Lederle)

Citracal + D Tablets (Mission)

Citrus Calcium + D Tablets (Rugby)

Daily Calcium + Vitamin D Tablets (Nature's Bounty)

Ferosul Tablets (Major Pharmaceuticals)

Florical Capsules (Mericon)

Florical Tablets (Mericon)

Healthy Woman Bone Health Supplement Tablets (Personal Products Company)

Liqua-Cal Capsules (Key Company)

Liquid Calcium Capsules (Major Pharmaceuticals)

Liquid Calcium Plus Vitamin D Capsules (Mason)

Magnebind 200 Tablets (Nephro-Tech)

Magnebind 300 Tablets (Nephro-Tech)

Magnebind 400 Rx Tablets (Nephro-Tech)

Marblen Suspension (Fleming)

Marblen Tablets (Fleming)

Monocal Tablets (Mericon)

One-A-Day Bone Strength Tablets (Bayer)

◆ One-A-Day Calcium Plus Chewable Tablets (Bayer) .. **G-3**

◆ Os-Cal 250 + D Tablets (SmithKline Beecham) **G-5**

◆ Os-Cal 500 + D Tablets (SmithKline Beecham) **G-5**

Oysco 500 + D Tablets (Rugby)

Oysco D Tablets (Rugby)

Oyst-Cal-D 500 Tablets (Zenith Goldline)

Oyst-Cal-D Tablets (Zenith Goldline)

Oyster Shell Calcium 500 w/D Tablets (Medicine Shoppe)

Oyster Shell Calcium 1000/ Vitamin D Tablets (Mason)

Oyster Shell Calcium 1000/ Vitamin D Tablets (Rexall Consumer)

Oyster Shell Calcium Natural/Vit D Tablets (Cardinal)

Oyster Shell Calcium/ Vitamin D Tablets (American Pharmacal)

Oyster Shell Calcium/ Vitamin D Tablets (Basic Vitamins)

Oyster Shell Calcium/ Vitamin D Tablets (Bergen Brunswig)

Oyster Shell Calcium/ Vitamin D Tablets (Dixon-Shane)

Oyster Shell Calcium/ Vitamin D Tablets (Major Pharmaceuticals)

Oyster Shell Calcium/ Vitamin D Tablets (Mason)

Oyster Shell Calcium/ Vitamin D Tablets (McKesson)

Oyster Shell Calcium/ Vitamin D Tablets (National Vitamin)

Oyster Shell Calcium/ Vitamin D Tablets (Perrigo)

Oyster Shell Calcium/ Vitamin D Tablets (Reese)

Oyster Shell Calcium/ Vitamin D Tablets (Rexall Consumer)

Oyster Shell Calcium/ Vitamin D Tablets (Vanguard)

Oystercal-D 250 Tablets (Nature's Bounty)

Oystercal-D 500 Tablets (Nature's Bounty)

Parva-Cal 250 Tablets (Freeda)

Super Calcium w/Vitamin D Tablets (Mason)

Viactiv Chewable Tablets (Mead Johnson)

Vita-Calcium Wafers (Vitaline)

SINUSITIS

May be treated with amoxicillin, amoxicillin-clavulanate, cefprozil, cefuroxime axetil, clarithromycin or loracarbef. The following products may be recommended for relief of symptoms:

BROMELAIN **70**

Bromanase Tablets (Kramer-Novis)

Bromelain 2400 Maximum Strength Tablets (Vitaline)

SKIN IRRITATION

May result from the use of transdermal drug delivery systems. The following products may be recommended:

DIMETHYL SULFOXIDE (DMSO) **132**

Catalytic Formula Tablets (Vitaline)

Rimso-50 Tablets (Edwards)

TUBERCULOSIS, NUTRIENTS DEFICIENCY SECONDARY TO

Tuberculosis may be treated with capreomycin sulfate, ethambutol hydrochloride, ethionamide, isoniazid, pyrazinamide, rifampin or streptomycin sulfate. The following products may be recommended for relief of nutrients deficiency:

MULTIVITAMIN PRODUCTS **550t**

BEC w/Zinc Tablets (Bergen Brunswig)

◆ Bugs Bunny Plus Extra C Chewable Tablets (Bayer) . . **G-3**

◆ Bugs Bunny Plus Iron Chewable Tablets (Bayer) . . **G-3**

Cardiotek Tablets (Stewart-Jackson)

Cefol Tablets (Abbott Hospital)

Circus Chews Children's Chewable Tablets (Rexall Consumer)

Daily Multiple Vitamins Tablets (Marlex)

Daily Multiple Vitamins Tablets (Rexall Consumer)

Daily Multiple Vitamins w/ Iron Tablets (Rexall Consumer)

Daily Multivitamins Tablets (Sky)

◆ Flintstones Original Children's Chewable Tablets (Bayer) **G-3**

◆ Flintstones Plus Calcium Chewable Tablets (Bayer) . . **G-3**

◆ Flintstones Plus Extra C Chewable Tablets (Bayer) . . **G-3**

◆ Flintstones Plus Iron Chewable Tablets (Bayer) . . **G-3**

Key-Plex Injection (Hyrex)

M.V.I. Pediatric Powder for Injection (AstraZeneca LP)

M.V.I.-12 Injection (AstraZeneca LP)

Multi-Vitamins Tablets (Rugby)

Multivitamin Capsules (Numark)

Once Daily Tablets (Prime Marketing)

◆ One-A-Day Essential Tablets (Bayer) **G-3**

Poly Vitamin Chewable Tablets (Rugby)

Stress Formula Plus Zinc Tablets (Rexall Consumer)

Stress Formula Tablets (Cardinal)

Stress Formula Tablets (Rexall Consumer)

Therapeutic Multivitamin Tablets (Bergen Brunswig)

Ultra Tabs Tablets (Major Pharmaceuticals)

Vitamins Children's Chewable Tablets (Prime Marketing)

MULTIVITAMIN AND MINERAL PRODUCTS **553t**

◆ Alpha Betic Tablets (Abkit) **G-3**

B-C w/Folic Acid Plus Tablet (Geneva)

B-Complex Plus Tablets (United Research)

B-Complex Vitamins Plus Tablets (Teva)

B-Plex Plus Tablets (Zenith Goldline)

Bacmin Tablets (Marnel)

Becomax RX Tablets (Ampharco)

Berocca Plus Tablets (Roche)

◆ Bugs Bunny Complete Children's Chewable Tablets (Bayer) **G-3**

Cerovite Senior Tablets (Rugby)

Circavite T Tablets (Circle)

Clusinex Syrup (Pharmakon)

Daily Multiple Vitamins/ Minerals Tablets (Vanguard)

Dr. Art Ulene's Vitamin Formula Packets (Feeling Fine)

Equi-Roca Plus Tablets (Equipharm)

Ferrex PC Tablets (Breckenridge)

◆ Flintstones Complete Children's Chewable Tablets (Bayer) **G-3**

Formula B Plus Tablets (Major Pharmaceuticals)

Glutofac-ZX Capsules (Kenwood)

Hematin Plus Tablets (Cypress)

Iromin-G Tablets (Mission)

Manly Machovites Tablets (Neurovites)

Mega-Multi Capsules (Innovative Health)

Niferex-PN Tablets (Schwarz)

O-Cal FA Tablets (Pharmics)

◆ One-A-Day 50 Plus Tablets (Bayer) **G-3**

◆ One-A-Day Antioxidant Capsules (Bayer) **G-3**

◆ One-A-Day Kids Complete Chewable Tablets (Bayer) . . **G-3**

◆ One-A-Day Maximum Tablets (Bayer) **G-3**

◆ One-A-Day Men's Tablets (Bayer) **G-3**

◆ One-A-Day Women's Tablets (Bayer) **G-3**

PMS Formula Tablets (Neurovites)

Poly Vitamin w/Iron Chewable Tablets (Rugby)

Protect Plus Capsules (Gil)

Protect Plus Liquid (Gil)

Strovite Forte Tablets (Everett)

Sunvite Platinum Tablets
(Rexall Consumer)
Sunvite Tablets (Rexall
Consumer)
Super Plenamins Extra
Strength Tablets (Rexall
Consumer)
Super Plenamins Tablets
(Rexall Consumer)
Support 500 Capsules
(Marin)
Support Liquid (Marin)
Thera Vite M Tablets
(PDK)
Thera-M w/Minerals
Tablets (Prime
Marketing)
♦ Theragran-M Tablets
(Bristol-Myers Products) G-3
Therapeutic Plus Vitamin
Tablets (Rugby)
Therobec Plus Tablets
(Qualitest)
Total Formula Original
Tablets (Vitaline)
V-C Forte Capsules
(Breckenridge)
Vicap Forte Tablets (Major
Pharmaceuticals)
Vicon Forte Tablets (UCB)
Vita-Min Rx Tablets (Bio-
Tech)
Vitacon Forte Tablets
(Amide)
Vitaplex Plus Tablets
(Amide)
Vitelle Nesentials Tablets
(Fielding)

VITAMIN B COMPLEX PRODUCTS .. *558t*
B-50 Complex Tablets
(Rexall Consumer)
B-100 Complex Tablets
(Rexall Consumer)
B-Ject-100 Injection
(Hyrex)
B-Plex Tablets (Contract
Pharmacal)
B-Plex Tablets (Zenith
Goldline)
Berocca Tablets (Roche)
Dialyvite Tablets
(Hillestad)
Formula B Tablets (Major
Pharmaceuticals)
Marlbee w/C Capsules
(Marlex)
Nephplex Rx Tablets
(Nephro-Tech)
Nephro-Vite Rx Tablets
(R&D)
Nephrocaps Capsules
(Fleming)
Primaplex Injection
(Primedics)
Stress B Complex with
Vitamin C Tablets
(Mission)
Strovite Tablets (Everett)
Therobec Tablets
(Qualitest)
Thex Forte Tablets (Lee)
Vicam Injection (Keene)
Vita-Bee w/C Tablets
(Rugby)
Vitamin B Complex 100
Injection (Hyrex)
Vitamin B Complex 100
Injection (McGuff)

Vitamin B Complex 100
Injection (Torrance)
Vitamin B Complex 100
Injection (Truxton)
Vitamin B Complex
Capsules (Rugby)
Vitamin B Complex w/
Vitamin C & B12
Injection (McGuff)
Vitamin B-100 Natural
Tablets (Cardinal)
Vitaplex Tablets (Amide)
Vitaplex Tablets (Medirex)

VAGINOSIS, BACTERIAL

May be treated with metronidazole
or sulfabenzamide/sulfacetamide/
sulfathiozole. The following
products may be recommended for
relief of symptoms:

PROBIOTICS 377
Acidophilus Lactocacilli w/
Pectin Capsules (Source)
Lacto Brev Capsules
(Source)
Life Flora Capsules
(Source)
Longest Living Acidophilus
Capsules (Freelife)
NutraFlora Tablets (Source)
♦ Probiata Tablets
(Wakunaga) G-6
YOGURT 532

VULVOVAGINITIS, CANDIDAL

May result from the use of
estrogen-containing oral
contraceptives, immunosuppressants
or recent broad-spectrum antibiotic
therapy. The following products may
be recommended:
YOGURT 532

Manufacturers Index

This index provides you with contact information for each supplier of supplements discussed in this book. A list of the company's nutritional products follows the contact information. Brands pictured in the Product Identification Guide are marked with a [♦] symbol and a page number giving the location of the photo.

ABBOTT HOSPITAL PRODUCTS
Div. of Abbott Labs.
1 Abbott Park Road D-R10
Abbott Park, IL 60064-3500

Direct Inquiries to:
(800) 222-6883
FAX: (847) 938-7935
www.abbott.com

Nutritional Products Available:
Calcium Acetate Injection
Calcium Chloride Injection
Cefol Tablets
Cenolate Injection
Magnesium Sulfate
  Injection
Zinc Chloride Injection
Zinc Injection

ABBOTT PHARMACEUTICAL
Div. of Abbott Labs.
1 Abbott Park Road
Abbott Park, IL 60064-3500

Direct Inquiries to:
(800) 255-5162
FAX: (847) 937-1862
www.abbott.com

Nutritional Products Available:
Cecon Liquid
Fero-Folic 500 Extended
  Release Tablets
Fero-Grad-500 Extended
  Release Tablets
Iberet-Folic-500 Extended
  Release Tablets

ABKIT
207 East 94th Street
New York, NY 10128

Direct Inquiries to:
(800) 226-6227
FAX: (212) 860-8323

Nutritional Products Available:
♦ Alpha Betic Tablets **G-3**

ACTION LABS, INC.
280 Adams Boulevard
Farmingdale, NY 11735

Direct Inquiries to:
(800) 932-2953
FAX: (516) 694-6493

Nutritional Products Available:
Wild Oats Liquid
Wild Oats Tablets

ADH HEALTH PRODUCTS INC.
215 North Route 303
Congers, NY 10920-1726

Direct Inquiries to:
(914) 268-0027
FAX: (914) 268-2988

Nutritional Products Available:
Borage Oil Capsules
Evening Primrose Oil
  Capsules
Ferrous Sulfate Tablets
Folic Acid Tablets
Niacin Capsules
Niacin Tablets
Pantothenic Acid Tablets
Soytein Natural Soy
  Protein Non-Gmo Powder

Vitamin C Chewable
  Tablets
Vitamin C/Rose Hips
  Tablets
Zinc Gluconate Tablets
Zinc Lozenges
Zinc Tablets

ADVANCE PHARMACEUTICAL INC.
2201-F 5th Avenue
Ronkonkoma, NY 11779

Direct Inquiries to:
(631) 981-4600
FAX: (631) 981-4112

Nutritional Products Available:
Antacid Multi-Symptom
  Tablets
Calcium Carbonate Tablets
Ferrous Sulfate Tablets

**ADVANCED NUTRITIONAL
TECHNOLOGY, INC.**
6988 Sierra Court
Dublin, CA 94568

Direct Inquiries to:
(800) 624-6543
(925) 828-2128
FAX: (925) 828-6848

Nutritional Products Available:
Alpha-E Capsules
DHEA Capsules
Flaxseed Oil Capsules
Garlic Oil Capsules
Lecithin Capsules
Liqui-Cal Chewable Tablets
Melatonin Tablets

N'Odor Capsules

Nutr-E-Sol Capsules

Nutr-E-Sol Liquid

Sharkare Capsules

Squalene Capsules

Super Choline Capsules

Super EPA Capsules

AK PHARMA INC.
P.O. Box 111
Pleasantville, NJ 08232-0111

Direct Inquiries to:
(609) 645-5100
FAX: (609) 645-0767

Nutritional Products Available:
Prelief Granules

Prelief Tablets

ALPHARMA
U.S. Pharmaceuticals Division
7205 Windsor Blvd.
Baltimore, MD 21244

Direct Inquiries to:
(800) 638-9096

Nutritional Products Available:
Constulose Solution

Enulose Solution

ALRA LABORATORIES
3850 Clearview Court
Gurnee, IL 60031

Direct Inquiries to:
(800) 248-2572

Nutritional Products Available:
Cholac Syrup

Constilac Syrup

ALVIN LAST, INC.
425 Saw Mill River Road
Ardsley, NY 10502

Direct Inquiries to:
(914) 479-0900
FAX: (914) 479-0901
E-mail: last@alast.com
www.alast.com

Nutritional Products Available:
Born Again Vitamin E Oil

Revelation Powder

ALVITA TEA COMPANY
600 East Quality Drive
American Fork, UT 84003-3302

Direct Inquiries to:
(800) 258-4828
FAX: (801) 763-0789
www.alvita.com

Nutritional Products Available:
Chinese Green Tea Bags

Irish Moss Tea Bags

Melatonin Peppermint Tea
Bags

AMERICAN CHICLE GROUP
201 Tabor Road
Morris Plains, NJ 07950

Direct Inquiries to:
(973) 540-2000
FAX: (973) 540-5966

Nutritional Products Available:
Rolaids Chewable Tablets

AMERICAN PHARMACAL, INC.
1201 Douglas Avenue
Kansas City, KS 66103

Direct Inquiries to:
(800) 349-4923
FAX: (210) 349-9043

Nutritional Products Available:
Calcium Lactate Tablets

Calcium-600 w/D Tablets

DSS w/Iron Extended
Release Capsules

Ferrous Sulfate T.D.
Capsules

Ferrous Sulfate Tablets

Niacin Capsules

Niacin Tablets

Oyster Shell Calcium
Tablets

Oyster Shell Calcium/
Vitamin D Tablets

Vitamin C Capsules

Vitamin C Chewable
Tablets

Vitamin C Tablets

Vitamin C w/Rose Hips
Tablets

Vitamin E Capsules

Zinc Gluconate Tablets

AMERICAN REGENT LABORATORIES, INC.
Sub. of Luitpold Pharm. Inc.
One Luitpold Drive
Shirley, NY 11967

Direct Inquiries to:
(631) 924-4000
FAX: (631) 924-1731
www.luitpold.com

Nutritional Products Available:
Ascorbic Acid Injection

Calcium Chloride Injection

Calcium Gluconate
Injection

Dexferrum Injection

Magnesium Chloride
Injection

Magnesium Sulfate
Injection

AMIDE PHARMACEUTICALS
101 E. Main Street
Little Falls, NJ 07424

Direct Inquiries to:
(973) 890-1440
FAX: (973) 890-7980

Nutritional Products Available:
Multiret Folic-500
Extended Release Tablets

Vitacon Forte Tablets

Vitaplex Plus Tablets

Vitaplex Tablets

AMPHARCO, INC.
International Pharm. Distrib. Co.
9549 A. Bolsa Avenue
Westminster, CA 92683

Direct Inquiries to:
(714) 531-3560

Nutritional Products Available:
Becomax RX Tablets

Calfort Tablets

APOTHECARY PRODUCTS
11750 12th Avenue S.
Burnsville, MN 55337-1297

Direct Inquiries to:
(800) 328-2742
FAX: (800) 328-1584
www.pillminder@aol.com

Nutritional Products Available:
Bee Pollen Chewable
Tablets

Beta Carotene Capsules

Brewer's Yeast Tablets

Calcium 600 Tablets

Calcium Antacid Tablets

Charcoal Capsules

Choline Bitartrate Tablets

Cod Liver Oil Capsules

Coenzyme Q10 Capsules

Fish Oil Concentrate
Capsules

Folic Acid Tablets

Garlic Oil Capsules

Garlic Tablets

Kelp Natural Iodine Tablets

Melatonin Capsules

Niacin Time-Release
Capsules

Oyster Shell Calcium
Tablets

Rutin Tablets

Selenium Tablets

Shark Cartilage Capsules

Vitamin C Chewable
Tablets

Vitamin C Tablets

Vitamin C Timed-Release
Tablets

Vitamin E Capsules

Vitamin E Natural
Capsules

Wheat Germ Oil Capsules

Zinc Gluconate Tablets

APOTHECON
A Bristol-Myers Squibb
Company
P.O. Box 4500
Princeton, NJ 08543-4500

Direct Inquiries to:
(800) 321-1335
(609) 818-3737

Nutritional Products Available:

Niacin Tablets

Theragran Hematinic
Tablets

ASCHER, B.F. & CO., INC.
15501 West 109th Street
Lenexa, KS 66219-1308

Direct Inquiries to:
(800) 324-1880
(913) 888-1880
FAX: (913) 888-2250
Email: bfascher@msn.com
www.bfascher.com

Nutritional Products Available:

Tolfrinic Tablets

ASTRAZENECA LP
1800 Concord Pike
Wilmington, DE 19850-5437

Direct Inquiries to:
(800) 236-9933
www.astrazeneca-us.com

Nutritional Products Available:

Aquasol E Liquid

M.V.I. Pediatric Powder for
Injection

M.V.I.-12 Injection

AVENTIS PHARMACEUTICALS
P.O. Box 663
399 Interpace Parkway
Parsippany, NJ 07054

Direct Inquiries to:
(800) 207-8049
(800) 633-1610

Nutritional Products Available:

Cephulac Syrup

Chronulac Syrup

BALAN, J.J. INC.
5725 Foster Avenue
Brooklyn, NY 11234

Direct Inquiries to:
(800) 552-2526
FAX: (718) 251-0024

Nutritional Products Available:

Ferrous Gluconate Tablets

Niacin Capsules

Vitamin C Tablets

BASIC VITAMINS
P.O. Box 412
Vandalia, OH 45377

Direct Inquiries to:
(800) 782-2742
FAX: (937) 898-0500
www.basicvitamins.com

Nutritional Products Available:

Bee Pollen Tablets

Beta Carotene Tablets

Biotin Tablets

Brewer's Yeast Tablets

Calcium 500 w/Vitamin D
Tablets

Calcium 600 Tablets

Calcium 600/Vitamin D
Tablets

Calcium Citrate 950
Tablets

Chromium Picolinate
Tablets

Cod Liver Oil Capsules

Coenzyme Q10 Capsules

Folic Acid Tablets

Garlic Oil Capsules

Garlic Tablets

Iron Tablets

Kelp Tablets

Lecithin Capsules

Magnesium Oxide Tablets

Niacin Capsules

Niacin Tablets

Oyster Shell Calcium/
Vitamin D Tablets

Pantothenic Acid Tablets

Selenium Tablets

Vitamin C Capsules

Vitamin C Chewable
Tablets

Vitamin C Tablets

Vitamin C w/Rose Hips
Natural Tablets

Vitamin E Capsules

Vitamin E Natural
Capsules

Zinc Tablets

**BAUSCH & LOMB PHARMACEUTICAL,
INC.**
8500 Hidden River Parkway
Tampa, FL 33637

Direct Inquiries to:
(800) 323-0000
(813) 975-7700

Nutritional Products Available:

Ocuvite Lutein Capsules

**BAYER CORP., CONSUMER CARE
DIVISION**
P.O. Box 1910
36 Columbia Road
Morristown, NJ 07962-1910

Direct Inquiries to:
(800) 348-2240

Nutritional Products Available:
♦ Alka-Mints Chewable
Tablets G-3
♦ Bugs Bunny Complete
Children's Chewable
Tablets G-3

♦ Bugs Bunny Plus Extra C
   Chewable Tablets **G-3**
♦ Bugs Bunny Plus Iron
   Chewable Tablets **G-3**
♦ Fergon Tablets **G-3**
♦ Flintstones Complete
   Children's Chewable
   Tablets **G-3**
♦ Flintstones Original
   Children's Chewable
   Tablets **G-3**
♦ Flintstones Plus Calcium
   Chewable Tablets **G-3**
♦ Flintstones Plus Extra C
   Chewable Tablets **G-3**
♦ Flintstones Plus Iron
   Chewable Tablets **G-3**
♦ One-A-Day 50 Plus Tablets ... **G-3**
♦ One-A-Day Antioxidant
   Capsules **G-3**
   One-A-Day Bone Strength
   Tablets
♦ One-A-Day Calcium Plus
   Chewable Tablets **G-3**
♦ One-A-Day Essential
   Tablets **G-3**
♦ One-A-Day Kids Complete
   Chewable Tablets **G-3**
♦ One-A-Day Maximum
   Tablets **G-3**
♦ One-A-Day Men's Tablets **G-3**
♦ One-A-Day Women's
   Tablets **G-3**

BEDFORD LABORATORIES
A Division of Ben Venue
   Laboratories, Inc.
300 Northfield Road
Bedford, OH 44146

Direct Inquiries to:
(800) 562-4797
FAX: (440) 232-6242

Nutritional Products Available:
   Folic Acid Tablets

BERGEN BRUNSWIG DRUG COMPANY
4000 Metropolitan Drive
Orange, CA 92868

Direct Inquiries to:
(714) 385-4000
FAX: (714) 385-8830

Nutritional Products Available:
   Antacid Chewable Tablets
   Antacid Ultra Strength
      Chewable Tablets
   BEC w/Zinc Tablets
   Bee Pollen Natural Tablets
   Beta Carotene Capsules
   Brewer's Yeast Natural
      Tablets
   Calcium 500 Supplement
      Chewable Tablets
   Calcium 600/Vitamin D
      Tablets
   Calcium Citrate Tablets
   Calcium Citrate/Vitamin D
      Tablets
   Calcium Lactate Tablets
   Calcium Tablets
   Chromium Picolinate
      Tablets
   Cod Liver Oil Capsules
   Coenzyme Q10 Capsules
   Evening Primrose Oil
      Capsules
   Ferrous Sulfate Liquid
   Ferrous Sulfate Tablets
   Fish Oil Concentrate
      Capsules
   Folic Acid Tablets
   Garlic Capsules
   Garlic Oil Capsules
   Grape Seed Extract
      Capsules
   Green Tea Capsules
   Iodine Tincture
   Iron Carbonyl Tablets
   L-Lysine Natural Tablets
   Lecithin Natural Capsules
   Magnesium Tablets
   Melatonin Tablets
   Niacin Capsules
   Niacin Tablets
   Niacinamide Tablets
   Oyster Shell Calcium
      Tablets
   Oyster Shell Calcium/
      Vitamin D Tablets
   Therapeutic Multivitamin
      Tablets

   Vitamin C Liquid
   Vitamin C Natural
      Chewable Tablets
   Vitamin C Tablets
   Vitamin C w/Rose Hips
      Natural Tablets
   Vitamin E Capsules
   Vitamin E Natural
      Capsules
   Vitamin E Oil
   Vitamin E w/s Capsules
   Zinc Gluconate Lozenges
   Zinc Gluconate Tablets

BIO-TECH PHARMACAL, INC.
P.O. Box 1992
Fayetteville, AR 72702

Direct Inquiries to:
(800) 345-1199
FAX: (501) 443-5643

Nutritional Products Available:
   Arginine Capsules
   B-3-50 Tablets
   B-3-500-GR Tablets
   C-500-GR Tablets
   C-Max Tablets
   Cal-Citrate Capsules
   Cal-Citrate Tablets
   Cal-Co3Y Capsules
   Cal-Glu Capsule
   Cal-Lac Tablets
   Cal-Mincol Capsules
   Cu-5 Capsules
   DL-PA-500 Capsules
   E-400-Mixed Capsules
   E-Max-1000 Capsules
   FA-8 Tablets
   Fe-40 Tablets
   Glutamine Capsules
   Green Tea Rx Tablets
   Ornithine Capsules
   Panto-250 Tablets
   Vita-Min Rx Tablets
   Zincolate Capsules
   Zn-50 Tablets

BIOTHERAPIES USA INC.
9 Commerce Road
Fairfield, NJ 07004

Direct Inquiries to:
(800) 700-7325

Nutritional Products Available:

Cartilade Capsules

Genista Soy Protein
Powder

Soy Isoflavones Tablets

BLAINE PHARMACEUTICALS
1515 Production Drive
Burlington, KY 41005

Direct Inquiries to:
(800) 633-9353
(859) 283-9437
FAX: (859) 283-9460
www.blainepharma.com

Nutritional Products Available:

Mag-Ox 400 Tablets

Uro-Mag Capsules

BOCA PHARMACAL, INC.
6601 Lyons Road
Suite I-10
Coconut Creek, FL 33073

Direct Inquiries to:
(800) 354-8460
FAX: (954) 426-0828

Nutritional Products Available:

Vitamin E Aqueous Liquid

BOIRON USA
6 Campus Boulevard
Newtown Square, PA 19073

Direct Inquiries to:
(800) 264-7661
FAX: (610) 325-7480

Nutritional Products Available:

Arnica Pellets

Arnicalm Arthritis Pellets

Arnicalm Trauma Pellets

Oscillococcinum Tablets

BRAINTREE LABORATORIES, INC.
P.O. Box 850929
Braintree, MA 02185-0929

Direct Inquiries to:
(781) 843-2202

Nutritional Products Available:

Phoslo Tablets

BRECKENRIDGE PHARMACEUTICAL, INC.
P.O. Box 206
Boca Raton, FL 33429

Direct Inquiries to:
(800) 367-3395
(561) 367-8512
FAX: (561) 367-8107

Nutritional Products Available:

Calciquid Syrup

Ferocon Capsules

Ferrex 150 Forte Capsules

Ferrex PC Tablets

V-C Forte Capsules

BRISTOL-MYERS PRODUCTS
A Bristol-Myers Squibb
Company
345 Park Avenue
New York, NY 10154

Direct Inquiries to:
(800) 468-7746

Nutritional Products Available:

♦ Theragran-M Tablets **G-3**

CAMBRIDGE NUTRACEUTICALS
294 Washington Street
Suite 601
Boston, MA 02108

Direct Inquiries to:
(617) 695-1255

Nutritional Products Available:

Glutamine Powder

Glutamine Rapid Release
Formula Powder

CARDINAL HEALTH, INC.
5555 Glendon Court
Dublin, OH 43016

Direct Inquiries to:
(614) 757-5000

Nutritional Products Available:

Antacid Chewable Tablets

Antacid Extra Strength
Chewable Tablets

Calcium 600/Vitamin D
Tablets

Calcium Tablets

Calcium Citrate + D
Tablets

Calcium/Magnesium/Zinc
Tablets

Chromium Picolinate
Tablets

Ferrous Sulfate Tablets

Fiber Powder

Folic Acid Tablets

Garlic Capsules

Garlic Oil Natural Capsules

Grape Seed Extract
Capsules

Multivitamins w/Iron
Children's Chewable
Tablets

Niacin Capsules

Oyster Shell Calcium
Natural Tablets

Oyster Shell Calcium
Natural/Vit D Tablets

Selenium Tablets

Slow Release Iron Tablets

Stress Formula Tablets

Stress Formula + Iron
Tablets

Vitamin B-100 Natural
Tablets

Vitamin C Chewable
Tablets

Vitamin C Tablets

Vitamin C w/Rose Hips
Natural Tablets

Vitamin E Capsules

Vitamin E Natural
Capsules

Zinc Natural Tablets

J.R. CARLSON LABS, INC.
15 College Drive
Arlington Heights, IL 60004-1985

Direct Inquiries to:
(888) 234-5656
FAX: (847) 255-1605
E-mail: carlson@carlsonlabs.com
www.carlsonlabs.com

Nutritional Products Available:

Golden Primrose Capsules

L-Ornithine Powder

Liquid Bone Meal Capsules

Reguloid Powder

Soy Isoflavones Tablets

CELESTIAL SEASONINGS, INC.
4600 Sleepytime Drive
Boulder, CO 80301-3292

Direct Inquiries to:
(303) 530-5300
FAX: (303) 581-1294
www.celestialseasonings.com

Nutritional Products Available:

Authentic Green Tea Bags

Grape Seed Capsules

Green Tea Bags

Green Tea Capsules

CENTURY PHARMACEUTICALS, INC.
10377 Hague Road
Indianapolis, IN 46256

Direct Inquiries to:
(317) 849-4210
FAX: (317) 849-4263
E-mail:
info@centurypharmaceuticals.com
www.centurypharmaceuticals.com

Nutritional Products Available:

Ferrous Sulfate Tablets

CIRCLE PHARMACEUTICALS, INC.
4136 North Keystone Avenue
Indianapolis, IN 46205

Direct Inquiries to:
(317) 568-0392
FAX: (317) 377-1961

Nutritional Products Available:

Circavite T Tablets

COLGATE ORAL PHARMACEUTICALS, INC.
A subsidiary of Colgate-
Palmolive Company
One Colgate Way
Canton, MA 02021

Direct Inquiries to:
(800) 226-5428

Nutritional Products Available:

Luride Chewable Tablets

Luride Liquid

Phos-Flur Gel

Phos-Flur Solution

Prevident 5000 Plus Cream

Prevident Cream

Prevident Solution

Thera-Flur-N Gel

COMPUMED PHARMACEUTICALS INC.
1517 Edwards Avenue
New Orleans, LA 70123

Direct Inquiries to:
(800) 443-9218
(504) 733-4254
FAX: (504) 734-0432
www.compumedph.com

Nutritional Products Available:

Calcium Carbonate/Vitamin
D Tablets

CONSOLIDATED MIDLAND CORP.
20 Main Street
Brewster, NY 10509

Direct Inquiries to:
(845) 279-6108
FAX: (845) 279-6109

Nutritional Products Available:

Ascorbic Acid Injection

Ascorbic Acid Tablets

Calcium Chloride Solution
Injection

Calcium Gluconate
Injection

Calcium Gluconate Tablets

Calcium Lactate Tablets

Ferrous Fumarate Tablets

Ferrous Gluconate Tablets

Ferrous Sulfate Elixir

Ferrous Sulfate Liquid

Ferrous Sulfate Tablets

Folic Acid Tablets

Iodine Tincture

Magnesium Sulfate
Injection

Nicotinic Acid Tablets

Sodium Flouride Chewable
Tablets

Vitamin E Capsules

CONTRACT PHARMACAL CORPORATION
160 Commerce Drive
Hauppauge, NY 11788

Direct Inquiries to:
(631) 231-4610
FAX: (631) 231-4156

Nutritional Products Available:

B-Plex Tablets

Ferotrinsic Capsules

COVEX
Sector Oficios 33, 1-3
28760 Tres Cantos
Madrid, Spain

Direct Inquiries to:
34-91-804-4545
FAX: 34-91-804-3030
E-mail: vinpocetin@covex.es

Nutritional Products Available:

♦ Intelectol Tablets G-4

CYPRESS PHARMACEUTICAL INC.
135 Industrial Blvd.
Madison, MS 39110

Direct Inquiries to:
(800) 856-4393
FAX: (601) 853-1567

Nutritional Products Available:

APF Gel

Aquavit-E Liquid

Hematin Plus Tablets

Hematin-F Tablets

Mag-Gel 600 Capsules

Mag-SR Tablets

Magnesium Oxide Tablets

Prenafort Tablets

Vitamin C Liquid

D'FRANSSIA CORP
4635 Mission Gorge Place
Suite B
San Diego, CA 92120-4133

Direct Inquiries to:
(323) 461-3444
FAX: (323) 461-9403

Nutritional Products Available:

Desempacho Tablets

DAWN PHARMACEUTICALS INC.
4555 West Addison
Chicago, IL 60641

Direct Inquiries to:
(800) 745-3296
FAX: (773) 481-2411

Nutritional Products Available:

Ferrous Sulfate Tablets

DAYTON LABORATORIES, INC.
3307 N.W. 74th Avenue
Miami, FL 33122

Direct Inquiries to:
(800) 446-0255
FAX: (305) 477-6506
E-mail: dayton@daytonlab.com
www.daytonlab.com

Nutritional Products Available:

Irofol Tablets

DENISON PHARMACEUTICALS, INC.
P.O. Box 1305
60 Dunnell Lane
Pawtucket, RI 02860

Direct Inquiries to:
(401) 723-5500
FAX: (401) 725-9972

Nutritional Products Available:

Burow's Solution Powder

Iodine Decolorized Tincture

Iodine Tincture

DERMARITE INDUSTRIES LLC
168 East Main Street
Prospect Park, NJ 07508

Direct Inquiries to:
(973) 595-5599
FAX: (973) 595-0095

Nutritional Products Available:

Dermamed Ointment

DERMASCIENCES, INC.
214 Carnegie Center
Suite 100
Princeton, NJ 08540

Direct Inquiries to:
(800) 825-4325
FAX: (800) 825-4325

Nutritional Products Available:

Dermagran Ointment

DIXON-SHANE DRUG COMPANY
256 Geiger Road
Philadelphia, PA 19115

Direct Inquiries to:
(800) 262-7770
FAX: (215) 673-8054
www.dixonshane.com

Nutritional Products Available:

Calcium Gluconate Tablets

Calcium Lactate Tablets

Ferrous Sulfate Tablets

Niacin Capsules

Niacin Tablets

Oyster Shell Calcium
Tablets

Oyster Shell Calcium/
Vitamin D Tablets

Thera Hematinic Tablets

Vitamin C Capsules

Vitamin C Tablets

Vitamin E Capsules

Vitamin E Natural
Capsules

DREIR PHARMACEUTICALS, INC.
8479 East San Daniel Drive
Scotsdale, AZ 85258

Direct Inquiries to:
(480) 607-3584
FAX: (480) 607-0731
www.dreirpharmaceuticals.com

Nutritional Products Available:

Lozengesi-Flur Lozenge

EARTHRISE NUTRITIONALS
424 Payran Street
Petaluma, CA 94952

Direct Inquiries to:
(800) 949-7473
FAX: (707) 778-9028
www.Earthrise.com

Nutritional Products Available:

Chlorella Powder

Chlorella Tablets

Spirulina Capsules

Spirulina Tablets

Sun Chlorella Granules

ECONOLAB
P.O. Box 85543
Westland, MI 48185-0543

Direct Inquiries to:
(561) 391-5245
FAX: (561) 391-2349

Nutritional Products Available:

Calciquid Syrup

ECONOMED PHARMACEUTICALS, INC.
4305 Sartin Road
Burlington, NC 27217

Direct Inquiries to:
(800) 327-6007
FAX: (336) 227-3636

Nutritional Products Available:

C-Tym Capsules

Calbon Tablets

EDWARDS LIFESCIENCES RESEARCH MEDICAL, INC.
One Edwards Way
Irvine, CA 92614

Direct Inquiries to:
(800) 453-8432
FAX: (801) 565-6209
www.edwards.com

Nutritional Products Available:

Rimso-50 Tablets

EDWARDS PHARMACEUTICALS, INC.
111 Mulberry Street
Ripley, MS 38663

Direct Inquiries to:
(800) 543-9560
(662) 837-8182
FAX: (662) 837-1473

Nutritional Products Available:

Ed Cyte F Tablets

Ed-In-Sol Elixir

EDYN CORP.
Box 6261
Newark, NJ 07106-0261

Direct Inquiries to:
(973) 399-0995
FAX: (973) 364-0437

Nutritional Products Available:

Vitedyn-Slo Capsules

ELI LILLY AND COMPANY
Lilly Corporate Center
Indianapolis, IN 46285

Direct Inquiries to:
(800) 545-5979
(317) 276-2000

Nutritional Products Available:

Calcium Carbonate Tablets

ENZYMATIC THERAPY
825 Challenger Drive
Green Bay, WI 54311

Direct Inquiries to:
(800) 783-2286
E-mail: etmail@enzy.com
www.enzy.com

Nutritional Products Available:

Grape Seed Phytosome
Capsules

Soy Essentials Tablets

EON LABS MANUFACTURING, INC.
227-15 North Conduit Avenue
Laurelton, NY 11413

Direct Inquiries to:
(800) 526-0225
FAX: (718) 949-3120

Nutritional Products Available:

Ferrous Sulfate Tablets

Foltrin Capsules

EQUIPHARM CORP.
P.O. Box D3700
Pomona, NY 10970

Direct Inquiries to:
(914) 354-8787
FAX: (914) 354-8703

Nutritional Products Available:

Equi-Cyte F Tablets

Equi-Roca Plus Tablets

E.R.B.L. (EUROPEAN REFERENCE BOTANICAL LABORATORIES)
P.O. Box 131135
Carlsbad, CA 92013-1135

Direct Inquiries to:
(760) 599-6088
FAX: (760) 599-6089

Nutritional Products Available:

♦ Coromega Packets G-4

Ferro-DSS Extended
Release Tablets

ETHEX CORPORATION
10888 Metro Court
Maryland Heights, MO 63043-2413

Direct Inquiries to:
(800) 321-1705
FAX: (314) 567-0701

Nutritional Products Available:

Anemagen Capsules

Anemagen FA Capsules

Conison Capsules

Fe-Tinic 150 Forte
Capsules

Nutrinate Chewable Tablets

EVERETT LABORATORIES, INC.
29 Spring Street
West Orange, NJ 07052

Direct Inquiries to:
(973) 324-0200
FAX: (973) 324-0795

Nutritional Products Available:

Strovite Forte Tablets

Strovite Tablets

FEELING FINE COMPANY
13160 Mindanao Way
Suite 270
Marina Del Ray, CA 90292

Direct Inquiries to:
(310) 822-1331
FAX: (310) 822-2331

Nutritional Products Available:

Dr. Art Ulene's Vitamin
Formula Packets

FIELDING PHARMACEUTICAL COMPANY
P.O. Box 2186
11551 Adie Road
Maryland Heights, MO 63043

Direct Inquiries to:
(314) 567-5462

Nutritional Products Available:

Vitelle Irospan Extended
Release Tablets and
Extended Release
Capsules

Vitelle Nesentials Tablets

FLEMING & COMPANY
1600 Fenpark Drive
Fenton, MO 63026

Direct Inquiries to:
(636) 343-8200
FAX: (636) 343-8203
www.flemingcompany.com

Nutritional Products Available:

Magonate Liquid

Magonate Natal Liquid

Magonate Tablets

Marblen Suspension

Marblen Tablets

Nephrocaps Capsules

Nicotinex Elixir

FLUORITAB CORP.
8151 Brentwood Lane
Temperance, MI 48182-0507

Direct Inquiries to:
(734) 847-3985

Nutritional Products Available:

Flouritab Chewable Tablets

Flouritab Liquid

FOREST PHARMACEUTICALS, INC.
Subsidiary of Forest
Laboratories, Inc.
13600 Shoreline Drive
St. Louis, MO 63045

Direct Inquiries to:
(800) 678-1605

Nutritional Products Available:

Almora Tablets

Feostat Chewable Tablets

Feostat Suspension

FREEDA VITAMINS, INC.
36 E. 41st Street
New York, NY 10017

Direct Inquiries to:
(800) 777-3737
(212) 685-4980
FAX: (212) 685-7297

Nutritional Products Available:

Apple Pectin Tablets

Bromelain Tablets

C-Gram Tablets

Cal-Mint Tablets

Cal/Mag Chelated Tablets

Cal/Mag Chewable Tablets

Calcium Ascorbate Powder

Calcium Ascorbate Tablets

Calcium Carbonate
Chewable Tablets

Calcium Carbonate Powder

Calcium Chelated Tablets

Calcium Citrate Tablets

Calcium Gluconate Powder

Calcium Gluconate Tablets

Calcium Lactate Tablets

Calcium Pantothenate
Tablets

Calcium Phosphate Powder

Chlorophyll Tablets

Copper Tablets

D-Biotin Tablets

Dull-C Powder

Folic Acid Tablets

Fruit C Chewable Tablets

Garlic Tablets

L-Carnitine Tablets

L-Glutamine Powder

L-Glutamine Tablets

L-Lysine Tablets

L-Phenylalanine Tablets

L-Tyrosine Tablets

Liquid E Liquid

Lycopene Tablets

Magnesium Carbonate
Powder

Magnesium Gluconate
Tablets

Magnesium Oxide Powder

Niacin Tablets

Octacosanol Tablets

Parva-Cal 250 Tablets

Quercetin Tablets

Rutin Tablets

Vita-C Powder

Vitamin C Tablets

Vitamin C w/Rose Hips
Tablets

Vitamin E Mixed Tablets

Vitamin E Tablets

Zinc Chelated Tablets

Zinc Elemental Lozenges

Zinc Elemental Tablets

Zinc Gluconate Tablets

FREELIFE INTERNATIONAL
333 Quarry Road
Milford, CT 06460

Direct Inquiries to:
(800) 882-7240
www.freelife.com

Nutritional Products Available:

CholesteSoy Caplets

DHEA Ultra Tablets

Longest Living Acidophilus
Capsules

MSM Ultra Caplets

MSM Ultra Powder

Melatonin Ultra Tablets

FRONTIER
P.O. Box 299
Norway, IA 52318

Direct Inquiries to:
(800) 786-1388
FAX: (800) 717-4372

Nutritional Products Available:

Psyllium Husks Vegetarian
Capsules

Spirulina Powder

FUTUREBIOTICS
145 Ricefield Lane
Hauppauge, NY 11788

Direct Inquiries to:
(800) 367-5433
www.futurebiotics.com

Nutritional Products Available:

Barley Grass Tablets

Bovine Cartilage Capsules

Colloidal Silver Liquid

DHEA Capsules

Grape Seed Extract
Capsules

Green Tea Extract Tablets

Pycnogenol Capsules

Shark Cartilage Capsules

Zinc Lozenges

GENERAL NUTRITION CORP.
921-T Penn Avenue
Pittsburg, PA 15222

Direct Inquiries to:
(412) 288-4600
FAX: (412) 288-4743

Nutritional Products Available

Apple Pectin Tablets

Arginine Tablets

Brewer's Yeast Powder

Brewer's Yeast Tablets

Fingerprinted Chlorophyll
Capsules

Fingerprinted Spirulina
Capsules

Isolated Soy Protein
Powder

Modified Citrus Pectin
Tablets

T.J. Clark's Legendary
Colloidal Mineral
Formula Liquid

Tokyo Green Tea Bags

Wellness Colloidal Silver
Nasal Spray

GENEVA PHARMACEUTICALS, INC.
2655 West Midway Boulevard
P.O. Box 446
Broomfield, CO 80038-0446

Direct Inquiries to:
(800) 525-8747
(303) 466-2400
FAX: (303) 727-4656

Nutritional Products Available:

B-C w/Folic Acid Plus
Tablet

Contrin Capsules

Ferrous Sulfate Tablets

Niacin Capsules

GERI-CARE PHARMACEUTICALS
1650 63rd Street
Brooklyn, NY 11204

Direct Inquiries to:
(718) 382-5000
FAX: (718) 382-5001

Nutritional Products Available:

Ferrous Sulfate Tablets

GERITREX CORPORATION
2 East Sandford Boulevard
Mount Vernon, NY 10550-4510

Direct Inquiries to:
(914) 668-4003
FAX: (914) 668-4047
E-mail: geritrex@aol.com
www.geritrex.com

Nutritional Products Available:

Vitamin E Natural Liquid

GIL PHARMACEUTICAL CORPORATION
P.O. Box 1645
Ponce, PR 00733-1645

Direct Inquiries to:
(787) 848-9114
FAX: (787) 848-8459

Nutritional Products Available:

Protect Plus Capsules

Protect Plus Liquid

GLOBAL SOURCE MANAGEMENT & CONSULTING, INC.
5371 N. Hiatus Road
Sunrise, FL 33351-8718

Direct Inquiries to:
(954) 747-8977
FAX: (954) 747-8660

Nutritional Products Available:

Calcium Gluconate Tablets

HALSEY DRUG CO., INC.
695 North Perryville Road
Rockford, IL 61107

Direct Inquiries to:
(815) 399-2060
FAX: (815) 399-9710
www.halseydrug.com

Nutritional Products Available:

Iron Sol Elixir

HART HEALTH AND SAFETY
P.O. Box 94044
Seattle, WA 98124

Direct Inquiries to:
(800) 234-4278
FAX: (206) 431-9828

Nutritional Products Available:

Nutralox Chewable Tablets

HAWTHORN PHARMACEUTICALS
135 Industrial Blvd.
Madison, MS 39110

Direct Inquiries to:
(800) 856-4393
FAX: (601) 853-1567

Nutritional Products Available:

Icar-C Plus Tablets

Icar-C Tablets

HEALTH FROM THE SUN
P.O. Box 179
Newport Beach, NH 03773

Direct Inquiries to:
(800) 447-2249
FAX: (603) 763-9159
www.hfts.com

Nutritional Products Available:

Arkopharma Exolise Green
Tea Extract Capsules

Bee Pollen Power Extract
Liquid

Borage Liquid Gold Liquid

Borage Oil Gla 240
Capsules

Borage Seed Oil Capsules

Evening Primrose De
Luxe-Hexan Capsules

Evening Primrose Oil
Capsules

Maxilife Mega Soy
Capsules

Vanadyl Sulfate Tablets

Veg Evening Primrose Oil
Capsules

HEALTH PRODUCTS CORPORATION
1060 Nepperhan Avenue
Yonkers, NY 10703-1432

Direct Inquiries to:
(914) 423-2900

Nutritional Products Available:

Bee Pollen Tablets

Calcium Carbonate Tablets

Niacin Tablets

Oyster Shell Calcium
Tablets

Vitamin C Chewable
Tablets

Vitamin C Tablets

Vitamin C w/Rose Hips
Tablets

Vitamin E Capsules

Vitamin E DL Alpha
Capsules

Zinc Lozenges

Zinc Tablets

HEARTLAND HEALTHCARE SERVICES
4755 South Avenue
Toledo, OH 43615

Direct Inquiries to:
(800) 270-6351
FAX: (419) 535-5682

Nutritional Products Available:

Ascorbic Acid Tablets

Calcium Carbonate
Chewable Tablets

Calcium Carbonate Tablets

Calcium Carbonate/
Vitamin D Tablets

Ferrous Gluconate Tablets

Ferrous Sulfate Capsules

Ferrous Sulfate Elixir

Ferrous Sulfate Tablets

Folic Acid Tablets

Oyster Shell Calcium
Tablets

Vitamin E Capsules

HERB PHARM
P.O. Box 116
Williams, OR 97544

Direct Inquiries to:
(800) 599-2392
(541) 846-6262
FAX: (800) 545-7392
E-mail: Herbpharm@aol.com
www.herb-pharm.com

Nutritional Products Available:

Proanthodyn Grape Seed
Extract Tablets

**HERITAGE CONSUMER PRODUCTS,
LLC**
246 Federal Road
Suite CL-41
Brookfield, CT 06804

Direct Inquiries to:
(800) 797-7969
FAX: (203) 740-8005

Nutritional Products Available:

Chooz Tablets

HILLESTAD PHARMACEUTICALS, INC.
178 U.S. Highway 51 North
P.O. Box 1700
Woodruff, WI 54568

Direct Inquiries to:
(800) 535-7742
(715) 358-2113
FAX: (715) 358-7812
E-mail: hill@newnorth.net

Nutritional Products Available:

Dialyvite Tablets

HI-TECH PHARMACAL CO., INC.
369 Bayview Avenue
Amityville, NY 11701-2801

Direct Inquiries to:
(631) 789-8228
FAX: (516) 789-8429
E-mail: hitechpharm.com

Nutritional Products Available:

Calcionate Syrup

Ferrous Sulfate Elixir

Ferrous Sulfate Liquid

Sodium Fluoride Solution

Vitamin C Liquid

HUMCO
7400 Alumax Drive
Texarkana, TX 75501

Direct Inquiries to:
(800) 662-3435
FAX: (903) 831-7736

Nutritional Products Available:

Ascorbic Acid Granules

Burow's Solution

Dewee's Carminative
Liquid

HYREX PHARMACEUTICALS
3494 Democrat Road
P.O. Box 18385
Memphis, TN 38181-0385

Direct Inquiries to:
(800) 238-5282
FAX: (901) 794-9051

Nutritional Products Available:

B-Ject-100 Injection

Calcium Gluconate
Injection

Key-Plex Injection

Vitamin B Complex 100
Injection

INNOVATIVE HEALTH PRODUCTS, INC.
695 Bryan Dairy Road
Largo, FL 33777

Direct Inquiries to:
(800) 654-2347
FAX: (727) 544-4386

Nutritional Products Available:

Mega-Multi Capsules

INVERNESS MEDICAL, INC.
200 Prospect Street
Waltham, MA 02453

Direct Inquiries to:
(800) 899-7353
FAX: (781) 647-3939

Nutritional Products Available:

Ferro-Sequels Extended
    Release Tablets

Posture Tablets

**JOHNSON & JOHNSON • MERCK
CONSUMER PHARMACEUTICALS CO.**
7050 Camp Hill Road
Ft. Washington, PA 19034

Direct Inquiries to:
(800) 469-5268

Nutritional Products Available:

Alternagel Suspension

Mylanta Calci Tabs Extra
    Strength

Mylanta Calci Tabs Ultra
    Chewable Tablets

Mylanta Children's
    Chewable Tablets

KAL, INC.
1104-T Country Hills Drive
Ogden, UT 84403

Direct Inquiries to:
(801) 626-4900
FAX: (801) 621-2961

Nutritional Products Available:

Apple Pectin Tablets

Argentine Liver
    Concentrate Capsules

Bovine Cartilage Capsules

Brewer's Yeast High
    Potency Tablets

Charcoal Capsules

Chlorella Tablets

Chlorophyll Tablets

Cod Liver Oil Capsules

D-Ribose Powder

Dolomite Powder

Green Tea Extract Capsules

L-Lysine Capsules

Modified Citrus Pectin
    Powder

Pycnogenol Capsules

Rutin Tablets

Shark Cartilage Tablets

KEENE PHARMACEUTICALS, INC.
303 S. Mockingbird Street
P.O. Box 7
Keene, TX 76059

Direct Inquiries to:
(800) 541-0530
FAX: (817) 517-5435

Nutritional Products Available:

Vicam Injection

KENWOOD THERAPEUTICS
Div. of Bradley Pharm., Inc.
383 Route 46 West
Fairfield, NJ 07004-2402

Direct Inquiries to:
(800) 929-9300
(973) 882-1505
FAX: (973) 575-5366
E-mail:
    bradpharm@worldnet.att.net
www.bradpharm.com

Nutritional Products Available:

Glutofac-ZX Capsules

Ircon Tablets

Ircon-FA Tablets

KENYON DRUG CO., INC.
207 2nd Avenue S.W.
Cedar Rapids, IA 52404

Direct Inquiries to:
(800) 553-7907
FAX: (319) 363-9132

Nutritional Products Available:

Ken-Zinc Lozenges

THE KEY COMPANY
P.O. Box 220370
1313 W. Essex Avenue
St. Louis, MO 63122

Direct Inquiries to:
(800) 325-9592
(314) 965-6699
FAX: (314) 965-7629

Nutritional Products Available:

Alph-E Capsules

Alph-E-Mixed Capsules

Asco-Caps Capsules

Asco-Tabs-1000 Tablets

Ascocid Powder

Ascocid Tablets

Ascocid-500-D Tablets

Cal-C-Caps Capsules

Cal-Cee Tablets

Cal-G Capsules

Cal-Lac Capsules

Calcimin-300 Tablets

Calcium & Magnesium
    Chelate Capsules

Calcium-600 Tablets

Chew-C Chewable Tablets

Coppermin Tablets

DI-Phen-500 Capsules

Ex-L Tablets

Fibro-XI Capsules

Folacin-800 Tablets

Germanium Forte Tablets

Kelp-Tabs

L-Ornithine Capsules

Lipo-Caps Capsules

Liqua-Cal Capsules

Magimin Tablets

Magimin-Forte Tablets

Magnacaps Capsules

Quest Soy Protein Powder

Spirulina Crystal Flakes

Taurine Capsules

Tyrosine Capsules

Zinc-15 Tablets

Zinc-50 Tablets

Zinimin Tablets

KIRKMAN LABORATORIES, INC.
P.O. Box 1009
Wilsonville, OR 97070-1009

Direct Inquiries to:
(503) 694-1600
FAX: (503) 682-0838
E-mail:
    kirkman@kirkmanlabs.com
www.kirkmanlabs.com

Nutritional Products Available:

Flura-Loz Chewable
    Tablets

KONSYL PHARMACEUTICALS
4200 South Hulen
Fort Worth, TX 76109

Direct Inquiries to:
(800) 356-6795
(817) 763-8011
FAX: (817) 731-9389
www.konsyl.com

Nutritional Products Available:

Konsyl Powder

Konsyl-D Powder

KOS PHARMACEUTICALS, INC.
1001 Brickell Bay Drive
25th Floor
Miami, FL 33131

Direct Inquiries to:
(888) 4-LIPIDS
(888) 454-7437

Nutritional Products Available:
Niaspan Tablets

KRAMER-NOVIS
P.O. Box 191775
San Juan, PR 00919-1775

Direct Inquiries to:
(787) 767-2072
FAX: (787) 767-7281

Nutritional Products Available:
Bromanase Tablets

LANE LABS-USA, INC.
100 Commerce Drive
Allendale, NJ 07401

Direct Inquiries to:
(201) 236-9090

Nutritional Products Available:
♦ AdvaCal Capsules **G-4**
Advanced Shark Cartilage
From Japan Powder
Benefin Shark Cartilage
Tablets

LASER, INC.
P.O. Box 905
2200 W. 97th Place
Crown Point, IN 46308

Direct Inquiries to:
(219) 663-1165

Nutritional Products Available:
Fumatinic Extended
Release Capsules

LEDERLE CONSUMER HEALTH
A Division of Whitehall-Robins
Healthcare
Five Giralda Farms
Madison, NJ 07940

Direct Inquiries to:
(800) 282-8805

Nutritional Products Available:
Caltrate 600 Tablets
Caltrate 600 + D Tablets

LEDERLE STANDARD PRODUCTS
P.O. Box 41502
Philadelphia, PA 19101

Direct Inquiries to:
(800) 934-5556
(610) 688-4400

Nutritional Products Available:
Folic Acid Injection

LEE PHARMACEUTICALS
P.O. Box 3836
1434 Santa Anita Avenue
South El Monte, CA 91733-3312

Direct Inquiries to:
(800) 950-5337
FAX: (626) 442-6994

Nutritional Products Available:
Cevi-Bid Tablets
Thex Forte Tablets

LEMAX PHARMACEUTICAL CORP.
6915 S.W. 92 CT.
Miami, FL 33173

Direct Inquiries to:
(305) 598-2333
FAX: (305) 596-9314

Nutritional Products Available:
Pellets C Capsules

**LEX PHARMACEUTICALS MFG. &
PACKAGING**
7155 N.W. 77th Terrace
Medley, FL 33166

Direct Inquiries to:
(305) 888-7375
FAX: (305) 883-8328

Nutritional Products Available:
Iodine Decolorized Tincture
Iodine Tincture
Maglex Tablets
Oyster Shell Calcium
Tablets
Vitamin C Tablets
Vitamin E Capsules
Zinc Gluconate Tablets

LORANN OILS
P.O. Box 22009
Lansing, MI 48909

Direct Inquiries to:
(800) 248-1302
FAX: (517) 882-0507

Nutritional Products Available:
Ascorbic Acid Powder

LUNSCO, INC.
4657 Wurno Road
Pulaski, VA 24301

Direct Inquiries to:
(800) 624-8614
(540) 980-4358
FAX: (540) 980-4484
E-mail: lunsco@i-plus.net

Nutritional Products Available:
Fetrin Extended Release
Capsules

3M HEALTH CARE
Bldg. 304-1-01
St. Paul, MN 55144-1000

Direct Inquiries to:
(800) 537-2191
(651) 733-2882

Nutritional Products Available:
Titralac Chewable Tablets
Titralac Extra Strength
Chewable Tablets

3M PHARMACEUTICALS
3M Center 275-2E-13
P.O. Box 33275
St. Paul, MN 55133-3275

Direct Inquiries to:
(800) 328-0255
(651) 736-4930
www.3M.com/pharma

Nutritional Products Available:
Alu-Cap Capsules

MAJOR PHARMACEUTICALS
31778 Enterprise Drive
Livonia, MI 48150

Direct Inquiries to:
(800) 875-0123
FAX: (734) 762-9730

Nutritional Products Available:
Antacid Chewable Tablets
Bee Pollen Tablets
Brewer's Yeast Powder
Calcitrate Tablets
Calcium Antacid Extra
Strength Chewable
Tablets
Calcium Antacid Ultra
Strength Chewable
Tablets
Calcium Carbonate
Chewable Tablets
Calcium Carbonate/
Vitamin D Tablets
Calcium Chewable Tablets
Calcium Lactate Tablets

Chewable Calcium
  Capsules
Evening Primrose Capsules
Ferosul Tablets
Ferrous Sulfate Elixir
Ferrous Sulfate Tablets
Folic Acid Tablets
Formula B Plus Tablets
Formula B Tablets
Iron-Folic 500 Tablets
L-Arginine Tablets
Liquid Calcium Capsules
Mag Delay Tablets
Magnesium Oxide Tablets
Niacin Capsules
Niacin Tablets
Oat Bran Tablets
Oyster Shell Calcium
  Tablets
Oyster Shell Calcium/
  Vitamin D Tablets
Pantothenic Acid Tablets
Sodium Fluoride Chewable
  Tablets
Ultra Tabs Tablets
Vicap Forte Tablets
Vitamin C Chewable
  Tablets
Vitamin C Tablets
Vitamin C w/Rose Hips
  Tablets
Vitamin E Capsules
Vitamin E Oil
Zinc Gluconate Lozenges
Zinc Gluconate Tablets

MANNE
P.O. Box 825
Johns Island, SC 29457

Direct Inquiries to:
(803) 768-4080
FAX: (216) 452-4692

Nutritional Products Available:
  Magnesium Oxide Tablets

A.G. MARIN PHARMACEUTICAL
1730 N.W. 79th Avenue
Miami, FL 33126

Direct Inquiries to:
(305) 593-5333
FAX: (305) 593-8333

Nutritional Products Available:
  Siderol Pediatric Tablets
  Support 500 Capsules
  Support Liquid

MARLEX PHARMACEUTICALS, INC.
50 McCullough Drive
Southgate Center
New Castle, DE 19720

Direct Inquiries to:
(302) 328-3355
FAX: (302) 328-6968

Nutritional Products Available:
  Ascorbic Acid Tablets
  Calcium Carbonate Tablets
  Calcium Gluconate Tablets
  Daily Multiple Vitamins
    Tablets
  Ferrous Sulfate Tablets
  Folic Acid Tablets
  Marlbee w/C Capsules
  Niacin Capsules
  Niacin Tablets
  Trinsicon Capsules
  Vitamin E Capsules
  Vitamins w/Iron Children's
    Chewable Tablets
  Zinc Gluconate Tablets

MARLOP PHARMACEUTICALS, INC.
230 Marshall Street
Elizabeth, NJ 07206

Direct Inquiries to:
(908) 355-8854
FAX: (908) 355-1419

Nutritional Products Available:
  Calcio Del Mar Tablets
  Martinic Capsules
  Promar Capsules

MARNEL PHARMACEUTICALS, INC.
206 Luke Drive
Lafayette, LA 70506

Direct Inquiries to:
(318) 232-1396
FAX: (318) 232-1491
E-mail:
  marnelpharm@worldnet.att.net

Nutritional Products Available:
  Bacmin Tablets

MASON VITAMINS, INC.
5105 N.W. 159th Street
Miami Lakes, FL 33014

Direct Inquiries to:
(800) 327-6005
FAX: (800) 328-3944
www.masonvitamins.com

Nutritional Products Available:
  Bee Pollen Tablets
  Brewer's Yeast Tablets
  C500 Capsules
  C500 Plus Rose Hips/
    Bioflavonoids Tablets
  C1000 Ascorbic Acid
    Tablets
  C1000 Plus Rose Hips/
    Bioflavonoids Tablets
  C1000 Tablets
  C1500 Plus Rose Hips/
    Bioflavonoids Tablets
  Calcium 500 Chewable
    Tablets
  Calcium 500 w/Vitamin D
    Tablets
  Calcium Antacid Chewable
    Tablets
  Calcium Citrate w/Vitamin D
    Tablets
  Calcium Gluconate
    Chewable Tablets
  Calcium Lactate Tablets
  Charcoal Capsules
  DL-Alpha Tocopheryl E400
    Capsules
  E1000 D-Alpha Capsules
  Evening Primrose Oil
    Capsules
  Ferrous Gluconate Tablets
  Ferrous Sulfate Tablets
  Folic Acid Tablets
  Glucomannan Capsules
  Iron Tablets
  L-Arginine Tablets
  L-Glutamine Tablets
  L-Ornithine Capsules
  L-Phenylalanine Capsules
  Liquid Calcium Plus
    Vitamin D Capsules
  Magnesium Tablets
  Niacin Capsules
  Niacin Tablets
  Oat Bran Tablets

Oyster Shell Calcium 1000/
   Vitamin D Tablets
Oyster Shell Calcium
   Tablets
Oyster Shell Calcium/
   Vitamin D Tablets
Pantothenic Acid Tablets
Royal Jelly Capsules
Super Calcium Extra
   Strength Chewable
   Tablets
Super Calcium Tablets
Super Calcium w/Vitamin D
   Tablets
Vitamin C Chewable
   Tablets
Vitamin C Plus Rose Hips
   Tablets
Vitamin C Tablets
Vitamin C500 Plus Tablets
Vitamin E Capsules
Vitamin E D-Alpha
   Capsules
Vitamin E DL-Alpha
   Capsules
Vitamin E Mixed Capsules
Vitamin E Oil
Zinc Gluconate Tablets
Zinc Lozenges
Zinc Picolinate Tablets

MATRIX HEALTH PRODUCTS INC.
8400 Magnolia Avenue, Suite N
Santee, CA 92071

Direct Inquiries to:
(800) 736-5609
FAX: (619) 448-2995
www.matrixhealth.com

Nutritional Products Available:
♦ Earth's Bounty Noni Caps **G-4**
♦ Earth's Bounty Noni Juice ... **G-4**
♦ Longevitrol Spray **G-4**

MCGUFF CO.
3524 West Lake Center Drive
Santa Ana, CA 92704

Direct Inquiries to:
(800) 854-7220
FAX: (714) 540-5614

Nutritional Products Available:
Ascorbic Acid Injection

Calcium Gluconate
   Injection
Dimethyl Sulfoxide
   Injection
Folic Acid Tablets
Magnesium Chloride
   Injection
Magnesium Sulfate
   Injection
Niacin Tablets
Vitamin B Complex 100
   Injection
Vitamin B Complex w/
   Vitamin C & B12
   Injection
Vitamin C Granules
Vitamin C Powder
Vitamin C w/Rose Hips
   Capsules
Zinc Chelated Tablets

MCKESSON DRUG COMPANY
One Post Street
San Francisco, CA 94104-5296

Direct Inquiries to:
(415) 983-8300
FAX: (415) 983-7160

Nutritional Products Available:
Antacid Extra Strength
   Tablets
Antacid Tablets
Calcium 600 Capsules
Calcium Tablets
Calcium/Vitamin D Tablets
Folic Acid Tablets
Iodine Tincture
Niacin Tablets
Oyster Shell Calcium
   Capsules
Oyster Shell Calcium
   Tablets
Oyster Shell Calcium/
   Vitamin D Tablets
Vitamin C Chewable
   Tablets
Vitamin C Tablets
Vitamin C w/Rose Hips
   Tablets
Vitamin E Capsules
Vitamin E Natural
   Capsules

MCNEIL CONSUMER HEALTHCARE
Division of McNeil-PPC, Inc.
Camp Hill Road
Fort Washington, PA 19034

Direct Inquiries to:
(215) 273-7000

Nutritional Products Available:
♦ Lactaid Tablets and Drops **G-4**

ME PHARMACEUTICALS
Div. of Vesco, Inc.
2800 S.E. Pkwy., Box 565
Richmond, IN 47374

Direct Inquiries to:
(765) 962-4410
FAX: (765) 966-5158

Nutritional Products Available:
Myferon 150 Forte
   Capsules

MEAD JOHNSON & COMPANY
A Bristol-Myers Squibb
   Company
2400 W. Lloyd Expressway
Evansville, IN 47721-0001

Direct Inquiries to:
(812) 429-5599

Nutritional Products Available:
Fer-In-Sol Liquid
Viactiv Chewable Tablets

THE MEDICINE SHOPPE
1100 North Lindbergh
St. Louis, MO 63132

Direct Inquiries to:
(800) 325-1397
(314) 993-6000
FAX: (314) 872-5500

Nutritional Products Available:
Calcium Antacid Chewable
   Tablets
Calcium Antacid Extra
   Strength Chewable
   Tablets
Calcium Formula Tablets
Magnesium Tablets
Niacin Tablets
Oyster Shell Calcium 500
   Tablets
Oyster Shell Calcium 500
   w/D Tablets
Oyster Shell Calcium
   Tablets

Vitamin C Chewable
Tablets
Vitamin C Tablets
Vitamin C w/Rose Hips
Tablets
Vitamin E Capsules
Vitamin E Natural Blend
Capsules

MEDIREX, INC.
20 Chapin Road, Unit H
P.O. Box 731
Pine Brook, NJ 07058

Direct Inquiries to:
(800) 343-3848
FAX: (973) 227-0779

Nutritional Products Available:
Ascorbic Acid Tablets
Ferrous Gluconate Tablets
Ferrous Sulfate Tablets
Folic Acid Tablets
Oyster Shell Calcium
Tablets
Vitaplex Tablets

MERICON INDUSTRIES, INC.
8819 N. Pioneer Road
Peoria, IL 61615-1561

Direct Inquiries to:
(800) 242-6464
FAX: (309) 693-2158
E-mail: monocal@aol.com

Nutritional Products Available:
Florical Capsules
Florical Tablets
Monocal Tablets
Zinc Lozenges
Zinc Tablets

MERIT PHARMACEUTICALS
2611 San Fernando Road
Los Angeles, CA 90065

Direct Inquiries to:
(800) 421-9657
(323) 227-4833

Nutritional Products Available:
Ascorbic Acid Injection
Chloromag Injection
Ferrous Sulfate Tablets
Mega-C Tablets
Mega-C/A Plus Injection
Ortho/CS Injection
Sulfa-Mag Injection

Vitamin C Injection

MERZ PHARMACEUTICALS
Division of Merz, Inc.
P.O. Box 18806
4215 Tudor Lane (27410)
Greensboro, NC 27419

Direct Inquiries to:
(336) 856-2003
FAX: (336) 856-0107

Nutritional Products Available:
Nu-Iron Plus Elixir

MET-RX
17861 Von Karman Avenue
Irvine, CA 92614-6213

Direct Inquiries to:
(800) 92-met-rx
FAX: (949) 955-3705

Nutritional Products Available:
Andros (4-Androstenedione)
Capsules
HMB Capsules
Pyruvate Capsules

MILLER PHARMACAL GROUP INC.
350 Randy Road, Unit 2
Carol Stream, IL 60188

Direct Inquiries to:
(630) 871-9557

Nutritional Products Available:
Calcium Ascorbate Liquid
Calcium Ascorbate Powder
Cemill 500 Tablets
Cemill 1000 Tablets
Elite Magnesium Capsules
Formula E 400 Capsules
Glutathione Tablets
L-Phenylalanine Capsules
L-Tyrosine Capsules
M2 Calcium Tablets
M2 Magnesium Capsules
M2 Zinc 50 Capsules
Taurine Tablets
Zinc Aspartate Tablets
Zn Plus Protein Tablets

MISSION PHARMACAL COMPANY
10999 IH 10 West, Suite 1000
San Antonio, TX 78230-1355

Direct Inquiries to:
(800) 292-7364
(210) 696-8400
FAX: (210) 696-6010

Nutritional Products Available:
Calcet Tablets
Citracal + D Tablets
Citracal Economy Tablets
Citracal Tablets
Iromin-G Tablets
Magtrate Tablets
Stress B Complex with
Vitamin C Tablets

MLO PRODUCTS
2351 N. Watney Way, Suite C
Fairfield, CA 94533

Direct Inquiries to:
(800) 228-4MLO
E-mail: sales@mloproducts.com
www.mloproducts.com

Nutritional Products Available:
Hard Body BCAA Powder

MORTON GROVE PHARMACEUTICALS
6451 W. Main Street
Morton Grove, IL 60053

Direct Inquiries to:
(800) 346-6854

Nutritional Products Available:
Acidulated Phosphate
Fluoride Liquid
Ferrous Sulfate Elixir
Ferrous Sulfate Liquid
Lithium Citrate Syrup

MYLAN PHARMACEUTICALS INC.
P.O. Box 4310
781 Chestnut Ridge Road
Morgantown, WV 26504-4310

Direct Inquiries to:
(877) 446-3679
(304) 599-2595

Nutritional Products Available:
Lactulose Solution

NATIONAL VITAMIN COMPANY, INC.
2075 West Scranton Avenue
Porterville, CA 93257-8358

Direct Inquiries to:
(800) 538-5828
FAX: (209) 781-8878

Nutritional Products Available:
Bee Pollen Capsules
Beta Carotene Capsules
C Complex Tablets

Calcium 500 Chewable
Tablets
Calcium Carbonate Tablets
Calcium Carbonate/Vitamin
D Tablets
Calcium Citrate Tablets
Calcium Lactate Tablets
Chromium Picolinate
Capsules
Cod Liver Oil Capsules
Evening Primrose Oil
Capsules
Ferrous Gluconate Tablets
Folic Acid Tablets
Garlic Capsules
Lecithin Capsules
Life-Line Co-Co Bear
Chewable Tablets
Lysine Tablets
Magnesium Elemental
Tablets
Nature's Blend Coenzyme
Q10 Capsules
Nature's Blend DHEA
Tablets
Nature's Blend
Glucosamine Sulfate
Capsules
Nature's Blend Royal Jelly
Capsules
Nature's Blend Shark
Cartilage Capsules
Niacin Tablets
Oat Bran Chewable Tablets
Oyster Shell Calcium
Tablets
Oyster Shell Calcium/
Vitamin D Tablets
PABA Tablets
Pantothenic Acid Tablets
Vitamin C Capsules
Vitamin C Chewable
Tablets
Vitamin C Powder
Vitamin C Tablets
Vitamin C w/Rose Hips
Tablets
Vitamin E Capsules
Vitamin E MTC Capsules
Vitamin E Oil

Vitamin E Water Soluble
Capsules
Vitamin E400 D Alpha
Capsules
Zinc Gluconate Tablets
Zinc Lozenges

NATROL
21411 Prairie Street
Chatsworth, CA 91311

Direct Inquiries to:
(800) 326-1520
www.natrol.com

Nutritional Products Available:
5-HTP Capsules
Alpha Lipoic Acid
Capsules
Beta Glucan Capsules
Beta Sitosterol Tablets
Bio-Cell Collagen Tablets
Bovine Cartilage Capsules
Calcium Cocoa Chewable
Calcium Pyruvate Capsules
China Chlorella Tablets
Chitosan Capsules
Chondroitin Sulfate
Capsules
CoQ10 Capsules
Collagen II Tablets
Creatine Powder
DHEA Tablets
Evening Primrose Oil
Capsules
Flax Seed Oil Capsules
Glucomannan Capsules
Grape Seed Extract
Capsules
Green Tea Bags
Green Tea Capsules
Green Tea Extract Liquid
L-Carnitine Capsules
Lycopene Tablets
MSM Capsules
Magnesium Tablets
Melatonin Tablets
My Favorite Borage Oil
Capsules
My Favorite Evening
Primrose Oil Capsules
Oat Bran Tablets

Oats Extract Liquid
PC Soy Isoflavones
Pycnogenol Capsules
Pyruvate Capsules
Resveratrol Capsules
SAMe Tablets
Shark Cartilage Tablets
Soy Protein Powder
Thera-Zinc Lozenges
Tototrien-All Capsules
Vitamin E Capsules

NATURAL BALANCE, INC.
3155 N. Commerce Court
Castle Rock, Colorado 80104

Direct Inquiries to:
(800) 833-8737
www.naturalbalance.com

Nutritional Products Available:
5-HTP Capsules
AndroMax Capsules
Chitosan Capsules
Creatine Capsules
Huperzine Capsules
MSM Tablets
PS Capsules
Pyruvate Capsules

NATURALIFE CORPORATION
10 Mountain Springs Parkway
Springville, UT 84663

Direct Inquiries to:
(800) 531-3233
FAX: (800) 489-3302

Nutritional Products Available:
Bee Pollen Premium
Capsules
Original Primrose For
Women Capsules

NATURE'S ANSWER
320 Oser Avenue
Hauppauge, NY 11788

Direct Inquiries to:
(800) 439-2324
(516) 231-7492
FAX: (516) 951-2499
www.naturesanswer.com

Nutritional Products Available:
Bee Propolis Tablets
Evening Primrose Oil
Capsules
Glucosamine Liquid

Green Tea Extract Liquid

Lycopene Drops

♦ Lycopene Liquid G-4

♦ Maitake Bio-Beta-Glucan
   Liquid G-4

Oats Extract Liquid

Propolis Alcohol Free
   Liquid

Propolis Drops

♦ Soy & Red Clover
   Isoflavones Liquid G-4

NATURE'S BOUNTY, INC.
90 Orville Drive
Bohemia, NY 11716

Direct Inquiries to:
(631) 567-9500
FAX: (631) 244-2136

Nutritional Products Available:

Bee Pollen Chewable
   Tablets

Biotin Tablets

Brewer's Yeast Tablets

C250 Chewable Tablets

C250 w/Rose Hips Tablets

C500 Capsules

C500 w/Rose Hips Tablets

C1000 Tablets

C1500 Tablets

Calcium 600 Plus
   Vitamin D Tablets

Calcium 600 Tablets

Calcium Citrate Tablets

Chromium Picolinate
   Tablets

Cod Liver Oil Capsules

Coenzyme Q10 Capsules

Daily Calcium +
   Vitamin D Tablets

Dolomite Tablets

E100 Capsules

E200 Capsules

E400 Capsules

E1000 Capsules

EPA Fish Oil Capsules

Evening Primrose Oil
   Capsules

Ferro-Caps Capsules

Ferrous Sulfate Tablets

Folic Acid Tablets

Garlic Extract Tablets

Garlic Oil Capsules

Glucosamine Sulfate
   Capsules

Grapeseed Extract Capsules

Inositol Tablets

Iron Tablets

Iron w/Docusate Sodium
   Extended Release Tablets

Kelp Tablets

L-Carnitine Capsules

L-Carnitine Liquid

L-Lysine Tablets

Lecithin Granules

Magnesium Chelated
   Tablets

Magnesium Tablets

Niacin Capsules

Niacin Tablets

Oat Bran Tablets

Oyster Shell Calcium
   Tablets

Oystercal 500 Tablets

Oystercal-D 250 Tablets

Oystercal-D 500 Tablets

Pantothenic Acid Tablets

Primrose Oil Capsules

Pure Vitamin C-Crystals
   Powder

Pycnogenol Capsules

Royal Brittany Evening
   Primrose Oil Capsules

Royal Jelly Capsules

Shark Cartilage Capsules

Soy Protein Powder

Vitamin C Buffered Tablets

Vitamin C Tablets

Vitamin C w/Rose Hips
   Liquid

Vitamin C500 Chewable
   Tablets

Vitamin E Cream

Vitamin E Lotion

Vitamin E Oil

Zinc Chelated Tablets

Zinc Gluconate Tablets

NATURE'S CODE
QVC, Inc.
Studio Park
1200 Wilson Drive
West Chester, PA 19380

Direct Inquiries to:
(800) 345-1515

Nutritional Products Available:

♦ Nutritional System For
   Men Over 50 . . . . G-4

♦ Nutritional System For
   Men Under 50 . . . . G-4

♦ Nutritional System For
   Women Over 50 . . . . G-4

♦ Nutritional System For
   Women Under 50 . . . . G-4

♦ Nutritional System Mix For
   Men Over 50 . . . . G-4

♦ Nutritional System Mix For
   Women Over 50 . . . . G-4

NATURE'S HERBS
150 Motor Parkway
Hauppauge, NY 11788

Direct Inquiries to:
(516) 467-3140
www.naturesherbs.com

Nutritional Products Available:

Barley Grass Capsules

Bee Pollen Capsules

Beta Sitosterol Capsules

Borage Power Capsules

Charcoal Activated
   Capsules

Chloraid Internal Deodorant
   Capsules

Chlorella Capsules

Curcumin-Power Capsules

Grape Seed Phytosome
   Capsules

Grape Seed Power
   Capsules

Green Tea Power Caffeine
   Free Capsules

Green Tea Power Capsules

Modified Citrus Pectin
   Power Capsules

Primrose Power Capsules

Propolis Plus Capsules

Propolis Ultra Mega
   Capsules

Psyllium Seed Capsules

Pycnogenol Plus Tablets

Pycnogenol Power
   Standardized Capsules

NATURE'S PLUS
548 Broadhollow Road
Melville, NY 11747-3708

Direct Inquiries to:
(631) 293-0030
FAX: (631) 293-0349
E-mail: Info@naturesplus.com
www.naturesplus.com

Nutritional Products Available:
Apple Pectin Tablets

Bee Pollen Tablets

Borage Oil Capsules

Chinese Green Tea
   Capsules

Flax Oil Capsules

Tyrosine-500 Tablets

Ultra EPO 1500 Capsules

NATURE'S WAY
10 Mountain Springs Parkway
Springville, UT 84663

Direct Inquiries to:
(800) 962-8873
FAX: (801) 489-1700
www.naturesway.com

Nutritional Products Available:
Activated Charcoal
   Capsules

Barley Grass Capsules

Barley Grass Powder

Bee Pollen Capsules

Borage Oil Omega-6
   Capsules

Chinese Spirulina Capsules

Chlorella Capsules

Cod Liver Oil Capsules

Evening Primrose Oil
   Capsules

Grape Seed Extract
   Standardized Capsules

Green Tea Standardized
   Extract Capsules

Psyllium Husk Powder

Psyllium Seed Capsules

Pycnogenol Capsules

Pyconogenol Tablets

Soy Isoflavones Capsules

NEPHRO-TECH, INC.
P.O. Box 16106
Shawnee, KS 66203

Direct Inquiries to:
(800) 879-4755
FAX: (913) 248-8809
E-mail: nephrotec@aol.com

Nutritional Products Available:
Calphron Powder

Magnebind 200 Tablets

Magnebind 300 Tablets

Magnebind 400 Rx Tablets

Nephplex Rx Tablets

Nephron FA Tablets

NEUROVITES
P.O. Box 180
Rockaway Beach, OR 97136

Direct Inquiries to:
(503) 228-4119

Nutritional Products Available:
L-Arginine Tablets

L-Lysine Tablets

L-Tyrosine Capsules

Manly Machovites Tablets

PMS Formula Tablets

Vitamin C Chewable
   Tablets

Vitamin C Cream

NICHE PHARMACEUTICALS, INC.
P.O. Box 449
200 N. Oak Street
Roanoke, Texas 76262

Direct Inquiries to:
(817) 491-2770
FAX: (817) 491-3533

Nutritional Products Available:
Mag-Tab Sr Tablets

NOVARTIS CONSUMER HEALTH, INC.
560 Morris Avenue
Summit, NJ 07901-1312

Direct Inquiries to:
(800) 452-0051
FAX: (800) 635-2801

Nutritional Products Available:
Fiberall Powder

Fiberall Wafers

♦ Perdiem Granules G-5

♦ Slow Fe w/Folic Acid
   Extended Release Tablets . . . G-3

♦ Slow Fe Tablets G-5

Sunkist Vitamin C
   Chewable Tablets

Vitron-C Plus Tablets

Vitron-C Tablets

NOVARTIS PHARMACEUTICALS CORPORATION
59 Route 10
East Hanover, NJ 07936

Direct Inquiries to:
(888) 669-6682
www.novartis.com

Nutritional Products Available:
Neo-Calglucon Syrup

NUMARK LABORATORIES, INC.
164 Northfield Avenue
Edison, NJ 08837

Direct Inquiries to:
(800) 331-0221
FAX: (732) 225-0066

Nutritional Products Available:
Hydrocil Powder

Multivitamin Capsules

NUTRICOLOGY/ALLERGY RESEARCH GROUP
30806 Santana Street
Hayward, CA 94544

Direct Inquiries to:
(800) 545-9960
www.nutricology.com

Nutritional Products Available:
Evening Primrose Oil
   Capsules

Germanium (Ge-132)
   Powder

Germanium Capsules

Grape Pips Tablets

L-Arginine Capsules

L-Lysine Capsules

L-Methionine Capsules

Liver Tablets

Modified Citrus Pectin
   Capsules

Taurine Capsules

OAKHURST COMPANY
3000 Hempstead Turnpike
Levittown, NY 11756

Direct Inquiries to:
(800) 831-1135

Nutritional Products Available:
Ennds Tablets

OHM LABORATORIES, INC.
600 College Road East
Princeton, NJ 08540

Direct Inquiries to:
(800) 527-6481
FAX: (732) 297-3884

Nutritional Products Available:
Calcium Lactate Tablets

OPTIMOX CORPORATION
2720 Monterey Street
Suite 406
Torrance, CA 90503

Direct Inquiries to:
(800) 722-9040

Nutritional Products Available:
Mag-200 Tablets

ORACHEM PHARMACEUTICALS
Div. of Medical Products Labs.
9990 Global Road
Philadelphia, PA 19115

Direct Inquiries to:
(800) 654-3997
FAX: (215) 677-7736

Nutritional Products Available:
Nafrinse Chewable Tablets
Nafrinse Solution

ORAL B LABORATORIES
Div. Gillette Company
600 Clipper Drive
Belmont, CA 94002

Direct Inquiries to:
(800) 446-7252

Nutritional Products Available:
Fluorinse Liquid
Neutracare Gel

ORPHAN MEDICAL, INC.
13911 Ridgedale Drive
Suite 250
Minnetonka, MN 55305

Direct Inquiries to:
(612) 513-6900
FAX: (612) 541-9209
E-mail: marketing@orphan.com
www.orphan.com

Nutritional Products Available:
Cystadane Powder

PADDOCK LABORATORIES, INC.
3940 Quebec Avenue North
Minneapolis, MN 55427

Direct Inquiries to:
(612) 546-4676
FAX: (612) 546-4842

Nutritional Products Available:
Ferrous Gluconate Tablets
Ferrous Sulfate Tablets

PASCAL CO., INC.
2929 N.E. Northrup Way
P.O. Box 1478
Bellevue, WA 98009-1478

Direct Inquiries to:
(425) 827-4694
FAX: (425) 827-6893
E-mail:
pascaldental@pascaldental.com
www.pascaldental.com

Nutritional Products Available:
Neutragard Fluoride Rinse
Solution

PDK LABS, INC.
145 Ricefield Lane
Hauppauge, NY 11788

Direct Inquiries to:
(800) 221-0855
(631) 273-2630
FAX: (631) 434-9145
E-mail: info@pdklabs.com

Nutritional Products Available:
Cal-600 Tablets
Cal-600 w/Vitamin D
Tablets
Thera Vite M Tablets
Vitamin C w/Rose Hips
Tablets

PD-RX PHARMACEUTICALS INC.
727 North Ann Arbor Avenue
Oklahoma City, OK 73127

Direct Inquiries to:
(800) 299-7379
FAX: (405) 942-5471

Nutritional Products Available:
Calcium Carbonate/Vitamin
D Tablets
Calcium/Vitamin D Tablets

PECOS PHARMACEUTICAL
25301 Cabot Road
Suite 212-213
Laguna Hills, CA 92653

Direct Inquiries to:
(800) 732-6796
FAX: (949) 837-6376

Nutritional Products Available:
Ferragen Capsules

PERRIGO
117 Water Street
Allegan, MI 49010

Direct Inquiries to:
(800) 827-2296
FAX: (616) 673-9122

Nutritional Products Available:
Calcium 600 + Vitamin D
Tablets
Calcium Antacid Chewable
Tablets
Calcium Antacid Extra
Strength Tablets
Calcium Antacid Ultra
Strength Chewable
Tablets
Calcium Chewable Tablets
Calcium Tablets
Niacin Tablets
Oyster Shell Calcium
Tablets
Oyster Shell Calcium/
Vitamin D Tablets
Vitamin C Chewable
Tablets
Vitamin C Tablets
Vitamin C w/Rose Hips
Tablets
Vitamin E Capsules
Vitamin E Natural Blend
Capsules
Vitamin E400 D-Alpha
Capsules

PERRY MEDICAL PRODUCTS
P.O. Box 1009
Wilsonville, OR 97070-1009

Direct Inquiries to:
(503) 694-1600
FAX: (503) 682-0838
E-mail:
kirkman@kirkmanlabs.com
www.kirkmanlabs.com

Nutritional Products Available:
Fluorabon Chewable
Tablets
Fluorabon Solution
Sodium Fluoride Chewable
Tablets

PERSONAL PRODUCTS COMPANY
A Division of Johnson & Johnson
199 Grandview Avenue
Skillman, NJ 08558

Direct Inquiries to:
(877) 678-4769

Nutritional Products Available:

Healthy Woman Bone
Health Supplement
Tablets

♦ Healthy Woman Soy
Menopause Tablets **G-5**

PHARMACEUTICAL ASSOCIATES, INC.
A Subsidiary of Beach Products,
Inc.
201 Delaware Street
Greenville, SC 29605

Direct Inquiries to:
(800) 845-8210
(864) 277-7282
FAX: (864) 277-8045

Nutritional Products Available:

Aluminum Hydroxide Gel
Concentrate

Antacid Suspension

Ferrous Sulfate Liquid

PHARMACEUTICAL CORP. OF AMERICA
12348 Hancock Street
Carmel, IN 46032

Direct Inquiries to:
(800) 722-0772
FAX: (800) 443-7134
E-mail: repackager@aol.com

Nutritional Products Available:

Folic Acid Tablets

PHARMACEUTICAL LABORATORIES, INC.
1170 Corporate Drive W.
Suite 102
Arlington, TX 76006-6813

Direct Inquiries to:
(817) 633-1461
FAX: (817) 633-8146

Nutritional Products Available:

Vitamin E Liquid

Zinc Drops

PHARMAKON LABS, INC.
6050 Jet Port Industrial Blvd.
Tampa, FL 33634

Direct Inquiries to:
(800) 888-4045
FAX: (813) 887-3028

Nutritional Products Available:

Clusinex Syrup

PHARMASCIENCE LABORATORIES, INC.
175 Rano Street
Buffalo, NY 14207

Direct Inquiries to:
(716) 871-9376
FAX: (716) 871-3415
www.pharmascience.com

Nutritional Products Available:

Fluor-A-Day Chewable
Tablets

Fluor-A-Day Liquid

Fluor-A-Day Lozenges

PHARMAVITE CORPORATION
15451 San Fernando Mission Blvd.
Mission Hills, CA 91345

Direct Inquiries to:
(800) 423-2405
FAX: (818) 837-6129

Nutritional Products Available:

Folic Acid Tablets

Magnesium Tablets

Niacin Tablets

Pantothenic Acid Tablets

Vitamin C Tablets

Vitamin C w/Rose Hips
Tablets

Vitamin E800 D-Alpha
Capsules

PHARMICS, INC.
2350 S. Redwood Road
P.O. Box 27554
Salt Lake City, UT 84127-0554

Direct Inquiries to:
(800) 456-4138
(801) 972-4138
FAX: (801) 972-4139
E-mail: pharmics@aros.net

Nutritional Products Available:

Ferretts Tablets

O-Cal FA Tablets

Pharmaflur Chewable
Tablets

PHYTOPHARMICA
825 Challenger Drive
Green Bay, WI 54311

Direct Inquiries to:
(800) 553-2370 (Doctors and
Pharmacists)
(800) 644-0799 (Consumers)

Nutritional Products Available:

B12-Active Tablets

CoQ10 Capsules

DHEA-25 Capsules

DLPA Capsules

Flush-Free Inositol
Hexaniacinate Capsules

Glucosamine Sulfate
Capsules

Green Tea Extracts
Capsules

Krebs Ionized Calcium
Tablets

Krebs Ionized Zinc Tablets

Ostivone Capsules

Pantechol Tablets

Soy Extract Capsules

PINES INTERNATIONAL
P.O. Box 1107
1992 East 1400 Road
Lawrence, KS 66044

Direct Inquiries to:
(800) 697-4637
FAX: (785) 841-1252
www.wheatgrass.com

Nutritional Products Available:

Barley Grass Powder

Barley Grass Tablets

Wheat Grass Capsules

Wheat Grass Tablets

PRIME MARKETING
1175 John Road
Troy, MI 48083

Direct Inquiries to:
(800) 222-5609
FAX: (248) 526-3751

Nutritional Products Available:

Calcium 600 Tablets

Feronate Tablets

Ferrousal Tablets

Once Daily Tablets

Oyster Shell Calcium
Tablets

Thera-M w/Minerals
Tablets

Vitamin C Tablets

Vitamin E Capsules

Vitamins Children's
Chewable Tablets

PRIMEDICS LABORATORIES
Ethical Div., Irenda Corp.
14131 S. Avalon Blvd.
Los Angeles, CA 90061

Direct Inquiries to:
(800) 533-0173

Nutritional Products Available:

Primaplex Injection

PROCTER & GAMBLE DISTRIBUTING COMPANY
P.O. Box 599
1 Procter & Gamble Plaza
Cincinatti, OH 45201-0599

Direct Inquiries to:
(513) 983-1100

Nutritional Products Available:

♦ Metamucil Powder and
Wafers **G-5**

Vicks Vitamin C Lozenge

PROLAB NUTRITION
11 Britton Drive
Bloomfield, CT 06002

Direct Inquiries to:
(800) prolab-1
www.prolabnutrition.com

Nutritional Products Available:

5-Androstenediol Capsules

19-Norandrostenedione
Capsules

Chrysin Capsules

Glutamine Powder

Whey Protein Powder

PROPHARMA INC.
3307 N.W. 74th Avenue
Miami, FL 33122

Direct Inquiries to:
(800) 446-0255
FAX: (305) 477-6506

Nutritional Products Available:

Ferrous Sulfate Tablets

QUALITEST PRODUCTS, INC.
1236 Jordan Road
Huntsville, AL 35811

Direct Inquiries to:
(800) 444-4011
(256) 859-4011
FAX: (256) 859-4021

Nutritional Products Available:

Calcium Antacid Chewable
Tablets

Calcium Antacid Extra
Strength Chewable
Tablets

Ferrous Sulfate Elixir

Fluoride Chewable Tablets

Fluoride Liquid

Folic Acid Tablets

Niacin Capsules

Therobec Plus Tablets

Therobec Tablets

Vitamin C Tablets

Vitamin E Capsules

QUALITY CARE PHARMACEUTICALS, INC.
3000 W. Warner Avenue
Santa Ana, CA 92704

Direct Inquiries to:
(714) 754-5800
(714) 754-5745

Nutritional Products Available:

Ferrous Sulfate Tablets

Folic Acid Tablets

Slow-Mag Tablets

Sodium Fluoride Chewable
Tablets

Vitamin E Capsules

THE QUIGLEY CORPORATION
P.O. Box 1349
10 South Clinton Street
Doylestown, PA 18901

Direct Inquiries to:
(215) 345-0919
FAX: (215) 345-5920
www.quigleyco.com

Nutritional Products Available:

Cold-Eeze Lozenges

R&D LABORATORIES, INC.
4640 Admiralty Way, Suite 710
Marina del Rey, CA 90292

Direct Inquiries to:
(800) 338-9066
(310) 305-8053, ext. 227
FAX: (310) 305-8103

Nutritional Products Available:

Calci-Chew Tablets

Calci-Mix Capsules

Mag-Carb Capsules

Nephro-Calci Tablets

Nephro-Fer Rx Tablets

Nephro-Fer Tablets

Nephro-Vite Rx Tablets

Nephro-Vite + FE Tablets

R.I.D., INC.
609 N. Mednik Avenue
Los Angeles, CA 90022-1326

Direct Inquiries to:
(323) 268-0635
FAX: (323) 268-1336

Nutritional Products Available:

Ridactate Tablets

Ridosol Tablets

Yieronia Elixir

Yierro-Gota Liquid

RAHWAY PHARMACAL INC.
15 Granit Road
Accord, NY 12404

Direct Inquiries to:
(914) 626-8133
FAX: (914) 626-8134

Nutritional Products Available:

Ascorbic Acid Injection

Ascorbic Acid Tablets

Calcium Chloride Solution
Injection

Calcium Gluconate
Injection

Ferrous Sulfate Tablets

Folic Acid Injection

Folic Acid Tablets

Magnesium Sulfate
Injection

Niacin Tablets

RAINBOW LIGHT NUTRITIONAL SYSTEMS
125 McPherson Street
Santa Cruz, CA 95060

Direct Inquiries to:
(800) 635-1233
(831) 429-9089
FAX: (831) 429-0189

Nutritional Products Available:

Grape Seed Supercomplex
Tablets

Hawaiian Spirulina Tablets

Propolis Herb Liquid

RECSEI LABORATORIES
330 S. Kellogg Avenue
Building M
Goleta, CA 93117-9973

Direct Inquiries to:
(805) 964-2912

Nutritional Products Available:
Vitamin C Granules

REESE PHARMACEUTICAL COMPANY
10617 Frank Avenue
P.O. Box 1957
Cleveland, OH 44106

Direct Inquiries to:
(800) 321-7178
FAX: (216) 231-6444
E-mail: reese@apk.net
www.reesechemical.com

Nutritional Products Available:
Oyster Shell Calcium Tablets
Oyster Shell Calcium/ Vitamin D Tablets
Zinc Preferred Capsules

REPUBLIC DRUG COMPANY, INC.
175 Great Arrow
Buffalo, NY 14207

Direct Inquiries to:
(800) 828-7444
FAX: (716) 874-6060

Nutritional Products Available:
Iron Tablets
Zinc-Ease Lozenges

REQUA, INC.
P.O. Box 4008
1 Seneca Place
Greenwich, CT 06830

Direct Inquiries to:
(800) 321-1085

Nutritional Products Available:
Charcoaid Granules
Charcoal Tablets
Charcocaps Capsules

REXALL CONSUMER PRODUCTS
Div. of Rexall Sundown, Inc.
6111 Broken Sound Parkway, NW
Boca Raton, FL 33487-3693

Direct Inquiries to:
(800) 255-7399
FAX: (561) 995-6881
www.rexallsundown.com

Nutritional Products Available:
B-50 Complex Tablets
B-100 Complex Tablets
C500 Tablets
C500 w/Rose Hips Chewable Tablets
C500 w/Rose Hips Tablets
C1000 Plus Rose Hips Tablets
C1000 Tablets
C1000 w/Rose Hips Tablets
Calcium 500 w/Vitamin D Tablets
Calcium 900 w/Vitamin D Capsules
Calcium 1200 w/Vitamin D Capsules
Calcium/Magnesium/Zinc Tablets
Circus Chews Children's Chewable Tablets
Daily Multiple Vitamins Tablets
Daily Multiple Vitamins w/ Iron Tablets
E200 Mixed Capsules
E400 Mixed Capsules
E400 Natural Capsules
E1000 Mixed Capsules
Folic Acid Tablets
Iron Advanced Tablets
Niacin Capsules
Niacin Tablets
Oyster Shell Calcium 1000/ Vitamin D Tablets
Oyster Shell Calcium Tablets
Oyster Shell Calcium/ Vitamin D Tablets
Stress Formula Plus Zinc Tablets
Stress Formula Tablets
Sunvite Platinum Tablets
Sunvite Tablets
Super Plenamins Extra Strength Tablets
Super Plenamins Tablets
Zinc Chelated Tablets

ROCHE LABORATORIES
340 Kingsland Street
Nutley, NJ 07110-1199

Direct Inquiries to:
(800) 526-6367

Nutritional Products Available:
Berocca Plus Tablets
Berocca Tablets

ROSS PRODUCTS DIVISION
Division of Abbott Laboratories Inc.
625 Cleveland Avenue
Columbus, Ohio 43215-1724

Direct Inquiries to:
(800) 227-5767

Nutritional Products Available:
Pediaflor Drops

ROXANE LABORATORIES, INC.
1809 Wilson Road
Columbus, OH 43228-8601

Direct Inquiries to:
(800) 962-8364

Nutritional Products Available:
Calcium Carbonate Suspension
Calcium Carbonate Tablets
Calcium Gluconate Tablets
Lactulose Solution
Lithium Carbonate Capsules
Lithium Citrate Syrup

RUGBY LABORATORIES, INC.
2725 Northwoods Parkway
Norcross, GA 30071-1533

Direct Inquiries to:
(800) 645-2158
FAX: (770) 840-9040

Nutritional Products Available:
Aluminum Hydroxide Gel Suspension
Cal-Gest Chewable Tablets
Calcionate Syrup
Calcium 600 Tablets
Calcium 600-D Tablets
Calcium Carbonate Tablets
Calcium Chewable Tablets
Calcium Gluconate Tablets
Calcium Lactate Tablets
Cerovite Senior Tablets
Citrus Calcium Tablets

Citrus Calcium + D
  Tablets
Fer-Iron Liquid
Ferrous Sulfate Elixir
Ferrous Sulfate Tablets
Folic Acid Tablets
L-Tyrosine Tablets
Magnesium Chelated
  Tablets
Multi-Vitamins Tablets
Niacin Capsules
Niacin Tablets
Oysco 500 Tablets
Oysco 500 + D Tablets
Oysco D Tablets
Pantothenic Acid Tablets
Poly Vitamin Chewable
  Tablets
Poly Vitamin w/Iron
  Chewable Tablets
Reguloid Powder
Therapeutic Plus Vitamin
  Tablets
Vita-Bee w/C Tablets
Vitamin B Complex
  Capsules
Vitamin C Chewable
  Tablets
Vitamin C Tablets
Vitamin C w/Rose Hips
  Tablets
Vitamin E Capsules
Vitamin E Oil
Zinc Chelated Tablets

SAVAGE LABORATORIES
A division of Altana Inc.
60 Baylis Road
Melville, NY 11747

Direct Inquiries to:
(800) 231-0206
FAX: (631) 454-0732

Nutritional Products Available:
Chromagen Capsules
Chromagen FA Tablets
Chromagen Forte Capsules
Modane Bulk Powder

SCHEIN PHARMACEUTICAL, INC.
100 Campus Drive
Florham Park, NJ 07932

Direct Inquiries to:
(800) 356-5790
FAX: (800) 760-9224

Nutritional Products Available:
Folic Acid Tablets
Infed Injection
Lactulose Syrup

SCHERING-PLOUGH HEALTHCARE PRODUCTS
3 Oak Way
Berkeley Heights, NJ 07922

Direct Inquiries to:
(908) 679-1983
FAX: (908) 679-1776

Nutritional Products Available:
Mol-Iron Tablets

SCHWARZ PHARMA, INC.
6140 W. Executive Drive
Mequon, WI 53092

Direct Inquiries to:
(800) 558-5114
(262) 238-9994

Nutritional Products Available:
Niferex-150 Forte Capsules
Niferex-PN Tablets

SHIRE U.S.
7900 Tanners Gate Dr., Suite 200
Florence, KY 41042

Direct Inquiries to:
(859) 282-2100
FAX: (859) 282-2127
www.shire.com

Nutritional Products Available:
Slow-Mag Tablets

SIGMA-TAU CONSUMER PRODUCTS
A division of Sigma-Tau
  Pharmaceuticals, Inc.
Gaithersburg, MD 20877

Direct Inquiries to:
(888) 818-5448
(301) 948-5450
FAX: (301) 948-5452
Email: info@sigmatau.com
www.proxeed.com

Nutritional Products Available:
♦ ProXeed Packets G-5

SILARX PHARMACEUTICALS, INC.
19 West Street
P.O. Box 449
Spring Valley, NY 10977

Direct Inquiries to:
(914) 352-4020
FAX: (914) 352-4037

Nutritional Products Available:
Ferrous Sulfate Elixir
Ferrous Sulfate Liquid
Vitamin E Aqueous Liquid

SKY PHARMACEUTICALS PACKAGING, INC.
2865 Armentrout Drive
Concord, NC 28025

Direct Inquiries to:
(888) 680-4759
(270) 784-4301
FAX: (270)788-4555

Nutritional Products Available:
Calcium Carbonate
  Chewable Tablets
Calcium Carbonate/Vitamin
  D Tablets
Daily Multivitamins Tablets
Ferrous Sulfate Tablets

SMITHKLINE BEECHAM PHARMACEUTICALS
P.O. Box 7929
One Franklin Plaza
Philadelphia, PA 19101

Direct Inquiries to:
(800) 366-8900

Nutritional Products Available:
Eskalith Capsules
Eskalith-CR Tablets
♦ Feosol Caplets G-5
♦ Feosol Elixir G-5
♦ Feosol Tablets G-5
♦ Os-Cal 250 + D Tablets G-5
♦ Os-Cal 500 + D Tablets G-5
♦ Os-Cal 500 Chewable
  Tablets G-5
♦ Os-Cal 500 Tablets G-5
Tums 500 Chewable
  Tablets
♦ Tums Chewable Tablets G-5
♦ Tums E-X Chewable
  Tablets G-5
♦ Tums Ultra Chewable
  Tablets G-5

SOLARAY
Division of Nutraceutical
   Corporation
1400 Kearns Blvd.
Park City, UT 84060

Direct Inquiries to:
(800) 669-8877
FAX: (800) 767-8514
www.nutraceutical.com

Nutritional Products Available:
Activated Charcoal
   Capsules
Beta Glucan Support
   Healthy Macrophage
   Activity Capsules
Borage Oil Capsules
Evening Primrose Oil
   Capsules
Free-Form L-Arginine
   Capsules
Free-Form L-Glutamine
   Capsules
Free-Form L-Lysine Tablets
Free-Form L-Tyrosine
   Capsules
Grapenol Capsules
Green Tea Extract Capsules
Primosa Capsules
Propolis Liquid Extract
   Liquid
Proven Pure 19-
   Norandrostenedione
   Capsules
Psyllium Seed Capsules
Soy Protein Bar For
   Women
Spirulina Tablets

**SOLGAR VITAMIN AND HERB
COMPANY, INC.**
500 Willow Tree Road
Leonia, NJ 07605

Direct Inquiries to:
(201) 944-2311
FAX: (201) 944-7351
www.solgar.com

Nutritional Products Available:
Bee Pollen Nuggets
   Powder
Bee Pollen Tablets
Calcium Citrate Tablets
Evening Primrose Oil
   Capsules

Flaxseed Oil Capsules
Folic Acid Tablets
Gentle Iron Capsules
Ipriflavone Capsules
L-Arginine Capsules
L-Methionine Capsules
L-Ornithine Capsules
Rutin Tablets
Sharkilage Shark Cartilage
   Capsules
Super GLA Capsules
Vitamin B-6 Tablets
Vitamin B-12 Nuggets
Vitamin K Tablets

SOLVAY PHARMACEUTICALS, INC.
901 Sawyer Road
Marietta, GA 30062

Direct Inquiries to:
(800) 241-1643
(770) 578-9000
FAX: (770) 578-5901

Nutritional Products Available:
Duphalac Syrup
Lithobid Tablets

SOURCE NATURALS
19 Janis Way
Scotts Valley, CA 95066

Direct Inquiries to:
(800) 815-2333
FAX: (831) 438-7410
www.sourcenaturals.com

Nutritional Products Available:
Acetyl L-Carnitine Tablets
Acidophilus Lactocacilli w/
   Pectin Capsules
Active A Tablets
Alpha-Lipoic Acid Tablets
Arthred Hydrolyzed
   Collagen Liquid
Benefin Shark Cartilage
   Powder
Beta Glucan Capsules
Beta Glucan From Yeast
   Capsules
Calcium Ascorbate Crystals
Charcoal Capsules
Chlorella Tablets
ColloidaLife Drops
Creatine Tablets
Diet Chitosan Capsules

Ester C Tablets
European Pine Pycnogenol
   Tablets
Evening Primrose Oil
   Capsules
Folic Acid Tablets
Genistein Soy Isoflavones
Genistein Tablets
Grapefruit Pectin Tablets
Green Tea Extract Tablets
Hawaiian Spirulina Tablets
Inosine Tablets
L-Arginine Powder
L-Aspartic Acid Powder
L-Cysteine Powder
L-Glutamine Tablets
L-Glutathione Tablets
L-Lysine Powder
L-Lysine Tablets
L-Methionine Powder
L-Ornithine Powder
L-Phenylalanine Tablets
L-Taurine Powder
L-Tyrosine Powder
L-Tyrosine Tablets
Lacto Brev Capsules
Life Flora Capsules
Lutein Capsules
Lycopene Capsules
MSM
   Methylsulfonylmethane
   Powder
MSM
   Methylsulfonylmethane
   Tablets
Mega Colloidal Silver
   Liquid
Mega GLA Capsules
Modified Citrus Pectin
   Powder
N-Acetyl L-Tyrosine
   Tablets
NADH Tablets
Nectar Pyruvate Powder
Niacin Tablets
No-Flush Niacin Tablets
NutraFlora Tablets
Oat Bran Soluble Fiber
   Tablets

PABA Tablets

Pantothenic Acid Tablets

Pregnenolone Tablets

Premium Soy Protein
Booster Powder

Propolis Extract Liquid

Propolis Power Capsules

Psyllium Husk Capsules

Pycnogenol Capsules

Pyruvate Burn Capsules

Pyruvate Fuel Capsules

Royal Jelly Capsules

Spirulina Capsules

Super Beta Carotene
Capsules

Tocotrienol Antioxidant
Complex Capsules

Ultra EPO 1500 Capsules

Vege Fuel Soy Protein
Powder

Vitamin B-1 Tablets

Vitamin B-2 Tablets

Vitamin B-6 Tablets

Vitamin B-12 Sublingual
Tablets

Vitamin E Capsules

Wellness Colloidal Silver
Spray

SPECTRUM ORGANIC PRODUCTS, INC.
1304 South Point Blvd.
Suite 280
Petaluma, CA 94952

Direct Inquiries to:
(800) 995-2705
FAX: (707) 765-8470
spectrumnaturals@netdex.com

Nutritional Products Available:

Evening Primrose Oil
Capsules

STANDARD HOMEOPATHIC COMPANY
P. O. Box 61067
210 West 131 Street
Los Angeles, CA 90061

Direct Inquiries to:
(310) 768-0700

Nutritional Products Available:

Arnicaid Tablets

Arsenicum Album Pellets

Arsenicum Album
Sublingual Tablets

STEWART-JACKSON PHARMACAL, INC.
4200 Lamar, Suite 103
Memphis, TN 38118

Direct Inquiries to:
(800) 367-1395
FAX: (901) 362-9102

Nutritional Products Available:

Cardiotek Tablets

SUPERIOR PHARMACEUTICAL COMPANY
Subsidiary of Dynagen Inc.
1385 Kemper Meadow Drive
Cincinnati, OH 45240-1635

Direct Inquiries to:
(800) 826-5035
FAX: (513) 742-6473

Nutritional Products Available:

Dibetex Power Packets

Ferrous Sulfate Elixir

SWANSON HEALTH PRODUCTS
1318 39th Street N.W.
Fargo, ND 58108

Direct Inquiries to:
(800) 451-9304
FAX: (800) 726-7691

Nutritional Products Available:

Copper Tablets

Ester-C Capsules

Ester-C Tablets

Niacin Capsules

Niacin Tablets

Vitamin C Capsules

Vitamin C w/Rose Hips
Capsules

Vitamin C w/Rose Hips
Tablets

Vitamin E Capsules

Vitamin E Dry Capsules

Vitamin E Mixed
Tocopherols Capsules

Zinc Lozenges

SYNERGY PLUS
500 Halls Mill Road
Freehold, NJ 07728

Direct Inquiries to:
(800) 375-8482

Nutritional Products Available:

Evening Primrose Oil
Capsules

Gelatin Capsules

Liver Tablets

Ribose Ribomax Powder

Rutin Tablets

TEVA PHARMACEUTICALS USA
650 Cathill Road
Sellersville, PA 18960

Direct Inquiries to:
(888) TEVA USA

Nutritional Products Available:

Acidulated Phosphate
Fluoride Chewable
Tablets

B-Complex Vitamins Plus
Tablets

Copper Sulfate Solution

Sodium Fluoride Chewable
Tablets

Sodium Fluoride Liquid

TEXTILEASE MEDIQUE
900 Lively Blvd.
Wood Dale, IL 60191

Direct Inquiries to:
(630) 694-4100
FAX: (630) 694-4140
E-mail: khurley@textilease.com
www.textileasemedique.com

Nutritional Products Available:

Alcalak Chewable Tablets

Mallamint Chewable
Tablets

TIME-CAP LABORATORIES, INC.
7 Michael Avenue
Farmingdale, NY 11735

Direct Inquiries to:
(631) 753-9090
FAX: (631) 753-2220

Nutritional Products Available:

C-Time Capsules

Ferro-Time Capsules

Ferrous Sulfate Tablets

Niacin Capsules

TOM'S OF MAINE
P.O. Box 710
Kennebunk, ME 04043

Direct Inquiries to:
(800) 367-8667
(207) 985-2944
FAX: (207) 985-2196
www.toms-of-maine.com

Nutritional Products Available:
♦ Natural Echinacea Tonic
   Concentrate G-5
♦ Natural Echinacea Tonic
   With Green Tea G-5
♦ Natural Ginseng Tonic G-5
♦ Natural Green Tea Tonic G-5
♦ Natural Liquid Extracts G-6
♦ Natural Valerian Tonic G-6

THE TORRANCE COMPANY
800 Lenox Avenue
Portage, MI 49024

Direct Inquiries to:
(800) 327-0722
FAX: (616) 327-0763

Nutritional Products Available:
Ascorbic Acid Injection
Magnesium Chloride
   Injection
Vitamin B Complex 100
   Injection

TRADITIONAL MEDICINALS
4515 Ross Road
Sebastopol, CA 95472

Direct Inquiries to:
(707) 823-8911
www.traditionals.com

Nutritional Products Available:
Earl Green Tea Bags
Golden Green Tea Bags

TREE OF LIFE
P.O. Box 410
1750 Tree Boulevard
St. Augustine, FL 32086-5174

Direct Inquiries to:
(904) 824-4699
FAX: (904) 825-2013
www.treeoflife.com

Nutritional Products Available:
Bee Pollen Caplets
Beta Carotene Capsules
Calcium Citrate Tablets
Chitosan Tablets
Chondroitin Sulfate Tablets
Chromium Picolinate
   Tablets

CoQ10 Capsules
Evening Primrose Capsules
Flaxseed Oil Capsules
Folic Acid Tablets
Iron Tablets
MSM Tablets
Magnesium Tablets
Niacin Vitamin B-3 Tablets
Pantothenic Acid Tablets
Potassium Gluconate
   Tablets
Pycnogenol Tablets
Pyruvate Tablets
Shark Cartilage Capsules
Vitamin B-1 Tablets
Vitamin B-12 Tablets
Vitamin D Tablets
Vitamin E Capsules

TRI-MED LABORATORIES, INC.
68 Veronica Avenue
Somerset, NJ 08873

Direct Inquiries to:
(732) 249-6363
FAX: (732) 214-1152

Nutritional Products Available:
Multi-Vitamin w/Iron
   Children's Liquid

TRIMEDICA INTERNATIONAL, INC.
1895 South Los Feliz Drive
Tempe, AZ 85282

Direct Inquiries to:
(800) 800-8849
www.trimedica.com

Nutritional Products Available:
Colloidal Silver Pro Spray

TRUXTON CO., INC.
136 Harding Avenue
P.O. Box 1081
Bellmawr, NJ 08099

Direct Inquiries to:
(800) 257-7704
FAX: (856) 933-0631

Nutritional Products Available:
Ascorbic Acid Chewable
   Tablets
Ascorbic Acid Tablets
Ferrous Gluconate Tablets
Ferrous Sulfate Capsules
Ferrous Sulfate Tablets

Folic Acid Tablets
Niacin Tablets
Oyster Shell Calcium
   Tablets
Vitamin B Complex 100
   Injection
Vitamin E Capsules
Zinc Gluconate Tablets

TWINLAB
150 Motor Parkway
Hauppauge, NY 11788

Direct Inquiries to:
(516) 467-3140
www.twinlab.com

Nutritional Products Available:
Advanced Shark Cartilage
   From Japan Capsules
Apple Pectin Capsules
Bee Propolis Tablets
Cartilade Shark Cartilage
   Capsules
Easysoy Gold Super
   Isoflavone Concentrate
   Tablets
Evening Primrose Oil
   Capsules
Glutamine Fuel Capsules
Glutamine Fuel Powder
Glycerol Fuel Liquid
Grape Seed Extract
   Capsules
HMB Fuel Capsules
Inosine Capsules
Isoflavone Capsules
Kic Fuel-Anti-Catabolic
   Amino Acid Capsules
L-Arginine Capsules
L-Lysine Tablets
L-Methionine Tablets
L-Ornithine Capsules
L-Tyrosine Capsules
L-Tyrosine Tablets
Maxilife Chicken Collagen
   Type II Capsules
Mega Charcoal Capsules
Mega Glutamine Fuel
   Capsules
Mega Primrose Oil
   Capsules

Mega Ribose Fuel Tablets

Mega Taurine Capsules

Methionine Free Form
   Capsules

Pinnacle Pyruvate Tablets

Pycnogenol Capsules

Pyruvate Diet Capsules

Pyruvate Fuel Capsules

Ribose Fuel Powder

Ribose Fuel Tablets

Ribose Powder

Serutan Granules

Shark Cartilgae Capsules

Veg Borage Oil Capsules

Whey Ahead Powder

TYLER ENCAPSULATIONS, INC.
2204 NW Birdsdale
Gresham, OR 97030

Direct Inquiries to:
(503) 661-5401
FAX: (503) 666-4913
www.tyler-inc.com

Nutritional Products Available:
   Niacinol Capsules

TYSON NEUTRACEUTICALS, INC.
12832 Chadron Avenue
Hawthorne, CA 90250-5525

Direct Inquiries to:
(800) 367-7744

Nutritional Products Available:
   Glutathione Powder
   L-Arginine Capsules
   L-Arginine Powder
   L-Ornithine Capsules
   L-Ornithine Powder
   L-Phenylalanine Capsules
   L-Phenylalanine Powder
   Royal Jelly Peking Liquid
   Zinc Picolinate Capsules

**U.S. PHARMACEUTICAL
CORPORATION**
2401-C Mellon Court
Decatur, GA 30035

Direct Inquiries to:
(800) 330-3040
FAX: (404) 987-4806

Nutritional Products Available:
   Hemocyte Injection
   Hemocyte Tablets

Hemocyte-F Tablets

UCB PHARMA, INC.
1950 Lake Park Drive
Smyrna, GA 30080

Direct Inquiries to:
(800) 477-7877

Nutritional Products Available:
   Vicon Forte Tablets

UDL LABORATORIES, INC.
1718 Northrock Court
Rockford, IL 61103

Direct Inquiries to:
(815) 282-1201
FAX: (815) 282-9391

Nutritional Products Available:
   Folic Acid Tablets

ULTIMATE NUTRITION, INC.
P.O. Box 643
7 Corporate Avenue
Farmington, CT 06034

Direct Inquiries to:
(860) 409-7373
FAX: (860) 793-5006
www.ultimatenutrition.com

Nutritional Products Available:
   Argentine Beef Liver
      Tablets
   BCAA Tablets
   HMB Capsules
   L-Lysine Premium
      Capsules
   Vanadyl Sulfate Capsules

**UNITED RESEARCH LABORATORIES,
INC.**
1100 Orthodox Street
Philadelphia, PA 19124

Direct Inquiries to:
(800) 523-3684
FAX: (215) 807-1090
www.urlmutual.com

Nutritional Products Available:
   B-Complex Plus Tablets
   Calcium Lactate Tablets
   Ferrous Gluconate Tablets
   Ferrous Sulfate Elixir
   Ferrous Sulfate Tablets
   Folic Acid Tablets
   Multi-Ferrous Folic
      Extended Release Tablets
   Niacin Capsules

Sodium Fluoride Chewable
   Tablets

Vitamin C Tablets

Vitamin E Capsules

UPSHER-SMITH LABORATORIES, INC.
14905 23rd Avenue North
Minneapolis, MN 55447

Direct Inquiries to:
(800) 654-2299

Nutritional Products Available:
   Feratab Tablets
   Ferrous Gluconate Tablets
   Niacor Tablets
   Slo-Niacin Tablets

VANGARD LABS, INC.
835 North L. Rogers Wells
   Blvd.
Glasgow, KY 42141

Direct Inquiries to:
(800) 825-4123
(270) 651-6188
FAX: (270) 651-6414

Nutritional Products Available:
   Calcium/Vitamin D Tablets
   Daily Multiple Vitamins/
      Iron Tablets
   Daily Multiple Vitamins/
      Minerals Tablets
   Ferrous Gluconate Tablets
   Ferrous Sulfate Tablets
   Folic Acid Tablets
   Oyster Shell Calcium
      Tablets
   Oyster Shell Calcium/
      Vitamin D Tablets
   Vitamin C Tablets

VINTAGE PHARMACEUTICALS, INC.
1236 Jordan Road
Huntsville, AL 35811

Direct Inquiries to:
(256) 859-4011
FAX: (256) 859-2903

Nutritional Products Available:
   Fluoride Liquid

VITALINE CORPORATION
385 Williamson Way
Ashland, OR 97520

Direct Inquiries to:
(800) 648-4755
(541) 482-9231
FAX: (541) 482-9112

Nutritional Products Available:

Bromelain 2400 Maximum
   Strength Tablets

Cal-Carb Forte Tablets

Cal-Carb Forte Wafers

Calcium Citrate Tablets

Catalytic Formula Tablets

E-Pherol Tablets

Pantothenic Acid Tablets

Resveratrol Tablets

Total Formula Original
   Tablets

Vita-Calcium Wafers

Vitamin C Powder

Vitamin C Tablets

Vitamin E Capsules

VITANICA
P.O. Box 1285
Sherwood, Oregon 97140

Direct Inquiries to:
(800) 572-4712
FAX: (503) 625-7192
E-mail: Vitanica@aol.com
www.vitanica.com

Nutritional Products Available:

Soy Isoflavones Capsules

VITA-RX CORP.
P.O. Box 8229
4625 Warm Springs Road
Columbus, GA 31908

Direct Inquiries to:
(800) 241-8276
FAX: (706) 568-1886

Nutritional Products Available:

Ferrous Fumarate DS
   Extended Release
   Capsules

Ferrous Gluconate Tablets

Ferrous Sulfate Capsules

Ferrous Sulfate Tablets

WAKUNAGA OF AMERICA CO.
23501 Madero
Mission Viejo, CA 92691

Direct Inquiries to:
(800) 527-5200

Nutritional Products Available:

Kyo-Chlorella Tablets

♦ Probiata Tablets G-6

WALKER PHARMACAL CO.
4200 Laclede Avenue
St. Louis, MO 63108

Direct Inquiries to:
(800) 325-8080

Nutritional Products Available:

Arnica Tablets

WALLACE LABORATORIES
P.O. Box 1001
Half Acre Road
Cranbury, NJ 08512

Direct Inquiries to:
(800) 526-3840
(609) 655-6000

Nutritional Products Available:

Super Whey Pro Powder

WARNER-LAMBERT COMPANY
Consumer Health Products
   Group
201 Tabor Road
Morris Plains, NJ 07950

Direct Inquiries to:
(800) 223-0182

Nutritional Products Available:

♦ Halls Defense Lozenges G-6

WESTERN RESEARCH LABORATORIES
12208 North 32nd Street
Phoenix, AZ 85032

Direct Inquiries to:
(877) 797-7997
FAX: (623) 879-8683

Nutritional Products Available:

Magnesium Gluconate
   Tablets

Vitamin E Capsules

WESTLAKE LABORATORIES, INC.
24700 Center Ridge Road
Cleveland, Ohio 44145

Direct Inquiries to:
(888) WSTLAKE (978-5253)
FAX: (440) 835-2177
www.westlake-labs.com

Nutritional Products Available:

Pantethine 500 Capsules

Total E-400 Capsules

WEST-WARD PHARMACEUTICAL CORP.
465 Industrial Way West
Eatontown, NJ 07724

Direct Inquiries to:
(800) 631-2174
FAX: (732) 542-0940

Nutritional Products Available:

Folic Acid Tablets

WYETH-AYERST PHARMACEUTICALS
Division of American Home
   Products Corporation
P.O. Box 8299
Philadelphia, PA 19101

Direct Inquiries to:
(800) 934-5556
(610) 688-4400

Nutritional Products Available:

Amphojel Suspension

Basaljel Capsules

Basaljel Tablets

YERBA PRIMA
740 Jefferson Avenue
Ashland, OR 97520-3743

Direct Inquiries to:
(800) 488-4339
FAX: (541) 488-2443

Nutritional Products Available:

Colon Care Formula
   Psyllium Seed Capsules

Great Plains Bentonite Clay
   Liquid

Psyllium Husks 100% Pure
   Powder

ZAND HERBAL FORMULAS
1722 14th Street, Suite #230
Boulder, CO 80302

Direct Inquiries to:
(800) 731-8420
E-mail: info@zandboulder.com
www.zand.com

Nutritional Products Available:

Green Tea Tablets

Spirulina-500 Tablets

ZENITH GOLDLINE PHARMACEUTICALS
4400 Biscayne Boulevard
Miami, FL 33137

Direct Inquiries to:
(800) 327-4114
FAX: (954) 575-4319

Nutritional Products Available:

Aluminum Hydroxide Gel
  Suspension
Antacid Chewable Tablets
Antacid Extra Strength
  Chewable Tablets
Ascorbic Acid Tablets
B-Plex Plus Tablets
B-Plex Tablets
Beta Carotene Capsules
Calcarb 600 Tablets
Calcarb 600 w/Vitamin D
  Tablets
Calcium Citrate Tablets
Calcium Lactate Tablets

Chondroitin Sulfate
  Capsules
Evening Primrose Oil
  Capsules
Fer-Gen-Sol Liquid
Ferrous Gluconate Tablets
Ferrous Sulfate Elixir
Ferrous Sulfate Tablets
Folic Acid Tablets
Garlic Oil Capsules
Genfiber Powder
Grape Seed Extract
  Capsules
Green Tea Extract Capsules
Lactulose Syrup

Lecithin Capsules
Magnesium Tablets
Niacin Capsules
Niacin Tablets
One Tablet Daily w/Iron
  Tablets
Oyst-Cal 500 Tablets
Oyst-Cal-D 500 Tablets
Oyst-Cal-D Tablets
Shark Cartilage Capsules
Vitamin C Chewable
  Tablets
Vitamin C Tablets
Vitamin E Capsules
Zinc Tablets

Product Identification Guide

In this section, you'll find full-color photos of some of the more popular nutritional products currently available on retail shelves. The photos are arranged alphabetically by manufacturer and brand name. The company's name appears above the product; its brand name below.

ABKIT

ABKIT

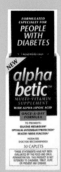

Multi-Vitamin Supplement
with Alpha Lipoic Acid

Alpha Betic™

BAYER CORPORATION

BAYER CORPORATION
CONSUMER CARE DIVISION

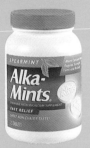

Spearmint and Assorted
Chewable Antacid and
Calcium Supplement

Alka-Mints®

BAYER CORPORATION
CONSUMER CARE DIVISION

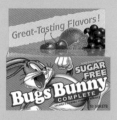

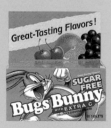

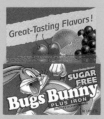

Sugar Free Children's Chewable Vitamins
Complete, with Extra C and Plus Iron

Bugs Bunny™ Vitamins

BAYER CORPORATION
CONSUMER CARE DIVISION

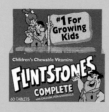

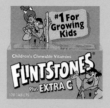

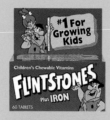

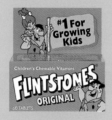

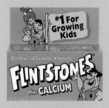

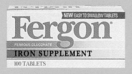

Complete, Plus Extra C, Plus Iron,
Original and Plus Calcium

**Flintstones® Children's
Chewable Vitamins**

BAYER CORPORATION
CONSUMER CARE DIVISION

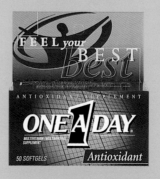

Ferrous Gluconate
Iron Supplement

Fergon®

BAYER CORPORATION
CONSUMER CARE DIVISION

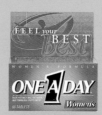

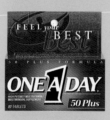

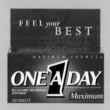

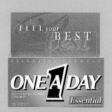

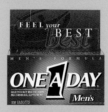

Women's, Men's, 50 Plus,
Maximum and Essential.

One-A-Day® Vitamins

BAYER CORPORATION
CONSUMER CARE DIVISION

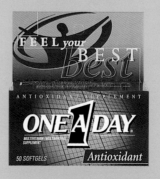

**One-A-Day®
Antioxidant Plus**

BAYER CORPORATION
CONSUMER CARE DIVISION

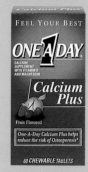

500 mg Calcium Carbonate
Plus Vitamin D and Magnesium

One-A-Day® Calcium Plus

BAYER CORPORATION
CONSUMER CARE DIVISION

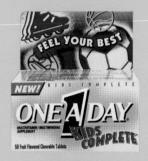

**One-A-Day®
Kids Complete**

FOR MORE INFORMATION...

...on these products,
check the Brand Name Index
for the location of the
monograph or table that
covers each brand.

BRISTOL-MYERS PRODUCTS

BRISTOL-MYERS PRODUCTS

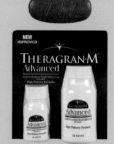

High Potency Multivitamins with Minerals
Available in 100 plus 30, and 220 caplets.

Theragran-M® Advanced

COVEX

COVEX

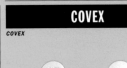

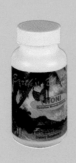

Powerful Memory Enhancer

Intelectol™

ERBL, INC.

ERBL, INC.

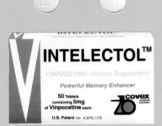

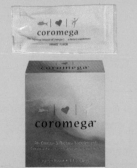

Available in 14 ct and 28 ct

Coromega™
omega-3 (Fish Oil)

LANE LABS

LANE LABS

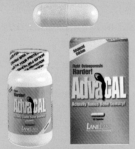

Advanced Calcium Complex
that builds bone density

AdvaCal™

MATRIX

MATRIX HEALTH PRODUCTS

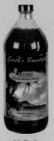

32 Fl. Oz

**Earth's Bounty®
Noni Juice**
(morinda citrifolia)

MATRIX HEALTH PRODUCTS

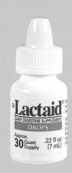

**Earth's Bounty®
Noni Caps**
(morinda citrifolia)

MATRIX HEALTH PRODUCTS

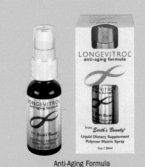

Anti-Aging Formula

Longevitrol™
(velvet antler)

MCNEIL

LACTAID INC. MARKETED BY
MCNEIL CONSUMER HEALTHCARE

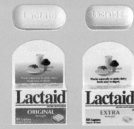

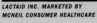

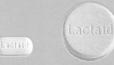

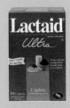

ORIGINAL STRENGTH available
in bottles of 120

EXTRA STRENGTH available
in bottles of 50

ULTRA CAPLETS available in
single serve packets of 12, 32
and 60 counts

ULTRA CHEWABLE TABLETS available in bottles
of 12 and 32 counts

**Lactaid® Caplets and
Chewable Tablets**

LACTAID INC. MARKETED BY
MCNEIL CONSUMER HEALTHCARE

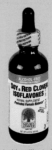

Available in 30 qt. supply

Lactaid® Drops

TO CHECK YOUR OPTIONS...

**...turn to the Indications Index.
There you'll find all the
supplements customarily
used for a particular
problem or purpose.**

NATURE'S ANSWER

NATURE'S ANSWER

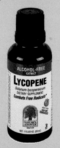

Supplied with orifice dropper;
Each serving guaranteed to contain a
minimum of 5 mg of Lycopene per dose
Available in a 1 ounce size

Lycopene

NATURE'S ANSWER

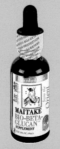

Supplied with calibrated dropper;
Each serving guaranteed to contain a
minimum of 14 mg of Beta-1,6-Glucan
with Beta 1, 3 branches per dose
Available in 1, 2 or 4 ounce sizes

**Maitake
Bio-Beta-Glucan™**

NATURE'S ANSWER

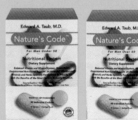

Supplied with calibrated dropper;
Each serving guaranteed to contain a total
minimum of 40 mg of isoflavones including
Genistein, Daidzein, Glycitein, Biochanin-A
and Formononetin per dose
Available in a 2 ounce size

**Soy & Red Clover
Isoflavones**

NATURE'S CODE

NATURE'S CODE

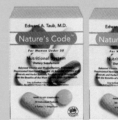

Women under 50   Women over 50

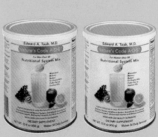

Men under 50   Men over 50

Nature's Code™ is an age and gender
specific balanced nutritional system with essential
vitamins, minerals and herbs in daily dose packets.
Formulated according to latest scientific research
with USP quality nutrients. Release Assured®.

**Nature's Code™
Nutritional System
Dietary Supplement**

NATURE'S CODE

Men over 50   Women over 50

**Nature's Code ADS™
Nutritional System
Powdered Dietary Supplement**

NOVARTIS CONSUMER HEALTH

NOVARTIS CONSUMER HEALTH, INC.

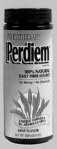

100% Natural Daily Fiber Source
available in 250 gm

Perdiem® Fiber Therapy

NOVARTIS CONSUMER HEALTH, INC.

Slow Release Iron available
in 30, 60 and 90 ct.
Slow Release Iron & Folic Acid
available in 20 ct.

Slow Fe®

PERSONAL PRODUCTS

PERSONAL PRODUCTS COMPANY

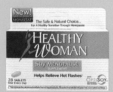

Soy Menopause Supplement

Healthy Woman™

PROCTER & GAMBLE

PROCTER & GAMBLE

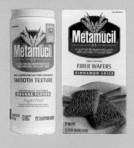

Available in 48, 72, 114 and 180 dose
canisters and cartons of 30 one-dose packets.
Also available in sugar free.
Cinnamon Spice and Apple Crisp Wafers
available in 12-dose cartons.

Metamucil®

SIGMA-TAU

SIGMA-TAU PHARMACEUTICALS, INC.

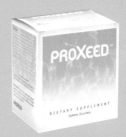

Dietary Supplement
Promotes optimum sperm quality

proXeed™

SMITHKLINE BEECHAM

*SMITHKLINE BEECHAM
CONSUMER HEALTHCARE, L.P.*

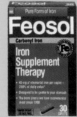

Packages of 30 caplets

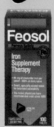

Packages of 100 tablets

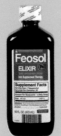

16 oz. bottle (Elixir)

Feosol®

SMITHKLINE BEECHAM
CONSUMER HEALTHCARE, L.P.

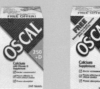

Calcium Supplement

Os-Cal®

*SMITHKLINE BEECHAM
CONSUMER HEALTHCARE, L.P.*

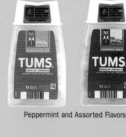

Peppermint and Assorted Flavors

Tums®

*SMITHKLINE BEECHAM
CONSUMER HEALTHCARE, L.P.*

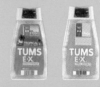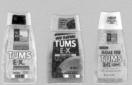

Tropical Fruit, Wintergreen,
Assorted Flavors, Assorted Berry
and SugarFree Orange Cream

Tums E-X®

*SMITHKLINE BEECHAM
CONSUMER HEALTHCARE, L.P.*

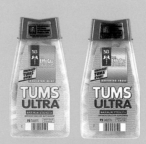

Assorted Mint and Fruit Flavors.
Also available in Tropical Fruit,
Assorted Berries and Spearmint flavors

Tums® Ultra™

TOM'S OF MAINE

TOM'S OF MAINE

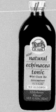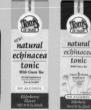

Elderberry and hibiscus flavors

**Natural Echinacea
Tonic Concentrate**

TOM'S OF MAINE

Ginger-orange and elderberry flavors

**Natural Echinacea
Tonic with Green Tea**

TOM'S OF MAINE

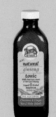

Cinnamon and ginger flavors

Natural Ginseng Tonic

TOM'S OF MAINE

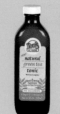

Ginger and lemongrass flavors

Natual Green Tea Tonic

TOM'S OF MAINE

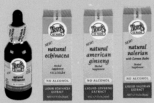

Hibiscus and elderberry flavors

Natural Liquid Extracts

TOM'S OF MAINE

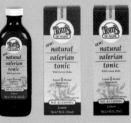

Lemon flavor

Natural Valerian Tonic

WAKUNAGA

WAKUNAGA CONSUMER PRODUCTS

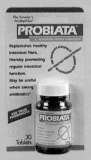

L. acidophilus

PROBIATA®

WARNER-LAMBERT CO.

WARNER-LAMBERT CO.

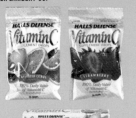

100% Daily Value Vitamin C in each drop.
Available in Assorted Citrus, Strawberry and
Harvest Cherry flavors.

Halls® Defense

Supplement Monographs

This section contains comprehensive profiles of virtually all the most popular nutritional supplements on retail shelves today. Included are an extensive array of amino acids and oligopeptides, fatty acids and other lipids, metabolites and cofactors, nucleic acids, proteins, glycosupplements, phytosupplements, hormonal products, and probiotics.

The monographs on these supplements are designed to arm you with all the information you need to forge rational recommendations and protect your patients' health. In addition to providing a penetrating summary of significant clinical research, they address all the practical issues encountered during routine use, from proper dosage to crucial precautions. Each monograph includes up to eleven standard sections. Here's a closer look at what they contain.

■ **Trade Names:** Listed here are the most widely distributed brands of the various formulations of the nutrient.

■ **Description:** This section provides a detailed discussion of the nature of the substance and its place in human biochemistry, along with its precise chemical structure.

■ **Actions and Pharmacology:** Here you'll find an overview of the nutrient's better documented actions,

the proposed or verified mechanisms through which it exerts its effects, and its pharmacokinetics, including absorption, metabolism, and excretion.

■ **Indications and Usage:** Described here are the specific therapeutic uses proposed for the supplement, ranging from the accepted indications to the more speculative possibilities.

■ **Research Summary:** This section enumerates the leading claims made for the substance and evaluates the merits of each. Included are the most significant findings, both pro and con, drawn from retrospective reviews, meta-analyses, and controlled clinical trials.

■ **Contraindications, Precautions, Adverse Reactions:** Here you'll find the important safety considerations to remember when recommending the supplement and while monitoring the patient's progress.

■ **Interactions:** Listed here are the drugs, herbs, foods, and supplements with which the substance may interact. The effect of each combination is summarized, along with the appropriate action to take as a result.

■ **Overdosage:** This section presents the warning signs of overdose (if any are known) and summarized emergency treatment measures.

■ **Dosage and Administration:** Described here are typical dosage recommendations for each formulation of the substance, together with any special measures to be taken during administration.

■ **How Supplied:** This section lists available dosage forms and strengths of each formulation and salt.

■ **Literature:** Here you'll find relevant citations from the clinical literature.

PDR for Nutritional Supplements is the product of one of the most thorough and inclusive examinations of the literature ever undertaken. Nevertheless, it's important to remember that it merely summarizes and synthesizes key data from the underlying reports, and of necessity includes neither every published report nor every recorded fact.

As in all scientific investigation, conclusions regarding the effectiveness of the supplements discussed in this compendium are based on the preponderance of current evidence and cannot be considered firm or final. The publisher does not warrant that any substance will unfailingly and uniformly exhibit the properties ascribed to it by researchers in the field.

Also, please remember that the products discussed in this book are marketed under the provisions of the Dietary Supplement and Health Education Act of 1994, which prohibits their sale for the diagnosis, treatment, cure, or prevention of any disease. The monographs in this compendium discuss scientific findings regarding the substance itself, and should not be construed as recommending any specific commercial preparation. Enumeration of specific products within a monograph implies no claim or warranty of their efficacy for any purpose, by either the manufacturer or the publisher. Furthermore, it should be understood that, just as omission of a product does not signify rejection, inclusion of a product does not imply endorsement, and that the publisher is not advocating the use of any product or substance described herein.

Please remember, too, that the potency and the purity of nutritional supplements are subject to substantial variation. Dosage ranges set forth in the monographs must therefore be considered nothing more than general guidelines. Likewise, safety information found in the monographs applies only to the substance itself, and does not allow for the effects of adulterants and variations in the manufacturing process.

In addition, the publisher does not guarantee that every possible hazard, adverse effect, contraindication, precaution, or consequence of overdose is included in the summaries presented here. The publisher has performed no independent verification of the data reported herein, and expressly disclaims responsibility for any error, whether inherent in the underlying literature or resulting from erroneous translation, transcription, or typography.

5-Hydroxytryptophan (5-HTP)

DESCRIPTION

5-Hydroxytryptophan is the immediate precursor in the biosynthesis of the neurotransmitter 5-hydroxytryptamine (5-HT or serotonin). 5-HT itself is derived biochemically from the essential protein amino acid L-tryptophan.

5-HTP, along with carbidopa, is used in Europe as a pharmaceutical agent for the treatment of depression. It has also been used in the treatment of Gilles de la Tourette syndrome and for the treatment of the self-mutilation symptoms of Lesch-Nyhan syndrome. 5-HTP is an orphan drug in the U.S. for the treatment of postanoxic intention myoclonus, a rare complication of CPR (cardiopulmonary resuscitation). It is used in this disorder in combination with carbidopa.

Until November, 1989, L-tryptophan was a popular nutritional supplement in the U.S. In November, 1989, the FDA recalled supplementary L-tryptophan because of several reports associating the amino acid with some severe side effects. These side-effects were part of a syndrome called the eosinophilia-myalgia syndrome. As it turned out, the cause of the syndrome was due to a contaminant in a batch of L-tryptophan that was produced from a genetically modified microorganism (GMO), and not L-tryptophan itself. However, the supplemental use of L-tryptophan never recovered following this tragic incident. 5-HTP was intended to fill the supplemental gap created by the removal of L-tryptophan from the nutritional supplement marketplace.

Unfortunately, a few cases of eosinophilia-myalgia syndrome have now been reported associated with the use of 5-HTP and once again, the problem appears to be due to contaminants in the supplement, and not to 5-HTP itself. However, 5-HTP suffers from another problem. High doses of 5-HTP are metabolized peripherally to serotonin and this can result in elevated serum levels of serotonin, with consequent adverse reactions related to the elevated levels (see Adverse Reactions). In Europe, where 5-HTP is used for the treatment of depression, it is used in combination with carbidopa, which inhibits the peripheral conversion of 5-HTP to serotonin. This is similar to the situation with the use of levodopa in the treatment of Parkinson's disease. For levodopa to be effective in this disorder, its peripheral conversion to dopamine must be prevented. This is the reason why L-dopa is combined with carbidopa and carbidopa is used in the treatment of Parkinson's disease. Carbidopa inhibits this conversion.

5-Hydroxytryptophan or 5-HTP is also known as L-5-HTP, L-5-hydroxytryptophan, oxitriptan and L-2-amino-3-(5-hydroxy-1-H-indol-3-yl)propionic acid. Its molecular formula is $C_{11}H_{12}N_2O_3$ and its molecular weight is 220.23 daltons. The structural formula of 5-Hydroxytryptophan is:

5-Hydroxytryptophan

A major commercial source of 5-HTP is the African plant *Griffonia simplicfolia*, a relative of carob. Small amounts of 5-HTP, as well as serotonin, are found in food sources, including bananas, tomatoes, plums, avocados, eggplant, walnuts and pineapples.

ACTIONS AND PHARMACOLOGY

ACTIONS

5-HTP may have antidepressant activity. It has putative analgesic and bariatric actions.

MECHANISM OF ACTION

The mechanism of the possible antidepressant activity of 5-HTP is accounted for by its conversion to the neurotransmitter serotonin which plays a central role in the affective state. Antidepressants may work by either binding to one or more of the family of serotonin 5-HT receptors (5-HT$_1$ - 5-HT$_7$) or by inhibiting the reuptake of serotonin. The tricyclic antidepressants may work, in part, by binding to the serotonin 5-HT$_6$ receptor, a member of the G protein superfamily which is positively coupled to an adenylate cyclase second-messenger system. The selective serotonin reuptake inhibitors (SSRIs) selectively inhibit the reuptake of serotonin. 5-HTP most likely binds to one or more of the 5-HT receptors, although which one(s) in not known for sure.

There is some evidence that 5-HTP has some analgesic activity in those with fibromyalgia, and in one study, 5-HTP was found to have some beneficial effect in those with chronic tension headache. The possible analgesic effect of 5-HTP may be accounted for, in part, by its conversion to serotonin. 5-HTP has also been found to increase plasma beta-endorphin and platelet met-enkephalin levels, which may signify a reinforcing effect upon an endogenous analgesic effect.

The mechanism of the putative bariatric action of 5-HTP is not well understood. Serotonin is known to regulate feeding behavior and decrease food intake in humans and rodents. A recent study suggests that this effect may be mediated via leptin. Serum leptin levels in mice were found to increase following systemic injection of 5-HTP. Leptin, an adipocyte-derived protein product of the ob (obesity) gene, is a multifunctional polypeptide associated with the development of obesity-related disorders in humans.

PHARMACOKINETICS

A significant amount of an ingested dose of 5-HTP is decarboxylated in the small intestine to 5-hydroxytryptamine (5-HT or serotonin). Carbidopa, if administered with 5-HTP, inhibits this decarboxylation which is catalyzed by a vitamin B_6-dependent decarboxylase. Peripheral decarboxylation of 5-HTP occurs to a much lesser extent in those with low vitamin B_6 status, and most likely to a greater extent, in those who take concurrent vitamin B_6 supplements of doses 5 milligrams or greater.

The efficiency of absorption of 5-HTP, as well as its decarboxylation product serotonin, is approximately 47% to 84%. Absorption of 5-HTP occurs by an active transport process. 5-HTP is transported by the portal circulation to the liver where approximately 25% of an administered dose is metabolized via vitamin B_6-dependent L-aromatic amino acid decarboxylase to 5-HT. 5-HT is subsequently metabolized to 5-hydroxyindole acetaldehyde which is rapidly metabolized to 5-hydroxyindoleacetic acid (5-HIAA). 5-HTP that is not metabolized in the liver is transported by the general circulation to the various tissues of the body, including the brain. 5-HTP readily crosses the blood-brain barrier, and is converted to serotonin in brain cells. 5-HIAA is the principal renal excretion product of 5-HTP.

INDICATIONS AND USAGE

5-HTP has shown some usefulness in some conditions characterized, in part, by serotonin deficits, principally depression. It has also been shown to be useful in some with obesity, insomnia, fibromyalgia and chronic tension headache.

RESEARCH SUMMARY

Scattered studies have shown that supplemental 5-HTP has significant anti-depressant effects in some. In one double-blind, multi-center study, 5-HTP was said to have antidepressant effects slightly better than the SSRI fluvoxamine. Other studies have been more equivocal. One study indicated that 5-HTP is not effective in those whose depression is not responsive to serotonin reuptake inhibitors (SSRIs). More rigorous, longer term studies are needed.

In a double-blind, placebo-controlled crossover study of 19 obese female subjects given 5-HTP (8 milligrams per kilogram of body weight daily) for five weeks, significant weight loss (about 5 percent) was recorded in 5-HTP treated subjects, compared with controls. No dietary prescriptions were prescribed during the course of this study.

These findings were confirmed in a second double-blind, placebo-controlled, randomized study conducted over a longer period of time—two consecutive six-week periods.

In a more recent double-blind study, subjects with non-insulin dependent diabetes were randomized to receive either placebo or 750 milligrams of 5-HTP daily for two weeks without dietary restrictions. Significant weight loss was achieved in the 5-HTP group. A 5-HTP-inhibiting effect on carbohydrate intake was noted.

There is preliminary, dated (1977) evidence that 5-HTP can be of benefit in those described as "mildly insomniac."

Evidence that 5-HTP might be helpful in fibromyalgia is also preliminary but more recent. In a 90-day open trial, 50 patients with primary fibromyalgia were reported to achieve significant improvement in all clinical variables measured, including tender points, anxiety, quality of sleep and fatigue.

There is evidence in some animal work, as well as some *in vitro* work, that 5-HTP is radioprotective. Combined with a thiol compound, 5-HTP protected peripheral blood and sperm cells.

In a recently reported randomized, double-blind, placebo-controlled trial, subjects who took 300 milligrams daily of 5-HTP were found to have a significant decrease in their use of analgesics for chronic tension-type headache, and also a significant decrease in the number of days with headaches following the conclusion of the trial.

CONTRAINDICATIONS, PRECAUTIONS, ADVERSE REACTIONS

CONTRAINDICATIONS

5-HTP is contraindicated in those hypersensitive to any component of a 5-HTP-containing product. It is also contraindicated in those with carcinoid tumors, and during or within 2 weeks after discontinuing MAOIs (type A).

PRECAUTIONS

Large doses of 5-HTP can trigger excess serotonin formation in tissues other than the target organ and cause significant adverse reactions.

5-HTP should not be used concurrently with any antidepressant, including selective serotonin reuptake inhibitors (SSRIs), tricyclic antidepressants or monoamine oxidase inhibitors (MAOIs). Concurrent use of 5-HTP with an antidepressant may increase the risk of adverse reactions.

5-HTP should not be used concurrently with serotonin $5-HT_1$ receptor agonists, including naratriptan, sumatriptan and zolmitriptan. Such use may increase the risk of adverse reactions.

5-HTP should be avoided by those with ischemic heart disease (history of myocardial infarction, angina pectoris, documented silent ischemia), coronary artery spasm (e.g., Prinzmetal's angina), uncontrolled hypertension and any other significant cardiovascular disease.

5-HTP should be avoided by pregnant women and nursing mothers.

ADVERSE REACTIONS

Eosinophilia and eosinophilia-myalgia syndrome (EMS) have been reported in those taking 5-HTP. The eosinophilia-myalgia syndrome is similar to that caused by L-tryptophan and was linked to contaminants in the 5-HTP preparation, rather than 5-HTP itself. Changing the 5-HTP lot in one group of patients resolved the eosinophilia. A scleroderma-like skin condition has been reported in some taking a combination of 5-HTP and carbidopa.

Other reported side effects, include nausea, diarrhea, loss of appetite, vomiting and difficult breathing. Neurological side effects, including dilation of the pupils, abnormally sensitive reflexes, loss of muscle coordination and blurring of vision, have been reported in those taking large doses of 5-HTP. Cardiac dysrhythmias have also been reported.

Large doses of 5-HTP may significantly increase serum levels of serotonin, and theoretically, this may result in the serotonin syndrome. Symptoms and signs of the serotonin syndrome, include confusion, agitation, diaphoresis, tachycardia, myoclonus and hyperreflexia. In addition, hypertension, coma/unresponsiveness, seizures, and death may occur if the syndrome is not promptly recognized and treated. There are no reports of the serotonin syndrome occurring with use of 5-HTP in humans. However, it could occur and the combination of 5-HTP with another serotonergic agent can increase the risk of it occurring. As a side note, there are 21 cases of 5-HTP toxicosis reported in dogs. Accidental ingestion of 5-HTP by dogs resulted in a serotonin-like syndrome. Three of the dogs died.

INTERACTIONS

DRUGS

5-HT antagonists (methysergide, cyproheptadine): 5-HTP may decrease the effectiveness of methysergide and cyproheptadine.

5-HT₁ receptor agonists (naratriptan, sumatriptan, zolmitriptan): Concurrent use of 5-HTP with a 5-HT₁ agonist may increase the risk of adverse reactions.

Carbidopa: Carbidopa suppresses peripheral 5-HTP metabolism, allowing greater amounts of 5-HTP to reach the brain.

Methyldopa: Methyldopa inhibits the enzymatic conversion of 5-HTP to serotonin.

Moroamine oxidase inhibitors (MAOIs; isocarboxazid, phenelzine sulfate, tranylcypromine): Concurrent use of 5-HTP with an MAOI (type A) may increase the risk of adverse reactions.

Phenoxybenzamine: Phenoxybenzamine inhibits the conversion of 5-HTP to serotonin.

Selective serotonin reuptake inhibitors (SSRIs; citalopram, fluvoxamine maleate, fluoxetine, paroxetine, sertraline, venlafaxine): Concurrent use of 5-HTP with a SSRI may potentiate the antidepressant effect of the SSRI and may also increase the risk of adverse reactions.

NUTRITIONAL SUPPLEMENTS

Vitamin B₆: Concurrent intake of 5-HTP and doses of vitamin B₆ 5 milligrams or greater, may enhance the peripheral decarboxylation of 5-HTP to serotonin.

HERBS

Saint John's wort: Theoretically, concurrent use of 5-HTP and Saint John's wort may both potentiate the possible antidepressant activity of the herbal product and increase the risk of adverse reactions.

OVERDOSAGE

There are no overdosage reports in humans. There are reports of overdosage and subsequent serotonin-like syndrome in dogs. Some of these overdosages resulted in death to the animals.

DOSAGE AND ADMINISTRATION

Supplemental 5-HTP is not recommended. In Europe, a combination of 5-HTP with carbidopa is available, and this combination appears to have a safer profile. However, those who wish to use this combination product, must do so only under medical supervision and prescription. It has been found that doses of 100 milligrams to 2 grams daily are required to observe any desired effect. These doses, without concomitant carbidopa, can be dangerous in some (see Precautions). Lower doses, which are available as dietary supplements, are unlikely to have any desirable effect.

LITERATURE

Boiardi A, Picotti GB, Di Giulio AM, et al. Platelet met-enkephalin immunoreactivity and 5-hydroxytryptamine concentrations in migraine patients: effects of 5-hydroxytryptophan, amitriptyline and chlorimipramine treatment. *Cephalalgia.* 1984; 4:81-84.

Byerley WF, Judd LL, Reimherr FW, et al. 5-Hydroxytryptophan: a review of its antidepressant efficacy and adverse effects. *J Clin Psychopharmacol.* 1987; 7:127-137.

Cangiano C, Ceci F, Cascino A, et al. Eating behavior and adherence to dietary prescriptions in obese adult subjects treated with 5-hydroxytryptophan. *Am J Clin Nutr.* 1992; 56:863-867.

Cangiano C, Laviano A, Del Ben M, et al. Effects of oral 5-hydroxytryptophan on energy intake and macronutrient selection in non-insulin dependent diabetes mellitus. *Int J Obes Relat Metab Disord*. 1998; 22:648-654.

Caruso I, Sarzi Puttini P, Cazzola M, Azzolini V. Double-blind study of 5-hydroxytryptophan versus placebo in the treatment of primary fibromyalgia syndrome. *J Int Med Res*. 1990; 18:201-209.

Ceci F, Cangiano C, Cairella M, et al. The effects of oral 5-hydroxytryptophan administration on feeding behavior in obese adult female subjects. *J Neural Transm*. 1989; 76:109-117.

Genazzani AR, Sandrini G, Facchinetti F, et al. Effects of L-5HTP with and without carbidopa on plasma beta-endorphin and pain perception. Possible implications in migraine prophylaxis. *Cephalalgia*. 1986; 6:241-245.

Gwaltney-Brant SM, Albertsen JC, Khan SA. 5-Hydroxy-trytophan toxicosis in dogs: 21 cases (1989-1999). *J Am Vet Med Assoc*. 2000; 216:1937-1940.

Imeri L, Mancia M, Bianchi S, Opp MR. 5-Hydroxytryptophan, but not L-tryptophan, alters sleep and brain temperature in rats. *Neuroscience*. 2000; 95:445-452.

Klarskov K, Johnson KL, Benson LM, et al. Eosinophilia-myalgia syndrome case-associated contaminants in commercially available 5-hydroxytryptophan. *Adv Exp Med Biol*. 1999; 467:461-468.

Michelson D, Page SW, Casey R, et al. An eosinophilia-myalgia syndrome related disorder associated with exposure to L-5-hydroxytryptophan. *J Rheumatol*. 1994; 21:2261-2265.

Nicoladi M, Sicuteri F. L-5-hydroxytryptophan can prevent nociceptive disorders in man. *Adv Exp Med Biol*. 1999; 467:177-182.

Puttini PS, Caruso I. Primary fibromyalgia syndrome and 5-hydroxy-L-tryptophan: a 90-day open study. *J Int Med Res*. 1992; 20:182-189.

Ribeiro CA. L-5-Hydroxytryptophan in the prophylaxis of chronic tension-type headache: a double-blind, randomized, placebo-controlled study. For the Portuguese Head Study. *Headache*. 2000; 40:451-456.

Sternberg EM, Van Woert MH, Young SN, et al. Development of a scleroderma-like illness during therapy with L-5-hydroxytryptophan and carbidopa. *N Eng J Med*. 1980; 303:782-787.

Williamson BL, Klarskov K, Tolminson A J, et al. Problems with over-the-counter 5-hydroxy-L-tryptophan. *Nat Med*. 1998; 4:983.

Yamada J, Ujikawa M, Sugimoto Y. Serum leptin levels after central and systemic injection of a serotonin precursor, 5-hydroxytryptophan, in mice. *Eur J Pharmacol*. 2000; 406:159-162.

Zhou SY, Goshgarian HG. 5-Hydroxytryptophan-induced respiratory recovery after cervical spinal cord hemisection in rats. *J Appl Physiol*. 2000; 89:1528-1536.

19-Norandrostenedione

TRADE NAMES

Bolandione (Syntrax Innovations), 19-N-Andro (MuscleLinc), Proven Pure 19-Norandrostenedione (Proven).

DESCRIPTION

19-Norandrostenedione refers to two steroid isomers that are marketed as dietary supplements and mainly used by body builders. The difference between the two 19-norandrostenedione isomers is in the position of the double bond in the cyclopentanoperhydrophenanthrene ring structure. The delta4 isomer has a double bond between carbons 4 and 5; the delta5 isomer has a double bond between carbons 5 and 6.

The delta4 isomer is also known as 19-nor-4-androstene-3, 17-dione. The delta5 isomer is also known as 19-nor-5-androstene-3, 17-dione. The delta4 isomer is sometimes referred to as 19-nor and is the more popular of the two substances. Nor refers to the absence of a 19 methyl group on the steroid ring structure. 19-Norandrostenedione is synthesized in the adrenal gland and gonads from androstenedione. It is metabolized by the aromatase complex to estrone. The delta4, as well as delta5, 19-norandrostenedione may also be metabolized by the enzyme 17 beta-hydroxy steroid dehydrogenase to 19-nortestosterone, also known as nandrolone. In this monograph, 19-norandrostenedione will generally be used in the singular to refer to both the delta4 and delta5 isomers.

ACTIONS AND PHARMACOLOGY

ACTIONS

Supplemental 19-norandrostenedione is a putative anabolic substance.

MECHANISM OF ACTION

19-Norandrostenedione may be metabolized to 19-nortestosterone in both men and women. 19-Norandrostenedione, also known as nandrolone, is the basic substance of some very popular injectable anabolic steroids. 19-Norandrostenedione is not metabolized to testosterone. Whether increases in 19-nortestosterone levels that may be produced by taking oral 19-norandrostenedione would be sustained long enough to show increase in nitrogen retention and muscle strength and mass is unknown.

PHARMACOKINETICS

There is scant human pharmacokinetic data on 19-norandrostenedione. Absorption appears variable, but some absorption does occur. Following ingestion of 19-norandrostenedione, metabolites, including 19-norandrosterone and 19-noretiocholanolone, appear in the urine. 19-Norandrostenedione and 19-noretiocholanolone are detectable in the urine for seven to 10 days after a single 50-mg oral dose. Specific metabolites of 19-nor-5-androstene-3, 17-dione are 19-nordehydroandrosterone and 19-nordehydroepiandrosterone. In the later stages of excretion, higher levels of 19-noretiocholanolone relative to 19-norandrosterone indicate intake of 19-nor delta5 steroids.

INDICATIONS AND USAGE

The claim that supplemental 19-norandrostenedione has anabolic effects is unsubstantiated. The use of this substance may pose serious health risks in some.

RESEARCH SUMMARY

There is no research showing that either oral or injectable 19-norandrostenedione has significant anabolic effects.

CONTRAINDICATIONS, PRECAUTIONS, ADVERSE REACTIONS

CONTRAINDICATIONS

19-Norandrostenedione is contraindicated in those with prostate, breast, ovarian and uterine cancer and those at risk for these cancers. 19-Norandrostenedione is also contraindicated in those who are hypersensitive to any component of a 19-norandrostenedione-containing preparation.

PRECAUTIONS

Children, adolescents, pregnant women and nursing mothers should avoid 19-norandrostenedione supplements. Women generally should be cautious in the use of 19-norandrostenedione because of possible virilizing effects

ADVERSE REACTIONS

No data are available on the long-term safety of taking supplemental 19-norandrostenedione. Adverse effects of exogenous testosterone in men include acne, testicular atrophy, gynecomastia, behavioral changes and possibly an increased risk of prostate cancer. Adverse effects of exogenous testosterone in women include hirsutism, deepening of the voice, acne, clitoral hypertrophy, amenorrhea, male-patten baldness and coarsening of the skin. In adolescents, exogenous testosterone can lead to early closing of bone growth plates and decreased adult height. Other adverse effects of testosterone include hepatic failure and increased platelet aggregation.

Many, if not all, of the above adverse reactions may occur with long-term use of 19-norandrostenedione.

INTERACTIONS

No drug, nutritional supplement, food or herb interactions have yet been reported.

OVERDOSAGE

No reports of overdosages.

DOSAGE AND ADMINISTRATION

Those who use 19-norandrostenedione typically take 100 mg daily.

HOW SUPPLIED

Capsules — 50 mg, 100 mg

Powder

LITERATURE

Uralets VP, Gillette PA. Over-the-counter anabolic steroids 4-androsten-3, 17-dione; 4-androsten-3beta, 17beta-diol; and 19-nor-4-androstene-3, 17-dione: excretion studies in men. *J Anal Toxicol.* 1999; 23:357-366.

Uralets VP, Gillette PA. Over-the-counter delta5 anabolic steroids 5-androsten-3, 17-dione, 5-androsten-3beta, 17 beta-diol; dehydroxyepiandrosterone; and 19-nor-5-androstene-3, 17-dione: excretion studies in men. *J Anal Toxicol.* 2000; 24:188-193.

7-Oxo-Dehydroepiandrosterone (7-Oxo-DHEA)

TRADE NAMES

7-Keto Fuel (Twinlab)

DESCRIPTION

7-Oxo-dehydroepiandrosterone, abbreviated as 7-oxo-DHEA, is a natural substance produced in the adrenal gland, gonads and brain. 7-Oxo-DHEA is a metabolite of the steroid hormone DHEA (see DHEA). DHEA and its metabolite dehydroepiandrosterone-3-sulfate, or DHEAS, are the major secretory steroidal products of the adrenal gland. DHEA is believed to have great importance in human physiology. However, to date, its exact role is unknown. 7-Oxo-DHEA has been studied to better understand, among other things, the biological role of DHEA. A major biochemical difference between 7-oxo-DHEA and DHEA is that DHEA is metabolized to the sex hormones while 7-oxo-DHEA does not appear to be metabolized to these hormones.

7-Oxo-DHEA is being studied for its possible cognition-enhancing and thermogenic activities. Steroids that are made in the brain are referred to as neurosteroids; steroids that may have thermogenic activity are referred to as ergosteroids. 7-Oxo-DHEA is also known as 3beta-hydroxyandrost-5-ene-7,17-dione, delta5-androstene-3beta-ol-7,17-dione and 7-keto-DHEA. The structural formula is:

7-Oxo-Dehydroepiandrosterone

7-Oxo-DHEA is marketed as a nutritional supplement. The form of 7-oxo-DHEA most commonly marketed is the 3-acetyl ester of 7-oxo-DHEA, also known as 3-acetyl-7-oxo-DHEA.

ACTIONS AND PHARMACOLOGY

ACTIONS

Supplemental 7-oxo-DHEA has putative cognition-enhancing, thermogenic and immunomodulatory activities.

MECHANISM OF ACTION

7-Oxo-DHEA was found to reverse scopolamine-induced cholinergic dysfunction in mice. It is speculated that 7-oxo-DHEA's effect on memory is via antagonizing the $GABA_A$ receptor.

7-Oxo-DHEA has been demonstrated to induce liver mitochondrial *sn*-glycerol 3 -phosphate dehydrogenase and cytosolic malic enzyme in rats. It is thought that the induction of these enzymes may account for the thermogenic effect of 7-oxo-DHEA in animal models.

7-Oxo-DHEA has been reported to augment interleukin 2 (IL-2) production by human lymphocytes *in vitro*. The mechanism of this effect is unknown.

PHARMACOKINETICS

There is little on the pharmacokinetics of 7-oxo-DHEA in humans. Preliminary studies indicate that it is absorbed following ingestion. However, the efficiency of its absorption, as well as its distribution, metabolism and excretion, need to be elucidated. It does not appear that 7-oxo-DHEA is converted to the sex hormones testosterone and estrogens; DHEA, on the other hand, is.

INDICATIONS AND USAGE

Claims for 7-oxo-DHEA include metabolic enhancements that help promote weight loss and increase lean body mass, favorable effects on immunity, improved memory and various anti-aging effects. These claims are largely extravagant extrapolations from very preliminary animal and *in vitro* studies. Some claim that 7-oxo-DHEA is superior to DHEA itself because 7-oxo-DHEA appears not to be converted to sex hormones (see DHEA).

RESEARCH SUMMARY

In a recent animal study, 7-oxo-DHEA was tested for its possible ability to reverse chemically induced memory abolition in young mice and for its effects on memory in old mice. Significant positive effects were reported in both test groups, compared with controls. A single dose of 7-oxo-DHEA reportedly completely reversed scopolamine-induced memory impairment in the young mice. And, in the old mice, single doses resulted in significant memory retention, as measured by water maze training, through a four-week test period. Memory retention was not improved in controls or in those animals given DHEA itself.

Several experimental studies have suggested that 7-oxo-DHEA might enhance thermogenesis. Some researchers have concluded that it is a more effective inducer of thermogenic enzymes than its parent steroid, DHEA. In large doses, DHEA has been shown to induce weight loss in genetically obese and in some normal animals without affecting food intake, but similar effects in humans have not been reliably confirmed. Similarly, there is no credible evidence that 7-oxo-DHEA significantly decreases weight or increases lean muscle mass in humans.

There are some data indicating that 7-oxo-DHEA might favorably impact some immune activities, such as stimulation of interleukin-2 and increased production of CD-4 and CD-8 cells *in vitro*.

CONTRAINDICATIONS, PRECAUTIONS, ADVERSE REACTIONS

CONTRAINDICATIONS

7-Oxo-DHEA is contraindicated in those hypersensitive to any component of a 7-oxo-DHEA-containing product.

PRECAUTIONS

7-Oxo-DHEA supplementation should be avoided by pregnant women and nursing mothers.

OVERDOSAGE

No reports.

DOSAGE AND ADMINISTRATION

7-Oxo-DHEA has recently been introduced in the nutritional supplement marketplace. It is marketed as the 3-acetyl ester of 7-oxo-DHEA. Those who use this supplement use from 50 milligrams to 100 milligrams daily.

HOW SUPPLIED

Capsules — 25 mg, 50 mg

LITERATURE

Bobyleva V, Bellei M, Kneer N, Lardy H. The effects of the ergosteroid 7-oxo-dehydroepiandrosterone on mitochondrial membrane potential: possible relationship to thermogenesis. *Arch Biochem Biophys.* 1997; 341:122-128.

Lardy H, Partridge B, Kneer N, Wei Y. Ergosteroids: induction of thermogenic enzymes in liver of rats treated with steroids derived from dehydroepiandrosterone. *Proc Natl Acad Sci USA.* 1995; 92:6617-6619.

Rose KA, Stapleton G, Dott K, et al. Cyp7b, a novel brain cytochrome P450, catalyzes the synthesis of neurosteroids 7alpha-hydroxy dehydroepiandrosterone and 7alpha-hydroxy pregnenolone. *Proc Natl Acad Sci USA.* 1997; 94:4925-4930.

Shi J, Schulze S, Lardy HA. The effect of 7-oxo-DHEA acetate on memory in young and old C57BL/6 mice. *Steroids.* 2000; 65:124-129.

Acetyl-L-Carnitine

DESCRIPTION

Acetyl-L-Carnitine is the acetyl ester of L-carnitine. It occurs naturally in animal products. Chemically, acetyl-L-carnitine is known as beta-acetoxy-gamma-N, N, N-trimethylamino-butyrate and is represented by the following chemical structure:

$$(CH_3)_3\overset{+}{N}\!-\!\!CH_2\text{-}CH\!-\!\!CH_2\text{-}COO^-$$

Acetyl-L-Carnitine

Acetyl-L-carnitine is also known as acetyl-carnitine, L-acetycarnitine, acetylcarnitine, acetyl levocarnitine, ALC and ALCAR.

Acetyl-L-carnitine is a delivery form for both L-carnitine and acetyl groups.

ACTIONS AND PHARMACOLOGY

ACTIONS

Supplemental acetyl-L-carnitine may have neuroprotective activity. In addition, it, like L-carnitine, may have cardioprotective activity and may beneficially affect cardiac function. It may enhance sperm motiliy. Acetyl-L-carnitine may also have cytoprotective, antioxidant and anti-apoptotic activity.

MECHANISM OF ACTION

Acetyl-L-carnitine is a delivery form for L-carnitine and acetyl groups. The functions of L-carnitine include transport of long-chain fatty acids across the mitochondrial membranes into the mitochondria (wherein their metabolism produces bioenergy) and transport of small-chain and medium-chain fatty acids out of the mitochondria in order to, among other things, maintain normal coenzyme A levels in these organelles. It may also have antioxidant activity.

The acetyl component of acetyl-L-carnitine provides for the formation of the neurotransmitter acetylcholine. Abnormal acetylcholine metabolism in the brain, leading to acetylcholine deficits in certain brain regions, is thought to be associated with age-related dementias, including Alzheimer's disease.

Acetyl-L-carnitine has been found to decrease glycation of lens proteins *in vitro*. It is thought to do so by acetylating certain lens proteins called crystallins. In so doing it protects them from glycation-mediated damage.

Many biochemical changes occur during the aging process. These include decreased cardiolipin synthesis in the heart and impaired mitochondrial function. Cardiolipin is a key phospholipid necessary for mitochondrial transport processes in the heart. Mitochondria are vital for the production of cellular energy. Experiments in aged rats have shown that acetyl-L-carnitine supplementation leads to improved mitochondrial function and increased cardiolipin production.

Acetyl-L-carnitine serves as a readily accessible energy pool for use in both activation of respiration and motility in human spermatozoa.

PHARMACOKINETICS

The pharmacokinetics of acetyl-L-carnitine are similar to L-carnitine (see L-carnitine). There is speculation that it is better absorbed than L-carnitine, but this has not yet been established.

INDICATIONS AND USAGE

Acetyl-L-carnitine has recently demonstrated some efficacy as a possible neuroprotective agent and may be indicated for use in strokes, Alzheimer's disease, Down's syndrome and for the management of various neuropathies. It may also have anti-aging properties. Research regarding acetyl-L-carnitine's possible beneficial effect on sperm motility is early-stage but promising.

RESEARCH SUMMARY

Several studies have now demonstrated some positive effects of acetyl-L-carnitine supplementation in Alzheimer's patients especially with regard to tasks involving attention and concentration. In a double-blind, parallel design, placebo-controlled pilot study of 30 patients whose mild-to-moderate dementias were believed to be symptoms of Alzheimer's disease, there were significant, positive results as measured by some of the neuropsychological tests used in the study.

In another early double-blind, placebo-controlled study of 130 patients with clinical diagnoses of Alzheimer's disease, a slower rate of deterioration was observed in 13 of 14 outcome measures at the end of this one-year study. Some of these measures reached statistical significance, including measures of logical intelligence, long-term verbal memory and selective attention.

More recent studies continue to show beneficial effects in Alzheimer's disease. Younger patients seem to benefit most.

It has been suggested that cognitive function may be improved in subjects with Alzheimer's disease by acetyl-L-carnitine's hypothesized ability to inhibit apoptosis of cerebral nerve cells.

Significant improvement in visual memory and attention in Down's syndrome subjects treated with acetyl-L-carnitine has also been reported. These researchers hypothesized that acetyl-L-carnitine's positive actions in both Alzheimer's disease and Down's syndrome result from its direct and indirect cholinomimetic effects.

There is also preliminary evidence that acetyl-L-carnitine can slow mental decline in the elderly who are not afflicted with dementias.

Neuroprotective effects of acetyl-L-carnitine have been reported after stroke in both animal models and in humans. Cerebral blood flow reportedly improves in acetyl-L-carnitine treated subjects with cerebrovascular disease.

Peripheral nerve function has been improved with the use of acetyl-L-carnitine in experimental diabetes. There is also early clinical evidence that acetyl-L-carnitine may be helpful in various peripheral neuropathies, and it has been suggested that this supplement might be helpful in alleviating the neurotoxicity associated with the nucleoside analogues used in the treatment of AIDS. This latter hypothesis has yet to be tested.

There is some evidence in animal work that acetyl-L-carnitine might have anti-aging effects. Mitochondrial function and ambulatory activity were assessed in a study of old rats fed acetyl-L-carnitine. Ambulatory activity was significantly increased in the old rats, and an examination of liver cells in the treated animals showed a significant reversal of age-associated decline of mitochondrial membrane potential. Cardiolipin, which declines with age, was significantly restored.

Finally, acetyl-L-carnitine has been reported to increase sperm motility *in vitro*, and in one human trial, 4 grams daily of this substance given to 20 oligoasthenospermic men, produced increased progressive sperm motility which was associated with a greater number of pregnancies.

CONTRAINDICATIONS, PRECAUTIONS, ADVERSE REACTIONS

CONTRAINDICATIONS

None Known.

PRECAUTIONS

Because of lack of long-term safety studies, acetyl-L-carnitine is not advised for pregnant women or nursing mothers. Those with seizure disorders should only use acetyl-L-carnitine under medical advisement and supervision.

ADVERSE REACTIONS

Mild gastrointestinal symptoms may occur in those taking acetyl-L-carnitine supplements. These include nausea, vomiting, abdominal cramps and diarrhea.

Increased agitation has been reported in some with Alzheimer's disease when taking oral acetyl-L-carnitine. In those with seizure disorders, an increase in seizure frequency and/ or severity has been reported in some taking this substance. The incidence of this in this population is low.

INTERACTIONS

Therapy with the nucleoside analogues didanosine (ddI), zalcitabine (ddC) and stavudine (d4T) may lead to decreased acetyl-L-carnitine levels.

Therapy with valproic acid and the pivalic acid-containing antibiotics may lead to secondary L-carnitine deficiencies (see L-carnitine).

OVERDOSAGE

There are no reports of overdosage.

DOSAGE AND ADMINISTRATION

Typical doses of supplemental acetyl-L-carnitine are 500 milligrams to 2 grams daily in divided doses.

LITERATURE

Brooks JO 3d, Yesavage JA, Carta A, Bravi D. Acetyl-L-carnitine slows decline in younger patients with Alzheimer's disease: a reanalysis of a double-blind, placebo-controlled trial using the trilinear approach. *Int Psychogeriatr.* 1998; 10:193-203.

Chuang WW, Lin WW, Lamb DJ, Lipshultz LI. Effect of acetylcarnitine on sperm motility. *J Urol.* 2000; 163(4 Suppl):Abstract1324.

Famularo G, Morreti S, Marcellini S, et al. Acetyl-carnitine deficiency in AIDS patients with neurotoxicity on treatment with antiretroviral nucleoside analogues. *AIDS.* 1997; 11:185-190.

Gorini A, D'Angelo A, Villa RF. Action of L-acetylcarnitine on different cerebral mitochondrial populations from cerebral cortex. *Neurochem Res.* 1998; 23:1485-1491.

Hagen TM, Ingersoll RT, Wehr CM, et al. Acetyl-L-carnitine fed to old rats partially restores mitochondrial function and ambulatory activity. *Proc Natl Acad SciUSA.* 1998; 95:9562-9566.

Hagen TM, Wehr CM, Ames BN. Mitochondrial decay in aging. Reversal through supplementation of acetyl-L-carnitine and N-tert-butyl-alpha-phenyl-nitrone. *Ann NYAcad Sci.* 1998; 854,214-223.

Lolic MM, Fiskum G, Rosenthal RE. Neuroprotective effects of acetyl-L-carnitine after stroke in rats. *Ann Emerg Med.* 1997; 29:758-765.

Moncada ML, Vicari E, Cimino C, et al. Effect of acetylcarnitine treatment in oligoasthenospermic patients. *Acta Eur Fertil.* 1992: 23:221-224.

Onofrj M, Fulgente T, Melchiadona D, et al. L- acetylcarnitine as a new therapeutic approach for peripheral neuropathies with pain. *Int J Clin Pharmacol Res.* 1995; 15:9-15.

Pettegrew JW, Klunke WE, Panchalingam K. Clinical and biochemical effects of acetyl-L-carnitine in Alzheimer's disease. *Neurobiol Aging.* 1995; 16:1-4.

Piovesan P, Quatrini G, Pacifici L, et al. Acetyl-L-carnitine restores choline acetyltransferase activity in the hippocampus of rats with partial unilateral fimbria-fornix transection. *Int J Dev Neurosci.* 1995; 13:13-19.

Salvioli G, Neri M. L-acetylcarnitine treatment of mental decline in the elderly. *DrugsExp Clin Res.* 1994; 20:169-176.

Sano M, Bell K, Cote L, et al. Double-blind parallel pilot study of acetyl levocarnitine in patients with Alzheimer's disease. *Arch Neurol.* 1992; 49:1137-1141.

Thal LJ, Carta A, Clarke WR, et al. A one year multicenter placebo-controlled study of acetyl-L-carnitine in patients with Alzheimer's disease. *Neurology.*1996; 47:705-711.

White HL, Scates PW. Acetyl-L-carnitine as a precursor of acetylcholine. *Neurochem Res.* 1990; 15:597-601.

Acetylcysteine

TRADE NAMES

N-acetylcysteine (NAC) is available generically from numerous manufacturers as a dietary supplement. Branded products include NAC fuel (Twinlab), N-A-C Sustain (Jarrow Formulas). Acetylcysteine is available as a prescription in the U.S. for use as an inhalant or as an I.V. infusion. Branded products include Mucomyst (Apothecon).

DESCRIPTION

Acetylcysteine, or N-acetylcysteine, commonly abbreviated as NAC, is the N-acetyl derivative of the protein amino acid L-cysteine (see L-Cysteine). NAC is available as a nutritional supplement and as a drug. It is given orally or by slow intravenous infusion in the treatment of acetaminophen (known as paracetamol in Europe) overdose. NAC is also used in the treatment of respiratory disorders, such as acute and chronic bronchitis associated with the production of excessive or viscous mucus. For such respiratory disorders, it is delivered as an inhalant.

NAC is a delivery form of L-cysteine. L-cysteine is hygroscopic and slowly decomposes and oxidizes. NAC is more stable than L-cysteine, and it may be better absorbed. NAC, in addition to being known as N-acetylcysteine, is known as acetylcysteine and N-acetyl-L-cysteine. It is represented by the following chemical structure:

$$HS—CH_2-CH \begin{matrix} COOH \\ \\ NH-\underset{\underset{O}{\|}}{C}—CH_3 \end{matrix}$$

N-acetyl-L-cysteine

ACTIONS AND PHARMACOLOGY

ACTIONS

NAC is a reducing agent and has antioxidant activity. It is also a mucolytic and a hepatoprotectant, and it may have anti-apoptotic activity.

MECHANISM OF ACTION

NAC's efficacy in the treatment of acetaminophen overdose is due mainly to its ability to regenerate liver stores of glutathione. NAC is a delivery form of L-cysteine, which serves as a major precursor to the antioxidant glutathione. An overdose of acetaminophen leads to its metabolism to large quantities of N-acetyl-benzoquinoneimine or NABQI in the liver. NABQI depletes hepatic glutathione stores, placing an enormous oxidative stress on the liver, which can lead to hepatic failure and be life-threatening.

NAC's mucolytic activity is believed to be due to its ability to reduce disulfide bonds in mucoproteins found in mucus, liquifying this viscous substance.

The hepatoprotectant activity of NAC is also due to its ability to serve as a precursor to glutathione. A major role of glutathione is the maintenance of a normal redox state of the liver. A normal redox state is vital to normal hepatic function.

There is some evidence that NAC may have anti-apoptotic activity, particularly in pancreatic beta-cells and nerve cells. This research is still preliminary, but it is believed that the possible anti-apoptotic effect of NAC is due to its antioxidant activity. Specifically, it is thought that NAC, in its role as a precursor to L-cysteine and glutathione, may protect cell membranes against lipid peroxidation and protein oxidation.

PHARMACOKINETICS

NAC is rapidly absorbed from the gastrointestinal tract and transported to the liver via the portal circulation, where it undergoes extensive first-pass metabolism. Peak plasma concentrations are observed approximately 0.5 to 1 hour following oral administration of doses of 200 to 600 milligrams. NAC is metabolized to N-acetylcysteine, N, N-diacetylcystine and L-cysteine. L-cysteine itself is metabolized to glutathione, protein, taurine and sulfate. NAC has low bioavailability, probably because of its extensive first-pass metabolism in the liver. The terminal half-life of total NAC is approximately 6.25 hours after ingestion.

INDICATIONS AND USAGE

Broad claims are made for NAC. There is some support for claims that it is hepatoprotective, that it is of benefit in some with early adult respiratory distress syndrome and chronic obstructive pulmonary disease and that it might help protect against cardiovascular disease. There is also some preliminary suggestion that it might have some usefulness in the treatment of diabetes, some cancers and some immune disorders. A recent study suggests that NAC might have some favorable impact on age-related memory loss. Its benefit in reversing tolerance to nitrates in patients with coronary artery disease remains controversial.

RESEARCH SUMMARY

High-dose NAC has been used successfully as an antidote for acetaminophen poisoning and *Amanita phalloides* intoxication. In one series of 11 patients with *Amanita phalloides* poisoning, a detoxifying regimen that included NAC produced successful recovery in all but one subject without need of liver transplantation. Fulminant hepatic failure induced by acetaminophen overdose has similarly been significantly ameliorated by NAC treatment. It is believed that NAC accomplishes these benefits by preventing hepatic necrosis through replenishment of glutathione and, possibly, through enhanced oxygen delivery and consumption.

Given that acetaminophen overdose is the most common cause of calls to poison control centers in the United States, NAC's contribution is quite significant in this context. It has been suggested that NAC might also be useful in some infectious liver disorders, such as hepatitis C. As of yet, there is no evidence of efficacy in those diseases.

Several studies have indicated that NAC might be helpful in treating chronic obstructive pulmonary disease (COPD). In an open, controlled multicenter study of 169 patients with moderate-to-severe COPD, subjects were randomized to receive standard treatment plus 600 milligrams of NAC once daily or standard therapy alone for a six-month period. Exacerbations of COPD were reduced 41% in the NAC-treated group, compared with the standard therapy-only group. There was also a significant reduction in number of sick days among the NAC-treated. Another study found benefit from NAC and rutin in protecting the lungs of patients, with early adult respiratory distress syndrome ARDS. However, not all with ARDS benefit from NAC.

NAC has improved myocardial contraction in an animal model of myocardial ischemia. It has also been shown to inhibit platelet aggregation; and it has lowered lipoprotein (a) levels to a degree not previously achieved by either drugs or diet, according to some researchers. Additionally, some recent clinical studies have demonstrated that intravenous infusion of NAC during thrombolysis is associated with decreased size of infarct and increased rescue of left ventricular function.

One group of researchers concluded: "Short-and long-term studies indicated that also on patients with unstable angina pectoris and threat of infarct, the intravenous or oral administration of N-acetylcysteine in association with nitroglyceren is highly effective in decreasing the risk of worsening, mainly by preventing the occurrence of acute myocardial infarction."

Animal model work has produced preliminary evidence that NAC, apparently more than either vitamins C or E, or both, can be of some benefit in insulin-dependent diabetes mellitus. NAC reportedly inhibits pancreatic beta-cell apoptosis without affecting the rate of beta-cell proliferation. NAC has also been shown to moderately decrease blood glucose levels and to retain glucose-stimulated insulin secretion.

There is some interest in NAC as a possible anti-cancer agent. There is some preliminary work indicating that it might be helpful in the early stages of some cancers. It is hypothesized to be a logical chemopreventive agent in some cancers based on its properties and some experimental data demonstrating, among other things, extracellular inhibition of mutagenic agents, protection of DNA and nuclear enzymes, and dampening of reactive oxygen species.

One group of researchers, however, claims to have found some evidence of NAC-induced DNA damage in a human leukemia cell line and has cautioned that NAC "may have the dual function of carcinogenic and anti-carcinogenic potentials." More research is needed.

NAC's therapeutic role, if any, in the treatment of immune disorders is similarly undecided. NAC has been shown to inhibit factors that are believed to stimulate HIV; this inhibition has been attributed to NAC-induced increases in intracellular thiol levels. These *in vitro* findings have not yet been demonstrated in clinical trials.

Recently, NAC was administered to eight patients with steroid-resistant acute graft-versus-host disease. Prompt significant response was seen in six of these subjects, four complete and two partial responses. More studies are needed.

A recent study of aged mice found some evidence that NAC can help prevent apoptotic death of neuronal cells and help protect against oxidative damage in synaptic mitochondria. NAC-supplemented mice were compared with unsupplemented mice fed standard food pellets. After 23 weeks, there was significant correction of some memory deficits in the aged mice receiving NAC, compared with those on the standard diet. And there were significant reductions in lipid peroxide and protein carbonyl levels in the synaptic mitochondria of the NAC-supplemented mice.

Finally, while some studies suggest that NAC can reverse tolerance to nitrates in patients with coronary artery disease, other studies have failed to demonstrate any benefit.

CONTRAINDICATIONS, PRECAUTIONS, ADVERSE REACTIONS

CONTRAINDICATIONS

There are no known contraindications to NAC used for nutritional supplementation.

PRECAUTIONS

Supplemental NAC should be avoided by nursing mothers and should only be used by pregnant women if prescribed by a physician.

N-acetylcysteine clearance is reduced in those with chronic liver disease as well as in pre-term newborns.

NAC may be harmful if administered early in the treatment of critically ill patients.

NAC may intensify headaches in those taking nitrates for the treatment of angina.

Although the incidence of cystine renal stones is low, they do occur. Those who do form renal stones, particularly cystine stones, should avoid NAC supplements.

NAC and its sulfhydryl metabolites, like other sulfhydryl-containing substances, could produce a false-positive result in the nitroprusside test for ketone bodies used in diabetes.

NAC should be used with caution in those with a history of peptic ulcer disease, since mucolytic agents may disrupt the gastric mucosal barrier.

ADVERSE REACTIONS

Adverse reactions reported with oral NAC include nausea, vomiting, diarrhea, headache (especially when used along with nitrates) and rashes. There are rare reports of renal stone formation.

Adverse reactions reported with intravenous NAC include bronchospasm, nausea, vomiting, stomatitis, rhinorrhea, headache, tinnitus, urticaria, rashes, chills and fever. There are rare reports of anaphylactic reactions. The most common symptoms of those experiencing anaphylactoid reactions are rash, pruritis, flushing, nausea, vomiting, angioedema, tachycardia, bronchospasm, hypotension, hypertension and ECG change. The anaphylactoid reactions are pseudo-allergic rather than immunologic.

INTERACTIONS

Nitrates: Use of supplemental NAC along with nitrates may cause headaches.

Carbamazepine: Use of supplemental NAC along with carbamazepine may cause reduced serum levels of carbamazepine.

No interactions with nutritional supplements, food or herbs are known.

OVERDOSAGE

There are no reports of overdosage with oral, supplemental NAC. There are reports of overdosage when using intravenous NAC for treatment of acetaminophen poisoning. Symptoms of overdosage are similar to those of anaphylaxis (rash, pruritis, flushing, nausea, vomiting, angioedema, tachycardia, bronchospasm, hypotension, hypertension, ECG abnormalities) but have been more severe. Hypotension appears to be a major symptom of overdosage. Other symptoms include respiratory depression, hemolysis, DIC (disseminated intravascular coagulation) and renal failure. It is unclear whether some of these symptoms may have been due to acetaminophen poisoning. Death has occurred in three patients receiving an overdosage of NAC while being treated for acetaminophen poisoning. The role of NAC in these deaths was unclear in two of the patients.

DOSAGE AND ADMINISTRATION

Use of NAC for mucus liquification in severe broncho-pulmonary disease or acetaminophen overedosage should be dosed according to instructions in the package insert.

Supplemental intake ranges from 600 milligrams once to three times daily. Those who supplement with NAC should drink 6 to 8 glasses of water daily in order to prevent cystine renal stones. Cystine renal stones are rare but do occur.

HOW SUPPLIED

Capsules — 500 mg, 500 mg, 750 mg
Solution — 10%, 20%
Tablets — 500 mg, 600 mg

LITERATURE

Ahola T, Fellman V, Laaksonen R, et al. Pharmacokinetics of intravenous N-acetylcysteine in pre-term new-born infants. *Eur J Clin Pharmacol.* 1999; 55:645-650.

Ardissino D, Melini PA, Savonitto S, et al. Effect of transdermal nitroglycerin or N-acetylcysteine, or both, in the long-term treatment of unstable angina pectoris. *J Am Coll Cardiol.* 1997; 29:941-947.

Bongers V, de Jong J, Steen I, et al. Antioxidant-related parameters in patients treated for cancer chemoprevention with N-acetylcysteine. *Europ J Cancer.* 1995; 31A:921-923.

Colombo AA, Alessandrino EP, Bernasconi P, et al. N-acetylcysteine in the treatment of steroid-resistant acute graft-versus-host-disease: preliminary results. Gruppo Italiano Trapianto di Midollo Osseo (GITMO) *Transplantation.* 1999; 68:1414-1416.

Dawson AH, et al. Adverse reactions to N-acetylcysteine during treatment for paracetamol poisoning. *Med J Aust.* 1989; 150:329-331.

De Flora S, Grassi C, Carati L. Attenuation of influence-like symptomatology and improvement of cell-mediated immunity with long-term N-acetylcysteine treatment. *Eur RespirJ.* 1997; 10:1535-1541.

DeVries N, De Flora S. N-acetyl-L-cysteine. *J Cell Biochem.* 1993; Supp 17F:270-277.

Gavish D, Breslow JL. Lipoprotein (a) reduction by N-acetylcysteine. *Lancet.* 1991; 337:203-204.

Harrison PM, Wendon JA, Gimson AES, et al. Improvement by acetylcysteine of hemodynamics and oxygen transport in fulminant hepatic failure. *N Engl J Med.* 1991; 324:1852-1857.

Ho E, Chen G, Bray TM. Supplementation of N-acetylcysteine inhibits NFkappaB activation and protects against alloxan-induced diabetes in CD-1 mice. *FASEB J.* 1999; 13:1845-1854.

Hogan JC, Lewis MJ, Henderson AH. N-acetylcysteine fails to attenuate haemodynamic tolerance to glyceryl trinitrate in healthy volunteers. *Br J Clin Pharmacol.* 1989; 28:421-426.

Hogan JC, Lewis MJ, Henderson AH. Chronic administration of N-acetylcysteine fails to prevent nitrate tolerance in patients with stable angina pectoris. *Br J Clin Pharmacol.* 1990; 30:573-577.

Holdiness MR. Clinical pharmacokinetics of N-acetylcysteine. *Clinical Pharmacokinet.* 1991; 20:123-134.

Horowitz JD, Henry CA, Syrjanen ML, et al. Nitroglycerine/N-acetylcysteine in the management of unstable angina pectoris. *Eur Heart J.* 1988; 9 Suppl A:95-100.

Iversen HK. N-acetylcysteine enhances nitroglycerin-induced headache and cranial artieral response. *Clin Pharmacol Ther.* 1992; 52:125-133.

Jones AL, Jarvie DR, Simpson D, et al. Pharmacokinetics of N-acetylcysteine are altered in patients with chronic liver disease. *Aliment Pharmacol Ther.* 1997; 11:787-791.

Kelebic T, Kinter A, Poli G, et al. Suppression of human immunodeficiency virus expression in chronically infected monocyte cells by glutathione, glutathione ester, and N-acetylcysteine. *Proc Natl Accd Sci.* 1991; 88:986-990.

Louwerse ES, Weverling GJ, Bossuyt PM, et al. Randomized double-blind controlled trial of acetylcysteine in amyotrophic lateral sclerosis. *Arch Neurol.* 1995; 52:559-564.

Mani TGK, et al. Adverse reactions to acetylcysteine and effects of overdose. *Br Med J.* 1984; 289:217-219.

Marchetti G, Lodola E, Licciardello L, Colombo A. Use of N-acetylcysteine in the management of coronary artery diseases. *Cardiologia.* 1999; 44:633-637.

Martinez M, Hernandez AI, Martinez N. N-acetylcysteine delays age-associated memory impairment in mice: role in synaptic mitochondric. *Brain Res.* 2000; 855:100-106.

Molnar Z, Schearer E, Lowe D. N-acetylcysteine treatment to prevent the progression of multisystem organ failure: a prospective, randomized placebo-controlled study. *Crit Care Med.* 1999; 27:1100-1104.

Montanini S, Sinardi D, Pratico C, et al. Use of acetylcysteine as the life-saving antidote in Amanita phalloides (death cap) poisoning. Case report on 11 patients. *Arzneimittel-forschung.* 1999; 49:1044-1047.

Oikawa S, Yamada K, Yamashita N, et al. N-acetylcysteine, a cancer chemopreventive agent, causes oxidative damage to cellular and isolated DNA. *Carcinogenesis.* 1999; 20:1485-1490.

Ortolani O, Conti A, De Gaudio AR, et al. Protective effects of N-acetylcysteine and rutin on the lipid peroxidation of the lung epithelium during the adult respiratory distress syndrome. *Shock.* 2000; 13:14-18.

Pela R, Calcagni AM, Subiaco S, et al. N-acetylcysteine reduces the exacerbation rate in patients with moderate to severe COPD. *Respiration.* 1999; 66:495-500.

Roederer M, Staal FJT, Raju PA, et al. Cytoline-stimulated human immunodeficiency virus replication is inhibited by N-acetyl-L-cysteine. *Proc Natl Accd Sci.* 1990; 87:4884-4888.

Sala R, Moriggi E, Corvasce G, Morelli D. Protection by N-acetylcysteine against pulmonary endothelial cell damage induced by oxidant damage. *Eur Respir J.* 1993; 6:440-446.

Unverferth DV, Jagadeesh JM, Unverferth BJ, et al. Attempt to prevent doxorubicin-induced acute human myocardial morphologic damage with acetylcysteine. *J Natl Canc Inst.* 1983; 71:917-920.

Activated Charcoal

TRADE NAMES

Activated charcoal is available from numerous manufacturers generically. Branded products include Liqui-Char (Jones Pharma), Kerr Insta-Char (Kerr), Charcoal Plus DS (Kramer labs), Actidose-Aqua (Paddock Labs), Charcoaid G (Requa), Charcocaps (Requa) and Mega charcoal (Twinlab).

DESCRIPTION

Activated charcoal is a type of amorphous carbon prepared by destructive distillation of such materials as wood, vegetables and coconut shells, materials that have much higher surface areas than charcoal itself. It is a fine, black powder of largely pure carbon. The large surface area of activated charcoal confers a great adsorptive capacity to this material. It is this great adsorptive capacity that is the basis for its many industrial as well as medical uses. There are different types of activated charcoal with different adsorption characteristics. The adsorptive characteristics are determined by the configuration of the surface of activated charcoal.

Activated charcoal is widely used in the treatment of acute poisoning (overdose) with such substances as acetaminophen, salicylates, barbiturates and tricyclic antidepressants. Activated charcoal strongly adsorbs aromatic substances such as the above, reducing their absorption from the gastrointestinal tract. Most inorganic poisons are not significantly adsorbed by activated charcoal. A major industrial use of activated charcoal is as a decolorizer. For example, it is used in the late stages of sugar refining to produce white sugar. Activated charcoal is commonly used in air and water filters.

Activated charcoal, in addition to some other substances, has been used in Russia for the treatment of a number of disorders and diseases, including hyperlipidemia, liver, biliary tract and renal diseases. The practice is known as enterosorption and carbon sorption therapy, when activated charcoal is the principle therapeutic component. Oral activated charcoal is known to lower cholesterol levels.

Activated charcoal is also known as active carbon, activated carbon, adsorbent charcoal, carbo activatus, carbo medicinalis, carbon active, carbon attivo, decolorizing charcoal, activkohle (German) and medicinal charcoal.

ACTIONS AND PHARMACOLOGY

ACTIONS
Activated charcoal is a gastrointestinal adsorbent. It may also have hypocholesterolemic activity.

MECHANISM OF ACTION
The large surface area of activated charcoal confers a great adsorptive capacity to this material. The adsorptive capacity of this substance differs for various chemical entities. Activated charcoal is most effective in adsorbing aromatic or benzenoid-type substances. Less well adsorbed are non-aromatic (non-benzenoid) substances, such as the various fatty acids and fatty alcohols. Inorganic substances are poorly adsorbed by activated charcoal. Aromatic substances, such as acetaminophen, salicylates, barbiturates and tricyclic antidepressants, are very strongly adsorbed by activated charcoal, and that is why activated charcoal is commonly used in the management of overdosage of these substances. Adsorption of these drugs reduces their absorption from the gastrointestinal tract.

The mechanism of the hypocholesterolemic effect of activated charcoal is not entirely clear. It is thought that the cholesterol-lowering effect of activated charcoal is caused by its interference with the enterohepatic circulation of bile acids.

PHARMACOKINETICS
Activated charcoal is not absorbed via the gastrointestinal tract, and all ingested activated charcoal is excreted in the feces.

INDICATIONS AND USAGE
Results have been mixed in studies using charcoal in patients with gas complaints. There is some evidence that activated charcoal can favorably affect lipids and that it might be helpful in alleviating symptoms associated with cholestasis of pregnancy. Activated charcoal looks promising for the treatment of uremic pruritis, as well as for congenital erythropoietic porphyria.

RESEARCH SUMMARY
There are inconsistent results in studies related to activated charcoal's efficacy in reducing intestinal gas and symptoms related thereto. In one double-blind study, the substance significantly reduced bloating and abdominal cramps associated with gaseousness. Some other studies have confirmed this effect, and some others have not, discrepancies that may be related to dosing and sampled populations. One researcher reported that activated charcoal effectively adsorbs intestinal gas in healthy subjects but that it "has not been properly investigated in patients with gas complaints."

Oral activated charcoal has significantly lowered plasma total cholesterol and LDL-cholesterol in both animals and humans. It has also raised HDL-cholesterol in some studies. In one crossover study of seven subjects ingesting 4, 8, 16 or 32 grams per day of activated charcoal, serum total and LDL-cholesterol were decreased (maximum 29% and 41% respectively) and the ratio of HDL/LDL-cholesterol was increased (maximum 121%) by activated charcoal in a dose-dependent pattern.

Ten additional subjects with severe hypercholesterolemia took daily, in random order, for three weeks, 16 grams of activated charcoal, 16 grams of cholestyramine or 8 grams of activated charcoal plus 8 grams of cholestyramine. Activated charcoal reduced total and LDL-cholesterol concentrations 23% and 29%, respectively; cholestyramine reduced them 32% and 39%; in combination, they reduced them 30% and 38%. The ratio of HDL/LDL-cholesterol increased from 0.13 to 0.23 with activated charcoal, to 0.29 with cholestyramine and to 0.25 with the combination. Cholestyramine increased serum triglycerides, but activated charcoal did not. Research is ongoing.

Given that elevated serum bile acid levels are thought to play a role in cholestasis of pregnancy, activated charcoal was administered to women with this condition to see if it could decrease these levels. The women were given 50 grams of the substance three times a day for eight days. By day eight, serum total bile acid concentrations were significantly reduced. Outcome of pregnancy was good. This preliminary study needs followup to see whether activated charcoal might be an option in the treatment of entrahepatic cholestasis of pregnancy.

Activated charcoal given as an oral dose of 6 grams provided symptomatic relief in nearly 50% of patients with uremic pruritis, a poorly understood symptom of uremia. The studies have, however, been limited. More research is needed.

Finally, activated charcoal was more effective in reducing plasma porphyrin levels than oral cholestyramine in a patient with congenital erythropoietic porphyria or Gunther's disease. Again, more research is needed.

CONTRAINDICATIONS, PRECAUTIONS, ADVERSE REACTIONS

CONTRAINDICATIONS

Activated charcoal is contraindicated in those whose gastrointestinal tract is not anatomically intact.

PRECAUTIONS

Activated charcoal adsorbs a wide range of drugs and nutrients. Those using activated charcoal should avoid using it within two hours of drug, food, nutritional supplement or herb intake or within two hours before their intake.

ADVERSE REACTIONS

Black stools (from the activated charcoal) occur frequently. Other reported adverse reactions include nausea, vomiting, blackening of the teeth and mouth, abdominal discomfort, diarrhea (more frequent) and constipation (less frequent).

There are occasional reports of drug failure in those who use activated charcoal concomitantly with a drug.

INTERACTIONS

Activated charcoal adsorbs a wide range of drugs and nutrients. Therefore, those using activated charcoal should avoid using it within two hours of drug, food, nutritional supplement or herb intake or within two hours before their intake.

OVERDOSAGE

None reported.

DOSAGE AND ADMINISTRATION

Those who use activated charcoal as an antflatulant typically use 500 to 1000 milligrams as needed. Those who use activated charcoal for its possible cholesterol-lowering effect take 5 to 8 grams two to three times daily. Those who use activated charcoal combine it with plenty of water and must not use it within two hours before or after ingesting any drug, food, nutritional supplement or herb.

HOW SUPPLIED

Capsules — 250 mg, 260 mg, 280 mg, 350 mg

Enteric Coated Tablets — 250 mg

Granules

Liquid — 15 g/75 ml, 25 g/120 ml, 30 gm/120 ml

Tablets — 250 mg

LITERATURE

Friedman EA, Saltzman MJ, Delano BG, Bayer MM. Reduction in hyperlipidemia in hemodialysis patients treated with charcoal and oxidized starch (oxystarch). Am J Clin Nutr. 1978; 31:1903-1914.

Giovannetti S, Barsotti G, Cupisti A, et al. Oral activated charcoal in patients with uremic pruritus. Nephron. 1995; 70:193-196.

Kaaja RJ, Kontula KK, Raiho A, Laatikainen T. Treatment of cholestasis of pregnancy with peroral activated charcoal. A preliminary study. Scand J Gastroenterol. 1994; 29:178-181.

Korkushko OV, Bogatskaia LN, Novikova SN, et al. [Use of enterosorption for correction of dyslipoproteinemias in patients with ischemic heart disease in geriatric patients]. [Article in Russian]. Klin Med (Mosk). 1991; 69:51-53.

Kuusisto P, Vapaatalo H, Manninen V, et al. Effect of activated charcoal on hypercholesterolaemia. Lancet. 1986; 2(8503):366-367.

Neuvonen PJ, Kuusisto P, Manninen V, et al. The mechanism of the hypocholesterolaemic effect of activated charcoal. Eur J Clin Invest. 1989; 19:251-254.

Neuvonen PJ, Kuusisto P, Vapaatalo H, Manninen V. Activated charcoal in the treatment of hypercholesterolaemia: dose-response relationships and comparison with cholestyramine. Eur J Clin Pharmacol. 1989; 37:225-230

Nikolaev VG. Peroral application of synthetic activated charcoal in USSR. Biomater Artif Cells Artif Organs. 1990; 18:555-568.

Pimstone NR, Gandhi SN, Mukerji SK. Therapeutic efficacy of oral charcoal in congenital erythropoietic porphyria. N Engl J Med. 1987; 316:390-393.

Robertson KE, Mueller BA. Uremic pruritis. Am J Health Syst Pharm. 1996; 53:2159-2170.

Suarez FL, Furne J. Springfield J, Levitt MD. Failure of activated charcoal to reduce the release of gases produced by the colonic flora. Am J Gastroenterol. 1999; 94:208-212.

Windrum P, Hull DR, Morris TCM. Herb-drug interactions. Lancet. 2000; 355:1019-1020.

Alkoxyglycerols

DESCRIPTION

Alkoxyglycerols are ether-linked glycerols derived from shark liver oil. They include such substances as batyl alcohol, chimyl alcohol and selachyl alcohol. They are also known as alkylglycerols, ether lipids and dietary ether lipids. The terms alkoxyglycerols and shark liver oil are frequently used interchangeably. Alkoxyglycerols are found naturaly in shark liver oil in the form of fatty acid esters. These fatty acid esters are called 1-O-alkyl-2,3-diacyl-sn-glycerols and are represented by the following chemical structure:

$$H_2C\!-\!\!-OH$$
$$HO\!-\!\!-CH$$
$$H_2C\!-\!\!-OR$$

Alkoxyglycerol

ACTIONS AND PHARMACOLOGY

ACTIONS
Alkoxyglycerols have putative antiproliferative and immuno-modulatory activities.

MECANISM OF ACTION
The mechanism of the putative antiproliferative and immu-nomodulatory actions of alkoxyglycerols is not known. Speculative mechanisms include protein kinase C inhibition, macrophage activation and natural killer cell activation.

PHARMACOKINETICS
Ether glycerols, when absorbed, may be incorporated into plasmalogens and alkylacyl glycerophospholipids. Little is available on the specific pharmacokinetics of the shark oil alkoxyglycerols in humans.

INDICATIONS AND USAGE
Support for claims that the alkoxyglycerols are indicated for the prevention and treatment of any cancer or for the treatment of wounds and inflammatory conditions in humans is limited and unsystematic. There is little support for claims that they are immune-enhancing in humans.

RESEARCH SUMMARY
This shark-liver oil derivative has been touted as an effective anti-cancer treatment. Unfortunately, there is little evidence to support this claim, at least for humans. There is scant evidence it inhibits tumor growth or reduces cancer mortality in humans. It should in no way be relied upon in the treatment of any form of cancer. Similarly, there is little evidence to support claims that this substance is useful for treating wounds and inflammatory conditions. Neither has it been demonstrated in appropriate human clinical studies that it has immune-enhancing effects. There are some *in vitro* and animal studies reporting antiproliferative and immunomodu-latory effects for these substances, and perhaps alkoxygly-cerols may eventually have a role to play in adjuvant management of certain types of cancer. However, this would need to be established by well-designed, double-blind, placebo-controlled trials, which have not yet been done.

CONTRAINDICATIONS, PRECAUTIONS, ADVERSE REACTIONS

CONTRAINDICATIONS
None known.

PRECAUTIONS
Those with cancer who are interested in alkoxyglycerols should discuss their use with their physicians. Under no circumstance should they be relied upon as principle elements in the management of their disease. Pregnant women and nursing mothers should avoid alkoxyglycerol supplements.

ADVERSE REACTIONS
Mild gastrointestinal symptoms, including diarrhea, have been reported.

DOSAGE AND ADMINISTRATION
There are no typical doses. Those who use shark liver oil products are cautioned that some prepartions may contain high amounts of vitamins A and D.

LITERATURE
Brohult A, Brohult J, Brohult S, Joelsson I. Reduced mortality in cancer patients after administration of alkoxyglycerols. *Acta Obstet Gynecol Scand.* 1986; 65:779-785.

Das AK, Holmes RD, Wilson GN, Hajra AK. Dietary ether lipid incorporation into tissue plasmologens of humans and rodents. *Lipids.* 1992; 27:401-405.

Hallgren B, Niklasson A, Stallberg G, Thorin H. On the occurrence of 1-O-(2-methoxyalkyl)glycerols and 1-O-phytanylglycerol in marine animals. *Acta Chem Scand B.* 1974; 28:1035-1040.

Hasle H, Rose C. [Shark liver oil (alkoxyglycerol) and cancer treatment]. [Article in Danish]. *Ugesk Laeger.* 1991; 153:343-346.

Oh SY, Jadhav LS. Effects of dietary alkoxyglycerols in lactating rats on immune responses in pups. *Pediatr Res.* 1994; 36:300-305.

Alpha-Lipoic Acid

TRADE NAMES
Alpha-lipoic acid is available generically from numerous manufacturers. Branded products include Ultra-Lipoic Forte (Westlake Labs).

DESCRIPTION
Alpha-lipoic acid, also known as thioctic acid, is a disulfide compound that is a cofactor in vital energy-producing reactions in the body. It is also a potent biological antioxidant. Alpha-lipoic acid was once thought to be a vitamin for animals and humans. It is made endogenously in humans—the details of its synthesis are still not fully understood—and so it is not an essential nutrient. There are, however, certain situations, for example, diabetic polyneuro-pathy, where alpha-lipoic acid might have conditional essentiality. And recent research indicates that the antioxi-dant roles of alpha-lipoic acid may confer several health benefits. Alpha-lipoic acid is found widely in plant and animal sources.

Most of the metabolic reactions in which alpha-lipoic acid participates occur in mitochondria. These include the oxida-tion of pyruvic acid (as pyruvate) by the pyruvate dehydro-genase enzyme complex and the oxidation of alpha-ketoglutarate by the alpha-ketoglutarate dehydrogenase enzyme complex. It is also a cofactor for the oxidation of branched-chain amino acids (leucine, isoleucine and valine) via the branched-chain alpha-keto acid dehydrogenase enzyme complex.

Alpha-lipoic acid is approved in Germany as a drug for the treatment of polyneuropathies, such as diabetic and alcoholic polyneuropathies, and liver disease.

Alpha-lipoic acid contains a chiral center and consists of two entantiomers, the natural R- or D- entantiomer and the S- or L- entantiomer. Commercial preparations of alpha-lipoic acid consist of the racemic mixture, i.e. a 50/50 mixture of the R- and E-entantiomers. It is represented by the following chemical structure:

Alpha-Lipoic acid

Alpha-lipoic acid has a variety of names. In addition to being known as alpha-lipoic acid and thioctic acid, it is also known as lipoic acid, 1,2-dithiolane-3-pentanoic acid; 1,2-ditholane-3-valeric acid; 6,8-thiotic acid; 5-[3-C1,2-dithiolanyl)]-pentanoic acid; delta-[3-(1,2-dithiacyclopentyl)] pentanoic acid; acetate replacing factor and pyruvate oxidation factor. Alpha-lipoic acid is water-insoluble.

Although the details of its synthesis have yet to be worked out, alpha-lipoic acid is synthesized in mitochondria; octanoic acid and L-cysteine (for its sulfur) are precursors in its synthesis.

ACTIONS AND PHARMACOLOGY

ACTIONS
Alpha-lipoic acid has biological antioxidant activity, antioxidant recycling activity and activity in enhancing biological energy production.

MECHANISM OF ACTION
Alpha-lipoic acid and its reduced metabolite, dihydrolipoic acid (DHLA), form a redox couple and may scavenge a wide range of reactive oxygen species. Both alpha-lipoic acid and DHLA can scavenge hydroxyl radicals, the nitric oxide radical, peroxynitrite, hydrogen peroxide and hypochlorite. Alpha-lipoic acid, but not DHLA, may scavenge singlet oxygen, and DHLA, but not alpha-lipoic acid, may scavenge superoxide and peroxyl reactive oxygen species.

Alpha-lipoic acid has been found to decrease urinary isoprostanes, O-LDL and plasma protein carbonyls, markers of oxidative stress. Further, alpha-lipoic acid and its redox couple DHLA have been found to have antioxidant activity in aqueous, as well as in lipophilic regions, and in extracellular and intracellular environments. Finally, with regard to alpha-lipoic acid's antioxidant activity, alpha-lipoic acid appears to participate in the recycling of other important biologic antioxidants, such as vitamins E and C, ubiquinone and glutathione.

Exogenous alpha-lipoic acid has been shown to increase ATP production and aortic blood flow during reoxygenation after hypoxia in a working heart model. It is thought that this is due to its role in the oxidation of pyruvate and alpha-ketoglutarate in the mitochondria, ultimately enhancing energy production. This activity, and possibly its antioxidant activity, may account for its possible benefit in diabetic polyneuropathy.

PHARMACOKINETICS
Most pharmacokinetic studies have been performed in animals. Alpha-lipoic acid is absorbed from the small intestine and distributed to the liver via the portal circulation and to various tissues in the body via the systemic circulation. The natural R-entantiomer is more readily absorbed than the L-entantiomer and is the more active form. Alpha-lipoic acid readily crosses the blood-brain barrier. It is found, after its distribution to the various body tissues, intracellularly, intramitochondrialy and extracellularly.

Alpha-lipoic acid is metabolized to its reduced form, dihydrolipoic acid (DHLA), by mitochondrial lipoamide dehydrogenase. DHLA, together with lipoic acid, form a redox couple. It is also metabolized to lipoamide, which functions as the lipoic acid cofactor in the multienzyme complexes that catalyze the oxidative decarboxylations of pyruvate and alpha-ketoglutarate. Alpha-lipoic acid may be metabolized to dithiol octanoic acid, which can undergo catabolism.

INDICATIONS AND USAGE
Lipoic acid shows evidence of being effective in the treatment of diabetic neuropathy and may be useful in treating some other aspects of diabetes. It may help prevent the oxidation of LDL cholesterol and may be protective, generally, against oxidative stress and, specifically, against atherosclerosis, ischemia-reperfusion injury and various radiologic and chemical toxins. It may also be useful in some inborn metabolic disorders. There is less evidence that it might be helpful in some neurodegenerative conditions. There is preliminary evidence that it might have some immune-modulating effects. It has been suggested that lipoic

acid may slow aging of the brain and that it may be an anti-aging substance, in general.

RESEARCH SUMMARY

Lipoic acid is an approved treatment for diabetic neuropathy in Germany. Numerous studies in both animals and humans have produced promising results with lipoic acid in this neuropathy. In animal models and culture studies, lipoic acid has demonstrated antioxidant properties that help reduce or eliminate a sequence of events that include reduced endoneural blood flow and oxygen tension, which are pre-requisites of neuropathy. In addition, some of these studies have revealed favorable lipoic acid effects that appear to be independent of its antioxidant properties, including increased glucose uptake, promotion of new neurite growth and chelation of transition metals thought to play a role in diabetic neuropathy.

In some animal experiments, lipoic acid, administered for up to three months, significantly reversed the increase in nerve vascular resistance and the decrease in nerve blood flow in diabetic rats. Nerve conduction velocity was entirely restored in some nerve groups after three months of treatment.

Human clinical trials have been similarly encouraging. In one of these studies, subjects received 200 milligrams of intravenous lipoic acid daily. After 21 days, significant pain reduction was achieved in most subjects.

In a larger, multi-center, double-blind, randomized, placebo-controlled study of 328 patients with type 2 diabetes, significant improvements were recorded in several clinical measures of diabetic polyneuropathy, including pain, numbness, paresthesia and burning sensations. These results were evident after three weeks of intravenous lipoic acid given five times weekly in doses of 600 and 1200 milligrams.

Nerve conduction velocity has not been shown to improve in the short-term human studies conducted so far. One group of researchers has suggested that proof of neurophysiological improvement in these neuropathies may emerge from long-term lipoic acid supplementation studies, as has been the case in some animal model studies. ''A period of several years,'' they have observed, ''is required to slow progress of diabetic neuropathy due to normalization of blood glucose levels.''

There is evidence, too, that lipoic acid may help prevent or slow the development of the atherosclerosis for which diabetics are at higher risk. It may do this, in part, through a gene-regulatory mechanism that helps prevent endothelial cell activity that has been implicated in the progression of atherosclerosis.

With respect to atherosclerosis, in general, lipoic acid's antioxidant and metabolic effects appear to offer some protection, as demonstrated in various animal models. Recently, researchers demonstrated, in a 16-week randomized trial, that lipoic acid, in oral doses of 600 milligrams daily for eight weeks, significantly inhibits the oxidation of LDL-cholesterol in healthy human subjects. The supplements also significantly reduced levels of F-2 isoprostanes, markers of oxidative stress. In this study, lipoic acid proved to be superior to vitamin E in decreasing levels of plasma protein carbonyls. Protein oxidation and LDL-cholesterol oxidation are implicated in heart disease.

Various animal studies have suggested that lipoic acid can prevent or reduce cell and tissue damage in heart attacks and stroke. There is extensive animal work showing that lipoic acid can exert significant protective effects against ischemia-reperfusion injury.

Lipoic acid is believed to work in this context, at least in part, through its antioxidant properties and its reported ability to increase cellular levels of glutathione that are typically depleted by the reactive oxygen species formation that characterizes ischemia-reperfusion. More research is needed to further elucidate these mechanisms and determine whether these results will apply in humans.

Animal work is also suggestive of some modest benefit from lipoic acid in the treatment of various neurodegenerative disorders, including Parkinson's disease, Alzheimer's disease, amyotrophic lateral sclerosis and Huntington's disease. Results to date, however, remain inconclusive. Clinical studies are needed.

There is some evidence that children afflicted with inborn errors of pyrurate metabolism may derive some benefit from lipoic acid treatment. Those with Wilson's disease, a genetic disorder characterized by disturbed copper metabolism, may be helped by lipoic acid as well. The supplement has also proved useful in conferring some protection against cadmium poisoning and hexane inhalation. It has also been used in some liver toxicities, such as *Amanita phalloides* mushroom poisoning.

Lipoic acid's role in immunity is not well understood. There are reports that it can augment antibody response in some animal models of immunosuppression. This research warrants followup.

Claims that lipoic acid slows aging of the brain and is an anti-aging substance generally seem to be related to its potent antioxidant properties. Direct proof of anti-aging is lacking, but there is some animal work suggestive of some possible anti-aging effects.

Rats were fed a lipoic-acid supplemented diet to see whether the substance can reverse age-related declines in metabolism and mitochondrial function. Unsupplemented aged rats (24 to 26 months) exhibited ambulatory activity, said to be a general measure of metabolic activity, that was threefold lower than that of young controls. But this decline was significantly reversed in similarly aged rats supplemented with lipoic acid for two weeks.

Hepatocytes from untreated aged rats, compared with hepatocytes of young controls (three to five months), had significantly lower oxygen consumption and mitochondrial membrane potential. But in supplemented aged rats, hepatocytes, by the same measures, were comparable to those of the young controls.

Lipoic acid supplementation was reported to completely reverse age-related declines in hepatocyte ascorbic acid and glutathione levels. There was additional evidence of decreased oxidative damage in the lipoic-acid supplemented aged rats. The researchers concluded: "Little is known about whether lipoic acid may be an effective anti-aging supplement...in humans. Our present findings using rats would suggest that lipoic acid supplementation may be a safe and effective means to improve general metabolic activity and increase antioxidant status, affording increased protection against external oxidative and xenobiotic insults with age.'' Again, further study is needed.

CONTRAINDICATIONS, PRECAUTIONS, ADVERSE REACTIONS

CONTRAINDICATIONS

None known.

PRECAUTIONS

Because of lack of long-term safety data, alpha-lipoic acid should be avoided by pregnant women and nursing mothers.

Those with diabetes and problems with glucose intolerance are cautioned that supplemental alpha-lipoic acid may lower blood glucose levels. Blood glucose should be monitored and antidiabetic drug dose adjusted, if necessary, to avoid possible hypoglycemia.

ADVERSE REACTIONS

To date, alpha-lipoic acid in doses up to 600 milligrams daily has been well tolerated.

INTERACTIONS

Supplemental alpha-lipoic acid may lower blood glucose levels. Those with diabetes on antidiabetic medication should have their blood glucose monitored and antidiabetic drug dose appropriately adjusted, if necessary, to avoid possible hypoglycemia.

OVERDOSAGE

There are no reports of alpha-lipoic acid overdosage.

DOSAGE AND ADMINISTRATION

Alpha-lipoic acid is available as a racemic mixture of D- and L- entantiomers. Some studies showing significant antioxidant effects have used doses of the racemic mixture of 600 milligrams daily.

Alpha-lipoic acid is available in Germany as a drug to treat polyneuropathy, such as diabetic polyneuropathy, and liver disorders. It is available for oral and parenteral use. Those with diabetic neuropathy use 300 milligrams daily of the oral preparation, taken in divided doses.

HOW SUPPLIED

Capsules — 100 mg, 330 mg
Powder
Tablets — 50 mg

LITERATURE

Hagen TM, Ingersoll RT, Lykkesfeldt J, et al. (R)-alpha-lipoic acid-supplemented old rats have improved mitochondrial function, decreased oxidative damage, and increased metabolic rate. *FASEB J. 1999;* 13:411-418.

Lykkesfeldt J, Hagen TM, Vinarsky V, Ames BN. Age-associated decline in ascorbic and concentration, recycling and biosynthesis in rat hepatocytes-reversal with (R)-alpha-lipoic acid supplementation. *FASEB J.* 1998; 12:1183-1189.

Marangon K, Devaraj S, Tirosh O, et al. Comparison of the effect of alpha-lipoic acid and alpha-tocopherol supplementation on measures of oxidative stress. *Free Rad Biol Med.* 1999; 27:1114-1121.

Natrej CV, Gandhi VM, Melon KKG. Lipoic acid and diabetes: effect of dihydrolipoic acid administration in diabetic rats and rabbits. *J Biosci* 1984; 6:37-46.

Nickander KK, McPhee BR, Low PA, Tritschler H. Alpha-lipoic acid: antioxidant potency against lipid peroxidation of neural tissues in vitro and implications for diabetic neuropathy. *Free Rad Biol Med.* 1996; 21:631-639.

Ohmori H, Yamauchi T, Yamamoto I. Augmentation of the antibody response by lipoic acid in mice II. Restoration of the antibody response in immunosuppressed mice. *Japan J Pharmacol* 1986; 42:275-280.

Packer L, Tritschler HJ, Wessel K. Neuroprotection by the metabolic antioxidant alpha-lipoic acid. *Free Rad Biol Med.* 1997; 22:359-378.

Packer L, Witt EH, Tritschler, HJ. Alpha-lipoic as a biological antioxidant. *Free Rad Biol Med.* 1995; 19:227-250.

Reed LJ. The chemistry and function of lipoic acids. *Adv Enzymol.* 1957; 18:319-347.

Sachse G, Willms B. Efficacy of throctic acid in the therapy of peripheral diabetic neuropathy. *Horm Metab Res Suppl.* 1980; 9:105-107.

Tirosh O, Sen CK, Roy S, et al. Neuroprotective effects of alpha-lipoic acid and its positively charged amide analogue. *Free Rad Biol Med.* 1999; 26:1418-1426.

Wagh SS, Natraj CV, Menon KKG. Mode of action of lipoic acid in diabetes. *J Biosci.* 1987; 11:59-74.

Ziegler D, Hanefeld M, Ruhnau KJ, et al. Treatment of symptomatic diabetic peripheral neuropathy with the antioxidant alpha-lipoic acid. A three-week multicentre randomized controlled trial (ALADIN study). *Diabetologia.* 1995; 38:1425-1433.

Zimmer G, Beikler TK, Schneider M, et al. Dose/response curves of lipoic acid R- and S- forms in the working rat heart during reoxygenation: superiority of the R-entantiomer in the enhancement of aortic flow. *J Mol Cell Cardiol.* 1995; 27:1895-1903.

Alpha-Tocopherol Polyethylene Glycol Succinate (TPGS)

DESCRIPTION

Alpha-tocopheryl polyethylene glycol succinate, abbreviated as TPGS, is a water-soluble derivative of d-alpha-tocopheryl succinate. TPGS is used as a water-soluble delivery form of vitamin E for those with fat malabsorption syndromes, such as chronic childhood cholestasis. It is also used as an absorption and bioavailability enhancer for certain water-insoluble drugs (e.g. the HIV protease inhibitor amprenavir) and fat-soluble vitamins such as vitamin D.

TPGS is synthesized by esterifying d-alpha tocopheryl succinate with polyethylene glycol (PEG) 1000 (the molecular weight of PEG 1000 is approximately 1,000 daltons). It is a pale yellow, waxy solid substance that is amphipathic and hydrophilic. Its molecular weight is approximately 1,513 daltons. d-alpha-tocopherol comprises 26% of TPGS. TPGS is also known as d-alpha-tocopheryl polyethylene glycol 1000 succinate and d-alpha-tocopheryl PEG 1000 succinate. Since there are eight stereoisomers of alpha-tocopherol, the designation d-alpha-tocopherol, although commonly used, is chemically incorrect. Correct chemical names for TPGS include RRR-alpha-tocopheryl polyethylene glycol 1000 succinate, 2R, 4'R, 8'R-alpha-tocopheryl polyethylene glycol 1000 succinate and 2, 5, 7, 8-tertramethyl-2-(4',8',12'-trimethyltridecyl)-6-chromanyl polyethylene glycol 1000 succinate.

ACTIONS AND PHARMACOLOGY

ACTIONS

TPGS is a water-souble delivery form of d-alpha-tocopherol. See Vitamin E for actions of this vitamin. TPGS may also enhance the absorption and bioavailability of certain drugs and nutritional substances.

MECHANISM OF ACTION

In contrast to other forms of vitamin E which require emulsification and micelle formation by bile salts for their absorption, TPGS, because of its amphipathic nature (has both hydrophilic and lipophilic ends), forms its own micelles and thus does not require bile salts to do so. This makes it an excellent alpha-tocopherol substance for those who have problems secreting bile salts into the intestine (e.g., those with chronic childhood cholestasis).

TPGS may enhance the absorption of lipophilic drugs if formulated together with them. For this reason, the HIV protease inhibitor amprenavir is formulated with TPGS. Further, the enhancement of the oral bioavailability of some drugs when co-administered with TPGS may, in part, be due to inhibition of P-glycoprotein in the intestine. P-glycoprotein is the multidrug resistance transporter and is involved in the mediation of multidrug resistance.

PHARMACOKINETICS

The pharmacokinetics of TPGS are still being worked out. TPGS is more efficiently absorbed from the lumen of the small intestine following ingestion than other forms of vitamin E. As mentioned above, TPGS forms micelles in the small intestine and does not require bile salts to do so. The mechanism of it's absorption into enterocytes remains unclear. A few possibilities exist. TPGS is hydrolyzed within the lumen of the small intestine to form d-alpha-tocopherol; it is hydrolyzed by lipase on the surface of the enterocytes to form d-alpha-tocopherol; or the entire TPGS micelle is taken up by the enterocytes and it is hydrolyzed within them to alpha-tocopherol. Whichever the case, alpha-tocopherol is secreted by the enterocytes into the lymphatics and is processed in a similar manner to other forms of vitamin E. (See Vitamin E.)

INDICATIONS AND USAGE

TPGS is indicated in some with chronic cholestatic liver disease of infancy and childhood. It may be helpful in some other forms of liver disease and in fat-soluble vitamin deficiency generally. It is useful in treating vitamin E malabsorption in short-bowel syndrome. It may protect the liver against some toxins. There is evidence that when co-administered it can enhance the absorbability of some pharmaceutical drugs. It has been suggested that it might be helpful in treating some of the malabsorption problems associated with Crohn's disease, HIV disease, ulcerative colitis, cystic fibrosis and others, but this hypothesis has not been adequately tested.

RESEARCH SUMMARY

There is considerable research supporting the use of TPGS in chronic childhood cholestasis and in some forms of liver disease characterized by significantly reduced bile acid secretion into the intestine. In a multicenter study, children with chronic cholestasis unresponsive to other forms of vitamin E were given TPGS supplements. All of the children experienced normalization of vitamin E status. Improvements were noted in the neurological function, which had deteriorated prior to the study's onset, in 25 of the subjects. Neurological function stabilized in 27 others and worsened in only two of the subjects; functions were measured after a mean of 2.5 years of TPGS therapy.

In addition, TPGS has been used with some preliminary success to help overcome the difficulty those with cholestasis have in absorbing other fat-soluble vitamins (A, D, K). Through admixture and co-administration of these other fat-soluble vitamins in TPGS preparations, absorption has reportedly been enhanced.

Similarly, co-administration of some poorly absorbed drugs with TPGS has enhanced the absorption of those drugs even in healthy volunteers. Recently TPGS, used in this context, was shown to increase the absorbability of the protease inhibitor amprenavir. TPGS has improved the absorbability of cyclosporin in children receiving liver transplants. It is useful in combating vitamin E malabsorption in short-bowel syndrome. It has also demonstrated hepatoprotective effects against carbon tetrachloride in animal studies.

CONTRAINDICATIONS, PRECAUTIONS, ADVERSE REACTIONS

CONTRAINDICATIONS

TPGS is contraindicated in those with known hypersensitivity to the substance.

PRECAUTIONS

Typically, TPGS is prescribed and monitored by a physician. Those on warfarin need to be aware that high doses of TPGS (greater than 500 milligrams daily, equivalent to 130 milligrams of d-alpha-tocopherol) may enhance the anticoagulant effect of warfarin, and therefore they should have their INRs carefully monitored and their warfarin doses appropriately adjusted if indicated. Those with vitamin K deficiencies should be aware that high doses of TPGS may have anticoagulant activity. TPGS should be used with caution in those with lesions with a propensity to bleed (e.g., bleeding peptic ulcers), those with a history of hemorrhagic stroke and those with inherited bleeding disorders (e.g., hemophilia).

High dose TPGS should be stopped about one month before surgical procedures, unless a physician advises otherwise.

Those on the HIV protease inhibitor amprenavir need to be aware that, if they are taking the recommended daily adult dose of this drug, they are receiving 1,168 milligrams (1,744 IUs) daily of d-alpha-tocopherol.

ADVERSE REACTIONS

No adverse reactions have been reported.

INTERACTIONS

DRUGS

Antiplatelet drugs, such as aspirin, dipyridamole, eptifibatide, clopidogrel, ticlopidine, tirofiban and abciximab: High doses of TPGS may enhance the effects of these antiplatelet drugs.

Cyclosporine and other lipophilic drugs: TPGS may increase absorption if taken concomitantly.

Warfarin: High dose (greater than 500 milligram daily) of TPGS may enhance the anticoagulant response of warfarin. Monitor INRs and appropriately adjust dose of warfare if necessary.

NUTRITIONAL SUPPLEMENTS

Flavonoids, polyphenols, CoQ₁₀: TPGS may increase the absorption of these supplements if taken concomitantly.

Selenium: may function synergistically with alpha-tocopherol.

Vitamin C: may help maintain alpha-tocopherol in its reduced (antioxidant) form.

Vitamin A, D and K: TPGS may increase the absorption of vitamins A, D and K if taken concomitantly. It may also increase the absorption of all forms of vitamin E (gamma-tocopherol, tocotrienol) if taken concomitantly.

FOODS

High doses of TPGS may cause decreased gamma-tocopherol and tocotrienol plasma levels.

HERBS

Some herbs, such as garlic and ginkgo, possess antithrombotic activity. High doses of TPGS used concomitantly with these herbs may enhance antithrombotic activity.

OVERDOSAGE

No reports of TPGS overdosage appear in the literature.

DOSAGE AND ADMINISTRATION

TPGS is typically used for the treatment of vitamin E deficiency states due to fat malabsorption, such as chronic childhood cholestasis. Doses used for this condition range from 10 to 17 milligrams (as d-alpha-tocopherol) per kilogram daily. Doses of up to 670 milligrams (as d-alpha-tocopherol) daily for up to three years have been used in the treatment of vitamin E deficiency secondary to short-bowel syndrome. Use of TPGS in these disorders, as well as other disorders of fat malabsorption, such as cystic fibrosis, requires medical supervision. It is unclear if TPGS offers any advantages, as a vitamin E supplement, to those without vitamin E deficiencies.

LITERATURE

Dintaman JM, Silverman JA. Inhibition of P-glycoprotein by d-alpha-tocopheryl polyethylene glycol 1000 succinate (TPGS). *Pharm Res.* 1999; 16:1550-1556.

Socha P, Koletzko B, Pawlowska J, et al. Treatment of cholestatic children with water-soluble vitamin E (alpha-tocopheryl polyethylene glycol succinate): effects on serum vitamin E, lipid peroxides, and polyunsaturated fatty acids. *J Pediatr Gastroenterol Nutr.* 1997; 24:189-193.

Sokol RJ, Butler-Simon N, Conner C, et al. Multicenter trial of d-alpha-tocopheryl polyethylene glycol 1000 succinate for treatment of vitamin E deficiency in children with chronic cholestasis. *Gastroenterology.* 1993; 104:1727-1735.

Traber MG, Shiano TD, Steephen AC, et al. Efficacy of water-soluble vitamin E in the treatment of vitamin E malabsorption in short-bowel syndrome. *Am J Clin Nutr.* 1994; 59:1270-1274.

Traber MG, Thellman CA, Rindler MJ, Kayden HJ. Uptake of intact TPGS (d-alpha-tocopheryl polyethylene glycol 1000 succinate) a water-miscible form of vitamin E by human cells in vitro. *Am J Clin Nutr.* 1998; 48:605-611.

Alpha-Tocopheryl Nicotinate

DESCRIPTION

Alpha-tocopheryl nicotinate is a synthetic ester formed from dl-alpha-tocopherol and nicotinic acid. It is a delivery form of nicotinic acid and is used in Europe and Japan for the treatment of hyperlipidemia. It is marketed in the United States as a nutritional supplement, usually in a combination formula.

Alpha-tocopheryl nicotinate is also known as vitamin E nicotinate and tocopheryl nicotinate.

ACTIONS AND PHARMACOLOGY

ACTIONS

Alpha-tocopheryl nicotinate may have triglyceride- and cholesterol-lowering activity in some.

MECHANISM OF ACTION

See the monograph on nicotinic acid for mechanism of action information.

PHARMACOKINETICS

There is little information on the pharmacokinetics of alpha-tocopheryl nicotinate. Absorption from the lumen of the small intestine is dependent on the presence or the absence of food. Absorption is much higher with food. Alpha-tocopheryl nicotinate appears to be transported by the lymphatics to the systemic circulation. It is taken up by the liver where it is hydrolyzed to dl-tocopherol and nicotinic acid.

See the Vitamin E and Nicotinic Acid monographs for information on these metabolites of alpha-tocoperyl nicotinate.

INDICATIONS AND USAGE

Alpha-tocopheryl nicotinate has shown some experimental antiarrhythmic activity and is used in Europe and Japan as a lipid-lowering agent.

RESEARCH SUMMARY

Alpha-tocopheryl nicotinate demonstrated an ability to significantly inhibit experimentally induced antiarrhythmic activity in isolated animal atria, as well as *in vivo* in an animal model. Of three substances tested (the other two were dodecanoic acid and alpha-tocopherol), alpha-tocopheryl nicotinate showed the greatest inhibiting activity.

Alpha-tocopheryl nicotinate is a delivery form of nicotinic acid which does possess hypocholesterolemic and hypotriglyceridemic activities. However, there is no evidence that it is superior to nicotinic acid itself in this regard (see Nicotinic Acid). Further, the doses typically used are unlikely to have hypolipidemic activity in most people.

CONTRAINDICATIONS, PRECAUTIONS, ADVERSE REACTIONS.

See Nicotinic Acid.

OVERDOSAGE

The literature does not contain reports of alpha-tocopheryl nicotinate overdosage.

DOSAGE AND ADMINISTRATION

Typical dosing is 100 to 200 milligrams three times a day. This dose is equivalent to about 120 to 240 milligrams of d-alpha-tocopherol daily and about 60 to 120 milligrams of nicotinic acid daily.

LITERATURE

Aigner O, Schlick W. [Effect of tocopherol nicotinate on serum lipids]. [Article in German]. *Int J Clin Pharmacol.* 1974; 10:216-219.

Hasegawa J, Tomono Y, Fujita T, et al. The effect of food on the absorption of alpha-tocopheryl nicotinate in beagle dogs and human volunteers. *Int J Clin Pharmacol Ther Toxicol.* 1981; 19:216-219.

Iino K, Abe K, Kariya S, et al. A controlled double-blind study of dl-alpha-tocopheryl nicotinate (Juvela-Nicotinate) for treatment of symptoms in hypertension and cerebral arteriosclerosis. *Jpn Heart J.*1977; 18:277-283.

Noma A, Maseda S, Okuno M, et al. Reduction of serum lipoprotein(a) levels in hyperlipidaemic patients with alpha-tocopheryl nicotinate. *Atherosclerosis.* 1990; 84:213-217,

Suzuki N, Nakamura T. Metabolism of the nicotinic acid moiety of dl-alpha tocopheryl nicotinate. *J Nutr Sci Vitaminol.* 1983; 29:93-103.

Aluminum

TRADE NAMES

Aluminum containing antacids include Basaljel (Wyeth-Ayrest), Alternagel (J&J/Merck Consumer), Amphojel (Wyeth-Ayrest) and Alu-Tab (3M Pharmaceutical). Aluminum-containing antiperspirants include Xerac AC (Person & Covey), Certain Dri (Numark Laboratories) and Drysol (Person & Covey).

DESCRIPTION

Aluminum is a light, ductile and malleable metal with atomic number 13 and symbol Al. Bound as oxides and complex aluminosilicates, it is the most abundant metal in the earth's crust. Aluminum is not considered an essential nutrient for humans. However aluminum deficiency states have been reported in some animals.

Goats fed diets low in aluminum have been reported to have depressed growth, an increased number of spontaneous abortions, decreased life expectancy, and incoordination and weakness in their hind legs. Chicks fed low-aluminum diets have been reported to have depressed growth.

Typical daily dietary intake of aluminum ranges from about 2 to 8 milligrams. The major source of aluminum in foods is food additives, such as sodium aluminum phosphates in cake mixes, frozen dough, self-rising flour and processed cheese, as well as sodium aluminum sulfate in baking powder. Aluminum is found in a number of commercial teas. However, the absorption of aluminum from tea may be quite low.

Aluminum-containing compounds are widely used in medicine and are found in many consumer products. Aluminum hydroxide is used as a phosphate binder in the treatment of hyperphosphatemia and to control renal osteodystrophy and secondary hyperphosphatemia in patients with end stage renal disease on hemodialysis. Sucralfate is used in the treatment of peptic ulcer disease. Aluminum and magnesium hydroxide mixtures are commonly used antacids. Aluminum-containing compounds are used as astringents, as antiperspirants and in underarm deodorants.

Toxic effects of aluminum—encephalopathy, osteomalacia and microcytic anemia—can occur in patients with chronic renal failure. The aluminum comes from excessive amounts of this substance in dialysis fluids and/or from its absorption from the oral doses of aluminum-containing medications given for the treatment of hyperphosphatemia. Aluminum is also neurotoxic in experimental animals, premature infants and those with chronic renal failure who are not on dialysis.

This neurotoxic activity of aluminum raised the concern of whether aluminum intake in healthy individuals could be a contributing factor to such disorders as Alzheimer's disease. Although aluminum has not been ruled out as playing some role in Alzheimer's disease, aluminum accumulation does not appear to occur to any appreciable extent in those with normal renal function who use aluminum-containing antacids. Consequently, it does not appear that dietary intake of aluminum would increase the risk of Alzheimer's disease in the general population. However, this remains a controversial topic.

ACTIONS AND PHARMACOLOGY

The actions and pharmacology of dietary aluminum are not known.

INDICATIONS AND USAGE

There are no indications for the supplemental use of aluminum.

RESEARCH SUMMARY

While there is no research relevant to the use of supplemental aluminum, current research has found that aluminum toxicity is rare in the general population and that aluminum intake from the use of aluminum cookware does not pose risks of aluminum toxicity. On the other hand, the prolonged use of antacids may result in aluminum intake high enough to produce adverse effects in those with kidney disorders and in low-birth-weight infants.

CONTRAINDICATIONS, PRECAUTIONS, ADVERSE REACTIONS

None known for dietary aluminum. See *Physicians' Desk Reference* and *Physicians' Desk Reference For Nonprescription Drugs* for information on aluminum-containing antacids and other aluminum-containing compounds.

OVERDOSAGE

None known for dietary aluminum.

DOSAGE AND ADMINISTRATION

No recommended dosage. Aluminum is present in colloidal or liquid minerals.

HOW SUPPLIED

Aluminum carbonate antacids are available in the following forms and strengths:

Capsules — 500 mg
Tablets — 500 mg

Aluminum hydroxide antacids are available in the following forms and strengths:

Capsules — 475 mg
Suspension — 320 mg/5 ml
Tablets — 600 mg

Aluminum chloride antiperspirants are available in the following forms and strengths:

Solution — 6.25%, 12.5%, 20%

LITERATURE

Jeffery EH, Abreo K, Burgess E, et al. Systemic aluminum toxicity: effects on bone, hematopoietic tissue and kidney. *J Toxicol Environ Health.* 1996; 48:649-665.

Lukiw WJ, Le Blanc HJ, Carver LA, et al. Run-on gene transcription in human neocortical nuclei. Inhibition by nanomolar aluminum and implications for neurodegenerative disease. *J Mol Neurosci.* 1998; 11:67-78.

Nielsen FH. Other trace elements. In: Ziegler EE, Filer LL Jr, eds. *Present Knowledge in Nutrition.* 7th ed. Washington, DC: ILSI Press; 1996:353-377.

Nielsen FH. Ultratrace minerals. In: Shils ME, Olson JA, Shike M, Ross AC, eds. *Modern Nutrition in Health and Disease.* 9th ed. Baltimore MD: Williams and Wilkins; 1999:283-303.

Rogers MA, Simon DG. A preliminary study of dietary aluminum intake and risk of Alzheimer's disease. *Age Aging.* 1999; 28:205-209.

Savory J, Exley C, Forbes WF, et al. Can the controversy of the role of aluminum in Alzheimer's disease be resolved? What are the suggested approaches to this controversy and methodological issues to be considered? *J Toxicol Environ Health.* 1996; 48:615-635.

Androstenediol

TRADE NAMES

Tetrabol (Syntrax Innovations), Pentabol (Syntrax Innovations), Mirabol (Syntrax Innovations), Andro-4-Diol Stack (Value Nutrition).

DESCRIPTION

Androstenediol refers to two steroid isomers that are marketed as dietary supplements and mainly used by body builders. The two androstenediol isomers are delta4-androstenediol and delta5-androstenediol. The difference between the two isomers is in the position of the double bond in the cyclopentanoperhydrophenanthrene ring structure. Delta4-androstenediol has a double bond between carbons 4 and 5; delta5-androstenediol has a double bond between carbons 5 and 6.

Delta4-androstenediol is also known as 4-androstene-3beta, 17beta-diol and (3beta, 17beta)-androst-4-ene-3, 17-diol. Delta5-androstenediol is also known as 5-androstene-3beta, 17beta-diol, androst-5-ene-3beta, 17beta-diol, (3beta, 17beta)-androst-5-ene-3, 17-diol and Adiol. The molecular formula of both delta4-androstenediol and delta5-androstenediol is $C_{19}H_{30}O_2$, and the molecular weight of these substances is 290.45 daltons.

Delta4-androstenediol and delta5-androstenediol are synthesized in the adrenal gland and gonads from dehydroepiandrosterone (DHEA) via the enzyme 17beta-hydroxysteroid dehydrogenase. They are metabolized to testosterone via the enzyme 3beta-hydroxysteroid dehydrogenase. Delta5-androstenediol is similar in structure to methandriol. Androstenediol is represented by the following structural formula:

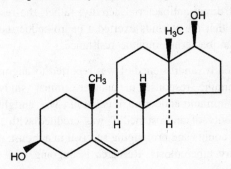

Androstenediol

ACTIONS AND PHARMACOLOGY

ACTIONS

Supplemental delta4- and delta5-androstenediol have putative anabolic activity. Delta5-androstenediol may have immunomodulatory activity.

MECHANISM OF ACTION

Supplemental delta4- and delta5-androstenediol may be metabolized to testosterone in both men and women. Whether increases in testosterone levels that may be produced by taking oral delta4- or delta5-androstenediol would be sustained long enough to show increases in nitrogen retention and muscle strength and mass is unknown. Delta5-androstenediol is similar in structure to methandriol, a one-time popular injectable anabolic steroid.

Delta5-androstenediol has been demonstrated to enhance the immune response against infection in mice. It is thought that this is due, in part, to delta5-androstenediol's possible role in counter-regulating the immunosuppressive effects of glucocorticoids. That is, delta5-androstenediol may have antiglucocorticoid activity.

PHARMACOKINETICS

There are scant human pharmacokinetic data on the androstenediol isomers. Absorption is variable following ingestion, but some absorption does occur. First-pass metabolism appears to render much of an oral dose of delta4-androstenediol into the inactive metabolites androsterone and etiocholanolone. Androsterone and etiocholanolone are found in the urine after ingestion of delta4-androstenediol and delta5-androstenediol. Both delta4- and delta5-androstenediol may be metabolized to testosterone.

INDICATIONS AND USAGE

The claim that oral androstenediol has anabolic effects is unsubstantiated. There is preliminary evidence that androstenediol hay have some immunomodulating effects. Use of androstenediol may pose health hazards in some.

RESEARCH SUMMARY

Androstenediol significantly protected mice from lethal bacterial infections (*Enterococcus faecalis* and *Pseudomonas veruginosa*) in one recent experiment. There was no evidence of direct antibacterial activity; rather, the researchers believed that the steroids exerted a neuro-endocrine regulation of antibacterial immune resistance.

Subsequently, androstenediol was reported to augment antiviral immune response in another animal study, again through immuno-endocrine regulation. The antiglucocorticoid activity of androstenediol was credited with reducing bacterial counts and prolonging survival in a mouse model of pulmonary tuberculosis. Research is ongoing.

CONTRAINDICATIONS, PRECAUTIONS, ADVERSE REACTIONS

CONTRAINDICATIONS

Delta4-androstenediol and delta5-androstenediol are contraindicated in those with prostate, breast, ovarian and uterine cancer and in those at risk for these cancers. Delta4-androstenediol and delta5-androstenediol are also contraindicated in those who are hypersensitive to any component of a delta4- or delta5-androstenediol-containing product.

PRECAUTIONS

Children, adolescents, pregnant women and nursing mothers should avoid delta4- and delta5-androstenediol supplements. Women generally should exercise caution in the use of delta4- and delta5-androstenediol supplements because of possible virilizing effects.

ADVERSE REACTIONS

No data are available on the long-term safety of supplemental 4delta- or 5delta-androstenediol. Adverse effects of exogenous testosterone—to which androstenediol may be metabolized—in men include acne, testicular atrophy, gynecomastia, behavioral changes and possibly an increased risk of prostate cancer. Adverse effects of exogenous testosterone in women include hirsutism, deepening of the voice, acne, clitoral hypertrophy, amenorrhea, male-pattern baldness and coarsening of the skin. In adolescents, exogenous testosterone can lead to early closing of bone growth plates and decreased adult height. Other adverse effects of testosterone include hepatic failure and increased platelet aggregation.

INTERACTIONS

No drug, nutritional supplement, food or herb interactions have been reported.

OVERDOSAGE

No reports of overdosage.

DOSAGE AND ADMINISTRATION

There are no typical doses and no recommended doses.

HOW SUPPLIED

Capsules — 50 mg, 100 mg

Powder

LITERATURE

Ben-Nathan D, Padgett DA, Loria RM. Androstenediol and dehydroepiandrosterone protect mice against lethal bacterial infections and lipopolysaccharide toxicity. *J Med Microbiol.* 1999; 48:425-431.

Earnest CP, Olson MA, Broeder CE, et al. In vivo 4-androstene-3,17-dione and 4-androstene-3beta, 17beta-diol supplementation in young men. *Eur J Appl Physiol.* 2000; 81:229-232.

Hernandez-Pando R, De La Luz Streber M, Orozco H, et al. The effects of androstenediol and dehydroepiandrosterone on the course and cytokine profile of tuberculosis in BALB/c mice. *Immunology.* 1998; 95:234-241.

Miyamoto H, Yeh S, Lardy H, et al. Delta5-androstenediol is a natural hormone with androgenic activity in human prostate cancer cells. *Proc Natl Acad Sci USA.* 1998; 95:11083-11088.

Padgett DA, Loria RM, Sheridan JF. Endocrine regulation of the immune response to influenza virus infection with a metabolite of DHEA-androstenediol. *J Neuroimmunol.* 1997; 78:203-211.

Padgett DA, Sheridan JF. Androstenediol (AED) prevents neuroendocrine-mediated suppression of the immune response to an influenza viral infection. *J Neuroimmunol.* 1999; 98:121-129.

Uralets VP, Gillette PA. Over-the-counter delta5 anabolic steroids 5-androsten-3, 17-dione; 5-androstene-3beta, 17beta-diol; dehydroepiandrosterone; and 19-nor-5-androstene-3, 17-dione: excretion studies in men. *J Anal Toxicol.* 2000; 24:188-193.

Androstenedione

TRADE NAMES

Androstenedione is available from numerous manufacturers generically. Branded products include Andro-Gen (Gen) and Andro (AST Sports Science).

DESCRIPTION

Androstenedione, a steroid hormone, is a natural substance made in the adrenal gland and the gonads. It is also found in small amounts in some plants. Androstenedione, commonly known as andro, became popular because of its use by the baseball player Mark McGwire. McGwire stopped using androstenedione in May, 1999.

Androstenedione is synthesized in the adrenal gland and gonads from dehydroepiandrosterone. It is metabolized by the enzyme 17 beta-hydroxy steroid dehydrogenase to testosterone, and by the aromatase enzyme complex to estrone. Estrone is metabolized to estradiol.

Androstenedione is also known as 4-androstenedione and chemically as 4-androstene-3,17-dione. The chemical structure is:

Androstenedione
(4-Androstene-3,17-dione)

The marketed supplement is synthetic. It is a solid lipophilic substance nearly insoluble in water. Use of androstenedione, like testosterone, is banned by the IOC (International Olympic Committee), NCAA (National Collegiate Athletic Association), NFL (National Football League) and other athletic organizations.

ACTIONS AND PHARMACOLOGY
ACTIONS
Androstenedione is a putative anabolic substance.

MECHANISM OF ACTION
Androstenedione is metabolized to testosterone in both men and women. Supraphysiologic doses of testosterone have been reported to increase nitrogen retention and increase muscle mass and strength. Women taking 100-milligram oral doses of androstenedione have had significant increases in serum testosterone. The results with men have been variable. One study reported that an androstenedione dose of 300 milligrams daily led to significant elevation of serum testosterone. The elevation was not seen, in the same study, in those receiving daily doses of 100 milligrams. Another study reported that neither 100- nor 300-milligram daily doses of androstenedione led to significant increases in serum testosterone. In any case, whether increases in testosterone levels that may be produced by taking oral androstenedione would be sustained long enough to show increases in nitrogen retention and muscle strength and mass is unknown.

PHARMACOKINETICS
There is scant pharmacokinetic data on orally administered androstenedione. Absorption appears variable, but some absorption does occur. Androstenedione is distributed to various tissues of the body and is metabolized to testosterone

and estrone. The amount of testosterone produced per given dose of androstenedione appears to vary. Typically, a greater increase in serum testosterone is found in women compared to men, following intake of oral androstenedione.

INDICATIONS AND USAGE
It has been claimed that supplemental androstenedione can significantly increase blood testosterone levels and build muscle. Recent research is conflicting with respect to the testosterone effect, but is unified in suggesting that prolonged use of this steroid could result in serious health risks.

RESEARCH SUMMARY
A very small 1962 study is often cited by those who claim that androstenedione can significantly boost serum testosterone. Marketers often neglect to mention, however, that this study involved only two subjects—both women.

Recently, for the first time, androstenedione was tested in healthy young men. This was a well-designed, double-blind, placebo-controlled study. The 30 subjects, aged 19 to 29, all had normal testosterone levels and were not taking nutritional supplements or anabolic steroids at baseline. Nor were they, at the outset, engaged in resistance training. Subjects were randomized to receive 300 milligrams of androstenedione daily or placebo and, concurrently, entered an eight-week program of whole-body resistance.

The researchers found that androstenedione exerted no effect on serum free and total testosterone levels. Nor was there any difference in lean body mass between those taking the steroid and those receiving placebo.

On the other hand, the researchers reported that serum estradiol and estrone levels increased significantly in those taking androstenedione, and serum HDL-cholesterol levels dropped by 12 percent in those receiving the steroid. The researchers expressed concern over these findings, noting that there is considerable research suggesting that increased estrogen levels may be associated with increased risk of gynecomastia, cardiovascular disease, breast cancer (in women) and pancreatic cancer (in men). Increased levels of androstenedione itself have been associated in some, but not all, studies with increased risk of prostate and pancreatic cancers.

The reduction in HDL-cholesterol seen in this study did not reach the level that is regarded as a risk factor for cardiovascular disease. Nonetheless, the researchers regarded the observed reduction as clinically relevant, and others have observed that the higher doses used by many body builders and athletes over longer periods of time could result in significant cardiovascular risk.

The dose of androstenedione used in this study exceeds the 100 to 200 milligram dose typically recommended by manufacturers of this supplement. But many athletes are reported to be taking far higher doses, often 500 to 1200 milligrams daily.

Two more recent studies, one using 100 milligrams of androstenedione for five days and the other (a randomized placebo-controlled, double-blind study) also using 100 milligrams daily over a 12-week period, similarly found no increase in testosterone levels and no anabolic effect in healthy males.

Another recent study, however, did find increased testosterone levels in those taking 300 milligrams of androstenedione daily. This study did not measure athletic performance. It also found that the steroid in these doses significantly increased estradiol levels. More research is needed to resolve the testosterone issue.

Some have suggested that more research is also needed to determine whether androstenedione may have some usefulness in those with low and declining testosterone levels, such as some women and older men. There is some evidence that supplementation with the steroid in doses under 300 milligrams a day might increase serum testosterone levels in those who are hypotestosterogenic.

CONTRAINDICATIONS, PRECAUTIONS, ADVERSE REACTIONS
CONTRAINDICATIONS
Androstenedione is contraindicated in those with prostate, breast and uterine cancer.

PRECAUTIONS
Children, adolescents, pregnant women and nursing mothers should avoid androstenedione supplements.

ADVERSE REACTIONS
No data are available on the long-term safety of taking supplemental androstenedione. Adverse effects of exogenous testosterone in men include acne, testicular atrophy, gynecomastia, behavioral changes and possibly an increased risk of prostate cancer. Adverse effects of exogenous testosterone in women include hirsutism, deepening of the voice, acne, clitoral hypertrophy, amenorrhea, male-pattern baldness and coarsening of the skin. In adolescents, exogenous testosterone can lead to early closing of bone growth plates and decreased adult height. Other adverse effects of testosterone include hepatic failure and increased platelet aggregation.

Oral androstenedione has been found to decrease HDL-cholesterol levels, which may increase risk of cardiovascular disease.

OVERDOSAGE
There are no reports of overdosage.

DOSAGE AND ADMINISTRATION
There is a wide range of doses taken by those who use androstenedione for "anabolic" purposes. Doses range from 50 milligrams to 100 to 200 milligrams daily and in some cases much higher. The safety of taking androstenedione, at any dose, especially long-term, is unknown.

HOW SUPPLIED
Capsules — 100 mg

Tablets — 50 mg

LITERATURE
King DS, Sharp RL, Vukovich MD, et al. Effect of oral androstenedione on serum testosterone and adaptations to resistance training in young men. A randomized controlled trial. *J Am Med Assoc.* 1999; 281:2020-2028.

Leder BZ, Longcope C, Catlin DH, et al. Oral androstenedione administration and serum testosterone concentrations in young men. *J Am Med Assoc.* 2000; 283:779-782.

Rasmussen BB, Volpi E, Gore DC, Wolfe RR. Androstenedione does not stimulate protein metabolism anabolism in young healthy men. *J Clin Endocrin Metab.* 2000; 85:55-59.

Wallace MB, Lim J, Cutler A, Bucci L. Effects of dehydroepiandrosterone vs. androstenedione supplementation in men. *Med Sci Sports Exerc.* 1999; 31:1788-1792.

Yesalis III CE. Medical, legal, and social implications of androstenedione use. *J Am Med Assoc.* 1999; 281:2043-2044.

Arginine Pyroglutamate

DESCRIPTION
Arginine pyroglutamate is the L-arginine salt of pyroglutamic acid. It is also known as pirglutargine and arginine pidolate. It is represented by the following chemical structure:

Arginine pyroglutamate

Arginine pyroglutamate is a delivery form of pyroglutamate. Pyroglutamate is formed in the body by the cyclization of the amino acid glutamic acid and is found naturally in plant and animal products, including the brain. Pyroglutamate is also known as 2-oxo-pyrrolidone carboxylic acid or PCA and 5-oxoproline. Pyroglutamate is an intermediate of the gamma-glutamyl cycle of glutathione synthesis and degradation.

Arginine pyroglutamate, which is comprised of the amino acid L-arginine and the imino acid pyroglutamate, is a water-soluble substance.

ACTIONS AND PHARMACOLOGY

ACTIONS

Arginine pyroglutamate is reputed to have cognition-enhancing activity. The activity is attributed to pyroglutamate.

MECHANISM OF ACTION

Since the action of arginine pyroglutamate is unclear, its mechanism of action is entirely speculative. However, pyroglutamate is structurally related to the drug piracetam, and more is known about piracetam's activity. Piracetam belongs to a class of drugs known as nootropics. The term "nootropic," from the Greek, means "acting on the mind." Piracetam, like pyroglutamate, is a pyrrolidone. Piracetam and related nootropics facilitate learning and memory in animal models, although human studies give mixed results except perhaps in dyslexia.

The effects of piracetam are thought to be mediated through effects on membrane fluidity in the brain. Further, some pyrrolidone-nootropic agents appear to interact with metabotropic glutamate receptors. It is not known whether pyroglutamate has any of these activities.

PHARMACOKINETICS

Little is known in detail about the pharmacokinetics of arginine pyroglutamate. Arginine pyroglutamate gets absorbed across the small intestine and is transported by the portal circulation to the liver, where both L-arginine and pyroglutamate enter into various metabolic pathways. Some pyroglutamate appears to pass into the brain.

INDICATIONS AND USAGE

Arginine pyroglutamate may help improve cognition (e.g. verbal memory) in the aged, though more research is required to confirm this.

RESEARCH SUMMARY

The primary claim made for this arginine salt of pyroglutamic acid relates to cognitive enhancement. It is asserted by some that this substance can help overcome memory defects induced by alcohol abuse and in those with some forms of dementia. Some use the supplement in Italy to treat alcoholism, senility and mental retardation. While such sweeping use is unwarranted based on current findings, there are data that suggest a cognitive-enhancing role for arginine pyroglutamate, though how significant a role is far from established. Some animal studies show that the substance has positive effects in cortical and cholinergic mechanisms and that it has cognition-enhancing properties. And in one double-blind study of aged human subjects, verbal memory was said to be improved in those taking arginine pyroglutamate compared with controls who received placebo.

CONTRAINDICATIONS, PRECAUTIONS, ADVERSE REACTIONS

CONTRAINDICATIONS

Hypersensitivity to any component of the preparation.

PRECAUTIONS

Children, pregnant women and nursing mothers should avoid taking arginine pyroglutamate supplements.

ADVERSE REACTIONS

Arginine pyroglutamate is generally well tolerated. Minor gastrointestinal complaints have been noted.

OVERDOSAGE

There are no known reports of overdosage.

DOSAGE AND ADMINISTRATION

The usual recommended dose is 500 to 1000 milligrams daily. A 500 milligram dose delivers about 150 milligrams of L-arginine and about 350 milligrams of pyroglutamate.

LITERATURE

Barone D, Spignal G. Investigations on the binding properties of the nootropic agent pyroglutamic acid. *Drugs Exp Clin Res.* 1990; 16:85-99.

Drago F, Valerio C, D'Agata V, et al. Pyroglutamic acid improves learning and memory capacities in old rats. *Funct Neurol.* 1988; 3:137-143.

Moos WH, Hershenson FM. Potential therapeutic strategies for senile cognitive disorders. *Drug News Perspect.* 1989; 2:397-409.

Provenzano PM, Brucato A, Gianguzza S, et al. Chemistry and pharmacology of arginine pyroglutamate. Analysis of its effects on the CNS. *Arzneimittelforschung.* 1977; 27:1553-1557.

Sinforiani E, Trucco M, Cavalline A, et al. Reversibility of cognitive disorders among chronic alcoholics in phases of withdrawal. Effect of arginine pyroglutamate. *Minerva Psichiatr.* 1985; 26:339-346.

Spignoli G, Magnani M, Giovannini MG, Pepeu G. Effect of pyroglutamic acid stereoisomers on ECS and scopalamine-induced memory disruption and brain acetylcholine levels in the rat. *Pharmacol Res Commun.* 1987; 19:901-912.

Arnica

TRADE NAMES

Arniflora Gel (Boericke & Tafel), Arnica Massage Oil (Weleda), Arnicalm Arthritis (Boiron), Arnicalm Trauma (Boiron) and Arnicaid (Standard Homeopathic).

DESCRIPTION

Arnica is perhaps best known as a homeopathic remedy for muscle strain and soreness. Arnica, also known as leopard's bane, mountain tobacco, mountain daisy and wolf's bane, is made from the dried flowers and sometimes roots of a few members of the daisy *(Asteraceae/Compositae)* family. These members include *Arnica montana L.,* the major source of arnica in Europe, *Arnica chamissonis* ssp foliosa, *Arnica fulgens* Pursh, *arnica soraria* Greene, *Arnica cordifolia* Hook and *Arnica latifolia* Bong. The dried flowers of another member of the daisy family, *Heterotheca inuloides,* also called arnica, are used in Mexico as a folk remedy.

In the United States, arnica is listed by the FDA as an unsafe herb and is only allowed for food use in alcoholic beverages, where it serves as a flavoring agent. Arnica contains some highly poisonous compounds, such as helenalin, and is considered unsafe for oral use. In addition to the sesquiterpenoid lactone helenalin, arnica contains carbohydrates, such as inulin; amines, such as betaine and choline; coumarins; flavonoids, such as quercetin, kaempferol, isorhamnetin and luteolin; thymol; caffeic acid; phytosterols; and other sesquiterpenoid lactones, such as 11alpha, 13-dihydrohelenalin and chamissonolid. Arnica from the Mexican medicinal plant *Heterotheca inuloides* also contains the sesquiterpenoids 7-hydroxy-3, 4-dihydrocadalin and 7-hydroxycadalin.

Arnica is available in homeopathic preparations, in herbal tinctures and in topical products. Externally applied tinctures of arnica are commonly used in countries such as Germany to treat contusions, sprains, hematomas, rheumatic disorders and superficial inflammations of the skin.

ACTIONS AND PHARMACOLOGY

ACTIONS
Arnica has putative analgesic and anti-inflammatory activities.

MECHANISM OF ACTION
The sesquiterpenoid lactone helenalin and, to lesser degrees, the sesquiterpenoid lactones 11alpha, 13-dihydrohelenalin and chamissonolid are reported to inhibit the activation of the transcription factor NF-kappa B by directly modifying this factor. Activation of NF-kappa B leads to inflammatory activity. This could account, at least in part, for the possible anti-inflammatory and analgesic actions of topical arnica preparations. There is no credible research supporting anti-inflammatory and/or analgesic activity for ingested arnica.

The sesquiterpenoids isolated from *Heterotheca inuloides*—7-hydroxy-3, 4-dihydrocadalin and 7-hydroxycadalin—have been reported to have activity against Gram-positive bacteria, including methicillin-resistant *Staphylococcus aureus* (MRSA). The mechanism of this antibacterial activity is unknown. Similarly unknown is how the antibacterial activities of the compounds relate to any possible action of Mexican arnica. In fact, one study reported only slight *in vitro* activity of arnica against oral pathogens.

PHARMACOKINETICS
There are no reports on the pharmacokinetics of arnica.

INDICATIONS AND USAGE

Claims that oral arnica is helpful in relieving pain and stiffness of muscle soreness and useful, generally, in tissue trauma are not supported by credible research.

RESEARCH SUMMARY

A recent review of all placebo-controlled studies related to the clinical efficacy of oral arnica found that the homeopathic remedy is no more efficacious than placebo.

A placebo-controlled study examining the possible ameliorative effect of oral arnica on the tissue trauma following removal of impacted wisdom teeth found more pain and swelling in the arnica-treated group than in the placebo group. A double-blind, placebo-controlled, randomized trial of its use in treating pain and infection after total hysterectomy found no significant difference between it and placebo. In another double-blind, placebo-controlled study, arnica-treated participants in a marathon race were no different than controls in terms of post-race cell damage and restitution time. There was some positive effect in the arnica group with respect to muscle stiffness. A subsequent study of long-distance runners, however, found arnica ineffective in reducing muscle soreness.

There is some positive evidence that arnica has some anti-inflammatory activity when applied externally. On the other hand, arnica is also reported to cause contact allergies in some.

CONTRAINDICATIONS, PRECAUTIONS, ADVERSE REACTIONS

CONTRAINDICATIONS
Oral use of arnica is considered unsafe. Topical use of arnica on broken skin and open wounds is also considered unsafe.

Arnica is contraindicated in those who are allergic to it or who have known allergies or hypersensitivity to other members of the daisy family, such as chamomile and marigolds. It is contraindicated in pregnant women and nursing mothers.

PRECAUTIONS
Sesquiterpenoid lactones in arnica, such as helenalin, are intensely poisonous and cardiotoxic. Therefore, oral use of arnica is considered unsafe, as is topical use of arnica on broken skin and open wounds. Those with hypertension, cardiac arrythmias, and those taking drugs known to cause a prolonged QT interval or drugs known to be potentially cardiotoxic, should be extremely cautious about the use of arnica (see Interactions).

ADVERSE REACTIONS
Ingested arnica may cause nausea, vomiting, abdominal pain, diarrhea, coma and death. Those allergic or hypersensitive to

arnica or to other members of the daisy family can develop rhinitis, conjunctivitis, urticaria, bronchospasm, asthmatic attacks and anaphylaxis.

Topical arnica can cause contact dermatitis manifested as pruritis and erythema.

INTERACTIONS
DRUGS
Arnica may potentiate the adverse effects of drugs known to cause a prolonged QT interval. Such drugs include quinidine, procainamide, disopyramide, sotalol, amiodarone, chlorpromazine, prochlorperazine, haloperidol, pentamidine, amitryptyline, desipramine and doxepim.

Arnica may potentiate the cardiotoxicity of such drugs as doxorubicin.

OVERDOSAGE
Overdosage can cause cardiac arrhythmias, coma and death.

DOSAGE AND ADMINISTRATION
No recommended dose.

Arnica is available in homeopathic preparations, herbal tinctures and topical ointments, gels and creams. Arnica is listed in the Homeopathic Pharmacopeia of the United States (HPUS).

HOW SUPPLIED
Cream

Gel — 7%

Ointment

Pellets

Tablets

Tincture

Topical Spray

LITERATURE
Ernst E, Pittler MH. Efficacy of homeopathic arnica: a systematic review of placebo-controlled clinical trials. *Arch Surg.* 1998; 133:1187-1190.

Hart O, Mullee MA, Lewith G, Miller J. Double-blind, placebo-controlled, randomized clinical trial of homeopathic arnica C30 for pain and infection after total abdominal hysterectomy. *J R Soc Med.* 1997; 90:73-78.

Hausen BM. [Arnica allergy.] [Article in German.] *Hautartz.* 1980; 31:10-17.

Lyss G, Knorre A, Schmidt TJ, et al. The anti-inflammatory sesquiterpene lactone helenalin inhibits the transcription factor NF-kappa B by directly targeting p65. *J Bio Chem.* 1998; 273:33508-33516.

Lyss G, Schmidt TJ, Merfort I, Pahl HL. Helenalin, an anti-inflammatory sesquiterpene lactone from arnica, selectively inhibits transcription factor NF-kappa B. *Biol Chem.* 1997; 378:951-961

Schroder H, Losche W, Strobach H, et al. Helenalin and 11alpha, 13-dihydrohelenalin, two constituents from *Arnica montana* L., inhibit human platelet function via thiol-dependent pathways. *Thromb Res.* 1990; 57:839-845.

Tveiten D, Bruseth S, Borchgrevink CF, Lohne K. [Effect of Arnica D 30 during hard physical exertion. A double-blind randomized trial during the Oslo Marathon 1990]. [Article in Norwegian]. *Tidsskr Nor Laegeforen.* 1991; 111:3630-3631.

Vickers AJ, Fisher P, Smith C, et al Homeopathic Arnica 30X is ineffective for muscle soreness after long-distance running: a randomized, double-blind, placebo-controlled trial. *Clin J Pain.* 1998; 14:227-231.

Arsenic

DESCRIPTION
Arsenic is a metalloid with atomic number 33 and symbol As. It occurs in many ores and is widely distributed in nature, being present in minute quantities in the soil, the sea and in living matter, such as the human body. Arsenic occurs mainly in the trivalent and pentavalent states as compounds of arsenite and arsenate. Arsenic-containing ribofuranosides (arsenosugars) have been identified in living matter. Methyl-containing arsenic compounds, such as arsenocholine and arsenobetaine, are also found in living organisms.

Arsenic is presently not considered an essential nutrient for humans. However, arsenic deficiency states have been reported in some animals. Goats, miniature pigs and rats fed low-arsenic diets were reported to have depressed growth, impaired fertility and increased perinatal mortality. In addition, goats fed arsenic-deficient diets have been found to have depressed triglyceride concentrations and an increased death rate during lactation. Lactating goats on low-arsenic diets suffer myocardial damage, which is associated with injury to the mitochondria.

Worldwide, the daily dietary intake of arsenic ranges from 12 to 60 micrograms. In the United States, the average daily dietary intake of arsenic is approximately 30 micrograms. This figure excludes any contribution from shellfish. Major sources of dietary arsenic are fish, grain and cereal products.

Arsenic is best known as a deadly poison. To a large degree this reputation derived from a 1944 film classic, *Arsenic and Old Lace*. In the movie, two spinsters, as acts of charity, murder lonely old men with their homemade elderberry wine laced with arsenic. Less known is the fact that the wine was also laced with strychnine and cyanide. The fact is that the manifestations of arsenic poisoning, except in very high doses, are typically not acute. However, arsenic can be toxic and is a known carcinogen and teratogen, and high dietary intake of arsenic is a serious public health problem in certain parts of the world, such as Bengal and Bangladesh.

Arsenic has a special role in medical history. Paul Ehrlich, considered the father of modern chemotherapy, discovered the first treatment for syphilis, which he called 606 (salvarsan), an arsenic-containing compound. The trivalent arsenical melarsoprol is used in the treatment of protozoal diseases. Arsenic preparations are widely used in homeopathy. And recently, intravenous arsenic trioxide was found to induce complete remission in patients with acute promyelocytic leukemia, apparently by upregulating apoptosis.

ACTIONS AND PHARMACOLOGY

ACTIONS
The actions of dietary arsenic are unknown.

PHARMACOKINETICS
Water-soluble arsenic acids and their salts are more rapidly absorbed from the gastrointestinal tract than poorly soluble arsenicals such as arsenic trioxide. Following absorption, arsenic is stored mainly in the liver, kidneys, heart and lungs, with smaller amounts in the muscle and nervous tissue. A couple of weeks following ingestion, arsenic is deposited in the hair and nails, and remains fixed to the keratin for years. Arsenic is also deposited in the bones and teeth.

In the liver, pentavalent arsenic is reduced to some degree to the more toxic trivalent form, and trivalent arsenic is slowly and extensively oxidized to pentavalent arsenic. Both pentavalent and trivalent arsenic are methylated with S-adenosylmethione to relatively non-toxic derivatives. These metabolites of arsenic are excreted in the urine mainly as dimethylarsinic acid and smaller amounts of monomethylarsinic acid and inorganic arsenic compounds. Approximately 50% of ingested arsenic is eliminated within three to five days. Small amounts may continue to be excreted for several weeks following a single dose. Small amounts of arsenic are excreted in the feces, sweat, lungs and skin. Arsenic is excreted in breast milk and readily crosses the placenta.

INDICATIONS AND USAGE
There are no indications for the use of supplemental arsenic. Homeopathic claims made for the use of arsenicum album are not supported by credible research. There is preliminary evidence that arsenic trioxide as a drug may be beneficial in the treatment of acute promyelocytic leukemia and possibly some other cancers.

RESEARCH SUMMARY
Complete remission in up to 90% of patients with acute promyelocytic leukemia, including some resistant to standard treatments, has been reported in recent studies. Clinical, randomized, controlled studies are ongoing, investigating the potential use of arsenic trioxide in acute promyelocytic leukemia and in various other tumors. Arsenic trioxide, however, is not a dietary supplement, and physicians should caution patients who hear about these studies not to take arsenic supplements.

CONTRAINDICATIONS, PRECAUTIONS, ADVERSE REACTIONS

CONTRAINDICATIONS
None known. Supplemental arsenic is not recommended.

PRECAUTIONS
Supplemental arsenic is not recommended for anyone. Arsenic trioxide is presently in clinical trials for the treatment of cancer, particularly acute promyelocytic leukemia. Under no circumstance should cancer patients self-medicate with arsenic trioxide or any other form of arsenic.

ADVERSE REACTIONS
Toxicity from dietary intake of arsenic—up to 60 micrograms daily—is relatively low. Intakes of higher amounts of arsenic on a chronic basis may cause hyperkeratosis, especially of the palms and soles, skin pigmentation, eczematous or follicular dermatitis, edema (especially of the eyelids), alopecia, muscle-aching and weakness, stomatitis, excessive salivation, anemia, leukopenia, thrombocytopenia, jaundice, cirrhosis, ascites, peripheral neuropathy, paresthesias, proteinuria, hematuria and anuria. Chronic-high arsenic ingestion has been associated with various cancers, such as basal cell carcinoma and bladder, liver and lung cancers. The nail changes associated with arsenic toxicity are known as Mees' lines or transverse striate leukonychia.

Ingested arsenic salts cause oral irritation and a sensation of burning in the mouth and throat.

OVERDOSAGE
Intake of 70 to 300 milligrams of arsenic trioxide may be fatal. Death typically occurs between 12 to 48 hours but can occur within one hour. Those who survive arsenic trioxide poisoning may develop encephalopathy or severe peripheral neuropathies. Toxicity of inorganic arsenic increases with greater solubility. Trivalent compounds (e.g., arsenic trioxide) are more toxic than pentavalent compounds. Some organic arsenic compounds, such as arsenobetaine, are significantly less toxic. Symptoms of acute poisoning usually occur within one hour of ingestion but may be delayed for up to 12 hours, particularly in the presence of food. The principle toxic effects are hemorrhagic gastro-enteritis, profound dehydration, cardiac arrhythmias, convulsions, muscle cramps, shock and death.

DOSAGE AND ADMINISTRATION
No recommended dosage of supplemental arsenic.

Small amounts of arsenic may be found in colloidal or liquid minerals. Arsenic is also found in several homeopathic remedies, including arsenicum album (arsenic trioxide), arsenicum bromatum, arsenicum vodatum, arsenicum metallicum and arsenicum sulfuratum flavum-arsenic trisulph.

HOW SUPPLIED
Arsenicum album is available in the following forms and homeopathic strengths:

Liquid

Pellets

Sublingual Tablets — 6X, 30X, 30C

LITERATURE
Hei TM, Liu SX, Waldren C. Mutagenicity of arsenic in mammalian cells: role of reactive oxygen species. *Proc Natl Acad Sci.* 1998; 95:8103-8107

Hertz-Picciotto I, Arrighi HM, Hu SW. Does arsenic exposure increase the risk for circulatory disease? *Am J Epidemiol.* 2000; 151:174-181.

Lehmann S, Paul C. [Arsenic efficient in acute promyelocytic leukemia.] [Article in Swedish.] *Lakartidningen.* 1999; 96:5626-5628.

Mazunder DN, Das Gupta J, Santra A, et al. Chronic arsenic toxicity in west Bengal—the worst calamity in the world. *J Indian Med Assoc.* 1998; 96:4-7,18.

Nielsen FH. Ultratrace minerals. In: Shils ME, Olson JA, Shike M, Ross AC, eds. *Modern Nutrition in Health and Disease.* 9th ed. Baltimore, MD: Williams and Wilkins; 1999; 283-303.

Pergantis SA, Wangkarn S, Francesconi KA, Thomas-Oates JE. Identification of arsenosugars at the picogram level using nanoelectrospray quadropole-time-of-flight mass spectrometry. *Anal. Chem.* 2000; 72:357-366.

Shen ZY, Shen J, Cai WJ, et al. The alteration of mitochondria is an early event of arsenic trioxide induced apoptosis in esophageal carcinoma cells. *Int J Mol Med.* 2000; 5:155-158.

Soignet SL, Maslak PM, Wang Z-G, et al. Complete remission after treatment of acute promyelocytic leukemia with arsenic trioxide. *N Eng J Med.* 1998; 339:1341-1348.

Ascorbyl Palmitate

DESCRIPTION
Ascorbyl palmitate is a synthetic ester comprised of the 16-carbon chain saturated fatty acid palmitic acid and L-ascorbic acid. The ester linkage is at the 6 carbon of ascorbic acid. It is used as an antioxidant in foods, pharmaceuticals and cosmetics, and is also used as a preservative for the natural oils, oleates, fragrances, colors, vitamins and other edible oils and waxes which are used in pharmaceuticals, cosmetics and foods.

Ascorbyl palmitate is a white or yellowish powder having a slight odor. It is very slightly soluble in water and in vegetable oils. Ascorbic acid comprises 42.5% of the weight of ascorbyl palmitate. Its molecular weight is 414.54 daltons and its empirical formula is $C_{22}H_{38}O_7$. Ascorbyl palmitate is also known as vitamin C palmitate, L-ascorbyl-6-palmitate and 3-oxo-L-gulofuranolactone 6-palmitate.

Ascorbyl palmitate is marketed as a nutritional supplement and claimed by some to be a superior delivery form of vitamin C. Since ascorbyl palmitate is a fat-soluble derivative of ascorbic acid, theoretically it can concentrate into the lipid domains of biological systems and protect cell membranes and low density lipoproteins (LDL) against oxidation.

ACTIONS AND PHARMACOLOGY
ACTIONS
Ascorbyl palmitate is a delivery form of ascorbic acid. Refer to the vitamin C monograph for the action of ascorbic acid.

MECHANISM OF ACTION
If ascorbyl palmitate is absorbed intact, it may be expected to be a better antioxidant in the lipid domains of the cell membranes and in LDL than is ascorbic acid. It may also be expected to be a more efficient partner with d-alpha-tocopherol than is ascorbic acid with regard to sparing vitamin E, as well as regenerating it from its radical form. However, to date, little is known of the pharmacokinetics of ascorbyl palmitate. Refer to the vitamin C monograph for details on the mechanism of action of ascorbic acid.

PHARMACOKINETICS
As mentioned above, little is known of the pharmacokinetics of ascorbyl palmitate. For details on the pharmacokinetics of ascorbic acid, refer to the vitamin C monograph.

INDICATIONS AND USAGE
Ascorbyl palmitate has indications similar to those of vitamin C. (See Vitamin C.) There is one report suggesting that it might be more effective than other forms of vitamin C in protecting against lipid peroxide-induced endothelial injury.

RESEARCH SUMMARY
There is one preliminary *in vitro* study suggesting that ascorbyl palmitate can protect cultured human umbilical vein endothelial cells from the cytotoxicity of linoleic acid hydroperoxide in circumstances where ascorbic acid itself failed to perform the same protective function. At this early state, however, there is no reason to recommend preferential use of ascorbyl palmitate. See the monograph for vitamin C for the research summary of ascorbic acid.

CONTRAINDICATIONS, PRECAUTIONS, ADVERSE REACTIONS
See Vitamin C.

INTERACTIONS
See Vitamin C.

DOSAGE AND ADMINISTRATION

Multiply ascorbyl palmitate dose by 0.425 to derive the amount of ascorbic acid in the preparation. For recommended dosage and administration, refer to the vitamin C monograph.

LITERATURE

Kaneko T, Kaji K, Matsuo M. Protective effects of lipophilic derivatives of ascorbic acid on lipid peroxide-induced endothelial injury. *Arch Biochem Biophys*. 1993; 304:176-180.

Perricone N, Nagy K, Horvath F, et al. The hydroxyl free radical reactions of ascorbyl palmitate as measured in various in vitro models. *Biochem Biophys Res Commun*. 1999; 262:661-665.

Refer to the vitamin C monograph to review further literature references for ascorbic acid.

Bee Pollen

TRADE NAMES

Bee Pollen is available generically from numerous manufacturers. Some common brand names include Bee Pollen Power Extract (Bee Pollen from England), Bee Pollen Nuggets (Mason) and Super Bee Pollen Complex (Basic Vitamins).

DESCRIPTION

Bee pollen consists of plant pollens collected by worker bees combined with plant nectar and bee saliva. The material is compacted into pellets, which are used as food for drone bees. Pollen consists of the male germ seeds of plants, flowers or blossoms on trees. As plants flower, pollen is transferred from the anther of a stamen to the stigma of a pistil; on reaching the ovary it brings about fertilization of the ovules and the growth of seeds. Flowers are mainly pollinated by insects, such as beetles, butterflies and bees. Palynology is the study of pollen.

Bee pollen is comprised of proteins (about 25-30%), carbohydrates (about 30-55%), lipids (about 1-20%), minerals, vitamins and trace amounts of other organic substances.

Bee pollen became popular as a nutritional supplement in the 1970s following testimonials by athletes claiming that its use increased stamina and improved athletic ability.

ACTIONS AND PHARMACOLOGY

ACTIONS

No known actions.

PHARMACOKINETICS

Proteins, carbohydrates and lipids in bee pollen should be digested, absorbed and metabolized, as are similar substances found in foods. However, the shells of the individual grains of pollen are not readily digestible, and only a small percentage of the above substances may actually be processed by the body.

INDICATIONS AND USAGE

There is insufficient clinical research to suggest any indication for supplemental bee pollen. A few *in vitro* and animal studies suggest that it might protect against some forms of radiation damage, that it might have some immunomodulating effects and that it might have some benefit in pregnancy.

RESEARCH SUMMARY

In vitro studies indicate that bee pollen exerts protective effects against radiation in some animal tissues. A study of pregnant rats associated the addition of bee pollen to diet with improved body weight, hemoglobin levels and total protein, serum iron and albumin levels in the mother, as well as greater body weight and decreased fatality in the fetuses, compared with controls. Some favorable immunomodulating effects were seen in other very preliminary animal work.

CONTRAINDICATIONS, PRECAUTIONS, ADVERSE REACTIONS

CONTRAINDICATIONS

Bee pollen is contraindicated in those with pollen allergies. It is also contraindicated in those hypersensitive to bee pollen. (There are other proteins in bee pollen in addition to those from pollen.)

Children, pregnant women and nursing mothers should avoid bee pollen.

ADVERSE REACTIONS

Those who are allergic or hypersensitive to bee pollen can develop symptoms, including pruritis, rhinitis, conjunctivitis and bronchospasm and, in some cases, urticaria and anaphylaxis. Two cases of hepatitis have been reported following ingestion of bee pollen for several weeks. Hypereosinophilia, neurologic symptoms (decreased memory, headache) and gastrointestinal symptoms (nausea, abdominal pain, diarrhea) have also been reported following bee pollen ingestion.

OVERDOSAGE

No reported overdosage of bee pollen.

DOSAGE AND ADMINISTRATION

Typical doses used are 1 to 1.5 grams daily in divided doses.

HOW SUPPLIED

Capsules — 580 mg

Chewable Tablets — 500 mg, 1000 mg

Granules

Liquid

Powder

Tablets — 500 mg, 1000 mg

LITERATURE

Anan'eva TV, Dvoretskii AI. [Effect of beta-carotene oil and bee pollen on ion transport in rat brain slices following radiation-chemical exposure.] [Article in Russian.] *Radiats Biol Radioecol.* 1999; 39:341-344.

Bevzo VV, Grygor'eva NP. [Effect of bee pollen extract on glutathione system activity in mice liver under X-ray irradiation.] [Article in Ukrainian.] *Ukr Biokhim Zh.* 1999; 69:115-117.

Cohen SH, Yunginger JW, Rosenberg N, Fink JN. Acute allergic reaction after composite pollen ingestion. *J Allergy Clin Immunol.* 1979; 64:270-274.

Dudov IA, Morenets AA, Artiukh VP, Starodub NF. [Immunotherapy effect of honeybee flower pollen load.] [Article in Russian.] *Ukr Biokhim Zh.* 1994; 66:91-93.

Geyman JP. Anaphylactic reaction after ingestion of bee pollen. *J Am Board Fam Pract.* 1994; 7:250-252.

Lin FL, Vaughan TR, Vandewalker ML, Weber RW. Hypereosinophilia, neurologic, and gastrointestinal symptoms after bee pollen ingestion. *J Allergy Clin Immunol.* 1989; 83:793-796.

Puente S, Iniquez A, Subirats M, et al. [Eosinophilic gastroenteritis caused by bee pollen sensitization.] [Article in Spanish.] *Med Clin (Barc).* 1997; 108:698-700.

Shad JA, Chinn CG, Brann OS. Acute hepatitis after ingestion of herbs. *South Med J.* 1999; 92:1095-1097.

Williams MH. Ergogenic and ergolytic substances. *Med Sci Sports Exerc.* 1992; 24 (9 Suppl):S344-S348.

Xie Y, Wan B, Li W. [Effect of bee pollen on maternal nutrition and fetal growth.] [Article in Chinese.] *Hua Hsi I Ko Hsueh Hsueh Pao.* 1994; 25:434-437.

Bentonite

TRADE NAMES

Bentonite #7 liquid (Sonne's) and Great Plains Bentonite Clay (Yerba Prima Botanicals).

DESCRIPTION

Bentonite is occasionally used in nutritional supplements as a source of trace minerals. It is a type of clay, the major constituent of which is a hydrated aluminum silicate called montmorillonite. Minor constituents found in bentonite include calcium, magnesium and iron. Bentonite is found in certain areas of the United States and Canada. Wyoming bentonite, found in Wyoming and South Dakota, contains sodium and is composed of alternating layers of aluminum oxide and silicon dioxide. It is also known as sodium montmorillonite. Bentonite found in Mississippi is known as calcium montmorillonite.

Bentonite absorbs water readily to form highly viscous suspensions or gels. Bentonite itself is practically insoluble in water. Because of its water-absorbing property, bentonite has been used as a bulk laxative and is used in the pharmaceutical industry as a suspending and stabilizing agent, as well as an adsorbent or clarifying agent. A derivative of bentonite is used to block urushiols from the skins. Urushiols are the etiological factors causing contact dermatitis from poison ivy, poison oak and poison sumac. Bentonite itself may bind to some toxins, such as paraquat, by adsorbing them.

ACTIONS AND PHARMACOLOGY

ACTIONS

Bentonite may be a delivery form of small amounts of certain trace minerals and small amounts of magnesium and calcium. It may also bind to some toxins, such as pesticides.

MECHANISM OF ACTION

Certain toxins, such as paraquat, may be adsorbed by bentonite.

PHARMACOKINETICS

Little is reported on the pharmacokinetics of bentonite. Following ingestion, there is probably very little to no absorption of bentonite from the gastrointestinal tract, and it is excreted in the feces. Small amounts of trace minerals and small amounts of calcium and magnesium may be absorbed.

INDICATIONS AND USAGE

It is claimed that bentonite binds to a number of toxins and thus renders them harmless. There is some evidence of this effect in animal studies.

RESEARCH SUMMARY

Bentonite has been shown to protect against the effects of aflatoxins in broiler chickens and rats but did not alleviate locoweed toxicosis in rats. Bentonite has also been shown to prevent high radiocesium levels in animal products. Clinical trials are lacking.

CONTRAINDICATIONS, PRECAUTIONS, ADVERSE REACTIONS

CONTRAINDICATIONS

Bentonite is contraindicated in those who are hypersensitive to any component of a bentonite-containing product. It is also contraindicated in those whose gastrointestinal tract is not anatomically intact.

PRECAUTIONS

Pregnant women, nursing mothers and the elderly should avoid using bentonite.

Those who do use bentonite should ingest plenty of fluid (water, juice) concomitantly in order to avoid possible intestinal obstruction.

Bentonite should not be used concomitantly with drugs or nutritional supplements.

There is no documentation in humans that bentonite has any benefit as a trace mineral source or as an aid in removing toxins from the colon.

ADVERSE REACTIONS

At doses usually used in nutritional supplements—5 to 10 mg—there are no reports of adverse reactions. Higher doses, e.g., greater than 10 grams daily, may have a laxative effect—bentonite was used as a bulk laxative—and if not taken with plenty of fluids may cause intestinal obstruction.

INTERACTIONS

DRUGS

Bentonite may adsorb certain drugs. Bentonite should not be taken concomitantly with any drugs.

NUTRITIONAL SUPPLEMENTS

Bentonite may adsorb certain nutritional supplements and should not be used concomitantly with them.

FOODS

Bentonite may adsorb certain food components.

HERBS

Bentonite may adsorb certain herb components.

DOSAGE AND ADMINISTRATION

Bentonite is available in some nutritional supplements as a trace mineral source. Dosage is usually 5 to 10 mg daily. Those who use bentonite as a ''colon cleanser'' use one tablespoon once or twice a day, which must be taken with at least one glass of water or juice. This is not recommended. Drugs and nutritional supplements should not be used concomitantly with the higher doses.

HOW SUPPLIED

Liquid

LITERATURE

Abdel-Wahhab MA, Nada SA, Farag IM, et al. Potential protective effect of HSCAS and bentonite against dietary aflatoxicosis in rat: with special reference to chromosomal aberrations. *Nat Toxins*.1998; 6:211-218.

Santurio JM, Mallmann CA, Rosa AP, et al. Effect of sodium bentonite on the performance and blood variables of broiler chickens intoxicated with aflatoxins. *Br Poult Sci*. 1999; 40:115-119.

Beta-Carotene

TRADE NAMES

A-Caro-25 (The Key Company), Caroguard (Bio-Tech Pharmacal), B-Caro-T (Bio-Tech Pharmacal), Biotene (Advanced Nutritional Technology), Lumitene (Tishcon Corp.), Eye Bright (Advanced Nutritional Technology), Oceanic Beta Carotene (Solgar), Dry Beta Carotene (Solgar), Mega Carotene (Twinlab), Marine Carotene (Twinlab), Ultra Beta Carotene (Nature's Plus), Superbeta Carotene (Source Naturals), Caro-Plete (Carlson).

DESCRIPTION

Beta-carotene is a member of a class of substances called carotenoids. Beta-carotene, similar to the other carotenoids, is a natural fat-soluble pigment found principally in plants, algae *(Dunaliella salina, Dunaliella bardawil)* and photosynthetic bacteria, where it serves as an accessory light-gathering pigment and to protect these organisms against the toxic effects of oxygen. Carotenoids are polyisoprenoids which typically contain 40 carbon atoms and an extensive system of conjugated double bonds. They usually show internal symmetry and frequently contain one or two ring structures at the ends of their conjugated chains. Beta-carotene contains a cyclic structure at each end of its conjugated chain. The structural formula for beta-carotene is:

Beta-Carotene

Carotenoids are the principal pigments responsible for the red, orange, yellow and green colors of vegetables and fruits. Beta-carotene is responsible for the color of carrots.

Beta-carotene along with alpha-carotene, lycopene, lutein, zeaxanthin and beta-cryptoxanthin are the principal dietary carotenoids. Three of these carotenoids, alpha-carotene, beta-carotene and beta-cryptoxanthin, can serve as dietary precursors of retinol (all-*trans* retinol, vitamin A). Collectively, these carotenoids are called provitamin A carotenoids or provitamin A. Dietary carotenoids that are not converted into retinol (lutein, zeaxanthin, lycopene) are referred to as nonprovitamin A carotenoids.

Beta-carotene occurs naturally as all-*trans* beta-carotene and 9-*cis* beta-carotene. Smaller amounts of 13-*cis* beta-carotene are also found naturally. Synthetic beta-carotene consists mainly of all-*trans* beta-carotene with smaller amounts of 13-*cis* beta-carotene and even smaller amounts of 9-*cis* beta-carotene. Carrots are the major contributors of beta-carotene in the diet. Beta-carotene is also found in cantaloupe, broccoli, spinach and collard greens. Palm oil, which is used as a food colorant, is rich in beta-carotene as well as alpha-carotene. Dietary intake of beta-carotene in the American diet ranges from 1.3 to 2.9 milligrams daily. The consumption of five or more servings of fruits and vegetables per day—which is recommended by a number of federal agencies and other organizations, including the National Cancer Institute—would provide 3 to 6 milligrams daily of beta-carotene.

Beta-carotene is considered a conditionally essential nutrient. Beta-carotene becomes an essential nutrient when the dietary intake of retinol (vitamin A) is inadequate. It is unclear whether beta-carotene has any biological function for humans other than as a precursor for vitamin A. There is some evidence that beta-carotene may play a beneficial role in human nutrition beyond its provitamin A function. Beta-carotene has antioxidant activity, at least *in vitro*, and it may enhance intercellular communication and may have immunomodulatory and anticarcinogenic activities in certain circumstances. However, the evidence for a unique role in human nutrition beyond its provitamin A function is, to date, not compelling.

The absorption efficiency of beta-carotene and the other carotenoids from food sources is highly variable. For this reason, it has been difficult to define a general numerical factor for converting provitamin A carotenoids to vitamin A. There are two systems of units which are currently used which do not agree with each other and which have caused confusion. In the first system, 1 IU (international unit) is equal to 0.6 micrograms of all-*trans* beta-carotene or 1.2 micrograms of mixed other provitamin A carotenoids. In this system, which is the one generally used for nutritional labeling, 3 milligrams of beta-carotene is equal to 5,000 IU. The U.S. RDA for vitamin A is 5,000 IU. The second system uses retinol equivalents in place of international units. In the second system, one retinol equivalent (RE) is defined as one microgram of all-*trans* retinol (vitamin A), six micrograms of all-*trans* beta-carotene or 12 micrograms of other provitamin A carotenoids. In the first system, two micrograms of all-*trans* beta-carotene are defined as being equal to one microgram of all-*trans* retinol. In the second system, six micrograms of dietary all-*trans* beta-carotene are assumed to be nutritionally equivalent to one microgram of all-*trans* retinol. It is clear that these two systems do not agree with each other. In any case, all-*trans* carotene, as found in nutritional supplements, should be converted according to the first system. That is, two micrograms of all-*trans* carotene are equal to one microgram of all-*trans* retinol (vitamin A) or 3.33 IU.

ACTIONS AND PHARMACOLOGY
ACTIONS
Beta-carotene may have antioxidant activity. It may also have immunomodulatory, anticarcinogenic and antiatherogenic activities in some cases.

MECHANISM OF ACTION
Beta-carotene has been found to have antioxidant activity *in vitro*. It has been demonstrated to quench singlet oxygen ($^1O_2$), scavenge peroxyl radicals and inhibit lipid peroxidation. The mechanism of beta-carotene's antioxidant activity is not clearly understood. Some, but not all, studies have shown a difference in the *in vitro* activities of the beta-carotene isomers. One study showed that 9-*cis* beta-carotene—a naturally occurring form of beta-carotene—protected methyl linoleate from oxidation more efficiently than all-*trans* beta-carotene. However, another study demonstrated that 9-*cis* beta-carotene and all-*trans* beta-carotene had equal antioxidant activities when assessed by enhanced human neutrophil chemiluminescence. Whether beta-carotene has significant antioxidant activity *in vivo* is unclear. Results from some human studies have shown improvement of measures of antioxidant activity (decreased copper-induced LDL oxidation, decreased DNA strand breaks and oxidized pyrimidine bases in lymphocytes, decreased serum lipid peroxide levels, decreased breath pentane, decreased serum malondialdehyde, increased red blood cell copper/zinc-superoxide dismutase activity) in those receiving relatively high intakes of beta-carotene. Studies of those receiving relatively low to modest levels of beta-carotene have shown no changes or inconsistent changes in the same antioxidant activities. Administration of beta-carotene to cystic fibrosis subjects was found to decrease serum malondialdehyde, in one study. Beta-carotene may have antioxidant activity in some with conditions of increased oxidative stress. Retinol itself appears to have low antioxidant activity. Therefore, possible *in vivo* antioxidant activity of beta-carotene is unlikely to be a consequence of its conversion to retinol.

Beta-carotene has demonstrated some immunomodulatory effects. In healthy male nonsmokers, beta-carotene supplementation (15 mg/day) was found to significantly increase the percentage of monocytes expressing the major histocompatibility complex class II molecule HLA-DR, to increase the expression of the adhesion molecules, intercellular adhesion molecule-1 and leukocyte function-associated antigen-3, and to increase *ex vivo* secretion of tumor necrosis factor (TNF)-alpha by blood monocytes. Beta-carotene supplementation has also been found to enhance natural killer cell activity in elderly men, to increase lymphocyte response to mitogens in healthy male cigarette smokers and to increase the CD4 lymphocyte count in some subjects with AIDS. The mechanism of the possible immunomodulatory activity of beta-carotene is not known. It is thought that the possible immunomodulatory activity may be independent of beta-carotene's role as a precursor of retinol.

Beta-carotene has been found to inhibit the growth of some malignant cells, including human prostate cancer cells, *in vitro*. The mechanism of this activity is not well understood. It is speculated that beta-carotene may increase cellular differentiation, down-regulate epidermal growth factor receptors, reduce adenyl cyclase activity, enhance expression of gap junctional proteins and protect against oxidative damage. The ability of beta-carotene to modulate the carcinogenic process, at least *in vitro*, may be due, in part, to its conversion to retinoids. In this regard, there is evidence that beta-carotene may be converted to retinol and other related metabolites (e.g., retinoic acid) in human prostate cell lines.

Several observational epidemiological studies have shown an inverse association between dietary beta-carotene intake and a number of cancers, in particular lung cancer. Intervention trials, however, have not found beta-carotene to be protective against lung cancer. In fact, two intervention trials, the Alpha-Tocopherol, Beta-Carotene (ATBC) Cancer Prevention Study (the ''Finnish study''), and the Carotene and Retinol Efficacy Trial (CARET), both reported an unexpected increase in the number of lung cancer cases in the groups that received supplemental beta-carotene. The subjects in the ATBC and CARET studies were smokers. In the case of these studies, the mechanism, not of the possible anticarcinogenic activity of beta-carotene, but of its possible procarcinogenic activity, at least for smokers, requires elucidation. Several possible explanations have been proposed to explain the unexpected increase in lung cancer in these studies. Beta-carotene may act as a prooxidant when present in high concentrations in an oxidative environment such as the lungs of smokers in the advanced promotional stage of the neoplastic process. (Beta-carotene may be effective in the prevention of lung cancer if chronically present before or during the phases of initiation and early promotion of the process). Supplemental beta-carotene is known to inhibit the absorption of the carotenoid lutein which itself may have chemopreventive activity. Beta-carotene may have a co-carcinogenic effect. Beta-carotene has been found in the rat lung to produce a booster effect on phase I carcinogen-bioactivating enzymes, including activators of polycyclic aromatic hydrocarbons (PAHs). Finally, oxidative metabolites of beta-carotene may diminish retinoid signaling and eventually enhance carcinogenesis. The mechanism of the possible effect of beta-carotene in enhancing lung cancer in smokers remains a mystery. The general opinion is that the effect is related to prooxidant activity of beta-carotene or oxidative metabolites of beta-carotene in the context of increased partial pressure of oxygen in smokers' lungs.

Beta-carotene may have anticarcinogenic activity in the case of prostate cancer. In the Physicians' Health Study, it was found that men with low baseline beta-carotene levels at the beginning of the study experienced a decreased risk of developing prostate cancer when supplemented with 50 milligrams of beta-carotene every other day. The mechanism of this possible anticarcinogenic effect is unclear. A review of the postulated mechanisms of possible anticarcinogenic activity in certain circumstances is as follows: beta-carotene may be metabolically converted to retinoids which modulate the gene expression of factors linked to differentiation and cell proliferation via retinoic acid. Beta-carotene may modulate the activity of enzymes that metabolize xenobiotics. The carotenoid has been found to increase the levels of phase II detoxifying enzymes such as glutathione S-transferase mu (GST-mu) and glutathione peroxidase. Beta-carotene's possible immunomodulatory activity may also play a role. Its possible antioxidant activity may result in prevention of oxidative damage to DNA and inhibition of lipid peroxidation as well as regulation of the expression of genes sensitive to the intracellular redox state that may be involved in carcinogenesis. Beta-carotene may modulate the gene expression of connexin 43 resulting in the induction of gap junctions with a consequent inhibition of neoplastic transformations. Finally, in animals, beta-carotene has been found to modulate the gene expression of the enzyme HMG-CoA reductase. This would inhibit the endogenous synthesis of cholesterol resulting in possible inhibition of cell proliferation and malignant transformation.

Epidemiological studies and some, but not all, intervention studies suggest an inverse association between coronary artery disease and beta-carotene intake. The possible antiatherogenic activity of beta-carotene may be accounted for, in part, by its possible antioxidant activity. Humans supplemented with beta-carotene, but not lycopene, were found to have low-density lipoproteins that were less oxidized than did controls using endothelial cell-initiated autoxidation.

PHARMACOKINETICS
The efficiency of absorption of beta-carotene is highly variable. The efficiency of absorption of beta-carotene from carrots and other beta-carotene containing raw foods is less than 5%. On the other hand, the efficiency of absorption of beta-carotene from beta-carotene-containing nutritional supplements can be as high as 70% or more. In foods, beta-carotene exists either as a solution in oil (e.g., red palm oil) or as part of a matrix within the vegetable or fruit. For example, in carrots, beta-carotene exists in a complex matrix, comprised of indigestible polysaccharides, digestible polysaccharides and protein. Only a small percentage of beta-carotene is released from the matrix during the passage of foods such as carrots, through the gastrointestinal tract.

Beta-carotene from supplements, oils or foods is either solubilized in the lipid core of micelles (formed from bile salts and dietary fat) in the lumen of the small intestine or forms clathrate complexes with conjugated bile salts. Micelles and clathrate complexes deliver beta-carotene to the enterocytes. All of the beta-carotene isomers—all-*trans* beta-carotene, 9-*cis* beta-carotene and 13-*cis* beta-carotene—are absorbed from the lumen of the small intestine into the enterocytes. Within the enterocytes, a fraction of all-*trans* beta-carotene is oxidized to retinal and then reduced to retinol. Retinol is then esterified to form retinyl esters. It appears that 9-*cis* carotene is isomerized to the all-trans form before being released into the lymphatics. The principal enzyme involved in the oxidation of beta-carotene is called beta-carotene 15, 15^1 dioxygenase.

Beta-carotene and retinyl esters are released from the enterocytes into the lymphatics in the form of chylomicrons. (See Vitamin A for the pharmacokinetics of that substance.) Beta-carotene is transported by the lymphatics to the general circulation via the thoracic duct. In the circulation, lipoprotein lipase hydrolyzes much of the triglycerides in the chylomicrons, resulting in the formation of chylomicron remnants. Chylomicron remnants retain apolipoproteins E and B48 on their surfaces and are mainly taken up by hepatocytes and to smaller degrees by other tissues. Within hepatocytes, beta-carotene is incorporated into lipoproteins. Beta-carotene is released into the blood from the hepatocytes in the form of very low-density lipoproteins (VLDL) and low-density lipoproteins (LDL). In the plasma, VLDLs are converted by lipoprotein lipase to LDLs. Beta-carotene is transported in the plasma predominantly in the form of LDLs.

INDICATIONS AND USAGE

Beta-carotene may be protective against some forms of cancer in some populations. It may also play a role in protecting against heart disease in some. Beta-carotene has demonstrated positive effects in the immune system. Diminished beta-carotene status has been observed in subjects with noninsulin-dependent diabetes, but supplementation with beta-carotene has so far produced no notable benefits in diabetic patients. Benefits sometimes attributed to beta-carotene in the prevention of cataracts and age-related macular degeneration may actually be due to other carotenoids, notably lutein and zeaxanthin.

RESEARCH SUMMARY

The epidemiologic evidence is overwhelming that those who consume three or more servings of fruits and vegetables daily have significantly lower risk of many forms of cancer and heart disease. The protective association is particularly strong for dietary carotenoids, especially with respect to protection against lung cancer in both men and women, smokers and non-smokers.

These epidemiologic findings have been fortified by other studies in which levels of carotenoids in blood and tissue have shown consistent inverse associations with cancer risks, especially lung-cancer risk. Plausible mechanisms of action in this context have further buttressed the case for a useful role of beta-carotene in cancer prevention.

Additionally, beta-carotene supplements have significantly inhibited oral leucoplakia and such other precancerous lesions as buccal cell micronuclei in subjects at risk of oral cancer. In the Linxian Interventive Trial, only a combination of beta-carotene, vitamin E and selenium, of four dietary regimens tested against placebo, had significant protective effects (principally against gastric and esophogeal cancers). *In vitro* and animal studies have also shown significant beta-carotene anticancer effects. Recently it was shown *in vitro* that beta-carotene significantly inhibited growth of three different human prostate cancer cell lines.

While the large Linxian Intervention Trial found that a supplementary regimen that included beta-carotene, as noted above, significantly reduced mortality from gastric and total cancer in marginally malnourished subjects, three other large intervention studies in normally nourished subjects, long-term smokers, former smokers and those exposed to asbestos found no overall benefit from high-dose beta-carotene. Moreover, in one of these studies, there was a significant 18% excess incidence of lung cancer among those who received beta-carotene supplements.

These contrary and unexpected findings initially caused great consternation among researchers and physicians and provoked "panic" headlines in the lay press, leaving many with the impression that beta-carotene was categorically of no value and that it most likely was hazardous to health. As the dust from this uproar has begun to settle, some plausible explanations for the overall failure of beta-carotene in these particular studies have begun to emerge along with a rationale for the continued use of beta-carotene supplementation in some circumstances.

The study that most surprised the research and medical communities was the Alpha-Tocopherol, Beta-Carotene Prevention study (ATBC). This randomized, double-blind, placebo-controlled study tested beta-carotene (20 milligrams daily) or 50 milligrams of alpha-tocopherol, or both, against placebo in Finnish smokers aged 50-69 years of age over a period of five to eight years, primarily to see what impact, if any, supplementation might have on the incidence of lung cancer. Not only was no protective effect demonstrated but there was a significant increase in lung cancer incidence and mortality among the supplemented group. (Alpha-tocopherol also failed overall to protect smokers against lung cancer, except in the case of those who took it for five or more years.

It was, however, associated with a significant reduction in risk of prostate cancer, a lesser reduction in colon cancer and increased risk of hemorrhagic stroke in smokers. See Vitamin E for more details.) It should be noted that there was evidence in this study that those with low beta-carotene status at baseline who received beta-carotene supplements had a 35% reduced incidence of pancreatic cancer, compared with controls who received placebo.

Another large intervention trial, the Beta-Carotene and Retinol Efficacy Trial (CARET), was halted prematurely in view of the ATBC findings and preliminary results demonstrating no benefit from supplemental beta-carotene and retinol in smokers, former smokers and those exposed to asbestos. Non-significant increases in cancer and cardiovascular incidence and mortality were noted. Doses used were 30 milligrams of beta-carotene and 25,000 IUs of retinyl palmitate.

In the Physicians' Health Study (PHS) which lasted 12 years, 22,071 healthy physicians, 11% of whom were current smokers and 39% of whom were former smokers, took high doses of beta-carotene, 50 milligrams every other day, or placebo. This was for a considerably longer period than supplements were taken in either the CARET or ATBC trials. Supplementation neither decreased nor increased overall risk of cancer. There was a non-significant decrease in the incidence of lung cancer among the smokers in this group receiving beta-carotene. In a subset of this population with low baseline blood levels of beta-carotene, there was, with supplements, a lower rate of total cancer and a 32% reduction in risk of prostate cancer. No toxic side effects were reported in this study.

How does one reconcile these confounding results? It appears, some researchers have concluded, that beta-carotene supplementation, even long-term and at doses as high as those used in these studies, while possibly not advisable or optimal, appears non-toxic in non-smoking and non-asbestos-exposed populations. Why even smokers in the PHS study suffered no harm, in contrast to some apparent harm in the CARET and ATBS studies, is unknown. It is possible that they smoked less, and that this well-educated, health-conscious population may have eaten more fruits and vegetables and may have more regularly consumed other vitamin-mineral preparations that favorably altered the activity of beta-carotene or that conferred some protection by themselves. Additionally, some others have pointed out that long-term, high-dose use of beta-carotene produced no toxic effects in the treatment of some with skin disorders.

As for why no overall benefit, as opposed to harm, was seen in the PHS group, some argue that this was due, in part, to the fact that this was a healthy, well-nourished population to begin with. In the Linxian Study, by contrast, the large number of subjects studied suffered from poor nutrition and showed significant benefit (in terms of cancer protection) from supplementation with beta-carotene, selenium and vitamin E. Even in the PHS study those with low baseline blood levels of beta-carotene apparently had some supplementation-associated reduction in prostate cancer risk.

Why might high-dose beta-carotene be helpful in some but harmful in smokers and others with significant lung impairment, such as that caused by asbestos exposure? Several researchers have now suggested that high concentrations of beta-carotene oxidize in the free-radical-rich milieu of the lungs of cigarette smokers and asbestos sufferers. More physiologic amounts of beta-carotene, such as that derived from diet, appear to have antioxidant effects, whereas, these researchers assert, the very high doses of beta-carotene used in these studies turned pro-oxidant in the lungs of smokers. Some experimental evidence *in vitro* and in animal models lends preliminary support to this hypothesis. Thus, the argument is made that doses of beta-carotene used were inappropriately high and that beta-carotene, without other nutrients to protect it against oxidation, could not be expected to have a beneficial effect in the lungs of long-term smokers.

It has been pointed out that other factors also may have conspired against beta-carotene in these studies. In the ATBC trial, for example, apparent adverse effects of beta-carotene were seen primarily in those who smoked and also consumed high quantities of alcohol, which also produces significant oxidative stress. In addition, others have noted that subjects studied in these largely negative interventive trials were mostly heavy smokers aged 50 or older who had been smoking for many years or were workers with long-term exposure to asbestos and were thus likely to be in the advanced promotional phase of carcinogenesis at the outset of the study. Many of these subjects had been smoking for decades, and the intervention, the argument goes, came too late and with doses so high they became pro-oxidant rather than antioxidant in these highly oxidative conditions.

Various researchers have proposed that beta-carotene be tested in more physiological doses and in combination with vitamins E and C and possibly some other antioxidant nutrients. In one recent study, the oxidative stress of environmental tobacco smoke was said to be reduced in humans supplemented with 3 milligrams of beta-carotene, 60 milligrams of vitamin C, 30 milligrams of alpha-tocopherol, 40 milligrams of zinc, 40 milligrams of selenium and 2 milligrams of copper. In another study, this one conducted double-blind, smokers and non-smokers received another mixture of antioxidants (35 milligrams of beta-carotene, 100 milligrams of vitamin C and 280 milligrams of vitamin E daily) for 20 weeks. Notable reductions were observed in endogenous oxidative base damage in the lymphocyte DNA of both smokers and non-smokers.

Others insist that more animal work should be done before more large interventive beta-carotene trials are launched.

One reviewer has stated that "the results of the major trials do not prove or disprove the value of antioxidant vitamins nor do they incriminate them as harmful." Another reviewer concurs, observing that "these results cannot be used as evidence to suggest that low-dose supplementation with beta-carotene would be harmful (or beneficial), but point out our lack of knowledge regarding the dose/response/toxicity of most prevention agents (certainly dietary supplements)." Both reviewers also note that the trials nonetheless signal caution. Other reviewers, while noting that beta-carotene has exhibited considerable, credible anti-cancer activity in a number of studies, conclude that "chronic pharmacological supplementation is not recommended for healthy populations, and the carotenoid may actually be deleterious to smokers."

Finally, another reviewer of the lung cancer research observes that recent data from followup in the same interventive trials that reported negative supplementation results show that "regardless of their intervention assignment, study participants with highest intake and serum concentrations of beta-carotene at baseline developed fewer subsequent lung cancers." Viewed in that epidemiological light, these negative interventive studies assume a positive shading. Research continues.

The situation with respect to beta-carotene and heart disease roughly parallels the beta-carotene-cancer story. A number of epidemiological studies, including several cohort and case-control studies, have reported significantly diminished risk of cardiovascular disease in those with high plasma/serum levels and/or high dietary intake of beta-carotene. Case-control studies showed significant protective effects in both smokers and non-smokers.

In the large interventive trials, however, no significant protective effects were seen with respect to heart disease. Some of the same arguments used in an attempt to explain inconsistent results in the beta-carotene cancer research have been put forward to try to explain inconsistencies in the heart-disease results. Obviously, more research is needed to resolve the issue.

Some animal, *in vitro* and human research persuasively suggests that beta-carotene has immune enhancing and anti-mutagenic effects independent of any vitamin A activity. Beta-carotene for example, had helped protect bone-marrow cells against mutagens in experiments in which vitamin A

did not provide the same protection. Beta-carotene activity independent of any provitamin A activity has been credited in other experiments with enhancing both T- and B-lymphocyte proliferative responses in mice fed nutritionally complete diets supplemented with beta-carotene.

T-helper cell counts were significantly increased in humans given very high dose (180 milligrams daily) beta-carotene for two weeks. Production of macrophage cytokines has been increased and tumor cell cytotoxicity enhanced in an animal model using beta-carotene supplementation. More tumor cells were killed by natural killer cells from human peripheral blood when incubated with beta-carotene, compared to killer cells not exposed to beta-carotene.

In another study, vegetarians were found to have twice the natural killer cell activity of non-vegetarians. Serum levels of vitamins A, E and C were equal in the two groups, but beta-carotene levels were about twice as high in the vegetarians as in the non-vegetarians.

Some effects have also been seen in autoimmune conditions. In one experiment, giving beta-carotene to autoimmune-prone mice resulted in reduced lymphodenopathy and prolonged lifespan.

Healthy non-smoking men receiving 15 milligrams of beta-carotene daily exhibited enhanced immune function of blood monocytes. Ultraviolet light suppression of one type of immune function was significantly inhibited in a randomized trial of healthy older men taking 30 milligrams of beta-carotene daily for 47 days while simultaneously consuming a low-carotenoid diet.

Though relationships have been reported between diminished beta-carotene status and increased risk of diabetes mellitus, supplementation with beta-carotene has so far not been found to reduce the incidence of this disease.

Again, low beta-carotene status has been associated with higher risk of developing cataracts, but, once more, supplementation with beta-carotene has not been shown to reduce the incidence of cataracts. In the 12-year followup of the Nurses Health Study, involving 77,488 women aged 45-71 years, beta-carotene intake had no apparent impact on cataracts, but other carotenoids (lutein, zeaxanthin) were associated with a significant reduction in cataract risk.

With respect to age-related macular degeneration, higher dietary intake of carotenoids is associated with reduced risk. Again, lutein and zeaxanthin are the carotenoids that appear to provide the most protection. Beta-carotene is largely absent in the macula, whereas lutein and zeaxanthin are the dominant pigments of the macula.

CONTRAINDICATIONS, PRECAUTIONS, ADVERSE REACTIONS

CONTRAINDICATIONS

Beta-carotene is contraindicated in those hypersensitive to any component of a beta-carotene-containing preparation.

PRECAUTIONS

Pregnant women and nursing mothers should try to obtain an intake of beta-carotene from 3 to 6 milligrams daily from the consumption of five or more servings daily of fruits and vegetables. Pregnant women and nursing mothers should avoid intakes of beta-carotene greater than 6 milligrams/day from nutritional supplements.

Smokers should be made aware that supplemental intake of beta-carotene of 20 milligrams daily or greater were associated with a higher incidence of lung cancer in smokers. Smokers should avoid beta-carotene supplementation pending the establishment of a safe dose for smokers.

The use of beta-carotene for the treatment of vitamin A deficiency requires medical management.

ADVERSE REACTIONS

Beta-carotene is used for the treatment of erythropoietic protoporphyria. This is a photosensitivity disorder. Doses of up to 180 milligrams daily are used for the treatment of this disorder. No toxic effects are seen in those with this disorder taking this high dose. Doses of 30 milligrams/day or greater of beta-carotene taken for prolonged periods may cause carotenodermia. Carotenodermia is characterized by yellowish discoloration of the skin and is distinguished from jaundice by the absence of yellowed ocular sclerae, which are found in those with jaundice. Carotenodermia is considered harmless and reversible with the discontinuation of beta-carotene.

There is no evidence of hypervitaminosis A in those consuming high doses (up to 180 mg/d of beta-carotene).

There is an association of increased lung cancer in smokers taking 20 mg/d or greater of beta-carotene. In the Alpha-Tocopherol, Beta-Carotene (ATBC) Cancer Prevention Study, smokers supplemented with 20 mg/d of beta-carotene for five to eight years showed a higher incidence of lung cancer compared to the placebo group. In the Carotene and Retinol Efficacy Trial (CARET), smokers taking 30 milligrams of beta-carotene daily and 25,000 IUs/d of retinol were found to have a higher incidence of lung cancer when compared to the placebo group. It is at present unclear if there is a true link between increased lung cancer incidence in smokers taking beta-carotene supplements.

INTERACTIONS

DRUGS

Cholestyramine: Concomitant intake of cholestyramine and beta-carotene may decrease the absorption of beta-carotene.

Colestipol: Concomitant intake of colestipol and beta-carotene may decrease the absorption of beta-carotene.

Mineral Oil: Concomitant intake of mineral oil and beta-carotene may reduce the absorption of beta-carotene.

Orlistat: Orlistat may decrease the absorption of beta-carotene.

NUTRITIONAL SUPPLEMENTS

Lutein: Concomitant intake of the carotenoid lutein and beta-carotene may decrease the absorption of lutein.

Pectin: Concomitant intake of pectin and beta-carotene may decrease the absorption of beta-carotene.

FOODS

Olestra: Concomitant intake of olestra and beta-carotene may decrease the absorption of beta-carotene.

OVERDOSAGE

Beta-Carotene overdosage is not reported in the literature.

DOSAGE AND ADMINISTRATION

Beta-carotene supplements are available as synthetic beta-carotene and natural beta-carotene. Synthetic beta-carotene is comprised mainly of all-*trans* beta-carotene with smaller amounts of 13-*cis* beta-carotene and even smaller amounts of 9-*cis* beta-carotene. Natural beta-carotene is principally derived from the algae *Dunaliella salina* and is comprised of all-*trans* beta-carotene and 9-*cis* beta-carotene. Three milligrams of beta-carotene is equal to 5,000 IUs. Supplemental intake of beta-carotene ranges from 3-15 milligrams/day.

HOW SUPPLIED

Capsules — 30 mg, 60 mg, 5,000 IU, 10,000 IU, 25,000 IU

Tablets — 10,000 IU, 25,000 IU

LITERATURE

Albanes D. Beta-carotene and lung cancer: a case study. *Am J Clin Nutr.* 1999; 69:1345S-1350S.

Albanes D, Heinonen OP, Taylor PR, et al. Alpha-tocopherol and beta-carotene supplements and lung cancer incidence in the alpha-tocopherol, beta-carotene cancer prevention study: effects of base-line characteristics and study compliance. *J Natl Cancer Inst.* 1996; 88:1560-1570.

Bendich A. Beta-carotene and the immune response. *Proc Nutr Soc.* 1991; 50:263-274.

Blot WJ, Li JY, Taylor PR, et al. Nutrition intervention trials in Linxian, China: supplementation with specific vitamin/mineral combinations, cancer incidence, and disease-specific mortality in the general population. *J Natl Cancer Inst.* 1993; 15:1483-1492.

Dietary Reference Intakes for Vitamin C, Vitamin E, Selenium, and Carotenoids. Washington, DC: National Academy Press; 2000.

Frieling UM, Schaumberg DA, Kupper TS, et al. A randomized, 12 year primary-prevention trial of beta carotene supplementation for nonmelanoma skin cancer in the Physicians' Health Study. *Arch Dermatol.* 2000; 136:179-184.

Garewal HS, Katz RV, Meyskens F, et al. Beta-carotene produces sustained remissions in patients with oral leukoplakia. *Arch Otolaryngol Head Neck Surg.* 1999; 125:1305-1310.

Gaziano JM. Antioxidants in cardiovascular disease: randomized trials. *Nutr Rev.* 1996; 54:175-177.

Goodman GE. Prevention of lung cancer. *Crit Rev Oncol Hematol.* 2000; 33:187-197.

Hennekens CH, Buring JE, Manson JE, et al. Lack of effect of long-term supplementation with beta carotene on the incidence of malignant neoplasms and cardiovascular disease. *N Engl J Med.* 1996; 334:1145-1149.

Hughes DA, Wright AJ, Finglas PM, et al. The effect of beta-carotene supplementation on the immune function of blood monocytes from healthy male nonsmokers. *J Lab Clin Med.* 1997; 129:309-317.

Lee I-M, Cook NR, Manson JE, et al. Beta-carotene supplementation and incidence of cancer and cardiovascular disease: The Women's Health Study. *J Natl Cancer Inst.* 1999; 91:2102-2106.

Liu S, Ajani U, Chae C, et al. Long-term beta-carotene supplementation and risk of type 2 diabetes mellitus. A randomized controlled trial. *JAMA.* 1999; 282:1073-1075.

Liu Q, Suzuki K, Nakaji S, Sugawara K. Antioxidant activities of natural 9-*cis* and synthetic all-*trans* beta-carotene assessed by human neutrophil chemiluminescence. *Nutr Res.* 2000; 20:5-14.

Naves MMV, Moreno FS. Beta-carotene and cancer chemoprevention: from epidemiological associations to cellular mechanisms of action. *Nutr Res.* 1998; 18:1807-1824.

Omenn GS, Goodman GE, Thornquist MD, et al. Effects of the combination of beta carotene and vitamin A on lung cancer and cardiovascular disease. *N Engl J Med.* 1996; 334:1150-1155.

Omenn GS, Goodman GE, Thornquist MD, et al. Risk factors for lung cancer and for intervention effects in CARET, the Beta-Carotene and Retinol Efficacy Trial. *J Natl Cancer Inst.* 1996; 88:1550-1559.

Paolini M, Cantelli-Forti G, Perocco P, et al. Co-carcinogenic effect of beta-carotene. *Nature.* 1999; 398:760-761.

Peto R, Doll R, Buckley JD, Sporn MB. Can dietary beta-carotene materially reduce human cancer rates? *Nature.* 1981; 290:201-208.

Prabhala RH, Braune LM, Garewal HS, Watson RR. Influence of beta-carotene on immune functions. *Ann NY Acad Sci.* 1993; 691:262-263.

Pryor WA, Stahl W, Rock CL. Beta carotene: from biochemistry to clinical trials. *Nutr Rev.* 2000; 58:39-53.

Rapola JM, Virtamo J, Ripatti S, et al. Randomized trial of alpha-tocopherol and beta-carotene supplements on incidence of major coronary events in men with previous myocardial infarction. *Lancet.*1997; 349:1715-1720.

Rapola JM, Virtamo J, Ripatti S, et al. Effects of alpha tocopherol and beta carotene supplements on symptoms, progression, and prognosis of angina pectoris. *Heart.* 1998; 79:454-458.

Redlich CA, Chung JS, Cullen MR, et al. Effect of long-term beta-carotene and vitamin A on serum cholesterol and triglyceride levels among participants in the Carotene and Retinol Efficacy Trial (CARET). *Atherosclerosis.* 1999; 145:425-432.

Santos MS, Gaziano JM, Leka LS, et al. Beta-carotene-induced enhancement of natural killer cell activity in elderly men: an investigation of the role of cytokines. *Am J Clin Nutr.* 1998; 68:164-170.

Santos MS, Meydani SN, Leka L, et al. Natural killer cell activity in elderly men is enhanced by beta-carotene supplementation. *Am J Clin Nutr.* 1996; 64:772-777.

Tavani A, La Vecchia C. Beta-carotene and risk of coronary heart disease. A review of observational and intervention studies. *Biomed Pharmacother.*1999; 53:409-416.

The Alpha-Tocopherol, Beta Carotene Cancer Prevention Study Group. The effect of vitamin E and beta-carotene on the incidence of lung cancer and other cancers in male smokers. *N Engl J Med.* 1994; 330:1029-1035.

van Poppel G, Spanhaak S, Ockhiuizen T. Effect of beta-carotene on immunological indexes in healthy male smokers. *Am J Clin Nutr.* 1993; 57:402-407.

Virtano J, Rapola JM, Ripatti S, et al. Effect of vitamin E and beta carotene on the incidence of primary nonfatal myocardial infarction and fatal coronary heart disease. *Arch Intern Med.* 1998; 158:668-675.

Wang X-D, Liu C, Bronson RT, et al. Retinol signaling and activator protein-1 expression in ferrets given beta-carotene supplements and exposed to tobacco smoke. *J Natl Cancer Inst.* 1999; 91:60-66.

Williams AW, Boileau T W-M, Zhou JR, et al. Beta-carotene modulates human prostate cancer cell growth and may undergo intracellular metabolism to retinol. *J Nutr.* 2000; 130:728-732.

Beta-Hydroxy-Beta-Methylbutyrate (HMB)

TRADE NAMES

HMB Fuel Plus (Twinlab) and HMB Fuel Mega 750 (Twinlab).

DESCRIPTION

Beta-hydroxy-beta-methylbutyrate, abbreviated HMB, is found naturally in living matter as a metabolite of the essential amino acid L-leucine. There is preliminary evidence suggesting HMB may have anticatabolic, as well as immunomodulatory, properties. As a nutritional supplement, it is popular among athletes engaged in strenuous physical activity.

HMB is also known as hydroxymethylbutyrate, beta-hydroxyisovalerate and 3-hydroxyisovalerate.

ACTIONS AND PHARMACOLOGY

ACTIONS

HMB has putative anticatabolic and immunomodulatory activities.

MECHANISM OF ACTION

The mechanism of HMB's possible actions is unknown. There is, however, speculation. The branched-chain amino acids L-leucine, L-isoleucine and L-valine are known to be beneficial to catabolic patients (sepsis, trauma, burns, etc.) by improving hepatic protein synthesis and nitrogen economy. These amino acids make up about one-third of muscle protein. Of these amino acids, L-leucine has the highest oxidation rate. Further, L-leucine has been shown to stimulate protein synthesis in muscle, and decreases in leucine levels in skeletal muscle and in serum have been noted following exhaustive exercise. However, L-leucine supplementation has not been found to have a significant effect on athletic performance. It has been speculated that the L-leucine metabolite HMB may be responsible for the inhibitory effect of L-leucine on protein breakdown. How this may happen is unknown.

In pigs, HMB is produced from alpha-ketoisocaproate, a metabolite of L-leucine, via the enzyme alpha-ketoisocarproate dioxygenase, an enzyme that requires oxygen and iron for its activity. This pathway, located in the cytosol, may also exist in humans. L-leucine is also metabolized in mitochondria to produce HMB in the form of HMB-coenzyme A (HMB-CoA), rather than free HMB.

HMB has been found to induce chicken macrophage growth and enhance chicken macrophage function in culture. It has also been found to enhance both humoral and cellular immunity in young broilers. The mechanism of these immunomodulatory activities is unknown.

PHARMACOKINETICS

Little is reported on the pharmacokinetics of HMB in humans. Apparently, HMB is absorbed, and about 50% of an ingested dose is excreted unchanged in the urine. HMB may be metabolized to beta-hydroxy-beta-methylglutaryl-CoA, which is, in turn, metabolized to acetyl-CoA and acetoacetate.

INDICATIONS AND USAGE

It is claimed that HMB can increase lean muscle mass and exercise performance, but this is far from conclusively established. There is the suggestion in some preliminary research that HMB may have some immunomodulating effects.

RESEARCH SUMMARY

One study has reported that HMB-supplemented subjects (receiving 1.5 or 3 grams daily) lifted more weight compared with unsupplemented subjects. The researchers concluded that either dose of HMB "can partly prevent exercise-induced proteolysis and /or muscle damage and result in larger gains in muscle function associated with resistance training."

Because the subjects in the above-described study were initiating training, another group of researchers sought to determine whether HMB might have effects similar to those reported in the first study — but this time in trained athletes. This was a double-blind study in which 40 experienced resistance-trained athletes were randomized to receive 0, 3 or 6 grams of HMB daily for 28 days. No significant differences were noted in whole body anabolic/catabolic status, muscle and liver enzyme efflux, fat/bone-free mass, fat mass, percent body fat, or leg press one repetition maximums(1RM) strength. More research is needed.

Very preliminary research in some animal models suggests that HMB supplementation may improve several immunological functions that may result in decreased mortality in these animals.

CONTRAINDICATIONS, PRECAUTIONS, ADVERSE REACTIONS

CONTRAINDICATIONS

None known.

PRECAUTIONS

Pregnant women and nursing mothers should avoid supplemental HMB.

ADVERSE REACTIONS

None reported.

OVERDOSAGE

No reported overdosage.

DOSAGE AND ADMINISTRATION

Some athletes use 3 grams of HMB daily during periods of training.

HOW SUPPLIED

Capsules — 250 mg, 500 mg, 750 mg

Tablets

LITERATURE

Kreider RB, Ferreira M, Wilson M, Almada AL. Effects of calcium-beta hydroxy-beta-methylbutyrate (HMB) supplementation during resistance-training on markers of catabolism, body composition and strength. *Int J Sports Med.* 1999; 20:503-509.

Mero A. Leucine supplementation and intensive training. *Sports Med.* 1999; 27:345-358.

Nissen S, Sharp R, Ray M, et al. Effect of leucine metabolite beta-hydroxy-beta-methylbutyrate on muscle metabolism during resistance exercise testing. *J Am Physiol.* 1996; 81:2095-2104.

Peterson AL, Qureshi MA, Ferket PR, Fuller JC Jr. Enhancement of cellular and humoral immunity in young broilers by the dietary supplementation of beta-hydroxy-beta-methylbutyrate. *Immunopharmacol Immunotoxicol.* 1999; 21:307-330.

Peterson AL, Qureshi MA, Ferket PR, Fuller JC Jr. In vitro exposure with beta-hydroxy-beta-methylbutyrate enhances chicken macrophage growth and function. *Vet Immunol Immunopathol.* 1999; 67:67-78.

Beta-Sitosterol

TRADE NAMES

Beta Sitosterol Power (Nature's Herbs). Combination products include Phytosterol Complex w/ Beta Sitosterol (Source Naturals), Cholestrex (Source Naturals), Beyond Cholesterol (Twinlab) and Super Prostate Power (Nature's Herbs).

DESCRIPTION

Beta-sitosterol is the most abundant phytosterol in the diet. (See Phytosterols.) It is also widely distributed in the plant kingdom and found in such botanicals as *Serenoa repens* (saw palmetto), *Curcurbita pepo* (pumpkin seed) and *Pygeum africanum.* These three botanicals are used in the herbal management of benign prostatic hypertrophy (BPH). There is some belief that beta-sitosterol plays some role in the possible benefits of these herbs in BPH. Beta-sitosterol itself is used as a medicine in Europe for BPH.

Chemically, beta-sitosterol is a very close relative of cholesterol. It differs from cholesterol by the presence of an ethyl group at the 24th carbon position of the side chain. It is also known as (3beta)-stigmast-5-en-3-ol; 22:23-dihydrostigmasterol; alpha-dihydrofucosterol; delta 5-stigmasten-3beta-ol; 24beta-ethyl-delta 5-cholesten-3beta-ol; alpha-phytosterol; cinchol; cupreol; rhamnol; quebrachol; and sitosterin. Beta-sitosterol is extremely insoluble in aqueous media and poorly soluble in lipid media. It is found in nature in ester and glycoside forms, both of which forms are more soluble than beta-sitosterol itself. The chemical structure is:

Beta-Sitosterol

ACTIONS AND PHARMACOLOGY

ACTIONS

Beta-sitosterol has possible activity in promoting prostate health. It also has cholesterol-lowering activity.

MECHANISM OF ACTION

See Phytosterols for cholesterol discussion.

The mechanism of its possible action in promoting prostate health is unknown. In one report, beta-sitosterol was found to activate the sphingomyelin cycle and induce apoptosis in LNCaP human prostate cancer cells *in vitro.* There are also reports suggesting it has some anti-inflammatory activity in the prostate.

PHARMACOKINETICS

About 5% of an ingested dose of supplemental beta-sitosterol is absorbed from the gastrointestinal tract and is transported via the portal circulation to the liver. Some beta-sitosterol is glucuronidated in the liver. A portion is also metabolized to cholic acid and chenodesoxycholic acid. Beta-sitosterol is transported via the systemic circulation to other tissues in the body. Excretion is mainly via the biliary route.

INDICATIONS AND USAGE

Beta-sitosterol may be helpful in some with BPH.

RESEARCH SUMMARY

A review of four double-blind, placebo-controlled studies that tested the efficacy of beta-sitosterol in men with symptomatic benign prostatic hyperplasia concluded that the phytosterol significantly improved urological symptoms and flow measure in those subjects. These trials included 519 men and lasted four to 26 weeks.

Three studies reviewed used nonglucoside beta-sitosterols, and one used a preparation of pure beta-sitosterol-beta-d-glucoside. The latter did not improve flow volume. The reviewers cautioned that, despite positive results to date, "the existing studies are limited by short treatment and lack of standardized beta-sitosterol preparations. Their long-term effectiveness, safety and ability to prevent the complications of benign prostatic hyperplasia are unknown."

CONTRAINDICATIONS, PRECAUTIONS, ADVERSE REACTIONS

CONTRAINDICATIONS

Beta-sitosterol is contraindicated in those with the genetic disorders sitosterolemia and cerebrotendinotic xanthomatosis, both rare conditions.

PRECAUTIONS

Beta-sitosterol supplements should be avoided by pregnant women and nursing mothers.

ADVERSE REACTIONS

Reported adverse reactions include gastrointestinal problems, such as indigestion, gas, diarrhea and constipation.

INTERACTIONS

NUTRITIONAL SUPPLEMENTS AND FOODS

Some randomized trials have indicated that phytosterols—beta-sitosterol was the most abundant phytosterol in these studies—may lower serum levels of alpha- and beta-carotene, lycopene and vitamin E, probably by interfering with their absorption.

OVERDOSAGE

No reports of overdoses.

DOSAGE AND ADMINISTRATION

Beta-sitosterol typically comes in mixtures with other phytosterols and also with substances such as pumpkin seed oil and saw palmetto extract. In Europe, doses used for BPH are 20 to 130 milligrams of beta-sitosterol three times daily with meals. Maintenance doses are 10 to 65 milligrams of beta-sitosterol two to three times daily with meals.

HOW SUPPLIED

Capsules — 60 mg

Tablets — 300 mg

LITERATURE

Berges RR, Windeler J, Trampisch HJ, Senge T. Randomized placebo-controlled, double-blind clinical trial of beta-sitosterol in patient with benign prostatic hyperplasia. Beta-sitosterol Study Group. *Lancet.* 1995; 345; 1529-1532.

Kobayashi Y, Sugaya Y, Tokue A. [Clinical effects of beta-sitosterol (phytosterol) on benign prostatic hyperplasia: preliminary study.] [Article in Japanese.] *Hinyokika Kiyo.* 1998; 44:865-868.

Normé n L, Dutta P, Lia A, Andersson H. Soy sterol esters and beta-sitostanol ester as inhibitors of cholesterol absorption in human small bowel. *Am J Clin Nutr.* 2000; 71:908-913.

Wilt TJ, Mac Donald R, Ishani A. Beta-sitosterol for the treatment of benign prostatic hyperplasia: a systematic review. *BMU Int.* 1999; 83:976-983.

von Holtz RL, Fink CS, Awad AB. Beta-sitosterol activates the sphingomyelin cycle and induces apoptosis in LNCaP human prostate cancer cells. *Nutr Cancer.* 1998; 32:8-12.

Betaine and Betaine Hydrochloride

DESCRIPTION

Betaine or trimethylglycine is a quarternary ammonium compound that was first discovered in the juice of sugar beets (*Beta vulgaris*). Betaine is a metabolite of choline (see Choline) and is a substrate in one of the two recycling pathways that convert homocysteine to L-methionine. The other and principal recycling reaction is catalyzed by the enzyme methionine synthase and uses methylcobalamin as a cofactor and 5-methyltetrahydrofolate as a cosubstrate (see Folate and Vitamin B_{12}).

Betaine, in the form of a white, granular, hygroscopic powder referred to as anhydrous betaine, is an orphan drug for the treatment of homocystinuria. Homocystinuria is a rare genetic disorder caused by any one of three inborn errors of metabolism. One type is known as cystathionine beta-synthase deficiency. Cystathionine beta-synthase is the enzyme that converts homocysteine to cystathionine, a precursor of cysteine. This is the most common genetic cause of homocystinuria. Cystathionine beta-synthase is a vitamin B_6-dependent enzyme, and deficiency of this enzyme may be responsive to treatment with vitamin B_6 (see Vitamin B_6).

A second type of inborn error of metabolism resulting in homocystinuria is due to deficiency of 5,10-methylenetetrahydrofolate reductase. This enzyme catalyzes the conversion of 5-methylenetetrahydrofolate to 5-methyltetrahydrofolate, the cosubstrate in the methionine synthase reaction mentioned above. The third type of inborn error of metabolism that can result in homocystinuria is due to a defect in the synthesis of methylcobalamin, the cofactor in the methionine synthase reaction. Betaine therapy may be effective in the treatment of all three of these primary types of homocystinuria.

Betaine is also known as trimethylglycine, N-trimethylglycine, glycine betaine, glycocoll betaine, oxyneurine and lycine. Its chemical name is 1-carboxy-N,N,N-trimethyl-methanaminium inner salt. The molecular formula of betaine is $C_5H_{11}NO_2$, its chemical formula is $(CH_3)_3N^+\text{-}CH_2COO^-$ and its molecular weight is 117.15 daltons. Betaine is very soluble in water and has a sweet taste. It is widely distributed in plants and animals. The hydrochloride of betaine is known as betaine hydrochloride, betaine HCL and pluchine. Its chemical name is 1-carboxy-N,N,N-trimethylmethanaminium chloride. The pH of a 5% aqueous solution of betaine hydrochloride is 1.

Betaine is represented by the following chemical structure:

Betaine

Both betaine and betaine hydrochloride are available as dietary supplements.

ACTIONS AND PHARMACOLOGY

ACTIONS

Betaine may lower elevated homocysteine levels in some. Betaine may also have lipotropic and hepatoprotective activity. Betaine hydrochloride is a delivery form of hydrochloric acid and may aid in digestion in some.

MECHANISM OF ACTION

Betaine-homocysteine methyltransferase (BHMT) is a zinc metalloenzyme which catalyzes the transfer of a methyl group from betaine to homocysteine in the formation of methionine. BHMT is found in the liver and kidneys and may also exist in brain tissue. Betaine acts to lower homocysteine levels in some with primary hyperhomocysteinemia/homocystinuria via this enzyme. Betaine has also been found to lower homocysteine levels in some animal studies, again, via BHMT. Mild to moderate elevation of homocysteine without homocystinuria is thought to be an independent risk factor for coronary heart disease. Betaine may lower elevated homocysteine levels in some with mild to moderate hyperhomocysteinemia, but this needs to be confirmed. A good group for such a study would be those with the C677T mutation for 5-methylenetetrahydrofolate reductase which occurs in approximately 10% of the population.

A lipotropic agent is defined as a substance that prevents the deposition of fat in the liver or accelerates its removal. The condition of fatty degeneration is called steatosis. Betaine, choline and L-methionine have been found to prevent or to reverse hepatic steatosis in experimental animals. It is thought that the lipotropic activity of betaine, choline and L-methionine is mediated via the body's principal transmethylating agent, S-adenosylmethionine (SAMe). SAMe is involved in a number of biochemical functions that may promote liver health, including its role in the formation of phospholipids which are essential for normal cell membrane formation and function (see S-Adenosyl-L-Methionine). SAMe's methyl group is derived from betaine via the betaine-homocysteine methyltransferase reaction which provides the immediate precursor of SAMe, L-methionine. Choline is metabolized to betaine via the enzymes choline dehydrogenase and betaine aldehyde dehydrogenase. Thus, through a couple of transmethylations, the methyl group in choline winds up as the methyl group in SAMe.

Betaine has been found to protect the livers of experimental animals against the hepatotoxins ethanol and carbon tetrachloride. The hepatoprotective effect of betaine is thought to be mediated via SAMe, as discussed above. Betaine may have hepatoprotective activity as well as lipotropic activity in humans, but this has not been confirmed. Another possible hepatoprotective mechanism of betaine, at least in animals, may be due to its osmolyte activity. Betaine has been shown to be an intracellular osmolyte in rat liver macrophages (Kupffer cells) and sinusoidal endothelial cells, and may play an important role in the functions of these cells.

As an interesting aside, the osmoprotective effect of betaine has been found to be cytoprotective in the deep freezing of stallion sperm and also has been found to protect salmon from the physiological stress induced by transfer from fresh water to seawater. The osmoprotective effect of betaine may be due to an interaction between this substance and chloride ions. There is as yet no evidence that the osmoprotective effect of betaine has any consequence for humans.

Betaine hydrochloride is a delivery form of hydrochloric acid. Some with hypochlorhydria have used betaine hydrochloride alone, or in combination with pepsin, as a digestive aid.

PHARMACOKINETICS

Betaine is absorbed from the small intestines into the enterocytes. It is released by the enterocytes into the portal circulation which carries it to the liver where there is significant first-pass extraction and first-pass metabolism of betaine. The principal metabolic reaction is the transfer of a methyl group from betaine to homocysteine via the enzyme betaine-homocysteine methyltransferase. The products of the reaction are L-methionine and dimethylglycine. Betaine hydrochloride is converted to betaine in the alkaline environment of the small intestine.

INDICATIONS AND USAGE

Anhydrous betaine has been useful in the treatment of homocystinuria and betaine may be helpful in other conditions characterized by elevated plasma homocysteine levels. Betaine hydrochloride is used as a digestive aid in some. There is some suggestion in animal research that betaine may be hepatoprotective in some circumstances.

RESEARCH SUMMARY

Betaine has been shown in numerous studies to be of significant benefit in all three primary types of homocystinuria. Clinical improvement has been reported in about 75% of the cases treated with betaine in these studies.

It has been suggested but not yet demonstrated that betaine might also be useful in other conditions characterized by elevated plasma homocysteine levels, such as those that have been noted in some with premature vascular disease and chronic renal failure.

Since hyperhomocysteinemia is thought to be an independent cardiovascular risk factor, betaine's role as a potential cardioprotector is suggested but, again, not yet demonstrated. Recently it was hypothesized that some of red wine's putative cardioprotective activity could be due to the fact that betaine is added to some wines via beet sugar used to increase alcohol content. More research is needed.

Several animal studies have indicated that betaine exerts some hepatoprotective effects. In one of these studies, betaine significantly speeded recovery of carbon tetrachloride-injured liver. It has also been credited with helping to protect against alcoholic steatosis resulting from dietary ethanol. Whether it might help similarly protect against or reverse fatty infiltration of the liver in humans has not yet been studied.

Betaine hydrochloride has been used for some time as a digestive aid. Those with excessive stomach acid should avoid this use.

CONTRAINDICATIONS, PRECAUTIONS, ADVERSE REACTIONS

CONTRAINDICATIONS

Betaine and betaine hydrochloride are contraindicated in those hypersensitive to any component of a betaine- or betaine hydrochloride-containing product.

PRECAUTIONS

Pregnant women and nursing mothers should avoid the use of betaine and betaine hydrochloride supplements.

Those with gastritis, gastroesophageal reflux disease (GERD) or peptic ulcer disease should avoid the use of betaine hydrochloride supplements.

ADVERSE REACTIONS

Occasional nausea, vomiting and diarrhea have been reported.

INTERACTIONS

NUTRITIONAL SUPPLEMENTS

Folic acid: Concomitant use of betaine and folic acid may be additive with regard to the possible lowering of serum homocysteine levels.

OVERDOSAGE

There are no reports of betaine overdosage in the literature.

DOSAGE AND ADMINISTRATION

Betaine and betaine hydrochloride are available as dietary supplements.

There are no typical doses for the management of mild to moderate hyperhomocysteinemia. Three grams taken twice daily were used in one small preliminary study showing a serum homocysteine-lowering effect.

Those who use betaine hydrochloride as a digestive aid, typically take a dose of 600 to 650 milligrams (usually in a combination product with pepsin) following a meal.

HOW SUPPLIED

Capsules — 650 mg

Tablets — 300 mg, 350 mg, 600 mg

LITERATURE

Barak AJ, Tuma DJ. Betaine, metabolic by-product or vital methylating agent? *Life Sci.* 1983; 32:771-774.

Barak AJ, Beckenhauser HC, Tuma DJ. Betaine effects on hepatic methionine metabolism elicited by short-term ethanol feeding. *Alcohol.* 1996; 13:483-486.

Barak AJ, Beckenhauser HC, Tuma DJ. Betaine, ethanol and the liver: a review. *Alcohol.* 1996; 13:395-398.

Barak AJ, Beckenhauser HC, Badakhsh S, Tuma DJ. The effect of betaine in reversing alcoholic steatosis. *Alcohol Clin Exp Res.* 1997; 21:1100-1102.

Brower IA, Verhoef P, Urgert R. Betaine supplementation and plasma homocysteine in healthy volunteers. *Arch Inter Med.* 2000; 160:2546-2547.

Davies SEC, Chalmers RA, Randall EW, Iles RA. Betaine metabolism in human neonates and developing rats. *Clin Chim Acta.* 1988; 178:241-250.

Gahl WA, Bernardini I, Chen S, et al. The effect of oral betaine on vertebral body bone density in pyridoxine-non-responsive homocystinuria. *J Inher Metab Dis.* 1988; 11:291-298.

Holme E, Kjellman B, Ronge E. Betaine for treatment of homocystinuria caused by methylenetetrahydrofolate reductase deficiency. *Arch Dis Childhood.* 1989; 64:1064.

Junnila M, Barak AJ, Beckenhauer HC, Rahko T. Betaine reduces hepatic lipidosis induced by carbon tetrachloride in Sprague-Dawley rats. *Vet Hum Toxicol.* 1998; 40:263-266.

Junnila M, Rahko T, Sukura A, Lindberg L-A. Reduction of carbon tetrachloride-induced hepatotoxic effects by oral administration of betaine in male Han: Wistar rats. A morphometric histological study. *Vet Pathol.* 2000; 37:221-238.

Koskinen E, Junnila M, Katila T, Soini H. A preliminary study on the use of betaine as a cryoprotective agent in the deep freezing of stallion semen. *Zentralbl Veterinarmed A.* 1989; 36:110-114.

Millian NS, Garrow TA. Human betaine-homocysteine methyltransferase is a zinc metalloenzyme. *Arch Biochem Biophys.* 1998; 356:93-98.

Smolin LA, Benevenga NJ, Berlow S. The use of betaine for the treatment of homocystinuria. *J Pediatr.* 1981; 99:467-472.

Virtanen E, Junnila M, Soivio A. Effects of food containing betaine/amino acid additive on the osmotic adaptation of young Atlantic salmon, *Salmo Salar* L. *Aquaculture*. 1989; 83:109-122.

Wendel U, Bremer HJ. Betaine in the treatment of homocystinuria due to 5,10-methylenetetrahydrofolate reductase deficiency. *Eur J Pediatr*. 1984; 142:147-150.

Wettstein M, Haussinger D. Cytoprotection by the osmolytes betaine and taurine in ischemia-reoxygenation injury in the perfused rat liver. *Hepatology*. 1997; 26:1560-1566.

Wettstein M, Weik C, Holneicher C, Haussinger D. Betaine as an osmolyte in rat liver: metabolism and cell-to-cell interactions. *J Hepatol*. 1998; 27:787-793.

Wilcken DE, Dudman NP, Tyrrell PA. Homocystinuria due to cystathionine beta-synthase deficiency - - the effects of betaine treatment in pyridoxine-responsive patients. *Metabolism*. 1985; 34:1115-1121.

Wilcken DE, Wilcken B, Dudman NP, Tyrrell PA. Homocystinuria - - the effects of betaine in the treatment of patients not responsive to pyridoxine. *N Engl J Med*. 1983; 309:448-453.

Biochanin A

DESCRIPTION

Biochanin A belongs to the isoflavone class of flavonoids. It is also classified as a phytoestrogen since it is a plant-derived nonsteroidal compound that possesses estrogen-like biological activity. Biochanin A has been found to have weak estrogenic activity.

Biochanin A is found in certain legumes, most notably red clover or *Trifolium pratense*. Red clover contains, in addition to biochanin A, the isoflavones genistein, daidzein and formononetin (methoxy daidzein). These isoflavones are present in red clover in the form of glycosides. However, when the leaves are crushed during the preparation of red clover isoflavone extracts, the glycosides undergo enzymatic hydrolysis, and the final preparation principally contains the aglycones.

Biochanin A is a solid substance that is virtually insoluble in water. Its molecular formula is $C_{16}H_{12}O_5$. It is the 4'-methyl ether of genistein. Biochanin A is also known as 5, 7-dihydroxy-4'-methoxyisoflavone and 5, 7-dihydroxy-4' -methoxy-3- (4-hydroxyphenyl)-4*H*-1-benzopyran-4-one.

ACTIONS AND PHARMACOLOGY

ACTIONS

Biochanin A has estrogenic activity. It may also have antioxidant, anticarcinogenic, anti-atherogenic and anti-osteoporotic activities.

MECHANISM OF ACTION

Biochanin A has weak estrogenic activity as measured in *in vivo* and *in vitro* assays.

Structurally, biochanin A would be expected to be able to scavenge reactive oxygen species and inhibit lipid peroxidation. However, there are few studies demonstrating this.

There are cell culture and animal studies indicating that biochanin A has anticarcinogenic activity. It is unclear what the mechanism of the possible anticarcinogenic activity might be.

Biochanin A has been found to have hypolipidemic activity in some animal models. Again the mechanism of this possible effect, as well as the mechanism of any anti-atherogenic activity, is unclear.

In comparison with other isoflavones, such as genistein and daidzein, biochanin A might be expected to have possible anti-osteoporotic activity. This might be due, in part, to its weak estrogenic activity.

PHARMACOKINETICS

Little is known about the pharmacokinetics of biochanin A in humans. Inferences can be drawn from some animal studies. Biochanin A appears to be absorbed from the small intestine from whence it is transported to the systemic circulation by the lymphatics. There is little information available on the tissue distribution of biochanin A. It appears that biochanin A delivered to the liver undergoes extensive conjugation with glucuronate and sulfate via hepatic UDP-glucuronosyl-transferases and sulfotransferases. The glucuronate and sulfate conjugates of biochanin A are excreted in the urine and the bile.

It is likely that there is considerable variation in the absorption and metabolism of ingested biochanin A.

INDICATIONS AND USAGE

There is very preliminary evidence that biochanin A may have some anti-atherosclerotic and anticarcinogenic effects. There are anecdotal reports that it may be helpful in ameliorating some of the problems associated with menopause, including osteoporosis.

RESEARCH SUMMARY

Biochanin A significantly reduced the incidence of chemically induced rat mammary cancer in a recent study. Multiplicity of tumors was also significantly decreased in biochanin A-supplemented animals, compared with unsupplemented controls. There is, additionally, some preliminary evidence that biochanin A may have some hypolipidemic effects. Clinical studies are lacking.

CONTRAINDICATIONS, PRECAUTIONS, ADVERSE REACTIONS.

CONTRAINDICATIONS

Biochanin A is contraindicated in those who are hypersensitive to any component of a biochanin A-containing product.

PRECAUTIONS

Pregnant women and nursing mothers should avoid the use of biochanin A-containing supplements.

Women with estrogen receptor-positive tumors should exercise caution in the use of biochanin A-containing supplements and should use them only if they are recommended and monitored by a physician.

DOSAGE AND ADMINISTRATION

Biochanin A-containing supplements are derived from red clover and, in addition to biochanin A, usually contain the isoflavones genistein, daidzein and formononetin. A typical dose of such an isoflavone mixture—which also contains ingredients other than isoflavones—is 40 mg daily.

LITERATURE

Gotoh T, Yamada K, Yin H, et al. Chemoprevention of N-nitroso-N-methylurea-induced rat mammary carcinogenesis by soy foods or biochanin A. *Jpn J Cancer Res*. 1998; 89:137-142.

Lee YS, Kim TH, Cho KJ, Jang JJ. Inhibitory effects of biochanin A on benzo[a]pyrene induced carcinogenesis in mice. *In vivo*. 1992; 6:283-286.

Saloniemi H, Wä hä lä K, Nykä nen-Kurki P, et al. Phytoestrogen content and estrogenic effect of legume fodder. *Proc Soc Exp Biol Med*. 1995; 208; 13-17.

Siddiqui MT, Siddiqui M. Hypolipidemic principles of *Cicer Arietnum*: biochanin A and formononetin. *Lipids*. 1976; 11:243-246.

Yanagihara K, Ito A, Toge T, Numoto M. Antiproliferative effects of isoflavones on human cancer cell lines established from the gastrointestinal tract. *Cancer Res*. 1993; 53:5815-5821.

Biotin

TRADE NAMES

D-Biotin (Numerous manufacturers), Biotin Forte (Vitaline Corporation), Meribin (Mericon Industries).

DESCRIPTION

Biotin, a member of the B-vitamin family, is an essential nutrient in human nutrition. It is involved in the biosynthesis of fatty acids, gluconeogenesis, energy production, the metabolism of the branched-chain amino acids (L-leucine, L-isoleucine, L-valine) and the *de novo* synthesis of purine nucleotides. Recent research indicates that biotin plays a role in gene expression, both at the transcriptional and translational levels, and that it may also play a role in DNA replication.

Biotin is widely distributed in natural foodstuffs. However, the absolute amounts of biotin in foodstuffs is relatively low when compared with the other B vitamins. Some of the better food sources of biotin, are egg yolk, liver, kidney, pancreas, milk, soya and barley. Brewer's yeast or *Saccharomyces cerevisiae* (see Brewer's Yeast), which is used as a nutritional supplement, is one of the richest sources of biotin, as well as the other B vitamins. Royal jelly, also used as a nutritional supplement (see Royal Jelly), is another rich source of biotin. Mammals and many plant species are unable to synthesize biotin. Biotin is synthesized by bacteria, yeast and other fungi, algae and certain plant species. In fact, the microflora of the human large intestine appear to contribute to the biotin requirements of the body.

The first demonstration of biotin-deficiency in animals was observed in animals fed raw egg white. Rats fed egg white protein were found to develop dermatitis, hair loss and neuromuscular dysfunction. This syndrome was called egg white injury and was discovered to be caused by a glycoprotein found in egg white called avidin. It was subsequently found that egg white injury could be cured by a liver factor which was first called protective factor X and later determined to be biotin. Because biotin cured the skin disorder of egg white injury it was called vitamin H. H is for haut, the German word for skin. Avidin causes egg white injury because it binds very tightly to biotin, preventing its absorption. This is only true for native avidin, which is resistant to hydrolysis by proteolytic enzymes. When egg white is cooked, avidin is denatured and denatured avidin is digested by proteolytic enzymes.

Although clinical biotin deficiency in humans is rare, it does occur. Prolonged consumption of raw egg white, long-term total parenteral nutrition without biotin supplementation and malabsorption syndromes, such as short-gut syndrome, have resulted in biotin-deficiency states. The symptoms and signs of biotin-deficiency, include a generalized erythematous scaly skin eruption, alopecia, conjunctivitis and neurological abnormalities. The rash may be distributed around the eyes, nose, mouth, ears and perineal orifices. The facial appearance associated with the deficiency, with the rash around the eyes, nose and mouth along with an unusual distribution of facial fat, is called biotin deficiency facies. In biotin deficient infants, the neurological findings are hypotonia, lethargy and developmental delay. In adults, the neurological findings are lethargy, depression, hallucinations and paresthesias of the extremities. Marginal biotin status may occur under certain conditions, e.g., during the first trimester of pregnancy, and it is thought that this situation may be teratogenic. Functional biotin deficiency occurs in certain genetic disorders. These will be discussed below.

Biotin is the coenzyme for four carboxylases. Acetyl coenzyme A (CoA) carboxylase, found in both the mitochondria and cytosol, catalyzes the carboxylation of acetyl-CoA to malonyl-CoA. Malonyl-CoA is the immediate precursor of 14 of the 16 carbon atoms of the fatty acid palmitic acid. It is also the immediate precursor of all of the fatty acids up to palmitic acid. Further, the reaction catalyzed by acetyl-CoA carboxylase, a complex reaction, is the primary regulatory, or rate-limiting, step in the biosynthesis of fatty acids. Pyruvate carboxylase, which is located in the mitochondria, catalyzes the carboxylation of pyruvate to form oxaloacetate. Oxaloacetate can be metabolized in the tricarboxylic acid cycle or it can be converted to glucose in the liver and kidney and other tissues that are involved in gluconeogenesis. The formation of oxaloacetate from pyruvate is known as an anaplerotic reaction. Anaplerotic is from the Greek word anaplerosis, meaning filling up or restoration. The pyruvate carboxylate reaction is the principal reaction which replenishes tricarboxylic acid cycle intermediates. Methylcrotonyl-CoA carboxylase, also located in the mitochondria, is involved in the metabolism of L-leucine, while the mitochondrial enzyme propionyl-CoA carboxylase is involved in the metabolism of L-isoleucine and L-valine, as well as L-threonine and L-methionine.

All four of the carboxylase enzymes, which use bicarbonate as their one-carbon substrate, share a common biochemical mechanism. In all four carboxylases, biotin is covalently linked by an amide bond between the carboxyl group of the valeric side chain of biotin and an epsilon-amino group of a specific lysyl residue in the apocarboxylase. The enzyme that catalyzes the formation of the covalent bond is called holocarboxylase synthetase. Biotin is recycled by the enzyme biotinidase. Biotinidase, an hydrolase, functions to recycle biotin by cleaving biocytin (epsilon-N-biotinyl-L-lysine), or short-chain oligopeptides containing biotin-linked lysyl residues, products of the normal breakdown of the holocarboxylases, to free biotin. Biotinidase is also thought to play a critical role in the release of biotin from biotin-containing dietary proteins. Recently, biotinidase has been found to have biotinyl-transferase activity. All five classes of histones are selectively biotinylated via the biotinyl-transferase activity of biotinidase. It is thought that biotinylation of histones is involved in the regulation of gene transcription and may also play a role in the packaging of DNA. Interestingly, biotinylation is an important technique in molecular biology. Biotin can be covalently linked to both proteins and nucleic acids, and is used as a label in many molecular biology and biochemistry technologies.

Certain inborn errors of metabolism result in functional biotin deficiency. These disorders, include multiple carboxylase deficiency, holocarboxylase synthetase deficiency, biotinidase deficiency and propionic-CoA carboxylase deficiency. Those with these disorders require much greater cellular biotin levels than normal in order to activate these biotin-dependent enzymes. Biotinidase deficiency is the most common cause of late-onset multiple carboxylase deficiency. Features of late-onset multiple carboxylase deficiency, include skin rash, alopecia, seizures, hypotonia, ataxia, hearing loss, optic atrophy, developmental delay, immune deficiency and recurrent infections. Coma and death may occur if the disorder is not treated. The treatment is high-dose biotin, which results in pronounced, rapid clinical and biochemical improvement. Holocarboxylase deficiency is the most common form of multiple carboxylase deficiency in neonates. Features of neonatal multiple carboxylase deficiency, include lethargy, hypotonia, vomiting, alopecia, lactic acidosis, keratoconjunctivitis, perioral erosions and seizures. Again, the treatment is high-dose biotin, which may completely reverse the symptoms and signs of the disorder. There is a relatively high incidence or propionyl-CoA carboxylase deficiency among the Inuits of Greenland. Those with this deficiency may present early in life with a severe, often fatal metabolic acidosis, hyperglycinemia and hyperammonemia. The only known treatment for this disorder is high-dose biotin. All of the above inborn errors of metabolism are referred to as biotin-responsive disorders.

Biotin is a bicyclic compound. The tetrahydrothiophene ring contains sulfur and has a valeric acid side chain. The second ring contains a ureido group. Eight stereoisomers of biotin exist. However, only one is found naturally, and it is the only one that is enzymatically active. The natural stereoisomer of biotin is called d-(+)-biotin or just biotin. In addition to being known as vitamin H, biotin is also known as hexahydro-2-oxo-1*H*-thieno[3,4-*d*]imidazole-4-pentanoic acid; *cis* -5-(hexahydro-2-oxo-1*H*-thieno[3,4-*d*]imidazol-4-yl)valeric acid; *cis* -tetrahydro-2-oxothieno[3,4-*d*]imidazoline-4-valeric acid; *cis* -hexahydro-2-oxo-1*H*-thieno[3,4]imidazole-4-valeric acid; coenzyme R and bios IIb. Its molecular formula is $C_{10}H_{16}N_2O_3S$ and its molecular weight is 244.31 daltons. Biocytin or epsilon-N-biotinyl-L-lysine is a naturally occurring complex of biotin which has approximately the same biochemical activity as biotin.

ACTIONS AND PHARMACOLOGY
ACTIONS

Biotin is used for the treatment of biotin-responsive inborn errors of metabolism. It has putative glucose tolerance-modulating activity. It may also have activity in the management of brittle fingernails and the uncombable hair syndrome. There is some evidence that it may have antioxidant activity.

MECHANISM OF ACTIONS

Holocarboxylase synthetase catalyzes the biotinylation of the four biotin-dependent carboxylases in humans. Holocarboxylase synthetase deficiency is the most common cause of neonatal multiple carboxylase deficiency. Biotinidase catalyzes the recycling of biotin, among other reactions. Biotinidase deficiency is the most common cause of late-onset multiple carboxylase deficiency. Cellular biotin concentrations higher than are normally present, are required to activate the mutant holocarboxylase synthetase and biotinidase enzymes. Biotin does not bind to the mutant enzymes as strongly as it does to non-mutant enzymes and therefore, greater amounts of biotin are required for their activation. Biotin may also play a role in the regulation of the transcription of holocarboxylase synthetase.

Biotin supplementation has been found to improve glucose tolerance and decrease insulin resistance in a diabetic mouse model. It has also been found to influence hepatic glucokinase expression both at the transcriptional and translational levels in cell culture. More recently, biotin has been shown to affect pancreatic islet glucokinase activity and expression and insulin secretion in cultured rat islet cells. Glucokinase has a central regulatory role in glucose metabolism. The results of above studies suggest that the administration of supplementary biotin may improve the metabolism and/or utilization of glucose in those with type 2 diabetes mellitus. Clinical trials are needed.

Some studies have found that high doses of biotin are helpful in the management of brittle fingernails in women. The rationale to use biotin for this condition came from the finding that pathologic hoof changes in horses and swine can be treated with oral biotin. The mechanism of the possible effect of biotin in the management of brittle fingernails is not known. Biotin deficiency does cause skin changes. However, the subjects studied were not biotin deficient.

The uncombable hair syndrome, also known as spun-glass hair and cheveux incoiffables, is a rare congenital disorder. It is characterized by a longitudinal grooving of the hair shaft resulting in a triangular cross section (pili trianguli et canaliculi). There is a report of biotin reversing scaling, hair loss, hair fragility, and uncombability in a two-year old boy with the syndrome. The hair remained combable even after one year. The mechanism of action of biotin in this condition is not known. Perhaps some cases of uncombable hair syndrome are biotin-responsive. The uncombable hair syndrome should not be confused with cowlicks, localized patches of hair that will not comb down. The cowlick is not a forme fruste of the uncombable hair syndrome, nor is there any evidence that biotin has any effect on cowlicks.

Biotin has been found to inhibit the generation of reactive oxygen species, including superoxide anions, by neutrophils, *in vitro*. The mechanism of this antioxidant effect is unknown. Biotin does not appear to scavenge superoxide anions.

PHARMACOKINETICS

The intestine is exposed to biotin from a few sources: the diet, biotin supplements and biotin synthesized by bacteria in the large intestine. Dietary biotin exists in free and protein-bound forms. Protein-bound biotin is digested by proteases and peptidases to biotin-containing oligopeptides and biocytin (epsilon-N-biotinyl-L-lysine). Biocytin and the biotin-containing oligopeptides are converted to biotin via the enzyme biotinidase. Biotin—both dietary-derived biotin and supplementary biotin—is efficiently absorbed from the small intestine. At doses of biotin derived from food, biotin appears to be transported into enterocytes by a sodium-dependent carrier. At higher doses of biotin, absorption appears to occur by passive diffusion. Absorption of the biotin produced by the colonic microflora, appears to occur by a carrier mediated process in the proximal large intestine.

Biotin is transported to the liver via the portal circulation and by the systemic circulation, to the other tissues of the body. Biotin appears to be transported in the serum in both bound and unbound forms. Uptake of biotin by cells appears to occur by both a sodium-dependent carrier process and by passive diffusion. Transport of biotin across the blood-brain barrier appears to occur by a saturable transport mechanism. Placental transport of biotin appears to occur by a passive process. Within cells, the carboxylases (pyruvate carboxylase, acetyl-CoA carboxylase, methycrotonyl-CoA carboxylase, propionyl-CoA carboxylase) are biotinylated via holocarboxylase synthetase. Biotin and apocarboxylases are the substrates. ATP and magnesium also participate in the reaction. Biotin is recycled from the holocarboxylases via the action of proteolytic enzymes and biotinidase. Biotin is catabolized to a number of different metabolites, including bisnorbiotin, biotin sulfoxide, biotin sulfone, bisonorbiotin methylketone and tetranorbiotin-1-sulfoxide. Biotin is excreted in the urine as biotin, bisnorbiotin, biotin sulfoxide, biotin sulfone, bisnorbiotin methyl ketone and tetranobiotin-1-sulfoxide.

INDICATIONS AND USAGE

Biotin is used to treat the biotin-responsive inborn errors of metabolism holocarboxylase synthetase deficiency and biotinidase deficiency. Holocarboxylase deficiency is the most common cause of neonatal multiple carboxylase deficiency. Biotinidase deficiency is the most common cause of late-onset multiple carboxylase deficiency.

Recent studies have revealed that even marginal biotin deficiency is teratogenic in many mammals. This is of special concern since there is also now data showing that marginal biotin deficiency occurs in a significant proportion of pregnant women. It is too early to recommend widespread biotin supplementation during pregnancy, but the use of this vitamin might be indicated in some pregnant women whose physicians advise its use. There is very preliminary evidence that supplemental biotin might improve disordered glucose metabolism and thus might be helpful in some cases of diabetes. It may also be indicated in some cases of those on total parenteral nutrition and in some with brittle nails. There is some dated evidence that biotin can favorably affect lipids. There is no evidence that it can restore hair growth except in some cases of biotin deficiency. Nor will it reverse graying of hair. There is some evidence, however, that it may help manage the ''uncombable hair syndrome,'' a rare condition seen in children. There is no evidence that biotin improves exercise performance.

RESEARCH SUMMARY

Biotin deficiency has been shown to cause birth defects in several animal, including mammalian, species. The level of deficiency required to be teratogenic is marginal, insufficient to produce any of the typical cutaneous and behavioral manifestations of more pronounced deficiency. These findings, coupled with recent disclosures that marginal biotin deficiency occurs in a significant proportion of pregnant women, raises serious concern.

A recent analysis of data from a multivitamin supplementation study has led one research group to conclude that there is at least indirect evidence of teratogenicity due to marginal biotin deficiency in humans. Adding to the concern are further findings that biotin deficiency can occur spontaneously in normal human gestation, that biotin transport by the human placenta is mainly passive and that proliferating cells have increased biotin requirements.

More research is required before biotin can be recommended for pregnant women as an antiteratogen, but physicians may find it appropriate to recommend its use in individual cases.

There are some recent preliminary animal studies suggesting that biotin may help improve glucose metabolism in ways that might be beneficial in some with diabetes. In one experiment, biotin supplemented diabetic mice had, compared with controls, lowered post-prandial glucose levels, improved glucose tolerance and decreased insulin resistance. Similar results were obtained in another animal study, leading the researchers to conclude that biotin may be helpful to patients with non-insulin-dependent diabetes mellitus (type 2 diabetes mellitus).

It has been claimed that supplemental biotin can reverse loss and graying of hair. In fact, biotin and pantothenic acid are widely used in cosmetic hair products. Except in cases of frank biotin deficiency, there appears to be no basis for this claim. There is a report, however, that severe hair loss secondary to biotin deficiency occurs in some patients receiving total parenteral nutrition (TPN). Supplementation with 200 micrograms of biotin daily has resulted in gradual regrowth of healthy hair in some of these patients.

There is also a report that supplemental biotin can help tame ''uncombable hair syndrome'' characterized by hair loss, hair fragility and uncombability, a rare disorder of children.

Biotin reportedly benefits some with brittle nails, as well. Supplementation with biotin resulted in a significant thickening of nail plates in 63% of subjects in a Swiss study.

There is a dated (1980) report that 0.9 milligrams of biotin daily for 71 days significantly and favorably affected lipids in 40 subjects aged 30-60. This isolated report needs follow-up.

CONTRAINDICATIONS, PRECAUTIONS, ADVERSE REACTIONS

CONTRAINDICATIONS

Biotin is contraindicated in those hypersensitive to any component of a biotin-containing product.

PRECAUTIONS

Pregnant women and nursing mothers should avoid supplemental doses of biotin greater than the adequate intakes (AI) recommended by the Food and Nutrition Board, unless higher doses are prescribed by their physicians. The AIs are 30 micrograms/day for pregnant women and 35 micrograms/day for nursing mothers.

The use of biotin for the treatment of a biotin-responsive medical conditions requires medical supervision.

ADVERSE REACTIONS

There are no reports of adverse reactions associated with biotin supplementation in the literature.

INTERACTIONS

DRUGS

Antibiotics: Antibiotic use may decrease the biotin contribution to the body made by the microflora of the large intestine.

Anticonvulsants (carbamazepine, phenytoin, phenobarbital, primidone): Carbamazepine, phenytoin and phenobarbital can accelerate biotin metabolism and may cause reduced biotin status. Long-term use of carbamazepine, phenytoin, phenobarbital and primidone has been associated with reduced plasma concentrations of biotin.

NUTRITIONAL SUPPLEMENTS

Pantothenic Acid: High-doses of pantothenic acid may inhibit the absorption of biotin produced by the microflora in the large intestine. Pantothenic acid and biotin appear to use the same uptake carrier in colonocytes.

DOSAGE AND ADMINISTRATION

Biotin is available in multivitamin and multivitamin/multimineral products as well as in single ingredient products. In single ingredient products, biotin is available as lozenges, tablets and capsules. Few prenatal vitamin/mineral formulas contain biotin. Those that do, typically contain biotin in doses of about 30 micrograms daily. Biotin is present in several combination products at doses of 30 to 60 micrograms daily. Intakes of biotin range from 30 to 1,000 micrograms/day.

The Food and Nutrition Board of the Institute of Medicine of the National Academy of Sciences has recommended the following Dietary Reference Intakes (DRI) for biotin:

Infants	Adequate Intake (AI)
0 through 6 months	5 micrograms/day ≈ 0.7 micrograms/Kg
7 through 12 months	6 micrograms/day ≈ 0.7 micrograms/Kg
Children	
1 through 3 years	8 micrograms/day
4 through 8 years	12 micrograms/day
Boys	
9 through 13 years	20 micrograms/day
14 through 18 years	25 micrograms/day
Girls	
9 through 13 years	20 micrograms/day
14 through 18 years	25 micrograms/day
Men	
19 years and older	30 micrograms/day
Women	
19 years and older	30 micrograms/day
Pregnancy	
14 through 50 years	30 micrograms/day
Lactation	
14 through 50 years	35 micrograms/day

The optimal intake values for biotin are not known. Those receiving hemodialysis, peritoneal dialysis or who have genetic abnormalities of biotin-dependent enzymes, such as biotinidase deficiency, have increased requirements for biotin. There are probably other such situations.

The U.S. RDA for biotin, the value used for nutritional supplement and food labeling purposes, is 300 micrograms/day.

HOW SUPPLIED

Capsules — 600 mcg, 1 mg, 5 mg

Lozenges — 1 mg

Tablets — 300 mcg, 600 mcg, 2.5 mg, 3 mg, 5 mg, 10 mg

LITERATURE

Bonjour J-P. Biotin. In: Machlin, LJ, ed. *Handbook of Vitamins. Nutritional, Biochemical and Clinical Aspects.* New York, NY: Marcel Dekker, Inc; 1984:403-435.

Borboni P, Magnaterra R, Rabini RA, et al. Effect of biotin on glucokinase activity, mRNA expression and insulin release in cultured beta-cells. *Acta Diabetologica.* 1996; 33:154-158.

Casado de Frias E, Campos-Castello J, Careaga Maldonado J, Perez Cerda C. Biotinidase deficiency: result of treatment with biotin from age 12 years. *Europ J Paedriatr Neurol.* 1997; 1:173-176.

Colombo VE, Gerber F, Bronhofer M, Floersheim GL. Treatment of brittle fingernails and onychoschizia with biotin: scanning electron microscopy. *J Am Acad Dermatol.* 1990; 23(6 Pt 1):1127-1132.

Dabbaugh O, Brismar J, Gascon GC, Ozand PT. The clinical spectrum of biotin-treatable encephalopathies in Saudi Arabia. *Brain Dev.* 1994; 16Suppl:72-80.

Diamantopoulos N, Painter MJ, Wolf B, et al. Biotinidase deficiency: accumulation of lactate in the brain and response to physiologic doses of biotin. *Neurology.* 1986; 36:1107-1109.

Dietary Reference Intakes for Thiamin, Riboflavin, Niacin, Vitamin B_6, Folate, Vitamin B_{12}, Pantothenic Acid, Biotin, and Choline. Washington, DC: National Academy Press; 1998:374-389.

Dupuis L, Campeau E, Leclerc D, Gravel RA. Mechanism of biotin responsiveness in biotin-responsive multiple carboxylase deficiency. *Mol Genet Metab.* 1999; 66:80-90.

Floerscheim GL. [Treatment of brittle fingernails with biotin]. [Article in German]. *Z Hautkr.* 1989; 64:41-48.

Furukawa Y. [Enhancement of glucose-induced insulin secretion and modification of glucose metabolism by biotin]. [Article in Japanese]. *Nippon Rinsho.* 1999; 57:2261-2269.

Hochman LG, Scher RK, Meyerson MS. Brittle nails: response to daily biotin supplementation. *Cutis.* 1993; 51:303-305.

Hwu WL, Suzuki Y, Yang X, et al. Late-onset holocarboxylase synthetase deficiency with homologous R508W mutation. *J Formos Med Assoc.* 2000; 99:174-177.

Hymes J, Fleischauer K, Wolf B. Biotinylation of histones by human serum biotinidase: assessment of biotinyl-transferase activity in sera from normal individuals and children with biotinidase deficiency. *Biochem Mol Med.* 1995; 56:76-83.

Hymes J, Wolf B. Human biotinidase isn't just for recycling biotin. *J Nutr.* 1999; 129:485S-489S.

Innis SM, Allardyce DB. Possible biotin deficiency in adults receiving long-term total parenteral nutrition. *Am J Clin Nutr.* 1983; 37:185-187.

Jung U, Helbich-Endermann M, Bitsch R, et al. Are patients with chronic renal failure (CRF) deficient in biotin and is regular biotin supplementation required? *Z Ernä hrungswiss.* 1998; 37:363-367.

Keipert JA. Oral use of biotin in seborrhoeic dermatitis of infancy: a controlled trial. *Med J Aust.* 1976; 1:584-585.

Marshall MW, Kliman PG, Washington VA. Effects of biotin on lipids and other constituents of plasma of healthy men and women. *Artery.* 1980; 7:330-351.

Michalski AJ, Berry GT, Segal S. Holocarboxylase synthetase deficiency: 9-year follow-up of a patient on chronic biotin therapy and a review of the literature. *J Inher Metab Dis.* 1989; 12:312-316.

Mock DM. Biotin. In: Shils ME, Olson JA, Shike M, Ross AC, eds. *Modern Nutrition in Health and Disease.* Baltimore, MD: Williams and Wilkins; 1999:459-466.

Mock DM. Biotin status: which are valid indicators and how do we know? *J Nutr.* 1999; 129:498S-503S.

Mock DM, Mock NI, Nelson RP, Lombard KA. Disturbances in biotin metabolism in children undergoing long-term anticonvulsant therapy. *J Pediatr Gastroenterol Nutr.* 1998; 26:245-250.

Romero-Navarro G, Cabrera-Valladares G, German MS, et al. Biotin regulation of pancreatic glucokinase and insulin in primary cultured rat islets and in biotin-deficient rats. *Endocrinology.* 1999; 140:4595-4600.

Ravn K, Chloupkova M, Christensen E, et al. High incidence of propionic acidemia in Greenland is due to a prevalent mutation, 1540insCCC, in the gene for the beta-subunit of propionyl CoA carboxylase. *Am J Hum Genet.* 2000; 67:203-206.

Reddi A, DeAngelis B, Frank O, et al. Biotin supplementation improves glucose and insulin tolerances in genetically diabetic KK mice. *Life Sci.* 1988; 42:1323-1330.

Rodriguez Melendez R. [Importance of biotin metabolism]. [Article in Spanish]. *Rev Invest Clin.* 2000; 52:194-199.

Sekiguchi T, Nagamine T. Inhibition of free radical generation by biotin. *Biochem Pharmacol.* 1994; 47:594-596.

Shelley WB, Shelley ED. Uncombable hair syndrome: observations on response to biotin and occurrence in siblings with ectodermal dysplasia. *J Am Acad Dermatol.* 1985; 13:97-102.

Sweetman L, Surh L, Baker H, et al. Clinical and metabolic abnormalities in a boy with dietary deficiency of biotin. *Pediatrics.* 1981; 68:553-558.

Velazquez A, Baez TM, Gutierrez J, Rodriguez R. Biotin supplementation affects lymphocyte carboxylases and plasma biotin in severe protein-energy malnutrition. *Am J Clin Nutr.* 1995; 61:385-391.

Zempleni J, McCormick DB, Cook DM. Identification of biotin sulfone, bisnorbiotin methyl ketone, and tetranorbiotin-1-sulfoxide in human urine. *Am J Clin Nutr.* 1997; 65:508-511.

Zempleni J, Mock DM. Bioavailability of biotin given orally to humans in pharmacologic doses. *Am J Clin Nutr.* 1999; 69:504-508.

Zempleni J, Mock DM. Marginal biotin deficiency is teratogenic. *Proc Soc Exp Biol Med.* 2000; 223:14-21.

Zempleni J, Mock DM. Utilization of biotin in proliferating human lymphocytes. *J Nutr.* 2000; 130:335S-337S.

Blackcurrant Seed Oil

TRADE NAMES

Blackcurrant seed oil is available from numerous manufacturers generically. Branded products include Black Currant Power (Nature's Herbs).

DESCRIPTION

Blackcurrant seed oil (BSO) is derived from the seeds of the plant *Ribes nigrum.* It is a rich source of the n-6 (omega-6) polyunsaturated fatty acid gamma-linolenic acid (GLA). Blackcurrant seed oil contains about 15 to 20% GLA. The n-3 (omega-3) polyunsaturated fatty acid alpha-linolenic acid (ALA) is also present in blackcurrant seed oil (12 to 14%) as is the fatty acid linoleic acid. Also present, in smaller amounts, is stearidonic acid or SDA (2 to 4%), an 18 carbon n-3 polyunsaturated fatty acid containing four double bonds. The various fatty acids are found in blackcurrant seed oil in the form of triacylglycerols (TAGs), also known as triglycerides. The stereospecific position of GLA varies among different oil sources. GLA is concentrated in the sn-3 position in blackcurrant seed oil as it is in evening primrose oil. In the case of borage oil, it is concentrated in the sn-2 position. The terms blackcurrant seed oil and blackcurrant oil are used interchangeably. (Also see monograph on GLA.)

ACTIONS AND PHARMACOLOGY

ACTIONS

Blackcurrant oil, owing to its GLA, ALA and stearidonic acid content, may have antithrombotic and anti-inflammatory actions.

MECHANISM OF ACTION

Any anti-inflammatory or antithrombotic actions that blackcurrant oil possesses may be accounted for, principally, by the presence of GLA, ALA and SDA. GLA is a precursor in the synthesis of prostaglandin E_1 (PGE_1), and ALA is a precursor in the synthesis of eicosapentaenoic acid (EPA). EPA itself is a precursor of the series-3 prostaglandins, the series-5 leukotrienes and the series-3 thromboxanes. These eicosanoids possess antithrombotic and anti-inflammatory activity. Other mechanisms include inhibition of inflammatory cytokines.

PHARMACOKINETICS

GLA-, ALA- and linoleic acid-laden TAGs in blackcurrant oil following ingestion undergo hydroysis via lipases to form monoglycerides (MGs) and free fatty acids (FFAs). Once formed, the MGs and the FFAs are absorbed by the enterocytes. In the enterocytes, a reacylation takes place reforming TAGs, which are then assembled with phospholipids, cholesterol and apoproteins into chylomicrons (CM). The CM are released into the lymphatics and are transported to the systemic circulation. In the circulation the CM are degraded by lipoprotein lipase and the fatty acids are taken up in part by the endothelial tissues to be used for oxidation or for synthesis of phospholipids, components of cell membranes. GLA is metabolized to dihomo-gamma-linolenic acid, which is converted to prostaglandin E1. ALA is metabolized to EPA, which itself is a precursor in the synthesis of the series-3 prostaglandins, the series-5 leukotrienes and the series-3 thromboxanes. Linoleic acid, also contained in blackcurrant oil, is metabolized to ALA. Stearidonic acid is also metabolized to EPA. The metabolites of GLA and ALA are catabolized by oxidative processes, and the catabolic products are mostly excreted in the urine.

INDICATIONS AND USAGE

Blackcurrant seed oil may have cardioprotective effects as well as some efficacy in rheumatoid arthritis. It is not a useful cholesterol-lowering agent. (See GLA for other possible indications.)

RESEARCH SUMMARY

Claims made for blackcurrant seed oil are similar to those related to gamma-linolenic acid (GLA). But since blackcurrant seed oil is a source of both GLA and alpha-linolenic acid (ALA), it has carved out a separate niche for itself. Blackcurrant oil may be cardioprotective.

Many of the benefits noted with the use of GLA in rheumatoid arthritis may be observed with the use of blackcurrant oil.

CONTRAINDICATION, PRECAUTIONS, ADVERSE REACTIONS

CONTRAINDICATIONS

None known.

PRECAUTIONS

Pregnant women, nursing mothers and children should avoid use of blackcurrant oil unless it is recommended by a physician. Because of possible antithrombotic activity, those with hemophilia and those taking warfarin (Coumadin) should use blackcurrant oil with caution.

ADVERSE REACTIONS

No significant adverse effects have been reported. Those taking blackcurrant oil may experience mild gastrointestinal symptoms such as diarrhea. Some cannot tolerate the number of capsules required to receive any benefit.

INTERACTIONS

No interaction between blackcurrant oil and aspirin, other NSAIDs, or herbs, such as *Allium sativum* (garlic) and *Ginkgo biloba* (ginkgo) have been reported. Such interactions, if they were to occur, might be manifested by nosebleeds and/or increased susceptibility to bruising. If this does occur, the blackcurrant oil dose should be lowered or stopped.

OVERDOSAGE

There are no reports of overdosage.

DOSAGE AND ADMINISTRATION

There are several blackcurrant seed oil supplements available, each differing slightly in the amount of GLA and ALA in a capsule. GLA ranges in these capsules from 60 to 90 milligrams and ALA 70 to 90 milligrams. The usual dose consumed is from three to six capsules, containing these amounts, daily in divided doses.

HOW SUPPLIED

Capsules — 500 mg, 1000 mg

LITERATURE

Deferne JL, Leeds AR. Resting blood pressure and cardiovascular reactivity to mental arithmetic in mild hypertensive males supplemented with blackcurrant seed oil. *J Hum Hyperten.* 1996; 10:531-537.

Diboune M, Ferard G, Ingenbleek V, et al. Composition of phospholipid fatty acids in red blood cell membranes of patients in intensive care units: effects of different intakes of soybean oil, medium chain triglycerides and blackcurrant oil. *J Parent Enteral Nutr.* 1992; 16:136-141.

Watson J, Byars ML, Mc Gill P, Kelman AW. Cytokine and prostaglandin production by monocytes of volunteers and rheumatoid arthritis patients treated with dietary supplements of blackcurrant seed oil. *Br J Rheumatol.* 1993; 32: 1055-1058.

Wu D, Meydani M, Leka LS, et al. Effect of dietary supplementation with blackcurrant seed oil on the immune response of healthy elderly subjects. *Am J Clin Nutr.* 1999; 70: 536-543.

Bone Meal

TRADE NAMES

Bone meal is available from numerous manufacturers generically. Many products combine bone meal with vitamin

D. Brand-name products include Liquid Bone Meal (Carlson Labs).

DESCRIPTION

Bone meal is used as a supplement for calcium and phosphorus. It is composed of finely crushed, processed bone, usually from cattle but sometimes also from horses. Bone marrow may also be added to the product. Calcium in bone meal occurs as a calcium phosphate compound known as hydroxyapatite or hydroxylapatite. Hydroxyapatite is an inorganic compound found in the matrix of bone and the teeth; it confers rigidity to these structures. The formula of hydroxyapatite is $(Ca_3 (PO_4)_2)_3 \bullet Ca (OH)_2$ or $Ca_{10} (PO_4)_6 (OH)_2$.

Bone meal was at one time a popular nutritional supplement for calcium. It is still marketed as a nutritional supplement, but it is no longer popular. The reason for this is that in the 1980s analysis of bone meal supplements revealed them to contain substantial amounts of lead, as well as other toxic elements, such as arsenic, mercury and cadmium. A second-generation "bone meal" product called microcrystalline hydroxyapatite, or MCHA, is being marketed as a calcium supplement and is claimed to be free of contaminants. See Microcrystalline Hydroxyapatite.

Bone meal is also used as a high-phosphorus fertilizer and in some pet foods.

ACTIONS AND PHARMACOLOGY

MECHANISM OF ACTION
See Calcium.

PHARMACOKINETICS
See Calcium.

Hydroxyapatite is apparently well-absorbed from the gastrointestinal tract.

INDICATIONS AND USAGE

Bone meal is still sold as a "natural" source of calcium. Its use should be avoided owing to potential toxic-metal contamination.

RESEARCH SUMMARY

The use of bone meal as a calcium source is no longer recommended. Several researchers have reported that many bone meal preparations are contaminated with toxic metals. In one study, bone meal samples were contaminated with significant amounts of lead, arsenic, mercury and other metals. Dolomite and calcium carbonate supplements labeled "oyster shell" or "natural source" have also been found to be contaminated with these metals.

One researcher has advised that "physicians must consider the possibility of unrecognized self-poisoning from the consumption of such substances, especially in the context of unexplained neurologic, gastrointestinal, cutaneous and hematologic disorders."

The feeding of meat and bone meal to cattle contaminated with bovine spongiform encephalopathy (BSE) led to an epidemic in the British cattle population in the 1990s.

CONTRAINDICATIONS, PRECAUTIONS, ADVERSE REACTIONS

CONTRAINDICATIONS
Bone meal is contraindicated in those with hypercalcemia. Conditions that cause hypercalcemia include hyperparathyroidism, hypervitaminosis D, some granulomatous diseases, sarcoidosis and cancer. Bone meal is also contraindicated in those with calcium pyrophosphate dihydrate (CPPD) deposition disease.

PRECAUTIONS
Bone meal is no longer recommended as a calcium supplement because of possible presence of toxic substances, such as lead. Children are especially sensitive to the effects of lead. Children, pregnant women and nursing mothers should absolutely avoid bone meal supplements.

ADVERSE REACTIONS
See Calcium. Prolonged use of bone meal contaminated with toxic elements, such as lead, may cause the typical toxic effects of these substances. Lead may produce abdominal pain, anemia and central nervous system damage.

OVERDOSAGE

There are no known reports of overdosage of bone meal.

DOSAGE AND ADMINISTRATION

No recommended dose. Second-generation "bone meal" supplements known as microcrystalline hydroxyapatite, or MCHA, are available as calcium supplements and are claimed to be free of contaminants. See Microcrystalline Hydroxyapatite.

HOW SUPPLIED

Capsules — 600 mg
Tablets

LITERATURE

Boulos FM, von Smolinski A. Alert to users of calcium supplements as antihypertensive agents due to trace mineral contaminants. *Am J Hypterten.* 1988; 1(3 Pt 3):137S-142S.

Bourquin BP, Evans DR, Cornett JR, et al. Lead content of 70 brands of dietary calcium supplements. *Am J Public Health.* 1993; 83:1155-1160.

Groschup MH. [Bovine spongiform encephalopathy in ruminants and the new variant of Creutzfeldt-Jakob disease in humans.] [Article in German.] *DTW Dtsch Tierarzl Wochenschr.* 1999; 106:329-331.

Roberts HJ. Potential toxicity due to dolomite and bone meal. *South Med J.* 1983; 76:556-559.

Whiting SJ. Safety of some calcium supplements questioned. *Nutr Rev*. 1884; 52:95-97.

Borage Oil

TRADE NAMES

Borage Oil Gla 240 (Health From the Sun), Borage Oil Omega-6 (Nature's Way), Borage Power (Nature's Herbs), Borage Oil HA (Nutritional Dynamics), Veg Borage Oil (Health From the Sun), My Favorite Borage Oil (Natrol), Borage GLA, (Health From the Sun) and Borage Liquid Gold (Health From the Sun).

DESCRIPTION

Borage oil is derived from the seeds of the borage plant (*Borago officinalis*), a member of the Boraginaceae family. Borage oil, also known as starflower oil and borage seed oil, is a rich source of the long-chain polyunsaturated fatty acid gamma-linolenic acid (GLA). The possible health benefits of borage oil are attributed to GLA. GLA is an unusual constituent of living matter and is found in very few plants. These include, in addition to borage, evening primrose, blackcurrant and hemp. The amount of GLA in borage oil, as the percentage of total fatty acid content, ranges from about 20% to 27%. Typical borage oil supplements contain approximately 24% GLA.

GLA is an all cis n-6 long-chain polyunsaturated fatty acid. It is comprised of 18 carbon atoms and three double bonds. GLA is also known as GLA; 18: 3n-6 and gamolenic acid. Chemically, it is known as 6, 9, 12-octadecatrienoic acid; (Z, Z, Z)-6, 9, 12-octadecatrienoic acid, and cis-6, cis-9, cis-12-octadecatrienoic acid. GLA is present in borage oil in the form of triglycerides. GLA is concentrated in the sn-2 position in the triglycerides. GLA has the following chemical structure:

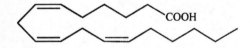

GLA (gamma-linolenic acid)

ACTIONS AND PHARMACOLOGY

ACTIONS

Borage oil may have anti-inflammatory and antithrombotic activities.

MECHANISM OF ACTION

The possible anti-inflammatory and anti-aggregatory actions of borage oil may be accounted for by examining the role of GLA in eicosanoid biochemistry. GLA is metabolized to the 20-carbon polyunsaturated fatty acid dihomo-gamma-linolenic acid (DGLA; 20: 3n-6), which is a precursor to the 1-series prostaglandins, such as prostaglandin E_1 (PGE_1). The action of PGE_1 on inflammatory cells (e.g. polymorphonuclear leukocytes or PMNs) is mostly inhibitory. PGE_1 increases intracellular cyclic AMP (cAMP). This increase reduces the release of lysosomal enzymes, PMN chemotaxis, and the margination and adherence of PMNs in the blood vessels. PGE_1 is also thought to inhibit lymphocyte function. PGE_1, in addition to its role in suppressing the inflammatory process, inhibits platelet aggregation and has vasodilatory activity.

GLA, via its metabolite DGLA, inhibits leukotriene (LT) synthesis. Leukotriene B_4 (LTB_4) is an inflammatory mediator. DGLA is metabolized to 15-hydroxyl DGLA, which blocks the conversion of arachidonic acid to LTs such as LTB_4.

In summary, GLA may suppress inflammation through its metabolism to DGLA, which in turn can competitively inhibit the pro-inflammatory 2-series prostaglandins and 4-series leukotrienes. The incorporation of GLA and its metabolites in cell membranes may also play a role in the possible anti-inflammatory, antithrombotic, anti-atherogenic and antiproliferative actions of borage oil.

PHARMACOKINETICS

GLA-laden triglycerides in borage oil are absorbed from the small intestine aided by bile salts. During this process, there is some deacylation of the fatty acid residues of the triglycerides. Reacylation takes place within the mucosal cells of the small intestine, and the GLA-laden triglycerides enter into the lymphatics in the form of chylomicrons. GLA-laden chylomicrons are transported from the lymphatics into the blood, where GLA is carried in lipid particles to the various tissues of the body.

GLA is metabolized to the 20-carbon polyunsaturated fatty acid dihomo-gamma-linolenic acid (DGLA), which is converted to prostaglandin E_1 (PGE_1). It may also be metabolized to eicosapentaenoic acid (EPA). GLA and DGLA are normally not found in cells as free fatty acids. They occur mainly in cell membranes as components of phopholipids, neutral lipids and cholesterol esters. PGE_1 is metabolized to smaller prostaglandin remnants, which are primarily polar dicarboxylic acids, most of which are excreted in the urine.

INDICATIONS AND USAGE

Borage oil appears to be effective in some cases of rheumatoid arthritis and may be indicated in some other inflammatory disorders, such as Sjogren's syndrome and ulcerative colitis. Possible other indications include osteoporosis, diabetic neuropathy, acute respiratory distress syndrome (ARDS), hypertension and elevated serum lipids. Borage oil has been used with some preliminary success in some cancers, principally cerebral gliomas. It has not proved useful for tardive dyskinesia, premenstrual syndrome or menopausal flushing. It may be indicated in some cases for atopic dermatitis, particularly to help with itching, as well as for uremic skin conditions in hemodialysis patients. It should probably not be used in efforts to enhance immunity, as it may be immunosuppressive.

RESEARCH SUMMARY
See GLA.

CONTRAINDICATIONS, PRECAUTIONS, ADVERSE REACTIONS
CONTRAINDICATIONS
None known.

PRECAUTIONS
Pregnant women and nursing mothers should avoid using borage oil supplements. Those with a history of partial complex seizure disorders, such as temporal lobe epilepsy, should avoid using borage oil. Likewise, those with other types of seizure disorders and schizophrenics who are being treated with certain neuroleptic drugs, such as aliphatic phenothiazines (e.g. chlorpromazine), which may lower seizure threshold, should avoid using borage oil. Because of possible antithrombotic activity of borage oil, those with hemophilia or other hemorrhagic diatheses and those taking warfarin should exercise caution in the use of this supplement. Borage oil supplementation should be halted before any surgical procedure.

Because of its possible inhibition of lymphocyte function, those with immune deficiency disorders, such as AIDS, should exercise caution in the use of borage oil.

Pyrrolizidine alkaloids, such as amabiline, lycopsamine and thesinine, are found in various parts of the borage plant. The unsaturated pyrrolizidine alkaloids, such as amabiline, are potentially hepatotoxic and carcinogenic. Amabiline has not been detected in borage oil supplements down to five parts per million. However, chronic consumption of borage oil containing levels of amabiline of one part per million may prove harmful. Those who use borage oil chronically should only use products that are certified free of unsaturated pyrrolizidine alkaloids.

ADVERSE REACTIONS
Borage oil may cause such gastrointestinal symptoms as nausea, vomiting, flatulence, diarrhea and bloating. Similar to evening primrose oil, borage oil may precipitate symptoms of undiagnosed complex partial seizures and should be used, if at all, with extreme caution in those with a history of seizure disorders or those taking drugs that lower the seizure threshold, such as aliphatic phenothiazines (e.g., chlorpromazine).

INTERACTIONS
DRUGS
Use of borage oil in schizophrenics who are being treated with certain neuroleptic agents that lower seizure threshold — e.g. aliphatic phenothiazines, such as chlorpromazine — may cause partial complex seizures and possibly other types of seizures. Interactions may occur between borage oil and anticoagulants, such as warfarin, as well as antiplatelet drugs, such as aspirin and NSAIDs. Such interactions may enhance the effects of the anticoagulants and antiplatelet drugs. Manifestations of such interactions, if they were to occur, include nosebleeds, hematuria and increased susceptibility to bruising. Borage oil intake should be stopped if these symptoms occur.

NUTRITIONAL SUPPLEMENTS
Interactions may occur if borage oil is used with supplements that have antithrombotic activity, such as fish oils. This may be manifested by nosebleeds and increased susceptibility to bruising.

HERBS
Interactions may occur if borage oil is used with such herbs as garlic (*Allium sativum*) and ginkgo (*Ginkgo biloba*). Such interactions may be manifested by nosebleeds and easy bruising.

OVERDOSAGE
There are no reports of overdosage with borage oil.

DOSAGE AND ADMINISTRATION
Borage oil is available in capsules and bottles. Capsules of borage oil typically contain about 24% GLA. Doses used for the management of rheumatoid arthritis range from about 360 milligrams to 2.8 grams daily in divided doses (expressed as GLA). For management of atopic dermatitis, doses of 320 to 480 milligrams (expressed as GLA) are used, taken daily in divided doses. Doses up to 2 grams daily (expressed as GLA) have been used by those with hypertriglyceridemia. For long-term use, borage oil should be certified free of unsaturated pyrrolizidine alkaloids. Borage oil supplements should contain an antioxidant, such as vitamin E, to protect the unsaturated fatty acids against oxidation.

HOW SUPPLIED
Capsules — 90 mg, 240 mg, 300 mg, 500 mg, 1000 mg, 1300 mg

Liquid

LITERATURE
For additional literature, see GLA and Evening Primrose Oil monographs.

Huang Y-S, Mills DE, eds. *Gamma-Linolenic Acid: Metabolism and its Roles in Nutrition.* Champaign, IL: American Oil Chemists Society Press; 1996.

Boron

TRADE NAMES

Boron is available generically from numerous manufacturers. Branded products include Boron Extra Strength (Vitaline), Tri-Boron (Twinlab), Tetra Boron (Solaray) and Boron 3 (GNC).

DESCRIPTION

Boron, the fifth chemical element, is a dietary trace mineral found primarily in plant foods. It is essential for plant growth. Recently it has been shown to be essential in an animal species (zebra fish), and evidence is mounting that boron is probably essential for humans, as well. The first edition of *The Merck Manual* (1899) credits boric acid, the most common form of boron, with being a useful treatment for amenorrhea, dysmenorrhea, epilepsy and elevated uric acid. Boric acid has, in fact, proved to be ineffective for all of those disorders, but recent research supports the use of boron for the promotion of bone and joint health. There is less evidence that it may be helpful in enhancing mental cognition.

ACTIONS AND PHARMACOLOGY

ACTIONS

Boron may have estrogen-mimetic and anti-osteoporotic activity. It may also participate in regulating the respiratory burst of neutrophils.

MECHANISM OF ACTION

The biochemical mechanism of boron is not yet known. Currently, two hypotheses have been advanced for the biochemical function of boron in animals, including humans. The first is that boron plays a role in cell-membrane functions that influence response to hormone action, trans-membrane signaling and trans-membrane movement of regulatory ions. Boron has been shown, in animal models, to influence the transport of extracellular calcium and the release of intracellular calcium in platelets activated by thrombin. It also influences redox actions involved in cellular membrane transport in plants.

A second hypothesis is that boron acts as a metabolic regulator in several enzymatic systems. Boron may play an important role in regulating the respiratory burst, which is the reactive-oxygen-species mechanism by which white blood cells kill micro-organisms. If boron does in fact regulate the respiratory burst, it assumes the role of a novel antioxidant, preventing some of the collateral damage that may occur when reactive oxygen species react with surrounding tissue.

The biochemistry of boron is essentially that of boric acid. Boric acid forms complexes with many of the chemical substances found in the body, such as carbohydrates (sugars and polysaccharides), nucleotides (such as adenosine mono-phosphate and niacinamide adenine dinucleotide) and vitamins (such as ascorbic acid, pyridoxine and riboflavin). Boric acid forms esters with hydroxyl groups found in many of these compounds. This occurs preferentially when the hydroxyl groups are next to each other and on the same side of the molecules. The most stable esters are those in which boric acid is the bridge between two carbohydrate molecules, e.g. fructose-boron-fructose. Such soluble boron complexes are found naturally in phloem saps and nectars in plants. Polysaccharides containing boron in similar linkages are found in plant cell walls in the form of pectins.

PHARMACOKINETICS

Nutritional forms of boron are readily and completely absorbed. They are either rapidly converted to boric acid and are absorbed as such or they are converted to boric acid following absorption. Absorbed boric acid is rapidly distributed throughout body water by passive diffusion. After being absorbed, boron's ratio of blood-to-soft-tissue concentration is approximately one. Concentrations of boron in bone, teeth and fingernails exceed those in blood by about a factor of four. Certain nutritional forms of boron (e.g., boron carbohydrate esters) are metabolized to boric acid. Boric acid itself does not undergo metabolism. It is eliminated unchanged in the urine. The half-life for elimination of boric acid, whether administered orally or intravenously, is about 21 hours.

INDICATIONS AND USAGE

Boron may be indicated for the promotion of bone and joint health, particularly in women. There is less evidence to support claims that boron enhances cognition and ameliorates the symptoms of arthritis. There is no evidence that it promotes the development of lean muscle mass.

RESEARCH SUMMARY

Boron's potential therapeutic value in promoting bone and joint health is underscored by the widespread incidence of osteoporosis. There are more than 100 million afflicted by this disease worldwide, eight million of them in the United States. Postmenopausal women are mostly affected, but osteoporosis is also found in some men as they age. In the United States, osteoporosis is responsible for 300,000 hip fractures, 700,000 spine fractures and 250,000 wrist fractures each year. Associated health care costs are in the billions of dollars annually.

Adequate intake and metabolism of minerals can largely prevent osteoporosis. Dietary boron has been shown to affect several aspects of mineral metabolism in animal studies. And in a human study, 12 postmenopausal women were fed a diet deficient in boron (0.25 mg daily) for 119 days followed by a 48-day period in which they received supplements of 3 mg daily. On the boron-deficient diet, the women experienced increased loss of both calcium and magnesium. On the boron-supplemented diet, the opposite was true. Urinary excretion of calcium and magnesium was significantly diminished, and serum concentrations of 17 beta-estradiol, as well as testosterone, increased. The findings of the study suggest that maintaining adequate levels of boron, particularly in the presence of adequate levels of magnesium, can help prevent calcium loss and bone demineralization in postmenopausal women and, perhaps, others. The boron effect on testosterone levels, while possibly significant for women, would be too low to have any significance for men.

In a subsequent human study, boron supplementation increased serum levels of 25-hydroxycholecalciferol, a metabolite of vitamin D important in mineral metabolism, in postmenopausal women who were deficient in boron. There were also findings suggesting that estrogen replacement therapy used in conjunction with boron may have a synergistic effect. There is evidence to support the assertion that boron can both mimic and enhance some of the effects of estrogen in post-menopausal women.

Findings to date suggest that boron and calcium actions are inter-related or that the two elements affect similar systems, including the modification of hormone action, the alteration of cell membrane characteristics and/or trans-membrane signaling. Boron appears to be a very important partner with calcium metabolism and as such should be expected to play an important role in the prevention of osteoporosis. Conclusive proof of this, however, remains to be demonstrated, though studies to date are highly suggestive of a positive effect.

Anecdotal reports, combined with some epidemiological findings, suggest that supplemental boron may alleviate the symptoms of osteoarthritis. There are reports that in those areas of the world where daily dietary intake of boron is 1 mg or less the estimated incidence of osteoarthritis ranges from 20 to 70%. In areas of the world where boron intakes are 3 to 10 mg daily, the estimated incidence of the disease ranges from 0 to 10%. This alone does not make a compelling argument for any role for boron in the prevention or treatment of osteoarthritis in the absence of clinical evidence. There is, however, one clinical study and one animal study that may justify further investigation.

The clinical trial involved 20 patients with radiographically confirmed osteoarthritis. This was a double-blind, placebo-controlled study in which half of the subjects were given 6 mg of boron daily while the other half received the placebo. The subjects were evaluated three times—prior to taking the tablets, after three weeks on the tablets and after eight weeks on the tablets. Patients were graded with respect to their symptoms as well as their use of a permitted analgesic. At the end of the eight-week period, 50% of those taking boron showed improvement, while only 10% of those on placebo showed similar improvement. The finding was declared statistically significant.

A recent study using rats indicated that dietary boron might be of benefit in adjuvant-induced arthritis. The benefits were evaluated by the amount of paw and joint swelling following adjuvant injection. A control group that did not receive boron was used for comparison. There was less swelling in the boron-supplemented animals. Measurements of natural killer cells, CD8 lymphocytes and neutrophils were also performed. The conclusion was that supplemental boron modulates the response to antigens of key immune cells and helps control the inflammatory process.

Further investigation is warranted and necessary before any conclusion can be made regarding the role of boron in the prevention and treatment of arthritis.

There is very preliminary evidence that supplemental boron may improve mental function. In one human study, subjects were first given a diet deficient in boron followed by a period in which they received supplemental boron in the amount of 3 mg daily. During the supplementation period, the subjects' electroencephalograms showed alterations suggesting improved behavioral activation (less drowsiness) and mental alertness. Improved psychomotor skills were also noted, along with improvement in attention and memory.

Studies have not supported the claim that boron can increase lean muscle mass. Studies show no effect on plasma testosterone levels or strength in male body builders. Claims to the contrary seem to have arisen from the studies on postmenopausal women, where boron may have induced a slight increase in plasma testosterone levels.

CONTRAINDICATIONS, PRECAUTIONS, ADVERSE REACTIONS

CONTRAINDICATIONS
None known.

PRECAUTIONS
None known.

ADVERSE REACTIONS
Doses up to 18 mg of boron daily appear to be safe for adults even if taken for prolonged periods of time. There is no evidence that boron is either carcinogenic or mutagenic. No adverse effects have been observed in either premenopausal or postmenopausal women using boron supplements.

OVERDOSAGE

The lowest levels at which boron supplementation may be toxic have not been established. In 1904, human volunteers consuming greater than 500 mg of boric acid daily (this is equivalent to about 180 mg of elemental boron) showed symptoms of poor appetite and digestive problems. Symptoms of acute toxicity typically include nausea, diarrhea and abdominal cramps. The symptoms of chronic toxicity include nausea, poor appetite and weight loss.

DOSAGE AND ADMINISTRATION

No DRI (dietary reference intake) has yet been established for boron. However, since there is mounting evidence for the essentiality of boron in humans, a DRI is likely to be established in the near future. The DRI that is likely to be established for boron will probably be an AI (adequate intake) rather than an RDA (recommended dietary allowance).

Fruits and vegetables are the most important dietary sources of boron. A vegetarian diet is higher in boron than the typical American diet. The range of intake in the American diet is 0.5 to 3 mg daily. The average intake is about 1 mg daily. It is lower in the elderly. There is some evidence that this average intake may be too low; a more optimal intake of boron may be 2 to 3 mg daily.

Dietary supplements of boron now available include the following forms: sodium borate, boron citrate, boron aspartate, boron glycinate. Once ingested, all of these forms are rapidly converted in the body to boric acid. Natural plant forms of boron or similar synthetic forms are not yet available, and whether they will have greater health benefits than the currently marketed forms remains to be seen.

Boron is often sold in supplements that combine a variety of nutrients. For example, it is found in products for bone and joint health that often combine such nutrients as vitamin D, calcium, magnesium, soy isoflavones, chondroitin sulfate, glucosamine, curcumin, boswellia, gelatin, ipriflavone, SAMe and others (see monographs on these substances). There's no evidence yet available that the therapeutic effects of boron are increased by such combinations.

HOW SUPPLIED

Capsules — 3 mg

Tablets — 3 mg, 6 mg

LITERATURE

Chapin RE, Ku WW, Kenny MA, Mc Coy H, Gladen B, Wine RN, Wilson R, Elwell MR. The effects of dietary boron on bone strength in rats. *Fundam Appl Toxical.* 1997; 35:205-215.

Green NR, Ferrando AA. Plasma boron and the effects of boron supplementation in males. *Environ Health Perspect.* 1994; 102 (Suppl 7):73-77.

Hu H, Penn SG, Lebrilla CB, Brown PH. Isolation and characterization of soluble boron complexes in higher plants. The mechanism of phloem mobility of boron. *Plant Physiol.* 1997; 113:649-655.

Hunt CD, Idso JP, Keehr KA. Dietary boron alleviates adjuvant-induced arthritis (AIA) and changes in the blood concentrations of neutrophil, CD8a, and natural killer cells in rats. *FASEBJ.* 1999; 13

Hunt CD. Biochemical effects of physiological amounts of dietary boron. *J Trace Elem Exp Med.* 1999; 9:185-213.

Linden CH, Hall AH, Kulig KW, Rumack BH. Acute ingestions of boric acid. *J Toxicol Clin Toxicol.* 1986; 24:269-279.

Moore JA. An assessment of boric acid and borax using the IEHR evaluative process for assessing human developmental and reproductive toxicity of agents. *Reproduct Toxical.* 1997; 11:123-160.

Murray FJ. A comparative review of the pharmacokinetics of boric acid in rodents and humans. *Biol Trace Elem Res.* 1998; 66:331-341.

Murray FJ. A human health assessment of boron (boric acid and borax) in drinking water. *Regulat Toxical Pharmicol.* 1995; 22:221-230.

Newnham RE. Essentiality of boron for healthy bones and joints. *Environ Health Perspect.* 102 (Suppl 7):83-85.

Nielsen FH. Ultratrace minerals in Modern Nutrition in Health and Disease. In: Shils ME, Olson JA, Shike M., Ross AC, eds. *Modern Nutrition in Health and Disease.* 9th ed. Baltimore, MD: Williams & Wilkins; 1999:283-303.

Nielsen FH. Facts and Fallacies about Boron. *Nutrition Today.* 1992; 27:6-12.

Nielsen FH. Biochemical and physiologic consequences of boron deprivation in humans. *Environ Health Perspect.* 1994; 102 (Suppl 7):59-63.

Nielsen FH, Gallagher SK, Johnson LK, Nielsen EJ. Boron enhances and mimics some effects of estrogen therapy in postmenopausal women. *J Trace Elem Exp Med.* 1992; 5: 237-246.

Nielsen FH, Hunt CD, Mullen LM, Hunt JR. Effect of dietary boron on mineral, estrogen, and testosterone metabolism in postmenopausal women. *FASEBJ.* 1987; 1:394-397.

Penland J.G. The importance of boron nutrition for brain and psychological function. *Biol Trace Elem Res.* 1998; 66:299-317.

Rainey CJ, Nyquist LA, Christensen RE, Strong PL, Culver BD, Coughlin JR. Daily boron intake from the American diet. *J Am Diet Assoc.* 1999; 99:335-340.

PDR for Dietary Supplements/BORON-12-

Further information in:

Proceedings of the 2nd International Symposium on the Health Effects of Boron and its Compounds. Irvine, California, U.S.A. October 22-24, 1997. *Biol Trace Elem Research.* 1998; 66:1-473

Health effects of boron. *Environmental Health Perspective Supplements*. 1994; 102(Suppl 7):1-141. suppl 7, 1994

Merck's 1899 Manual, Merck and Co., New York, 1899

Bovine Cartilage

DESCRIPTION
Bovine cartilage is mainly comprised of the protein collagen and proteoglycans. Proteoglycans are composed of a core protein to which polysaccharides, known as glycosaminoglycans (GAGs) or mucopolysaccharides, are attached. The main glycosaminoglycan in bovine cartilage is chondroitin sulfate.

In 1976, Judah Folkman and his colleagues reported on the isolation of a factor from the scapular cartilage of calves that inhibited the growth of new blood vessels supporting implanted tumors in rabbits. It also stopped the growth of the tumors.

Subsequently, it was found that factors in shark cartilage had similar effects (see Shark Cartilage). Bovine cartilage, marketed as a nutritional supplement and for other indications, is primarily derived from bovine trachea.

ACTIONS AND PHARMACOLOGY
ACTIONS
Bovine cartilage has putative antitumor and anti-arthritic actions. Topical bovine cartilage may have wound-healing activity.

MECHANISM OF ACTION
The mechanism of the putative antitumor activity of bovine cartilage is unknown. Substances in bovine cartilage may have some anti-angiogenic activity. It has been suggested that chondroitin sulfate in bovine cartilage may have immunomodulatory activity and that such activity may play some role as well.

Bovine cartilage's putative anti-arthritic activity may be accounted for, in part, by the presence of chondroitin sulfate (see Chondroitin Sulfate).

Topical bovine cartilage appears to have wound-healing activity by stimulating granulation within the wound, thus establishing a matrix that induces wound repair.

PHARMACOKINETICS
The pharmacokinetics of collagen in bovine cartilage should be similar to those of dietary proteins. See Chondroitin Sulfate for pharmacokinetics of that substance.

INDICATIONS AND USAGE
As with shark cartilage, claims for bovine cartilage include anticancer, anti-inflammatory and anti-arthritic effects. Ac-

celerated wound-healing effects are also claimed for oral bovine cartilage. There is little support for these claims. Topical bovine cartilage does appear to aid in wound healing.

RESEARCH SUMMARY
There are no well-controlled clinical studies showing efficacy of bovine cartilage in any cancer. There is one ongoing study on the effects of bovine cartilage in metastatic renal cell cancer. Similarly, there is no credible evidence that it is helpful in any form of arthritis. It contains chondroitin sulfate, which has been shown to be helpful in some with osteoarthritis, but studies showing similar activity with the use of bovine cartilage are lacking. Some anti-inflammatory and antitumor effects have been shown in animal and *in vitro* studies.

CONTRAINDICATIONS, PRECAUTIONS, ADVERSE REACTIONS
CONTRAINDICATIONS
Bovine cartilage supplements are contraindicated in those who are hypersensitive to any component of a bovine cartilage-containing product.

PRECAUTIONS
Pregnant women and nursing mothers should avoid using bovine cartilage supplements.

Those with renal failure or liver failure should exercise caution in the use of bovine cartilage.

Those with cancer who wish to try bovine cartilage must do so under medical supervision.

ADVERSE REACTIONS
These are occasional reports of gastrointestinal complaints, such as nausea, bloating and diarrhea. Also, fatigue has been associated with the use of this supplement.

DOSAGE AND ADMINISTRATION
Bovine cartilage is available in capsules and powders and in combination products. There are no typical doses. Bovine cartilage is also available as a wound dressing and as a dermatologic cream for skin care.

HOW SUPPLIED
Capsules — 750 mg

Powder

LITERATURE
Durie BG, Soehnlen B, Prudden JF. Antitumor activity of bovine cartilage extract (Catrix-S) in the human tumor stem cell assay. *J Biol Response Mod.* 1985; 4:590-595.

Langer R, Brem H, Falterman K, et al. Isolation of a cartilage factor that inhibits tumor neovascularization. *Science.* 1976; 193:70-72.

Prudden JF. The treatment of human cancer with agents prepared from bovine cartilage. *J Biol Response Mod.* 1985; 4:551-584.

Prudden JF, Balassa LL. The biological activity of bovine cartilage preparations. Clinical demonstration of their potent anti-inflammatory capacity with supplementary notes on certain relevant fundamental support studies. *Semin Arthritis Rheum.* 1974; 3: 287-321.

Puccio C, Mittelman A, Chun P, et al. Treatment of metastatic renal cell carcinoma with catrix. *Proc Amer Soc Clin Onc.* 1994; 13:A769.

Romano CF, Lipton A, Harvey HA, et al. A phase II study of Catrix-S in solid tumors. *J Biol Response Mod.* 1985; 4:585-589.

Rosen J, Sherman WT, Prudden JF, Thorbecke GJ. Immunoregulatory effects of catrix. *J Biol Resp Mod.* 1988; 7:498-512.

Sieper J, Kary S, Sorensen H, et al. Oral type II collagen treatment in early rheumatoid arthritis. A double-blind, placebo-controlled, randomized trial. *Arthritis Rheum.* 1996; 39:41-51.

Wolarsky ER, Finke SR, Prudden JF. Acceleration of wound healing with heterologous cartilage. Immunological considerations. *Proc Soc Exp Biol Med.* 1966; 123:556-561.

Bovine Colostrum

TRADE NAMES
Mega Bovine Colostrum (Bricker Labs)

DESCRIPTION
Colostrum is the pre-milk fluid produced from the mother's mammary glands during the first few days after birth. Bovine colostrum is derived from cows. Colostrum is a rich source of antibodies, growth factors and nutrients for the suckling neonate and may provide passive immunity to the newborn against various infectious microorganisms, particularly those that affect the gastrointestinal tract. It may also have other health benefits.

The protein content of bovine colostrum is three to four times higher—up to 150 grams per liter compared to 30 to 40 grams per liter—than it is in regular cow's milk.

The greater part of this protein is comprised of whey proteins (see Whey Proteins). Immunoglobulins, mainly IgG, make up about 75% of the whey proteins. Other substances found in bovine colostrum include casein, lactoferrin, alpha-lactalbumin, beta-lactoglobulin, and the growth factors insulin-like growth factor-1 (IGF-1), insulin-like growth factor-2 (IGF-2), transforming growth factor beta (TGFbeta) and epidermal growth factor (EGF). In addition, bovine colostrum contains vitamins, minerals, lipids and lactose. Bovine colostrum may also contain colostrinin, also known as

proline-rich polypeptide (PRP), a substance found in ovine (sheep) colostrum.

Bovine colostrum is marketed in several forms. Bovine colostrum prepared by microfiltration is mainly composed of whey proteins and their associated immunoglobulins and the growth factors IGF-1, IGF-2, TGFbeta and EGF.

Substances such as lactose, fats, casein and lactalbumin are significantly reduced in microfiltered bovine colostrum. Hyperimmune bovine colostrum is rich in immunoglobulins of the IgG type, which are protective against such infectious microorganisms as *Cryptosporidium parvum* (a major cause of AIDS-associated diarrhea), diarrheogenic *Escherichia coli* strains, *Shigella flexneri, Clostridium difficile,* and rotavirus, the most common cause of severe diarrhea in young children.

Hyperimmune bovine colostrum is prepared from cows previously immunized with specific antigens. Hyperimmune bovine colostrum IgG concentrate is an orphan drug for the treatment of diarrhea in AIDS patients caused by infection with *Cryptosporidium parvum.*

ACTIONS AND PHARMACOLOGY
ACTIONS
Bovine colostrum may have immunostimulatory and antimicrobial actions. It is reputed to have ergogenic activity as well.

MECHANISM OF ACTION
Hyperimmune bovine colostrum may have antimicrobial activity based on the ability of specific immunoglobulins of the IgG type to react with bacterial, viral and other microbiological antigens in the gut. Bovine colostrum contains a few immunostimulatory substances, including lactoferrin. It may also contain colostrinin or proline-rich polypeptide (PRP), another possible immunomodulatory substance. The combination of specific, as well as nonspecific, IgGs and such immunomodulatory factors as lactoferrin and PRP may afford general antimicrobial protection of the gastrointestinal tract.

Bovine colostrum's putative exercise-performance-enhancment is mainly attributed to such growth factors as IGF-1.

PHARMACOKINETICS
The pharmacokinetics of bovine colostrum, particularly with regard to the immunoglobulins, is unclear. It would be expected that immunoglobulins found in bovine colostrum would be rapidly inactivated by stomach acid and proteolytic action in the small intestine. Enteric coating would protect the proteins from acid in the stomach but not from proteolytic activity in the small intestine. However, following ingestion of bovine colostrum, some immunoglobulins are found to be excreted intact in the feces after a few days.

This suggests that some immunoglobulins may be more resistant to degradation in the gut.

Growth factors and other peptides and proteins in bovine colostrum are most likely degraded by proteolytic enzymes and absorbed, distributed and metabolized in the same fashion as similar dietary substances.

INDICATIONS AND USAGE

Claims made for bovine colostrum are mostly unsubstantiated. Some preparations may have some antimicrobial effects. There is no credible evidence to support claims that bovine colostrum burns fat, builds muscle, speeds healing of injuries, regulates blood sugars, improves mood and fights depression or that it has anti-cancer effects.

RESEARCH SUMMARY

Well-designed, controlled clinical trials of bovine colostrum are largely lacking. A few small, usually uncontrolled or poorly controlled human studies have suggested that some components of some bovine colostrum preparations have significant antimicrobial activity. Immunoglobulins in colostrum derived from cows immunized against particular pathogens may help protect against those specific pathogens in some instances, but bovine colostrum supplements may vary widely in terms of specific constituents.

A bovine colostrum product derived from cows immunized against *Candida albicans* was reported to be effective in reducing levels of this fungal pathogen in severely immuno-compromised patients. Similarly, AIDS patients with chronic *Cryptosporidium parvum* diarrhea were said to be helped by a formulation of concentrated bovine immunoglobulins given in dosages up to 40 grams daily.

Some bovine colostrum preparations pooled from many different cows may confer broad-spectrum antimicrobial activity, some animal research suggests. Better, designed, controlled clinical testing is needed to determine the safety and efficacy of bovine colostrum supplements.

CONTRAINDICATIONS, PRECAUTIONS, ADVERSE REACTIONS

CONTRAINDICATIONS

Bovine colostrum is contraindicated in those with hypersensitivity to any component of bovine colostrum-containing products.

PRECAUTIONS

Pregnant women and nursing mothers should avoid bovine colostrum supplements.

Bovine colostrum contains insulin-like growth factor-1 (IGF-1). IGF-1 levels are elevated in prostate, colorectal and lung cancer. Recent studies have found that IGF-1 levels correlate with risk of prostate cancer and colorectal cancer in men, premenopausal breast cancer in women and lung cancer in both men and women. Those with these types of cancer and those at risk for these cancers should exercise caution in the use of bovine colostrum supplements. It is unlikely that the amount of IGF-1 in bovine colostrum would be a problem, but caution should still be exercised.

ADVERSE REACTIONS

Adverse reactions to bovine colostrum supplements are mainly gastrointestinal and include nausea and vomiting, bloating and diarrhea. Bovine colostrum is generally well tolerated.

DOSAGE AND ADMINISTRATION

Bovine colostrum is available in several forms, including tablets, powders, bars and liquid solutions. Dosage is variable. Hyperimmune bovine colostrum used for AIDS-associated diarrhea usually caused by *Cryptosporidium parvum* is dosed at 10 grams four times daily for 21 days. This must only be taken under medical supervision.

HOW SUPPLIED

Powder

Tablets — 1000 mg

LITERATURE

Bitzan MM, Gold BD, Philpott DJ, et al. Inhibition of Heliobacter pylori and Helicobacter mustelae binding to lipid receptors by bovine colostrum. *J Infect Dis.* 1998; 177:955-961.

Greenberg PD, Cello JP. Treatment of severe diarrhea caused by Crytosporidium parvum with oral bovine immunoglobulin concentrate in patients with AIDS. *J Acquir Immune Defic Syndr Hum Rretrovirol.* 1996; 13:348-354.

Huppertz HI, Rutkowski S, Busch DH, et al. Bovine colostrum ameliorates diarrhea in infection with diarrheagenic Escherichia coli, shiga toxin-producing E. coli, and E. coli expressing intimin and hemolysin. *J Pediatr Gastroenterol Nutr.* 1999; 29:452-456.

Lissner R, Thurmann PA, Merz G, Karch H. Antibody reactivity and fecal recovery of bovine immunoglobulins following oral administration of a colostrum concentrate from cows (Lactobin) to healthy volunteers. *Int J Clin Pharmacol Ther.* 1998; 36:239-245.

Merendino N, Prosperi S, Franci O, et al. Immunomodulatory activity of bovine colostrum on human peripheral blood mononuclear cells. *J Nutr Immunol.* 1996; 4:5-21.

Mero A, Miikkulainen H, Riski J, et al. Effects of bovine colostrum supplementation on serum IGF-1, IgG, hormone and saliva IgA during training. *J Appl Physiol.* 1997; 83: 1144-1151.

Playford RJ, Floyd DN, Macdonald CE, et al. Bovine colostrum is a health food supplement which prevents NSAID induced gut damage. *Gut.* 1999; 44:653-658.

Petschow BW, Talbott RD. Reduction in virus-neutralizing activity of a bovine colostrum immunoglobulin concentrate by gastric acid and digestive enzymes. *J Pediatr Gastroenterol Nutr.* 1994; 19:228-235.

Popik P, Bobula B, Janusz M, et al. Colostrinin, a polypeptide isolated from early milk, facilitates learning and memory in rats. *Pharmacol Biochem Behav.* 1999; 64:183-189.

Sarker SA, Caswall TH, Mahalanabis D, et al. Successful treatment of rotavirus diarrhea in children with immunoglobulin from immunized bovine colostrum. *Pediatr Infect Dis J.* 1998; 17:1149-1154.

Tacket CO, Binion SB, Bostwick E, et al. Efficacy of bovine milk immunoglobulin concentrate in preventing illness after Shigellla flexneri challenge. *Am J Trop Med Hyg.* 1992; 47:276-283.

Tacket CO, Losonsky G, Livio S, et al. Lack of prophylactic efficacy of an enteric-coated bovine hyperimmuune milk product against enterotoxigenic Escherichia coli challenge administered during a standard meal. *J Infect Dis.* 1999; 180:2056-2059.

Warny M, Fatimi A, Bostwick EF, et al. Bovine immunoglobulin concentrate-*Clostridium difficile* retains *C. difficile* toxin neutralizing activity after passage through the human stomach and small intestine. *Gut.* 1999; 44:212-217.

Branched-Chain Amino Acids (L-Leucine, L-Isoleucine, L-Valine)

TRADE NAMES

Hi-Test Muscle Octane BCAA's (Anabol Naturals), Hard Body BCAA (MLO Products).

DESCRIPTION

The branched-chain amino acids (BCAAs) comprise the three essential amino acids L-leucine, L-isoleucine and L-valine. These amino acids are found in proteins of all life forms. Dietary sources of the branched-chain amino acids are principally derived from animal and vegetable proteins. Vegetables and juices contain small amounts of the free amino acids, which are also found in fermented foods like yogurt and miso.

Several years ago the branched-chain amino acids created some interest in the neurological research community when a pilot study indicated that amyotrophic lateral sclerosis (ALS) patients showed symptomatic improvement when given large doses of BCAAs. It was theorized that BCAAs may protect against neuronal damage from the neuroexcitatory neurotransmitter glutamate. Based on this pilot study, branched-chain amino acids received orphan drug approval for the treatment of ALS. Unfortunately, most of the followup

studies were negative, and one even suggested that BCAAs may increase mortality in those with ALS.

Branched-chain amino acids are sometimes used in enteral and parenteral feedings in the management of hepatic encephalopathy. They are also occasionally used enterally and parenterally in the management of extensive burns and other severe trauma conditions because of their possible anticatabolic action in these conditions.

L-leucine is also known as 2-amino-4-methylvaleric acid, alpha-aminoisocaproic acid and (*S*)-2-amino-4-methylpentanoic acid. It is abbreviated as Leu or by its one letter abbreviation L. Its molecular formula is $C_6H_{13}NO_2$, and its molecular weight is 131.17 daltons. The structural formula is:

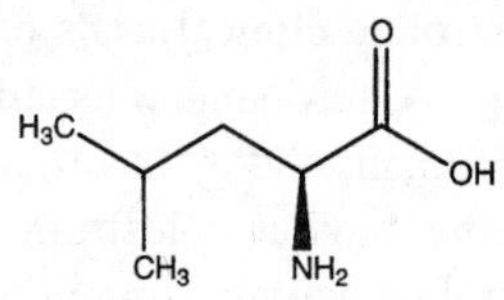

L-leucine

L-isoleucine is also known as 2-amino-3-methylvaleric acid, alpha-amino-beta-methylvaleric acid and (2*S*, 3*S*)-2-amino-3-methylpentanoic acid. It is abbreviated as Ile or by its one letter abbreviation I. Its molecular formula is $C_6H_{13}NO_2$, and its molecular weight is 131.17 daltons. The structural formula is:

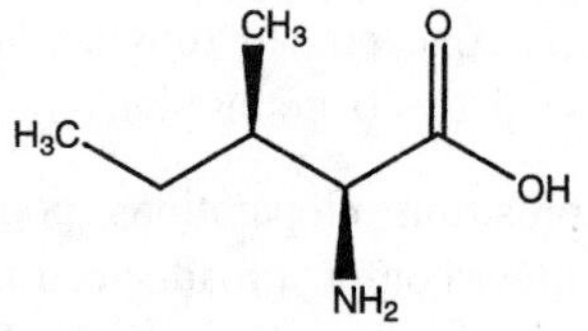

L-isoleucine

L-valine is also known as 2-aminoisovaleric acid, 2-amino-3-methylbutyric acid, alpha-aminoisovaleric acid and (*S*)-2-amino-3-methylbutanoic acid. It is abbreviated as Val, and its one letter abbreviation is V. Its molecular formula is $C_5H_{11}NO_2$, and its molecular weight is 117.15 daltons. The structural formula is:

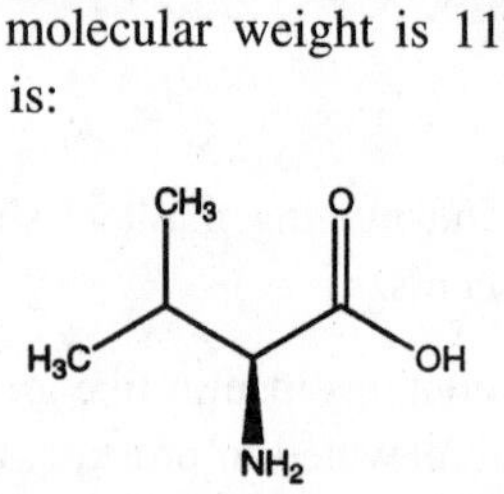

L-valine

The branched-chain amino acids are sometimes classified as large neutral amino acids or LNAAs.

ACTIONS AND PHARMACOLOGY

ACTIONS

The branched-chain amino acids may have antihepatic encephalopathy activity in some. They may also have anticatabolic and antitardive dyskinesia activity in some.

MECHANISM OF ACTION

It has been theorized that some of the symptoms of hepatic encephalopathy are due to the accumulation of false neurotransmitters in the brain resulting, in part, from alterations in plasma levels of BCAAs. BCAAs may improve encephalopathy symptoms in some by decreasing the accumulation of these false neurotransmitters and perhaps other substances involved in the encephalopathy. The pathogenesis of hepatic encephalopathy is very complex and still poorly understood.

Although amino acids are not considered important energy sources, BCAAs serve as important fuel sources for skeletal muscle during periods of metabolic stress. Under such conditions, BCAAs may promote protein synthesis, suppress protein catabolism and serve as substrates for gluconeogenesis. BCAAs are mainly catabolized in skeletal muscle, stimulating the production of, among other substances, L-alanine and L-glutamine.

The BCAAs' possible anti-tardive dyskinesia activity may be accounted for, in part, by decreasing the availability of L-phenylalanine in the brain.

PHARMACOKINETICS

Following ingestion, the BCAAs are absorbed from the small intestine by a sodium-dependent active-transport process and transported to the liver via the portal circulation. In the liver, the BCAAs can serve as substrates for protein synthesis. Some catabolism of the BCAAs occurs in the liver. The catabolism of L-leucine, L-isoleucine and L-valine initially involves the same three reactions: the conversion of the amino acids to their corresponding alpha-keto acids; the conversion of the alpha-keto acids to their corresponding acyl-CoA thioesters and carbon dioxide; and the conversion of the acyl-CoA thioesters to their corresponding alpha, beta-unsaturated acyl-CoA thioesters. The enzyme deficiency in the inborn error of metabolism maple syrup urine disease is in the conversion of the acyl-CoA thioesters to the alpha, beta-unsaturated acyl-CoA thioesters, via the enzyme branched-chain alpha-keto acid decarboxylase.

L-leucine, L-isoleucine and L-valine are catabolized differently starting from their corresponding acyl-CoA thioesters. L-leucine, which is a ketogenic amino acid, is converted via a number of metabolic steps to beta-hydroxy-beta-methyl-glutaryl-CoA, which in turn is converted to acetoacetic acid and acetyl-CoA. The B vitamin biotin participates in this pathway. L-isoleucine, which is both glycogenic and ketogenic, is converted via a number of metabolic steps to alpha-methyl-acetoacetyl-CoA, which in turn is converted to acetyl-CoA (ketogenic) and propionyl-CoA (glycogenic). Finally, the glycogenic L-valine is converted via a number of steps to methylmalonyl-CoA and then, with the assistance of vitamin B12, to succinyl-CoA.

The BCAAs are distributed to the various tissues of the body via the systemic circulation. The BCAAs appear to be preferentially taken up by skeletal muscle, where they undergo similar catabolic reactions to those described above. Skeletal muscle appears to be the major site of both BCAA transamination and oxidation in humans. BCAAs are also taken up by other organs, particularly the brain and kidney, where they also undergo oxidation.

INDICATIONS AND USAGE

BCAAs may be helpful in a minority of patients with hepatic encephalopathy. There is preliminary evidence that BCAAs may prevent muscle catabolism and promote protein synthesis in some trauma subjects and, possibly, in some exercises. There is no evidence that they are effective for enhancement of athletic performance. Neither have they proved useful in treating amotrophic lateral sclerosis (ALS). In one trial, BCAAs reduced symptoms of tardive dyskinesia. They have also been used with some benefit in some with phenylketonuria.

RESEARCH SUMMARY

Meta-analyses have produced conflicting and largely ambiguous results with respect to the role, if any, that BCAAs may play in the prevention or treatment of hepatic encephalopathy. One group of researchers concluded several years ago that BCAAs might be helpful in treating some with advanced cirrhosis who are intolerant to alimentary proteins. More recently, a consensus review written under the auspices of the European society for parenteral and enteral nutrition, similarly concluded that BCAAs might be indicated in that small number of patients intolerant to the supplementary dietary proteins needed to achieve nitrogen balance in this condition.

There is some preliminary evidence that BCAAs might help prevent muscle catabolism and promote protein synthesis in those with various forms of trauma. In one very small study, BCAAs were reported to inhibit protein breakdown in five men exercising the knee extensor muscles. Another very small study suggested that BCAAs might have inhibited muscle glycogen degradation during exercise.

On the other hand, there is no credible evidence that BCAAs have any significant effect on exercise performance. In a study of well-trained cyclists, BCAAs had no effect on performance in a 100-kilometer trial.

There were some early reports suggesting that BCAAs might help ameliorate some of the symptoms of amyotrophic lateral sclerosis (ALS). In one of these studies, ALS patients receiving 12 grams of L-leucine, 8 grams of L-isoleucine and 6.4 grams of L-valine daily for one year showed significant benefit, as measured by maintenance of muscle strength in extremities and walking ability. Those receiving placebo in this small study showed a linear decline in these parameters consistent with the normal course of this disease.

More recently, however, most studies have produced negative results with respect to BCAA use in ALS. In one double-blind, placebo-controlled trial on the safety and efficacy of BCAAs in the treatment of ALS, there was a significant excess mortality in subjects randomized to BCAAs versus placebo. This finding, coupled with lack of apparent BCAA efficacy, resulted in early termination of the study.

In a two-center, double-blind, placebo-controlled trial of BCAAs in ALS patients, six months of treatment failed to produce results better than placebo. In fact, treatment with BCAAs in this study was associated with increased loss of pulmonary function. Decline in forced vital capacity (FVC) was said to be 2.5 times greater than in subjects receiving placebo.

In one recent study, BCAAs significantly decreased symptoms of tardive dyskinesia in nine men who had used neuroleptics for prolonged periods.

In a preliminary study, adolescents and young adults with phenylketonuria were said to benefit from BCAA treatment over a period of several months. Those receiving BCAAs performed better on neuropsychologic tests than did unsupplemented controls. More research is needed.

CONTRAINDICATIONS, PRECAUTIONS, ADVERSE REACTIONS

CONTRAINDICATIONS
Branched-chain amino acids are contraindicated in those with the rare inborn errors of metabolism maple syrup urine disease and isovaleric acidemia. BCAAs are also contraindicated in those with hypersensitivity to any component of a BCAA-containing supplement.

PRECAUTIONS
Pregnant women and nursing mothers should avoid BCAA supplementation.

Treatment of hepatic encephalopathy, trauma and ALS or other diseases with BCAAs must only be done under qualified medical supervision.

Some recent research indicates that some ALS patients may get worse if treated with BCAAs.

ADVERSE REACTIONS
A recent study indicated increased mortality in ALS patients taking large doses of BCAAs.

OVERDOSAGE
No reports of overdosage.

DOSAGE AND ADMINISTRATION
Branched-chain amino acids are available for enteral and parenteral nutrition in the management of hepatic encephalopathy and metabolic stress conditions.

Nutritional supplements of BCAAs are available. Dosage is variable. Some combination BCAA products include other nutrients such as biotin and vitamin B12, which are involved in the metabolism of the BCAAs.

HOW SUPPLIED
Capsules

Powder

Tablets

LITERATURE
Abeta S, Inoue N, Matsui H, Yoshino Y. [Effect of branched-chain amino acids on glutamate neurotoxicity in primary cultured rat cerebral neurons.] [Article in Japanese.] *Rinsho Shinkeigaku.* 1995; 35:420-423.

Austic RE, Su C-L, Strupp BJ, Levitsky DA. Effects of dietary mixtures of amino acids on fetal growth and maternal and fetal amino acid pools in experimental maternal phenylketonuria. *Am J Clin Nutr.* 1999; 69:687-696.

Bastone A, Michel. A, Beghi E, Salmona M. The imbalance of brain large-chain amino acid availability in amyotrophic lateral sclerosis patients treated with high doses of branched-chain amino acids. *Neurochem Int.* 1995; 27:467-472.

Berry HK, Brunner RL, Hunt MM, White PP. Valine, isoleucine and leucine. A new treatment for phenylketonuria. *Am J Dis Child.* 1990; 144:539-543.

Fabbri A, Magrini N, Bianchi G, et al. Overview of randomized clinical trials of oral branched-chain amino acid treatment in chronic hepatic encephalopathy. *J Parenter Enteral Nutr. 1996; 20:159-164.*

MacLean DA, Graham TE, Saltin B. Stimulation of muscle ammonia production during exercise following branched-chain amino acid supplementation in humans. *J Physiol (Lond).* 1996; 493(Pt3):909-922.

Maddrey WC. Branched chain amino acid therapy in liver disease. *J Am Coll Nutr.* 1985; 4:639-650.

Madsen K, Maclean DA, Kiens B, Christensen D. Effects of glucose, glucose plus branched-chain amino acids, or placebo on bike performance over 100km. *J Appl Physiol.* 1996; 81:2644-2650.

Marchesini G, Bianchi G, Rossi B, et al. Nutritional treatment with branched-chain amino acids in advanced liver cirrhosis. *J Gastroenterol.* 2000; 35 Suppl 12:7-12.

Marchesini G, Zoli M, Dondi C, et al. Anticatabolic effect of branched-chain amino acid-enriched solutions with liver cirrhosis. *Hepatology.* 1982; 2:420-425.

Pelosi G, Proietti R, Magalini SI, et al. Anticatabolic properties of branched chain amino acids in trauma. *Resuscitation.* 1983; 10:153-158.

Plaitakis A, Smith J, Mandeli J, Yahr MD. Pilot trial of branched-chain amino acids in amyotrophic lateral sclerosis. *Lancet.* 1988; 1(8593):1015-1018.

Richardson MA, Bevans ML, Weber JB, et al. Branched chain amino acids decrease tardive dyskinesia symptoms. *Psychopharmacol.* 1999; 143:358-364.

Suryawan A, Hawes JW, Harris RA, et al. A molecular model of human branched-chain amino acid metabolism. *Am J Clin Nutr.* 1998; 68:72-81.

Tandan R, Bromberg MB, Forshew D, et al. A controlled trial of amino acid therapy in amyotropic lateral sclerosis: I. Clinical, functional, and maximum isometric torque data. *Neurology.* 1996; 47:1220-1226.

Testa D, Caraceni T, Fetoni V. Branched-chain amino acids in the treatment of amyotrophic lateral sclerosis. *J Neurol.* 1989; 236:445-447.

The Italian ALS Study Group. Branched-chain amino acids and amyotrophic sclerosis: a treatment failure? *Neurology.* 1993; 43:2466-2470.

Brewer's Yeast

DESCRIPTION

Brewer's yeast is derived from the unicellular fungus *Saccharomyces cerevisiae*, which causes the fermentation process basic to the brewing of beer. Different strains of this yeast are used in the production of the various types of beer. Still other strains are used in the fermentation of dough to produce bread. The strains of *Saccharomyces cerevisiae* that are used for the production of bread are collectively called baker's yeast.

Dried brewer's yeast is a rich source of several nutrients, including the B vitamins thiamin, riboflavin, niacin, pyridoxine, pantothenic acid, folate, vitamin B12 and biotin, and such trace minerals as chromium and selenium. It also contains beta-glucans (see Yeast Beta-Glucan), ribonucleic acid or RNA (see Nucleic Acids/Nucleotides), para-aminobenzoic acid and myo-inositol. A substance isolated from brewer's yeast called skin respiratory factor or SRF has found application in some cosmetic and wound-healing products, as well as in some hemorrhoidal preparations. The chemical identity of SRF is unknown.

Brewer's yeast has been a popular nutritional supplement for many years. Much of the brewer's yeast marketed for nutritional supplement use is grown specifically for that marketplace. The supplements are prepared from dry, crushed cells of *Saccharomyces cerevisiae*. The cells are not alive. There are other yeast preparations, such as *Saccharomyces boulardii*, in which the cells are alive; are used as probiotics. (See Probiotics.)

ACTIONS AND PHARMACOLOGY

ACTIONS

Brewer's yeast is a delivery form of the B vitamins and other nutrients, such as selenium and chromium. It is also a delivery form for beta-glucans and RNA. High-selenium brewer's yeast may have anticarcinogenic activity. High-chromium brewer's yeast has putative antidiabetic activity.

MECHANISM OF ACTION

High-selenium brewer's yeast given to deliver a daily dose of 200 micrograms of selenium was found to reduce the incidences of lung, prostate and colorectal cancer in one study. The mechanism of the possible anticarcinogenic activity is unclear. Selenium's antioxidant activity may account, in part, for its possible anticarcinogenic activity. (See Selenium.) The beta-glucans in yeast may also account, in part, for the possible anticarcinogenic activity via their possible immune-modulating activity. (See Yeast Beta-Glucan.)

High-chromium use has been found in a few, but not all, studies to improve glucose tolerance in those with hyperglycemia and in some with type 2 diabetes mellitus. Earlier, it was proposed that chromium acted via a so-called glucose tolerance factor, or GTF, in brewer's yeast. The chemical identity of this putative GTF has not been established. The mechanism of the putative antidiabetic effect of high-chromium yeast is unknown. (See Chromium.) RNA may also have immunomodulatory activity. (See Nucleic Acids/Nucleotides.)

PHARMACOKINETICS

See the various monographs on the B vitamins, as well as Selenium, Chromium, Yeast Beta-Glucan and Nucleic Acids and Derivatives, for pharmacokinetic information on these substances.

INDICATIONS AND USAGE

Claims that brewer's yeast is useful for diarrhea, acne, furunculosis, colds, coughs, dyspepsia, inflammatory conditions and various infections have little or no credible support.

Some have confused the brewer's yeast that is typically sold as a supplement with *Saccharomyces boulardii*, a probiotic (see Probiotics) that has demonstrated some of the benefits erroneously attributed to brewer's yeast, at least in very preliminary research. There is some suggestion that high-selenium brewer's yeast may have some anticarcinogenic effects and that high-chromium yeast might be helpful in some with type 2 diabetes.

RESEARCH SUMMARY

Supplementation with selenium-enriched brewer's yeast (delivering 200 micrograms of selenium a day) over a period of several years was associated, in one study, with significant reduction in the incidence of lung, colorectal, prostate and total cancer, as well as a reduction in total cancer mortality. It is not known with certainty which components in selenium-enriched brewer's yeast may exert anti-cancer effects. One recent animal study found that DL-selenomethionine lacked chemopreventive efficacy in colon carcinogenesis. (See Selenium.)

Some studies have shown that high-chromium brewer's yeast can improve glucose tolerance in some with type 2 diabetes. These results, however, are inconsistent. In one placebo-controlled study of elderly subjects with stable impaired glucose tolerance, chromium-rich yeast had no significant effects on glucose tolerance or serum lipids, compared with controls. In another study, brewer's yeast improved glucose tolerance and had beneficial effects on lipids in Chinese adults. More study is needed.

CONTRAINDICATIONS, PRECAUTIONS, ADVERSE REACTIONS

CONTRAINDICATIONS

Brewer's yeast is contraindicated in those hypersensitive to any component of a brewer's yeast containing-product. It is also contraindicated in those taking monoamine oxidase inhibitors.

PRECAUTIONS

Pregnant women and nursing mothers should avoid brewer's yeast supplements pending long-term safety studies.

ADVERSE REACTIONS

Brewer's yeast is generally well tolerated. Occasional allergic reactions have been reported. Some may develop flatulence when taking brewer's yeast. Some do not like the bitter taste.

INTERACTIONS

DRUGS

Monoamine oxidase (MAO) inhibitors: including phenelzine sulfate, tranylcypromine sulfate and pargyline HCl. Concomitant use of brewer's yeast and MAO inhibitors may cause hypertension.

OVERDOSAGE

No reports of overdosage.

DOSAGE AND ADMINISTRATION

Brewer's yeast is available as flakes, powder, tablets and capsules. These preparations are prepared from dried, crushed cells of *Saccharomyces cerevisiae*. Dosage is variable. Some marketed chromium and selenium preparations are derived from chromium-rich and selenium-rich baker's yeast, respectively. (See Chromium and Selenium.)

HOW SUPPLIED

Powder

Tablets — 486 mg, 500 mg

LITERATURE

See Chromium, Selenium, Yeast Beta-Glucan and Nucleic Acids/Nucleotides.

Also:

Clark LC, Combs GF Jr, Turnball BW, et al. Effects of selenium supplementation for cancer prevention in patients with carcinoma of the skin. A randomized controlled trial. Nutritional Prevention of Cancer Study Group. *JAMA.* 1996; 276:1957-1963.

Guan X, Matte JJ, Ku PK, et al. High chromium yeast supplementation improves glucose tolerance in pigs by decreasing hepatic extraction of insulin. *J Nutr.* 2000; 130:1274-1279.

Li YC. Effects of brewer's yeast on glucose tolerance and serum lipids in Chinese adults. *Biol Trace Elem Res.* 1994; 41:341-347.

Bromelain

TRADE NAMES

Bromanase (Kramer-Novis), Bromelain 2400 Maximum Strength (Vitaline Corp.).

DESCRIPTION

Bromelain is the collective term for enzymes (principally proteolytic enzymes) derived from the ripe and unripe fruit, as well as the stem and leaves, of the pineapple plant, *Ananas comosus*, a member of the Bromeliaceae family. Commercial bromelain is typically stem bromelain. Bromelain is mainly comprised of cysteine proteases, with smaller amounts of acid phosphatase, peroxidase, amylase and cellulase. Bromelain contains at least four distinct cysteine proteases. The principal stem protease is called stem bromelain or stem bromelain protease. Two additional proteases found in the stem are called ananain and comosain. Fruit bromelain is the name given to the principal protease found in the fruit. Stem protease is a basic glycoprotein with a molecular weight of 28,000 daltons.

Pineapple has been used as a folk medicine by the natives of the tropics for centuries. It has been used as a digestive aid, as a cleansing agent to improve the texture of the skin, and to promote the healing of wounds. It is used commercially in certain cosmetics and as a meat tenderizer and dietary supplement. Bromelain may have digestant activity and there is research suggesting that it may have wound healing, anti-inflammatory, antidiarrheal and anticarcinogenic effects, as well.

The activity of bromelain may be expressed in six different ways: Rorer units, FIP units, BTU (bromelain tyrosine units), CDU (casein digestion units), GDU (gelatin digestion units) or MCU (milk clotting units).

The most commonly used measures of activity are MCU or GDU. One GDU is equivalent to about 1.5 MCU.

An interesting aside, is that pineapple workers often have their fingerprints almost completely obliterated due to the proteolytic action of bromelain.

ACTIONS AND PHARMACOLOGY
ACTIONS
Bromelain may have digestant activity and has putative anti-inflammatory, immunomodulatory, antidiarrheal, anticarcinogenic and wound healing actions.

MECHANISM OF ACTION
Bromelain's digestant activity is based on its ability to hydrolyze proteins to oligopeptides and amino acids. Bromelain's proteolytic enzymes are cysteine proteases. Cysteine proteases cleave peptide bonds by nucleophilic attack via active-site cysteine residues. Other members of the cysteine protease family, include calpains and caspases.

The mechanism of the putative anti-inflammatory activity is not well understood. It may be accounted for, in part, by activation of plasmin production from plasminogen and reduction of kinin, via inhibition of the conversion of kininogen to kinin. Other possibilities, include proteolytic degradation of circulating immune complexes and inhibition of signaling by extracellular regulated kinase (ERK)-2 and p21^{ras}. It is speculated that the possible protective effect of bromelain in murine EAE (experimental allergic encephalomyelitis), the animal model of multiple sclerosis, is due to proteolytic cleavage of accessory molecules involved in the interaction of T lymphocytes and antigen presenting cells, thus increasing the activation threshold of the autoreactive T lymphocytes.

The mechanism of bromelain's putative immunomodulatory activity is likewise poorly understood. Bromelain has been shown to increase CD2-mediated T cell activation, to enhance antigen-independent binding to monocytes and to increase interferon (IFN)-gamma-dependent, tumor necrosis factor (TNF)-alpha, interleukin(IL)-1 beta, and interleukin(IL)-6 production in peripheral blood monocytes. These effects are thought to be due to bromelain's proteolytic activity at cell surfaces, whereby it either removes surface molecules or reveals ones that already exist on cell membranes, thereby altering receptor-ligand interactions. Recent studies have reported that bromelain proteolytically blocks activation of extracellular regulated kinase(ERK)-2 in T cells, resulting in inhibition of T cell signal transduction.

Bromelain has been found to reduce the incidence of enterotoxigenic *Escherichia coli* diarrhea in piglets. This effect is thought to be due to inactivation of enterotoxigenic *E. coli* receptors in the small intestine via proteolytic cleavage of the glycoprotein receptor.

The putative anticarcinogenic activity of bromelain is open to speculation. Possibilities include disruption of adhesion molecules on tumor and endothelial cells via its proteolytic activity and inhibition of signaling by ERK-2 and p21^{ras}. It has also been speculated that bromelain may play a role in the differentiation of malignant cells. Certain cysteine proteases (e.g., caspases) are involved in apoptosis. Were bromelain to enter cancer cells, one may speculate that it could induce apoptosis. On the other hand, bromelain entering normal cells does not appear to be desirable.

The putative wound healing activity of bromelain may be accounted for by its possible anti-inflammatory activity.

PHARMACOKINETICS
The pharmacokinetics of bromelain in humans are mostly unknown. Bromelain is active under a wide pH range (between pH3-10) and may not be inactivated by stomach acid. The putative anti-inflammatory, immunomodulatory and anticarcinogenic actions of bromelain most likely require that it gets absorbed from the intestine. It is conceivable that unabsorbed bromelain may mediate some of these possible effects via a signal transduction mechanism. However, this is entirely speculative. There is some evidence from tissue culture studies that bromelain may be able to enter cells and some bromelain may be absorbed via the enteropancreatic circulation. Research is very much needed on the pharmacokinetics of bromelain.

INDICATIONS AND USAGE
There is some evidence that bromelain may be useful in speeding the healing time of some injuries and surgical wounds, that it is a digestive aid in some conditions, that it inhibits platelet aggregation and is helpful in some with thromboses and angina, that it has positive effects in some respiratory tract diseases, dysmenorrhea and some forms of diarrhea. It has also exhibited some immune-enhancing and anticancer effects.

RESEARCH SUMMARY

Bromelain has been shown to speed healing time and reduce pain following various surgical procedures, including oral surgical procedures and episiotomy. It has also been used with significant positive results in the treatment of various athletic injuries. In one open case observation study, high-dose bromelain was administered to 59 patients with blunt injuries to the musculoskeletal system. A clear reduction in swelling, pain at rest and during movement and in tenderness was reported. Positive bromelain studies related to oral surgery and episiotomy have been double-blind and placebo-controlled. Positive effects have been attributed by some to anti-inflammatory activity, rather than to an analgesic effect.

Bromelain has been used with some success as a substitute for trypsin and pepsin in cases of pancreatic insufficiency and post-pancreatectomy.

In vitro and *in vivo* studies show some bromelain-induced inhibition of platelet aggregation, and some positive bromelain-related effects have been reported in patients with thromboses and angina. In one double-blind study of 73 patients with acute thrombophlebitis, bromelain, used with analgesics, reduced pain, edema, redness, tenderness, elevated skin temperature and disability. The effective doses ranged between 60-160 milligrams daily of 1,200 MCU bromelain.

Bromelain's reported mucolytic activity has prompted some use of it in respiratory tract diseases. It has shown some benefit in chronic bronchitis and, in a double-blind study, in acute sinusitis.

Bromelain's reported efficacy (in combination with papain) in easing dysmenorrhea symptoms has been attributed to a smooth-muscle-relaxant effect since it has been observed to decrease spasms of contracted cervixes in these patients. Some hypothesize that muscle-relaxing effects of bromelain on the uterus are due to modulation of various prostaglandins.

In animal models, bromelain has shown significant antidiarrheal activity. In these experiments, bromelain inhibited activity of enterotoxigenic *Escherichia coli* and *Vibrio cholerae*. It significantly reduced heat-stable and heat-labile enterotoxin-induced secretion, among other effects.

In the realm of immunity, bromelain is being tested for possible effects in T cell-mediated autoimmune diseases, including multiple sclerosis, type 1 diabetes and rheumatoid arthritis. In combination with trypsin and the flavonoid rutin, bromelain has been reported to protect against experimental allergic encephalomyelitis. This research is ongoing.

Bromelain has recently shown an ability to decrease lung metastases of Lewis lung cancer cells in mice. In another recent study, oral bromelain was administered to 16 breast cancer patients for ten days. The results of this study suggested that bromelain stimulated deficient monocyte cytotoxicity of mammary tumor patients. More research is needed.

CONTRAINDICATIONS, PRECAUTIONS, ADVERSE REACTIONS

CONTRAINDICATIONS

Bromelain is contraindicated in those hypersensitive to any component of a bromelain-containing product.

PRECAUTIONS

Bromelain supplements should be avoided by pregnant women and nursing mothers.

The use of bromelain for the treatment of any disorder must be medically supervised. The use of bromelain for the treatment of diarrhea caused by enteropathogenic *E. coli*, cancer or any inflammatory disorder is experimental.

Those on anticoagulants or antithrombotic agents should exercise caution in the use of bromelain. Bromelain may have blood-thinning activity in some.

ADVERSE REACTIONS

Gastrointestinal symptoms such as nausea and vomiting, diarrhea and cramping have been reported. There are occasional reports of metrorrhagia and menorrhagia.

INTERACTIONS

DRUGS

Antibiotics (amoxicillin, tetracycline): Concomitant use of bromelain and amoxicillin or tetracycline have been reported to increase the serum levels of these antibiotics.

Anticoagulants (e.g., warfarin): Bromelain may enhance the anticoagulant activity of such drugs as warfarin.

Antithrombotic agents (e.g., aspirin): Bromelain may enhance the antithrombotic activity of such drugs as aspirin.

OVERDOSAGE

There are no reports of bromelain overdosage in the literature.

DOSAGE AND ADMINISTRATION

Bromelain is available as a single ingredient product or in combination with other supplementary enzymes (see Supplementary Enzymes). Dosage ranges from 500-2,000 GDUs (gelatin digestion units) taken one to three times daily.

HOW SUPPLIED

Tablets — 100 mg, 250 mg, 500 mg

LITERATURE

Batkin S, Taussig SJ, Szekerezes J. Antimetastatic effect of bromelain with or without its proteolytic and anticoagulant activity. *J Cancer Res Clin Oncol.* 1988; 114:507-508.

Bock U, Kolac C, Borchard G, et al. Transport of proteolytic enzymes across Caco-2 cell monolayers. *Pharm Res.* 1998; 15:1393-1400.

Chandler DS, Mynott TL. Bromelain protects piglets from diarrhea caused by oral challenge with K88 positive enterotoxigenic Escherichia coli. *Gut.* 1998; 43:196-202.

Eckert K, Grabowska E, Strange R, et al. Effects of oral bromelain administration on the Impaired immunocytotoxicity of mononuclear cells from mammary tumor patients. *Oncol Rep.* 1999; 6:1191-1199.

Kumakura S, Yamashita M, Tsurufuji S. Effect of bromelain on kaolin-induced inflammation in rats. *Eur J Pharmacol.* 1988; 150:295-301.

Masson M. [Bromelain in blunt injuries of the locomotor system. A study of observed applications in general practice]. [Article in German]. *Fortschr Med.* 1995; 113:303-306.

Metzig C, Grabowska E, Eckert K, et al. Bromelain proteases reduce human platelet aggregation in vitro, adhesion to bovine endothelial cells and thrombus formation in rat vessels in vivo. *In Vivo.* 1999; 13:7-12.

Munzig E, Eckert K, Harrach T, et al. Bromelain protease F9 reduces the CD44 mediated adhesion of human peripheral blood lymphocytes to human umbilical vein endothelial cells. *FEBS Lett.* 1994; 351:215-218.

Mynott TL, Guandalini S, Raimondi F, Fasano A. Bromelain prevents secretion caused by Vibrio cholerae and Escherichia coli enterotoxins in rabbit ileum in vitro. *Gastroenterology.* 1997; 113:175-184.

Mynott TL, Ladhams A, Scarmato P, Engwerda CR. Bromelain from pineapple stems, proteolytically blocks activation of extracellular regulated kinase-2 in T cells. *J Immunol.* 1999; 163:2568-2575.

Rowan AD, Butte DJ, Barrett AJ. The cysteine proteinases of the pineapple plant. *Biochem J.* 1990; 266:869-875.

Targoni OS, Tary-Lehmann M, Lehmann PV. Prevention of murine EAE by oral hydrolytic enzyme treatment. *J Autoimmun.* 1999; 12:191-198.

Taussig SJ, Batkin S. Bromelain, the enzyme complex of pineapple (*Ananas comosus*) and its clinical application. *J Ethnopharmcol.* 1988; 22:191-203.

Bromine (Bromide)

DESCRIPTION

Bromine belongs to the halogen group of elements. Its atomic number is 35 and its symbol is Br. Bromine is a readily volatile, dark-reddish-brown liquid with a strong, disagreeable odor (*bromos* in Greek means stench) and an irritating effect on the eyes and throat. It is the only non-metallic element that is liquid under ordinary conditions. Many of the compounds of bromine are salts or bromides.

Halogen comes from the Greek word meaning salt-producer. Bromine occurs in the form of salts in sea and ocean water, mineral springs and natural salt deposits.

Bromine is not considered an essential nutrient for humans. A bromine-deficiency state has been reported in goats. Goats fed diets low in bromide were found to have depressed growth, fertility and life expectancy. Also observed in these animals were decreased red-blood-cell count, increased milk fat and a greater number of spontaneous abortions. Dietary bromide has also been found to alleviate growth retardation caused by hyperthyroidism in mice and chicks and to substitute for part of the chloride requirement for chicks. Insomnia in some hemodialysis patients has been associated with bromide deficiency.

Bromide is the fifth most abundant inorganic anion in human plasma and tissues, following chloride, bicarbonate, phosphate and sulfate. In plasma, it is present at a concentration of 20-150 micromolar.

Bromine may play a role in the respiratory burst of eosinophils. Eosinophils play a central role in host defenses against helminthic parasites and other large invading metazoan pathogens, and possibly against some cancers. This is in contrast to neutrophils, which primarily ingest and kill relatively small microbes Eosinophil peroxidase catalyzes the oxidation of bromide to hypobromous acid and hypobromite, which may participate in the killing role of eosinophils.There is some evidence that this may occur by oxidative damage to proteins through bromination of tyrosine residues. Brominating oxidants may also participate in allergen-induced asthma.

Daily dietary intake of bromide is about 2 to 8 milligrams. Fish, grains and nuts are rich sources of bromide.

Potassium bromide had been used as a sedative drug in the United States and is still occasionally used as a sedative and anticonvulsant in Europe. Prolonged intake of potassium bromide can lead to bromide intoxication or bromism. Bromo-Seltzer does not contain bromine. Bromides are used in some homeopathic remedies such as kali bromatum.

The terms bromine and bromide are sometimes used interchangeably. Bromine is usually found as its bromide form.

ACTIONS AND PHARMACOLOGY

ACTIONS

None known for dietary bromine.

INDICATIONS AND USAGE

There are no indications for the supplemental use of bromine (bromide).

RESEARCH SUMMARY

An association has been made between insomnia experienced by some hemodialysis patients and bromide deficiency. This warrants followup.

CONTRAINDICATIONS, PRECAUTIONS, ADVERSE REACTIONS

CONTRAINDICATIONS

None known.

PRECAUTIONS

Given our present state of knowledge regarding bromine, supplemental bromide is not recommended for anyone.

ADVERSE REACTIONS

Use of potassium bromide as a sedative drug may give rise to bromide intoxication or bromism. Symptoms include nausea, vomiting, slurred speech, memory impairment, drowsiness, irritability, ataxia, tremors, hallucinations, mania, delirium, psychoses, stupor and coma. Skin rashes of various types may occur, and toxic epidermal necrolysis has been reported.

OVERDOSAGE

Death after acute bromide poisoning is rare since vomiting follows the ingestion of large doses of potassium bromide. Ingestion of large doses of potassium bromide can lead to severe central nervous system depression, including coma.

DOSAGE AND ADMINISTRATION

No recommended dosage. Bromine as bromide may be found in colloidal or liquid mineral preparations and in some homeopathic remedies.

LITERATURE

Nielsen FH. Other trace elements. In: Ziegler EE, Filer LL Jr, eds. *Present Knowledge in Nutrition.* 7th ed. Washington, DC: ILSI Press; 1996:353-377.

Nielsen FH. Ultratrace minerals. In: Shils ME, Olson JA, Shike M, Ross AC, eds. *Modern Nutrition in Health and Disease.* 9th ed. Baltimore MD: Williams and Wilkins; 1999:283-303.

Thomas EL, Bozeman PM, Jefferson MM, King CC. Oxidation of bromide by the human leukocyte enzymes myeloperoxidase and eosinophil peroxidase. *J Biol Chem.* 1995; 270;2906-2913.

Wu W, Samoszuk MK, Comhair SAA, et al. Eosinophils generate brominating oxidants in allergen-induced asthma. *J Clin Invest.* 2000; 105:1455-1463.

Calcium

TRADE NAMES

Oyster Shell Calcium (Numerous manufacturers), Calci-Mix (R&D Laboratories), Liqui-Cal (Advanced Nutritional Technology), Tums (SmithKline Beecham Consumer), Mylanta Calci Tabs (J & J/Merck Consumer), Os-Cal (SmithKline Beecham Consumer), Gal-Gest (Rugby Labs), Calci-Chew (R&D Laboratories), Caltrate 600 (Lederle Consumer), Calcarb 600 (Zenith Goldline), Cal-Citrate (Bio-Tech Pharmacal), Cal-C-Caps (The Key Company), Citracal (Mission Pharmacal), Neo-Calglucon (Novartis Pharmaceutical), Calcionate (Rugby Labs), Calfort (Ampharco Inc.), Calbon (Economed Pharmaceuticals), Ridactate (R.I.D. Inc.), Posture (Inverness Medical).

DESCRIPTION

Calcium is an essential mineral with a wide range of biological roles. Apart from being a major constituent of bones and teeth, calcium is crucial for muscle contraction, nerve conduction, the beating of the heart, blood coagulation, glandular secretion, the production of energy and the maintenance of immune function, among other things. Calcium is an alkaline-earth metal with atomic number 20 and an atomic mass of 40.08 daltons. Its atomic symbol is Ca.

Calcium is found in bone and teeth primarily in the form of the calcium phosphate compound hydroxyapatite. The molecular formula of hydroxyapatite is $Ca_{10}(PO_4)_6(OH)_2$. Over 99% of the total body calcium is found in bone and teeth, and calcium makes up from 1% to 2% of adult body weight.

Milk products are the most calcium-dense foods. Other foods rich in calcium include the vegetables collard greens, Chinese cabbage, mustard greens, broccoli and bok choy, as well as tofu and sardines with bones included. About 25% of women in the United States take calcium supplements. The average intake of calcium in the American diet is approximately 800 milligrams daily. Calcium intake is typically higher in males than it is in females.

ACTIONS AND PHARMACOLOGY

ACTIONS

Calcium has anti-osteoporotic activity. It may also have anticarcinogenic, antihypertensive and hypocholesterolemic activity.

MECHANISM OF ACTION

Inadequate calcium intake results in reduced bone mass and osteoporosis. Calcium exists in bone primarily in the form of hydroxyapatite $(Ca_{10}(PO_4)_6(OH)_2)$. Hydroxyapatite comprises approximately 40% of the weight of bone. The skeleton has an obvious structural requirement for calcium. The skeleton also serves as a reservoir for calcium.

A number of studies suggest that calcium may reduce the risk of colorectal cancer. Calcium supplementation has been found to reduce colonic mucosal proliferation. Greater colonic mucosal proliferation is observed in those at high risk for colon cancer when compared with those at low risk. Calcium ions may precipitate bile acids and fatty acids that can stimulate the proliferation of colon cells.

Calcium supplementation has been found to have a modest effect on the reduction of systolic blood pressure in those with hypertension. Diastolic blood pressure does not appear to be affected by calcium, and calcium does not affect blood pressure in normotensives. The mechanism of the possible systolic blood pressure-lowering effect of supplemental calcium is unclear.

Some, but not all, studies have found supplemental calcium to lower serum cholesterol levels. A mechanism of this possible effect may be the binding of calcium ions with bile acids to form insoluble soaps, thus removing cholesterol entering the gut via the enterohepatic circulation.

PHARMACOKINETICS

Calcium is absorbed from the small intestine by both active and passive mechanisms. At low and moderate intakes of calcium, calcium is absorbed via active transfer. Active transfer depends on the action of the active form of vitamin D,1,25-dihydroxycholecalciferol or $1,25(OH)_2D_3$. Vitamin D-induced calcium transport involves the synthesis of the calcium-binding protein, calbindin. Calbindin serves as a calcium translocator. It also serves as a cytosolic calcium buffer. Calcium is typically freed from calcium complexes during digestion and is released in a soluble and probably ionized form for absorption. Low molecular weight complexes, such as calcium carbonate, may be absorbed intact.

As calcium intakes increase, the active transfer mechanism becomes saturated and an increasing proportion of calcium is absorbed via passive diffusion.

The absorption efficiency of calcium varies throughout the life span. It is highest during infancy when it is about 60%. In prepubertal children, it is about 28%. During early puberty, at the time of the growth spurt, it increases to about 34% and then drops to 25% two years later where it remains for several years. Absorption efficacy increases during the last two trimesters of pregnancy. It does decline with aging. In postmenopausal women, fractional absorption of calcium declines on the average of 0.21% yearly. Men lose absorption efficiency at about the same rate as women.

Absorption efficiency appears to vary with the different calcium complexes. In one study, absorption efficiency from a 250 milligram dose of calcium citrate malate was found to be 35%; from calcium carbonate, 27%; and from tricalcium phosphate, 25%. For comparison, calcium absorption efficiency from milk was found to be 29%. Some, but not all, studies suggest that calcium is more efficiently absorbed from calcium citrate and calcium citrate malate than it is from calcium carbonate. The efficiency of absorption of calcium from a calcium supplement is greatest when calcium is taken at doses of 500 milligrams or lower. Individuals with achlorhydria absorb calcium from calcium carbonate poorly unless the calcium carbonate supplement is taken with food.

Calcium that is unabsorbed from the intestine is excreted in the feces. Greater than 98% of calcium from the glomerular filtrate is reabsorbed. Renal reabsorption is primarily regulated by parathyroid hormone or PTH.

The colon plays an important role in calcium absorption after resection of the small intestine.

Approximately 40% of calcium in the plasma is bound to proteins, primarily albumin; about 50% of calcium in the plasma is diffusible ionic calcium and about 10% is diffusible, but is complexed with such anions as phosphate and citrate.

INDICATIONS AND USAGE

Calcium is useful in preventing and treating osteoporosis. It may also be effective in reducing the risk of colorectal cancer. It may be of benefit in some with hypertension and may diminish some of the symptoms of premenstrual syndrome (PMS). Results are mixed and weak with respect to claims that calcium has favorable effects on lipids. An association has been made between higher intakes of calcium and lower incidence of stroke among women. A recent preliminary study has suggested that calcium may help reduce the risk of obesity.

RESEARCH SUMMARY

In a review of 52 intervention trials investigating calcium's effects on osteoporosis, all but two were said to have shown beneficial effects, including better bone balance, greater bone gain during growth, reduced bone loss in the elderly and reduced risk of fracture. Observational studies have also, for the most part, associated higher calcium intake with enhanced bone health. Most of the intervention trials utilized calcium supplements; some used dairy products as the source of calcium. Most of these studies reported that high calcium intake augmented the osteoprotective effects of estrogen.

Some recent studies have suggested that calcium citrate is better absorbed than calcium carbonate and that the citrate form might thus be more effective in helping to prevent or ameliorate osteoporosis. An analysis of 15 randomized trials concluded that calcium citrate was absorbed 22% to 27% better than calcium carbonate, whether taken on an empty stomach or with food. More research will be needed, however, to demonstrate conclusively that calcium citrate is more beneficial than calcium carbonate in osteoporosis.

Calcium has shown benefit in individuals who have lost bone mineral density due to long term corticosteroid therapy. In a double-blind, placebo-controlled study of subjects with rheumatoid arthritis, many of whom were being treated with corticosteroids, a combination of 1,000 milligrams of calcium carbonate and 500 IUs of vitamin D₃ daily was found to confer significant benefits. While subjects receiving placebo and prednisone lost bone mineral density in the lumbar spine and trochanter at a rate of 2% and 0.9%, respectively, per year, those getting prednisone and calcium gained bone mineral density in the lumbar spine and trochanter at a rate of 0.72% and 0.85% per year, respectively. No calcium-related improvements were seen, however, at any site in subjects who did not receive corticosteroids.

An inverse relationship has been noted in epidemiological studies between colon cancer incidence and calcium intake. In the four-year, multicenter Calcium Polyp Prevention study, calcium supplementation was associated with a significant reduction in the risk of recurrent colorectal adenomas. This double-blind, randomized trial enrolled 930 subjects with a history of colorectal adenomas. Mean age was 61, and 72% of the subjects were men. Calcium was supplied in the carbonate form in a dose of 1,200 milligrams of elemental calcium daily. Follow-up continued for four years after initial examination.

Some other intervention trials, as well as several experimental studies, have provided further support for calcium benefit in modulating the rate of human colon cell proliferation and reducing the rate of colonic adematous polyps. It should be noted, however, that while many positive significant results have been reported, reduction in ademona incidence has generally been modest in these studies.

There is some preliminary evidence that calcium supplementation may help some with PMS. A pilot study suggested that calcium might diminish some PMS symptoms. Subsequently, a placebo-controlled, multicenter study produced results showing that calcium-supplemented women had an overall reduction of 48% in severity of PMS symptoms, compared with a 30% reduction in those on placebo. Those in the calcium group reported a 54% reduction in aches and pains, compared with a 15% increase in pains reported by the placebo group. One of the researchers has speculated that women with PMS may have a functional hypocalcemia in which urine and blood levels of calcium are normal—but only because abnormally high levels of parathyroid hormone constantly extract calcium from bone. More research is needed.

In a recent, randomized, double-blind, placebo-controlled study of the effects of calcium supplementation on serum cholesterol and blood pressure in 193 men and women aged 30 to 74 years, treatment with 1 and 2 grams daily of calcium for four months conferred no significant benefits, compared with placebo. No significant effects were seen with respect to blood pressure, total or HDL-cholesterol levels. In some earlier trials, however, some modest hypocholesterolemic

effects were observed. And in an analysis of 14 studies, calcium supplementation in women (1.5 to 2 grams daily) was associated with a reduction of 5.40 mmHg in systolic blood pressure and a reduction of 3.44 mmHg in diastolic blood pressure, compared with controls. Some associated but inconclusive reduction in the incidence of preterm delivery, cesarean delivery, intrauterine growth retardation, perinatal death and preeclampsia has been reported.

In the ongoing Nurse's Health Study, with 86,000 participants, supplementary intake of 400 or more milligrams daily of calcium has been associated with a significantly reduced risk of stroke among women. Supplementary intakes higher than 600 milligrams daily did not appear to confer further benefit. Authors of the study hypothesized that a possible hypocholesterolemic effect or some anti-clotting mechanism might account for the protective association observed in this population. Magnesium and potassium intakes were not associated with reduced risk of stroke in this study, although they have been thus associated in some other studies.

One group of researchers has recently reported that increasing the dietary calcium of obese subjects for one year produced a 4.9 kilogram loss of body fat. Experiments in mice showed that high calcium diets could reduce weight gain and foot pad mass by 26% to 39%. The same researchers examined epidemiological data in which they found a significant association between higher levels of body fat and lower intake of calcium. They concluded that "increasing dietary calcium suppresses adipocyte intracellular calcium and thereby modulates energy metabolism and attenuates obesity risk."

Prior laboratory research has shown that increased adipocyte intracellular calcium produces both stimulation of lipogenesis and inhibition of lipolysis. The high-calcium diets used in the studies of mice produced a 51% inhibition of adipocyte fatty acid synthase expression and activity and a 3.4- to 5.2-fold increase in lipolysis. More research is warranted.

CONTRAINDICATIONS, PRECAUTIONS, ADVERSE REACTIONS
CONTRAINDICATIONS
Calcium supplementation is contraindicated in those with hypercalcemia. Conditions causing hypercalcemia include sarcoidosis, hyperparathyroidism, hypervitaminosis D and cancer.

Calcium supplementation is contraindicated in those hypersensitive to any component of a calcium-containing supplement.

PRECAUTIONS
Supplemental calcium taken without food may increase the risk of kidney stones in women and possibly also in men. It is thought that taking supplemental calcium without food

limits the opportunity for the beneficial effect that calcium may have in binding oxalate in the intestine. Therefore, it is advisable that supplemental calcium be taken with food.

Those who form calcium-containing kidney stones are generally advised not to take supplemental calcium.

Those with achlorhydria should take calcium carbonate with food.

ADVERSE REACTIONS

Calcium supplements are generally well tolerated. Use of calcium carbonate may cause such gastrointestinal side reactions as constipation, bloating, gas and flatulence. Prolonged use of large doses of calcium carbonate—greater than 12 grams daily (about 5 grams of elemental calcium)—may lead to the milk-alkali syndrome, nephrocalcinosis and renal insufficiency.

INTERACTIONS

DRUGS

Biphosphonates (alendronate, etidronate, risedronate): Concomitant intake of a bisphosphonate and calcium may decrease the absorption of the bisphosphonate.

H_2 blockers (cimetidine, famotidine, mizatidine, ranitidine): Concomitant use of H_2 blockers and calcium carbonate or calcium phosphate can cause decreased absorption of these calcium salts.

Levothyroxine: Concomitant intake of levothyroxine and calcium carbonate was found to reduce levothyroxine absorption and to increase serum thyrotropin levels. Levothyroxine may adsorb to calcium carbonate in an acidic environment, which may block its absorption. There is no evidence that other forms of calcium block levothyroxine absorption if taken concomitantly.

Proton Pump Inhibitors (lansoprazole, omeprazole, rabeprazole sodium): Concomitant use of proton pump inhibitors and calcium carbonate or calcium phosphate can cause decreased absorption of these calcium salts.

Quinolones (ciprofloxacin, gatifloxacin, levofloxacin, lomefloxacin, moxifloxacin, norfloxacin, ofloxacin, sparfloxacin, trovafloxacin): Concomitant use of a quinolone and calcium may decrease the absorption of the quinolone.

Tetracyclines (doxycycline, minocycline, tetracycline): Concomitant intake of a tetracycline and calcium may decrease the absorption of the tetracycline. Tetracyclines may form nonabsorbable complexes with calcium.

Vitamin D Analogues (calcitriol, alfacalcidol): Concomitant use of these vitamin D analogues and calcium can cause increased absorption of calcium.

NUTRITIONAL SUPPLEMENTS

Inositol Hexaphosphate: Concomitant use of inositol hexaphosphate (phytic acid) and calcium may decrease the absorption of calcium.

Minerals (iron, fluoride, magnesium, phosphorous): Concomitant use of iron and calcium may inhibit the absorption of iron. Similarly, concomitant use of fluoride, magnesium, phosphorous or zinc and calcium may decrease the absorption of these minerals. However, these possible mineral interactions have not been shown to be of clinical significance.

Non-digestible oligosaccharides (fructo-oligosaccharides, inulin): Concomitant use of these oligosaccharides and calcium may increase the absorption of calcium in the colon.

Sodium Alginate: Concomitant intake of sodium alginate and calcium may decrease the absorption of calcium.

Vitamin D: Concomitant use of vitamin D and calcium may increase the absorption of calcium.

FOODS

Calcium may be poorly absorbed from foods rich in oxalic acid (spinach, sweet potatoes, rhubarb and beans) or phytic acid (unleavened bread, raw beans, seeds, nuts and grains and soy isolates). Concomitant intake of a calcium supplement with foods rich in oxalic acid or phytic acid may decrease the absorption of calcium. The phytate associated with dietary fiber appears to be the major factor involved in depressing absorption of calcium.

OVERDOSAGE

Overdosage has not been reported with calcium supplements.

DOSAGE AND ADMINISTRATION

There are several different calcium salts available as supplements. These include calcium carbonate, calcium citrate, calcium phosphate, calcium lactate and calcium gluconate. Calcium carbonate and calcium phosphate contain approximately 40% elemental calcium; calcium citrate, approximately 21% elemental calcium; calcium lactate, approximately 13% elemental calcium; calcium gluconate, approximately 9% elemental calcium. Some calcium preparations also contain vitamin D.

Adequate intake of calcium for women and men 19 through 50 years is 1,000 milligrams daily. Adequate intake of calcium for men and women 31 years through greater than 70 years is 1,200 milligrams daily. Adequate intake of vitamin D for women and men 19 to 50 years is 200 IU or 5.0 micrograms daily. Adequate intake of vitamin D for men and women 51 through 70 years is 400 IU or 10 micrograms daily. Adequate intake of vitamin D for men and women over 70 years is 600 IU or 15 picograms daily.

Absorption of calcium is greatest in doses of 500 milligrams or less and when taken with food.

There are several food products, including orange juice, that are now available which have added calcium. The salt calcium citrate malate is used to fortify some foods. Some physicians recommend 1,000 milligrams of supplement calcium daily for postmenopausal women taking estrogen replacement therapy (ERT) and 1,500 milligrams daily for postmenopausal women not taking ERT. An intake of 1,200 milligrams daily appears to be adequate for both groups. The Food and Nutrition Board of the Institute of Medicine of the U.S. National Academy of Sciences has recommended the following adequate intakes (AI) for calcium:

Infants	(AI)
0-6 months	200 mg/day
7-12 months	270 mg/day
Children	
1-3 years	500 mg/day
4-8 years	800 mg/day
Boys	
9-13 years	1,300 mg/day
14-18 years	1,300 mg/day
Girls	
9-13 years	1,300 mg/day
14-18 years	1,300 mg/day
Men	
19-30 years	1,000 mg/day
31-50 years	1,000 mg/day
51-70 years	1,200 mg/day
> 70 years	1,200 mg/day
Women	
19-30 years	1,000 mg/day
31-50 years	1,000 mg/day
51-70 years	1,200 mg/day
> 70 years	1,200 mg/day
Pregnancy	
14-18 years	1,300 mg/day
19-30 years	1,000 mg/day
31-50 years	1,000 mg/day
Lactation	
14-18 years	1,300 mg/day
19-30 years	1,000 mg/day
31-50 years	1,000 mg/day

A LOAEL (lowest-observed-adverse-effect level) in the range of 4 to 5 grams can be identified for adults. Based on this LOAEL and an uncertainty factor (UF) of 2 the Food and Nutrition Board of the Institute of Medicine has recommended the following tolerable upper intake levels (UL) for calcium:

Infants	(UL)
0-12 months	Not possible to establish for supplementary calcium
Children	
1-18 years	2,500 mg/day
Adults	
19-70 years	2,500 mg/day
> 70 years	2,500 mg/day
Pregnancy	
14-50 years	2,500 mg/day
Lactation	
14-50 years	2,500 mg/day

HOW SUPPLIED

Calcium Carbonate is available in the following forms and strengths:

Capsules — 250 mg, 500 mg
Chewable Tablets — 500 mg, 750 mg, 1000 mg
Liquid
Powder
Suspension — 500 mg/5 mL
Tablets — 250 mg, 500 mg, 600 mg, 650 mg
Wafers — 500 mg

Calcium Citrate is available in the following forms and strengths:

Capsules — 150 mg, 800 mg
Effervescent Tablets — 500 mg
Granules
Tablets — 200 mg, 250 mg, 950 mg, 1150 mg

Calcium Glubionate is available in the following forms and strengths:

Capsules — 500 mg, 700 mg
Chewable Tablets — 650 mg
Powder
Syrup — 1.8 Gm/5 mL
Tablets — 486 mg, 500 mg, 650 mg, 975 mg

Calcium Lactate is available in the following forms and strengths:

Capsules
Tablets — 325 mg, 500 mg, 650 mg

Calcium Phosphate is available in the following forms and strengths

Powder

Tablets — 600 mg

LITERATURE

Allender PS, Cutler JA, Follman D, et al. Dietary calcium and blood pressure: meta—analysis of randomized clinical trials. *Ann Intern Med.* 1996; 124:825-831.

Baron JA, Beach M, Mandel JS, et al. Calcium supplements for the prevention of colorectal adenomas. *N Engl J Med.* 1999; 340:101-107.

Bell L, Halstenson CE, Halstenson CJ, et al. Cholesterol-lowering effects of calcium carbonate in patients with mild to moderate hypercholesterolemia. *Arch Intern Med.* 1992; 152:2441-2444.

Bostick RM, Fosdick L, Grandits GA, et al. Effect of calcium supplementation on serum cholesterol and blood pressure. A randomized, double-blind, placebo-controlled, clinical trial. *Arch Fam Med.* 2000; 9:31-39.

Bronner F, Pansu D. Nutritional aspects of calcium absorption. *J Nutr.* 1999; 129:9-12.

Butner LE, et al. Calcium carbonate induced hypothyroidism. *Ann Intern Med.* 2000; 132:595.

Buckley LM, Leib ES, Cartularo KS, et al. Calcium and vitamin D_3 supplementation prevents bone loss in the spine secondary to low-dose corticosteroids in patients with rheumatoid arthritis. *Ann Intern Med.* 1996; 125:961-968.

Curhan GC, Willett WC, Speizer FE, et al. Comparison of dietary calcium with supplemental calcium and other nutrients as factors affecting the risk of kidney stones in women. *Ann Intern Med.* 1997; 126:497-504.

Dawson-Hughes B, Harris SS, Krall EA, Dallal GE. Effect of calcium and vitamin D supplementation on bone density on men and women 65 years of age and older. *N Engl J Med.* 1997; 337:670-676.

Dietary Reference Intakes For Calcium, Phosphorous, Magnesium, Vitamin D, and Fluoride. Washington, DC: National Academy Press; 1997.

Garland CF, Garland FC, Gorham ED. Calcium and vitamin D. Their potential roles in colon and breast cancer prevention. *Ann NY Acad Sci.* 1999; 889:107-119.

Heaney RP. Calcium, dairy products and osteoporosis. *J Am Coll Nutr.* 2000; 19(2 Suppl):83S-99S.

Heaney RP, Dowell MS, Barger-Lux MJ. Absorption of calcium as the carbonate and citrate salts, with some observations on method. *Osteoporosis Int.* 1999; 9:19-23.

Heller HJ, Stewart A, Haynes S, Pak CY. Pharmacokinetics of calcium absorption from two commercial calcium supplements. *J Clin Pharmacol.* 1999; 39:1151-1154.

Levine RJ, Hauth JC, Curet LB, et al. Trial of calcium to prevent preeclampsia. *N Engl J Med.* 1997; 337:69-76.

Lipkin M, Newmark H. Effect of added dietary calcium on colonic epithelial-cell proliferation in subjects at high risk for familial colonic cancer. *N Engl J Med.* 1985; 313:1381-1384.

Oginni LM, Sharp CA, Worsfold M, et al. Healing of rickets after calcium supplementation. *Lancet.* 1999; 353:296-297.

Recker RR. Calcium absorption and achlorhydria. *N Engl J Med.* 1985; 313:70-73.

Reid IR, Ames RW, Evans MC, et al. Effect of calcium supplementation on bone loss in postmenopausal women. *N Engl J Med.* 1993; 328:460-464.

Singh N, Singh PN, Hershman JM. Effect of calcium carbonate on the absorption of levothyroxine. *JAMA.* 2000; 283:2822-2825.

Talbot JR, Guardo P, Seccia S, et al. Calcium bioavailability and parathyroid hormone acute changes after oral intake of dairy and nondairy products in healthy volunteers. *Osteoporosis Int.* 1999; 10:137-142.

Wargovich MJ, Eng VWS, Newmark HL. Calcium inhibits the damaging and compensatory proliferative effects of fatty acids on mouse colon epithelium. *Cancer Lett.* 1984; 23:253-258.

Weaver CM, Heaney RP. Calcium. In: Shils ME, Olson JA, Shike M, Ross AC, eds. *Modern Nutrition in Health and Disease.* 9th ed. Baltimore, MD: Williams and Wilkins; 1999:141-155.

Wolf RL, Cauley JA, Baker CE, et al. Factors associated with calcium absorption efficiency in pre- and perimenopausal women. *Am J Clin Nutr.* 2000; 72:466-471.

Zemel MB, Shi H, Greer B, et al. Regulation of adiposity by dietary calcium. *FASEB J.* 2000; 14:1132-1138.

Caprylic Acid

TRADE NAMES

Caprylic acid is available generically from numerous manufacturers. Branded products include Capryl (Solaray) and Caprinol (Nature's Herbs).

DESCRIPTION

Caprylic acid is a medium-chain 8-carbon saturated fatty acid. It is also known as octanoic acid. It occurs naturally in butterfat and palm and coconut oils in the form of triacylglcerols (TAG). It is represented by the following chemical structure:

$$CH_3(CH_2)_5CH_2 - \overset{\displaystyle O}{\overset{\displaystyle \|}{C}} - OH$$

Caprylic acid

ACTIONS AND PHARMACOLOGY
ACTIONS
Caprylic acid was reported many years ago to have some antifungal activity *in vitro*. Other *in vitro* studies showed some activity against some viruses and bacteria. The monoglyceride of caprylic acid, monooctanin, given as an infusion into the bile duct, has been used for gallstone dissolution.

MECHANISM OF ACTION
The mechanism of caprylic acid's possile actions is unclear. Caprylic acid may affect the fluidity of viral and fungal cell membranes.

PHARMACOKINETICS
Caprylic acid is absorbed from the intestine and, in contrast with long-chain fatty acids, immediately enters into the portal circulation. It is carried by blood lipids. Most ingested caprylic acid undergoes beta-oxidation in the liver.

INDICATIONS AND USAGE
There is no significant clinical evidence to support an indication for the use of caprylic acid in the treatment or prevention of fungal infections such as *Candida albicans*.

RESEARCH SUMMARY
Some rather old studies reported antifungal activity of caprylic acid *in vitro*. However, clinical use of caprylic acid has not proved to be effective against *Candida albicans* or any other fungi. This is most likely due to the fact that caprylic acid is rapidly metabolized in the usual fatty acid pathways.

CONTRAINDICATIONS, PRECAUTIONS, ADVERSE REACTIONS
CONTRAINDICATIONS
None known.

PRECAUTIONS
Infants, children, pregnant women, nursing mothers and those prone to stomach upsets should avoid caprylic acid supplementation.

ADVERSE REACTIONS
Caprylic acid has an unpleasant rancid taste and may cause mild gastrointestinal symptoms such as nausea and diarrhea.

DOSAGE AND ADMINISTRATION
The usual doses that are taken orally are 300 to 1200 milligrams daily.

HOW SUPPLIED
Capsules — 325 mg
Tablets — 365 mg

LITERATURE
Abate MA, Moore TL. Monooctanin use for gallstone dissolution. *Drug Intell Clin Pharm.* 1985; 19:708-713.

Kabara JJ. Fatty acids and derivatives as antimicrobial agents. In: Kabara JJ, ed. *The Pharmacological Effect of Lipids I.* Champaign, IL: American Oil Chemists' Society; 1978; 1-14.

Wyss O, Ludwig BJ, Joiner RR. The fungistatic and fungicidal action of fatty acids and related compounds. *Arch Biochem.* 1943;7,415.

CDP-Choline

DESCRIPTION
CDP-choline is a naturally occurring substance found in most life forms. It is an intermediate metabolite in the major pathway for the synthesis of phosphatidylcholine. Phosphatidylcholine is a phospholipid that is a major component of cell membranes. Phosphatidylcholine is necessary for the structure and function of all cells and is crucial for sustaining life.

CDP-choline is synthesized in cells by the reaction of the nucleotide cytidine triphosphate or CTP with phosphocholine. The enzyme catalyzing the reaction is called CTP:phosphocholine cytidyltransferase. This reaction is the rate-limiting step in the synthesis of phosphatidyl choline.

Phosphocholine is synthesized from choline, and, for the synthesis of phosphatidylcholine, CDP-choline reacts with diacylglyceride, catalyzed by the enzyme CDP-choline: 1,2-diacylglycerol cholinephosphotransferase.

CDP-choline is also known as cytidine-5'-diphosphate choline and citicholine, and has the following structural formula:

CDP-Choline

ACTIONS AND PHARMACOLOGY
ACTIONS
CDP-choline has putative activity as a cognition enhancer and in cell-membrane repair.

MECHANISM OF ACTION
Since the action of CDP-choline either as a pharmaceutical or nutraceutical agent has yet to be clarified, discussion of its mechanism of action is speculative. However, much is

known about the biochemistry of endogenous CDP-choline. CDP-choline is an intermediate metabolite in the major pathway for the synthesis of the membrane phospholipid, phosphatidylcholine. Phosphatidylcholine is crucial for the maintenance of cell-membrane fluidity and cellular integrity. CDP-choline, hypothetically, may aid in cell-membrane repair, particularly neuronal cell membranes that have been damaged by trauma, ischemic events, toxins, infections or during the course of aging.

CDP-choline is also a delivery form of choline and cytidine. Choline is a precursor of acetylcholine and betaine. Acetylcholine is a neurotransmitter whose deficiency in certain regions of the brain is believed to be an etiological factor in certain dementia syndromes, including Alzheimer's disease. Betaine is involved in the conversion of the amino acid homocysteine to the essential amino acid L-methionine. L-methionine is a protein amino acid. Cytidine, following conversion to cytidine triphosphate, participates in a few reactions, including the formation of CDP-choline and nucleic acids.

PHARMACOKINETICS

Most pharmacokinetic studies have been performed in animals. Following oral intake, most CDP-choline is hydrolyzed in the small intestine to choline and cytidine. Choline and cytidine are absorbed and transported to the liver via the portal circulation. In the liver, choline may enter various metabolic pathways, resulting in the biosynthesis of various substances, including CDP-choline, betaine and phosphatidylcholine. Cytidine enters the cytidine nucleotide pool and may be incorporated into nucleic acids. Choline and cytidine not metabolized in the liver are distributed to various tissues in the body, where they undergo further metabolism. The uptake of CDP-choline by the brain is low. However, choline and cytidine may be taken up by the brain. Within the brain, cytidine and choline may be metabolized via a few steps to CDP-choline, which can serve as a substrate for phosphatidylcholine synthesis.

INDICATIONS AND USAGE

CDP-choline may be useful in the treatment of stroke and brain injury. There is some preliminary evidence that CDP-choline may be helpful in some with tardive dyskinesia, Parkinson's disease, Alzheimer's disease and other conditions characterized by impaired cognitive function, including memory loss. An indication may emerge for it to help improve visual acuity in those with amblyopia.

RESEARCH SUMMARY

In numerous studies of CDP-choline, favorable results have been obtained in cerebral ischemia and traumatic head injury. Its efficacy in these studies has been attributed to its apparent ability to increase phosphatidylcholine synthesis in the brain. In animal studies, it has been shown to enhance cell-membrane formation and repair, to restore intracellular enzyme function, to limit nerve damage and decrease edema.

The same mechanisms, generally, are said to account for favorable effects reported for it in the treatment of Parkinson's disease, Alzheimer's disease and a variety of cognitive disorders, including impaired memory associated with aging.

In a randomized, double-blind, placebo-controlled study, 259 patients with ischemic stroke received placebo or 500 to 2000 milligrams of CDP-choline daily for six weeks commencing within 24 hours of stroke. Among subjects who received 500 milligrams of CDP-choline daily, 53 percent achieved full or nearly-full recovery as measured by tests of neurolgic function. Among those receiving placebo, 33 percent achieved similar levels of recovery in the same time frame. The 500 milligram dose was as efficacious as higher doses and produced no significant side effects. Higher doses produced dizziness in some. Research continues.

In one study, CDP-choline, given in a daily dose of 1000 milligrams for a month, slightly improved mental performance in subjects with Alzheimer's disease. Better results have been reported with similar doses of CDP-choline in patients with early-onset Alzheimer's disease. Both favorable immunogenic and neurotrophic effects are reported in many of these CDP-choline/Alzheimer's studies.

In a randomized, double-blind, placebo-controlled study, subjects, aged 50 to 85, received placebo or varying doses of CDP-choline, generally 1000 to 2000 milligrams a day, for several months. A subgroup of these subjects, shown to have relatively inefficient memories, benefited the most from CDP-choline, as measured by tests of logical memory. The researchers concluded: "Citicholine may prove effective in treating age-related cognitive decline that may be the precursor of dementia."

There is preliminary evidence that CDP-choline might be useful in some disorders of vision. Statistically significant vision improvement was noted in a study of 50 patients with amblyopia treated with CDP-choline for 15 days. The improvement was sustained at a four-month follow-up. More research is warranted.

CONTRAINDICATIONS, PRECAUTIONS, ADVERSE REACTIONS

CONTRAINDICATIONS

None known.

PRECAUTIONS

Because of lack of long-term safety studies, CDP-choline should be avoided by children, pregnant women and nursing mothers.

ADVERSE REACTIONS

Adverse reactions reported include epigastric distress, nausea, rash, headache and dizziness.

DOSAGE AND ADMINISTRATION

A parenteral form of CDP-choline (citicoline) is marketed as a drug in Europe, and an oral form is being developed as a drug in the United States for treatment of ischemic stroke. CDP-choline is also being marketed along with other ingredients as a nutritional supplement. Doses of 500 to 2000 milligrams daily are used. Choline makes up approximately 21 percent of CDP-choline.

Stability is a concern with CDP-choline. Long-alkyl chain sulfonate salts of CDP-choline appear to show enhanced stability for oral use.

LITERATURE

Babb SM, Appelmans KE, Renshaw PF, et al. Differential effect of CDP-choline on brain cytosolic choline levels in younger and older subjects as measured by proton magnetic resonance spectroscopy. *Psychopharmacol.* 1996; 127:88-94.

Franco-Maside A, Coamano J, Gomez MJ, Cacabelos R. Brain mapping activity and mental performance after treatment with CDP-choline in Alzheimer's disease. *Methods Find Exp Clin Pharmacol.* 1994; 16:597-607.

Galletti P, DeRosa M, Cotticelli MG, et al (1991). Biochemical rationale for the use of CDPcholine in traumatic brain injury: pharmacokinetics of the orally administered drug. *J Neurol Sci.* 1991; 103 Suppl:S19-S25.

Gimenez R, Soler S, Aquilar J. Cytidine diphosphate choline administration activates brain cytidine triphosphate: phosphocholine cytidyltransferase in aged rats. *Neurosci Lett.* 1999; 273:163-166.

Spiers PA, Myers D, Hochanadel GS. Citicholine improves verbal memory in aging. *Arch Neurol.* 1996; 53:441-448.

Weiss GB. Metabolism and actions of CDP-choline as an endogenous compound and administered exogenously as citicholine. *Life Sci.* 1995; 56:637-660.

Cetyl Myristoleate

DESCRIPTION

Cetyl myristoleate is an ester comprised of the 16-carbon atom alcohol, cetyl alcohol, and the 14-carbon monounsaturated fatty acid cis-9 tetradecenoic acid, or myristoleic acid. It is a waxy, lipid substance with the following chemical structure:

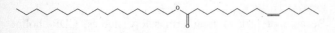

Cetyl myristoleate

ACTIONS AND PHARMACOLOGY

ACTIONS

None have been identified.

PHARMACOKINETICS

No reported pharmacokinetics. It is likely to be absorbed in the small intestine and transported from the lymph to the blood in lipid particles. Upon metabolism in the cells, it is likely that cetyl myristoleate undergoes enzymatic hydrolysis and that the component molecules, cetyl alcohol and myristoleic acid, are catabolized by normal cellular oxidative processes.

INDICATIONS AND USAGE

There is no credible support for claims that cetyl myristoleate is effective in arthritis, fibromyalgia, chronic fatigue syndrome and immune disorders.

RESEARCH SUMMARY

Claims for this substance have been sweeping—based upon an isolated finding that it provides protection against adjuvant-induced arthritis in rats. Until further positive research results are obtained from well-designed and executed clinical trials, the human use of cetyl myristoleate supplements has no scientific rationale. Claims that it is helpful in human arthritis, fibromyalgia, chronic fatigue syndrome and immune disorders have not been substantiated by credible research.

CONTRAINDICATIONS, PRECAUTIONS, ADVERSE REACTIONS

CONTRAINDICATIONS

None known.

PRECAUTIONS

Children, pregnant women and nursing mothers should avoid cetyl myristoleate supplements.

ADVERSE REACTIONS

May cause mild gastrointestinal symptoms.

DOSAGE AND ADMINISTRATION

There are no typical doses.

LITERATURE

Diehl HW, May EL. Cetyl myristoleate isolated from Swiss albino mice: an apparent protective agent against adjuvant arthritis in rats. *J Pharm Sci.* 1994; 83:296-299.

Chelated Minerals

DESCRIPTION

Chelated minerals are minerals complexed with various amino acids and/or oligopeptides.

It is believed by some that chelated minerals are better absorbed than non-chelated minerals. There may be certain minerals, e.g., trivalent chromium and zinc, where this is possibly the case. However, in most cases chelated and non-chelated minerals are absorbed with equivalent efficiency.

ACTIONS AND PHARMACOLOGY

ACTIONS

Chelated minerals are delivery forms of minerals.

MECHANISM OF ACTION

See monographs on individual minerals. Chelated chromium forms appear to be better absorbed than non-chelated forms. The mechanism of this is not entirely clear.

PHARMACOKINETICS.

See monographs on individual minerals.

INDICATIONS AND USAGE

See individual mineral monographs to determine whether chelated forms confer any advantage. The mere claim of "chelation" does not necessarily mean a superior product.

RESEARCH SUMMARY

The issue of mineral chelation is a complex one. See monographs on individual minerals.

CONTRAINDICATIONS, PRECAUTIONS, ADVERSE REACTIONS.

See monographs on individual minerals.

OVERDOSAGE

The only mineral in which overdosage is a significant problem is iron. See monograph on Iron.

DOSAGE AND ADMINISTRATION

See monographs on individual minerals.

LITERATURE

See monographs on individual minerals.

Chicken Collagen II

TRADE NAMES

Maxilife Chicken Collagen Type II (Twinlab), Bio-Cell Collagen II (Natrol), Collagen II (Natrol).

DESCRIPTION

Chicken collagen II is type II collagen derived from the sternum of chickens. Type II collagen is the most abundant collagen found in hyaline cartilage (in synovial joints, sternum, respiratory tract), comprising 80 to 90% of the total collagen content. Chicken collagen II is also known as type II chicken collagen and is abbreviated as CCII.

Type II chicken collagen shares some similar antigenic regions with type II human collagen. Autoimmune response to type II collagen is thought to be a significant factor in the pathogenesis of rheumatoid arthritis. A few studies suggest that oral type II chicken collagen may be beneficial to some

with rheumatoid arthritis, acting by a process known as oral tolerance.

ACTIONS AND PHARMACOLOGY

ACTIONS

Chicken collagen type II may have anti-rheumatoid arthritis activity in some.

MECHANISM OF ACTION

The mechanism of the possible anti-rheumatoid arthritis activity of chicken collagen type II may be through oral tolerance. Oral tolerance refers to the observation that if a protein is orally administered, subsequent immunization with the protein leads to a state of systemic hyporesponsiveness to it. Autoantibodies to type II collagen are thought to play a role in the pathogenesis of rheumatoid arthritis. Therefore, feeding antigenic type II collagen may be predicted to lead to the induction of immune tolerance to type II collagen, especially in the context of elevated autoantibodies to this substance.

The mechanism for oral tolerance appears to depend on the dose of the fed antigen. Low doses appear to induce active suppression, while high doses result in clonal anergy. Suppressive cytokines, such as interleukin-4 and transforming growth factor beta, appear to mediate active suppression. Studies in animals demonstrate the generation of regulatory lymphocytes in Peyer's patches, which subsequently migrate to mesenteric lymph nodes and spleen. Secretion of suppressive cytokines by these cells is believed to depend on antigen-specific stimulation with the fed antigen. Further, it is believed that active suppression of the inflammatory process by the regulatory lymphocytes requires their migration to the location where the fed antigen is present. Since the clinical studies to date indicate that low doses, but not high doses, have possible mild efficacy in rheumatoid arthritis, the mechanism responsible for oral tolerance would appear to be induction of active suppression, rather than clonal anergy.

PHARMACOKINETICS

There are no reports on the pharmacokinetics of chicken collagen type II. The pharmacokinetics of the substance should be similar to those of dietary proteins.

INDICATIONS AND USAGE

Chicken collagen II may offer some mild benefit for some with rheumatoid arthritis.

RESEARCH SUMMARY

A multicenter, randomized, controlled trial of oral type II collagen derived from chicken cartilage tested the substance in four different daily doses versus placebo in 273 rheumatoid arthritis patients. Various criteria were used to evaluate the results. The daily dose levels were 20 micrograms, 100 micrograms, 500 micrograms and 2,500 micrograms.

Results were negative at all dose levels except the lowest dose (20 micrograms daily). The difference in response between this dose level and placebo was significant only with respect to what was described as the weakest of the evaluative criteria. A *post hoc* analysis revealed that those who had antibodies reactive with type II collagen in their serum (at the baseline exam) were more likely to respond to collagen administration.

More research is needed, in part to investigate whether still lower doses might further improve efficacy of this antigenic substance.

CONTRAINDICATIONS, PRECAUTIONS, ADVERSE REACTIONS

CONTRAINDICATIONS
Chicken collagen II is contraindicated in those who are hypersensitive to any component of a chicken collagen II-containing product.

PRECAUTIONS
Because of lack of long-term safety studies, nutritional supplements containing chicken collagen II should be avoided by pregnant women and nursing mothers.

Those with rheumatoid arthritis who are interested in trying chicken collagen II should consult with their physicians before doing so.

ADVERSE REACTIONS
Chicken collagen type II supplements are generally well tolerated. There is one report of transient flushing in a patient with juvenile rheumatoid arthritis.

DOSAGE AND ADMINISTRATION
Chicken collagen II, derived from chicken sterum, is available as capsules and tablets. Some use 500 to 1000 mg daily. However, in the clinical trials showing possible mild effectiveness of chicken collagen type II, lower doses and different delivery forms were used. In these trials, the substance was first dissolved in 0.1 M acetic acid and added to orange juice prior to ingestion. The dose used in the trial of juvenile rheumatoid arthritics was 100 micrograms (0.1 mg) daily for one month followed by a dose of 500 micrograms (0.5 mg) daily. In a subsequent larger clinical trial involving rheumatoid arthritics, a dose of 20 micrograms (0.02 mg) daily appeared to have mild benefits in some. Higher doses did not.

HOW SUPPLIED
Capsules — 500 mg
Tablets — 500 mg

LITERATURE
Barnett ML, Combitchi D, Trentham DE. A pilot trial of oral type II collagen in the treatment of juvenile rheumatoid arthritis. *Arthritis Rheum.* 1996; 39:623-628.

Barnett ML, Kremer JM, St Clair EW, et al. Treatment of rheumatoid arthritis with oral type II collagen. Results of a multicenter, double-blind, placebo-controlled trial. *Arthritis Rheum.* 1998; 41:290-297.

Trentham DE. Evidence that type II collagen feeding can induce a durable therapeutic response in some patients with rheumatoid arthritis. In: Weiner HL, Mayer LF, eds. *Oral Tolerance: Mechanisms and Applications. Ann NY Acad Sci.* 1996; 778:306-314.

Trentham DE. Oral tolerization as a treatment of rheumatoid arthritis. *Rheum Dis Clinc North Am.* 1998; 24: 525-536.

Trentham DE, Dynesius-Trentham RA, Orav EJ, et al. Effects of oral administration of type II collagen on rheumatoid arthritis. *Science.* 1993; 261:1727-1730.

Watson WC, Cremer MA, Wooley PH, Townes AS. Assessment of the potential pathogenicity of type II collagen autoantibodies in patients with rheumatoid arthritis. *Arthritis Rheum.* 1986; 29:1316-1321.

Chitosan

TRADE NAMES
Chitosan is available generically from numerous manufacturers. Branded products include Diet Chitosan (Source Naturals) and Chitosan Support (Natural Treasures).

DESCRIPTION
Chitosan and chitin are polysaccharide polymers containing more than 5,000 glucosamine and acetylglucosamine units, respectively, and their molecular weights are over one million Daltons. Chitin is found in fungi, arthropods and marine invertebrates. Commercially, chitin is derived from the exoskeletons of crustaceans (shrimp, crab and other shellfish). Chitosan is obtained from chitin by a deacetylation process.

Chitin, the polysaccharide polymer from which chitosan is derived, is a cellulose-like polymer consisting mainly of unbranched chains of N-acetyl-D-glucosamine. Deacetylated chitin, or chitosan, is comprised of chains of D-glucosamine. When ingested, chitosan can be considered a dietary fiber. Chitosan has the following chemical structure:

Chitosan

Chitosan itself is the major source of the nutritional supplement glucosamine.

ACTIONS AND PHARMACOLOGY

ACTIONS

Chitosan may have hypocholesterolemic activity in some and may be beneficial in renal disease in some.

MECHANISM OF ACTION

Chitosan is, at the pH of the gastrointestinal tract, a positively charged polymer and can bind to negatively charged substances. It is believed that chitosan, similar to cholestryamine, has bile acid sequestration activity and that this may be the mechanism for its hypocholesterolemic effect. There is some evidence that chitosan binds to bile acids and some evidence that the polymer affects the metabolism of intestinal bile acids. However, in contrast to cholestyramine, chitosan does not have consistent hypocholesterolemic activity. There is also evidence that chitosan binds to fats in the intestine, blocking their absorption.

The mechanism of action of chitosan's possible beneficial effects on renal disease in some is unknown. Chitosan can absorb urea and ammonia, but it is unclear whether this mechanism has anything to do with its putative renal effects.

PHARMACOKINETICS

Ingested chitosan can be considered as a cellulose-like dietary fiber. After ingesting, there is minimal digestion and most of the ingested chitosan is excreted in the feces.

INDICATIONS AND USAGE

There is some evidence that supplemental chitosan may have favorable effects on lipids and may be of some use in renal failure. There is some suggestion from available research data that it might be helpful in preventing atherosclerosis and could play a role in wound healing, some types of diabetes and liver disease or injury. Claims that it can help reduce weight, fight cancer, heal ulcers, aid digestion and boost immunity are unsubstantiated.

RESEARCH SUMMARY

There are several studies, in both animals and humans, demonstrating chitosan's effect on lipids. These effects have generally been more dramatic in various animal models, possibly due to higher chitosan intake in many of those studies. Some of these animal studies show very dramatic reductions in cholesterol and in LDL-cholesterol. Some have observed increases in the HDL-cholesterol, as well.

In humans, results have been less clear-cut, though still suggestive of positive effects. In one recent placebo-controlled, double-blind study, there was a significant decrease in LDL-cholesterol among subjects receiving 2,400 milligrams of chitosan daily, compared with placebo subjects. Chitosan had no significant effect on serum total cholesterol or on HDL-cholesterol, but it slightly increased triglycerides. Others have reported similar effects: reduced LDL-cholesterol with little or no effect on HDL and total cholesterols. A few others, however, have reported no lipid effects. Differences may be due to dissimilar dosing.

In animal models of chronic renal failure, chitosan produced decreases in serum urea nitrogen, serum creatine and serum phosphate. It also ameliorated anemia and increased fecal weight, fecal water content, fecal nitrogen and fecal sodium. The apparent protein ratio was decreased in a dose-dependent pattern in some of these studies, and survival times were markedly and significantly extended.

In a human study of 80 patients with chronic renal failure, similarly encouraging results were obtained. Half of these patients received 30 chitosan tablets (each containing 45 milligrams of chitosan) three times a day for a total of 4,050 milligrams daily. After four weeks on this regimen, these subjects experienced significant reductions in urea and creatine levels in serum, compared with controls. Significant gains were also measured in physical strength, appetite and sleep patterns after 12 weeks of chitosan supplementation. It is interesting to note that chitosan at this dose also significantly reduced total serum cholesterol levels (and increased serum hemoglobin levels).

Favorable lipid results would suggest that supplemental chitosan might help prevent atherosclerosis. This idea has been tested in some animal models with promising results. Using the apolipoprotein E-deficient mouse model of atherosclerosis, for example, researchers recently showed that a 5% chitosan diet could produce "a highly significant inhibition of atherogenesis"—42% inhibition in the whole aorta and 50% inhibition in the aortic arch, compared with controls. These positive effects were attributed to a 65% reduction in blood cholesterol levels (after 20 weeks on the 5% chitosan diet).

Some research has demonstrated that topical preparations containing chitosan can help speed wound healing. Other preliminary studies suggest that chitosan might be useful in lean type non-insulin-dependent diabetes mellitus. In an animal model of this disease, chitosan significantly reduced blood glucose, cholesterol and triglycerides. (The same results, however, could not be obtained in obese type NIDDM.) Still other similarly preliminary studies suggest that chitosan might help protect the liver against some toxins. More research in these areas is needed.

Claims have been made that chitosan can help reduce weight. There is insufficient data to support this claim. Two recent studies failed to find any weight-loss effect from the use of chitosan in overweight subjects. In the larger and longer-term of these two studies, 51 healthy obese women were given either placebo or 2,400 milligrams of chitosan for eight weeks. No significant weight reduction was noted in the treatment group.

Similarly, there is insufficient data to support claims that chitosan fights cancer, heals ulcers, aids digestion, or boosts or otherwise modifies immunity.

CONTRAINDICATIONS, PRECAUTIONS, ADVERSE REACTIONS

CONTRAINDICATIONS
None known.

PRECAUTIONS
Children, pregnant women and nursing mothers should avoid using chitosan.

Those with shellfish allergies should exercise caution in taking chitosan supplements.

ADVERSE REACTIONS
Occasionally, gastrointestinal side effects, such as nausea and diarrhea have been reported.

INTERACTIONS

DRUGS
No interactions are known. However, chitosan might bind to certain drugs, especially lipophilic drugs.

NUTRITIONAL SUPPLEMENTS
Vitamin C is believed to enhance the putative benefits of chitosan. Chitosan might bind to the fat soluble vitamins A, D, E and K, as well as carotenoids and flavonoids. It might also bind with some minerals such as zinc.

FOODS
Chitosan might bind some dietary lipids. It may also bind the fat-soluble vitamins A, D, E and K, as well as flavonoids, carotenoids and some minerals, such as zinc, found in foods.

OVERDOSAGE
There are no reports of overdosage.

DOSAGE AND ADMINISTRATION
There are several chitosan supplements available. Those who use chitosan for cholesterol-lowering effects typically use 1000 to 1200 milligrams twice a day, taken before or after meals and with a glass of water. Chitosan can be contaminated with such metals as lead, mercury, iron, copper and arsenic.

Chitosan supplements should not be consumed within two hours of taking the fat-soluble vitamins A, D, E and K, carotenoids (e.g., lycopene, lutein), flavonoids (e.g., genistein, quercetin, ipriflavone) or prescription medication.

HOW SUPPLIED
Capsules — 500 mg, 1000 mg
Tablets — 500 mg

LITERATURE

Ebihara K, Schneeman BO. Interaction of bile acids, phospholipids, cholesterol and triglyceride with dietary fibers in the small intestine of rats. *J Nutr.* 1989; 119 006700-1106.

Fukada Y, Kimura K, Ayaki Y. Effect of chitosan feeding on intestinal bile acid metabolism in rats. *Lipids.* 1991;26:395-399.

Han LK, Kimura Y Okuda H. Reduction in fat storage during chitin-chitosan treatment in mice fed a high-fat diet. *Int J Obes Relat Metab Disord.* 1999;23:174-179.

Jing SB, Li L, Ji D, et al. Effect of chitosan on renal function in patients with chronic renal failure. *J. Pharm Pharmacol* 1997;49:721-723.

Lee JK, Kim SU, Kim JH. Modification of chitosan to improve its hypocholesterolemic capacity. *Biosci Biotechnol Biochem.* 1999;63:833-839.

LeHoux JG, Grondin F. Some effects of chitosan on liver function in the rat. *Endocrinology.* 1993; 132:1078-1084.

Miura T, Usami M, Tsuura Y, et al. Hypoglycemic and hypolipidemic effect of chitosan in normal and neonatal streptozotacin-induced diabetic mice. *Biol Pharm Bull.* 1995; 18:1623-1625.

Nagano N, Yoshimoto H, Nishitoba T, et al. Pharmacological properties of chitosan-coated dialdehyde cellulose (chitosan DAC), a newly developed oral adsorbent (II). Effect of chitosan DAC on rats with chronic renal failure induced by adriamycin. [Article in Japanese]. *Nippon Yakurigaku Zasshi.* 1995; 106:123-133.

Omrod DJ, Holmes CC, Miller, TE. Dietary chitosan inhibits hypercholesterolcemia and atherosclerosis in the apolipoprotein E-deficient mouse model of atherosclerosis. *Atherosclerosis.* 1998; 138:329-334.

Pittler MH, Abbot NC, Harkness EF, Ernst E. Randomized, double-blind trial of chitosan for body weight reduction. *Eur J Clin Nutr.* 1999;53:379-381.

Sugano M, Watanabe S, Kishi A, et al. Hypocholesterolemic action of chitosans with different viscosity in rats. *Lipids.* 1988;23:187-191.

Wuolijoki E, Hirvela T, Ylitalo P. Decrease in LDL-cholesterol with microcrystalline chitosan. *Methods Find Exp Clin Pharmacol.* 1999;21:357-361.

Yoshimoto H, Nagano N, Nishitoba N, et al. Pharmacological properties of chitosan-coated dialdehyde cellulose (chitosan DAC), a newly developed oral adsorbent (I). Effect of chitosan DAC in normal rats. [Article in Japanese]. *Nippon Yakurigaku Zasshi.* 1995; 106 00673-122.

Chlorella

TRADE NAMES
Spirulina Chlorella (Earthrise), Sun Chlorella Granules (Sun Wellness), China Chlorella (Natrol), Kyo-Chlorella (Kyolic).

DESCRIPTION

Chlorella is a genus of unicellular green algae belonging to the Phylum *Chlorophyta*. Chlorophytes comprise a major component of the phytoplankton. Chlorella is a popular food supplement in Japan and is marketed as a nutritional supplement in the United States. Chlorella, along with wheat grass, barley grass and spirulina, are sometimes referred to as "green foods." There are several species of chlorella. Those most commonly used in nutritional supplements are *Chlorella vulgaris* and *Chlorella pyrenoidosa*.

Chlorella is rich in protein. In addition, it is rich in chlorophyll, carotenoids, such as astaxanthin, canthaxanthin, flavoxanthin, loraxanthin, neoxanthin and violaxanthin. Chlorella also contains the xanthophyll, echinenone.

ACTIONS AND PHARMACOLOGY

ACTIONS

Chlorella has putative anticarcinogenic, immunomodulatory, hypolipidemic, gastric mucosal-protective and detoxification activities.

MECHANISM OF ACTION

Glycoprotein-rich extracts of *Chlorella vulgaris* have been found to have antitumor activity against both spontaneous and experimentally induced metastasis in mice. The antitumor activity is thought to be mediated by an immunopotentiation mechanism. The glycoprotein-rich extracts may enhance the migration of T cells to the tumor sites.

The mechanism of the putative hypolipidemic and gastric mucosal-protective activities of chlorella, which again have only been found in animal studies, is unknown.

In rats, chlorella was found to promote the excretion of dioxin in the feces. The mechanism of this action is unknown.

PHARMACOKINETICS

The pharmacokinetics of chlorella in humans have not been studied. However, the proteins, lipids and carbohydrates in chlorella should be digested, absorbed and metabolized by normal physiological processes.

INDICATIONS AND USAGE

A chlorella extract has demonstrated antitumor and antimetastatic effects in animal experiments. Chlorella has shown some experimental antiatherogenic activity and some radioprotective and chemo-detoxifying effects. It has shown some preliminary benefit in immune function and in some with fibromyalgia.

RESEARCH SUMMARY

An extract of chlorella markedly increased survival time in mice injected with Meth-a tumor cells. A glycoprotein constituent of chlorella demonstrated antitumor properties *in vitro*. Recently, a glycoprotein extract exerted a pronounced antitumor effect against spontaneous and experimentally induced metastasis in mice. Immune-enhancement appeared to play a central role, particularly T cell activation in the peripheral lymph nodes of the tumor-bearing mice.

Chlorella has demonstrated an ability to protect against gamma-radiation, as well as against a number of drugs and various toxic chemicals. In one animal experiment, it alleviated some of the side effects of 5-fluorouracil. In another study, chlorella helped prevent gastrointestinal absorption and promoted the excretion of dioxin already present in tissues in rats.

Chlorella has exhibited hypolipidemic and antiatherogenic effects in some animal experiments. Aortic atheromatous lesions were significantly inhibited by chlorella in rabbits on a high-cholesterol diet.

In one animal model of peptic ulcer, oral administration of dry powder chlorella helped protect gastric mucosa.

In a recent clinical trial of chlorella, some patients with moderately severe symptoms of fibromyalgia syndrome were said to derive significant benefit from consumption, over a two-month period, of 10 grams daily of Sun chlorella tablets and 100 ml of liquid Wakasa Gold, two commercial chlorella products. Evaluation of improvement was largely subjective.

CONTRAINDICATIONS, PRECAUTIONS, ADVERSE REACTIONS

CONTRAINDICATIONS

Chlorella is contraindicated in those who are hypersensitive to any component of a chlorella-containing nutritional supplement.

PRECAUTIONS

Pregnant women and nursing mothers should avoid chlorella-containing supplements.

Some chlorella-containing supplements may be rich in vitamin K. Therefore those on warfarin should be cautious in the use of chlorella supplements.

Allergic reactions have been reported in some using chlorella supplements. Therefore, those with allergic diatheses should exercise caution in the use of chlorella supplements.

ADVERSE REACTIONS

Allergic reactions and photosensitivity reactions have been reported in some using chlorella supplements.

INTERACTIONS

Some chlorella supplements may be rich in vitamin K and may affect the INR of those on warfarin. Animal studies suggest that certain substances in chlorella may ameliorate some of the side effects of 5-fluorouracil. There is no human documentation of this.

OVERDOSAGE

No reports of overdosage.

DOSAGE AND ADMINISTRATION

There are various forms of chlorella, including capsules, tablets, softgels and granules. Most chlorella marketed in the U.S. is grown in Japan and Taiwan and is processed into the various supplemental forms. Chlorella is marketed as a stand-alone supplement or combined with other so-called "green foods," such as wheat grass, barley grass and spirulina. There is no typical dosage.

HOW SUPPLIED

Capsules — 200 mg, 350 mg, 385 mg, 400 mg, 414 mg, 500 mg

Powder

Tablets — 200 mg, 400 mg, 500 mg

LITERATURE

Konishi F, Mitsuyama M, Okuda M, et al. Protective effect of an acidic glycoprotein obtained from culture of Chlorella vulgaris against myelosuppression by 5-fluorouracil. *Cancer Immunol Immunother.* 1996; 42:268-274.

Konishi F. Tanaka K, Kumamoto S, et al. Enhanced resistance against Escherichia coli infection by subcutaneous administration of the hot-water extract of Chlorella vulgaris in cyclophosphamide-treated mice. *Cancer Immunol Immunother.* 1990; 32:1-7.

Merchant RE, Carmack CA, Wise CM. Nutritional supplementation with Chlorella pyrenoidosa for patients with fibromyalgia syndrome: a pilot study. *Phytother Res.* 2000; 14:167-173.

Morita K, Matsueda T, Iida T, Hasegawa T. *Chlorella* accelerates dioxin excretion in rats. *J Nutr.* 1999; 129:1731-1736.

Noda K, Ohno N, Tanaka K, et al. A water-soluble antitumor glycoprotein from Chlorella vulgaris. *Planta Med.* 1996; 62:423-426.

Sano T, Kumanoto Y, Kamiya N, et al. Effect of lipophilic extract of Chlorella vulgaris on alimentary hyperlipidemia in cholesterol-fed rats. *Artery.* 1988; 15:217-224.

Sano T, Tanaka Y. Effect of dried, powdered Chlorella vulgaris on experimental atherosclerosis and alimentary hypercholesterolemia in cholesterol-fed rabbits. *Artery.* 1987; 76-84.

Tanaka K, Koga T, Konishi F, et al. Augmentation of host defense by unicellular green alga, Chlorella vulgaris, to Escherichia coli infection. *Infect Immun.* 1986; 53:267-271.

Tanaka K, Yamada A, Noda K, et al. Oral administration of a unicellular green algae, Chlorella vulgaris, prevents stress-induced ulcer. *Planta Med.* 1997; 63:465-466.

Tanaka K, Yamada A, Noda K, et al. A novel glycoprotein obtained from Chlorella vulgaris strain CK22 shows antimetastatic immunopotentiation. *Cancer Immunol Immunother.* 1998; 45:313-320.

Chlorophyll/Chlorophyllin

TRADE NAMES

Ennds (Oakhurst), Mega Cholorphyll (World Organics), Chlorocaps (World Organics), Chloraid Internal Deodorant (Nature's Herbs), Fingerprinted Chlorophyll (GNC), Triple Chlorophyll (GNC).

DESCRIPTION

Chlorophyll is the green pigment found in higher plants, as well as algae. Chlorophyll is the principal photoreceptor in photosynthesis, the light-driven process in which carbon dioxide is "fixed" to yield carbohydrates and oxygen. Chlorophyll is a cyclic tetrapyrolle, similar in structure to the heme group of globins (hemoglobin, myoglobin) and cytochromes. Chlorophyll differs from heme in a few major respects, most notably that the central metal ion in chlorophyll is magnesium while that in heme is iron.

There are a few types of chlorophyll. Higher plants and green algae, such as chlorella (see Chlorella) contain chlorophyll a and chlorophyll b in the approximate ratio of 3:1. The molecular formula of chlorophyll a is $C_{55}H_{72}MgN_4O_5$; the molecular formula of chlorophyll b is $C_{55}H_{70}MgN_4O_6$. The difference between the two chlorophylls is that a methyl side-chain in chlorophyll a is replaced by a formyl group in chlorophyll b. Chlorophyll a is found with chlorophyll c in many types of marine algae. Red algae contain principally chlorophyll a and also chlorophyll d.

Chlorophyllin is a semi-synthetic sodium/copper derivative of chlorophyll. In contrast to chlorophyll, chlorophyllin is water-soluble. Chlorophyllin, like chlorophyll, has deodorizing activity. It is used as an aid to reduce odor from a colostomy or ileostomy and also as an aid to reduce fecal odor due to incontinence. A topical ointment of chlorophyllin is used to reduce malodors in wounds and surface ulcers.

Chlorophyll and chlorophyllin are available as nutritional supplements. Preliminary evidence from *in vitro* and animal studies suggests that these substances may have anticarcinogenic activity.

ACTIONS AND PHARMACOLOGY

ACTIONS

Chlorophyll and chlorophyllin may have antimutagenic and anticarcinogenic activities.

MECHANISM OF ACTION

Chlorophyll and its metabolites pheophytin, pyropheophytin and pheophorbide, as well as chlorophyllin, have demonstrated antimutagenic effects *in vitro* against such mutagens as 3-methylcholanthrene, N-methyl-N'-nitro-N'-nitrosoguanidine (MNNG) and aflatoxin B1. Chlorophyll and chlorophyllin have also demonstrated anticarcinogenic effects in animal models against such carcinogens as aflatoxin B1, 1,2-dimethylhydrazine and dibenzo[*a,1*]pyrene.

The mechanism of the antimutagenic and anticarcinogenic activities of chlorophyll and chlorophyllin are unknown. It is speculated that antioxidant activity of chlorophyll/chlorophyllin may play a role in these activities. Another possible mechanism is the formation of complexes between the mutagen/carcinogen with chlorophyll/chlorophyllin through strong interactions between their planar unsaturated cyclic rings. The complexes would effectively inactivate the mutagens/carcinogens.

PHARMACOKINETICS

There is little on the pharmacokinetics of chlorophyll and its derivative chlorophyllin in humans. Some older studies showed that chlorophyll, following absorption, is converted into pheophytin, pyropheophytin and pheophorbide. These three derivatives of chlorophyll are tetrapyrolles.

INDICATIONS AND USAGE

Some experimental data suggests that chlorophyll and chlorophyllin may have some antimutagenic and anticarcinogenic potential, may help protect against some toxins, and may ameliorate some drug side effects. They are useful in reducing urinary and fecal odor in some circumstances. They may help ease constipation in some. There is some preliminary indication that they could be beneficial in the treatment of calcium oxalate stone disease and that they may have some anti-atherogenic activity.

RESEARCH SUMMARY

In one *in vitro* test, chlorophyllin demonstrated significant inhibition of several mutagens, including cigarette smoke, coal dust and diesel emission particles. Its antioxidant activity may have accounted for this effect. In another assay, chlorophyllin proved a more effective antimutagen than retinol, beta-carotene, vitamin C and vitamin E. In an animal study, chlorophyllin demonstrated both antimutagenic and anticarcinogenic activity, inhibiting 1,2-dimethylhydrazine-induced nuclear damage in rat colonic epithelium.

In another animal study, chlorophyllin significantly inhibited aflatoxin B1 hepatocacinogenesis. In a rainbow trout multi-organ tumor model, chlorophyllin markedly reduced liver, stomach and swimbladder cancer incidence.

Chlorophyllin has been used to reduce some of the side effects of cyclophosphamide. Chlorophyll consumption has been associated, in an animal study, with increased fecal excretion of polychlorinated dibenzo-p-dioxin (PCDD) con-

geners and polychlorinated dibenzofuran (PCDF). The researchers suggested that green vegetables rich in chlorophyll might be helpful in humans exposed to PCDD and PCDF congeners.

In a study of geriatric patients, chlorophyllin was said to be effective in helping control body and fecal odors and helped ease chronic constipation. It also reduced excessive flatus is some. In another study, this one involving incontinent geriatric patients, subjects received 100 mg of chlorophyllin daily or placebo for two weeks. A non-significant decrease in urinary odor was noted in those receiving chlorophyllin, compared with those on placebo.

One preliminary study indicated that chlorophyllin can inhibit the crystallisation and growth kinetics of calcium oxalate dihydrate in normal urine and that it might be helpful in the treatment of calcium oxalate stone disease.

Finally, chlorophyllin significantly decreased serum cholesterol and triglycerides in a study using rats with experimental atherogenesis. Followup is needed.

CONTRAINDICATIONS, PRECAUTIONS, ADVERSE REACTIONS

CONTRAINDICATIONS

Chlorophyll and chlorophyllin are contraindicated in those who are hypersensitive to any component in a chlorophyll-containing or chlorophyllin-containing preparation.

PRECAUTIONS

Supplemental chlorophyll and supplemental chlorophyllin should be avoided by pregnant women and nursing mothers.

ADVERSE REACTIONS

Use of chlorophyll and chlorophyllin supplements may cause discoloration of the urine (green urine), the feces (green stool) and the tongue (yellow to black tongue). There are occasional reports of diarrhea with use of these substances.

INTERACTIONS

In a mouse model, chlorophyllin ameliorated some of the side effects of cyclophosphamide.

OVERDOSAGE

No reports of overdosage.

DOSAGE AND ADMINISTRATION

There are a few chlorophyll and chlorophyllin nutritional supplements. Chlorophyllin is available as a liquid supplement. A typical dose is 100 mg daily. Those who use chlorophyllin to reduce fecal odor due to incontinence or to reduce odor from a colostomy or ileostomy typically take 100 mg daily.

HOW SUPPLIED

Capsules— 50 mg, 60 mg, 100 mg
Liquid— 45 mg/15 ml, 75 mg/5 ml

Tablets— 20 mg, 200 mg

LITERATURE

Breinholt V, Arbogast D, Loveland P, et al. Chlorophyllin chemoprevention: an evaluation of reduced bioavailability vs. target organ protective mechanisms. *Toxicol Appl Pharmacol.* 1999; 158:141-151.

Breinholt V, Hendricks J, Pereira C, et al. Dietary chlorophyllin is a potent inhibitor of aflatoxin B1 hepatocarcinogenesis in rainbow trout. *Cancer Res.* 1995; 55:57-62.

Chernomorsky S, Segelman A, Poretz RD. Effect of dietary chlorophyll derivatives on mutagenesis and tumor cell growth. *Teratogen Carcinogen Mutagen.* 1999; 19:313-322.

Dashwood RH, Breinholt V, Bailey GS. Chemopreventive properties of chlorophyllin: inhibition of aflatoxin B1 (AFB1)-DNA binding *in vivo* and antimutagenic activity against AFB1 and two heterocyclic amines in the Salmonella mutagenicity assay. *Carcinogenesis.* 1991; 12:939-942.

Nahata MC, Slencsak CA, Kamp J. Effect of chlorophyllin on urinary odor in incontinent geriartric patients. *Drug Intell Clin Pharm.* 1983; 17:732-734.

Ong TM, Whong WZ, Stewart J, Brockman HE. Chlorophyllin: a potent antimutagen against environmental and dietary complex mixtures. *Mutat Res.* 1986; 173:111-115.

Reddy AP, Harttig U, Barth MC, et al. Inhibition of dibenzo[*a,l*]pyrene-induced multi-organ carcinogenesis by dietary chlorophyllin in rainbow trout. *Carcinogenesis.* 1999; 20:1919-1926.

Robins EW, Nelson RL. Inhibition of 1,2-dimethylhydrazine-induced nuclear damage in rat colonic epithelium by chlorophyllin. *Anticancer Res.* 1989; 9:981-985.

Te C, Gentile JM, Baguley BC, et al. *In vivo* effects of chlorophyllin on the antitumot agent cyclophosphamide. *Int J Cancer.* 1997; 70:84-89.

Vlad M, Bordas E, Caseanu E, et al. Effect of cuprofilm on experimental atherosclerosis. *Biol Trace Elem Res.* 1995; 48:99-109.

Young RW, Beregi JS Jr. Use of chlorophyllin in the care of geriatric patients. *J Am Geriatr Soc.* 1980; 28:46-47.

Choline

DESCRIPTION

Choline is an essential nutrient that is widely distributed in foods, principally in the form of phosphatidylcholine but also as free choline. It is also found in foods in the form of the phospholipid sphingomyelin. Choline is necessary for the structure and function of all cells and is crucial for sustaining life.

Choline plays many roles in the body. The three major metabolic functions of choline are as a precursor for phosphatidylcholine biosynthesis, as a precursor for acetylcholine biosynthesis and as a methyl donor. In addition to serving as a precursor for phosphatidylcholine, choline is the precursor of the phospholipid sphingomyelin. Phosphatidylcholine and sphingomyelin are structural components of biological membranes. These phospholipids also serve as precursors for the intracellular messengers ceramide and diacylglycerol. Choline is also the precursor of the signaling lipids, platelet-activating factor (PAF) and sphingosylphosphoryl-choline.

An association between a low-choline diet and fatty infiltration of the liver in rats was first reported in 1935. Choline, as well as other substances, such as methionine, folic acid and vitamin B_{12}, that prevent deposition of fat in the liver are known as lipotropes. The primary criterion used to estimate the Adequate Intake (AI) for choline is the prevention of liver damage as assessed by measuring serum levels of the liver enzyme alanine aminotransferase or ALT. ALT was formerly called and is still referred to as SGPT (serum glutamate pyrutate transaminase).

The foods richest in phosphatidylcholine, the major delivery form of choline, are beef liver, egg yolks and soya. Beef liver, iceberg lettuce, peanut butter, peanuts and cauliflower are some foods that contain free choline.

Choline is also known as 2-Hydroxy-N,N,N-trimethylethanaminum; (beta-hydroxyethyl) trimethylammonium and bilineurine. The major commercial salts for supplementation are choline chloride and choline bitartrate. The chemical structure of Choline is:

$$CH_3 \mathrm{-\!\!\!-} \underset{\underset{CH_3}{|}}{\overset{\overset{CH_3}{|}}{N^+}} \mathrm{-\!\!\!-} CH_2\text{-}CH_2\text{-}OH$$

Choline

The major pathway for phosphatidylcholine synthesis in the body utilizes preformed or dietary choline. In an alternative pathway for phosphatidylcholine biosynthesis, phosphatidylcholine is sequentially methylated to form phosphatidylcholine, using S-adenosylmethionine as the methyl donor. This is probably the only pathway for *de novo* synthesis of choline in the body. However, *de novo* synthesis does not appear adequate to meet the demand for the nutrient.

ACTIONS AND PHARMACOLOGY

ACTIONS

Choline is a precursor for phosphatidylcholine, sphingomyelin, acetylcholine and the methyl donor betaine. Thus, choline is important for normal cellular membrane composition and repair, normal brain function and normal cardiovascular function.

MECHANISM OF ACTION

Choline is involved in several basic biological processes. Choline is a major part of the polar head group of phosphatidylcholine. Phosphatidylcholine's role in the maintenance of cell membrane integrity is vital to all of the basic biological processes: information flow, intracellular communication and bioenergetics. Inadequate choline intake would negatively affect all these processes. Choline is also a major part of another membrane phospholipid, sphingomyelin, also important for the maintenance of cell structure and function. It is noteworthy and not surprising that choline deficiency in cell culture causes apoptosis or programmed cell death. This appears to be due to abnormalities in cell membrane phosphatidylcholine content and an increase in ceramide, a precursor, as well as a metabolite, of sphingomyelin. Ceramide accumulation, which is caused by choline deficiency, appears to activate a caspase, a type of enzyme that mediates apoptosis.

Evidence is mounting that an elevated homocysteine level is a significant risk factor for atherosclerosis, as well as other cardiovascular and neurological disorders. Betaine or trimethylglycine is derived from choline via an oxidation reaction. Betaine is one of the factors that maintains low levels of homocysteine by resynthesizing L-methionine from homocysteine.

Acetylcholine is one of the major neurotransmitters and requires choline for its synthesis. Adequate acetylcholine levels in the brain are believed to be protective against certain types of dementia, including Alzheimer's disease. Human studies are needed to determine whether dietary choline might be useful in the prevention of dementia.

The mechanism of the carcinogenic actions of choline deficiency are not known.

PHARMACOKINETICS

Choline is absorbed from the small intestine by means of transporter proteins in the intestinal cells. Some choline is metabolized in the gut to betaine (trimethylglycine) and trimethylamine, which are also absorbed by the gut. Choline, as well as betaine and trimethylamine, are transported to the liver via portal circulation. All tissues accumulate choline by diffusion and mediated transport.

In the liver, choline participates in various metabolic reactions, including the formation of CDP-choline, which combines with diacylglycerol to form phosphatidylcholine. Through oxidation, it forms the methyl donor betaine. Trimethylamine, a choline metabolite, is oxidized to trime-

thylamine oxide in the liver. Choline is transported across the blood-brain barrier by a specific carrier mechanism. Within the brain and other nervous tissue, choline is converted to acetylcholine by the enzyme choline acetyltransferase. Only a small fraction of dietary choline goes to form acetylcholine. The kidney also accumulates choline. Some appears in the urine unchanged but most is oxidized to form betaine.

INDICATIONS AND USAGE

Increased choline intake has recently been recommended by the Food and Nutrition Board of the National Academy of Sciences for pregnant and nursing women to help ensure normal fetal brain development. And, like phosphatidylcholine (see Phosphatidylcholine), choline may be helpful in some liver diseases, manic conditions, cognitive disorders, tardive dyskinesia and, possibly, some cancers.

RESEARCH SUMMARY

There is some evidence, derived from animal studies, that choline, if present in adequate amounts during pregnancy and breast feeding, can help ensure healthy fetal brain development. These studies further suggest that adequate prenatal choline can have long-lasting positive effects on cognitive function, including memory.

In a series of studies, the diets of pregnant rats have been supplemented with varying amounts of choline for variable periods of time during gestation. Supplementation, especially during the second half of pregnancy, has been strongly associated with positive cognitive effects (which are not seen in control animals receiving little or no choline).

Tested as adults, rats that had received approximately three times control amounts of choline during gestation were significantly superior in tasks that assess attention and spatial and temporal memory. Offspring of mothers that received no choline during pregnancy had attention and memory task impairment. And, even though both control and experimental animals were given the same standardized normal diet after birth, those whose mothers got higher levels of choline during pregnancy continued to exhibit significant cognitive superiority over controls throughout life. "Thus," one of the researchers concluded, "prenatal supplementation with choline prevented the normally observed memory decline of old age."

These significant studies are buttressed by neuroanatomical, neurophysiological and neurochemical studies that have similarly shown that choline has positive, long-lasting effects on prenatal brain development at the cellular level. Some of these studies have produced direct evidence that choline supplementation stimulates cell division in the embryonic brain, while choline deficiency increases apoptosis in areas of the brain, principally the hippocampus and septum, associated with memory processing. It has been hypothe-sized that choline supplementation during gestation may exert its apparent long-term effects through cellular and synaptic modifications that permanently increase memory-processing capacity.

Human studies have yet to be conducted on choline's effects on the fetus, but one researcher concludes that there is hope that ''optimal dietary choline early in life may improve human cognitive development and slow cognitive declines associated with aging.''

The Food and Nutrition Board of the National Academy of Sciences is impressed enough with research to date that it has recently recommended that pregnant and nursing women increase their intake of choline. The board recommends 425 milligrams of choline daily for women who are not pregnant, 450 milligrams daily for pregnant women and 550 milli-grams daily for nursing women.

For information about other research related to choline, see Phosphatidylcholine.

CONTRAINDICATIONS, PRECAUTIONS, ADVERSE REACTIONS

CONTRAINDICATIONS
No contraindications are reported.

PRECAUTIONS
Trimethylaminuria or fish-odor syndrome: Trimethylamin-uria is a rare genetic metabolic disorder occurring in oil to 0.1 to 1% of the population. It is due to deficiency of the enzyme trimethylamine-N-oxide synthetase, which converts trimethylamine to trimethylamine-N-oxide. Trimethylamine, which is produced from choline, is excreted from the body via the urine, sweat, breath and other bodily secretions. It has a nauseating, rotten-fish-smelling odor. Trimethylamine-N-oxide, the metabolite of trimethylamine, is non-odorous. Those with primary genetic trimethyluria (the inherited enzyme deficiency) should restrict intake of choline. Also, those with certain types of liver disease caused by any of the hepatitis viruses or from other etiologies may develop fishy body odor when taking supplemental choline. Choline intake should be restricted in these cases.

ADVERSE REACTIONS
Choline doses of up to 3 grams daily are generally well tolerated with occasional reports of nausea, diarrhea and loose stools. Higher doses have been associated with fishy body odor—particularly in those with trimethylaminuria (fish-odor syndrome). Trimethylaminuria may also occur in those with liver damage who are using high doses of choline. High intakes of choline have been associated with excessive sweating and hypotension. There are some reports of depression or increased symptoms of depression in those using high doses of choline bitartrate.

There are no adequate data demonstrating a no-observed-adverse-effect level (NOAEL) for excess choline intake. Based on two clinical studies in humans, a lowest-observed-adverse-effect level (LOAEL) of 7.5 grams daily has been determined. At 7.5 grams of choline daily, nausea, diarrhea and a small decrease in blood pressure were reported in some patients. The upper limit (UL) for adults is 3.5 grams daily. Individuals that may be at increased risk of side effects with choline intakes at the UL include those with trimethylamin-uria, liver disease, renal disease, depression and Parkinson's disease.

INTERACTIONS

DRUGS
Methotrexate: Methotrexate may diminish pools of all choline metabolites. Choline supplementation reverses fatty liver caused by methotrexate administration in rats.

NUTRITIONAL SUPPLEMENTS
Choline, via its metabolism to betaine, works in concert with vitamins B_6, B_{12} and folic acid in the metabolism of the potentially atherogenic substance homocysteine.

DOSAGE AND ADMINISTRATION

Typical doses of choline intake range from 300 to 1,200 milligrams daily. The major choline salt forms available are choline chloride and choline bitartrate.

Phosphatidylcholine is a delivery form of choline (see Phosphatidylcholine).

Choline is also added to some infant formulas and to some TPN formulations.

Adequate intakes (AI) of choline have been established by the Food and Nutrition Board of the Institute of Medicine of the National Academy of Sciences. The AI for adults is 550 milligrams daily for men and 425 milligrams daily for women. A summary of AIs for various age groups is as follows:

	(AI)
Infants	0-5 months, 125 mg/day or 8 mg/kg; 6-11 months, 150 mg/day or 17 mg/kg.
Children	1-3 years, 200 mg/day; 4-8 years, 250 mg/day; 9-13 years, 375 mg/day.
Males Females	14-18 years, 550 mg/day; 14-18 years, 450 mg/day.
Men Women	19 and older, 550 mg/day; 19 and older, 425 mg/day.

Pregnant Women   450 mg/day.

Lactating Women
   All Ages   550 mg/day.

All of the above values are for the choline base. Values for choline salts are higher. For example, values for choline chloride would be 1.4 times as high and for choline bitartrate even higher. About 13 percent of phosphatidylcholine is choline.

HOW SUPPLIED

Capsules — 350 mg, 648 mg
Powder
Tablets — 250 mg, 500 mg, 648 mg, 650 mg

LITERATURE

Albright CD, Liu R, Berthea TC, et al. Choline deficiency induces apoptosis in SV 40-immortalized CW SV-1 rat hepatocytes in culture. *FASEB J.* 1996; 10:510-516.

Blusztajn JK. Choline, a vital amine. *Science.* 1998; 281:794-795.

Canty DJ, Zeisel SH. Lecithin and choline in human health and disease. *Nutr Rev.* 1994; 52:327-339.

Cohen BM, Renshaw PF, Stoll, AL. Decreased brain choline uptake in older adults. An in vivo magnetic resonance spectroscopy study. *J Amer Med Ass.* 1995; 274:902-907.

Food and Nutrition Board. Institute of Medicine. *Dietary Reference Intakes for Thiamin, Riboflavin, Niacin, Vitamin B6, Folate, Vitamin B12, Pantothenic Acid, Biotin, and Choline* (National Academy Press, Washington, DC, 1998).

Pyapili GK, Turner DA, Williams, CL. Prenatal dietary choline supplementation decreases the threshold for induction of long-term potentiation in young adult rats. *J Neurophysiol.* 1998; 79:1790-1796.

Schocke Z, J, Kohlmueller D, Quak E, et al. Mild trimethylaminuria caused by common variants in FMO3 gene. *Lancet.* 1997; 354:834-835.

Shelly EP, Shelley WB. The fish odor syndrome. Trimethyluria. *J Amer Med Ass.* 1984; 251:253-255.

Wurtman RJ, Hefti F, Melamed E. Precursor control of neurotransmitter synthesis. *Pharmacol Rev.* 1981; 32:315-335.

Yen C-L, E Mar, M-H, Zeisel SH. Choline deficiency-induced apoptosis in PC 12 cells is associated with diminished membrane phosphatidylcholine and sphingomyelin, accumulation of ceramide and ciccylglycerol, and activation of a caspace. *FASEB J.* 1999; 13:135-142.

Chondroitin Sulfate

TRADE NAMES

Chondroitin sulfate is available from numerous manufacturers generically. Branded products include Ramott (Key Company) Chondroitin Sulfate Support (Natural Treasures), CSA (Twinlab), Chonflex (American Health).

DESCRIPTION

Chondroitin sulfate belongs to a family of heteropolysaccharides called glycosaminoglycans or GAGs. Glycosaminoglycans were formerly known as mucopolysaccharides. GAGs in the form of proteoglycans comprise the ground substance in the extracellular matrix of connective tissue. Chondroitin sulfate is made up of linear repeating units containing D-galactosamine and D-glucuronic acid. Chondroitin sulfate is found in humans in cartilage, bone, cornea, skin and the arterial wall. This type of chondroitin sulfate is sometimes referred to as chondroitin sulfate A or galactosaminoglucuronoglycan sulfate. The amino group of galactosamines in the basic unit of chondroitin sulfate A is acetylated, yielding N-acetyl-galactosamine; there is a sulfate group esterified to the 4-position in N-acetyl-galactosamine. (Chondroitin sulfate A is also sometimes called chondroitin 4-sulfate.) The molecular weight of chondroitin sulfate ranges from 5,000 to 50,000 daltons and contains about 15 to 150 basic units of D-galactosamine and D-glucuronic acid. It is represented by the following structural formula:

Chondroitin sulfate A $R = SO_3H$ $R^1 = H$
Chondroitin sulfate C $R = H$ $R^1 = SO_3H$

Chondroitin sulfate C, primarily found in fish and shark cartilage, but also in humans, is also made up of linear repeating units of D-galactosamine and D-glucuronic acid. The amino group of D-galactosamine is acetylated to give N-acetyl-galactosamine, and, in the case of chondroitin sulfate C, the sulfate group is esterified to the 6-position in N-acetyl-galactosamine. Chondroitin sulfate C is sometimes called chondroitin 6-sulfate. Chondroitin sulfate B is also known as dermatan sulfate. It is abundant in skin and is also found in heart valves, tendons and arterial walls. Dermatan sulfate is made up of linear repeating units containing D-galactosamine and either L-iduronic acid or D-glucuronic acid. Its molecular weight ranges from 15,000 to 40,000 daltons.

The source of chondroitin sulfate used in nutritional supplements includes the cartilaginous rings of bovine trachea and pork byproducts (ears and snout). Shark cartilage and whale septum cartilage have also been used to obtain chondroitin sulfate. Chondroitin sulfate supplements are usually isomeric mixtures of chondroitin sulfate A(chondroitin 4-sulfate) and chondroitin sulfate C(chondroitin 6-sulfate).

ACTIONS AND PHARMACOLOGY

ACTIONS

The action of orally administered chondroitin sulfate has yet to be clarified. Possible actions include promotion and maintenance of the structure and function of cartilage (referred to as chondroprotection), pain relief of osteoarthritic joints and anti-inflammatory activity.

MECHANISM OF ACTION

Until the specific actions of supplemental chondroitin sulfate are determined, the mechanism of action is a matter of speculation. However, much is known about the biochemistry and physiology of chondroitin sulfate and similar molecules. Glycoproteins known as proteoglycans form the ground substance in the extracellular matrix of connective tissue. Proteoglycans are polyanionic substances of high molecular weight and contain heteropolysaccharide-side-chains covalently linked to a polypeptide-chain backbone. The polysaccharides, which include chondroitin sulfate and hyaluronic acid, make up as much as 95% of the proteoglycan structure.

The polysaccharides in proteoglycans are called glycosaminoglycans or GAGs. Chondroitin sulfate and hyaluronic acid are vital for the structure and function of articular cartilage. Chondroitin sulfate and hyaluronic acid are fundamental components of aggrecan found in articular cartilage. Aggrecan confers upon articular cartilage shock-absorbing properties. It does this by providing cartilage with a swelling pressure that is restrained by the tensile force of collagen fibers. This balance confers upon articular cartilage the deformable resilience vital to its function. Hyaluronic acid, which is also found in synovial fluid, has lubricating properties for the joint.

In the progression of degenerative joint disease or osteoarthritis, aggrecan synthesis is decreased, leading to the loss of cartilage resiliency and the pain and other symptoms that accompany osteoarthritis.

Intra-articular injections of hyaluronic acid, an FDA-approved drug, can relieve joint pain and improve mobility. This type of therapy is called viscotherapy and is believed to act by improving joint lubrication. If chondroitin sulfate were delivered into joints, some similar effects would be expected. Animal studies have shown that parenterally administered chondroitin sulfate does get into cartilage tissue as does orally administered chondroitin sulfate. There is some human data suggesting orally administered chondroitin

sulfate, particularly low-molecular-weight chondroitin sulfate, is also delivered to articular tissue. There is some indication that orally administered chondroitin sulfate leads to increases in hyaluronic acid and viscosity of synovial fluid, as well as decreases in collagenase in synovial fluid. That is, glucosamine delivered into joints may inhibit enzymes involved in cartilage degradation and enhance the production of hyaluronic acid.

PHARMACOKINETICS

Earlier studies using high-molecular-weight chondroitin sulfate, concluded that there was no significant absorption of this high-molecular-weight version of chondroitin sulfate. More recent studies demonstrate that there is probably significant absorption of low-molecular-weight chondroitin sulfate. Absorption appears to occur from the stomach and small intestine. There is also an indication that some chondroitin sulfate, after absorption, does enter the joint space. Studies of the pharmacokinetics of orally administered chondroitin sulfate are ongoing.

It is of interest to note that a molecule similar in many resects to chondroitin sulfate, pertosan polysulfate, FDA-approved for the treatment of interstitial cystitis, is given orally and is absorbed to some extent.

INDICATIONS AND USAGE

Low-molecular-weight oral chondroitin sulfate may be indicated for the treatment and prevention of osteoarthritis, either by itself or in combination with a glucosamine supplement (see Glucosamine). There is a suggestion that chondroitin sulfate may be helpful in atherosclerosis, but more research is needed to determine if this is the case.

RESEARCH SUMMARY

Two recent meta-analyses indicate that chondroitin sulfate may be useful in the treatment of osteoarthritis. One of these meta-analyses included all double-blind, placebo-controlled trials that lasted four weeks or longer. This meta-analysis also included trials that studied the effects of glucosamine (see Glucosamine) on osteoarthritis. In all, there were 13 of these studies (six involving glucosamine and seven involving chondroitin sulfate).

All 13 studies found positive results in hip or knee osteoarthritis. The authors of the meta-analysis judged a trial positive if there was 25% or more improvement in the treatment group compared with placebo. The Levesque Index and global pain scores were used to assess improvement. Very significant improvement was associated with both glucosamine (39.5%) and chondroitin (40.2%), compared with placebo.

In another recent meta-analysis of chondroitin sulfate, this one examining four randomized double-blind, placebo- or

NSAID-controlled studies of 227 patients, chondroitin sulfate supplemented subjects showed at least 50% improvement, compared with controls. Various studies have reported significant reduction in NSAID use among osteoarthritis subjects supplemented with chondroitin sulfate.

There is also radiological evidence of chondroitin's possible efficacy in osteoarthritis. Knee joint space decreased significantly in placebo subjects but remained unchanged in those receiving chondroitin sulfate for a year. And, in another study, those receiving chondroitin sulfate showed significantly fewer instances of erosive osteoarthritis (compared with placebo controls) on hand radiographs over a three-year period.

A significant synergistic effect has been reported recently using combined glucosamine hydrochloride and chondroitin sulfate in an experimental study. The combination was more effective than either substance alone in inhibiting progression of degenerative cartilage lesions. Longer term clinical studies are needed to confirm or refute this synergy effect. A large multi-center study directed by the National Institutes of Health is now underway and may shed further light on this issue.

It is believed that chondroitin sulfate's possible efficacy in osteoarthritis derives from the fact that it is one of the two most abundant glycosaminoglycans (GAGs) in articular cartilage. Supplementation with this GAG seems, in part at least, to confer chondroprotection through its inhibitory action on some of the enzymes that damage cartilage. Further, by inhibiting other enzymes that can block transport of nutrients that nourish cartilage, this GAG may promote cartilage replacement.

It has been known for some time that injections of hyaluronic acid into arthritic joints can bring significant pain relief and enhanced mobility. Thus it is logical to assume that chondroitin sulfate, if it can reach the joints, may have similar effects since this substance has the ability to bind to receptor sites on synovial cell surfaces and thus induce production of hyaluronic acid, crucial to joint mobility.

The question for some time was whether a large molecule like chondroitin sulfate could achieve this penetration. Recent studies demonstrate that a low-molecular-weight version of oral chondroitin sulfate, of the sort used in all of the U.S. clinical trials, is absorbed.

Some years ago, chondroitin sulfate was investigated for its possible use in atherosclerosis. There was some evidence that it could favorably lower lipid levels and protect against blood clotting. Atheromatous aortic lesions were prevented in animals on high-cholesterol diets.

In a clinical trial, 60 patients suffering from coronary artery disease received 2 grams of oral chondroitin sulfate daily for 900 days. During that period, 16 of 60 unsupplemented control patients suffered acute coronary incidents. Only one of the chondroitin sulfate-treated subjects had an acute coronary incident. The same research group later followed up with similarly positive results.

More research is needed before any conclusions can be drawn with respect to a possible role for chondroitin sulfate in the treatment or prevention of atherosclerosis.

CONTRAINDICATIONS, PRECAUTIONS, ADVERSE REACTIONS

CONTRAINDICATIONS
None known.

PRECAUTIONS
Because of insufficient safety data, children, pregnant women and nursing mothers should avoid using chondroitin sulfate. Because of the theoretical possibility that chondroitin sulfate may have antithrombotic activity, those taking warfarin and those with hemophilia should exercise caution in its use. Those who need to restrict their salt intake should , if they use chondroitin sulfate, use salt-free preparations.

ADVERSE REACTIONS
Side effects that have been reported are mostly of the mild gastrointestinal variety, such as epigastric distress, nausea and diarrhea. No sulfa-allergic reactions or other allergic reactions have yet been reported.

INTERACTIONS
There are no known drug, nutrient, food or herb interactions. Chitosan (see Chitosan) may form complexes with chondroitin sulfate decreasing its absorption. Therefore, chondroitin sulfate should not be used concomitantly with chitosan.

OVERDOSAGE
Overdosage of chondroitin has not been reported in the literature.

DOSAGE AND ADMINISTRATION
Low-molecular-weight chondroitin sulfate is available as a stand-alone supplement or in combination with glucosamine (see Glucosamine). The usual dose used by those with osteoarthritis is 1,200 milligrams daily in divided doses.

It usually takes several weeks of supplementation before effects, if any, are experienced.

Chondroitin sulfate in combination with hyaluronic acid is available as an FDA-approved drug. It is used as a viscoelastic agent in cataract surgery. Hyaluronic acid itself is FDA approved for the treatment of osteoarthritis. The two forms presently available, Hylan G-F 20 (Synvisc, Wyeth-Ayerst) and sodium hyaluronate (Hyalgan, Sanofi/Orthologic), are given by intra-articular injection.

HOW SUPPLIED

Capsules — 250 mg, 400 mg, 500 mg
Powder
Tablets — 250 mg, 400 mg, 600 mg

LITERATURE

Baici A, Horler D, Moser B, et al. Analysis of glycosaminoglycans in human serum after oral administration of chondroitin sulfate. *Rheum Int.*1992; 12:81-88.

Bartolucci C, Cellai L, Cordani D, et al. Chondroprotective action of chondroitin sulfate. Competitive action of chondroitin sulfate on the digestion of hyaluronan by bovine testicular hyaluronidase. *Int J Tiss Res*. 1991; 13:311-317.

Bourgeois P, Chales G, Dehais J, et al. Efficacy and tolerability of chondroitin sulfate 1,200 mg/day vs. chondroitin 400 mg/day vs placebo. *Osteoarthritis Cartilage*. 1998; 6 SupplA:25-30.

Busci L, Poor G. Efficacy and tolerability of oral chondroitin sulfate as a symptomatic slow-acting drug. for osteoarthritis (SYSADOA) in the treatment of knee osteoarthrosis. *Osteoarthritis Cartilage*. 1998; 6 SupplA:31-36.

Conte A, Volpi N, Palmiera L, et al. Biochemical and pharmacokinetic aspects of oral treatment with chondroitin sulfate. *Drug Res*. 1995; 45:918-925.

Deal CL, Moskowitz RW. Nutraceuticals as therapeutic agents in osteoarthritis. The role of glucosamine, chondroitin sulfate, and collagen hydrolysate. *Rheum Dis Clin North Am*. 1999; 25:379-395.

Leffler CT, Phillipi AF, Leffler SG, et al. Glucosamine, chondroitin, and manganese ascorbate for degenerative joint disease of the knee or low back: a randomized, double-blind, placebo-controlled pilot study. *Mil Med*. 1999; 164:85-91.

McAlindon TE, LaValley MP, Gulin JP, Felson DT. Glucosamine and chondroitin for treatment of osteoarthritis. A systematic quality assessment and meta-analysis. *JAMA*. 2000; 283:1469-1475.

Morrison LM, Enrick L. Coronary heart disease: reduction of death rate by chondroitin sulfate A. *Angiology*. 1973; 24:269-287.

Morrison LM, Bajwa GS, Alfin-Slater RB, Ershoff BH. Prevention of vascular lesions by chondroitin sulfate A in the coronary artery and aorta of rats induced by a hypervitaminosis D, cholesterol-containing diet. *Atherosclerosis*. 1972; 16:105-118

Pipitone VR. Chondroprotection with chondroitin sulfate. *Drugs Exp Clin Res*. 1991; 17:3-7.

Ronca F, Palmieri L, Panicucci P. Ronca G. Anti-inflammatory activity of chondroitin sulfate. *Osteoarthritis Cartilage*. 1998; 6 SupplA:14-21.

Towheed TE, Anastassiades TP. Glucosamine and chondroitin for treating symptoms of osteoarthritis. Evidence is widely touted but incomplete. *JAMA*. 2000; 283:1483-1484.

Uebelhart D, Thonar EJ, Delmas PD, et al. Effects of oral chondroitin sulfate on the progression of knee osteoarthritis: a pilot study. *Osteoarthritis Cartilage*. 1998; 6 SupplA:39-46.

Yamanashi S, Toyoda H, Furuya N, et al. Metabolic study on chondroitin sulfate in rabbits. *Yakugaku Zasshi*. 1991; 111:73-76.

Chromium

TRADE NAMES

Chromate (Western Research Labs), GTF Chromium (Swanson Health Products), M2 Chromium (Miller Pharmacal Group), Chromacaps (The Key Company), Amino-CR (Tyson Neutraceuticals), Chromax (Western Research Labs), Pichrome (Camall Company), Nia-Chrom (Miller Pharmacal), CR-GTF (Bio-Tech Pharmacal).

DESCRIPTION

Chromium is believed to be an essential trace mineral in human nutrition. Evidence suggests that it plays an important role in normal carbohydrate metabolism. In the 1950s it was found that chromium was necessary for the maintenance of normal glucose tolerance in rats; chromium-deficient rats had impaired glucose tolerance. Subsequently, it was found that patients receiving long-term total parenteral nutrition (TPN) without chromium developed glucose intolerance, weight loss and peripheral neuropathy. These symptoms were reversed when the patients were given intravenous chromium chloride.

Chromium is a metal with atomic number 24 and an atomic mass of 52 daltons. Its symbol is Cr. It occurs in nature chiefly as a chrome-iron ore. Chromium exists in several valence states, of which the trivalent and hexavalent states are the most common. Most chromium in the food supply is in the trivalent state. Hexavalent chromium compounds are recognized as toxic and are potential carcinogens. Chromium is found in many foods, typically in small amounts. Good food sources of chromium include whole grains, cereals, spices (black pepper, thyme), mushrooms, brown sugar, coffee, tea, beer, wine and meat products. Brewer's yeast is also a good source of chromium. Fruits and vegetables are generally poor sources of chromium, as are most refined foods.

ACTIONS AND PHARMACOLOGY

ACTIONS

Chromium may have glucose-regulatory activity. It may also have hypocholesterolemic and anti-atherogenic activities.

MECHANISM OF ACTION

The mechanism of chromium's possible glucose-regulatory activity is not well understood, but there are some theories. It is thought that the possible action of chromium on the control of blood glucose concentrations is the potentiation of insulin. One proposed mechanism involves increased insulin binding, increased insulin receptor number and increased insulin receptor phosphorylation. Chromium stimulates protein kinase activity of rat adipocytes in the presence of insulin. Chromium also inhibits phosphotyrosine phosphatase, a rat homolog of tyrosine phosphatase that inactivates the insulin receptor. The activation by chromium of insulin receptor kinase activity and the inhibition of insulin receptor tyrosine phosphatase would lead to increased phosphorylation of the insulin receptor, which is associated with increased insulin sensitivity.

It has also been suggested that chromium may decrease hepatic extraction of insulin and improve glucose tolerance by such a mechanism. Earlier, it was found that glucose tolerance could be restored in chromium-deficient rats by feeding them an extract of brewer's yeast. Brewer's yeast is rich in chromium, and it was proposed that it contained an organic factor which potentiated the action of insulin. This factor was called the glucose tolerance factor or GTF. GTF was hypothesized to contain trivalent chromium bound to nicotinic acid and the amino acids glycine, cysteine and glutamic acid. However, an organic glucose tolerance factor has, to date, not been isolated from brewer's yeast.

Recently, an oligopeptide low molecular-weight chromium-binding substance (LMWCr) has been isolated from animal tissues. The oligopeptide is comprised of the amino acids glycine, cysteine, glutamic acid, and aspartic acid, with the two carboxylic acids (glutamic, aspartic) comprising more than half the amino acid residues. It is proposed that LMWCr is part of an insulin signal amplification system. Its possible participation in the glucose-regulatory activity may be as follows: chromium ions are transferred from transferrin to LMWCr. LMWCr normally exists in insulin-dependent cells in the apo or inactive form. Binding to chromic ions converts the inactive form to its holo or active form. Chromic-containing LMWCr then binds to insulin-activated insulin receptor, stimulating its tyrosine kinase activity and potentiating the activity of insulin. LMWCr is also called chromodulin because its proposed action is similar to that of calmodulin.

The mechanism of the possible hypocholesterolemic activity of chromium is unknown. The possible anti-atherogenic activity of chromium may be accounted for by its possible glucose-regulatory activity.

PHARMACOKINETICS

Very little chromium in the form of inorganic compounds, such as chromic chloride, is absorbed. The efficiency of absorption of chromium from chromic chloride is less than 2%. The efficiency of absorption of chromium from organic compounds is higher. For example, approximately 2.8% of an ingested dose of chromium picolinate is absorbed.

Following absorption, chromium is bound to transferrin and albumin. Chromium is transported primarily by transferrin.

Chromium is distributed to various tissues of the body but appears to have a preference for bone, spleen, liver and kidney. Pharmacokinetic studies indicate that chromium is distributed into four different compartments that have rapid, medium, slow and very slow turnover, respectively. Bone, spleen, liver and kidney appear to contain all four compartments. The half-life of the rapid compartment is less than one day, that of the medium compartment approximately one week and that of the slow compartment from 7 to 12 weeks. The half-life of chromium in the compartment which appears to turn over most slowly is approximately one year. This compartment is probably related to long-term tissue deposition.

Most of an ingested dose of chromium is excreted in the feces. Chromium that has been absorbed is excreted mainly in the urine. Little excretion occurs via the biliary route.

There is much that remains unknown regarding the pharmacokinetics of chromium and its various trivalent forms in humans. More research in this area is needed.

INDICATIONS AND USAGE

There is some evidence that chromium may improve glucose tolerance and may be helpful in some with diabetes. There is preliminary evidence it may have some favorable effects on lipids. Claims that it boosts athletic performance, builds muscle and promotes weight loss have little, if any, credible support. The Federal Trade Commission has, in fact, declared such claims to be unsubstantiated and deceptive. Evidence is mixed and still inconclusive with respect to claims that chromium picolinate may be mutagenic. The suggestion that chromium is nephrotoxic is based on isolated case studies and requires further investigation.

RESEARCH SUMMARY

The American Diabetes Association asserted in 1996 that ''chromium supplementation has no known benefit in patients who are not chromium deficient.'' Some patients on long-term parenteral nutrition have developed chromium deficiency and diabetic symptoms that were reversed with chromium supplementation. In general, plasma chromium levels are about 40% lower in diabetic subjects, compared with healthy individuals.

Recently a double-blind, placebo-controlled study of 180 subjects with type 2 diabetes demonstrated that supplemental chromium significantly improved fasting glucose, postprandial glucose, insulin, hemoglobin A_{1c} and cholesterol levels. Subjects in this study, conducted in China, received placebo, 200 micrograms of chromium picolinate or 1,000 micrograms of chromium picolinate daily. Subjects had suffered from diabetes for five to eight years. Better results were achieved with the higher dose of chromium.

This trial, while encouraging, was flawed in that baseline chromium status was not assessed; neither was postsupplemental status evaluated. Extrapolation of these results to Western populations is not possible. Additionally, the best designed prior studies have failed to show consistent results. Two of the best studies were largely negative. Variations may be due to divergence in chromium status at baseline and to the type and dose of chromium used. No beneficial effect was seen in diabetic patients taking 200 micrograms of chromium chloride, for example, but some positive effects were noted in those getting 400 micrograms or more of chromium chloride daily. With respect to the study in China, some hypothesized that the more dramatic effects achieved in that trial may be due to possible greater chromium deficiency in that country. More research is needed.

Chromium picolinate supplementation (200 micrograms daily) significantly decreased levels of total cholesterol, LDL-cholesterol and apolipoprotein B, compared with controls, in one small study. There was no significant effect on HDL-cholesterol. In a subsequent trial, 600 micrograms of chromium daily reportedly increased serum levels of HDL-cholesterol in patients taking beta-blockers. Again, however, studies have produced mixed results so that no persuasive conclusion can yet be reached with respect to chromium's effects on lipids.

One study reported that six weeks of chromium supplementation resulted in a significant increase in lean body mass and a decrease in body fat among athletes. Numerous, better designed follow-up studies, however, failed to confirm this finding. The original study used skinfold measurements (anthropometry) to assess changes in body composition. The subsequent studies used more sensitive measures, e.g., dual x-ray absorptiometry (DXA) and underwater weighing (hydrodensitometry). Even a study using the same anthropometry measurements that were employed in the original study also produced negative results.

Claims that chromium can be useful in treating obesity have similarly met with largely negative results. In some of these studies subjects have actually gained weight. Claims related to obesity were fueled by a study in which 200 micrograms of chromium daily reportedly led to weight loss even without alterations in food intake and exercise. In fact, however, weight loss in this small study was very modest, with a consequent high dropout rate. The same researchers conducted another study in which greater weight loss was achieved, but in this study chromium supplementation was used in conjunction with caloric restriction, dietary fiber and other

nutritional support, making it impossible to assess the role of chromium, if any, in the final results.

There are two *in vitro* reports that, in high concentrations, chromium picolinate, but not chromium chloride or chromium nicotinate, is clastogenic. Thus some have concluded that picolinate, rather than chromium itself, might be mutagenic and should thus be avoided. Some have suggested that long-term use of chromium picolinate, particularly at doses higher than 200 micrograms daily, could be hazardous. More research is needed to clarify this issue.

Additional warnings have been issued based upon scattered case reports. In one of these cases, a 33-year-old woman taking 1,200-2,400 micrograms of chromium picolinate daily for four to five months in an effort to lose weight developed renal failure. In another case, a 49-year-old woman who took 600 micrograms of chromium picolinate daily for six weeks was also diagnosed with chronic renal failure.

It has not been demonstrated conclusively that chromium picolinate caused the renal failure, but some have speculated that the greater absorbability of the picolinate form of chromium may, when used at higher doses long term, increase the incidence of any possible side effects. One researcher has speculated that supplementation with 600 micrograms of chromium picolinate daily for five years could result in tissue accumulation of chromium picolinate possibly sufficient to cause chromosomal damage similar to that seen in *in vitro* studies.

Though these precautions need to be further investigated, the observation of one reviewer should also be noted. In reviewing the safety data, he concluded; ''in contrast, better evidence exists that chromium is safe rather than toxic at very high doses.'' In contrast with the *in vitro* studies showing clastogenic effects, experimental *in vivo* results have differed. In one of these experiments, rats were fed either chromium chloride or chromium picolinate at high doses for 20 weeks. These doses were calculated to be several thousand times greater than the ESSADI (Estimated Safe and Adequate Daily Dietary Intake) for humans. After being killed, the animals were examined for toxic effects. Whether the animals received 0, 5, 25, 50 or 100 mg/kg of chromium, there were no significant differences in body weight, organ weight or blood variables. Histologic evaluations of liver and kidneys of controls and those fed the highest chromium doses, whether chloride or picolinate, also failed to find significant differences. Again, more research is needed.

CONTRAINDICATIONS, PRECAUTIONS, ADVERSE REACTIONS
CONTRAINDICATIONS
Chromium is contraindicated in those hypersensitive to any component of a chromium-containing supplement.

PRECAUTIONS

Pregnant women and nursing mothers should avoid doses of chromium above the upper limit of the estimated safe and adequate daily dietary intake (ESADDI). The ESADDI for chromium is 50 to 200 micrograms daily.

Those with a history of hypoglycemia should exercise caution in the use of chromium supplements.

Those with a history of hyperglycemia or type 2 diabetes mellitus should only use chromium supplements for the possible management of abnormal glucose tolerance under medical supervision.

ADVERSE REACTIONS

Chromium supplements are generally well tolerated. There are a few reports of adverse reactions particularly with use of chromium picolinate. There is one report of a 24-year-old body builder who developed rhadomyolysis after ingesting 1,200 micrograms of chromium in the form of chromium picolinate. Acute generalized exanthematous pustulosis was reported to be associated with the use of chromium picolinate. A case of interstitial nephritis was reported to occur five months after a subject received a six-week course of 600 micrograms of chromium in the form of chromium picolinate daily. Another report described anemia, thrombocytopenia, hemolysis, liver dysfunction, renal failure and weight loss after the use of 1,200-2,400 micrograms of chromium picolinate daily for four to five months.

INTERACTIONS

DRUGS

Beta-Blockers: One study reported that those on beta-blockers who took 600 micrograms daily of chromium in the form of high-chromium yeast were found to have modestly elevated HDL-cholesterol levels after two months of chromium use.

NUTRITIONAL SUPPLEMENTS

Ascorbate: Concomitant intake of ascorbate and chromium may increase the absorption of chromium.

FOODS

Concomitant intake of chromium with foods rich in phytic acid (unleavened bread, raw beans, seeds, nuts and grains and soy isolates) may decrease the absorption of chromium.

DOSAGE AND ADMINISTRATION.

There are a few forms of chromium available for nutritional supplementation. They include chromium picolinate, chromium polynicotinate, chromium chloride and high-chromium yeast. These forms are available as stand-alone supplements or in combination products. Typical doses of chromium range from 50 to 200 micrograms daily, expressed as elemental chromium.

Dietary intake of chromium is approximately 25 micrograms daily. The Food and Nutrition Board of the U.S. National Academy of Sciences has recommended the following estimated safe and adequate daily dietary intake (ESADDI) values for chromium:

Age (years)	ESSADI (micrograms)
0-0.5	10-40
0.5-1	20-60
1-3	20-80
4-6	30-120
7-adults	50-200

HOW SUPPLIED

Capsules — 100 mcg, 500 mcg

Tablets — 100 mcg, 200 mcg, 400 mcg, 500 mcg, 1 mg

LITERATURE

Anderson RA. Chromium, glucose intolerance and diabetes. *J Amer Coll Nutr.* 1998; 17:548-555.

Anderson RA. Effects of chromium on body composition and weight loss. *Nutr Rev.* 1998; 56:266-270.

Anderson RA, Bryden NA, Polansky MM. Lack of toxicity of chromium chloride and chromium picolinate in rats. *J Amer Coll Nutr.* 1997; 16:273-279.

Anderson RA, Cheng N, Bryden NA, et al. Elevated intakes of supplemental chromium improve glucose and insulin variables in individuals with type II diabetes. *Diabetes.* 1997; 46:1786-1791.

Cerulli J, Grabe DW, Gauthier I, et al. Chromium picolinate toxicity. *Ann Pharmacother.* 1998; 32:428-431.

Donaldson RM Jr, Barreras RF. Intestinal absorption of trace quantities of chromium. *J Lab Clin Med.* 1966; 68:484-493.

Guan X, Matte JJ, Ku PK, et al. High chromium yeast supplementation improves glucose tolerance in pigs by decreasing hepatic extraction of insulin. *J Nutr.* 2000; 130:1274-1279.

International Symposium on the Health Effects of Dietary Chromium. J Trace Elem Exp Med. 1999; 12:53-169.

Jeejeebhoy KN. The role of chromium in nutrition and therapeutics and as a potential toxin. *Nutr Rev.* 1999; 57:329-335.

Kaats GR, Blum K, Fisher JA, Adelman JA. Effects of chromium picolinate supplementation on body composition: a randomized, double-masked, placebo-controlled study. *Curr Therap Res.* 1996; 57:747-756.

Lukaski HC. Chromium as a supplement. *Annu Rev Nutr.* 1999; 19:279-302.

Martin WR, Fuller RE. Suspected chromium picolinate-induced rhabdomyolysis. *Pharmacotherapy.* 1998; 18:860-862.

Merz W. Chromium in human nutrition: a review. *J Nutr.* 1993; 123:626-633.

Nielsen FH. Controversial chromium. *Nutr Today.* 1996; 31:226-233.

Press RI, Geller J, Evans GW. The effect of chromium picolinate on serum cholesterol and apolipoprotein fractions in human subjects. *West J Med.* 1990; 152:41-45.

Porter DJ, Raymond LW, Anastasio GD. Chromium: Friend or foe? *Arch Fam Med.* 1999; 8:386-390.

Roeback JR Jr, Hla KM, Chambless LE, Fletcher RH. Effects of chromium supplementation on serum high-density lipoprotein cholesterol levels in men taking beta-blockers. *Ann Int Med.* 1991; 115:917-924.

Speetjens JK, Collins RA, Vincent JB, Woski SA. The nutritional supplement chromium (III) tris (picolinate) cleaves DNA. *Chem Res Toxicol.* 1999; 12:483-487.

Stearns DM, Belbruno JJ, Wetterhahn KE. A prediction of chromium (III) accumulation in humans from chromium dietary supplements. *FASEB J.* 1995; 9:1650-1657.

Stearns DM, Wise JP Sr, Patierno SR, Wetterhahn KE. Chromium (III) picolinate produces chromosome damage in Chinese hamster ovary cells. *FASEB J.* 1995; 9:1643-1649.

Stoecker BJ. Chromium. In: Shils ME, Olson JA, Shike M, Ross AC, eds. *Modern Nutrition in Health and Disease.* 9th ed. Baltimore, MD: Williams and Wilkins; 1999:277-282.

Verhage AH, Cheong WK, Jeejeebhoy. Neurologic symptoms due to possible chromium deficiency in long-term parenteral nutrition that closely mimic metronidazole-induced syndromes. *J Parenter Enter Nutr.* 1996; 20:123-127.

Vincent J. The biochemistry of chromium. *J Nutr.* 2000; 130:715-718.

Vincent JB. Quest for the molecular mechanism of chromium action and its relationship to diabetes. *Nutr Rev.* 2000; 58:67-72.

Wasser WG, Feldman NS, D'Agati VD. Chronic renal failure after ingestion of over-the-counter chromium picolinate [letter]. *Ann Intern Med.* 1997; 126:410.

Young PC, Turiansky GW, Bonner MW, Benson PM. Acute generalized exanthematous pustulosis induced by chromium picolinate. *J Am Acad Dermatol.* 1999; 41(5 pt 2):820-823.

Chrysin

TRADE NAMES

Chrysinex (Pinnacle), Fx Chrysin (Genetic Evolutionary Nutrition).

DESCRIPTION

Chrysin belongs to the flavone class of flavonoids. Chrysin is found naturally in various plants including the *Pelargonium* species, which are germanium-like plants; the *Passiflora* or passion flower species, which include tropical passion fruit; and the *Pinaceae* species, including pine trees.

Chrysin, principally obtained from the plant *Passiflora coerulea*, is marketed as a nutritional supplement and is especially popular among male body builders and other athletes because of its possible action in inhibiting the conversions of androgens to estrogens.

Chrysin is a solid substance with the molecular formula $C_{15}H_{10}O_4$. Its molecular weight is 254.24 daltons. It is practically insoluble in water. Chrysin is also known as 5,7-dihydroxyflavone and 5,7-dihydroxy-2-phenyl-4*H*-1-benzo-pyran-4-one. Chrysin is found in plants as such but is mainly found naturally in the form of a glucoside. Chrysin has the following chemical structure:

Chrysin

ACTIONS AND PHARMACOLOGY

ACTIONS

Chrysin may have aromatase-inhibitory action. It may also have phytoestrogenic, antioxidant and anxiolytic activities.

MECHANISM OF ACTION

Aromatase is a cytochrome P-450 enzyme that catalyzes the rate-limiting step in estrogen synthesis, the conversion of androgens to estrogens. Androstenedione and testosterone serve as substrates for aromatase. Aromatase, also known as estrogen synthase or synthetase, is inhibited by chrysin *in vitro*.

Chrysin has been demonstrated to bind weakly to estrogen receptors alpha and beta, again *in vitro*.

Chrysin's antioxidant potential has been shown by its ability to inhibit xanthine oxidase and consequently suppress the formation of uric acid and certain reactive oxygen species. It may also, under some conditions, inhibit lipid peroxidation.

Other *in vitro* studies have shown that chrysin binds to an area of the $GABA_A$ receptor known as the benzodiazepine receptor.

PHARMACOKINETICS

Little is known of the pharmacokinetics of chrysin in humans. Intestinal and hepatic cell cultures indicate that chrysin can get into cells but that it undergoes extensive glucuronidation and sulfation within the cells. If oral chrysin were to be extensively metabolized following absorption, one would expect that it would be essentially inactivated.

Human pharmacokinetic studies are needed to clarify this. Chrysin does appear to be absorbed and to have activity in certain animal models.

INDICATIONS AND USAGE

Chrysin's aromatase-inhibiting effects have made it popular among some body builders and athletes who use androgens. Very preliminary research suggests that chrysin may emerge as a useful anxiolytic agent, that it might aid in the control of morphine withdrawl and that it might have some chemopreventive properties in cardiovascular disease and cancer.

RESEARCH SUMMARY

Chrysin's ability to inhibit the aromatization of androstenedione and testosterone to estrogens has been demonstrated in the laboratory. Chrysin has been shown to be among the most potent of the natural and synthetic flavone inhibitors of human estrogen aromatase. There are no studies directly demonstrating that chrysin makes the use of testosterone and related steroids less likely to produce estrogenic side effects.

A study using rats has shown that various flavonoids, including chrysin, can selectively bind to the central benzodiazepine receptor and thus exert potent anxiolytic and other benzodiazepine effects. More research is warranted.

Another study, this one *in vitro*, has suggested that chrysin might be helpful in controlling morphine withdrawal. Still other *in vitro* studies have found some chrysin-related chemopreventive effects in cardiovascular disease and cancer. No conclusions can yet be drawn from these very early studies.

CONTRAINDICATIONS, PRECAUTIONS, ADVERSE REACTIONS

CONTRAINDICATIONS

Chrysin is contraindicated in those with prostate cancer. It is also contraindicated in those hypersensitive to any component of a chrysin-containing product.

PRECAUTIONS

Pregnant women, nursing mothers, children and adolescents should avoid using chrysin. Women generally should avoid its use.

Hormonal manipulation may have unforeseen consequences. Those interested in chrysin supplementation should exercise caution in its use.

Women with hormone dependent malignancies (breast, uterine, ovarian) should only use chrysin if they are in a clinical study or if chrysin is prescribed and monitored by their physicians.

ADVERSE REACTIONS

No reported adverse reactions.

INTERACTIONS

Aromatase inhibitors: Chrysin may be addictive to the effects of such aromatase inhibitors as aminoglutethimide, anastrozole and letrozole.

OVERDOSAGE

There are no reports of overdosage.

DOSAGE AND ADMINISTRATION

Body builders and athletes—typically male—who use chrysin take about one gram daily during training.

HOW SUPPLIED

Capsules — 250 mg

Extended Release Tablets — 250 mg

LITERATURE

Capasso A, Piacente S, Pizza C, Sorrentino L. Flavonoids reduce morphine withdrawl *in vitro*. *J Pharm Pharmacol.* 1998; 50:561-564.

Galijatovic A, Otake Y, Walle UK, Walle T. Extensive metabolism of the flavonoid chrysin by human Caco-2 and Hep G2 cells. *Xenobiotica.* 1999; 29:1241-1256.

Jeong HJ, Shin YG, Kim IH, Pezzuto JM. Inhibition of aromatase activity by flavonoids. *Arch Pharm Res.* 1999; 22:309-312.

Kellis JT Jr, Vickery LE. Inhibition of human estrogen synthetase (aromatase) by flavones. *Science.* 1984; 225:1032-1034.

Kuiper GG, Lemmen JG, Carlsson B, et al. Interaction of estrogenic chemicals and phytoestrogens with estrogen receptor beta. *Endocrinology.* 1998; 139:4256-4263.

Nagao A, Seki M, Kobayashi H. Inhibition of xanthine oxidase by flavonoids. *Biosci Biotechnol Biochem.* 1999; 63:1787-1790.

Paladini AC, Marder M, Viola H, et al. Flavonoids and the central nervous system: from forgotten factors to potent anxiolytic compounds. *J Pharm Pharmacol.* 1999; 51:519-526.

Salgueriro JB, Ardenghi P, Dias M, et al. Anxiolytic natural and synthetic flavonoid ligands of the central benzodiazepine receptor have no effect on memory tasks in rats. *Pharmacol Biochem Behav.* 1997; 58:887-891.

Walle UK, Galijatovic A, Walle T. Transport of the flavonoid chrysin and its conjugated metabolites by the human intestinal cell line Caco-2. *Biochem Pharmacol.* 1999; 58:431-438.

Cocoa Flavonoids

TRADE NAMES

Calcium Cocoa Chewable (Natrol).

DESCRIPTION

Cocoa and chocolate are products derived from cacao beans, the seeds of the *Theobroma cacao* tree. Polyphenols comprise about 12 to 18% of the dry weight of cacao beans.

About 60% of the polyphenols are in the form of procyanidins (also known as leucocyanidins).

Procyanidins in cocoa and chocolate are mainly homodimers and homotrimers of (-)-epicatechin or heterodimers of (-)-epicatechin and (+)-catechin. (-)-Epicatechin and (+)-catechin belong to the flavan-3-ol class of flavonoids. Procyanidins containing up to 10 subunits (decamers) are found in fresh cacao beans and in dark chocolate. These are also called oligomeric procyanidins.

In addition to containing (-)-epicatechin, (+)-catechin and procyanidins, cocoa and chocolate contain other flavonoids, including other catechins and the flavanol quercetin and its glycosides. Collectively, these flavonoids are known as cocoa flavonoids or cocoa polyphenols.

Interestingly, the Mayans and Aztecs used cacao beans for the preparation of various remedies. The cocoa flavonoids appear to have potent antioxidant activity and may eventually turn out to have health-promoting benefits.

ACTIONS AND PHARMACOLOGY

ACTIONS

Cocoa flavonoids have antioxidant activity. They also may have anti-inflammatory and immunomodulatory activities.

MECHANISM OF ACTIONS

Cocoa flavonoids have been demonstrated to scavenge reactive oxygen and reactive nitrogen species. They may also chelate metals, such as ferrous cations, which participate in reactive oxygen species-generating reactions. Further, there is some evidence that the larger procyanidin oligomers have greater antioxidant potential.

Cocoa flavonoids have been shown to inhibit the oxidation of LDL. The oxidation of LDL is thought to be a crucial event in the pathogenesis of atherosclerosis.

Some of the cocoa flavonoids appear to reduce the expression of phytohemagglutinin-induced interleukin 2 (IL-2) mRNA, as well as the expression of interleukin 1beta (IL-1B), in peripheral blood mononuclear cells (PBMC).

Reduction of IL-2 and IL-1beta in PBMC could account, in part, for possible anti-inflammatory and immunomodulatory activities of cocoa flavonoids. The mechanism of these actions could again be due to the antioxidant action of cocoa flavonoids. Reactive oxygen species can activate nuclear transcription factor-Kappa B (NF-Kappa B). NF-Kappa B, in turn, may stimulate the production of such pro-inflammatory factors as IL-2 and IL-1 beta.

PHARMACOKINETICS

Little is known about the pharmacokinetics of cocoa polyphenols in humans. It appears that they do, at least partially, get absorbed. However, the extent of absorption appears to vary widely, not only among the different cocoa flavonoids, but also among subjects.

It also appears that the cocoa flavonoids undergo extensive glucuronidation, sulfation and methylation following and/or during absorption.

INDICATIONS AND USAGE

Cocoa flavonoids, in early-stage research, show some potential for the promotion of cardiovascular and immune health.

RESEARCH SUMMARY

Recent studies have shown that the cocoa bean is a rich source of polyphenols that exhibit significant antioxidant activity *in vitro*. These polyphenols are found in cocoa, baking chocolate and milk chocolate, among other foods. In one *in vitro* study, all three of these showed some ability to inhibit the oxidation of LDL-cholesterol. Cocoa was the most potent in this respect.

CONTRAINDICATIONS, PRECAUTIONS, ADVERSE REACTIONS

Cocoa polyphenols are contraindicated in those who are hypersensitive to any component of a cocoa polyphenol-containing product.

OVERDOSAGE

There are no reports of overdosage.

DOSAGE AND ADMINISTRATION

Products are currently under development. No dosage recommendations at this time.

HOW SUPPLIED

Chewable Tablets

LITERATURE

Arteel GE, Sies H. Protection against peroxynitrite by cocoa polyphenol oligomers. *FEBS Left.* 1999; 462:167-170.

Arts ICW, Hollman PCH, Kromhout D. Chocolate as a source of tea flavonoids. *Lancet.* 1999; 354:488.

Hammerstone JF, Lazarus SA, Mitchell AE, et al. Identification of procyanidins in cocoa (*Theobroma Cacao*) and chocolate using high-performance liquid chromatography/mass spectrometry. *J Agric Food Chem.* 1999; 47:490-496.

Lazarus SA, Hammerstone JF, Schmitz HA. Chocolate contains additional flavonoids not found in tea. *Lancet.* 1999; 354:1825.

Mao TK, Powell J, Van de Water J, et al. The effect of cocoa procyanidins on the transcription and secretion of interleukin 1beta in peripheral blood mononuclear cells. *Life Sci.* 2000; 66:1377-1386.

Mao TK, Powell JJ, Van de Water J, et al. The influence of cocoa procyanidins on the transcription of interleukin-2 in peripheral blood mononuclear cells. *Int J Immunotherapy.* 1999; 15:23-29.

Sanbongi C, Suzuki N, Sakane T. Polyphenols in chocolate, which have antioxidant activity, modulate immune function in humans *in vitro. Cell Immunol.* 1997; 177:129-136.

Vinson JA, Proch J, Zubik L. Phenol antioxidant quantity and quality in foods: cocoa, dark chocolate and milk chocolate. *J Agric Food Chem.* 1999; 47:4821-4824.

Coenzyme Q10 (CoQ10)

TRADE NAMES

Coenzyme Q10 (CoQ10) is available generically from numerous manufacturers. Branded products include Lynae CoQ10 (Boscogen), Natures Blend Coenzyme Q10 (National Vitamin Company) and Ultra CoQ10 (Twinlab).

DESCRIPTION

Coenzyme Q_{10} or CoQ_{10} belongs to a family of substances called ubiquinones. Ubiquinones, also known as coenzymes Q and mitoquinones, are lipophilic, water-insoluble substances involved in electron transport and energy production in mitochondria. The basic structure of ubiquinones consists of a benzoquinone "head" and a terpinoid "tail." The "head" structure participates in the redox activity of the electron transport chain. The major difference among the various coenzymes Q is in the number of isoprenoid units (5-carbon structures) in the "tail." Coenzymes Q contain one to 12 isoprenoid units in the "tail"; 10 isoprenoid units are common in animals.

Coenzymes Q occur in the majority of aerobic organisms, from bacteria to plants and animals. Two numbering systems exist for designation of the number of isoprenoid units in the terpinoid "tail": coenzyme Qn and coenzyme Q(x). N refers to the number of isoprenoid side chains, and x refers to the number of carbons in the terpinoid "tail" and can be any multiple of five. Thus, coenzyme Q_{10} refers to a coenzyme Q having 10 isoprenoid units in the "tail." Since each isoprenoid unit has five carbons, coenzyme Q_{10} can also be designated coenzyme Q(50). The structures of coenzymes Q are analogous to those of vitamin K2.

Coenzyme Q_{10} is also known as Coenzyme Q(5O), CoQ_{10}, CoQ(50), ubiquinone (50), ubiquinol — 10 and ubidecarerone. Chemically, CoQ_{10} is known as 2, 3-dimethyoxy-5-methyl-6-decaprenyl-1,4-benzoquinone, and its structural formula is:

CoEnzyme Q_{10}

It is a solid wax-like substance. CoQ_{10} is the predominant form in humans, and CoQ_9 is the predominant form in rats.

Supplemental CoQ_{10} is typically derived from tobacco leaf extracts and fermented sugar cane and beets.

ACTIONS AND PHARMACOLOGY

ACTIONS

Supplemental CoQ_{10} may have cardioprotective, cytoprotective and neuroprotective activities.

MECHANISM OF ACTION

Since the actions of supplemental CoQ_{10} have yet to be clarified, the mechanism of these actions is a matter of speculation. However, much is known about the biochemistry of CoQ_{10}. CoQ_{10} is an essential cofactor in the mitochondrial electron transport chain, where it accepts electrons from complex I and II, an activity that is vital for the production of ATP.

CoQ_{10} has antioxidant activity in mitochondria and cellular membranes, protecting against peroxidation of lipid membranes. It also inhibits the oxidation of LDL-cholesterol. LDL-cholesterol oxidation is believed to play a significant role in the pathogenesis of atherosclerosis.

CoQ_{10} is biosynthesized in the body and shares a common synthetic pathway with cholesterol. CoQ_{10} levels decrease with aging in humans. Why this occurs is not known but may be due to decreased synthesis and/or increased lipid peroxidation which occurs with aging.

PHARMACOKINETICS

CoQ_{10} is absorbed from the small intestine into the lymphatics; from there it enters the blood. Absorption of CoQ_{10} is poor. Well over 60% of an oral dose is excreted in the feces. Furthermore, absorption of CoQ_{10} is highly variable and depends not only on food intake but also on the amount of lipids present in the food. Absorption is lower on an empty stomach and greater when taken with food of high lipid content. In the blood, CoQ_{10} is partitioned into the various lipoprotein particles, including VLDL, LDL and HDL.

It takes about three weeks of daily dosing with CoQ_{10} to reach maximal serum concentrations, which then plateau with continuous daily dosing. CoQ_{10} is distributed to the various tissues of the body and is able to enter the brain. The main elimination of CoQ_{10} occurs via bile.

INDICATIONS AND USAGE

Coenzyme Q_{10} may be indicated in cardiovascular disease, particularly in congestive heart failure. It may also be indicated to correct reduced blood levels of CoQ_{10} that result from the use of HMG-CoA reductase inhibitors used to treat elevated cholesterol levels. It also appears to have usefulness in the management of periodontal disease in some. There is far less evidence to support claims that it has positive effects in cancer, muscular dystrophy and immune dysfunction. Similarly, there is as yet no reliable evidence that it can inhibit obesity or enhance athletic performance.

RESEARCH SUMMARY

There are many studies, spanning more than two decades, reporting positive results from the use of CoQ10 as adjunctive therapy in the treatment of congestive heart failure. CoQ10 has been an approved drug in Japan for use in congestive heart failure since 1974. It has also been approved for this use in some other countries. Several studies have demonstrated a strong correlation between severity of heart disease and severity of CoQ10 deficiency. Some have suggested that this deficiency is the primary cause of some variations of heart muscle dysfunction, while others believe it plays a secondary role in the etiology of heart failure.

Early studies of congestive heart failure focused on idiopathic dilated cardiomyopathy, testing CoQ10 against placebo using echocardiography to assess heart function. Echocardiographic improvement seen in these studies was generally slow but sustained and was accompanied by diminished fatigue, chest pain, dyspnea and palpitations. Normal heart size and function were restored in some patients using only CoQ10; this occurred primarily in patients with recent onset of congestive heart failure.

Subsequently, nearly all of the several placebo-controlled studies investigating CoQ10's effects on heart muscle function have reported significant positive results. One multi-center Italian study included 2,664 patients with congestive heart failure. No notable adverse effects on drug interactions have been reported in these studies except for one report that noted a slight diminution in coumadin activity.

Many studies to date have examined CoQ10 as an addition to standard medical treatments. In several studies involving hypertension and other manifestations of cardiovascular disease, there was a significant reduction in the use of concomitant drug therapies when CoQ10 was added to the treatment regimen.

It is now known that the HMG-CoA reductase inhibitors, while very effective in lowering cholesterol levels, also significantly lower levels of CoQ10. This may be particularly hazardous for patients with heart failure, suggesting a possible indication for CoQ10 in many, if not all, individuals using these cholesterol-lowering drugs. There has been some suggestion that CoQ10, especially if it could be more readily absorbed, might be a cholesterol-lowering agent itself. There is, however, no evidence for this.

Significant CoQ10 deficiencies have been noted in diseased gingiva. CoQ10's efficacy in reducing gingival inflammation and periodontal pocket-depth has been demonstrated in placebo-controlled trials. Claims that CoQ10 might be an effective anti-cancer agent are based upon a few suggestive case histories that will require far more rigorous clinical investigation before these claims can be properly evaluated. Similarly, claims that CoQ10 might be useful in AIDS and some other immune dysfunctions are premature.

It is not unreasonable to hypothesize that CoQ10 might be helpful in muscular dystrophy—and there is some very preliminary animal and clinical data suggesting that it might be. Muscular dystrophy is usually associated with cardiac disease. Research is ongoing but, to date, is inconclusive.

There is also some evidence that CoQ10 might boost energy and speed recovery of exercise-related muscle exhaustion and damage. This work, too, needs more rigorous followup.

There is no evidence that CoQ10 can inhibit obesity.

CONTRAINDICATIONS, PRECAUTIONS, ADVERSE REACTIONS

CONTRAINDICATIONS

None known.

WARNINGS AND PRECAUTIONS

There is one report of CoQ10 decreasing the effectiveness of warfarin. Those taking warfarin should be aware of this possibility.

Because of lack of long-term safety studies, pregnant women and nursing mothers should avoid CoQ10 supplements.

Clinical reports from Japan suggest that supplemental CoQ10 may improve beta-cell function and glycemic control in type II diabetics. CoQ10 does not appear to improve glycemic control in type I diabetics. Diabetics should be made aware of this possibility, and those diabetics who do use supplemental CoQ10 should determine by appropriate monitoring if they need to make any adjustments in their diabetic medications.

ADVERSE REACTIONS

Mild gastrointestinal symptoms such as nausea, diarrhea and epigastric distress have been reported, particularly with higher doses (200 milligrams or more daily).

INTERACTIONS

DRUGS

Warfarin: There is one report of CoQ10 decreasing the effectiveness of warfarin.

Statins: CoQ10 and cholesterol share the same metabolic pathways. Inhibition of the enzyme 3-hydroxyl-3-methylglutonyl coenzyme A (HMG-CoA) reductase would be expected to decrease CoQ10 levels. The statin drugs lovastatin, simvastatin and pravastatin are known to decrease CoQ$_{10}$ levels in humans. It is likely that all statins have this effect.

Doxorubicin: CoQ$_{10}$ may help ameliorate the cardiotoxicity of doxorubicin.

Antidiabetic medications: CoQ$_{10}$ may improve glycemic control in some type II diabetics. If this were to occur, antidiabetic medications might need appropriate adjusting.

Beta Blockers: Some beta blockers, in particular propanolol, have been reported to inhibit some CoQ$_{10}$-dependent enzymes

Piperine: Piperine, found in black pepper, may increase plasma levels of CoQ$_{10}$.

DOSAGE AND ADMINISTRATION

CoQ$_{10}$ is available in different formulations: oil-based capsules, powder-filled capsules, and tablets and solubilized softgels (microemulsions and others). The solubilized soft-gels are claimed to give higher absorption.

Daily doses of CoQ$_{10}$ range from 5 to 300 milligrams. Those who use CoQ$_{10}$ for periodontal health take 100 to 150 milligrams daily. Effectiveness, if any, is thought to be obtained with doses of 50 to 200 milligrams daily. The same dose range applies to those who take statin drugs for treatment of hypercholesterolemia.

CoQ$_{10}$ is best taken with food. About three weeks of daily dosing are necessary to reach maximal serum concentrations of CoQ$_{10}$.

CoQ$_{10}$ is also available topically in some toothpastes and skin creams.

HOW SUPPLIED

Capsules — 10 mg, 30 mg, 50 mg, 75 mg, 100 mg, 150 mg
Chewable Tablets — 100 mg, 200 mg
Liquid — 30 mg/5 mL
Powder
Tablets — 25 mg, 50 mg, 60 mg, 200 mg
Wafers — 60 mg, 200 mg

LITERATURE

Atar D, Mortensen SA, Flachs H, Herzog WR. Coenzyme Q$_{10}$ protects ischemic myocardium in an open-chart swine model. *Clin Investig.* 1993; 71(Suppl):S103-S111.

Baggio E, Gandini R, Plancher AC, et al. Italian multicenter study on the safety and efficacy of coenzyme Q$_{10}$ as adjunctive therapy in heart failure. *Mol Aspects Med.* 1994; 15(Suppl):287-294.

Bergossi AM, Grossi G, Fioletta PL, et al. Exogenous CoQ$_{10}$ supplementation prevents plasma ubiquone reduction induced by HMG-CoA reductase inhibitors. *Mol Aspects Med.* 1994; 15(Suppl):187-193.

Bliznakov EM, Wilkins DJ. Biochemical and clinical consequences of inhibiting coenzyme Q$_{10}$ biosynthesis by lipid-lowering HMG-CoA reductase inhibitors (statins). *Advanc Therap.* 1998; 15:218-228.

Chopra RK, Goldman R, Sinatra ST, Bhagavan HN. Relative bioavailability of coenzyme Q$_{10}$ formulations in human subjects. *Int J Vitam Nutr Res.* 1998; 68:109-113.

Crane FL, Sun IL, Sun EE. The essential functions of coenzyme Q. *Clin Investig.* 1993; 71(Suppl):S55-S59.

Folkers K, Mortensen SA, Littarru GP, Yamagami T, Lenaz G, eds. The biochemical and clinical aspects of coenzyme Q. *Clin Investig.* 1993; 71(Suppl):S51-S178.

Folkers K. Critique of 30 years of research on hematopoietic and immunological activities of coenzyme Q$_{10}$ and potentiality for therapy of AIDS and cancer. *Med Chem Res.* 1992; 2:48-60.

Folkers K, Hanioka T, Xia L-J, et al. Coenzyme Q$_{10}$ increase T4/T8 ratios of lymphocytes in ordinary subjects and relevance to patients having the AIDS related complex. *Biochem Biophys Res Comm.* 1991; 176:786-791.

Folkers K, Langsjoen P, Willis R, et al. Lovastatin decreases coenzyme Q levels in humans. *Proc Natl Acad Sci USA.* 1990; 87:8931-8934.

Folkers K, Vadhanavikit S, Mortensen SA. Biochemical rationale and myocardial tissue data on the protective therapy of cardiomyopathy with coenzyme Q$_{10}$. *Proc Natl Acad Sci USA.* 1985; 82:901-904.

Ghirlanda G, Oradei A, Manto A, et al. Evidence of plasma CoQ$_{10}$ -lowering effect by HMG-CoA reductase inhibitors: a double-blind, placebo-controlled study. *J Clin Pharmacol.* 1993; 33:226-229.

Hanioka T, Tanaka M, Oijima M, et al. Effect of topical application of coenzyme Q$_{10}$ on adult periodontitis. *Molec Aspects Med.* 1994; 15 (suppl):S241-S248.

Hanaki Y, Sugiyama S, Ozawa T, Ohno M. Coenzyme Q$_{10}$ and coronary artery disease. *Clin Investig.* 1993; 71 (suppl):S112-S115.

Henriksen JE, Andersen CB, Hother-Nielsen O, et al. Impact of ubiquinone (coenzyme Q10) treatment on glycaemic control, insulin requirement and well-being in patients with type 1 diabetes mellitus. *Diabet Med.* 1999; 16:312-318.

Hofman-Bang C, Rehnqvist N, Swedberg K, et al. Coenzyme Q$_{10}$ as an adjunctive in the treatment of chronic congestive heart failure. The Q$_{10}$ study group. *J Card Fail.* 1995; 1: 101-107.

Kishi H, Kishi T, Folkers K. Bioenergetics in clinical medicine. III. Inhibition of coenzyme Q10-enzymes by clinically used anti-hypertensive drugs. *Res Commun Chem Pathol Pharmacol.* 1975; 12:533-540.

Kishi T, Watanabe T, Folkers K. Bioenergetics in clinical medicine XV. Inhibition of coenzyme Q10-enzymes by clinically used adrenergic blockers of beta-receptors. *Rev Commun Chem Pathol Pharmacol.* 1977; 17:157-164.

Lampertico M, Comis S. Italian multicenter study on the efficacy and safety of coenzyme Q10 as adjuvant therapy in heart failure. *Clin Investig.* 1993; 71 (Suppl):S129-S133.

Lass A, Sohal RS. Effect of coenzyme Q10 and alpha-tocopherol content of mitochondria on the production of superoxide anion radicals. *FASEB J.* 2000; 14:87-94.

Lucker PW, Werzelberger N, Hennings G, Rehn D. Pharmacokinetics of coenzyme ubidecarenone in healthy volunteers. In: Folkers K, Yamamura Y, eds. *Biomedical and clinical aspects of coenzyme Q.* Vol 4. Amsterdam: Elsevier Sci. Publ. BV. 1984; 143-148.

Matthews RT, Yang L, Browne S, et al. Coenzyme Q10 administration increases mitochondrial concentrations and exerts neuroprotective effects. *Proc Natl Acad Sci USA.* 1998; 95:8892-8897.

Morisco C, Trimarco B, Condorelli M. Effect of coenzyme Q10 therapy in patients with congestive heart failure: a long-term multi-center randomized study. *Clinic Investig.* 1993; 71(Suppl):S134-S136.

Pozzi F, Longo A, Lazzarini C, Carenzi A. Formulations of ubidecarenone with improved bioavailabiltity. *Eur J Pharm Biopharm.* 1991; 37:243-246.

Spigset O. Reduced effect of warfarin caused by ubidecarenone. *Lancet.* 1994; 344:1372-1373..

Stocker R, Bowry VW, Frei B. Ubiquinol-10 protects human low-density lipoprotein more efficiently against lipid peroxidation than does alpha-tocopherol. *Proc Natl Acad Sci USA.* 1991; 88:1646-50.

Tomasetti M, Littaru GP, Stocker R, Alleva R. Coenzyme Q10 enrichment decreases oxidative DNA damage in human lymphocytes. *Free Rad Biol Med.* 1999; 27:1027-1032.

Tomono Y, Hasegawa J, Seki T, et al. Pharmacokinetic study of deuterium-labeled coenzyme Q10 in man. *Int J Clin Pharmacol Ther Toxicol.* 1986; 24:536-541.

Watts GF, Castellucio CLA, Riceevans CLA, et al. Plasma coenzyme Q (ubiquinone) concentration in patients treated with simvastatin. *J Clin Pathol.* 1995; 46:1055-1057.

Watts TLP. Coenzyme Q10 and periodontal treatment: is there any beneficial effect? *Br Dent J.* 1995; 178:209-213.

Colloidal Minerals

TRADE NAMES

T.J. Clark's Legendary Colloidal Mineral Formula (T.J. Clark), Virgin Earth Colloidal Minerals (American Longevity), Crystal Energy (New Tech Nutrition), Colloidal Grape Elixir (Cyber Strength Nutrition) and Ionic Colloidal Mineral (Active Life).

DESCRIPTION

Colloidal mineral supplements refer to liquid extracts of minerals mainly derived from humic shale deposits or from aluminosilicate-containing clays. Humic shale extracts predominantly contain sulfates of iron and aluminum and traces of colloidal metal hydroxides. The term colloidal mineral is derived from the presence in these preparations of colloidal metal hydroxides. However, many of the minerals are present in ionic forms.

In addition to the sulfates of iron and aluminum, colloidal minerals from humic shale deposits contain zinc, nickel, manganese, magnesium, calcium, chromium, boron, copper, lithium and silicon. They also contain traces of several other elements including arsenic, vanadium, strontium, selenium, iodine and praseodymium. Similar minerals may be found in colloidal minerals derived from clay and from plant sources. Humic and fulvic acids are found in some preparations. Interestingly, humic acids convert minerals into more useable forms for plants. It is believed by some that minerals in colloidal form are more easily absorbable than minerals in solid form (tablets and capsules).

Colloidal minerals are sometimes referred to as liquid minerals. However, some supplements marketed as liquid minerals are generally different from the so-called colloidal mineral supplements. They are liquid mixtures comprised of chelated minerals, ocean minerals and mineral citrates, as well as some colloidal minerals.

Note: Products called ''colloidal silver'' should not be confused with the colloidal mineral supplements. Colloidal silver may pose health threat and should be avoided (see Colloidal Silver).

ACTIONS AND PHARMACOLOGY

ACTIONS

Colloidal minerals are delivery forms of trace minerals. They have putative enhanced-absorption capability.

MECHANISM OF ACTION

It is speculated that because colloidal minerals do not have to undergo disintegration and dissolution, in contrast with minerals taken in the form of tablets and capsules, they are better absorbed.

PHARMACOKINETICS

There is little on the pharmacokinetics of colloidal minerals, and there are no adequate studies comparing mineral absorption in this form with minerals in tablet or capsule form.

INDICATIONS AND USAGE

There is no credible evidence to support claims that colloidal minerals are effective in the prevention and treatment of arthritis, diabetes, cancer, cardiovascular disease, immune disorders or any other disease condition. Safety data are lacking on most or all of them. Some have been found to contain varying levels of mercury, lead, aluminum, cadmium and arsenic, among other substances.

RESEARCH SUMMARY

There is no credible research showing benefits from colloidal minerals. Claims that they are more absorbable are also unsubstantiated.

CONTRAINDICATIONS, PRECAUTIONS, ADVERSE REACTIONS

CONTRAINDICATIONS

Colloidal minerals are contraindicated in those who are hypersensitive to any component of a colloidal mineral supplement.

PRECAUTIONS

Pregnant women and nursing mothers should avoid supplementing with colloidal minerals.

Those with hemochromatosis or those with any condition of iron overload should avoid colloidal mineral supplementation. Iron is one of the richest minerals in these supplements.

Those with hepatolenticular degeneration (Wilson's disease) should avoid colloidal mineral supplementation because of the presence of copper in these supplements.

Those who do use colloidal minerals should refrigerate the bottle after opening.

Those who require mineral supplementation should be aware of the great variability of minerals in these supplements from batch to batch.

ADVERSE REACTIONS

There are no reports of adverse reactions in those ingesting colloidal minerals. Earlier reports of colloidal minerals containing radioactivity and unusually high levels of strontium have not been confirmed. Some earlier preparations contained high levels of aluminum. Some preparations contain potentially toxic minerals (e.g., arsenic, lead), but in very small amounts.

INTERACTIONS

No known interactions with drugs, nutritional supplements, food or herbs.

OVERDOSAGE

There are no reports of overdosage.

DOSAGE AND ADMINISTRATION

No recommended dosage.

HOW SUPPLIED

Liquid

LITERATURE

Schauss A. Colloidal minerals: clinical implications of clay suspension products sold as dietary supplements. *Am J Nat Med.* 1997; 4:3-10.

Schrauzer GN. An evaluation of liquid vitamin-mineral supplement technology. *J Med Food.* 1998; 1:207-216.

Colloidal Silver

TRADE NAMES

Wellness Colloidal Silver Nasal Spray (Source Naturals), Wellness Colloidal Silver Throat Spray (Source Naturals), Colloidal Silver Silica Gold (Etherium Technology).

DESCRIPTION

Silver is a metallic element with atomic number 47 and atomic symbol Ag. It occurs in nature in ores and as a free metal and is also found in living matter. Ultratrace amounts of silver occur in the diet. The daily dietary intake of silver from food and water is approximately 300 micrograms. However, silver is not an essential nutrient for humans. Nor does it appear to be essential for any living organism.

Silver is highly toxic to most microbial cells and can be used as an antimicrobial agent. Silver-containing compounds, such as silver sulfadiazine, which has broad antimicrobial as well as antifungal activity, and silver nitrate, are used in medicine as topical agents. Colloidal silver is a suspension of extremely small silver particles and was used in medicine until the 1940s as both a topical and an internal antiseptic. Colloidal silver was also known as argentum colloidale, argentum credé and collargolum. Argentum is Latin for silver.

Colloidal silver no longer has a role in medicine but reappeared in the 1990s as a nutritional supplement. Neither colloidal silver nor any form of silver has any valid role in nutrition as a nutritional or dietary supplement.

ACTIONS AND PHARMACOLOGY

ACTIONS

There are no known actions of supplemental colloidal silver.

PHARMACOKINETICS

There are no reported studies on the pharmacokinetics of colloidal silver.

INDICATIONS AND USAGE

There are no indications for use of supplemental silver. In 1999, the Food and Drug Administration issued a final rule establishing that all over-the-counter products containing colloidal silver ingredients or silver salts for external or internal use are not generally recognized as safe and effective and are misbranded. These products are being marketed for numerous disease conditions, and the FDA states that it is ''not aware of any substantial scientific evidence that supports the use of OTC colloidal silver ingredients or silver salts for these disease conditions.''

RESEARCH SUMMARY

Silver has long been used as a topical antiseptic. Doses that could have internal antiseptic effects are not considered safe. There are many documented cases of argyria, a condition in which the skin of the entire body assumes a grayish-blue pigmentation that is irreversible and permanent. It is often attended by permanent discoloration of hair, nails and oral and gingival mucosae. Not only quantity of silver intake but also individual sensitivity to silver and other factors, such as exposure to sunlight, contribute to the appearance of argyriasis.

A number of case studies shed light on the etiology of this disfiguring condition. A 34-year old woman, for example, developed it when she took colloidal silver for 25 months in an effort to treat intestinal dyspepsia with diarrheic episodes. Some others have developed it after treating themselves with silver nitrate eye drops or to treat oral ulcers. Cases have resulted from the use of silver acetate chewing gum used as a putative, unproved smoking deterrent. One schizophrenic patient developed argyria and convulsive seizures, which some researchers also associated with prolonged silver use.

Current research makes it clear that there are no safe uses for over-the-counter silver products.

CONTRAINDICATIONS, PRECAUTIONS, ADVERSE REACTIONS

CONTRAINDICATIONS

Supplemental colloidal silver is not advised for anyone.

ADVERSE REACTIONS

Prolonged intake of colloidal silver can cause argyria, a condition in which the skin of the entire body assumes a blue-gray discoloration, particularly in areas exposed to light. Argyria is permanent and irreversible. Argyria also affects the lips, cheeks and gums.

OVERDOSAGE

There are no reports of overdosage of colloidal silver.

DOSAGE AND ADMINISTRATION

Supplemental colloidal silver is not recommended. Colloidal or liquid minerals often contain silver.

HOW SUPPLIED

Cream — 100 ppm
Liquid — 10 ppm, 24 ppm, 50 ppm
Nasal Spray — 10 ppm
Ointment
Throat Spray — 30 ppm

LITERATURE

Anon. Over the-counter drug products containing colloidal silver ingredients or silver salts. Department of Health and Human Services (HHS), Public Health Service (PHS), Food and Drug Administration (FDA). Final rule. *Fed Regist.* 1999; 64:44653-44658.

Fung MC, Bowen DL. Silver products for medical indications: risk-benefit assessment. *J Toxicol Clin Toxicol.* 1996; 34:119-126.

Hollinger MA. Toxicological aspects of topical silver pharmaceuticals. *Crit Rev Toxicol* 1996; 26:255-260.

Ohbo Y, Fukuzako H, Takeuchi K, Takigawa M. Argyria and convulsive seizures caused by ingestion of silver in a patient with schizophrenia. *Psychiatry Clin Neurosci.* 1996; 50:89-90.

Pardo-Peret P, Sans-Sebrafen J, Boleda Relats M. [Argyriasis. Report of a case.] [Article in Spanish.] *Med Clin (Barc).* 1979; 73:386-389.

Russell AD, Hugo WB. Antimicrobial activity and action of silver. *Prog Med Chem.* 1994; 31:351-370.

Slawson RM, Lee H, Trevors JT. Bacterial interactions with silver. *Biol Met.* 1990; 3:151-154.

Colosolic Acid

TRADE NAMES

Glucosol (Soft Gel Technologies)

DESCRIPTION

Colosolic acid, sometimes called corosolic acid, is a triterpene compound extracted from the leaves of the plant *Lagerstroemia speciosa*. The leaves of *Lagerstroemia speciosa* are used in Southeast Asia as an herbal remedy for a number of disorders, including diabetes and obesity. In the Phillipines, the plant is known by the Tagalog name of banaba.

Colosolic acid has been reported to activate glucose transport in cell cultures and to lower glucose in diabetic mice. There are a few reports that colosolic acid lowers blood glucose levels in type 2 diabetic subjects. However, none of these reports has appeared in peer-reviewed scientific literature.

Colosolic acid is also known as 2alpha-hydroxyursolic acid, corosolic acid and botanical insulin. A similar triterpene called corosolic acid has been isolated from the fruit of *Crataegus pinnatifida* var. pilosa, a member of the hawthorn family.

ACTIONS AND PHARMACOLOGY

ACTIONS

Supplemental colosolic acid is reputed to activate glucose transport, resulting in hypoglycemic activity.

MECHANISM OF ACTION

The mechanism of action of colosolic's putative hypoglycemic action is not known.

PHARMACOKINETICS

There are no reported pharmacokinetics on colosolic acid.

INDICATIONS AND USAGE

It is claimed that colosolic acid lowers blood glucose in type 2 diabetics, burns fat, lowers elevated blood pressure and boosts energy, among other things. Currently, there is no credible evidence to support any claim for the use of this substance in humans.

RESEARCH SUMMARY

Colosolic acid is reported to activate glucose transport in Ehrlich ascites tumor cells. Extracts from *Lagerstroemia speciosa*. Leaves have been reported to have hypoglycemic activity in genetically diabetic KK-AY mice. There are no credible reports that colosolic acid can lower blood glucose in type 2 diabetics, boost energy, burn fat or lower blood pressure in hypertensives.

CONTRAINDICATIONS, PRECAUTIONS, ADVERSE REACTIONS

CONTRAINDICATIONS

None known.

PRECAUTIONS

Children, pregnant women and nursing mothers should avoid using products called colosolic acid or corosolic acid. Those with diabetes should be extremely cautious about using colosolic/corosolic acid. Those with hypoglycemia should avoid using colosolic/corosolic acid.

ADVERSE REACTIONS

None reported.

INTERACTIONS

If colosolic acid were to lower blood glucose, it could have additive effects with drugs used in the management of diabetes, and therefore blood glucose must be closely monitored.

OVERDOSAGE

None reported.

DOSAGE AND ADMINISTRATION

No recommended dose. Colosolic acid is marketed in stand-alone supplements and in combination products. Colosolic acid in these products is usually from extracts of *Lagerstroemia speciosa* leaves.

HOW SUPPLIED

Capsules — 0.16 mg

LITERATURE

Ahn KS, Hahm MS, Park EJ, et al. Corosolic acid isolated from the fruit of *Crataegus pinnatifida* var. pilosa is a protein kinase inhibitor a well as a cytotoxic agent. *Planta Med.* 1998; 64:468-470.

Kakuda T, Sakane I, Takhara T, et al. Hypoglycemic effect of extracts from *Lagerstroemia speciosa* L. leaves in genetically diabetic KK-AY mice. *Biosci Biotechnol Biochem.* 1996; 60:204-208.

Murakami C, Myoga K, Kasai R, et al. Screening of plant constituents for effect on glucose transport activity in Ehrlich ascites tumour cells. *Chem Pharm Bull.* 1993; 41:2129-2131.

Conjugated Linoleic Acid (CLA)

DESCRIPTION

Conjugated linoleic acid or CLA refers to a group of positional and geometric octadecadienoic acid isomers of linoleic acid. CLA is not a single substance. In contrast to linoleic acid, all the CLA isomers have conjugated bonds. In an unsaturated organic compound, two double bonds separated by a single bond are said to be conjugated. CLA is represented by the following structural formulas:

Conjugated linoleic acid (CLA)

A. $CH_3(CH_2)_5$ ... COOH

trans,9-cix,11-octadecadienoic acid

B. $CH_3(CH_2)_4$ ... COOH

trans,10-cis,12-octadecadienoic acid

CLA is found naturally in animal tissues and food sources, including ruminant meats, poultry, eggs and dairy products, such as cheeses, milk and yogurt that have undergone heat processing treatments. Vegetable fats are generally poorer sources of CLA. However, CLA is produced from linoleic acid in safflower oil and sunflower oil by special treatment of these oils. CLA was originally found in milk fat where it exists in the form of phospholipids and triglycerides. Also, there is evidence that human milk contains CLA.

The principal dietary isomer of CLA is cis-9, trans-11 CLA, also known as rumenic acid and RA. This isomer is produced in the rumen of ruminant animals by microbial metabolism of linoleic and linolenic acids. Cis-9, trans-11 CLA may be absorbed directly or undergo further metabolism. Another CLA isomer, also found in ruminant tissue, is trans-10, cis-12 CLA. Most of the animal studies to date with CLA have used mixtures of CLA isomers that are mostly cis-9, trans-11 CLA and trans-10, cis-12 CLA in approximately equal amounts. Most commercial preparations of CLA contain cis-9, trans-11 CLA and trans-10, cis-12 CLA along with smaller amounts of other CLA isomers, including trans-9, cis-11 CLA, cis-10, cis-12 CLA, trans-9, trans-11 CLA, trans-10, trans-12 CLA and other isomers with conjugated double bonds at the 8, 10 and 11, 13 positions. The various isomers may produce different biologic effects.

Cis-9, trans-11 CLA is also known as c9, t11-octadecadien-oic acid; trans-10, cis-12 CLA is also known as t10, c12-octadecadienoic acid. The term octadecadienoates is sometimes used synonymously with CLA.

ACTIONS AND PHARMACOLOGY

ACTIONS

CLA may have anti-carcinogenic, anti-atherogenic, anti-diabetagenic and body composition-modifying activities in humans. These activities have been reported in experimental animals.

MECHANISM OF ACTION

The mechanism(s) of actions of CLA are not clearly understood. To reach a better understanding, it is necessary to determine the specific, possibly varying, effects of the different isomers. For example, the CLA-associated body composition changes observed in animals appear to be associated mainly with the trans-10, cis-12 CLA isomer. In mouse tissue culture, the trans-10, cis-12 CLA isomer was found to reduce lipoprotein lipase activity and concentrations of intracellular triglyceride. The trans-10, cis-12 isomer also decreased the expression of hepatic steroyl-CoA desaturase mRNA in one mouse study and the expression of stearoyl-CoA desaturase activity in mouse adipocytes in tissue culture in another study. Inhibition of stearoyl-CoA desaturase activity may depress fat synthesis.

Both cis-9, trans-11 and trans-10, cis-12 CLA isomers show anti-cancer activity. It is speculated that CLA may modulate eicosanoid activity as well as the activity of such cytokines as tumor necrosis factor-alpha. It is also speculated that activation of peroxisome proliferator-activated receptor-gamma (PPAR-gamma) may play some role in the putative anti-diabetic activity of CLA. Activation of PPAR-gamma and/or PPAR-alpha may account, in part, for the anti-carcinogenic, lipid-lowering and anti-atherogenic effects of CLA reported in animal studies. The enymes to produce the major isomers are being cloned in bacteria, and it is expected that with the availability of larger amounts of these materials, the effects and mechanisms of actions of these isomers, alone or in combination, will become clearer.

PHARMACOKINETICS

Little is currently known about the pharmacokinetics of CLA in humans. In experimental animals, the CLA isomers do get absorbed following digestion, but not much is known about CLA's metabolism subsequent to absorption. Some CLA appears to get incorporated into the phospholipids of cell membranes.

INDICATIONS AND USAGE

In vivo animal work, as well as *in vitro* studies, suggest that indications may emerge for the use of CLA in the management and prevention of various cancers, cardiovascu-lar disease, hypercholesterolemia, triglyceridemia and type 2 diabetes mellitus. It may also reduce body fat and promote lean body mass under certain conditions.

RESEARCH SUMMARY

CLA has exhibited promising anti-cancer effects in a number of recent animal and *in vitro* studies. Proliferation of human malignant breast, colorectal, prostate, melanoma and lung cell lines has been inhibited by CLA. CLA has inhibited mammary tumorogenesis in a number of studies that demonstrate its efficacy in animal models independent of the amount and type of fat in the diet. In other experimental animal studies, it has significantly inhibited mouse foresto-mach neoplasia, epidermal tumors in mice and aberrant crypt foci in rat colon.

The mechanisms by which CLA exerts its anti-cancer effects are not yet understood, but it is evident that, in some cases, it appears to interact directly with carcinogens to reduce their potency and that, in other instances, it protects specific tissues through its interaction with those tissues, independent of the carcinogen. It appears to modulate carcinogenesis in all of its separate stages: initiation, promotion, progression.

At one time it was believed that CLA's anti-cancer and other therapeutic effects were largely due to an anti-oxidant property. More recent research demonstrated no significant CLA anti-oxidant effect. Instead, it is now believed by some that CLA exerts beneficial complex regulatory effects at the molecular level through its influence, among other things, on peroxisome proliferator-activated receptors (PPAR). The PPARs are nuclear receptors that modulate gene expression in response to fatty acids, some drugs and other substances. It is also believed to modulate eicosanoid and cytokine activity as well.

One group of researchers recently reported that high-CLA diets reduce the quantity of terminal end buds out of which mammary tumors develop. They further observe that CLA seems to inhibit cancer by selectively inhibiting rapidly dividing cells and by promoting programmed cell death or apoptosis.

CLA's widely reported hypolipidemic effects (in animal studies) are also believed to be linked to the substance's influence on PPAR subtypes involved with lipid metaboliz-ing enzymes and the modulation of plasma triglyceride clearance, among other things. Beneficial effects on lipids have been reported in rats, mice, rabbits, chickens, hamsters and in other animal models. Atheromatous lesions have regressed significantly in CLA-supplemented animals. And CLA has significantly reduced free fatty acids and triglycer-ides in Zucker diabetic fatty rats compared with fatty rats on control diets.

CLA has also recently demonstrated an ability to normalize impaired glucose tolerance and improve hyperinsulinemia in a pre-diabetic animal model. Again, CLA's activation of a PPAR subtype is believed to play a central role in this beneficial activity. The effects of CLA in this study were significant enough that the researchers concluded: ''CLA may prove to be an important therapy for the prevention and treatment of NIDDM.''

CLA may attract attention for its reported ability (in animal models) to reduce body fat and increase lean body mass. In some of these studies, CLA-enriched diets resulted in reduced body weight independent of food intake. Whereas many of the beneficial effects of CLA were thought to be derived from the cis-9, trans-11 isomer, it has recently been reported that the trans-10, cis-12 isomer is perhaps more effective in reducing body weight. One of the researchers has asserted, ''This CLA makes big fat cells get little and stay that way.''

CONTRAINDICATIONS, PRECAUTIONS, ADVERSE REACTIONS

CONTRAINDICATIONS

CLA is contraindicated in those hypersensitive to any component of the preparation.

PRECAUTIONS

Because of lack of long-term safety data, CLA supplements should be avoided by children, pregnant women and nursing mothers.

ADVERSE REACTIONS

At doses of up to 2 grams daily, occasional gastrointestinal complaints, such as nausea, have been noted.

DOSAGE AND ADMINISTRATION

There are a few products with CLA available. The amounts of the two most studied isomers of CLA, cis-9, trans-11 and trans-10, cis-12 CLA, vary. Also, there are different amounts of other isomers of CLA in the various preparations. Typical doses are 1 to 2 grams daily. Some use doses up to 6 grams daily.

CLA is also being developed for use in functional foods.

LITERATURE

Banni S, Angioni E, Stefania M, et al. Conjugated linoleic acid and oxidative stress. *J Am Oil Chem Soc.* 1998; 75:261-267.

Belury MA. Conjugated linoleate: a polyunsaturated fatty acid with unique chemopreventive properties. *Nutr Rev.* 1995; 53:83-89.

Cesano A, Visonneau S, Scimeca JA, et al. Opposite effects of linoleic acid and conjugated linoleic acid on human prostate cancer in SCID mice. *Anticanc Res.* 1998; 18:833-38.

de Deckere EA, van Amelsvoort JM, Mc Neill GP, Jones P. Effects of conjugated linoleic acid (CLA) isomers on lipid levels and peroxisome proliferation in the hamster. *Br J Nutr.* 1999; 82:309-17.

Gavino VC, Gavino G, Leblanc MJ, Tuchweber B. An isomeric mixture of conjugated linoleic acids but not pure cis-9, trans-11-octadecadienoic acid affects body weight gain and plasma lipids in hamsters. *J Nutr.* 2000; 130:27-29.

Houseknecht KL, Vanden Heuvel JP, Moya-Camarena SY, et al. Dietary conjugated linoleic acid normalizes impaired glucose tolerance in the Zucker diabetic fatty fa/fa rat. *Biochem Biophys Res Commun.* 1998; 244:678-682.

Lee KN, Kritchevsky D, Pariza MW. Conjugated linoleic acid and atherosclerosis in rabbits. *Atherosclero.* 1994; 108:19-25.

Lee KN, Pariza MW, Ntambi JM. Conjugated linoleic acid decreases hepatic stearoyl-CoA desaturase mRNA expression. *Biochem Biophys Res Commun.* 1998; 248:817-821.

McCarty MF. Downregulaton of macrophage activation by PPAR gamma suggests a role for conjugated linoleic acid in prevention of Alzheimer's disease. *J Med Food.* 1998; 1:217-226.

Moya-Camarena SY, Belury MA. Species differences in the metabolism and regulation of gene expression by conjugated linoleic acid. *Nutr Rev.* 1999; 57:336-340.

Ostrowski E, Muralitharan M, Cross RF. Dietary conjugated linoleic acids increase lean tissue and decrease fat deposition in growing pigs. *J Nutr.* 1999; 129:2037-2042.

Pariza MW, Park Y, Cook ME. Mechanisms of action of conjugated linoleic acid: evidence and speculation. *Proc Soc Exp Biol Med.* 2000; 223: 8-13.

Pariza MW, Parks Y, Cook ME. Conjugated linoleic acid and the control of cancer and obesity. *Toxicol Sci.* 1999; 51 (2 Suppl):107-110.

Pariza MW, Park Y, Kim S, et al. Mechanism of body fat reduction by conjugated linoleic acid. *FASEB J.* 1997; 11:A139.

Park Y, Albright KJ, Liu W, et al. Effect of conjugated linoleic acid on body composition in mice. *Lipids.* 1997; 32:853-858.

van den Berg JJ, Cook NE, Tribble DL. Reinvestigation of the antioxidant properties of conjugated linoleic acid. *Lipids.* 1995; 30:599-605.

West DB, Delany JP, Camet PM, et al. Effects of conjugated linoleic acid on body fat and energy metabolism in the mouse. *Am J Physiol.* 1998; 275(3 Pt 2):R667-R672.

Yurawecz MP, Mossoba MM, Kramer JKG, Pariza MW, Nelson GJ, eds. *Advances in Conjugated Linoleic Acid Research.* Volume 1. Champaign, IL: AOCS Press; 1999.

Further information:

To keep track of CLA progress, an updated listing can be found on the Internet at http://www.wisc.edu/fri/clarefs.htm.

Copper

TRADE NAMES

CU-5 (Bio-Tech Pharmacal), Coppermin (The Key Company)

DESCRIPTION

Copper is an essential trace mineral in animal and human nutrition. Anemia, neutropenia and osteoporosis are found with frank copper deficiency. Copper deficiency in humans is rare but it does occur under certain circumstances, such as in patients receiving long-term total parenteral nutrition (TPN). Mild copper deficiency due to marginal copper intake over a long period may also occur. In addition to possible anemia, neutropenia and osteoporosis, manifestations of mild copper deficiency may include abnormal glucose tolerance, hypercholesterolemia, arthritis, myocardial disease, arterial disease, cardiac arrhythmias, loss of pigmentation and neurological problems.

Copper is a transition metal with atomic number 29 and an atomic weight of 63.55 daltons. Its symbol is Cu. Copper participates in metabolism as a component of many metalloenzymes, including ceruloplasmin or ferroxidase I, cytochromecoxidase, copper/zinc superoxide dismutase, dopamine beta-hydroxylase, tyrosinase, monoamine oxidase, diamine oxidase, lysyl oxidase (protein-lysine 6-oxidase), peptidylglycine-alpha-amidating monoxygenase and ferroxidase II.

Copper essentiality for humans was first demonstrated in malnourished children in Peru. The children had an anemia that was not responsive to iron therapy, as well as neutropenia and bone abnormalities. The anemia, neutropenia and bone abnormalities were responsive to copper supplementation. Copper is required for normal infant development, red and white blood cell maturation, iron transport, bone strength, cholesterol metabolism, myocardial contractility, glucose metabolism, brain development and immune function, among other things.

Although copper is clearly essential for a wide range of biochemical processes which are necessary for the maintenance of good health, copper is also a potentially toxic substance. Copper exists in the oxidation states Cu(I) or Cu^+(cuprous), and Cu(II) or Cu^{2+} (cupric) under physiological conditions. The shift back and forth between these two oxidation states via single-electron-transfer reactions is the property that makes copper such an essential component of the enzymes mentioned above. However, this redox property also contributes to its potential toxicity. Redox cycling between Cu^+ and Cu^{2+} can generate the highly reactive oxygen species hydroxyl radicals which can damage lipids, DNA and proteins. Recently, intracellular proteins have been discovered yhat protect against the potential toxicity of copper ions. These proteins escort copper ions directly to enzymes that require them in order to function. Free copper ions are involved in the formation of hydroxyl radicals. The proteins that protect cells from copper toxicity are called copper chaperones and essentially keep the cells free of free copper ions. Wilson's disease, or hepatolenticular degeneration, is an autosomal recessive disorder that results from pathological accumulation of copper, principally in liver and brain tissues.

The richest dietary sources of copper include nuts, seeds, legumes, the bran and germ portions of grains, liver, kidneys, shellfish, oysters and crustaceans. Cow's milk has little copper.

ACTIONS AND PHARMACOLOGY

ACTIONS

Copper may have antioxidant activity.

MECHANISM OF ACTION

Copper deficiency has been found to increase the susceptibility of lipoproteins to peroxidation in rats and to increase oxidative DNA damage in lymphocytes in culture. Supplemental copper was found to prevent oxidative DNA damage in lymphocytes in culture. Copper supplementation in middle-aged volunteers was found to protect red blood cells against oxidation. Copper is a cofactor for copper/zinc superoxide dismutase and ceruloplasmin, two important antioxidant enzymes, and the possible antioxidant activity of copper may be accounted for, at least in part, by its role in these enzymes. However, the study with human volunteers mentioned above did not show increased copper/zinc superoxide activity with copper supplementation. The mechanism of the possible antioxidant activity of supplemental copper is unclear.

PHARMACOKINETICS

Copper is principally absorbed in the small intestine. A small amount of copper is absorbed in the stomach. Copper appears to be absorbed by both active and passive processes. At low and moderate intakes of copper, it appears to be absorbed by a saturable active transport mechanism. At high copper intakes the active transport mechanism becomes saturated, and copper is absorbed by passive diffusion. The absorption efficiency of copper ranges from 15% to 97%. The absorption efficiency appears to depend on the level of dietary copper intake. As dietary copper increases, the fractional absorption of copper decreases.

Following absorption from the small intestine, copper is transported in the blood primarily bound to albumin. Copper is mainly taken up by the liver where it is principally incorporated into ceruloplasmin. Copper-containing ceruloplasmin is released from the liver into the blood and delivered to cells containing ceruloplasmin receptors.

Copper containing ceruloplasmin binds to these receptors and releases copper into the cell. The major route of copper excretion is via bile into the gastrointestinal tract.

INDICATIONS AND USAGE

There is some experimental indication that supplemental copper may have some anticancer effects and may be of benefit in some with arthritis. Claims that it is protective against cardiovascular disease apply primarily to those with copper deficiency. There is preliminary evidence that copper may have beneficial effects on immunity in those with copper deficiency and perhaps in those with marginal copper deficiency.

RESEARCH SUMMARY

There are some dated reports that supplementary copper significantly protected rats against chemically-induced cancers. Another study reported that a copper-salicylate derivative inhibited tumor promotion in mice. In an *in vitro* study, several copper-containing compounds prevented the malignant transformation of chick-embryo cells by the Rous sarcoma virus. Further research may be warranted.

Copper bracelets have been worn by many in an effort to ameliorate symptoms of arthritis. A study of this folk remedy found that some of those who had worn the bracelets for prolonged periods and then discontinued wearing them became significantly worse, compared with controls who wore placebo bracelets that also appeared to be made of copper. The subjects in this study suffered primarily from osteoarthritis. There was evidence that copper from the bracelets, dissolved in sweat, was absorbed through the skin.

There is also evidence from animal studies that copper complexes of aspirin, tryptophan and penicillamine have anti-inflammatory effects. Injections of copper/zinc superoxide dismutase directly into the joints of some patients with osteoarthritis and rheumatoid arthritis have reportedly produced some relief. More research is needed.

There is no doubt that copper deficiency can contribute to cardiovascular disease. It seems likely that supplemental copper might be helpful in preventing and treating cardiovascular disease even in those with marginal copper deficiency. This hypothesis needs further investigation. Animal studies have shown that copper deficiency increases the susceptibility of lipoproteins and tissues to peroxidation. There are also indications that copper deficiency may play a role in hypertension, in weakening of the structural integrity of the heart and blood vessels and in reduced ability of the heart to contract, among other negative effects.

Similarly, copper appears to play some important roles in immunity, and supplemental copper might thus be beneficial in even those with slight or marginal copper deficiency. Copper deficiency has been shown to increase vulnerability to and mortality from infection in some animal studies. Recently, it has been shown that neutrophils in human peripheral blood are significantly diminished both in number and in their ability to create superoxide anions and kill ingested micro-organisms in conditions of marginal, as well as overt, copper deficiency. Animal and *in vitro* studies have also demonstrated that even marginal copper deficiency reduces levels of interleukin 2 and diminishes T cell proliferation.

CONTRAINDICATIONS, PRECAUTIONS, ADVERSE REACTIONS

CONTRAINDICATIONS

Supplemental copper is contraindicated in those with Wilson's disease (hepatolenticular degeneration), a disease of abnormal copper accumulation.

Supplemental copper is also contraindicated in those hypersensitive to any component of a copper-containing nutritional supplement.

PRECAUTIONS

Pregnant women and nursing mothers should avoid doses of copper above the upper limit of the stated safe and adequate daily dietary intake (ESSADI). The ESSADI for copper for adults is 1.5 to 3.0 milligrams daily.

Those with chronic liver failure and chronic renal failure should exercise extreme caution in the use of copper supplements.

Copper in gram amounts is extremely toxic. Accidental copper poisoning has occurred among children. Others have ingested several grams in suicide attempts.

ADVERSE REACTIONS

Excessive copper intake produces nausea and vomiting, epigastric pain and diarrhea.

INTERACTIONS

DRUGS

Penicillamine: Concomitant use of penicillamine and copper can cause decreased absorption of both substances. Those who use penicillamine for the treatment of Wilson's disease should avoid the use of supplemental copper (see Contraindications).

NUTRITIONAL SUPPLEMENTS

Iron: Excessive intake of nonheme iron may decrease copper status.

Molybdenum: Excessive intake of molybdenum may decrease copper status.

Zinc: Excessive use of zinc may cause decreased absorption of copper. One explanation for this interaction is that high dietary zinc induces intestinal metallothionein. Copper has a stronger affinity for intestinal metallothionein than does zinc and displaces zinc in intestinal metallothionein and is trapped. Copper depletion was observed when supplements of 50 milligrams or more of zinc were given for extended periods. Copper absorption was not affected by zinc doses of 16.5 milligrams daily for extended periods.

Vitamin C: Vitamin C supplementation of 1,500 milligrams daily caused the activity of the copper transporting protein ceruloplasmin to decline. Vitamin C supplementation of 600 milligrams daily also caused a decline in ceruloplasmin, but copper absorption was not impaired.

FOODS

Concomitant intake of copper with foods rich in phytic acid (unleavened bread, raw beans, seeds, nuts and grains and soy isolates) may decrease the absorption of copper.

Diets high in fructose may decrease copper status.

OVERDOSAGE

Gram amounts of copper can cause coma, oliguria, hepatic necrosis, vascular collapse and death.

DOSAGE AND ADMINISTRATION

Copper supplements are available in several forms, including cupric oxide, copper gluconate, copper sulfate and copper amino acid chelates. Copper supplements are typically found in combination products. Typical doses range from 1.5 to 3.0 milligrams daily. There is no reason to use higher amounts of copper.

The Food and Nutrition Board of the U.S. National Academy of Sciences has recommended the following estimated safe and adequate daily dietary intake (ESSADI) values for copper:

Age (year)	ESSADI (milligrams)
Infants	0.4-0.7
1-3	0.7-1.0
4-6	1.0-1.5
7-10	1.0-2.0
11-18	1.5-2.5
Adults	1.5-3.0

HOW SUPPLIED

Capsules — 5 mg
Solution
Tablets — 2 mg, 5 mg

LITERATURE

Fields M, Lewis CG. Starch diets high in iron can duplicate the severity of copper deficiency in rats fed fructose. *J Med Food.* 1998; 1:193-199.

Harrison MD, Jones CE. Solioz M, Dameron CT. Intracellular copper routing: the role of copper chaperones. *Trends Biochem Sci.* 2000; 25:29-32.

Harris ED. Cellular copper transport and metabolism. *Annu Rev Nutr.* 2000; 20:291-310.

Johnson WT, Thomas AC. Copper deprivation potentiates oxidative stress in HL-60 cell mitochondria. *Proc Soc Exp Biol Med.* 1999; 221:147-152.

Klevay LM. Cardiovascular disease from copper deficiency — a history. *J Nutr.* 2000; 130:489S-492S.

Klevay LM. Coronary heart disease: the zinc/copper hypothesis. *Am J Clin Nutr.* 1975; 28:764-774.

Rayssiguier Y, Gueux E, Bussiere L, Mazur A. Copper deficiency increases the susceptibility of lipoproteins and tissues to peroxidation in rats. *J Nutr.* 1993; 123:1343-1348.

Rock E, Mazur A, O'Connor JM, et al. The effect of copper supplementation on red blood cell oxidizability and plasma antioxidants in Middle-aged healthy volunteers. *Free Rad Biol Med.* 2000; 28:324-329.

Saari JT, Sahuschke DA. Cardiovascular effects of dietary copper deficiency. *Biofactors.* 1999; 10:359-375.

Toyama T, Kubuki Y, Suzuki M. Tsubouchi H. [Copper deficiency anemia and neutropenia secondary to total gastrectomy]. [Article in Japanese]. *Rinsho Ketsueki.* 2000; 41:441-443.

Turnlund Jr. Copper. In: Shils ME, Olson JA, Shike M. Ross AC, eds. *Modern Nutrition in health and Disease,* 9th ed. Baltimore, MD: Williams and Wilkins; 1999:241-252.

Waggoner DJ, Bartnikas TB, Gitlin JD. The role of copper in neurodegenerative disease. *Neurobiology of Disease.* 1999; 6:221-230.

Creatine

TRADE NAMES

Creatine is available generically from numerous manufacturers. Branded products include Muscle Power (Mason Vitamins), Creatine Fuel (Twinlab), Creatine Booster (Champion Nutrition), Creatigen (Bricker Labs), CreaVate (Prolab Nutrition), Perfect Creatine (Nature's Best), Xtra Advantage Creatine Serum (Muscle Marketing USA), Micronized Creatine (Met-Rx), Creavescent (GEN), Power Creatine (Champion Nutrition), Phosphagen (GNC), Crea-Tek (Iron Tek), Effervescent Creatine Elite (Muscle Link).

DESCRIPTION

Creatine is a non-protein amino acid found in animals and, in much lesser amounts, plants. Creatine is synthesized in the kidney, liver and pancreas from the amino acids L-arginine, glycine and L-methionine. Following its biosynthesis, creatine is transported to the skeletal muscle, heart, brain and other tissues. Most of the creatine is metabolized in these tissues to phosphocreatine (creatine phosphate). Phosphocreatine is a major energy storage form in the body.

Creatine is known chemically as N-(aminoiminomethyl)-N-methyl glycine and its structural formula is:

$$HOOC-\underset{H_2}{C}-\underset{\underset{CH_3}{|}}{N}-\underset{\underset{NH_2}{|}}{C}=NH$$

Creatine

Supplemental creatine is typically a synthetic substance. It is a solid and is water-soluble.

ACTIONS AND PHARMACOLOGY

ACTIONS

Supplemental creatine may have an energy-generating action during anaerobic exercise and may also have neuroprotective and cardioprotective actions.

MECHANISM OF ACTION

Since the action of supplemental creatine has yet to be clarified, the mechanism of action is a matter of speculation. Much is known, however, about the biochemistry of endogenous creatine. Creatine is mainly synthesized in the kidney, liver and pancreas. In its synthesis, the guanidino group of L-arginine is transferred to glycine to form guanidinoacetate and ornithine by a transamidinase reaction, a reaction that takes place in the pancreas, liver and kidney. Guanidinoacetate is methylated by S-adenosylmethione (SAMe) to form creatine. About 1 to 2 grams of creatine are biosynthesized daily and another 1 to 2 grams are obtained from diet.

In muscle and nerve, most of the creatine is phosphorylated to phosphocreatine (PCr) in a reaction that is catalyzed by the enzyme creatine kinase (CK). There are three isoforms (isoenzymes) of CK. CK-MM is the skeletal muscle isoform; CK-BB, the brain isoform, and CK-MB, the isoform found in cardiac muscle. Most of the PCr in the body is in skeletal muscle.

Creatine, creatine kinase and phosphocreatine make up an intricate cellular energy buffering and transport system connecting sites of energy production in the mitochondria with sites of energy consumption. CK is a key enzyme involved in cellular energy homeostasis. It reversibly catalyzes the transfer of the high-energy phosphate bond in PCr to adenosine diphosphate (ADP) to form adenosine triphosphate (ATP), and it catalyzes the transfer of the high-energy phosphate bond in ATP to creatine to form PCr. During periods of intense exercise and skeletal muscle contraction, bioenergetic metabolism switches from one in which oxidative phosphorylation is the major pathway of ATP production to one in which so-called anaerobic glycolysis becomes dominant. Much less ATP would be generated during this period if it were not for phosphocreatine (PCr) being the only fuel available to regenerate ATP during this period. Thus the availability of PCr is the limiting factor of skeletal-muscle performance during high intensity and brief bursts (about 10 seconds) of activity. Supplemental creatine may increase PCr levels in skeletal muscle and hypothetically enhance ATP turnover during maximal exercise.

Creatine supplementation of transgenic amyotrophic lateral sclerosis (ALS) mice carrying the superoxide dismutase (SOD)1 mutation has reportedly produced improvement in motor performance and extension of survival, as well as protection against loss of both motor neurons and substantia nigra neurons. Mitochondrial dysfunction is among the earliest features found in these mice models of familial ALS. Creatine administration to these mice appears to stabilize mitochondrial CK and inhibits opening of the mitochondrial transition pores.

Creatine, as well as a creatine analogue called cyclocreatine, inhibit growth of a broad range of solid tumors in rat models of cancer; these tumors express high levels of CK. Although the mechanism of tumor inhibition is unknown, there is speculation about what it may be. Creatine feedback inhibits the transamidination step in its biosynthesis. This results in sparing L-arginine, the limiting precursor in creatine synthesis. More available L-arginine can lead to increased levels of nitric oxide (NO), which is a factor in macrophage activation. Another possibility is that glycolysis is inhibited in these tumors. Phosphocreatine inhibits enzymes in the glycolitic pathway, including glyceraldehyde-3-phosphate dehydrogenase, phosphofructokinase and pyruvate kinase.

PHARMACOKINETICS

Creatine is absorbed from the small intestine and enters the portal circulation and is transported to the liver. The ingested creatine, along with creatine made in the liver, is then transported into the systemic circulation and distributed to various tissues of the body, including muscle and nerves, by crossing the cell membrane via a specific creatine-transporter system against a 200:1 gradient. Chronic creatine supplementation in rats down-regulates creatine transporter protein expression. If this is also the case in humans, then chronic creatine supplementation would lead to lower amounts entering cells at any given time.

Within muscle and nerve cells, about 60 to 67% of the creatine entering the cells gets converted to phosphocreatine via the enzyme creatine kinase. About 2% of creatine is converted to creatinine, and both creatine and creatinine are excreted by the kidneys.

INDICATIONS AND USAGE

There is some evidence that supplemental creatine may enhance performance in a limited number of high-intensity, short-term physical activities, but the data are mixed, and no ergogenic effect has been convincingly demonstrated outside of laboratory settings. Adequate safety data are still lacking. There is some very preliminary data that creatine may be helpful in treating muscular dystrophy and amyotrophic lateral scleroses and may improve skeletal muscle function in some with congestive heart failure and gyrate atrophy of the retina. Creatine has inhibited the growth of some solid tumors in rats, but no human cancer data exist.

RESEARCH SUMMARY

Limited muscle function benefit has been noted in some early studies of creatine. All of these studies have been of short duration (mostly lasting one or two weeks and, in no case, more than eight weeks). Many other studies have found no benefit.

A recent review article summarized the results of 71 trials published between 1993 and 1997. Of those that studied effects of supplemental creatine (usually 20 grams daily for 4 to 21 days) on short term, high-intensity performance, 23 reported positive effects and 20 reported no effect. Studies examining the effects of creatine on oxidative energy systems, muscle isokinetic torque and isometric force produced similarly mixed results. Among the few field tests that have been conducted (all related to swim sprints) none detected any effect on athletic performance. Only among studies of cycle ergometer performance was there any superiority of creatine over placebo (11 trials reported improvement, while six others reported no improvement).

Since this review was published there have been a few more positive than negative reports, but, again, the positive effects are almost entirely seen in laboratory settings and are confined to short-term, high-intensity performance.

One author recently reviewed the creatine data and has concluded that supplemental creatine achieves an ergogenic effect, at least in the laboratory, in repeated stationary cycling sprints. But he found no convincing evidence that it does so in single sprints. He also discerned a possible ergogenic effect in weightlifting, but none in running or swimming sprints of any kind. He and others have speculated that the weight gain that typically accompanies creatine supplementation offsets any ergogenic effect that might otherwise benefit runners and swimmers.

Some have claimed that this weight gain, typically 0.5 to 1.6 kilograms occurring in the first few days to first two weeks

of creatine supplementation, is evidence of increased muscle mass. Most researchers, however, believe that this weight gain is accounted for by creatine-induced water retention. The longer-term studies needed to confirm or refute claims that chronic creatine supplementation can result in greater muscle mass have not been conducted.

Another caveat offered by several researchers is that almost all of the positive creatine effects so far noted have been achieved in laboratory tests of elite athletes and were observed only in the sort of maximal intermittent exercise that non-athletes can rarely achieve. No benefit for any aerobic activity has been demonstrated.

In addition, safety data are lacking and are urgently needed, especially for long-term use of creatine and for use among the pediatric population (including adolescents) and among those in poor health. There are some reports that long-term use of creatine may be nephrotoxic. This needs further investigation before long-term creatine supplementation can be recommended under any circumstance.

Possible additional uses for creatine have been suggested by preliminary work. There is some evidence of creatine synthesis in the retina, and supplementation with 1.5 grams of creatine daily for a year has been reported to bring improvement in genetic gyrate atrophy—not in the blindness that results from this condition but in the skeletal muscle abnormalities that also characterize it. Giving 5 grams of creatine four times a day for a period of five days has similarly been reported to improve skeletal muscle function in some with congestive heart failure. The effect was small.

In a mouse model of amyotrophic lateral sclerosis (ALS), supplemental creatine significantly prolonged survival. Improvement was seen on motor-performance tests, and there was histologic evidence of neuron protection associated with creatine supplementation. Because creatine protected neurons in the substantia nigra, there is speculation that the supplement could also have positive effects in Parkinson's disease.

These researchers have suggested that creatine may exert the favorable results seen in the mouse model through an intracellular energy-buffering effect that may help prevent the sort of mitochondrial dysfunction that they postulate plays a role in neuronal cell death. More research is needed.

Another recent, preliminary report asserts a positive role for supplemental creatine in the treatment of muscular dystrophy and some other neuromuscular disorders. This study tested 10 grams of creatine daily for five days, followed by 5 grams daily for an additional 5 to 7 days, against placebo. Increases were noted in handgrip, ankle and knee strength among those taking creatine. Again, more research is needed.

CONTRAINDICATIONS, PRECAUTIONS, ADVERSE REACTIONS

CONTRAINDICATIONS
Creatine is contraindicated in those with renal failure and renal disorders such as nephrotic syndrome.

PRECAUTIONS
Creatine supplements should be avoided by children, adolescents, pregnant women, nursing mothers and anyone at risk for renal disorders such as diabetics. Those taking creatine should have serum creatinine levels monitored.

ADVERSE REACTIONS
The deaths of three American college wrestlers had been linked to the use of creatine supplements. However, results of post mortem tests led to the conclusion that the deaths were caused by severe dehydration and renal failure, and were not due to creatine. Apparently, the wrestlers were trying to lose enough weight through perspiration to allow them to compete in lower-weight classes. Typical adverse effects are gastrointestinal and include nausea, diarrhea and indigestion. Also common are muscle cramping and strains. Weight gain may occur from water retention. During a five day loading period, weight gains of 1.1 to 3.5 pounds have been reported. There are reports of elevated serum creatinine, a metabolite of creatine and a marker of kidney function, in some who take creatine and have normal renal function. This is reversible upon discontinuation of creatine.

Anecdotal reports of adverse events to FDA have included rash, dyspnea, vomiting, diarrhea, nervousness, anxiety, migraine, fatigue, polymyositis, myopathy, seizures and atrial fibrillation.

INTERACTIONS
There are as yet no known drug, nutritional supplement or herb interactions. Caffeine (in coffee, tea and caffeinated beverages) appears to interfere with any beneficial effects of creatine supplementation.

DOSAGE AND ADMINISTRATION
The typical form of creatine available is a creatine monohydrate powder.

The dosing for those who use creatine to attempt to improve performance in brief, high-intensity activities, is a loading dose of 20 grams or 0.3 grams per kilogram in divided doses four times a day for two to five days, followed by a maintenance dose of no more than 2 grams daily or 0.03 grams per kilogram. Those who use creatine supplements should take them with adequate water, six to eight glasses per day.

HOW SUPPLIED
Capsules — 700 mg, 725 mg, 750 mg, 1200 mg
Effervescent Tablets — 5 gm
Effervescent Powder — 27 gm/packet
Powder — 5 gm/tsp
Wafers — 1000 mg

LITERATURE
Feldman EB. Creatine: a dietary supplement and ergogenic aid. *Nutr Rev.*1999; 57:45-50.

Greenhoff PL. Creatine and its application as an ergogenic aid. *Int J Sport Nutr.* 1995; 5:S100-S110.

Juhn MS. Oral creatine supplementation. *Phys Sports Med.* 1999; 27;47-45..

Klivenyi P, Ferrante RJ, Matthews RT, et al. Neuroprotective effects of creatine in a transgenic animal model of amyotrophic lateral sclerosis, *Nat Med.* 1999; 5:47-350.

Koshy KM, Griswald E, Sneeberger EE. Interstitial nephritis in a patient taking creatine. *N Engl J Med.* 1999; 340:814-815.

Miller EE, Evans AE, Cohn M. Inhibitions of rate of tumor growth by creatine and cyclocreatine. *Proc Natl Accd Sci USA.* 1993; 90:3304-3308.

Poortman JR, Augier H, Renaut V, et al. Effect of short-term creatine supplementation on renal responses in men. *Eur J Appl Physiol.* 1997; 76:566-567.

Sipila I, Rapola J, Simell O, et al. Supplemental creatine as a treatment for gyrate atrophy of the choroid and retina. *N Engl J Med.* 1981; 304:867-870.

Tarnopolsky M, Martin J. Creatine monohydrate increases strength in patients with neuromuscular disease. *Neurology.* 1999; 52:854-857.

Toler SM. Creatine is an ergogenic for anaerobic exercise. *Nutr Rev.* 1997; 55:21-23.

Vandenberghe K, Gillis N. Van Leemputte M, et al. Caffeine counteracts the ergogenic action of muscle creatine loading. *J Appl Physiol.* 1996; 80:452-457.

Williams MH, Branch JD. Creatine supplementation and exercise performance: an update. *J Am Coll Nutr.* 1998; 17:216-234.

Curcuminoids

TRADE NAMES
Curcumin is available as turmeric generically from numerous manufacturers. Branded products include Turmeric Special Formula (Solaray) and Turmeric Power (Nature's Herbs).

DESCRIPTION
Curcuminoids are polyphenolic pigments found in the spice turmeric. The term turmeric is used both for the plant *Curcuma longa* L. and the spice derived from the rhizomes of the plant. The major curcuminoids are curcumin, demethoxycurcumin and bisdemethoxycurcumin. These substances comprise 3 to 6% of *Curcuma longa*. Curcumin

makes up 70 to 75% of the curcuminoids, demethoxycurcumin 15 to 20% and bisdemethoxycurcumin about 3%.

Curcuma longa is a tropical plant native to south and southeast tropical Asia. It is a member of the ginger or *Zingiberaceae* family. Turmeric is widely consumed in the countries of origin for a variety of uses, including use as a dietary spice, as a dietary pigment and as an Indian folk medicine for the treatment of various illnesses. It is also used in Hindu religious ceremonies in one form or another as part of the religious rites.

Curcuminoids are responsible for the yellow color of turmeric, as well as the yellow color of curry.

Curcuminoids are derived from turmeric by extraction with ethanol. Curcumin is the most studied of the curcuminoids. In pure form, it is an orange-yellow, crystalline powder that is insoluble in water. It is also known as diferuloylmethane and turmeric yellow. Its chemical name is (E, E) —1, 7-bis(4-hydroxy-3- methoxyphenyl)-1,6-heptadiene-3, 5 dione. The molecular formula of curcumin is $C_{21}H_{20}O_6$, its molecular weight is 368.39 daltons, and its structural formula is:

Curcumin

Curcumin and the other curcuminoids have been found to have antioxidant and anti-inflammatory activities and have been entered into Phase I clinical trials for cancer chemoprevention by the National Cancer Institute.

ACTIONS AND PHARMACOLOGY

ACTIONS

Curcumin, demethoxycurcumin and bisdemethoxycurcumin have antioxidant activity. They may also have anticarcinogenic, anti-inflammatory, antiviral and hypocholesterolemic activities.

MECHANISM OF ACTION

The curcuminoids have been found to have a number of antioxidant activities, including scavenging of such reactive oxygen species as superoxide anions and hydrogen peroxide, inhibition of lipid peroxidation and inhibition of the oxidation of low-density lipoprotein (LDL). The reduced derivative of curcumin, tetrahydrocurcumin, has been found to have even stronger antioxidant activity. Tetrahydrocurcumin may be formed from curcumin following ingestion; however, this is unclear.

The possible anticarcinogenic activity of curcumin and the other curcuminoids may be accounted for by a few mechanisms. These include inhibition of angiogenesis, upregulation of apoptosis, interference with certain signal transduction pathways that are critical for cell growth and proliferation, inhibition of colonic mucosa cyclooxygenase (COX) and lipoxygenase (LOX) activities and inhibition of farnesyl protein transferase. In addition to its possible activity in preventing malignant transformation and inhibiting tumor growth, curcumin may have antimetastatic potential, as well. In this regard, curcumin has been found to inhibit matrix metalloproteinase-9 in a human hepatocellular carcinoma cell line. The possible anticarcinogenic activity of the curcuminoids may be attributed, at least in part, to their ability to inhibit activation of the transcription factors NF-KappaB and AP-1. Curcuminoids have also been found to target the fibroblast growth factor-2 (FGF-2) angiogenic signaling pathway and inhibit expression of gelatinase B in the angiogenic process.

In the final analysis, the curcuminoids' antioxidant activity may underlie many of the above mechanisms. Reactive oxygen species (ROS) can activate AP-1 and NF-KappaB. Further, FGF-2 induces AP-1 activation via ROS produced through NADPH oxidase. The curcuminoids, acting as antioxidants, may interfere with the ability of FGF-2 to stimulate AP-1, and they may generally inhibit the activation of NF-KappaB and AP-1.

The possible anti-inflammatory activity of the curcuminoids may also be accounted for by several mechanisms, including inhibition of COX and LOX, reduction of the release of ROS by stimulated neutrophils, inhibition of AP-1 and NF-KappaB, and inhibition of the activation of the pro-inflammatory cytokines TNF (tumor necrosis factor) -alpha and IL (interleukin)-1 beta.

Curcumin has modest anti HIV-1 activity. It has been found to inhibit HIV-1 and HIV-2 proteases, HIV-1 LTR (long terminal repeat)-directed gene expression, Tat-mediated transactivation of HIV-1-LTR and HIV-1 integrase. All of these actions have been demonstrated *in vitro*. There is no evidence that curcumin or the other curcuminoids significantly inhibit the replication of HIV-1 *in vivo*. The mechanism of the possible hypocholesterolemic effect of the curcuminoids is unclear.

PHARMACOKINETICS

The pharmacokinetics of the curcuminoids remain incompletely understood. Of the curcuminoids, curcumin has been most studied, mainly in animals. Curcumin is poorly absorbed following ingestion in mice and rats. In these animals, 38 to 75% of an ingested dose is excreted directly in the feces. Absorption appears to be better with food. In mice, the major metabolites of curcumin are curcumin glucuronoside, dihydrocurcumin glucuronoside, tetrahydrocurcumin glucuronoside and tetrahydrocurcumin. These metabolites are formed in the liver. Animal studies and the pharmacokinetics of curcumin are continuing. Human pharmacokinetic studies are needed.

INDICATIONS AND USAGE

The curcuminoids may have anticarcinogenic, anti-atherosclerotic, anti-inflammatory (including anti-arthritic), antiviral, antifungal and immune-modulating effects. They appear to help detoxify some drugs and other chemicals. There is some evidence the curcuminoids may help prevent cataracts and ameliorate chronic anterior uveitis. They may also help speed wound healing. Claims that the curcuminoids may be helpful in gall bladder disease are poorly supported. Credible clinical trials related to the curcuminoids in general are lacking.

RESEARCH SUMMARY

The curcuminoids have exhibited significant anticarcinogenic effects in numerous *in vitro* and animal studies. They have inhibited progression of chemically induced colon and skin cancers through, it has been suggested, their ability to inhibit angiogenesis, among other possible mechanisms. In some of these studies, curcumin has reduced both the size and number of tumors as well as the incidence of tumorigenesis. Curcumin appears to have significant inhibitory effects in both the promotional and progression stages of colon cancer.

In *in vitro* studies, curcumin has induced apoptosis in human leukemia cells, a variety of B lymphoma cells and others. It has been used topically *in vitro* and in some animal work to inhibit some skin cancers.

Turmeric, the activity of which may be due to constituents in addition to, or other than, the curcuminoids, has been used in various parts of the world to treat everything from abdominal bloating and flatulence to gonorrhea and hepatitis. Evidence in support of these uses is largely anecdotal. The German commission E, however, has approved turmeric for the treatment of liver and gall bladder disorders and for appetite loss.

Turmeric, administered in 1-gram doses daily for nine months, reportedly conferred significant protection against palatal cancer in a study of subjects at risk of this malignancy owing to reverse smoking. Significant regression of precancerous lesions was noted. Curcumin has also been reported to diminish the toxic effects of a number of cancer drugs and other chemicals, including cisplatin, doxorubicin, carbon tetrachloride, paraquat and ethanol. This work has been conducted using animals. Marked neuroprotective, hepatoprotective and pulmonary-protective effects have been seen.

In one recent study, curcumin significantly reduced the total amount of chromosomal damage in nontumor cells of rats given cisplatin. This effect was attributed to curcumin's free radical-scavenging activity. Similarly, curcumin was recently shown to significantly prevent the nephrotoxicity of doxorubicin in rats.

The anti-inflammatory properties of the curcuminoids have been demonstrated in a number of *in vitro* and in some animal studies. These substances are widely used in India and Indonesia for various inflammatory conditions. *In vitro*, curcumin inhibits the production of such pro-inflammatory cytokines as tumor necrosis factor-alpha (TNF-alpha), interleukin-1 beta (IL-1 beta) and interleukin-8, among other anti-inflammatory actions.

Some preliminary evidence that one or more constituents of turmeric may be helpful in some forms of arthritis has emerged from a few animal studies and some human work. Curcumin itself was administered to rheumatoid arthritis patients (400 milligrams of curcumin three times a day for a total daily dose of 1,200 milligrams) for two weeks in a randomized, double-blind, crossover study. Significant subjective improvement was reported in terms of morning stiffness, walking time and joint swelling. No significant improvement was observed, however, in any objective measurement. Some have suggested that curcuminoids might be helpful in osteoarthritis, but there is no supporting evidence.

Claims that the curcuminoids may have anti-atherosclerotic effects are supported by some preliminary animal studies. Curcumin has shown some antithrombotic, anti-platelet aggregating activity in some *in vitro* and animal studies. It has also inhibited vascular smooth muscle cell proliferation *in vitro*. A turmeric extract was recently shown to significantly inhibit LDL-cholesterol oxidation in rabbits with experimental atherosclerosis.

The curcuminoids have demonstrated antiviral, anti-fungal and immunomodulating effects, mostly *in vitro*. Curcumin has been described as having HIV-1-inhibiting effects *in vitro*. In a clinical trial of curcumin in 40 subjects with HIV-1 infection, however, the substance was ineffective in reducing viral load or increasing CD4 counts. The low bioavailability of curcumin may account, in part, for its lack of *in vivo* antiviral activity. There is no credible clinical data to support claims that curcumin is helpful in those with hepatitis C. Some of the curcuminoids and turmeric extracts have exhibited some *in vitro* anti-fungal activity, specifically against *Candida albicans, Candida kruseii* and *Candida parapsilosis*. Recently, curcumin was shown to have various immunomodulating effects *in vitro*, which the researchers concluded might indicate some therapeutic potential for curcumin in T helper 1(Th1)-mediated immune diseases. Research is ongoing.

Recently, curcumin was administered to subjects with chronic anterior uveitis (375 milligrams three times daily for 12 weeks). Significant improvement was noted beginning two weeks after beginning curcumin supplementation. Follow-up over three years showed there was a 55% recurrence rate. The response to curcumin was said, in this study, to be equivalent to that of corticosteroid therapy but, in contrast with the latter, there were no notable side effects associated with curcumin. The researchers have called for a double-blind, multi-center clinical follow-up trial.

Recently it was demonstrated in an animal study that naphthalene-initiated cataracts can be significantly prevented by curcumin. Naphthalene-initiated cataract is used as a model for studying senile human cataract. The study showed for the first time that these experimental cataracts are associated with apoptosis of lens epithelial cells and that curcumin prevents some of the apoptotic activity.

Finally, curcumin has recently enhanced cutaneous wound-healing in diabetic mice. Previous studies showed that curcumin could enhance cutaneous wound-healing in rats and guinea pigs. Both oral and topical curcumin were effective in the diabetic mice. Earlier re-epithelialization and improved neovascularization were among the healing processes observed in curcumin-treated animals. The researchers concluded that curcumin might be of benefit in helping to overcome diabetic-impaired healing processes.

CONTRAINDICATIONS, PRECAUTIONS, ADVERSE REACTIONS
CONTRAINDICATIONS
Curcuminoids should be avoided by those hypersensitive to any component of a curcuminoid-containing supplement.

Curcuminoids may stimulate bile production in some. The volatile oil of turmeric is thought to be responsible for the bile-stimulating activity of turmeric, but this has not been conclusively established. Therefore, curcuminoids are contraindicated in those with bile duct obstructions and those with gallstones.

PRECAUTIONS
Pregnant women and nursing mothers should avoid curcuminoid supplemention.

Those with gastroesophogeal reflux disease (GERD) and those with a history of peptic ulcer disease should exercise caution in the use of curcuminoid supplements.

Curcuminoids may have antithrombotic activity in some. Therefore, those on warfarin or anti-platelet drugs should exercise caution in their use. Cancer patients should only use curcuminoid supplements under medical supervision.

Curcuminoid supplements must be taken with food. Curcuminoids may cause gastric irritation and ulceration if taken on an empty stomach.

ADVERSE REACTIONS
Adverse reactions of supplements principally comprised of curcuminoids are mainly gastrointestinal and include epigastric distress and nausea. There is one report of transient giddiness following curcuminoid ingestion. Abnormal liver tests have been reported in rats but not humans, and transient hypotension has been reported in dogs but, again, not in humans.

Curcuminoids may cause gastritis and peptic ulcer disease if taken without food.

INTERACTIONS
DRUGS
Chemotherapeutic agents: In animal studies, curcumin was found to enhance the antitumor effect of cisplatin against fibrosarcoma. It was also found to decrease the clastogenic effect of cisplatin. Also in animal studies, curcumin was found to decrease the nephrotoxicity due to doxorubicin and to decrease chromosomal aberrations due to bleomycin.

Anti-platelet drugs: Curcuminoids may enhance the action of anti-platelet drugs.

Warfarin: Curcuminoids may enhance the anticoagulant effect of warfarin.

NUTRITIONAL SUPPLEMENTS
Bromelain: Bromelain (see Bromelain) is reputed to enhance the absorption of curcuminoids. However, there is no credible documentation of this.

Piperine: Piperine (see Piperine) may enhance the absorption of curcuminoids.

DOSAGE AND ADMINISTRATION
Curcuminoid supplements are available that contain curcumin at 70 to 75%, demethoxycurcumin at 15 to 20% and bisdemethoxycurcumin at about 3%. Doses used range from 500 to 4000 milligrams daily, and they are taken with meals.

Curcuminoids taken on an empty stomach may cause gastric distress.

HOW SUPPLIED
Most commercial products are standardized to 95% curcumin.

Capsules — 300 mg, 350 mg, 450 mg, 500 mg
Liquid
Tablets — 300 mg, 350 mg, 400 mg

LITERATURE
Antunes LMG, Araú jo MCP, Darin JD'AC, Bianchi MdeLP. Effects of the antioxidants curcumin and vitamin C on cisplatin-

induced clastogenesis in Wistar rat bone marrow cells. *Mutat Res.* 2000; 465:131-137.

Arbiser JL, Klauber N, Rohan R, et al. Curcumin is an in vivo inhibitor of angiogenesis. *Mol Med.* 1998; 4:376-383.

Barthelmy S, Vergnes L, Moynier M, et al. Curcumin and curcumin derivatives inhibit Tat-mediated transactivation of type 1 human immunodeficiency virus long terminal repeat. *Res Virol.* 1998; 149:43-52.

Chan MM-Y. Inhibition of tumor necrosis factor by curcumin, a phytochemical. *Biochem Pharmacol.* 1995; 49:1551-1556.

Hellinger JA, Cohen CJ, Dugan ME, et al. Phase I/II randomized, open-label study of oral curcumin safety, and antiviral effects on HIV-RT PCR in HIV+ individuals. Third Conference on Retroviruses and Opportunistic Infections. Washington, DC; 1996: Abstract # 140.

Huang MT, Newmark HL, Fenkel K. Inhibitory effects of curcumin on tumorigenesis in mice. *J Cell Biochem Suppl.* 1997; 27:26-34.

Kang BY, Song YJ, Kim KM, et al. Curcumin inhibits Th1 cytokine profile in CD4+ T cells by suppressing interleukin-12 production in macrophages. *BR J Pharmacol.* 1999:128:380-384.

Kawamori T, Lubet R, Steele VE, et al. Chemopreventive effect of curcumin, a naturally occurring anti-inflammatory agent, during the promotion/progression stages of colon cancer. *Cancer Res.* 1999; 59:597-601.

Khopde SM, Priyadarsini KI, Guha SN, et al. Inhibition of radiation-induced lipid peroxidation by tetrahydrocurcumin: possible mechanisms by pulse radiolysis. *Biosci Biotechnol Biochem.* 2000; 64:503-509.

Kuo ML, Huang TS, Lin JK. Curcumin, an antioxidant and anti-tumor promoter, induces apoptosis in human leukemia cells. *Biochim Biophys Acta.* 1996; 1317:95-100.

Mazumder A, Raghavan K, Weinstein J, et al. Inhibition of human immunodeficiency virus type-1 integrase by curcumin. *Biochem Pharmacol.* 1995; 49:1165-1170.

Mohan R, Sivak J, Ashton P, et al. Curcuminoids inhibit the angiogenic response stimulated by fibroblast growth factor-2, including expression of matrix metalloproteinase gelatinase B. *J Biol Chem.* 2000; 275:10405-10412.

Pan M-H, Huang T-M, Lin J-K. Biotransformation of curcumin through reduction and glucuronidation in mice. *Drug Metab Disp.* 1999; 27:486-494.

Pandya U, Saini MK, Jin GF, et al. Dietary curcumin prevents ocular toxicity of naphthalene in rats. *Toxicol Lett.* 2000; 115:195-204.

Park EJ, Jeon CH, Ko G, et al. Protective effect of curcumin in rat liver injury induced by carbon tetrachloride. *J Pharm Pharmacol.* 2000; 52:437-440.

Ramiré z-Tortosa MC, Mesa MD, Aguilera MC, et al. Oral administration of a turmeric extract inhibits LDL oxidation and has hypocholesterolemic effects in rabbits with experimental atherosclerosis. *Atherosclerosis.* 1999; 147:371-378.

Sidhu GS, Mani H, Gaddipati JP, et al. Curcumin enhances wound healing in streptozotocin induced diabetic rats and genetically diabetic mice. *Wound Rep Reg.* 1999; 7:362-374.

Venkatesan N. Pulmonary protective effects of curcumin against paraquat toxicity. *Life Sci.* 2000; 66:PL21-PL28.

Venkatesan N, Punithavathi D, Arumugam V. Curcumin prevents adriamycin nephrotoxicity in rats. *Br J Pharmacol.* 2000; 129:231-234.

Zhang F, Altorki NK, Mestre JR, et al. Curcumin inhibits cyclooxygenase-2 transcription in bile acid-and phorbol ester-treated human gastrointestinal epithelial cells. *Carcinogenesis.* 1999; 20:445-451.

Daidzein

DESCRIPTION

Daidzein belongs to the isoflavone class of flavonoids. It is also classified as a phytoestrogen since it is a plant-derived nonsteroidal compound that possesses estrogen-like biological activity. Daidzein has been found to have both weak estrogenic and weak anti-estrogenic effects.

Daidzein is the aglycone (aglucon) of daidzin. The isoflavone is found naturally as the glycoside daidzin and as the glycosides 6''-O-malonylgenistin and 6''-O-acetyldaidzin. Daidzein and its glycosides are mainly found in legumes, such as soybeans and chickpeas. Soybeans and soy foods are the major dietary sources of these substances. Daidzein glycosides are the second most abundant isoflavones in soybeans and soy foods; genistein glycosides are the most abundant. Nonfermented soy foods, such as tofu, contain daidzein, principally in its glycoside forms. Fermented soy foods, such as tempeh and miso, contain significant levels of the aglycone.

Daidzein and daidzin are also found in *Radix puerariae* (RP). RP is an herbal medicine prepared from the root of the legume *Pueraria labata,* commonly known as kudzu. RP has been used for centuries in traditional Chinese medicine for the treatment of a wide range of disorders. It has also been used in traditional Chinese medicine since 600 AD for its ''anti-drunkenness'' effect and is still used by traditional Chinese physicians for the treatment of those who abuse alcohol. It is thought that the antidipsotropic (anti-drinking) effect of RP is due to daidzein and daidzin.

Daidzein is a solid substance that is virtually insoluble in water. Its molecular formula is $C_{15}H_{10}O_4$, and its molecular weight is 254.24 daltons. Daidzein is also known as 7-hydroxy-3- (4-hydroxyphenyl)-4*H* -1-benzopyran-4-one and 4', 7-dihydroxyisoflavone. Daidzin, which has greater water solubility than daidzein, is the 7-beta glucoside of daidzein. The structural formula of daidzein is:

Daidzein

When marketed as a nutritional supplement, daidzein is mainly present in the form of its beta-glucoside, daidzin.

ACTIONS AND PHARMACOLOGY

ACTIONS

Daidzein has estrogenic activity. Daidzein may have antioxidant activity. It may also have antidipsotropic, anticarcinogenic, anti-atherogenic and anti-osteoporotic activity.

MECHANISM OF ACTION

Daidzein has weak estrogenic activity as measured *in vivo* and *in vitro* assays. *In vivo,* its estrogenic activity is the lowest of the soy isoflavones.

Daidzein is a scavenger of reactive oxygen species. Genistein is the most studied of the soy isoflavones with regard to antioxidant activity. It is thought that genistein may be a more potent antioxidant than daidzein. There are few studies comparing the antioxidant activity of the two isoflavones.

The proposed mechanism of daidzein's possible antidipsotropic activity is as follows. Daidzein inhibits the class I isoenzymes of human alcohol dehydrogenase (ADH), especially the gamma-type ADH. Inhibition of human class I ADH may suppress ethanol consumption by increasing the bioavailability of ingested ethanol. Daidzin is an inhibitor of human mitochondrial aldehyde dehydrogenase (ALDH)-2. Inhibition of ALDH-2 could also suppress ethanol consumption by increasing the bioavailability of ingested ethanol. Finally, daidzin has been found to inhibit the metabolism of serotonin via its inhibition of ALDH-2. This inhibition is accompanied by a concomitant accumulation of 5-hydroxy-indole-3-acetaldehyde (S-HIAL) and 3, 4-dihydroxyphenyla-cetaldehyde (DOPAL). 5-HIAL and DOPAL may be involved in mediating the possible antidipsotropic action of daidzein. In contrast to the broad-acting ALDH inhibitor disulfiram, daidzein/daidzin does not appear to block acetaldehyde metabolism.

The mechanism of daidzein's possible anticarcinogenic activity, as well as its possible anti-atherogenic activity, is unclear. Daidzein's weak estrogenic effect may play some role in the possible activity of soy isoflavones against prostate cancer. Likewise, daidzein's weak estrogenic effect, as well as its possible antioxidant activity, may contribute to its possible anti-atherogenic activity.

Daidzein's weak estrogenic effect may also be involved in its possible anti-osteoporotic activity. Daidzein has been found to have an anabolic effect in an osteoblastic cell line in culture, suggesting that it may be able to stimulate osteoblastic bone formation. Also, the major metabolite of the synthetic isoflavone ipriflavone is daidzein. Ipriflavone has demonstrated a significant ability to prevent osteoporosis in both animal models and humans.

PHARMACOKINETICS

The pharmacokinetics of daidzein in humans is complex and not well understood. Pharmacokinetics of daidzein and daidzin are available from animal models, and some inferences can be made. The aglycone daidzein may be absorbed from the small intestine from whence it is transported to the systemic circulation by the lymphatics. There is little information available on the tissue distribution of daidzein. That which is delivered to the liver mainly undergoes conjugation with glucuronate and sulfate via hepatic phase II enzymes (UDP-glucuronosyltransferases and sulfotransferases). The glucuronate and sulfate conjugates of daidzein are excreted in the urine and in the bile. The daidzein conjugates may be deconjugated to release daidzein, which may be reabsorbed via the enterohepatic circulation.

Most of ingested daidzin, the major dietary and supplemental form of daidzein, is delivered to the large intestine intact. In the large intestine, bacterial beta-glucosidases hydrolyze daidzin to daidzein. Daidzein is either absorbed and processed as described above or further metabolized in the large intestine to dihydrodaidzein, which is then metabolized to equol or O-desmethylangolensin.

There is considerable individual variation in the absorption and metabolism of ingested daidzein and daidzin. The extent of absorption of the daidzein beta-glucoside daidzin is also unclear.

INDICATIONS AND USAGE

Daidzein, like the other soy isoflavones, may have some anticancer and anti-atherogenic effects. It may also help to suppress ''hot flashes'' in some menopausal women and may help prevent osteoporosis. Preliminary animal work suggests that it might help curb ethanol intake in those who are alcohol-dependent.

RESEARCH SUMMARY

It has recently been demonstrated that daidzein can promote bone formation and mineralization *in vitro*. Its activity in this regard is similar to that of genistein, another soy isoflavone. It also has some of genistein's and glycitein's estrogenic effects, and may be helpful to some menopausal women, particularly with respect to ameliorating ''hot flashes.'' It also appears to share the anti-atherogenic and anticancer properties of the other soy isoflavones. (See Soy Isoflavones, Glycitein and Ipriflavone.)

Daidzein has been shown to suppress free-choice ethanol intake in Syrian Golden hamsters. *Radix puerariae,* a herb rich in daidzein and daidzin, the 7-glucoside of daidzein, has long been used in traditional Chinese medicine to treat those who are alcohol-dependent. Both daidzein and daidzin themselves were effective in significantly reducing ethanol intake by more than 50% in hamsters dependent on alcohol. The treatment did not significantly affect body weight, water or food intake.

More recent work has confirmed that daidzin, which is the major delivery form of daidzein, successfully and significantly suppresses ethanol intake in all rodent models tested. A recent study showed that daidzin inhibits serotonin and dopamine metabolism in isolated mitochondria. The researchers involved in this study believe this inhibition may be one of the mechanisms by which this soy isoflavone suppresses ethanol intake. Clinical testing is needed to evaluate the possible benefits of daidzein/daidzin in human dipsomaniacs.

CONTRAINDICATIONS, PRECAUTIONS, ADVERSE REACTIONS

CONTRAINDICATIONS

Daidzein is contraindicated in those who are hypersensitive to any component of a daidzin- or daidzein-containing product.

PRECAUTIONS

Pregnant women and nursing mothers should avoid the use of daidzein/daidzin-containing supplements pending long-term safety studies.

Men with prostate cancer should discuss the advisability of the use of daidzein/daidzin-containing supplements with their physicians before deciding to use them.

Women with estrogen receptor-positive tumors should exercise caution in the use of daidzein/dadzin-containing supplements and should only use them if they are recommended and monitored by a physician.

Daidzein/daidzin intake has been associated with hypothyroidism in some.

INTERACTIONS

Ethanol: Daidzein/daidzin may increase the bioavailability of ingested ethanol.

OVERDOSAGE

There are no reports of overdosage.

DOSAGE AND ADMINISTRATION

Daidzein is available in a few different isoflavone formulas. A standard soy isoflavone formula contains daidzein principally in the form of daidzin, as well as genistin and glycitin,

with much smaller amounts of the aglycones daidzein, genistein and glycitein. The percentages of the soy isoflavones present in such a supplement reflect the percentages of these substances as found in soybeans and are: daidzin, about 38%; genistin, about 50%; and glycitin, about 12%. A 50-mg dose of soy isoflavone supplement—a typical daily dose—delivers 19 mg of daidzin, 25 mg of genistin and about 6 mg of glycitin. Usually, 40% of the formula is comprised of soy isoflavones. Therefore, to get a dose of 50 mg of soy isoflavones, 125 mg of the soy preparation are required.

Smaller amounts of daidzein in the aglycone form are available in some red clover preparations (see Biochanin A).

LITERATURE

Keung W-M, Lazo O, Kunze L, Vallee B. Daidzin suppresses ethanol consumption by Syrian golden hamsters without blocking acetaldehyde metabolism. *Proc Natl Acad Sci USA.* 1995; 92:8990-8993.

Keung W-M, Lazo O, Kunze L, Vallee BL. Potentiation of the bioavailability of daidzin by an extract of *Radix puerariae. Proc Natl Acad Sci USA.* 1996; 93:4284-4288.

Keung W-M, Vallee BL. Daidzin and daidzein suppress free-choice ethanol intake by Syrian Golden hamsters. *Proc Natl Acad Sci USA.* 1993; 90:10008-10012.

Keung W-M, Vallee BL. Daidzin and its antidipsotropic analogs inhibit serotonin and dopamine metabolism in isolated mitochondria. *Proc Natl Acad Sci USA.* 1998; 95:2198-2203.

Sugimoto E, Yamaguchi M. Stimulatory effect of daidzein in osteoblastic MC3T3-E1 cells. *Biochem Pharmacol.* 2000; 59:471-475.

For additional references, see Soy Isoflavones.

Deanol

DESCRIPTION

Deanol or dimethylaminoethanol is presently marketed as a dietary supplement, but at one time it was used as a drug for the treatment of hyperactivity in children and was also used for such conditions as neuroleptic-induced tardive dyskinesia. Deanol was thought to affect tardive dyskinesia because it was believed to be a cholinergic precursor and to enhance acetylcholine synthesis in the brain. It is now known that, although deanol is a precursor to choline, very little of the choline formed from it is converted to acetylcholine in the brain.

Deanol or dimethylaminoethanol is also known as 2-(dimethylamino)ethanol, beta-dimethylaminoethyl alcohol and N, N-dimethyl-2-hydroxy ethylamine. It is abbreviated DMAE. When deanol was on the market as a drug, it was called Deaner and was in the form of deanol acetamidobenzoate.

Deanol is itself a liquid. The most common form of deanol supplement is deanol bitartrate.

Another deanol-containing substance, deanol 4-chlorphenoxyacetate hydrochloride or centrophenoxine hydrochloride, is used in Europe, Japan, Australia and Mexico as a cognition enhancer in the elderly.

ACTIONS AND PHARMACOLOGY

ACTIONS

Deanol may increase choline levels.

MECHANISM OF ACTION

Deanol is a precursor to choline.

PHARMACOKINETICS

There is limited information on the pharmacokinetics of deanol in humans. Deanol is absorbed from the small intestine from whence it is transported to the liver where much of it is metabolized to choline. Very little of this choline appears to be converted to acetylcholine in the brain. In fact, it is reported that deanol inhibits the uptake of choline into the brain. Deanol also appears to inhibit the oxidation of choline to betaine and may inhibit other reactions of choline metabolism.

INDICATIONS AND USAGE

Results with deanol in the treatment of tardive dyskinesia are mostly negative. Claims that deanol is helpful in Alzheimer's disease, age-related cognitive deficits and in aging itself are without foundation.

RESEARCH SUMMARY

Given the assumption that deanol is an acetylcholine precursor and that it might thus enhance the cholinergic neurotransmitter system, deanol has been used in numerous trials investigating it as a possible treatment for tardive dyskinesia. The results have been mixed but mostly negative. A recent meta-analysis showed that it is no more effective than placebo in this disorder.

Deanol has similarly been shown to have no significant effect in the treatment of Alzheimer's disease, amnesic disorders, age-related cognitive impairment and Tourette's syndrome. Effects on aging in animal models have been contradictory; one study showed decreased life span.

CONTRAINDICATIONS, PRECAUTIONS, ADVERSE REACTIONS

CONTRAINDICATIONS

Deanol should be avoided by pregnant women and nursing mothers. Deanol has also been reported to inhibit the oxidation of choline to betaine. Betaine is involved in the metabolism of homocysteine. Elevated homocysteine levels are associated with an increased risk of atherosclerosis. Those with elevated homocysteine levels should avoid deanol.

ADVERSE REACTIONS

Reported adverse reactions include headache, cramps, constipation, insomnia and the induction of lucid dreams. There is one report of a subject who was treated for 10 years with deanol for essential tremor who developed a marked dyskinesia syndrome affecting predominantly orofacial and respiratrory musculature. This was partially reversed upon discontinuation of deanol.

DOSAGE AND ADMINISTRATION

Deanol is available as a liquid or as deanol bitartrate. Typical doses are 100 milligrams daily.

LITERATURE

Andriamampandry C, Freysz L, Kanfer JN, et al. Conversion of ethanolamine, monomethylethanolamine and dimethylethanolamine to choline-containing compounds by neurons in culture and by the rat brain. *Biochem J.* 1989; 264:555-562.

Cherkin A, Exhardt MJ. Effects of dimethylaminoethanol upon life-span and behavior of aged Japanese quail. *J Geront.* 1977; 32:38-45.

de Montigny C, Chouinard G, Annable L. Ineffectiveness of deanol in tardive dyskinesia: a placebo-controlled study. *Psychopharmacology.* 1979; 65:219-223.

Fisman M, Mersky H, Holmes H. Double-blind trial of 2-dimethylaminoethanol in Alzheimer's disease. *Am J Psychiatry.* 1981; 138:970-972.

Haubrich DR, Gerber NH, Pflueger AB. Deanol affects choline metabolism in peripheral tissues of mice. *J Neurochem.* 1981; 37:476-482.

Jope RS, Jenden DJ. Dimethylaminoethanol (deanol) metabolism in rat brain and its effect on acetylcholine synthesis. *J Pharamacol Exp Ther.* 1979; 211:472-479.

Millington WR, Mc Call AL, Wurtman RJ. Deanol acetamidobenzoate inhibits the blood-brain barrier transport of choline. *Ann Neurol.* 1978; 4:302-306.

Penovich P, Morgan JP, Kerzner B, et al. Double-blind evaluation of deanol in tardive dyskinesia. *JAMA.* 1978; 239:1997-1998.

Sergio W. Use of DMAE (dimethylaminoethanol) in the induction of lucid dreams. *Med Hypotheses.* 1988; 26:255-257.

Soares KV, McGrath JJ. The treatment of tardive dyskinesia—a systematic review and meta-analysis. *Schizophr Res.* 1999; 39:1-16.

Zahniser NR, Chou D, Hanin I. Is 2-dimethylaminoethanol (deanol) indeed a precursor of brain acetylcholine? A gas chromotographic evaluation. *J Pharmacol Exp Ther.* 1977; 200:545-549.

Deglycyrrhizinated Licorice (DGL)

TRADE NAMES

DGL is available from numerous manufacturers generically. Branded products include DGL-Power (Nature's Herbs).

DESCRIPTION

Deglycyrrhizinated licorice, commonly abbreviated DGL, is an extract of the root of true licorice, *Glycyrrhiza glabra*, which has significantly reduced mineralocorticoid activity. Licorice has a number of medicinal properties, including peptic ulcer healing, anti-inflammatory, antimicrobial and antioxidant activities. Glycyrrhizinic acid and its metabolite, glycyrrhetinic acid, have mineralocorticoid-like, as well as testosterone-reducing, activities. The use of licorice for the management of peptic ulcer disease is associated with hypertension, water retension and hypokalemia. The removal of most of the glycyrrhizinic and glyceyrrhetinic acids yields a product without these undesirable effects.

ACTIONS AND PHARMACOLOGY

ACTIONS

DGL may have peptic ulcer-healing activity.

MECHANISM OF ACTION

The mechanism of action of the peptic ulcer-healing activity of DGL is not entirely understood. DGL was found to stimulate and/or accelerate the differentiation of glandular cells in the forestomach of the rat, as well as stimulate mucus formation and secretion. The stimulation of mucus secretion in the stomach is believed to account, at least in part, for the activity of DGL. DGL contains some flavonoids that have antimicrobial activity, including activity against the ulcer-causing bacterium *Helicobacter pylori*. This too could account, at least in part, for DGL's activity. New substances are continually being discovered in licorice, and it is possible that some of these may also play a role in DGL's activity.

PHARMACOKINETICS

There is very little known about the pharmacokinetics of DGL.

INDICATIONS AND USAGE

DGL has been shown to be useful in the management of gastric and duodenal ulcers.

RESEARCH SUMMARY

Several studies in animals and humans have demonstrated positive effects from the use of DGL in gastric and duodenal ulcer conditions. DGL, administered in chewable doses of 760 milligrams a day for one month, was significantly superior to placebo in reducing peptic ulcer size and in hastening healing in human subjects, compared with the placebo control subjects. DGL produced complete healing in 44% of those receiving it, compared with complete healing in 6% of controls.

Subsequent studies have shown that DGL is about as effective as cimetidine and ranitidine for both treatment and maintenance therapy of gastric ulcers. Comparison studies have not been made with DGL and famotidine, lansoprazole, omeprazole and other more recent anti-ulcer drugs.

DGL appears to confer significant protection against the gastric mucosal damage caused by aspirin and other nonsteroidal anti-inflammatory drugs. Gastric bleeding induced by aspirin intake can also be reduced with DGL supplementation.

DGL has also demonstrated significant efficacy in the treatment of duodenal ulcers. In one study, 40 patients who had suffered from severe duodenal ulcers for four to 12 years (and who had experienced more than six relapses in the previous year) were treated with either 3 grams of DGL daily for eight weeks or with 4.5 grams daily for 16 weeks. All showed significant improvement, but more improvement was seen with the higher-dose regimen. None of the patients required surgery during a one-year follow-up period. In other research, DGL had a therapeutic effect in duodenal ulcers equal to that of cimetidine.

DGL's protective activity is attributed by some to its ability to stimulate the formation and secretion of mucus. It has been shown, in rats, to stimulate epithelial proliferation in the forestomach. More recently, it has been demonstrated that several flavonoids that are present in DGL can inhibit *Helicobacter pylori* growth.

CONTRAINDICATIONS, PRECAUTIONS, ADVERSE REACTIONS

CONTRAINDICATIONS

None known.

PRECAUTIONS

Because of lack of long-term safety studies, DGL should be avoided by children, pregnant women and nursing mothers.

Those with hypertension, congestive heart failure, arrhythmias, water retention and low potassium and/or magnesium levels should discuss the use of DGL with their physicians and should be certain that any DGL they use is free of glycyrrhizinic acid.

ADVERSE REACTIONS

There are significant adverse effects with licorice extracts containing glycyrrhizinic and glycyrrhetinic acid when used for the management of peptic ulcer disease, including hypokalemia, hypomagnesemia, hypertension, headache, cardiac arrhythmias, water retention and congestive heart failure. DGL, however, should be free of these side effects.

There are occasional reports of gastrointestinal side effects, such as diarrhea and nausea.

INTERACTIONS

The excretion rate of nitrofurantoin was found to be significantly higher in patients receiving the drug along with DGL. No interactions with drugs used in the treatment of peptic ulcer disease are known.

OVERDOSAGE

There are no reports of overdosage with DGL.

DOSAGE AND ADMINISTRATION

In Europe, Canada and South Africa, DGL is available as a medicinal preparation called Caved-S. In the U.S., DGL is available as a nutritional supplement in the form of chewable tablets. Typically, those who use DGL for management of peptic ulcer disorders chew from one to four 380-milligram tablets or the equivalent before each meal.

HOW SUPPLIED

Chewable Tablets — 140 mg, 380 mg

Wafers — 380 mg

LITERATURE

Armanini D, Bonanni G, Palermo M. Reduction of serum testosterone in men by licorice. *N Eng J Med.* 1999; 341:1158.

Balackrishnan V, Pillai MV, Raveendran PM, Nair CS. Deglycyrrhizinated liquorice in the treatment of chronic duodenal ulcer. *J Assoc Physicians India.* 1978; 26:811-814.

Bardham KD, Cumberland DC, Dixon RA, Holdsworth CD. Proceedings: deglycyrrhizinated liquorice in gastric ulcer: a double-blind controlled study. *Gut.* 1976; 17:397

Beil W, Birkholz C, Sewing KF. Effects of flavonoids on parietal cell acid secretion, gastric mucosal prostaglandin production and *Helicobactee pylori* growth. *Arzneimittelforschung.* 1995; 45:697-700.

Bennett A, Clark-Wibberley T, Stamford IF, Wright JE. Aspirin-induced gastric mucosal damage in rats: cimetidine and deglycyrrhizinated liquorice together give greater protection than low doses of either drug alone. *J Pharm Pharmacol.* 1980; 32:151.

Dalta R, Rao SR, Murthy KJ. Excretion studies of nitrofurantoin and nitrofurantoin with deglycyrrhizinated liquorice. *Indian J Physiol Pharmacol.* 1981; 25:59-63.

Farese Jr RV, Biglieri EJ, Shackleton CHL, et al. Licorice-induced hypermineralocorticoidism. *N Engl J Med.* 1991; 325:1223-1227.

Glick L. Deglycyrrhizinated liquorice for peptic ulcer. *Lancet* 1982; 2:817.

Li W, Asada Y, Yoshikawa T. Antimicrobial compounds from *Glycyrrhiza glabra* hairy root cultures. *Planta Med.* 1998; 64:746-747.

Morgan AG, McAdam WA, Pascoo C, Darnborough A. Comparison between cimetidine and Caved-S in the treatment of gastric ulceration and subsequent maintenance therapy. *Gut.* 1982; 23:545-551.

Morgan AG, Pacsoo C, McAdam WA. Comparison between ranitidine and ranitidine plus Caved-S in the treatment of gastric ulceration. *Gut.* 1985; 26:1377-1379.

Morgan AG, Pacsoo C, McAdam WA. Maintenance therapy: a two year comparison between Caved-S and cimetidine treatment in the prevention of symptomatic gastric ulcer recurrence. *Gut.* 1985; 26:599-602.

Rees WD, Rhodes J, Wright JE, et al. Effect of deglycyrrhizinated liquorice on gastric mucosal damage by aspirin. *Scand J Gastroenterol.* 1979; 14:605-607.

Stewart PM, Wallace AM, Vallentino R, et al. Mineralocorticoid activity of liquorice: 11-beta-hydroxysteroid dehyrdogenase deficiency comes of age. *Lancet.* 1987; 2:821-824.

van Marle J, Aarsen PN, Lind A, van Weeren-Kramer, J. Deglycyrrhizinated liquorice (DGL) and the renewal of rat stomach epithelium. *Eur J Pharmacol.* 1981; 72:219-225.

D-Glucarate

DESCRIPTION

D-glucarate is the anionic form of D-glucaric acid, a dicarboxylic sugar acid derived from the oxidation of D-gluconic acid. It is naturally found in some vegetables and fruits, including cruciferous vegetables, bean sprouts and apples. D-glucarate may have cancer-chemopreventive activity.

D-glucarate is also known as D-saccharate. D-glucarate, in the form of its calcium salt, calcium D-glucarate, is marketed as a nutritional supplement. The molecular formula of calcium D-glucarate is $C_6H_8C_9O_8$, and its molecular weight is 248.20 daltons.

ACTIONS AND PHARMACOLOGY

MECHANISM OF ACTION

The mechanism of D-glucarate's possible anticarcinogenic activity is not entirely clear. One possibility is the inhibition of beta-glucuronidase via the D-glucarate derivative D-glucaro-1, 4-lactone (1, 4-GL). A major mechanism for the detoxification of certain carcinogens is via glucuronidation, which is catalyzed by glucuronyl transferase. The glucuronide conjugates are excreted in the urine and bile. However, deconjugation can occur via the enzyme beta-glucuronidase. Inhibition of beta-glucuronidase prevents deconjugation. D-glucarate may have anticarcinogenic activity independent of 1, 4-GL. D-glucarate has been demonstrated to inhibit protein kinase, and this is a possible mechanism for a direct anticarcinogenic effect of the substance.

D-glucarate has been shown to lower cholesterol in rats. The mechanism of this effect is unknown.

PHARMACOKINETICS

There is little on the pharmacokinetics of D-glucarate in humans. Rat studies indicate that D-glucarate is converted to 1, 4-GL in the stomach. 1, 4-GL, again in rats, appears to be absorbed, transported by the blood to various tissues and excreted in the urine and, to a lesser extent, in the bile. Calcium-D-glucarate is claimed to be a sustained or slow release precursor of 1, 4-GL, but there are few human data to substantiate this.

INDICATIONS AND USAGE

Animal and *in vitro* work suggest that D-glucarate may have some anticancer and lipid-lowering effects. Clinical data, however, are lacking.

RESEARCH SUMMARY

D-glucarate has exhibited significant anticarcinogenic effects in numerous *in vitro* and animal experiments. It has shown some efficacy when used alone or in combination with some other putative anticancer substances, notably some of the retinoids. It has shown preventive and therapeutic activity against a number of cancers, including mammary, liver, prostate and colon cancer. There is evidence it may protect against a number of chemical carcinogens.

In one experiment, D-glucarate was found to be particularly effective in inhibiting chemically induced cancer in animals when fed during the promotional phase of carcinogenesis, but it was also effective when fed during the initiation phase. A more recent study also found that D-glucarate seems to be most effective in the post-initiation phases of cancer, as assessed, in this study by its inhibiting effects on carcinogen-induced aberrant crypt foci in the colons of rats. Research is ongoing.

Data related to claims that D-glucarate is an effective lipid-lowering agent are not as plentiful as the cancer data. Some animal data, however, suggest that D-glucarate may reduce total cholesterol and LDL-cholesterol. It does not appear to affect HDL-cholesterol. More research is needed.

CONTRAINDICATIONS, PRECAUTIONS, ADVERSE REACTIONS

CONTRAINDICATIONS

D-glucarate is contraindicated in those hypersensitive to any component of a D-glucarate-containing product.

PRECAUTIONS

Pregnant women and nursing mothers should avoid D-glucarate supplementation pending long-term safety studies.

INTERACTIONS

DRUGS

Retinoids: D-glucarate has shown synergistic chemopreventive effects with retinoids in some tumor models.

5-Fluorouracil: D-glucarate and 5-fluorouracil exhibited synergistic antitumor activity in a rat-tumor model.

DOSAGE AND ADMINISTRATION

D-glucarate is available in supplemental form as calcium-D-glucarate. A usual dose is 200 mg once or twice daily.

LITERATURE

Abou-Issa H, Moeschberger M, el-Masry W, et al. Relative efficacy of glucarate on the initiation and promotion phases of rat mammary carcinogenesis. *Anticancer Res.* 1995; 15:805-810.

Curley RW Jr, Humphries KA, Koolemans-Beyman A, et al. Activity of D-glucarate analogues: synergistic antiproliferative effects with retinoid in cultured human mammary tumor cells appear to specifically require the D-glucarate structure. *Life Sci.* 1994; 54:1299-1303.

Dwivedi C, Heck WJ, Downie AA, et al. Effect of calcium glucarate on beta-glucuronidase activity and glucarate content of certain vegetables and fruits. *Biochem Med Metab Biol.* 1990; 43:83-92.

Heerdt AS, Young CW, Borgen PI. Calcium glucarate as a chemopreventive agent in breast cancer. *Isr J Med Sci.* 1995; 31:101-105.

Oredipe OA, Barth RF, Dwivedi C, Webb TE. Dietary glucarate-mediated inhibition of initiation of diethylnitrosamine-induced hepatocarcinogenesis. *Toxicology.* 1992; 74:209-222.

Schmittgen TD, Koolesmans-Beynen A, Webb TE, et al. Effects of 5-fluorouracil, leucovorin, and glucarate in rat colon-tumor explants. *Cancer Chemother Pharmacol.* 1992; 30:25-30.

Walaszek A, Szemraj J, Hanausek M, et al. D-glucaric acid content of various fruits and vegetables and cholesterol-lowering effects of dietary D-glucarate in the rat. *Nutr Res.* 1996; 16:673-682.

Walaszek Z. Potential use of D-glucaric acid derivatives in cancer prevention. *Cancer Lett.* 1990; 54:1-8.

Walaszek Z, Szemraj J, Narog M, et al. Metabolism, uptake, and excretion of D-glucaric acid salt and its potential use in cancer prevention. *Cancer Detect Prev.* 1997; 21:178-190.

DHEA (Dehydroepiandrosterone)

TRADE NAMES

DHEA is available generically from numerous manufactures. Branded products include Natures Blend DHEA (National Vitamin Company) and DHEA Max (Nutraceutics Corp.)

DESCRIPTION

Dehydroepiandrosterone, commonly abbreviated as DHEA, is a natural substance produced in the adrenal gland, gonads and brain. DHEA is a steroid hormone. DHEA and its metabolite dehydroepiandrosterone-3-sulfate or DHEAS are the major secretory steroidal products of the adrenal gland. The ratio of DHEAS to DHEA in serum is approximately 300 to 500 to one, and the concentration of DHEAS in the serum is approximately 20 times higher than any other steroid hormone. It is noteworthy that the mean concentration of DHEAS in serum decreases progressively from a peak at age 25 to less than 20% of that peak before the age of 70. Further, DHEAS serum levels are typically low in those with chronic diseases, such as cancer and AIDS. To date, the physiological roles of DHEA and DHEAS remain largely unknown.

DHEA is synthesized in the adrenal cortex in the region known as the zona reticularis. Cholesterol is the precursor to DHEA. Pregnenolone and 17-hydroxy pregnenolone are intermediates, and oxygen and cytochrome P450a17 are involved in the reaction. DHEA has weak androgenic activity. It is metabolized in the adrenal gland to other androgenic substances, including androstenediol, androstenedione and testosterone. It is also metabolized to the estrogens, estrone and estradiol. DHEA is reversibly converted to DHEAS. DHEA and DHEAS have also been found in the brain, and there appears to be synthetic pathways to their production present in the nervous system. Neurosteroids are steroids that accumulate in the nervous system independently, at least in part, of supply by the steroidogenic endocrine glands. These can be synthesized *de novo* in the nervous system from sterol precursors. DHEA and DHEAS in the nervous system are classified as neurosteroids.

DHEA and DHEAS are being developed by biotechnology companies as possible pharmaceuticals. DHEA is being developed as a treatment for systemic lupus erythematosus. Injectable DHEAS is being developed for the treatment of acute asthmatic attacks and severe burns. Injectable DHEA is being developed to preserve neuronal and myocardial tissue from the harmful effects of ischemia/reperfusion injury associated with heart attacks, stroke and cardiovascular surgery. Whether these drugs will prove effective and be marketed remains to be seen.

DHEA is known as dehydroepiandrosterone and prasterone. DHEAS is known as dehydroepiandrosterone sulfate, dehydroepiandrosterone-3-sulfate and prasterone sulfate. DHEA has the following structural formula:

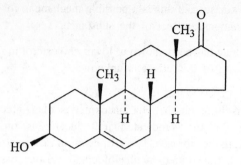

DHEA
(Dehydroepiandrosterone)

Extracts of the Mexican yam *Dioscorea mexicana* or the wild yam *Dioscorea villosa* are not converted to DHEA following ingestion.

ACTIONS AND PHARMACOLOGY

ACTIONS

Oral DHEA has weak and adrogenic activity. Otherwise, the action of oral DHEA is unknown. DHEA and DHEAS have several putative actions, including anti-inflammatory, anti-cancer, antiobesity, antidiabetogenic and antiaging.

MECHANISM OF ACTION

Some of the reported effects of oral DHEA may be due to its weak androgenic activity and to the fact that it is metabolized to androstenedione which, in turn, is metabolized to androgens and estrogens. The observed benefits of DHEA in post-menopausal women, for example, may be accounted for by this weak androgenic activity.

DHEA is an inhibitory modulator of the gamma-aminobutyric acid-benzodiazepine receptor complex in rats, and DHEA enhances the effect of excitatory amino acids on the NMDA receptors, also in rats. How this relates to any effect of oral DHEA in humans is entirely speculative.

PHARMACOKINETICS

DHEA is absorbed from the small intestine and is transported to the liver, where it is metabolized mainly to DHEAS by the enzyme sulfotransferase. DHEA and DHEAS are distributed to the various tissues in the body where metabolites, including androstenedione, testosterone, estrogens (estrone and estradiol), androstenediol and 7-oxo-DHEA, are synthesized. There is great individual variability in the metabolism of oral DHEA. Excretion of DHEA and its metabolites is primarily via the urinary route.

INDICATIONS AND USAGE

Regarded as a drug by many researchers and banned for all uses in the United Kingdom and Canada, the use of DHEA as a supplement is not indicated for the treatment or prevention of any condition without qualified medical recommendation and monitoring. The best available research suggests that DHEA, particularly at the high doses many have reported are being used, poses potentially serious health risks.

There is some evidence that DHEA, in monitored doses in selected subjects, may be of some help in easing some of the symptoms of systemic lupus erythematosus, may enhance immune response in some others and may be indicated in some women with adrenal insufficiency. There is very preliminary evidence that DHEA can have a positive impact on mood and memory. DHEA replacement after menopause has been proposed.

There is no credible evidence that DHEA can burn fat and build lean muscle mass, that it can boost sexual performance or that it can fight cancer, heart disease, fatigue, diabetes, osteoporosis and aging itself.

RESEARCH SUMMARY

Recent research has raised hopes that DHEA may provide some benefit to those with systemic lupus erythematosus. Studies, both completed and underway, indicate that DHEA, at dose levels that most researchers regard as risky for the general population, enabled some lupus patients to reduce their reliance on prednisone while still achieving equivalent relief from pain, fatigue and inflammation.

In vitro and animal studies have shown that DHEA can inhibit the cytokine molecular messaging that directs release of some of the inflammatory substances implicated in lupus. A synthesized DHEA product called GL701 is currently being tested as a drug for treatment of lupus.

DHEA may have other useful immune-modulating properties. In some studies of immune function in older humans, DHEA has boosted national killer-cell activity and has dampened immune-damaging interleukin-6 activity. It has also increased levels of circulating insulin-like growth factor-1 and, when given concomitantly with influenza vaccine, it has boosted antibody titers in an elderly subgroup with particularly low levels of DHEA to begin with. It did not have similar effects when combined with tetanus vaccine. More study is needed to see whether DHEA might be an effective vaccine adjuvant.

DHEA's use in adrenal insufficiency was tested recently in a double-blind study of 24 women with this disorder who were randomized to receive either placebo or 50 milligrams of oral DHEA daily for four months. These subjects were all DHEA-deficient at baseline. Treatment with DHEA normalized serum concentrations of DHEA, androstenedione and testosterone. Researchers noted a significant correlation between DHEA supplementation and overall ''well-being.'' DHEA-treated women were said to be significantly less depressed and anxious, compared with controls. Sexual thoughts and interest were also found to significantly increase.

Some androgenic effects were observed in this study, but only one subject had to be given a reduced dose of DHEA for this reason. The researchers noted, however, that lower doses in general might be required in the longer-term studies that will be needed to confirm the findings of this preliminary study. They cautioned that DHEA should be used only with medical supervision and carefully monitored to see whether it initiates or promotes breast or prostatic cancer.

In a few aged and severely depressed subjects with diminished baseline DHEA, supplemental DHEA (30 milligrams to 90 milligrams orally each day for four weeks) produced significant improvement. This open-label study involved only six subjects, but some other equally preliminary research, largely confined to animal models, similarly suggests that supplemental DHEA, in some subgroups, might elevate mood and improve age-related declines in memory. One study, however, in which subjects took 100 milligrams of DHEA daily for six months, found no mood-elevating effects. There is no evidence at this time that DHEA is useful in Alzheimer's disease.

It has been proposed that DHEA be used (much as estrogen replacement therapy is used) in post-menopausal women to compensate for endogenous age-related and menopause-accelerated declines in DHEA. A dose of 50 milligrams daily has been suggested for this purpose, but there are no clinical trials demonstrating that this regimen would either be effective or safe long-term. It has been noted that DHEA can bring estrogen levels in postmenopausal women to levels equal to that observed in standard hormone-replacement therapy. This may prove risky inasmuch as it has been shown that taking estrogen without concomitant use of progesterone is an established risk factor for uterine cancer.

A number of positive effects have been seen in some DHEA-treated animal models but usually at doses that are considered dangerous in humans. Additionally, these studies have been short-term for the most part, and animal models are considered by many researchers to be poor predictors of human effects since these animals, unlike humans, have little endogenous DHEA and do not exhibit the kind of age-related DHEA declines that are found in humans.

In any case, there is no convincing evidence that DHEA boosts sexual performance, retards aging in general, fights cancer, heart disease, diabetes and osteoporosis, or that it burns fat and builds muscle.

Several studies have failed to find any benefit from DHEA in breast cancer. On the contrary, two studies have found an association between higher levels of DHEA and higher incidence of breast cancer.

Another study has found no correlation between bone density and DHEA levels.

A 19-year followup study of nearly 2,000 people reported only a modest decrease in cardiac risk for men and a slight, nonsignificant increase in risk for women associated with DHEA levels. Some small studies have shown that DHEA can inhibit platelet aggregation. But other studies have also shown that supplemental DHEA can lower levels of HDL-cholesterol in some women.

A report in 1988 that high-dose DHEA could favorably affect lipids and induce weight loss in young males was not confirmed in two subsequent trials. In another trial, using the same 1,600-milligram daily dosage of DHEA used in the 1988 study but this time in women, there was, again, no weight loss. The women subjects suffered androgenic effects and developed insulin resistance and adverse changes in lipoprotein.

Other serious adverse effects noted in DHEA studies include transient jaundice and adverse hepatic effects, increased risk of uterine, breast, ovarian and prostate cancers.

CONTRAINDICATIONS, PRECAUTIONS, ADVERSE REACTIONS
CONTRAINDICATIONS
DHEA supplementation is contraindicated in those with prostate, breast, uterine and ovarian cancer.

PRECAUTIONS
DHEA supplementation should be avoided by children, adolescents, pregnant women and nursing mothers.

ADVERSE REACTIONS
Various androgenic effects, including acne, deepening of the voice, hirsutism and hair loss have been reported in women using supplemental DHEA. There is a report of transient hepatitis associated with DHEA use by a woman. Decreased HDL-cholesterol levels have been reported in women using oral DHEA. This could increase risk of cardiovascular disease. Elevated IGF (insulin-like growth factor)-1 levels have been noted in both men and women taking oral DHEA. Elevated IGF-1 levels have been associated with increased risk of certain types of cancer, e.g. prostate cancer. Oral DHEA has also been observed to increase insulin resistance when taken by women.

INTERACTIONS
In some individuals taking alprazolam, or diltiazem, serum DHEA and DHEAS levels may increase. These individuals could be at higher risk of any adverse effects from supplemental DHEA. Danazol, dexamethasone, insulin and morphine may lower endogenous DHEA and DHEAS levels.

DHEA may have additive adverse effects if used along with 4-androstenedione, 4-androstenediol, 5-androstenedione, 19-4-norandrostenedione and 19-5-norandrostenediol—all available as OTC sports supplements.

DHEA could have additive adverse effects if used along with testosterone replacement therapy.

OVERDOSAGE
There are no reports of overdosage.

DOSAGE AND ADMINISTRATION
Those who use oral DHEA typically dose at 25 to 50 milligrams daily. All who use DHEA must be under medical supervision and be closely monitored for any of the possible adverse effects mentioned above.

HOW SUPPLIED
Capsules — 25 mg, 50 mg
Cream — 1%
Powder
Tablets — 25 mg

LITERATURE
Araghiniknan M, Chung S, Nelson-White T, et al. Antioxidant activity of Dioscorea and dehydroepiandrosterone (DHEA) in older humans. *Life Sciences*. 1996; 59:147-157.

Arlt W, Callies F, van Vlijmen JC, et al. Dehydroepiandrosterone replacement in women with adrenal insufficiency. *N Engl J Med*. 1999; 341:1013-1020.

Barrett-Connor E, Khaw K-T, Yen SSC. A prospective study of dehydroepiandrosterone sulfate, mortality, and cardiovascular disease. *N Eng J Med*. 1986; 315:1519-1524.

Baulieu E-E, Robel P. Dehydroepiandrosterone (DHEA) and dehydroepiandrosterone sulfate (DHEAS) as neuroactive neurosteroids (Commentary). *Proc Natl Acad Sci*. 1998; 95:4089-4091.

Berr C, Lafont S, Debuire B, et al. Relationships of dehydroepiandrosterone sulfate in the elderly with functional, psychological, and mental status, and short-term mortality: a French community-based study. *Proc Natl Acad Sci*. 1996; 93:13410-13415.

Cardounel A, Regelson W, Kalimi M. Deyhydroepiandrosterone protects hippocampal neurons against neurotixin-induced cell death: mechanism of action. *Proc Soc Exp Biol Med*. 1999; 222:145-149.

Cleary, MP. The antiobesity effect of dehydroepiandrosterone in rats. *Proc Soc Exp Biol Med*. 1991; 196:8-16.

Compagnone NA, Mellon SH. Dehydroepiandrosterone: a potential signalling molecule for neocortical organizatin during development. *Proc Natl Acad Sci*. 1998; 95:4678-4683.

Dwell T, Norton SD, Araneo BA. Method for reducing mast cell medicted allergic reactions. 1999. U.S. Patent Number 585900. Issued Jan 12, 1999.

Ebeling P, Koivisto VA. Physiological importance of dehydroepiandrosterone. *Lancet.* 1994; 343:1479-1481.

Kimonides VG, Khatibi NH, Svendsen CN, et al. Dehydrocepiandrosterone (DHEA) and DHEA-sulfate (DHEAS) protect hippocampal neurons against excitatory amino acid-induced neurotoxicity. *Proc Natl Acad Sci.* 1998; 95:185-1857.

Kroboth PD, Salek FS, Pittenger AL, et al. DHEA and DHEA-S: A review. *J Clin Pharmacol.* 1999; 39:327-348.

McIntosh M, Bao, H Lee, C. Opposing actions of dehydroepiandrosterone and cortocosterone in rats. *Proc Soc Exp Biol Med.* 1999; 221:198-206.

Morales AJ, Nolan JJ, Nelson JC, Yen SCC. Effects of replacement dose of dehydroepiandrosterone in men and women of advancing age. *J Clin Endocrinol Metab.* 1994; 78:1360-1367.

Mortola JF, Yen SSC. The effects of oral dehydroepiandcosterone on endocrine-metabolic parameters in postmenopausal women. *J Clin Endocrinol Metab.* 1990; 71:696-704.

Oelkers W. Dehydroepiandrosterone for adrenal insufficiency (editorial). *N Engl J Med.* 1999; 341:1073-1074.

Skolnick AA. Scientific verdict still out on DHEA. *J Am Med Assoc.* 1996; 276:1365-1367.

Van Vollenhaven RF, Morabito LM, Engleman EG, et al. Treatment of systemic lupus erythematosus with dehydroepiandrosterone: 50 patients treated up to 12 months. *J Rheumatol.* 1998; .25:285-289.

Dimethylglycine (DMG)

DESCRIPTION

Dimethylglycine or DMG is a non-protein amino acid found naturally in animal and plant cells. DMG is produced in cells as an intermediate in the metabolism of choline to glycine.

There has been much confusion surrounding the history of DMG as a nutritional supplement. DMG appeared as a supplement in the 1960s under the names vitamin B15, pangamic acid and calcium pangamate. Calcium pangamate was originally a mixture of calcium gluconate and DMG. Calcium pangamate was intended as a delivery form of DMG. However, several products entered the supplement marketplace called pangamic acid or calcium pangamate, and these did not contain DMG. Some of these products contained, instead of DMG, a substance called diisopropylammonium dichloroacetate. At present, DMG supplements are available that do contain dimethylglycine.

DMG-containing calcium pangamate was popular with Russian athletes and cosmonauts because it was reputed to enhance oxygenation at the cellular level, reduce fatigue and enhance physical stamina. None of those claims, however, was ever substantiated. DMG is neither a vitamin nor an essential nutrient. DMG is also known as N, N-dimethylglycine, (dimethylamino)acetic acid and N-methylsarcosine. Its chemical structure is:

$$H_3C \diagdown \atop H_3C \diagup N\!-\!CH_2\!-\!\underset{\underset{O}{\|}}{C}\!-\!OH$$

Dimethylglycine (N,N-Dimethylglycine)

DMG is a solid, water-soluble substance. DMG should not be confused with TMG (trimethylglycine or betaine). TMG is involved in the methylation of homocysteine to form methionine (see Trimethylglycine).

ACTIONS AND PHARMACOLOGY

ACTIONS

There are no known actions of supplemental DMG.

PHARMACOKINETICS

DMG is absorbed from the small intestine and from there transported by the portal circulation to the liver. DMG is metabolized in the liver to monomethylglycine or sarcosine which, in turn, is converted to glycine. Dimethylglycine dehydrogenase, a flavoprotein, is the enzyme that catalyzes the oxidative demethylation of DMG to sarcosine. The methyl group produced in this reaction returns to the one carbon pool at the level of N^{10}-hydroxymethyl-tetrahydrofolic acid. DMG itself is formed from trimethylglycine or betaine. DMG that is not metabolized in the liver is transported by the circulatory system to various tissues in the body.

INDICATIONS AND USAGE

It is too early to say whether DMG might eventually be indicated as an immune enhancer or in the management of autism. It is not indicated as an anticonvulsant, in epilepsy or for any condition characterized by seizures. Nor is it indicated as an energy booster or athletic-performance enhancer.

RESEARCH SUMMARY

Based on claims that DMG is a highly potent "oxygenator" of body/brain tissues, this supplement has been touted as a panacea for years.

Several studies show that DMG has no anticonvulsant value and is thus of no help in epilepsy or other conditions characterized by seizures. Persistent claims that DMG is useful in autism are thus far anecdotal.

Claims that DMG can boost energy and athletic performance have been refuted by human and animal studies. Tests on exercising thoroughbred horses found "no beneficial effects on cardiorespiratory function or lactate production.'' And male track athletes supplemented with DMG exhibited no significant changes in short-term maximal treadmill performance.

On the other hand, an early finding that DMG can enhance both humoral and cell-mediated immune responses has been fortified by some subsequent research. This animal research needs to be extended to humans.

Early fears that DMG might be mutagenic now appear to be unfounded.

CONTRAINDICATIONS, PRECAUTIONS, ADVERSE REACTIONS

CONTRAINDICATIONS

Those with hypersensitivity to any component of the preparation should not use DMG.

PRECAUTIONS

DMG is not advised for pregnant women or nursing mothers and should only be used in children under medical supervision.

ADVERSE REACTIONS

Those with the rare disorder of dimethylglycine dehydrogenase deficiency may complain of a fish odor when taking DMG supplements. No other significant adverse reactions have been reported with DMG.

INTERACTIONS

There are no known drug, nutritional supplement, food or herb interactions. There is no known interaction with alcohol.

OVERDOSAGE

There are no known reports of overdose with DMG.

DOSAGE AND ADMINISTRATION

Use of DMG should be restricted to items specifically labeled DMG or dimethylglycine. Items labeled pangamic acid, calcium pangamate and vitamin B15 should be avoided. DMG comes in tablets, capsules and sublingual preparations, typically at a dose of 125 milligrams. The usual dose is 125 milligrams daily with meals.

LITERATURE

Bolman WM, Richmond JA. A double-blind, placebo-controlled crossover pilot trial of low dose dimethylglycine in patients with autistic disorder. *J Autism Dev Disord.* 1999; 29:191-194.

Gascon G, Patterson B, Yearwood K, Slotnick H. N, N-dimethylglycine and epilepsy. *Epilepsia.* 1989; 30:90-93.

Graber CD, Goust JM, Glassman AD, et al. Immunomodulating properties of dimethylglycine in humans. *J Infect Dis.* 1981; 143:101-105.

Gray ME, Titlow LW. The effect of pangamic acid on maximal treadmill performance. *Med Sci Sports Exerc.* 1982; 14:424-427.

Hoorn AJ. Dimethylglycine and chemically related amines tested for mutagenicity under potential nitrosation conditions. *Mutat Res.* 1989; 222:343-350.

Moolenaar SH, Paggi-Bach J, Engelke UF, et al. Defect in dimethylglycine dehydrogenase, a new inborn error of metabolism: NMR spectroscopy study. *Clin Chem.* 1999; 45:459-464.

Reap EA, Lawson JW. Stimulation of the immune response by dimethylglycine, a nontoxic metabolite. *J Lab Clin Med.* 1990; 115:481-486.

Rose RJ, Schlierf HA. Knight PK, et al. Effects of N, N-dimethylglycine on cardiorespiratory function and lactate performance in thoroughbred horses performing incremental treadmill exercise. *Vet Rec.* 1989; 125; 268-271.

Dimethyl Sulfoxide (DMSO)

TRADE NAMES

Rimso-50 (Edwards Lifesciences)

DESCRIPTION

Dimethyl sulfoxide or DMSO is a very hygroscopic, sulfur-containing organic compound. It is a colorless liquid with a faint scent of sulfur and mixes readily with a wide range of water-insoluble and water-soluble substances, including water itself. DMSO is rapidly absorbed into the body if ingested or even if touched by the hands, very quickly producing a garlic-like taste. It occurs naturally in small amounts in vegetables, grains, fruits and animal products. DMSO is formed as a byproduct of wood pulp processing and is used as an industrial solvent.

Up until the 1970s DMSO was sold in vitamin stores and used both externally and internally, primarily for various aches and pains. DMSO is approved by the FDA for the palliative treatment of interstitial cystitis and for limited veterinary use. It is not allowed for use as a dietary supplement. A second-generation DMSO, methylsulfonylmethane or MSM (see Methylsulfonylmethane), which is a metabolite of DMSO, is marketed as a dietary supplement.

DMSO is also known as sulfinylbismethane and methyl sulfoxide. The inclusion of DMSO, which is not a nutritional supplement in this PDR, is for historical and informational purposes, and because one of its metabolites, methylsulfonylmethane or MSM, is marketed as a nutritional supplement. The claims for MSM are related to claims made for DMSO.

ACTIONS AND PHARMACOLOGY

ACTIONS

DMSO may have anti-inflammatory, antioxidant and analgesic activities. DMSO also readily penetrates cellular membranes.

MECHANISM OF ACTION

The mechanism of DMSO's actions is not well understood. DMSO has demonstrated antioxidant activity in certain biological settings. For example, the cardiovascular protective effect of DMSO in copper-deficient rats is thought to occur by an antioxidant mechanism. It is also thought that DMSO's possible anti-inflammatory activity is due to antioxidant action. The membrane-penetrating ability of DMSO may enhance diffusion of other substances through the skin. For this reason, mixtures of idoxuridine and DMSO have been used for topical treatment of herpes zoster in the United Kingdom.

PHARMACOKINETICS

DMSO is readily and rapidly absorbed following administration by all routes and distributed throughout the body. It is metabolized in part by oxidation to methylsulfonylmethane and by reduction to dimethyl sulfide. These metabolites are excreted in the urine and feces. Most of administered DMSO is excreted in the urine as such. Dimethyl sulfide is excreted through the lungs and skin, producing a characteristic sulfuric odor.

Following ingestion by Rhesus monkeys, DMSO was rapidly absorbed, reached a steady state blood level after one day and was cleared from the blood within 72 hours after ending treatment. Urinary excretion of unmetabolized DMSO and methylsulfonylmethane accounted for about 60% and 16%, respectively, of the ingested dose.

INDICATIONS

The medical use of DMSO is currently restricted by the FDA to the palliative treatment of interstitial cystitis and to certain experimental applications. It may have shown some usefulness in some forms of arthritis and connective tissue injuries, in amyloidosis, in scleroderma, in the prevention of skin ulceration induced by some antineoplastic agents, in reversing cerebral edema and intracranial hypertension and in the topical treatment of herpes zoster. It may have some anti-cancer, neuroprotective and cardioprotective effects. It has not been established that it can halt progression of degenerative joint disease.

RESEARCH SUMMARY

DMSO has been used for years to treat the symptoms of interstitial cystitis. Dermal applications often bring quick relief from pain caused by arthritis and connective tissue injury. It has not been established, however, that DMSO has any effect on the degenerative processes of arthritis. There is some preliminary evidence that DMSO diminishes destructive changes in the joints in a spontaneous arthritis animal model. This warrants followup. In another animal model, DMSO did not suppress the clinical manifestations of arthritis.

DMSO has exerted favorable effects in the treatment of amyloidosis, possibly, it has been hypothesized, by helping to move amyloid deposits out of tissue and into urine. In one case study, a girl with secondary amyloidosis, which was a complication of juvenile rheumatoid arthritis, was treated with topical DMSO. Gastrointestinal symptoms and massive proteinuria improved. There was marked improvement of decreased left ventricular function and creatinine clearance.

Topical preparations containing high concentrations of DMSO have helped resolve cutaneous manifestations of scleroderma in some.

In a multi-center, placebo-controlled study, 157 patients with acute tenopathies were randomized to treatment with 10% DMSO gel applied three times daily or gel excipient for 14 days. Treatment in all cases started within 72 hours after onset of acute symptoms. Pain and mobility were significantly improved in the DMSO group, beginning as early as three days after onset of treatment. After 14 days, 44% of DMSO subjects were pain free, compared with 9% of placebo subjects.

Skin ulcers have been prevented by a topical application of DMSO and alpha-tocopherol in patients under treatment with anti-neoplastic agents that typically induce these ulcers. In other studies, topical DMSO has alleviated some of the symptoms of herpes zoster. It has demonstrated neuroprotective effects in experimental cerebral ischemia, significantly reducing infarction volume compared with controls. It has also demonstrated some efficacy in reversing cerebral edema and intracranial hypertension. Chronic treatment with DMSO has experimentally protected against cardiovascular—but not renal—effects of copper deficiency.

Some animal studies have further suggested that DMSO might have some anti-cancer effects. A 3% concentration of DMSO added to the drinking water of a strain of mice that spontaneously develop a series of diseases, including some cancers, had significant beneficial effects. Commencing at 10 weeks of age, mice were given the DMSO, and 90% of them were still alive at 40 weeks compared with 50% of controls. Incidence of tumors was far lower in 40-week-old treated mice than in 20-week-old untreated mice. Significant tumor regression has been seen in other DMSO-treated mice. Followup research is needed.

CONTRAINDICATIONS, PRECAUTIONS, ADVERSE REACTIONS

CONTRAINDICATIONS

None known.

PRECAUTIONS

DMSO is neither a nutritional supplement nor an over-the-counter product; its use for the treatment of interstitial cystitis—performed by interstitial instillation—requires a physician with expertise in this procedure. Bladder instillation may be harmful in patients with urinary-tract malignancy. Those who receive long-term treatment with intravesical DMSO should have liver and renal function tests as well as ophthalmologic evaluation performed every six months during treatment. DMSO has been associated with lens changes in animals.

Pregnant women and nursing mothers should avoid using DMSO.

DMSO used as an industrial solvent is not medical grade.

ADVERSE REACTIONS

Adverse reactions reported in those using DMSO for treatment of interstitial cystitis include garlic-like taste, transient chemical cystitis, bladder spasm, discomfort, allergic reactions and anaphylactoid reactions. Adverse reactions for topical use include garlic-like taste, local dermatitis, nausea, vomiting, headache, burning eyes and sedation. Concomitant use of DMSO and sulindac may cause peripheral neuropathy.

INTERACTIONS

Sulindac may decrease the pharmacologic effects of DMSO. DMSO may impair sulindac's conversion to its sulfide metabolite by competitive inhibition of sulfide reductase. Peripheral neuropathy has been reported with the simultaneous use of DMSO and sulindac.

DOSAGE AND ADMINISTRATION

No recommended dose. DMSO is not a nutritional supplement. It is used as a treatment for interstitial cystitis, and treatment must be performed by a qualified physician. DMSO is metabolized to methylsulfonylmethane, which is available as a nutritional supplement. See Methylsulfonylmethane.

DMSO sold as an industrial solvent is not medical grade.

HOW SUPPLIED

Cream — 70%

Gel — 70%, 90%

Injection — 50%, 100%

Liquid — 99%, 90%, 70%

Solution — 50%

LITERATURE

Eberhardt R, Zwingers T, Hoffman R. [DMSO in patients with active gonarthrosis. A double-blind, placebo-controlled phase III study.] [Article in German.] *Fortschr Med*. 1995; 113:446-450.

Jacob SW, Herschler R. Pharmacology of DMSO. *Cryobiology*. 1986; 23:14-27.

Jacob SW, Wood DC. Dimethyl sulfoxide (DMSO) toxicology, pharmacology and clinical experience. *Am J Surg*. 1967; 114:414-426.

Kolb KH, Jaenicke G, Kramer M, Schulze PE. Absorption, distribution and elimination of labeled dimethyl sulfoxide in man and animals. *Ann NY Acad Sci*. 1967; 141:85-95.

Layman DL, Jacob SW. The absorption, metabolism and excretion of dimethyl sulfoxide by Rhesus monkeys. *Life Sci*. 1985; 37:2431-2437.

Ludwig CU, Stoll HR, Obrist R, Obrecht JP. Prevention of cytotoxic drug induced skin ulcers with dimethyl sulfoxide (DMSO) and alpha-tocopherol. *Eur J Cancer Clin Oncol*. 1987; 23:327-329.

Milner LS, de Chadaré vian J-P, Goodyer PR, et al. Amelioration of murine lupus nephritis by dimethylsulfoxide. *Clin Immun Immunopathol*. 1987; 45:259-267.

Perez-Marrero R, Emerson LE, Feltis JT. A controlled study of dimethyl sulfoxide in interstitial cystitis. *J Urol*. 1988; 140:36-39.

Shimizu S, Simon RP, Graham SH. Dimethyl sulfoxide (DMSO) treatment reduces infarction volume after permanent focal cerebral ischemia in rats. *Neurosci Lett*. 1997; 239:125-127.

Swanson BN. Medical use of dimethyl sulfoxide (DMSO). *Rev Clin Basic Pharm*. 1985; 5:1-33.

Trentham DE, Rowland D. Dimethyl sulfoxide does not suppress the clinical manifestations of collagen arthritis. *J Rheumatol*. 1983; 10:114-116.

Yokoi K, Kimura M, Itokawa Y. Cardiovascular but not renal effects of copper deficiency are inhibited by dimethyl sulfoxide. *Nutr Res*. 1990; 10:467-477.

DL-Phenylalanine

TRADE NAMES

DL-Phen-500 (Key Company), DL-PA-500 (Bio-Tech Pharmacal), Endorphenyl (Tyson Neutraceuticals).

DESCRIPTION

DL-phenylalanine refers to a racemic mixture consisting of 50% D-phenylalanine and 50% L-phenylalanine. L-phenylalanine is an essential protein amino acid. (See L-Phenylalanine.) D-phenylalanine is the enantiomer of L-phenylalanine. D-phenylalanine is a nonprotein amino acid, meaning that it does not participate in protein biosynthesis. D-phenylalanine and other D-amino acids are, however, found in proteins, in small amounts, particularly aged proteins and food proteins that have been processed. The biological functions of D-amino acids remain unclear. Some D-amino acids, such as D-phenylalanine, may have pharmacologic activity.

DL-phenylalanine is marketed as a nutritional supplement for its putative analgesic and antidepressant activities. D-phenylalanine is not available as a nutritional supplement.

ACTIONS AND PHARMACOLOGY
DL-phenylalanine has putative analgesic and antidepressant activities.

MECHANISM OF ACTION
The putative analgesic activity of DL-phenylalanine may be explained by the possible blockage by D-phenylalanine of enkephalin degradation by the enzyme carboxypeptidase A.

The mechanism of DL-phenylalanine's putative antidepressant activity may be accounted for by the precursor role of L-phenylalanine in the synthesis of the neurotransmitters norepinephrine and dopamine. Elevated brain norepinephrine and dopamine levels are thought to be associated with antidepressant effects.

PHARMACOKINETICS
See L-Phenylalanine for the pharmacokinetics of this amino acid. D-phenylalanine is absorbed from the small intestine, following ingestion, and transported to the liver via the portal circulation. A fraction of D-phenylalanine appears to be converted to L-phenylalanine. D-phenylalanine is distributed to the various tissues of the body via the systemic circulation. D-phenylalanine appears to cross the blood-brain barrier with less efficiency than L-phenylalanine. A fraction of an ingested dose of D-phenylalanine is excreted in the urine. There is much about the pharmacokinetics in humans that is unknown.

INDICATIONS AND USAGE
There is very preliminary evidence that DL-phenylalanine might be helpful in some with depression. It may also have some analgesic properties. It has not shown benefit in the treatment of attention deficit disorder.

RESEARCH SUMMARY
In a small open trial, depressed subjects were treated with 75 to 200 mg of DL-phenylalanine daily for 20 days. Significant benefit was reported. The same researchers subsequently conducted a double-blind study in which depressed patients were given either 150 to 200 mg of DL-phenylalanine or 150 to 200 mg of imipramine daily for 30 days. There was no significant difference in the antidepressant activity of the two substances. Both of these studies are dated. There are a few studies showing that D-phenylalanine, not available as a supplement, has some analgesic effects. Thus, DL-phenylala-

nine, an equal mixture of D-phenylalanine and L-phenylalanine, may have some of the same activity, although this has not been persuasively demonstrated to date.

CONTRAINDICATIONS, PRECAUTIONS, ADVERSE REACTIONS
CONTRAINDICATIONS
DL-phenylalanine is contraindicated in those with phenylketonuria. It is also contraindicated in those taking non-selective monoamine oxidase (MAO) inhibitors. DL-phenylalanine is contraindicated in those hypersensitive to any component of a DL-phenylalanine-containing supplement.

PRECAUTIONS
Pregnant women and nursing mothers should avoid supplementation with DL-phenylalanine.

Tardive dyskinesia has been reported to be exacerbated after ingestion of L-phenylalanine by schizophrenics. Therefore, those with schizophrenia should exercise extreme caution in the use of DL-phenylalanine.

Those with hypertension should exercise caution in the use of DL-phenylalanine.

ADVERSE REACTIONS
L-phenylalanine will exacerbate symptoms of phenylketonuria if used by phenylketonurics. L-phenylalanine was reported to exacerbate tardive dyskinesia when used by some with schizophrenia.

INTERACTIONS
DRUGS
Non-selective monoamine oxidase (MAO) inhibitors: including phenelzine sulfate, tranylcypromine sulfate and pargyline HCl — Concomitant use of L-phenylalanine and non-selective MAO inhibitors may cause hypertension.

Selegiline: L-phenylalanine and the selective MAO inhibitor selegiline may have synergistic antidepressant activity if used concomitantly.

Neuroleptic drugs: L-phenylalanine may potentiate the tardive dyskinesia side effects of neuroleptic drugs if used concomitantly.

OVERDOSAGE
No reports of overdosage.

DOSAGE AND ADMINISTRATION
Those who use DL-phenylalanine supplements typically use 375 mg to 2.25 grams daily.

HOW SUPPLIED
Capsules — 200 mg, 500 mg, 600 mg
Powder
Tablets — 500 mg

LITERATURE

Beckman H, Athen D, Olteanu M, Zimmer R. DL-phenylalanine versus imipramine: a double-blind controlled study. *Arch Psychiatr Nervenkr.* 1979; 227:49-58.

Beckman H, Ludolph E. [DL-phenylalanine as an antidepressant. Open study.] [Article in German.] *Arzneimittelforschung.* 1978; 28:1283-1284.

Beckman H, Strauss MA, Ludolph E. DL-phenylalanine in depressed patients: an open study. *J Neural Transm.* 1977; 41:123-134.

Dove B, Morgenstern E, Gores E. [Analgesic effect, tolerance development and dependence potential of D-phenylalanine.] [Article in German.] *Pharmazie.* 1985; 40:648-650.

Ehrenpreis S. Pharmacology of enkephalinase inhibitors: animal and human studies. *Acupunct Electrother Res.* 1985; 10:203-208.

Halpern LM, Dong WK. D-phenylalanine: a putative enkephalinase inhibitor studied in a primate acute pain model. *Pain.* 1986; 24:223-237.

Lehmann WD, Theobald N, Fischer R, Heinrich HC. Stereospecificity of phenylalanine plasma kinetics and hydroxylation in man following oral application of a stable isotope-labeled pseudo-racemic mixture of L- and D-phenylalanine. *Clin Chim Acta.* 1983; 128:181-198.

Walsh NE, Ramamurthy S, Schoenfeld L, Hoffman J. Analgesic effectiveness of D-phenylalanine in chronic pain patients. *Arch Phys Med Rehabil.* 1986; 67:436-439.

Wood DR, Reimherr FW, Wender PH. Treatment of attention deficit disorder with DL-phenylalanine. *Psychiatry Res.* 1985; 16:21-26.

Docahexaenoic Acid (DHA)

DESCRIPTION

Docahexaenoic acid, or DHA, is a major component of fish oil. It is a long-chain polyunsaturated fatty acid (LCPUFA) of the n-3 or omega-3 type. DHA is an all cis polyunsaturated fatty acid containing 22 carbon atoms and 6 double bonds. It has the following structural formula:

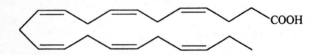

DHA (cis-4,7,10,13,16,19-Docosahexaenoic Acid)

DHA is also known as DHA; C22: 6n-3 and cis-4, 7, 10, 13, 16, 19-docosahexaenoic acid. DHA is a vital component of the phospholipids of human cellular membranes, especially those in the brain and retina. It is necessary for optimal neural development and visual acuity. DHA is the most abundant omega-3 fatty acid in human breast milk. DHA occurs naturally in the form of triacylglycerols (TAGs).

ACTIONS AND PHARMACOLOGY

ACTIONS

Supplemental DHA may lower triglyceride levels and in some, may elevate HDL-cholesterol levels. DHA is vital for normal brain development for the fetus and infant and for the maintenance of normal brain function throughout life. Supplemental DHA may have anti-inflammatory and immune-modulating activities.

MECHANISM OF ACTION

DHA's triglyceride-lowering property results from the combined effects of inhibition of lipogenesis and stimulation of fatty acid oxidation. Fatty acid oxidation of eicosapentaenoic (EPA) acid occurs mainly in the mitochondria, while DHA undergoes fatty acid oxidation in the peroxisomes.

DHA is taken up by the brain in preference to other fatty acids and is incorporated into the phospholipids of the cell membranes of brain cells and the retina. DHA-containing phospholipids in the cell membranes of the neurons appear to be necessary for neurite elongation and formation of synapses. DHA-containing phospholipids in these cells are believed to be vital for cell signaling. DHA is the prominent structural fatty acid in the gray matter of the brain and retinal tissues of humans, as well as other animals.

PHARMACOKINETICS

DHA-laden TAGs, following ingestion, undergo hydrolysis via lipases to form monoglycerides (MG) and free fatty acids (FFA). Once formed, the MG and the FFA are absorbed by the enterocytes. In the enterocytes, reacylation takes place reforming TAGs, which are then assembled with phospholipids, cholesterol and apoproteins into chylomicrons. The chylomicrons are released into the lymphatics and from there transported to the systemic circulation. In the circulation, the chylomicrons are degraded by lipoprotein lipase, and the fatty acids, including DHA, are taken up in part by the endothelial tissues. DHA is transported via the circulation to various tissues in the body, where it is used for the synthesis of phospholipids. These phospholipids are incorporated into the cell membranes of red blood cells, platelet cells and cells of the brain and retina. DHA is taken up by the brain in preference to other fatty acids. During fetal development, DHA is preferentially transported across the placenta into the fetal circulation. About 10% of DHA is retroconverted to eicosapentaenoic acid (EPA).

INDICATIONS AND USAGE

DHA is indicated to lower triglycerides in some hypertriglyceridemic individuals. It may also be indicated for pregnant women and nursing mothers, for those with peroxisomal disorders (such as Zellweger's syndrome), for cystic fibrosis sufferers, for those with attention deficit disorder, dyslexia and, possibly, those with cognitive impairment and dementia (including Alzheimer's disease).

RESEARCH SUMMARY

A double-blind placebo-controlled study was performed to determine the triglyceride-lowering effect of DHA compared with EPA. In this seven-week study, 234 healthy men were randomly given: DHA in the ethyl ester form at a dose of 3.6 grams daily, the ethyl ester of EPA at 3.18 grams daily or corn oil at 4 grams daily. Triglycerides decreased by 26% in the DHA group and 21% in the EPA group compared with placebo. Some retroconversion of DHA to EPA was noted, but no significant conversion of EPA to DHA was observed. A slight, but significant, increase in HDL-cholesterol was seen in the DHA group.

In another study on the effect of DHA on serum triglycerides, 27 hypertriglyceridemic subjects were randomized to receive either 1.25 grams of DHA daily, 2.5 grams of DHA daily or a vegetable oil placebo. The DHA was in the natural form derived from triglycerol microalgae, and the study lasted six weeks. Serum triglycerides decreased 17 to 21% and were of similar magnitude in both DHA groups. HDL-cholesterol increased by 6% and again were of similar magnitude in both DHA groups. LDL-cholesterol increased by 9.3% in the 1.25 gram DHA group. This was not significant. An increase of LDL-cholesterol of 13.6% was noted in the 2.5-gram DHA group, which was statistically significant.

DHA is essential for the growth and functional development of the fetal and infant brain and visual system. Human breast milk contains DHA but, unless supplemented with DHA, infant formulas in the U.S. do not contain any significant amounts. (The DHA level in the breast milk of the average American woman is among the lowest in he world.) In Europe and Japan, by contrast, infant formulas are routinely supplemented with DHA.

Whether to supplement these formulas in the U.S. continues to be a matter of considerable controversy. A recent double-blind, randomized, controlled efficacy and safety trial of infant formulas with and without DHA failed to resolve the controversy. No beneficial effects were noted, but more long-term studies are needed to settle the issue. No adverse safety outcomes, measured by growth, infection, atopy and gastrointestinal tolerance, were noted.

The data for supplementation of DHA in infant-formula milk for pre-term infants are more compelling. One study compared pre-term infants on formula without supplemental DHA with infants getting breast milk. The breast-fed infants had an IQ 8.3 points higher at 7½ to 8 years of age.

Another study comparing pre-term infants receiving formula supplemented with DHA with those receiving formula unsupplemented with DHA demonstrated a significantly higher Bayley Mental Development Index at 12 months in the infants receiving the DHA-supplemented formula. Large scale retrospective studies have shown that pre-term breast-fed infants have an average 5- to 12-point higher IQ later in life than babies fed formula milk without supplemental DHA. The difference in term infants is 2 to 5 IQ points.

Preliminary research suggests that some other therapeutic roles might emerge for DHA. There is some indication that, in both humans suffering from cystic fibrosis and in the cystic fibrosis mouse model, in cell membranes of the lung, pancreas and intestine (the organs most affected by this disease) there are abnormally elevated levels of arachidonic acid and abnormally diminished levels of DHA. In a pilot animal study, daily supplementation of the mouse diet with DHA corrected the lipid imbalance and reversed the progression of the disease after one week. These results have prompted a human clinical trial, the results of which are not yet available.

DHA is similarly deficient, this time in the brain, as well as in the blood and all body tissues, in those suffering from congenital peroxisomal disorders. This includes those with Zellweger cerebro-hepato-renal syndrome, neonatal adreno-leukodystrophy (made famous by the film Lorenzo's Oil) and infantile Refsum disease, characterized by severe psychomotor retardation, retinopathy, liver disease and early death.

In one very encouraging early study of Zellweger Syndrome patients, the ethyl ester of DHA in daily doses of 100 to 500 milligrams was given to 13 patients. Blood DHA levels became normal within a few weeks, liver enzymes returned nearly to normal, and most of the patients showed improvement in vision, liver function, muscle tone and social skill. Normalization of brain myelin was confirmed by MRI in three patients.

DHA deficiencies have been established in the plasma phospholipids of those with attention deficit disorder, and it has been suggested that such deficiencies may be a risk factor in those with Alzheimer's disease. Nutritional intervention trials are indicated.

A small study suggests that DHA might prove beneficial in the treament of dyslexia. Dark adaptation was found to be impaired in 10 dyslexic subjects—compared with a non-dyslexic control group. A fish oil high in DHA improved dark adaptation in five subjects after one month of supplementation.

CONTRAINDICATIONS, PRECAUTIONS, ADVERSE REACTIONS

CONTRAINDICATIONS

At present, DHA is contraindicated for hemophiliacs and those taking warfarin, since fish oils themselves are known to increase bleeding time and have anticoagulant properties.

PRECAUTIONS

Infants, pregnant women or nursing mothers should use DHA only if recommended and monitored by a physician.

Because DHA may have antithrombotic activity, those taking warfarin (Coumadin) and those with hemophilia should exercise caution in its use. Similarly, DHA supplementation should be stopped before any surgery.

ADVERSE REACTIONS

There have been no reports of serious adverse events in those taking DHA supplements. Those side effects that have been reported include mild gastrointestinal upsets such as nausea and diarrhea, eructation and "fishy" smelling breath. To date, there have been no significant reports of nosebleeds and easy bruising. One study performed in healthy adult male volunteers found no observable physiological changes in blood coagulation, platelet function or thrombotic tendencies in those consuming 6 grams daily of supplemental DHA for 90 days. Studies have not yet been done on those with hemophilia or those taking warfarin (Coumadin).

INTERACTIONS

No interactions between DHA and aspirin, other NSAIDs or herbs, such as *Allium sativum* (garlic) and *Ginkgo biloba* (ginkgo), have been reported. Such interactions, if they were to occur, might be manifested by nosebleeds and increased susceptibility to bruising.

OVERDOSAGE

None reported.

DOSAGE AND ADMINISTRATION

There are several forms of DHA supplements. These include DHA as the triacylglycerol ester derived from fish or from phytoplankton and DHA as the ethyl ester. Infant formulas containing DHA are available in Europe and Japan, but not yet approved in the U.S. Functional foods high in DHA, such as eggs, are now available.

Recommended DHA products should contain antioxidants, such as tocopherol, to protect against their oxidation.

Usual doses consumed by pregnant and nursing women are 100 to 200 milligrams daily. Doses of DHA for hypertriglyceridemics range from 1 to 4 grams. The dose needs to be determined by optimization of triglyceride levels. In those with elevated triglycerides and elevated cholesterol, doses of 1 to 2 grams daily may lower triglyceride levels and increase HDL-cholesterol levels in some. DHA is best tolerated with meals.

LITERATURE

Davidson MH, Maki KC, Kalkowski J, et al. Effects of docosahexaenoic acid on the serum lipoproteins with combined hyperlipidemia: a randomized, double-blind, placebo-controlled trial. *J Am Coll Nutr.* 1997; 16:236-243.

Eriksson PS, Perfilieva E, Bjork-Eriksson T, et al. Neurogenesis in the adult human hippocampus. *Nat Med.* 1998; 4:1313-1317.

Freedman SD, Katz MH, Parker EM, et al. A membrane lipid imbalance plays a role in the phenotypic expression of cystic fibrosis in aftr -/-mice. *Proc Natl Acad Sci USA.* 1999; 96:13995-14000.

Grimsgaard S, Bonaa KH, Hansen J-B, Nordoy A. Highly purified eicosapentaenoic acid and docosahexaenoic acid in humans have similar triacylglycerol- lowering effects but divergent effects on serum fatty acids. *Am J Clin Nutr.* 1997; 66:649-959.

Horrocks LA, Yeo YK. Health benefits of docosahexaenoic acid. *Pharma Res.* 1999; 40:211-225.

Lucas A, Stafford M, Morley R, et al. Efficacy and safety of long-chain polyunsaturated fatty acid supplementation of infant-formula milk: a randomized trial. *Lancet.* 1999; 354:1948-1954

Madsen L, Rustan AC, Vaagenes H, et al. Eicosapentaenoic and docosahexaenoic acid affect mitochondrial and peroxisomal fatty acid oxidation in relation to substrate preference. *Lipids.* 1999; 34:951-963..

Martinez M, Vazquez E, Garcia-Silva MT, et al. Therapeutic effects of docosahexaenoic acid ethyl ester in patients with generalized peroxisomal disorders. *Am J Clin Nutr.* 2000; 71:376S-385S.

Nelson GJ, Schmidt PS, Bartolini GL, et al. The effect of dietary docosahexaenoic acid on platelet function, platelet fatty acid composition, and blood coagulation in humans. *Lipids.* 1997; 32:1129-1136.

Soderberg M, Edlund C, Kristennson K, et al. Fatty acid composition of brain phospholipids in aging and Alzheimer's disease. *Lipids.* 1991; 26:421-415.

Stordy BJ. Dark adaptation, motor skills, docosahexaenoic acid, and dyslexia. *Am J Clin Nutr.* 2000; 71:323S-326S.

Dolomite

DESCRIPTION

Dolomite, named for the French geologist D.G. Dolomieu, is a mineral containing calcium and magnesium carbonate, as well as trace heavy metals. It is a double salt made up of approximately 60% calcium carbonate (equivalent to 24% calcium) and 40% magnesium carbonate (equivalent to 12% magnesium). Dolomite is also known as magnesium limestone and earlier was called compound-spar, bitter-spar, rhomb-spar and pearl-spar. The Dolomites, a mountain region in the South Tyrolese Alps, are named for the presence of dolomite in the mountains.

Dolomite was at one time a popular nutritional supplement for calcium and magnesium. It is still marketed as a nutritional supplement, but is no longer popular. The reason for this is that in the early 1980s analysis of dolomite nutritional supplements revealed them to contain substantial amounts of lead, as well as other toxic elements, such as mercury, arsenic and cadmium. In addition, much better supplementary forms of calcium and magnesium are available. Dolomite is still used in several parts of the world as a liming agent, to raise the pH of the soil, and as a fertilizer to maintain soil magnesium levels. It is also used to make magnesia, which has medical applications.

ACTIONS AND PHARMACOLOGY

ACTIONS

Dolomite is a delivery form of calcium and magnesium.

MECHANISM OF ACTION

See Calcium and Magnesium.

PHARMACOKINETICS

See Calcium and Magnesium. Noteworthy is that magnesium from magnesium carbonate is more poorly absorbed than it is from most other magnesium supplements.

INDICATIONS

Dolomite is no longer recommended as a calcium or magnesium source because it may be contaminated with toxic metals such as lead.

RESEARCH SUMMARY

Several studies have revealed significant toxic metal contamination of many randomly selected and analyzed dolomite supplements (the same is true of some other ''natural'' calcium sources, e.g., bonemeal and ''oyster shell'' or ''natural source'' calcium carbonate). In one study of randomly selected dolomite tablets, aluminum, arsenic, zinc, cadmium and lead were among the metals found. The researchers cautioned that ''these trace metals could pose health risks to the public such as lead poisoning, dementia and hypertension due to cadmium. Also, zinc can potentiate cadmium-hypertensive effects.''

Another researcher has pointed out that ''physicians must consider the possibility of unrecognized self-poisoning from the consumption of such substances, especially in the context of unexplained neurologic, gastrointestinal, cutaneous and hematologic disorders.''

CONTRAINDICATIONS, PRECAUTIONS, ADVERSE REACTIONS

CONTRAINDICATIONS

Those with hypercalcemia should not take calcium supplements. Conditions that cause hypercalcemia include hyper-

parathyroidism, hypervitaminosis D, some granulomatous diseases, sarcoidosis and cancer.

Those with renal failure and high-grade atrioventricular blocks should not take magnesium supplements.

PRECAUTIONS

Dolomite is no longer recommended as a calcium and magnesium supplement because of possible presence of toxic metals, such as lead, Children are especially sensitive to the effects of lead. Children, pregnant women and nursing mothers should absolutely avoid dolomite.

INTERACTIONS

See Calcium and Magnesium for adverse reactions of supplements containing these minerals. Prolonged use of dolomite containing toxic elements, such as lead, may cause the typical toxic effects of those substances.

OVERDOSAGE

There are no known reports of overdosage of dolomite.

DOSAGE AND ADMINISTRATION

No recommended dose.

HOW SUPPLIED

Powder

Tablets — 500 mg

LITERATURE

Boulos FM, von Smolinski A. Alert to users of calcium supplements as antihypertensive agents due to trace mineral contaminants. *Am J Hypterten.* 1988; 1(3 Pt 3):137S-142S.

Bourquin BP, Evans DR, Cornett JR, et al. Lead content of 70 brands of dietary calcium supplements. *Am J Public Health.* 1993; 83:1155-1160.

Roberts HJ. Potential toxicity due to dolomite and bone meal. *South Med J.* 1983; 76:556-559.

Whiting SJ. Safety of some calcium supplements questioned. *Nutr Rev.* 1884; 52:95-97.

D-Ribose

TRADE NAMES

Ribose Power (Champion Nutrition), Ribomax Ribose (Natural Balance), Ribose Fuel (Twinlab), Rx-Energy Ribose (Nutritional Dynamics) and Mega Ribose Fuel (Twinlab).

DESCRIPTION

D-ribose is a naturally occurring five-carbon sugar found in all living cells, as well as in RNA-containing viruses. It is not an essential nutrient, since it can be made in the body from other substances, such as glucose. D-ribose, however, is very essential for life. Some of the most important biological molecules contain D-ribose, including ATP (adenosine triphosphate), all the nucleotides and nucleotide coenzymes and all forms of RNA (ribonucleic acid). D-ribose, in the form of ribonucleoside diphosphates, is converted to deoxyribonucleoside diphosphates, precursor molecules for DNA. D-ribose in RNA and D-deoxyribose in DNA may be considered genetic sugars.

Since D-ribose is ubiquitous in living matter, it is ingested in our diets. Such nutritional substances as brewers yeast are rich in RNA and are thus rich sources of D-ribose. Some recent research suggests that supraphysiological amounts of this sugar may have cardioprotective effects, particularly for the ischemic heart.

D-ribose is a sweet, solid, water-soluble substance that is also known as alpha-D-ribofuranoside. L-ribose does not have biological activity. D-ribose is sometimes referred to as just ribose. Supplemental D-ribose is produced from the fermentation of corn syrup. D-ribose has the following structural formula:

D-ribose

ACTIONS AND PHARMACOLOGY

ACTIONS

Supplemental D-ribose may have metabolic cardioprotective activity. It may also enhance *de novo* purine biosynthesis.

MECHANISM OF ACTION

Following a cardiac ischemic event, ATP levels in the heart decline rapidly and are slow to rebound. 5-Phosphoribosyl 1-pyrophosphate (PRPP) is a key intermediate in the *de novo* and salvage pathways of purine nucleotide formation, as well as a key intermediate in synthesis of pyrimidine nucleotides. PRPP is the biochemically activated form of D-ribose and is synthesized from D-ribose-5-phosphate, which is produced in the oxidative pentose phosphate pathway (PPP). The limiting step in the PPP is the glucose-6-phosphate dehydrogenase (G-6-PD) reaction. The G-6-PD reaction can be bypassed with D-ribose. In supraphysiological amounts, D-ribose may serve as a precursor to PRPP, which then allows for *de novo* synthesis of purine nucleotides, including ATP. D-ribose infusion has been shown to significantly enhance the recovery of energy levels in the post-ischemic myocardium in animal models.

PHARMACOKINETICS

About 88% to 100% of an oral dose of D-ribose, up to 200 milligrams per kilogram per hour, is absorbed from the small intestine, from whence it is distributed to various tissues of the body, including cardiac muscle and skeletal muscle. Very little first-pass metabolism occurs in the liver. Following transport into cells, D-ribose is phosphorylated to D-ribose-5-phosphate. D-ribose-5-phosphate is metabolized via a number of pathways, including the pentose phosphate pathway and glycolytic pathway. Its metabolism is complex. It is also metabolized to PRPP, which is the precursor to purine nucleotides, as well as L-histidine and pyrimidine nucleotides. Those receiving very high doses of D-ribose excrete a small fraction of the administered dose unchanged in the urine.

INDICATIONS AND USAGE

D-ribose may have some protective effects in cardiac ischemia. Claims that it is an effective "energizer" and exercise-performance enhancer are not substantiated by credible evidence. D-ribose may also be beneficial in some rare genetic diseases, such as adenylosuccinase deficiency and myoadenylade deaminase deficiency.

RESEARCH SUMMARY

In a study of 20 men (aged 45 to 69 years) with documented severe coronary artery disease and a history of angina induced by normal daily activities, 60 grams of ribose (in four doses of 15 grams each) were tested against placebo. Treated subjects exhibited improvement as measured electro-cardiographically, and time to onset of moderate angina (during exercise testing) increased significantly in those ribose-treated subjects. There was no significant electrocardiograph improvement in the placebo group, and there was no significant difference between the groups in time to onset of moderate angina. The authors concluded: "In patients with CAD, administration of ribose by mouth for three days improved the heart's tolerance to ischemia. The presumed effects on cardiac energy metabolism offer new possibilities for adjunctive medical treatment of myocardial ischemia."

Claims that supplemental ribose is an energy booster and exercise/athletic-performance enhancer are unfounded. Studies sometimes cited in support of these claims fall far short of being substantiating. It has been shown that administration of ribose in patients with myoadenylate deaminase deficiency disease can reduce cramping and stiffness caused by exercise. On the other hand, in a double-blind, placebo-controlled crossover trial of ribose in McArdle's disease, 60 grams of ribose daily for seven days failed to improve exercise tolerance in these subjects. Finally, there is one case report of a patient with adenylosuccinate deficiency whose neurological symptoms (behavior and seizure frequency) improved with supplemental D-ribose.

CONTRAINDICATIONS, PRECAUTIONS, ADVERSE REACTIONS

CONTRAINDICATIONS

None known.

PRECAUTIONS

Pregnant women and nursing mothers should avoid supplemental D-ribose.

Supplemental D-ribose may cause hypoglycemia and elevation in uric acid levels. Those with gout should avoid supplemental D-ribose, and those with elevated uric acid levels and hypoglycemics should exercise extreme caution in its use. Those with diabetes should also exercise extreme caution in its use. And those diabetics who decide to try D-ribose must be under a physician's supervision and have their blood glucose levels closely monitored and their antidiabetic medications appropriately adjusted, if necessary.

ADVERSE REACTIONS

Reported adverse reactions include hypoglycemia, hyperuricemia, hyperuricosuria, diarrhea, nausea and headache.

INTERACTIONS

Antidiabetic drugs: D-ribose may cause hypoglycemia. Diabetics who use D-ribose must have their blood glucose levels closely monitored and their antidiabetic medicines appropriately adjusted, if necessary.

OVERDOSAGE

No reports of overdosage.

DOSAGE AND ADMINISTRATION

No typical dosage. Most experimental studies with ribose used very high doses, usually about 60 grams daily.

HOW SUPPLIED

Capsules — 500 mg

Powder

Tablets — 500 mg, 1000 mg

LITERATURE

Gross M, Dormann B, Zollner N. Ribose administration during exercise: effects on substrates and products of energy metabolism in healthy subjects and a patient with myoadenylate deaminase deficiency. *Klin Wochenschr.* 1991; 69:151-155.

Priml W, von Arnim T, Stablein A, et al. Effects of ribose on exercise-induced ischaemia in stable coronary artery disease. *Lancet.* 1992; 340:507-510.

Salerno C, D'Eufermia P, Finocchiaro R, et al. Effect of D-ribose on purine synthesis and neurological symptoms in a patient with adenylsuccinase deficiency. *Biochim Biophys Acta.* 1999; 1453:135-140.

Steele IC, Patterson VH, Nicholls DP. A double-blind, placebo-controlled, crossover trial of D-ribose in McArdle's disease. *J Neurol Sci.* 1996; 136:174-177.

Tullson PC, Terjung RL. Adenine nucleotide synthesis in exercising and endurance-trained skeletal muscle. *Am J Physiol.* 1991; 261:C342-C347.

Zimmer HG. The oxidative pentose phosphate pathway in the heart: regulation, physiological significance and clinical implications. *Basic Res Cardiol.* 1992; 87:3003-316.

Zimmer HG. Regulation of and intervention into the oxidative pentose phosphate pathway and adenine nucleotide metabolism in the heart. *Mol Cell Biochem.* 1996; 160/161:101-109.

Zimmer HG. Significance of the 5-phosphoribosyl-1-pyrophosphate pool for cardiac purine and pyrimidine nucleotide synthesis: studies with ribose, adenine, inosine, and orotic acid in rats. *Cardiovasc Drugs Ther.* 1998; 12 Suppl 2:179-187.

Zollner N, Reiter S, Gross M, et al. Myoadenylate deaminase deficiency: successful symptomatic therapy by high dose oral administration of ribose. *Klin Wochenschr.* 1986; 64:1281-1290.

Eicosapentaenoic (EPA)

DESCRIPTION

Eicosapentaenoic acid, or EPA, is a major component of fish oil. It is a long-chain polyunsaturated fatty acid of the n-3 or omega-3 type. EPA is an all cis polyunsaturated fatty acid containing 20 carbons and 5 double bonds. EPA is also known as EPA; C20: 5n-3 and cis-5, 8, 11, 14,17-eicosapentaenoic acid. The structural formula is as follows:

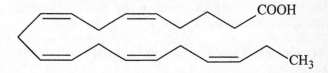

EPA (5,8,11,14,17-Eicosapentaenoic Acid)

EPA is a precursor of the series-3 prostaglandins, the series-5 leukotrienes and the series-3 thromboxanes, which are anti-artherogenic and antithrombogenic. EPA is found naturally in the form of triacylglycerols (TAGs).

ACTIONS AND PHARMACOLOGY

ACTIONS

Supplemental EPA may have anti-inflammatory, antithrombotic and immunomodulatory activities. It may also have triglyceride-lowering activity.

MECHANISM OF ACTION

The possible anti-inflammatory, antithrombotic and immunomodulatory actions of supplemental EPA are probably due mostly to EPA's role in eicosanoid physiology and biochemistry.

Eicosanoids are produced by the metabolism of the n-3 or omega-3 polyunsaturated fatty acids, and in particular the 20 carbon n-3 polyunsaturated fatty acid, arachidonic acid. These eicosanoids are of the leukotriene 4 series and thromboxane 2 series. Leukotriene B_4 (LTB$_4$) and thromboxane A$_2$ (TXA$_2$) stimulate leukocyte chemotaxis, platelet aggregation and vasoconstriction. These eicosanoids are thrombogenic and artherogenic.

On the other hand, EPA is metabolized to leukotriene B$_5$ (LTB$_5$) and thromboxane A$_3$ (TXA$_3$), eicosanoids that promote vasodilation, inhibit platelet aggregation and leukocyte chemotaxis and are anti-artherogenic and anti-thrombotic.

The triglyceride-lowering effect of EPA results from inhibition of lipogenesis and stimulation of fatty acid oxidation. Fatty acid oxidation of EPA occurs mainly in the mitochondria.

(For further discussion on the action of EPA, see the Fish Oil monograph.)

PHARMACOKINETICS
See the Fish Oil monograph.

INDICATIONS AND USAGE
EPA may be indicated for lowering elevated triglycerides in those who are hyperglyceridemic. EPA may play some therapeutic role in those with cystic fibrosis to reduce disease severity and may similarly play a role in type 2 diabetics in retarding the progression of diabetic nephropathy. However, the latter two indications require clinical trials and documentation to establish this.

See the monograph on Fish Oils for further information.

RESEARCH SUMMARY
A double-blind, placebo-controlled study was performed to determine the triglyceride-lowering effect of EPA and DHA by themselves. In the seven-week study, 234 healthy men were randomly given the following: EPA in the ethyl ester at a dose of 3.8 grams daily, the ethyl ester of DHA at 3.6 grams daily or corn oil at 4 grams daily as a placebo. Triglycerides decreased by 21% in the EPA group and by 26% in the DHA group when compared with placebo. Some retroconversion of DHA to EPA was found, but no significant conversion of EPA to DHA was observed. A small, but significant increase in HDL-cholesterol was seen in the DHA group, and a small, but significant, decrease of total cholesterol and apolipoprotein A1 (Apo A1) was noted in the EPA group.

A randomized, double-blind, placebo-controlled crossover trial comparing fish oil supplementation against placebo was performed to determine fish oil effects on markers of clinical state, neutrophil function and lung inflammation in 16 patients with cystic fibrosis who were colonized with *Pseudomonas aeruginosa*. The fish oil used in this trial contained 2.7 grams of EPA (the amount of DHA in the capsules was not mentioned), which the subjects received daily for a six-week period. The placebo group received olive oil. The fish oil-supplemented group showed a significant reduction in disease severity and sputum volume and in the pathogenesis of lung damage.

The study also showed that EPA-rich fish oil dampens the damaging effects of the circulating neutrophils in the chronic inflammatory process. There is a reduction of leukotriene B4, which is believed to play an important role in the pathogenesis of lung damage in cystic fibrosis.

The effect of EPA on the progression of diabetic nephropathy has been studied in rats and humans. Measurement of urinary albumin is a key marker in determining renal function in diabetics. In a six-month study with Wister rats made diabetic by administration of streptozotocin, the ethyl ester of EPA was given to 16 rats, while an equal number served as the control. The mean microalbuminuria of the EPA group was significantly lower than that of the control group after four months, and this significant difference persisted for the remaining two months of the trial.

In a human study with type 2 diabetics, administration of 900 milligrams daily of the ethyl ester of EPA resulted in a significant decrease in urinary albumin excretion at three months after start of treatment; this reduction was sustained for a year after the start of treatment. These studies suggest that EPA supplementation of diabetics with albuminuria might retard the progression of diabetic nephropathy.

See the monograph on Fish Oil for further discussion.

CONTRAINDICATIONS, PRECAUTIONS, ADVERSE REACTIONS.
CONTRAINDICATIONS
None known.

PRECAUTIONS
Because of possible antithrombotic activity of EPA, it should be used with caution in those who take warfarin (Coumadin) and by those with hemophilia. Similarly, EPA should be stopped before surgical procedures.

EPA supplements should be used by children, pregnant women and nursing mothers only if recommended and monitored by a physician.

ADVERSE REACTIONS
There have been no reports of serious adverse events in those taking EPA supplements, even up to 15 grams daily, for prolonged periods of time. Those side effects that have been reported include mild gastrointestinal upsets such as nausea and diarrhea, halitosis, eructation, "fishy" smelling breath, skin and even urine. The blood-thinning effects can cause occasional nosebleeds and easy bruising.

INTERACTIONS

Interactions may occur between EPA supplements and aspirin and other non-steroidal anti-inflammatory drugs and herbs such as garlic (*Allium sativum*) and ginkgo (*Ginkgo biloba*). Such interactions might be manifested by increased susceptibility to bruising, nosebleeds, hemoptysis, hematemesis, hematuria and blood in the stool. Most who take EPA supplements and the above drugs or herbs do not suffer from these problems and if they occur, they are rare. If they do occur, the EPA dose should be lowered or discontinued.

Conflicting results have been reported regarding the effects of EPA supplements on glycemic control in non-diabetics with glucose intolerance, and those with type 2 diabetes. Some early studies indicated that EPA supplements might have detrimental effects in those groups. Recent, better designed studies have not reported these adverse effects. There is no evidence that EPA supplements have detrimental effects on glucose tolerance, insulin secretion or insulin resistance in non-diabetic subjects. Diabetics should discuss the use of these supplements with their physicians and note if the supplements affect their glycemic control. Diabetics who take EPA supplements should be monitored by their physicians.

OVERDOSAGE

None known.

DOSAGE AND ADMINISTRATION

EPA is typically available in fish oil in combination with DHA. The usual ratio of EPA to DHA in these preparations is about 1.5. Fish oil preparations are available with higher ratios up to about 3. There is an ethyl ester form of EPA.

See Fish Oil monograph for further discussion.

LITERATURE

Fujikawa M, Yamazaki K, Hamazaki T, et al. Effect of eicosapentaenoic acid ethyl ester on albuminuria in streptozotocin-induced diabetic rats. *J Nutr Sci Vitaminol.* 1994; 40: 49-61.

Grimsgaard S, Bønaa KH, Hansen JB, Nordøy A. Highly purified eicosapentaenoic acid and docosahexaenoic acid in humans have similar triacylglycerol-lowering effects but divergent effects on serum fatty acids. *Am J Clin Nutr.* 1997; 66:649-659.

Lawrence R, Sorrell T. Eicosapentaenoic acid in cystic fibrosis: evidence of a pathogenic role for leukotriene B₄. *Lancet.*1993; 342:465-469.

Madsen L, Rustan QC, Vaagenes H, et al. Eicosapentaenoic and docosahexaenoic acid affect mitochondrial and peroxisomal fatty acid oxidation in relation to substrate preference. *Lipids.* 1999; 34:951-963.

Shimizu H, Ohtani K, Tanaka Y, et al. Long-term effect of eicosapentaenoic acid ethyl (EPA-E) on albuminuria of non-insulin dependent diabetic patients. *Diabetes Res Clin Pract.* 1995; 28:35-40.

Terano T, Hira A, Hamazaki T, et al. Effect of oral administration of highly purified eicosapentaenoic acid on platelet function, blood viscosity and red blood cell deformability in healthy human subjects. *Atheroscler.* 1983; 46: 321-331.

See Fish Oil monograph for further literature.

Evening Primrose Oil

TRADE NAMES

Primosa (Solaray), Golden Primrose (Carlson Laboratories), Mega Primrose Oil (Twinlab), Ultra EPO (Nature's Plus), Veg Evening Primrose Oil (Health From the Sun), My Favorite Evening Primrose Oil (Natrol), Royal Brittany Evening Primrose Oil (American Health).

DESCRIPTION

Evening primrose oil (EPO) is derived from the seeds of the evening primrose plant also known as *Oenthera biennis*. The evening primrose is native to North America, where it is regarded as a weed. This biennial plant is thought to be a complex of several closely related species belonging to the *Onagraceae* family.

EPO is a rich source of the long-chain fatty acid gamma-linolenic acid (GLA). The health benefits of EPO are attributed to GLA. GLA is an unusual constituent of living matter and is found in very few plants. These include, in addition to evening primrose, black currant, borage and hemp. GLA content in EPO ranges from approximately 7 to 14%. Typical EPO supplements contain about 9% GLA.

GLA is an all cis n-6 long-chain polyunsaturated fatty acid. It is comprised of 18 carbon atoms and three double bonds. GLA is also known as GLA; 18: 3n-6 and gamolenic acid, and chemically it is known as 6, 9, 12-octadecatrienoic acid; (Z, Z, Z)-6, 9, 12-octadecatrienoic acid, and cis-6, cis-9, cis-12-octadecatrienoic acid. GLA is present in EPO in the form of triglycerides. One such triglyceride in EPO contains two linoleic acid residues and one of GLA. This triglyceride, called di-linoleoyl-mono-gamma-linenyl-glycerol (DLMG), makes up about 18 to 19% of the triglycerides in EPO. GLA is concentrated in the sn-3 position in the triglycerides. GLA is represented by the following chemical structure:

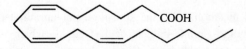

GLA (gamma-linolenic acid)

EPO is approved in the United Kingdom as a pharmaceutical treatment for atopic dermatitis and mastalgia.

ACTIONS AND PHARMACOLOGY
ACTIONS
EPO may have anti-inflammatory and antithrombotic activities.

MECHANISM OF ACTION
The possible anti-inflammatory and anti-aggregatory actions of EPO may be accounted for by examining the role of GLA in eicosanoid biochemistry. GLA is metabolized to the 20-carbon polyunsaturated fatty acid dihomo-gamma-linolenic acid (DGLA; 20: 3n-6), which is a precursor to the 1-series prostaglandins, such as prostaglandin E_1 (PGE_1). The action of PGE_1 on inflammatory cells (e.g., polymorphonuclear leukocytes or PMNs) is mostly inhibitory. PGE_1 increases intracellular cyclic AMP (cAMP). This increase reduces the release of lysosomal enzymes, PMN chemotaxis and the margination and adherence of PMNs in the blood vessels. PGE_1 is also thought to inhibit lymphocyte function.

PGE_1, in addition to its role in suppressing the inflammatory process, inhibits platelet aggregation and has vasodilatory activity.

GLA, via its metabolite DGLA, has an inhibitory effect on leukotriene (LT) synthesis. Leukotriene B_4 (LTB_4) is an inflammatory mediator. DGLA is metabolized to 15-hydroxyl DGLA, which blocks the conversion of arachidonic acid to LTs, such as LTB_4.

In summary, GLA may suppress inflammation through its metabolism to DGLA, which, in turn, can competitively inhibit the pro-inflammatory 2-series prostaglandins and 4-series leukotrienes. The incorporation of GLA and its metabolites in cell membranes may also play a role in the possible anti-inflammatory, antithrombotic, anti-atherogenic and antiproliferative actions of EPO.

PHARMACOKINETICS
GLA-laden triglycerides in EPO are absorbed from the small intestine aided by bile salts. During this process, there is some deacylation of the fatty acids of the triglycerides. Reacylation takes place within the mucosal cells of the small intestine, and the GLA-laden triglycerides enter into the lymphatics in the form of chylomicrons. GLA-laden chylomicrons are transported from the lymphatics into the blood where GLA is carried in lipid particles to the various tissues of he body.

GLA is metabolized to the 20-carbon polyunsaturated fatty acid dihomo-gamma-linoleic acid (DGLA), which is converted to prostaglandin E_1 (PGE_1). It may also be metabolized to eicosapentaenoic acid (EPA). GLA and DGLA are normally not found as free fatty acids in cells. They occur mainly in cell membranes as components of phospholipids, neutral lipids and cholesterol esters. PGE_1 is metabolized to smaller prostaglandin remnants, which are primarily polar dicarboxylic acids, most of which are excreted in the urine.

INDICATIONS AND USAGE
EPO appears to be effective in some cases of rheumatoid arthritis and may be indicated in some other inflammatory disorders, such as Sjogren's syndrome and ulcerative colitis. Possible other indications include diabetic neuropathy, osteoporosis, acute respiratory distress syndrome (ARDS), hypertension and elevated serum lipids. EPO has been used with some preliminary success in some cancers, principally cerebral gliomas. It has not proved useful for tardive dyskinesia, premenstrual syndrome or menopausal flushing. It may be indicated in some cases for atopic dermatitis, particularly to help with itching, as well as for uremic skin conditions in hemodialysis patients. It should probably not be used in efforts to enhance immunity as it may be immunosuppressive.

RESEARCH SUMMARY
See GLA.

CONTRAINDICATIONS, PRECAUTIONS, ADVERSE REACTIONS
CONTRAINDICATIONS
None known.

PRECAUTIONS
Pregnant women and nursing mothers should avoid EPO supplements. Those with a history of partial complex seizure disorders, such as temporal lobe epilepsy, should avoid using EPO. Likewise, those with other types of seizure disorders and schizophrenics who are being treated with certain neuroleptic drugs, such as aliphatic phenothiazines (e. g., chlorpromazine), which may lower seizure threshold, should avoid using EPO. Because of possible antithrombotic activity of EPO, those with hemophilia or other hemorrhagic diatheses and those taking warfarin should exercise caution in the use of this supplement.

EPO supplementation should be halted before any surgical procedure. Because of its possible inhibition of lymphocyte function, those with immune deficiency disorders, such as AIDS, should exercise caution in the use of EPO.

ADVERSE REACTIONS
EPO may cause gastrointestinal symptoms like nausea, vomiting, flatulence, diarrhea and bloating. Headaches have also been reported in those taking EPO. It may precipitate symptoms of undiagnosed complex partial seizures and should be used, if at all, with extreme caution in those with a history of seizure disorder or those taking drugs that lower the seizure threshold, such as aliphatic phenothiazines.

INTERACTIONS

DRUGS

Use of EPO in schizophrenics who are being treated with certain neuroleptic agents which lower seizure threshold e.g., aliphatic phenothiazines, such as chlorpromazine may cause partial complex seizures (e. g., temporal lobe epilepsy), as well as other types of seizures. Interactions may occur between EPO and warfarin, aspirin and NSAIDs. Such interactions, if they were to occur, might be manifested by nosebleeds, increased susceptibility to bruising and hematuria. If these symptoms occur, EPO intake should be stopped.

NUTRITIONAL SUPPLEMENTS

Interactions may occur if EPO is used with supplements that have antithrombotic activity, such as fish oils. This may be manifested by nosebleeds and increased susceptibility to bruising.

HERBS

Interactions may occur if EPO is used with such herbs as garlic (*Allium sativa*) and ginkgo (*Ginkgo biloba*). Such interactions may be manifested by nosebleeds and easy bruising.

OVERDOSAGE

There are no reports of overdosage with EPO.

DOSAGE AND ADMINISTRATION

EPO is available in capsules and also in topical preparations for cosmetic use. A capsule of EPO typically contains about 9% GLA. Doses used for the management of rheumatoid arthritis range from about 360 milligrams to 2.8 grams daily in divided doses (expressed as GLA). For management of atopic dermatitis, doses of 320 to 480 milligrams daily are used in divided doses (expressed as GLA). Doses of up to 2 grams daily (expressed as GLA) have been used by those with hypertriglyceridemia. EPO supplements should contain an antioxidant, such as vitamin E, to protect the unsaturated fatty acids against oxidation.

HOW SUPPLIED

Capsules — 500 mg, 1200 mg, 1300 mg

Liquid

Tablets — 500 mg

LITERATURE

See GLA monograph for additional literature.

Belch JJF, Hill A. Evening primrose oil and borage oil in rheumatologic conditions. *Am J Clin Nutr.* 2000; 71(suppl):352S-355S.

Holman CP, Bell AFJ. A trial of evening primrose oil in the treatment of chronic schizophrenia. *J Orthomol Psychiatry.* 1983; 12; 302-304.

Huang Y-S, Mills DE, eds. *Gamma-linolenic Acid: Metabolism and its Roles in Nutrition.* Champaign IL: American Oil Chemists Society Press; 1996.

Newall CA, Anderson LA, Phillipson, JD. Herbal Medicines: *A Guide for Health-Care Professionals.* London: The Pharmaceutical Press; 1996, pp110-113.

Vaddahi KS. The use of gamma-linolenic acid and linoleic acid to differentiate between temporal lobe epilepsy and schizophrenia. *Prostaglandins Med.* 1981; 6:375-379.

Fish Oils

TRADE NAMES

Fish oil is available generically from numerous manufacturers. Branded products include MaxEPA, Super EPA, Omega 3 (several manufacturers), Sof-Gel E.P.A. (Tyson Neutraceuticals), Marine Lipid Concentrate (Vitaline), Formula 3/6/9 (Advanced Nutritional), Prolinic (Key Company), Sam-E.P.A. (Bio-tech Pharmacal), Sea Omega (Rugby), Twin-EPA (Twinlab), Ultra 30/20 (Health From the Sun), Norwegian Fish Oil (Spectrum Naturals).

DESCRIPTION

Fish oils, also known as marine oils, are lipids found in fish, particularly cold water fish, and other marine life such as phytoplankton. These oils are rich sources of long-chain polyunsaturated fatty acids (LCPUFA) of the n-3 (omega-3) type. The two most studied fish oils are the 20 carbon eicosapentaenoic acid (EPA; C20:5n-3) and the 22-carbon docosahexaenoic acid (DHA; C22:6n-3). EPA contains five double bonds and DHA, six double bonds. These double bonds are all in the cis configuration. DHA is a vital component of the phospholipids of human cellular membranes, especially those in the brain and retina.

Both EPA and DHA are found naturally in the form of tiacylglycerols or TAGs. The docosahexaenate in the triacylglycerols of fish oil appears to be primarily in the sn-2 position (the middle carbon) of glycerol whereas there is more random distribution of eicosapantaenoate over all three positions of glycerol.

ACTIONS AND PHARMACOLOGY

ACTIONS

Supplemental fish oils have triglyceride-lowering activity. They may also have anti-inflammatory, anti-thrombotic and immunomodulatory actions.

MECHANISM OF ACTION

EPA and DHA have several actions in a number of body systems. EPA and DHA lower elevated triglyceride levels. In the cardiovascular system, EPA and DHA have anti-arrythmic properties. EPA and DHA have anti-inflammatory and immune-modulating properties and are beneficial for the musculoskeletal, gastrointestinal and immune systems. EPA and DHA are also important for maintenance of normal blood flow as they lower fibrinogen levels and prevent platelets from sticking to each other. DHA is vital for normal brain development for the fetus and infant and for the maintenance of normal brain function throughout life. DHA appears to be a major determinant of membrane fluidity in brain cells, and this could play a major role in the maintenance of normal cognition and mood.

The triglyceride-lowering effect of EPA and DHA appears to result from the combined effects of inhibition of lipogenesis and stimulation of fatty acid oxidation in liver. EPA and DHA inhibit the transcription of genes coding for lipogenesis enzymes and increase the transcription of the regulatory enzymes of fatty acid oxidation. Stimulation of fatty acid oxidation is through activation of PPAR (peroxisome proliferator-activated receptor)- alpha. Inhibition of lipogenesis is through down-regulation of SREBP (sterol regulatory element binding protein) -1c messenger RNA.

Several mechanisms are believed to account for the anti-inflammatory activity of EPA and DHA. The two competitively inhibit the conversion of arachidonic acid to the pro-inflammatory eicosanoids PG (prostaglandin)E_2 and LT(leukotiene)B_4, thus reducing their synthesis. EPA and DHA also inhibit the synthesis of the inflammatory cytokines TNF (tumor necrosis factor)-alpha and IL(interleukin)-1 beta in both healthy volunteers and rheumatoid arthritis patients. EPA and DHA inhibit the 5-LOX (lipoxygenase) pathway responsible for the conversion of arachidonic acid to inflammatory leukotrienes in neutrophils and monocytes and can suppress phopholipase C-mediated signal transduction, also involved in inflammatory events. EPA and DHA may possess disease-modifying activity. Incorporation of EPA and DHA into articular cartilage chondrocyte membranes results in a dose-dependent reduction in the expression and activity of the proteoglycan-degrading enzymes known as aggrecanases. This similarly results in decreased expression of interleukin IL-1 alpha and TNF-alpha as well as COX (cyclooxygenase) -2, but not COX-1.

EPA and DHA have both similar and dissimilar physiologic roles. EPA appears to be more important in those roles where the eicosanoids are involved, whereas DHA seems to play its most important roles in the membranes of CNS cells and in the PPAR system. EPA is the precursor to series-3 prostaglandins (PG), the series-5 leukotrienes (LT) and the series-3 thromboxanes (TX). Specifically, EPA is the precursor of TXA_3 and LTB_5, eicosanoids, which reduce platelet aggregation and increase vasodilation. This could account in part for those fish oil effects that may lead to reduced clotting activity and decreased blood pressure.

Fish oils appear to have mood-stabilizing properties when used in the treatment of bipolar disorder. Overactive cell-signaling pathways may be involved in the pathophysiology of bipolar disorder. EPA and DHA may dampen signal transduction associated with phosphatidylinositol and arachidonic acid. These LCPUFAs, especially DHA, are incorporated into the phospholipids of the membranes of cells involved in cell-signaling pathways.

The mechanism by which fish oils appear to prevent cardiac arrythmia is unclear but also may have something to do with the incorporation of these LCPUFAs into the cell membranes of the heart.

Fish oils may have cancer chemopreventive effects, but clinical chemoprevention studies are needed to determine if this is the case. *In vitro* and animal studies have shown EPA and DHA to suppress neoplastic transformation, inhibit cancer growth, enhance apoptosis or programmed cell death and to have anti-angiogenic activity. A common mechanism underlying all of the above activity could be the role of the LCPUFAs in modulating eicosanoid production and activity. Fats other than from fish sources are known risk factors for cancer as well as cardiovascular disease. Those fats may direct the eicosanoid pathways toward situations in which cancer cells can flourish, whereas the opposite may be the case for the fish oils.

PHARMACOKINETICS
Different forms of fish oil are commercially available. The natural forms of EPA and DHA, as found in fish and phytoplankton, exist in the form of triacylglycerols (TAGs). These are the forms most commonly available at present. More concentrated forms of EPA and DHA are the EPA and DHA ethyl esters and free (i.e. unesterified) EPA and DHA. The pharmacokinetics of these forms are similar.

EPA- and DHA-laden triacylglycerols, following ingestion, undergo hyrolysis via lipases to form monoglycerides and free fatty acids. In the enterocytes, reacylation takes place reforming TAGs, which are then assembled with phospholipids, cholesterol and apoproteins into chylomicrons. The chylomicrons are released into the lymphatics from whence they are transported to the systemic circulation. In the circulation, the chylomicrons are degraded by lipoprotein lipase, and EPA and DHA are transported by the circulation to various tissues of the body where they are used mainly for the synthesis of phospholipids. These phospholipids are incorporated into the cell membranes of red blood cells, platelets and CNS cells, among others. EPA and DHA are mainly found in the phospholipid components of the cell membranes. DHA is taken up by the brain in preference to other fatty acids. DHA can partially retroconvert to EPA, and EPA may partially convert to DHA.

Enteral absorption of EPA and DHA is at least as good from semi-synthetic ethyl esters as it is from the natural forms.

INDICATIONS AND USAGE

Fish oils may primarily be indicated to lower triglyceride levels in those with hypertriglyceridemia. Another important indication may be to prevent death in those who have suffered myocardial infarctions. Fish oils are used to decrease clotting tendencies of the blood. They may also be indicated for lowering blood pressure, for preventing restenosis following coronary angioplasty, for alleviating some of the symptoms of rheumatoid arthritis and ulcerative colitis and for helping to prevent relapse in Crohn's disease. They may help stabilize mood in bipolar disorder and may have beneficial effects in IgA nephropathy. There is evidence they may help prevent rejection in renal transplant patients, and they are used in enteral feeding of various patient categories.

There is very little evidence in support of an indication for use in angina and no convincing evidence to support claimed indications for asthma, hay fever and psoriasis. There is insufficient data to make any judgment about possible use of fish oil in cancer.

RESEARCH SUMMARY

A meta-analysis of several studies to determine the effect of fish oil supplementation on serum triglyceride levels consistently shows a significant triglyceride-lowering effect. Doses of fish oil in the studies ranged from 0.5 grams to 25 grams daily with an average intake of about 6 grams daily. These numbers refer to the amount of EPA and DHA received. The average ratio of EPA to DHA in these studies was about 1.5, and the studies lasted from two weeks to two years. The triglyceride-lowering effect was dose-related. Overall, cholesterol levels did not change. Some of the studies reported an increase in LDL cholesterol and some showed an increase in HDL cholesterol.

A double-blind, placebo-controlled study was performed to determine the triglyceride-lowering effect of EPA and DHA by themselves. In this seven-week study, 234 healthy men were randomly given the following: EPA, in the ethyl ester at a dose of 3.8 grams daily, the ethyl ester of DHA at 3.6 grams daily or corn oil at 4 grams daily. Triglycerides decreased by 21% in the EPA group and by 26% in the DHA group when compared to placebo. Some retroconversion from DHA to EPA was noted, but no significant conversion of EPA to DHA was observed. A slight, but significant, increase in HDL-cholesterol was seen in the DHA group, and a slight, but significant, decrease of total cholesterol and apolipoprotein A1 was noted in the EPA group.

Another study looked at the effect on serum lipids of fish oil supplements by themselves and in combination with fish oils and garlic powder. Fifty men with moderately elevated cholesterol were assigned to one of four treatment groups and followed for 12 weeks. The fish oil used in this study was a natural triacylglycerol, and those receiving fish oil took 12 grams containing 30% of a mixture of EPA and DHA in a 1.5 ratio for a total of 2.16 grams of EPA and 1.44 grams of DHA daily. One group received fish oil and garlic powder, another group received fish oil and a placebo powder, a third group received powder and a placebo oil, and the remaining group was given a placebo oil and a placebo powder.

The fish oil group registered a 3.73% lowering of serum triglycerides, no significant change in total cholesterol and an 8.5% increase in LDL-cholesterol. No significant changes were noted in this group in the ratios of total cholesterol over HDL-cholesterol and LDL-cholesterol over HDL-cholesterol. The fish oil and garlic powder group were found to have a 34.3% lowering of triglycerides, a 12% lowering of total cholesterol, a 9.5% decrease in LDL cholesterol, a 16% decrease in the total cholesterol over HDL-cholesterol ratio and a 19% decrease in the LDL-cholesterol over HDL-cholesterol ratio. The garlic group showed no change in the serum triglyceride value, and 11.5% decrease in total cholesterol, a 14% decrease in LDL cholesterol, a 12.5% decrease in the total cholesterol to HDL-cholesterol ratio and a 15% decrease in the LDL-cholesterol ratio. No change in HDL-cholesterol was observed in the fish oil group. A slight non-significant increase in HDL-cholesterol was noted in the garlic group.

The GISSI-Prevenzione study examined the effect of dietary fish oil and vitamin E supplementation on mortality and morbidity in over 11,000 subjects who had suffered a myocardial infarction within three months of entering the trial. The subjects (85% men, 51% younger than 60) were randomly assigned to one of four groups. One group, consisting of 2,836 subjects, received 1 gram of fish oil daily containing 850 to 882 milligrams of EPA and DHA in the form of the ethyl esters and in a ratio of EPA to DHA of 1 to 2. A second group, consisting of 2,830 subjects, received 300 milligrams of vitamin E in the form of synthetic D alpha-tocopherol. A third group of 2,830 subjects received both the fish oils and vitamin E, while the fourth group of 2,828 acted as the control. The trial lasted for 42 months.

The primary combined endpoint was death, non-fatal myocardial infarction and stroke. Treatment with fish oil, but not vitamin E, significantly lowered the risk of the primary endpoint. The effect of the combined treatment was similar to that of fish oil alone. Although vitamin E did show a trend toward a reduction in mortality, the trend did not show significance. No adverse effects were reported except for some mild gastrointestinal symptoms. The dose of fish oil used in the trial lowered serum triglycerides by 3.4%.

The most significant result of this trial was the reduction in risk for overall and sudden cardiac death. It is believed that the reduction of sudden cardiac death was due to the anti-arrythmic effect of the LCPUFAs. The study suggests that up to 20 lives per 1,000 post-MI patients could be saved by consuming daily doses of less than 1 gram of EPA and DHA.

Meta-analysis of 17 controlled studies with fish oil indicates that supplementation with 3 or more grams of fish oil daily can lead to clinically relevant systolic and diastolic blood pressure reductions in individuals with untreated hypertension but not in normotensives. The EPA plus DHA doses used in these trials ranged from 1 to 15 grams with an EPA to DHA ratio of about 1.5.

A meta-analysis of the effect of fish oils following coronary angioplasty indicated that subjects who had undergone successful angioplasty had a significantly lower rate (13.9%) of restenosis when given 4 to 5 grams daily of mixtures of EPA and DHA for three months to one year following the angioplasty.

Daily ingestion of at least 3 grams of EPA and DHA mixtures for a period of 12 weeks or longer has been found to reduce the number of tender joints and amount of morning stiffness in subjects with rheumatoid arthritis. Those with rheumatoid arthritis consuming these supplements have been reported to lower or discontinue use of nonsteroidal anti-inflammatory drugs or disease-modifying anti-rheumatic drugs. The supplements appeared to be well tolerated in these individuals, and no serious toxicity was reported.

A one year double-blind trial of subjects with Crohn's disease randomized these subjects into two groups. One group received a mixture of 2.7 grams of EPA and DHA daily. The fish oil was in the form of enterically coated free fatty acids and provided 1.8 grams of EPA and 0.9 grams of DHA daily. It was noted that the subjects taking the fish oil supplement had a significantly reduced relapse rate. No significant adverse effects were reported.

Supplementation of fish oils in subjects with ulcerative colitis has shown some encouraging trends. In one study, six patients with active ulcerative colitis were given 3 to 4 grams of a mixture of EPA and DHA daily in the form of natural triacylglycerols for a period of 12 weeks. Significant results were reported regarding the subjects' symptoms and histological appearance of the rectal mucosa by the end of the 12 weeks.

A few open studies with few subjects have suggested that fish oil supplements positively affect the clinical course of psoriasis. The best study to date, a double-blind, placebo-controlled, multi-center trial of 155 subjects with moderate-to-severe psoriasis showed no clinically important difference between subjects receiving 5 grams daily of EPA and DHA in ethyl ester form and the placebo group over a four-month period.

A four-month double-blind, placebo-controlled study of 30 subjects with bipolar disorder compared the effects of fish oil supplements with placebo. Fourteen subjects received 9.6 grams daily of fish oil consisting of 6.2 grams of EPA and 3.4 grams of DHA, and 16 subjects received olive oil as a placebo. This study showed improvement in the short-term course of the disorder with fish oil supplementation. Among those taking fish oils, longer periods of remission were observed in nearly every outcome category, and the results were statistically significant. Mild gastrointestinal side effects were reported in the fish oil group.

Immunoglobulin (Ig) A nephropathy is the most common glomerular disease worldwide. Beneficial effects with fish oil supplements have been reported in two studies, while two other studies showed no beneficial effects. In the largest and longest study to date, daily supplementation with fish oil showed protection against progressive renal disease. This blinded, placebo-controlled trial included 51 subjects who received a daily mixture of EPA and DHA at 1.87 grams and 1.36 grams, respectively. The study lasted two years, and the placebo group used olive oil as the control. It was concluded that fish oil retarded the rate of renal function loss.

CONTRAINDICATIONS, PRECAUTIONS, ADVERSE REACTIONS

CONTRAINDICATIONS
None known.

PRECAUTIONS
Fish oil supplements should be used by children, pregnant women and nursing mothers only if recommended and monitored by a physician. Because of the possible anti-thrombotic effect of fish oil supplements, hemophiliacs and those taking warfarin (Coumadin) should exercise caution in their use. Fish oil supplements should be stopped before any surgical procedure. Conflicting results have been reported regarding the effects of fish oil supplements on glycemic control in those with glucose intolerance including type 2 diabetics. Some early studies indicated that fish oil supplements might have detrimental effects in those groups. Recently, better designed studies have not reported these adverse effects. There is no evidence that fish oil supplements have detrimental effects on glucose tolerance, insulin secretion or insulin resistance in non-diabetic subjects. Diabetics should discuss the use of these supplements with their physicians and note if the supplements affect their glycemic control. Diabetics who take fish oil supplements should be monitored by their physicians.

ADVERSE REACTIONS

There have been no reports of serious adverse events in those taking fish oil supplements, even up to 15 grams daily for prolonged periods of time. Those side effects that have been reported include mild gastrointestinal upsets such as nausea and diarrhea, halitosis, eructation and "fishy" smelling breath, skin and even urine. The blood-thinning effects can cause occasional nosebleeds and easy bruising.

INTERACTIONS

Interactions may occur between fish oil supplements and aspirin and other non-steroidal anti-inflammatory drugs and herbs such as garlic (*Allium sativum*) and ginkgo (*Ginkgo biloba*). Such interactions might be manifested by increased susceptibility to bruising, nosebleeds, hemoptysis, hematemesis, hematuria and blood in the stool. Most who take fish oil supplements and the above drugs or herbs do not suffer from these problems, and, if they occur, they are rare. If they do occur, the dose should be lowered or discontinued.

OVERDOSAGE

Not reported.

DOSAGE AND ADMINISTRATION

There are several forms of fish oil supplements. The most common form is natural fish oil, usually produced from the body of cold-water fish. These fish oils are, typically, 30% EPA and DHA with a ratio of EPA to DHA of 1.5. A typical 1 gram softgel capsule of fish oil contains 180 milligrams of EPA and 120 milligrams of DHA. Natural EPA and DHA are chemically triacylglycerols. Natural fish oil capsules containing 50% EPA and DHA in a 1.5 ratio are now available. Some natural fish oil supplements contain EPA and DHA in a higher ratio, i.e. higher EPA. There are also fish oil supplements with a lower ratio, i.e. higher DHA.

A more concentrated form of fish oil is the semi-synthetic ethyl ester product containing 85% EPA/DHA. One such product contains 490 milligrams of EPA ethyl ester and 350 milligrams of DHA ethyl ester per 1 gram capsule.

Enteric coated EPA and DHA as the free fatty acids are also available. These capsules are more concentrated in EPA and DHA. Emulsions of fish oils are now available that can be used as constituents for salad dressings and other foods. Functional foods, including bars containing fish oil, are becoming available. Infant formulas containing DHA are available in Europe and Japan. Certain enteral supplements contain EPA and DHA as well as other immune-modulating nutrients such as L-arginine, L-glutamine and RNA.

Recommended fish oil products must contain antioxidants such as tocopherol to protect against their oxidation. Further, fish oil products that contain high quantities of vitamin A and D, which could be toxic, should not be used.

The usual oral dose of fish oil for use in hypertriglyceridemia is about 5 grams of combined EPA/DHA daily. The values expressed in this section refer to the amounts of EPA plus DHA. The actual weight of the capsule is typically much higher. Labels should be checked in order to determine the actual EPA/DHA content. The daily intake should be taken in divided doses; the supplements are best tolerated with meals. The usual dose for hypertensives who have not previously been treated is about 3 grams of EPA/DHA daily. About 3 grams daily is also the usual dose for those with rheumatoid arthritis, Crohn's disease and ulcerative colitis. Those who have had successful angioplasty and are trying to prevent restenosis might use 4 to 5 grams daily. Based on the GISSI-Prevenzione trial, a dose of 1 gram daily of EPA and DHA might have protective value for those who have had an MI.

HOW SUPPLIED

Capsules — 400 mg, 500 mg, 1000 mg, 1200 mg, 2000 mg

LITERATURE

Adler AJ, Holub BJ. Effect of garlic and fish-oil supplementation on serum lipid and lipoprotein concentrations in hypercholesterolemic men. *Am J Clin Nutr*. 1997; 65:445-450.

Appel LJ, Miller ER III, Seidler AJ, Whelton PK. Does supplementation of diet with 'fish oil' reduce blood pressure? A meta-analysis of controlled clinical trials. *Arch Intern Med*. 1993; 153:1429-1438.

Ariza-Ariza R, Mestanza-Peralta M, Cardiel MH. Omega-3 fatty acid in rheumatoid arthritis: an overview. *Semin Arthritis Rheum*. 1998; 27:366-370.

Belluzi A, Brignola C, Campieri M, et al. Effect of an enteric-coated fish-oil preparation on relapses in Crohn's disease. *N Engl J Med*. 1996; 334:1557-1560.

Connor WE, Prince MJ, Ullman D, et al. The hypotriglyceridemic effect of fish oil in adult-onset diabetes without adverse glucose control. *Ann NY Acad Sci*. 1993; 683: 337-340.

Curtis CL, Hughes CE, Flannery CR, et al. n-3 Fatty acids specifically modulate catabolic factors involved in articular cartilage degradation. *J Biol Chem*. 2000; 275:721-724.

Donadia Jr, JV, Bergstralh MS, Offard MS, et al. A controlled trial of fish oil in Iga nephropathy. *N Engl J Med*. 1994; 331:1194-1199.

GISSI-Prevenzione Investigators. Dietary supplementation with n-3 polyunsaturated fatty acids and vitamin E after myocardial infarction: results of the GISSI-Prevenzione trial. *Lancet*. 1999; 354:447-455.

Gapinski JP, VanRuiswyk JV, Heudebert GR, Schectman GS. Preventing restenosis with fish oils following coronary angioplasty: a meta-analysis. *Arch Intern Med*. 1993; 153:1595-1601.

Grimsgaard S, Bonaa KH, Hansen J-B, Nordoy A. Highly purified eicosapentaenoic acid and docosahexaenoic acids in humans have similar triacylglycerol-lowering effects but divergent effects on serum fatty acids. *Am J Clin Nutr*. 1997; 66:649-659.

Harris WS. Fish oils and plasma lipid and lipoprotein metabolism in humans: a critical review. *J Lipid Res*. 1989; 30:785-807.

Homan van der Heide JJ, Bilo HGJ, Donker JM, et al. Effect of dietary fish oil on renal function and rejection in cyclosporine-treated recipients of renal transplants. *N Engl J Med*. 1993; 329:769-763.

Kim H-J, Takahashi M, Ezaki O. Fish oil feeding decreases mature sterol regulatory element-binding protein 1 (SREBP-1) by down-regulation of SREBP-1c mRNA in mouse liver. *J Biol Chem*. 1999; 274:25892-25898.

Kremer JM. n-3 Fatty acid supplements in rheumatoid arthritis. *Am J Clin Nutr*. 2000; 71:349s-351s.

McManus RM, Jumpson J, Finegood DT, et al. A comparison of the effects of n-3 fatty acids from linseed oil and fish oil in well-controlled type II diabetes. *Diabetes Care*. 1996; 9:463-467.

Stoll AL, Severus WE, Freeman MP, et al. Omega 3 fatty acids in bipolar disorder. *Arch Gen Psychiatry*. 1999; 56:407-412.

Toft I, Bonaa KH, Ingebresten OC, et al. Effects of n-3 polyunsaturated fatty acids on glucose homeostasis and blood pressure in essential hypertension. *Ann Intern Med*. 1995; 123:911-918.

Von Schacky C, Angerer P, Kothny W, et al. The effect of dietary omega-3 fatty acids on coronary atherosclerosis. A randomized, double-blind, placebo-controlled trial. *Ann Intern Med*. 1999; 130:554-562.

Flaxseed Oil

TRADE NAMES

Flaxseed oil is available from numerous manufacturers generically. Branded products include Tona-lean 1000 CLA (Action Labs), New Energy (Advanced Nutritional), Bioflax (Bio-tech Pharmacal), FiProFlax (Health From the Sun), BioEFA Flax 1000 (Health From the Sun) and Linum-20 (Key Company).

DESCRIPTION

Flaxseed, also known as flax oil and linseed oil, is derived from the seeds of the plant *Linium usitatissimum*. Flaxseed oil is a very rich source of alpha-linolenic acid. Alpha-linolenic acid concentration in flaxseed oil ranges from approximately 40 to 60%. Lower amounts of linoleic acid and oleic acid (each about 15%) are also present in flaxseed

oil. In addition, flaxseed oil contains varying amounts of the lignan, secoisolariciresinol diglycoside (SDG).

Alpha-linolenic acid (ALA) is an n-3(omega-3), all-cis polyunsaturated fatty acid containing 18 carbon atoms and three double bonds. It is also known as ALA; ALA, 18:3n-3; 9,12,15-octadecatrienoic acid and (Z, Z, Z)-9, 12, 15 octadecatrienoic acid. ALA has the following structural formula:

$$H_3C \diagdown\!=\!\diagdown\!=\!\diagdown\!=\!(CH_2)_6COOH$$

Alpha-linolenic acid

ALA is present in flaxseed oil in the form of a triglyceride. The Mediterranean diet, high in ALA, appears to lower the risk of coronary artery disease and certain types of cancer.

The lignan SDG belongs to a group of plant substances known as phytoestrogens.

ACTIONS AND PHARMACOLOGY

ACTIONS

Flaxseed oil may have anti-inflammatory, anti-thrombotic and anti-proliferative activities.

MECHANISM OF ACTION

ALA is metabolized to eicosopentaenoic acid (EPA). EPA is a precursor of the series-3 prostaglandins, the series-5 leukotrienes and the series-3 thromboxanes. These eicosanoids have anti-inflammatory and anti-atherogenic properties. ALA metabolites may also inhibit the production of the pro-inflammatory eicosanoids, prostaglandin E_2 (PGE2) and leukotriene B4 (LTB4), as well as the pro-inflammatory cytokines, tumor necrosis factor-alpha (TNF-alpha) and interleukin-1 beta (IL-1 beta). Incorporation of ALA and its metabolites in cell membranes can affect membrane fluidity and may play a role in anti-inflammatory activity, inhibition of platelet aggregation and possibly in anti-proliferative actions of ALA.

Secoisolaricoresinol diglycoside (SDG) is metabolized to enterolactone and enterodiol. These substances may have anti-platelet-activating factor activity, which would produce anti-thrombotic activity. SDG metabolites may also block some of the cancer-inducing effects of estrogen and may have selective estrogen receptor modulating (SERM) activity.

PHARMACOKINETICS

ALA-laden triglycerides in flaxseed oil are absorbed from the small intestine aided by bile salts. During this process, there is some deacylation of the fatty acids of the triglycerides. Reacylation takes place within the mucosal cells of the small intestine, and the ALA-laden triglycerides enter the lymph system in the form of chylomicrons. ALA-laden chylomicrons are transported from the lymph into the blood, where ALA is then carried in various lipid particles to the various cells of the body, where it gets metabolized to EPA and series-3 prostaglandins, series-5 leukotrienes and series-3 thromboxanes.

The flaxseed oil lignan SDG is metabolized by bacteria in the colon to enterolactone and enterodiol. These substances are absorbed from the colon and metabolized to several hydroxylated metabolites in the body.

INDICATIONS AND USAGE

Flaxseed and flaxseed oil may be indicated in hyperlipidemia, to decrease platelet aggregation, to lower blood pressure, to help prevent heart attacks and stroke, and to ameliorate some of the symptoms of arthritis. There is a suggestion that it may be helpful in some cancers. Claims that it can be useful in the treatment of anxiety, benign prostatic hyperplasia, constipation, vaginitis and weight loss are unsubstantiated.

RESEARCH SUMMARY

Though high in alpha-linolenic acid (ALA), flaxseed and flaxseed oil may have beneficial effects that may sometimes be independent of their ALA content. In animal models, flaxseed-enriched diets have significantly reduced hypercholestemic atherosclerosis; this has been true even when CDC-flaxseed (Type II flaxseed), which contains quantities of oil and lignan similar to that of standard flaxseed but with very little ALA content, has been used. Lignan content could be responsible for some of the positive effects. Lignans have been shown, in various studies, to contain anti-platelet-activating factor activity and possess antioxidant properties. Development of atherosclerosis has been reduced by up to 69% in some of these studies using flaxseed-enriched diets.

To what extent research findings using flaxseed itself can be extended to the use of flaxseed oil remains to be determined. There is preliminary clinical evidence suggesting that the oil can decrease platelet aggregation, that it may lower cholesterol (but probably not triglycerides) and that it might have some ability to lower blood pressure and have some anti-inflammatory effects in some with arthritis.

Some animal studies have suggested a possible role for flaxseed in the treatment of some cancers, particularly mammary cancers. Lignans have been shown to block some of the cancer-inducing effects of endogenous estrogens. Human trials are underway.

Recently, some poultry farmers have begun feeding chickens diets rich in flaxseed, boosting the omega-3 fatty acid content of the eggs of these chickens to levels eight to 10 times that of regular eggs. These functional foods have already captured four percent of the Canadian egg market. It has been reported that two of these eggs supply half of Health Canada's recommended daily intake of omega-3 fatty acids for adults.

A researcher at the Center for Genetics, Nutrition and Health, Washington, D.C., has concluded: "The availability of omega-3 fatty acid-enriched products should lead to improvements in the food supply...studies with omega-3-enriched eggs lower cholesterol levels, platelet aggregation and blood pressure."

Claims that flaxseed and flaxseed oil are useful in treating anxiety, prostate problems, vaginitis and weight loss are not substantiated by the available research data. Veterinarians reportedly use these products to treat some animals for constipation, but human data are lacking. And, regarding animals, flaxseed oil fed to broiler chickens has been found to reduce pulmonary hypertension and right ventricular hypertrophy in birds raised under hypoxic conditions. No human data are available.

CONTRAINDICATIONS, PRECAUTIONS, ADVERSE REACTIONS
CONTRAINDICATIONS
Women who are pregnant should not use supplemental flaxseed oil or flaxseed because of the theoretical possibility that these lignan-containing substances might induce menstruation.

PRECAUTIONS
Infants, young children, and nursing mothers should avoid supplemental flaxseed oil. Because of possible antithrombotic activity, those with hemophilia and those taking warfarin should be cautious about the use of supplemental flaxseed oil or flaxseed. Flaxseed oil intake should be halted in those having surgical procedures.

ADVERSE REACTIONS
Flaxseed oil may cause mild gastrointestinal symptoms, such as diarrhea.

INTERACTIONS
DRUGS
Interactions may occur between flaxseed oil-ALA and its metabolites and warfarin, aspirin and NSAIDs. Such interactions, if they were to occur, might be manifested by nosebleeds and increased susceptibility to bruising. If this does occur, consideration should be given to lowering or stopping intake.

NUTRITIONAL SUPPLEMENTS
Interactions may occur if flaxseed oil is used with other nutritional supplements, such as fish oils, which have antithrombotic activity.

HERBS

Interactions may occur between ALA and its metabolites with such herbs as garlic (*Allium sativa*) and ginkgo (*Ginkgo biloba*). Such interactions might be manifested by nosebleeds and easy bruising.

OVERDOSAGE

There are no reports of flaxseed oil overdosage.

DOSAGE AND ADMINISTRATION

Flaxseed oil comes in a few forms: capsules containing from 40-60 percent ALA, oils and in functional foods. Regarding the latter, ALA-laden eggs are available from laying hens fed flaxseed diets.

Three to four grams of ALA is approximately equivalent to the 0.3 grams of EPA, which one would derive from a fish-rich diet. Six 1-gram capsules of flaxseed oil that are 50% ALA contains 3 grams of ALA. A tablespoon of 50% ALA-containing flaxseed oil provides about 7.5 grams of ALA.

Many use flaxseed oil as a component in salad dressings. Since flaxseed oil is easily oxidized, it is important that it contains an antioxidant, such as vitamin E.

The amounts of flaxseed lignan in flaxseed oil are highly variable.

HOW SUPPLIED

Capsules — 1000 mg, 1130 mg, 1250 mg, 1300 mg

Oil

Tea

LITERATURE

Allman MA, Penna MM, Pang D. Supplementation with flaxseed oil versus sunflower seed oil in healthy young men consuming a low fat diet: effects on platelet composition and function. *Eur J Clin Nutr*. 1995; 49:169-178.

Fisher S, Honigmann, G, Hora C, et al. Results of linseed oil and olive oil therapy in hyperlipoproteinemia patients. [Article in German]. *Dtsch Z Verdau Stoffwechselkr*. 1984; 44:245-251.

Indu M, Ghafoorunissa. n-3 fatty acids in Indian diets: comparison of the effects of precursor (alpha-linolenic acid) vs. product (long-chain n-3 polyunsaturated fatty acids). *Nutr Res*. 1992; 12:569-582.

James MJ, Gibson RA, Cleland LG. Dietary polyunsaturated fatty acids and inflammatory mediator production. *Am J Clin Nutr*. 2000; 71(Suppl):343S-348S.

Jenkins DJ, Kendall CW, Vidgen E, et al. Health aspects of partially defatted flaxseed, including effects on serum lipids, oxidative measures, and ex vivo androgen and progestin activity: a controlled crossover trial. *Am J Clin Nutr*. 1999; 69:395-402.

Prasad K, Mantha SV, Muir AD, Westcott ND. Reduction of hypercholesterolemic atherosclerosis by CDC-flaxseed with very low alpha-linolenic acid. *Atherosclerosis*. 1998; 136:367-375.

Prasad K. Dietary flaxseed in prevention of hypercholesterolemic atherosclerosis. *Atherosclerosis*. 1997; 132:69-76.

Rozanova IA, Pogozheva AV, Kupakova SN, et al. Effect of anti-atherosclerotic diet, containing polyunsaturated fatty acids of the omega-3 family from flax oil, on fatty acid composition of cell membranes of patients with ischemic heart disease, hypertensive disease and hyperlipoproteinemia. [Article in Russian]. *Vopr Pitan*. 1997; (5):15-17.

Simopoulos AP. New products from the agri-food industry: the return of n-3 fatty acids into the food supply. *Lipids*. 1999; 34 Suppl:S297-S301.

Singer P, Wirth M, Berg, I. A possible contribution of decrease in free fatty acids to low serum triglyceride after diets supplemented with n-6 and n-3 polyunsaturated fatty acids. *Atherosclerosis*. 1990; 83:167-175.

Tou JC, Thompson LU. Exposure to flaxseed or its lignan component during different developmental stages influences rat mammory gland structures. *Carcinogenesis*. 1999; 20:1831-1835.

Walton JP, Bond JM, Julian RJ, Squires EJ. Effect of dietary flax oil and hypobaric hypoxia on pulmonary hypertension and haematological variables in broiler chickens. *Br Poult Sci*. 1999; 40:385-391.

Flower Pollen

DESCRIPTION

The supplement flower pollen is an extract of pollen. Pollen consists of the male germ seeds of plants, flowers or blossoms on trees. As plants flower, pollen is transferred from the anther of a stamen to the stigma of a pistil; on reaching the ovary it brings about fertilization of seeds. Entomophilus pollen refers to pollen that is spread by insects such as bees; anemophilous pollen refers to pollen spread by wind.

In contrast to bee pollen, which is collected from bees (see Bee Pollen), flower pollen is harvested directly from plants. The major flower pollen supplement in the marketplace is harvested from a number of organically grown specially selected flowers. The harvested pollen then undergoes extraction and fermentation processes in order to produce a better-absorbable product. Substances found in this product include vitamins, carotenoids, minerals, amino acids, lipids, enzymes, flavonoids, long-chain alcohols and phytosterols, among others.

ACTIONS AND PHARMACOLOGY

ACTIONS

Supplemental flower pollen may promote prostate health and may have anti-inflammatory activity.

MECHANISM OF ACTION

The mechanism of these possible activities is not known.

PHARMACOKINETICS

There is little information on the pharmacokinetics of flower pollen in humans. The various components present in flower pollen should be digested, absorbed and metabolized as are similar substances found in food.

INDICATIONS AND USAGE

Flower pollen may have some effectiveness in benign prostatic hyperplasia and in prostatitis. It has reported hepato and gastroprotective effects and may have some ability to inhibit some cancers, ameliorate symptoms of rheumatoid arthritis and protect against cardiovascular disease.

RESEARCH SUMMARY

Several studies have demonstrated positive effects for flower pollen extracts in the management of benign prostatic hyperplasia. In one double-blind, placebo-controlled study, a flower pollen extract taken for six months achieved significant subjective improvement in 69% of patients receiving it, compared with 30% improvement in placebo subjects. Treated subjects had significantly decreased residual urine and significantly decreased antero-posterior diameter of the prostate on ultrasound. In some other studies, average and maximum urine flow rates have also significantly improved with flower pollen supplementation.

In an open British study, 13 of 15 patients with chronic abacterial prostatitis and prostatodynia that had resisted other treatments enjoyed marked-to-complete relief of symptoms with flower pollen extract treatment. Experimental studies suggesting that flower pollen has anti-inflammatory and anti-androgenic properties may explain some of its apparent efficacy in these prostatic disorders.

There have also been numerous studies indicating that flower pollen and its extracts have hepatoprotective effects and have increased survival rates in animals exposed to such potential toxins as acetaminophen, organic solvents, ammonium fluoride, methionine, carbon tetrachloride, galactosamine and allyl alcohol. Protective effects in the lungs have been seen with exposure to ammonium fluoride. Gastroprotective effects of flower pollen have been seen in some with gastroduodenal disorders.

Some improvement in clinical manifestations of rheumatoid arthritis has been reported in one study using flower pollen. There are a few *in vitro* studies indicating that flower pollen extracts may inhibit prostate cancer cells. And in animals with experimental atherosclerosis, pollen extracts have been reported to significantly lower serum lipid levels and to decrease arterial lipid deposits.

CONTRAINDICATIONS, PRECAUTIONS, ADVERSE REACTIONS

CONTRAINDICATIONS

Flower pollen is contraindicated in those allergic or hypersensitive to flower pollen.

PRECAUTIONS

Flower pollen supplements should be avoided by pregnant women and nursing mothers.

ADVERSE REACTIONS

No adverse reactions have been reported. However, those who are allergic or hypersensitive to flower pollen may develop symptoms, including rhinitis, conjunctivitis, pruritis and bronchospasm and, in some cases, urticaria and anaphylaxis.

OVERDOSAGE

No reports of overdosage.

DOSAGE AND ADMINISTRATION

Those who take flower pollen for prostate health typically use about 360 milligrams daily taken in divided doses.

LITERATURE

Buck AC, Cox R, Rees RW, et al. Treatment of outflow tract obstruction due to benign-prostatic hyperplasia with the pollen extract, cernilton. A double-blind, placebo-controlled study. *Br J Urol.* 1990; 66:398-404.

Buck AC, Rees RW, Ebeling L. Treatment of chronic prostatitis and prostadynia with pollen extract. *Br J Urol.* 1989; 64:496-499.

Czarnecki R, Librowski T, Polanski M. [Hepatoprotective effect of flower pollen lipid extract in paracetamol-induced hepatotoxicity in mice.] [Article in Polish.] *Folia Med Cracov.* 1997; 38:53-61.

Dutkiewicz S. Usefulness of Cernilton in the treatment of benign prostatic hyperplasia. *Int Urol Nephrol.* 1996; 28:49-53.

Habib FK, Ross M, Buck AC, et al. *In vitro* evaluation of the pollen extract, cernitin T-60, in the regulation of prostate cell growth. *Br J Urol.* 1990; 66:393-397.

Habib FK, Ross M, Lewenstein A, et al. Identification of a prostate inhibitory substance in a pollen extract. *Prostate.* 1995; 26:133-139.

Polanski M, Czarnecki R, Woron J. [The hepatoprotective and hypolipidemic effect of flower pollen lipid extract in androgenized rats.] [Article in Polish.] *Folia Med Cracov.* 1996; 37:89-95.

Roberts KP, Iyer RA, Prasad G, et al. Cyclic hydroxamic inhibitors of prostate cell growth: selectivity and structure activity relationships. *Prostate.* 1998; 34; 92-99.

Voloshym OI, Pishak OV, Seniuk BP, Cherniavs'ka NB. [The efficacy of flower pollen in patients with rheumatoid arthritis and concomitant diseases of the gastrointestinal and hepatobiliary systems.] [Article in Ukrainian.] *Lik Sprava.* 1998; 4:151-154.

Yasumoto R, Kawanishi H, Tsujino T, et al. Clinical evaluation of long-term treatment using cernitin pollen extract in patients with benign prostatic hyperplasia. *Clin Ther.* 1995; 17:82-87.

Fluoride

TRADE NAMES

Neutracare (Oral B Laboratories), Fluorigard (Colgate Oral Pharmaceuticals), Neutragard Fluoride Rinse (Pascal Co.), Phos-Flur (Colgate Oral Pharmaceuticals)

DESCRIPTION

In the 1930s, it was discovered that high fluoride intake was responsible for a dental condition which is characterized by mottled enamel and which is known as dental fluorosis. Observational studies at the time led to the conclusion that those who lived in areas with a high incidence of dental fluorosis also had a lower incidence of caries than those who lived in areas where the fluoride intake was low.

In 1945, water fluoridation began in Grand Rapids, Michigan as a public health measure to reduce the incidence of caries. Presently, approximately 60% of community water supplies in the United States contain fluoride from 0.7 to 1.2 parts per million or 0.7 to 1.2 milligrams per liter.

Fluoride is the anionic form of fluorine. Fluorine is a halogen gas with atomic number 9 and an atomic weight of 19 daltons. Its symbol is F. Fluorine is the most electronegative element in the periodic table and, in size, it is very similar to the first element, hydrogen.

Even though fluoride has a beneficial role in the protection against caries, there is no evidence that fluoride is an essential nutrient for humans. The only evidence that it may be essential for higher animals is a recent report that fluoride deficiency in goats decreased life expectancy and caused pathological findings in the kidneys and endocrine organs. Fluoride, in addition to being found in municipal drinking water, is found in many foods. Particularly rich sources of fluoride are teas and marine fish.

ACTIONS AND PHARMACOLOGY

ACTIONS

Fluoride may have cariostatic and anti-osteoporotic activities.

MECHANISM OF ACTION

The mechanism of the cariostatic activity of fluoride is not completely understood. It is thought that fluoride interacts with hydroxyapatite to form the less acid soluble fluorhydroxyapatite. Fluorhydroxyapatite is believed to be more resistant to dissolution by the acids produced by bacteria found in plaque. Fluoride may also promote the remineralization of enamel in early caries. Finally fluoride may reduce oral concentrations of cariogenic bacteria or reduce the metabolism of bacteria in plaque.

The mechanism of the possible anti-osteoporotic activity of fluoride is also incompletely understood. Fluoride is thought to have osteoblastic activity and, in partnership with calcium, stimulates the production of new bone. Insufficient intake of calcium at the time that fluoride is administered could lead to osteoid formation and osteomalacia. Fluoride is incorporated in the crystalline structure of bone as fluoroapatite. Fluoride may also slow the resorptive phase of the remodeling process and promote calcification.

PHARMACOKINETICS

Approximately 75% to 90% of ingested fluoride is absorbed from the gastrointestinal tract. About 50% of ingested fluoride is absorbed after 30 minutes. Absorption appears to occur by passive diffusion. A large fraction of ingested fluoride is absorbed from the stomach. Fluoride absorbed from the stomach appears to be absorbed as hydrofluoric acid. Fluoride absorbed from the small intestine is absorbed as fluoride. Slow-release sodium fluoride preparations are principally absorbed from the small intestine as fluoride. Concomitant intake of fluoride with antacids of the aluminum hydroxide type or high doses of calcium can cause decreased absorption of fluoride. Fluoride may form insoluble compounds with aluminum hydroxide and calcium.

For healthy, young, or middle aged adults, approximately 50% of absorbed fluoride is deposited in calcified tissues and 50% is excreted in the urine. For young children, up to 80% is deposited in bone and developing teeth. From 5% to 10% of ingested fluoride is excreted in the feces.

INDICATIONS AND USAGE

Fluoride, in appropriate doses, protects against dental caries. Its use in the treatment of osteoporosis remains controversial and experimental. A trend toward increased fluoride exposure has heightened concerns related to enamel and skeletal fluorosis, the incidences of which, however, still remain low.

RESEARCH SUMMARY

Sodium fluoride is approved by the Food and Drug Administration (FDA) for the prevention of dental caries. Fluoride is often added to public water supplies to achieve concentrations of 0.7 to 1.2 ppm. Higher concentrations (in the maximum 1.2 ppm range) are used in colder climates and lower concentrations in warmer climates where more water is typically consumed.

Epidemiological data show that low fluoride consumption is significantly associated with a higher incidence of dental caries. Experimental and clinical studies provide further substantial support for these epidemiologic findings. Numerous studies have shown that benefits are greatest when teeth get adequate pre-eruptive, as well as posteruptive, fluoride exposure.

Concerns have grown in recent years, however, that some children may be over-exposed to fluoride. Despite some reduction in exposure levels recommended by the American Academy of Pediatrics, incidence of dental fluorosis, while small, has continued to increase, a finding that some attribute to increased opportunities for fluoride exposure, not only from water but also from oral supplements, toothpastes, rinses, gels and some processed foods and beverages. Further modifications in recommended exposure levels are under consideration.

Because it is an effective osteoblast stimulator, fluoride has been investigated as a treatment for osteoporosis. It has shown some usefulness in this regard, particularly when given in the earliest stages of osteoporosis and particularly in patients with intact trabecular bone. Its effectiveness appears to be enhanced when combined in low doses with vitamin D and calcium.

Fluoride's efficacy in osteoporosis, however, is far from established. Where benefit has been demonstrated it has often been modest. Some studies have shown that it has no benefit. In one study, fluoride plus calcium decreased vertebral fracture rates, compared with calcium alone, in postmenopausal women with moderate osteoporosis. The dose of fluoride was 20 milligrams per day. In another recent study, a fluoride/calcium/vitamin D regimen was no more effective than a calcium/vitamin D regimen in preventing new vertebral fractures in women with postmenopausal osteoporosis.

Some have reported that fluoride-stimulated bone has abnormal texture and is less mineralized and durable than healthy bone. In some studies, despite increased bone mineral density, an increased incidence of fracture has been reported. Additionally, some have reported upper gastrointestinal discomfort and, of greater concern, lower extremity pain syndrome said to be caused by stress fractures. Thus, the benefits of fluoride in the treatment of osteoporosis remain in doubt. And its use in this context remains experimental.

There have been some cases of skeletal fluorosis associated with fluoride supplementation, particularly in those with various forms of renal failure. Two cases of bilateral hip fracture were reported involving women (aged 69 and 78) receiving 40 to 60 milligrams of fluoride daily for 11 to 21 months, in combination with calcium and vitamin D. Both women had moderate renal failure. Histological examination of a bone specimen from the 69-year-old patient revealed severe fluorosis. A specimen from the 78-year-old patient revealed osteomalacia and skeletal fluorosis. Researchers concluded that the fractures were caused by excessive fluoride retention due to renal insufficiency.

CONTRAINDICATIONS, PRECAUTIONS, ADVERSE REACTIONS

CONTRAINDICATIONS

Use of fluoride supplements is contraindicated in areas where fluoride water content is greater than 0.6 parts per million (ppm) or 0.6 milligrams per liter.

Fluoride supplements are contraindicated in those who are hypersensitive to any component of a fluoride-containing supplement.

PRECAUTIONS

Fluoride supplementation is not recommended in children under six months of age.

Excess fluoride intake may result in dental fluorosis in children and skeletal fluorosis in children and adults. Fluoride is not presently approved for the prevention or treatment of osteoporosis.

Pregnant women and nursing mothers should avoid intake of fluoride greater than adequate intake (AI) amounts.

ADVERSE REACTIONS

At the amounts recommended for fluoridation of drinking water and at the recommended doses used for caries prophylaxis, fluoride (sodium fluoride) is generally well tolerated and has not been found to have significant adverse reactions.

Recommended adequate intake for adult males is 4 milligrams daily and for adult females, 3 milligrams daily.

Adverse reactions are occasionally reported at doses of 5 to 10 milligrams daily and are more frequently reported at doses of 10 to 20 milligrams daily and higher. Adverse reactions include nausea, vomiting, mouth sores, rashes, and upper gastrointestinal complaints, such as abdominal distress. Gastrointestinal side effects (nausea, vomiting, abdominal distress) are generally less frequent with slow-acting fluoride preparations than with immediate-release preparations.

A single dose of sodium fluoride of 5 to 10 grams may be lethal. Less than one gram of sodium fluoride has caused serious poisoning.

Chronic fluoride poisoning may result in dental fluorosis and skeletal fluorosis. Symptoms of skeletal fluorosis include bone pain, stiffness and limited movement. A so-called lower extremity pain syndrome has been reported which was caused by stress fractures. Dental fluorosis is characterized by mottled enamel.

INTERACTIONS

DRUGS

Aluminum hydroxide: Concomitant intake of aluminum hydroxide antacids and fluoride can cause decreased absorption of fluoride.

NUTRITIONAL SUPPLEMENTS

Calcium: Concomitant intake of a calcium supplement and fluoride can cause decreased absorption of fluoride.

FOODS

Concomitant intake of foods rich in calcium, such as milk or dairy products, can cause decreased absorption of fluoride.

OVERDOSAGE

Symptoms of acute overdosage include nausea, bloody vomiting, increased salivation, watery eyes, weakness, tremors, tarry stools, drowsiness, faintness, shallow breathing, hypocalcemia, hyperkalemia, convulsions, cardiac arrhythmias, shock, respiratory arrest and cardiac arrest. Death may occur within two to four hours. A single oral dose of 5 to 10 grams of sodium fluoride may be lethal.

DOSAGE AND ADMINISTRATION

Sodium fluoride is available as a prescription supplement, either as a stand-alone product or in combination with vitamins and other minerals. High-fluoride waters are also available containing up to 3 parts per million (3 milligrams per liter) of fluoride. Intakes of fluoride of higher than 4 milligrams daily for adult males and 3 milligrams daily for adult females are not recommended.

The recommendations for fluoride supplementation by the Council on Dental Therapeutics of the American Dental Association are as follows:

Fluoride supplements are not recommended for infants under six months of age. If the fluoride content of the drinking water contains less than 0.3 parts per million (ppm) or 0.3 mg per liter, children aged six months to three years may be given 0.25 mg of fluoride daily; those aged three to six years, 0.5 mg of fluoride daily, and those aged six years and older, 1 mg daily. When the drinking water contains 0.3 to 0.6 ppm or 0.3 to 0.6 mg per liter of fluoride, lower doses should be considered. Specifically, it is recommended that no additional fluoride should be given to children less than three years of age. For children aged three to six years, 0.25 mg of fluoride daily is recommended, and for those aged six years and older, 0.5 mg daily is recommended. Again, if the fluoride content of the drinking water is greater than 0.6 ppm, fluoride supplementation is not recommended.

For calculation purposes, 1.1 milligrams of sodium fluoride are equivalent to 0.5 milligram of fluoride. Fluoride comprises approximately 45% of sodium fluoride.

The Food and Nutrition Board of the Institute of Medicine of the U.S. National Academy of Sciences has recommended the following adequate intakes (AI) for fluoride:

Infants	(AI)
0 through 6 months	0.01 mg/day
7 through 12 months	0.5 mg/day
Children	
1 through 3 years	0.7 mg/day
4 through 8 years	1 mg/day
Boys	
9 through 13 years	2 mg/day
14 through 18 years	3 mg/day
Girls	
9 through 13 years	2 mg/day
14 through 18 years	3 mg/day
Males	
19 and over	4 mg/day
Females	
19 and over	3 mg/day
Pregnancy	
14 through 18 years	3 mg/day
19 through 50 years	3 mg/day
Lactation	
14 through 18 years	3 mg/day
19 through 50 years	3 mg/day

The Food and Nutrition Board of the Institute of Medicine has recommended the following tolerable upper limits (UL) for fluoride.

Infants	(UL)
0 through 6 months	0.7 mg/day
7 through 12 months	0.9 mg/day
Children	
1 through 3 years	1.3 mg/day
4 through 8 years	2.2 mg/day
Children and Adults	
More than 8 years	10 mg/day
Pregnancy and Lactation	
14 through 50 years	10 mg/day

HOW SUPPLIED

Sodium Fluoride is available in the following forms and strengths for Rx use:

Chewable Tablet — 0.25 mg, 0.5 mg, 1 mg
Cream — 1.1%
Gel — 1.1%

Liquid — 0.125 mg/drop, 0.25 mg/0.6 mL, 0.25 mg/drop, 0.5 mg/mL

Lozenge — 1 mg

Solution — 0.05%, 0.2%, 1 mg/5 mL

Sodium Fluoride is available in the following forms and strengths for OTC use:

Gel

Paste

Solution — 0.5%, 1 mg/5 mL

LITERATURE

Adair SM. Overview of the history and current status of fluoride supplementation schedules. *J Public Health Dent.* 1999; 59:252-258.

Angelillo IF, Torre I, Nobile CG, Villari P. Caries and fluorosis prevalence in communities with different concentrations of fluoride in the water. *Caries Res.* 1999; 33:114-122.

Dietary Reference Intakes for Calcium Phosphorus, Magnesium, Vitamin D, and Fluoride. Washington, DC: National Academy Press; 1997.

Guañabens N, Farrerons J, Perez-Edo L, et al. Cyclical etidronate versus sodium fluoride in established postmenopausal osteoporosis: a randomized 3 year trial. *Bone.* 2000; 27:123-128.

Hillier S, Cooper C, Kelligray S, et al. Fluoride in drinking water and risk of hip fracture in the UK: a case-control study. *Lancet.* 2000; 355:265-269.

Horowitz HS. The role of dietary fluoride supplements in caries prevention. *J Public Health Dent.* 1999; 59:205-210.

Leverett DH, Adair SM, Vaughan BW, et al. Randomized clinical trial of the effect of prenatal fluoride supplements in preventing dental caries. *Caries Res.* 1997; 31:174-179.

Lips P. [Fluoride in osteoporosis: still an experimental and controversial treatment]. [Article in Dutch]. *Ned Tijdschr Geneeskd.* 1998; 142:1913-1915.

Meunier PJ, Sebert JL, Reginster JY, et al. Fluoride salts are no better at preventing new vertebral fracture than calcium-vitamin D in postmenopausal osteoporosis: the FAVO Study. *Osteoporosis Int.* 1998; 8:4-12.

Nielsen FH. Ultratrace minerals. In: Shils ME, Olson JA, Shike M, Ross AC, eds. *Modern Nutrition in Health and Disease,* 9th ed. Baltimore, MD: Williams and Wilkins; 1999:283-303.

Pak CYC, Sakhaee K, Adams-Huet B, et al. Treatment of postmenopausal osteoporosis with slow-release sodium fluoride. *Ann Int Med.* 1995; 123:401-408.

Pak CYC, Sakhaee K, Piziak V, et al. Slow-release sodium fluoride in the management of postmenopausal osteoporosis. *Ann Int Med.* 1994; 120:625-632.

Reginster JY, Meurmans L, Zegels B, et al. The effect of sodium monofluorophosphate plus calcium on vertebral fracture rate in postmenopausal women with moderate osteoporosis. A randomized, controlled trial. *Ann Intern Med.* 1998; 129:1-8.

Schulz W. [Fluoride treatment of osteoporosis]. [Article in German]. *Wien Med Wochenschr.* 2000; 150:42-52.

Folate

TRADE NAMES

Folic Acid (folate) is available generically from numerous manufacturers. Brand name products include: Folacin-800 (The Key Company), FA-8 (Bio Tech Pharmacal).

DESCRIPTION

The term folate is used in two different ways. Folate, a member of the B-vitamin family, is a collective term for a number of chemical forms which are structurally related and which have similar biological activity to folic acid. Folate is also the term which is used for the anionic form of folic acid. Folic acid or pteroylglutamic acid (PGA) is comprised of *para*-aminobenzoic acid linked at one end to a pteridine ring and at the other end to glutamic acid. The pteridine-*para*-aminobenzoic acid portion of the molecule is called the pteroyl group. Folic acid is a synthetic folate form which is used for food fortification and nutritional supplements. It is not one of the principal naturally occurring forms of folate, used in the collective sense.

The naturally occurring forms of folate differ in the extent of the reduction state of the pteroyl group, the nature of the substituents on the pteridine ring and the number of glutamyl residues attached to the pteroyl group. The naturally occurring folates, include 5-methyltetrahydrofolate (5-MTHF), 5-formyltetrahydrofolate (5-formyl-THF), 10-formyltetrahydrofolate (10-formyl-THF), 5,10-methylenetetrahydrofolate (5,10-methylene-THF), 5,10-methenyltetrahydrofolate (5,10-methenyl-THF), 5-formiminotetrahydrofolate (5-formimino-THF), 5,6,7,8-tetrahydrofolate (THF) and dihydrofolate (DHF). Most naturally occurring folates are pteroylpolyglutamates, containing two to seven glutamates joined in amide (peptide) linkages to the gamma-carboxyl of glutamate. The principal intracellular folates are pteroylpentaglutamates, while the principal extracellular folates are pteroylmonoglutamates. Pteroylpolyglutamates with up to 11 glutamic acid residues exist naturally. Folate is represented by the following chemical structure.

Folic Acid

Folate participates in several key biological processes, including the synthesis of DNA, RNA and proteins. It is necessary for DNA replication and repair, the maintenance of the integrity of the genome, and is involved in the regulation of gene expression, among other things. Folate deficiency leads to an anemia, called megaloblastic anemia, which is very similar to that caused by vitamin B_{12}. However, folate deficiency does not result in the neurological symptoms and signs that occur with vitamin B_{12} deficiency. Other symptoms and signs of folate deficiency, include weakness, fatigue, irritability, headache, difficulty concentrating, cramps, palpitations, shortness of breath and atrophic glossitis. Laboratory findings of folate deficiency, include decreased serum folate and erythrocyte folate concentrations, elevated serum homocysteine concentration, hypersegmentation of the neutrophils, decreased hemoglobin and erythrocyte concentrations, decreased hematocrit and macrocytic, hyperchromic erythrocytes. Marginal folate deficiency appears to increase the risk of cardiovascular disease, certain types of cancer, Alzheimer's disease and depression. Marginal folate deficiency in pregnant women results in an increased incidence of neural tube defects, including meningomyelocele (e.g., spina bifida), anencephaly, meningocele and craniorachischisis, in their neonates.

A number of conditions can lead to folate deficiency. Chronic alcohol users can become deficient in the vitamin secondary to inadequate intake as well as to ethanol's impairment of folate absorption and hepatobiliary metabolism, as well as to increased renal folate excretion caused by ethanol. Malabsorption syndromes, including Crohn's disease, lymphoma or amyloidosis of the small intestine, diabetic enteropathy, tropical sprue and non-tropical sprue (gluten-sensitive enteropathy), can result in folate deficiency secondary to inadequate absorption of the vitamin, as can small intestinal resections or diversions for the same reason. Some conditions or situations, such as chronic hemolytic anemias (e.g., sickle cell disease), chronic hemodialysis or peritoneal dialysis, chronic exfoliative skin disorders and pregnancy, cause increased demand for folate and folate deficiency will result if the increased demand is not met. Certain drugs, e.g., methotrexate, trimethoprim, pyrimethamine, sulfasalazine and phenytoin, interfere with folate metabolism and may cause functional folate deficiencies. In fact, the mechanism of action of certain antimetabolites, including methotrexate, 5-fluoruracil and the newer multitargeted antifolates, depends on their creating a functional folate deficiency. Some genetic disorders result in folate deficiency and are responsive to folate treatment. Folate-induced remission has been reported in aplastic anemia with familial defect of cellular folate uptake.

Recognizing the increased demand of folate during pregnancy and the increased risk of neural tube defects in neonates born to pregnant women with marginal folate status, the United States Food and Drug Administration (FDA) mandated that folic acid be added to all enriched cereal grains in order to prevent neural tube defects. The mandate became effective on January 1, 1998. The level of folic acid adopted for enriched cereal grain fortification was 140 micrograms per 100 grams. The U.S. Public Health Service recommends that all women of childbearing age in the U.S. consume 400 micrograms of folic acid daily to reduce their risk of having a baby affected with spina bifida or other neural tube defects. This is one of the few health claims allowed by the FDA for nutritional supplementation. The FDA determined 400 micrograms of folic acid daily to be an optimal dose for the prevention of neural tube defects. Those women who already have had a child with a neural tube defect require higher doses.

Natural folates are found in dark green leafy vegetables (spinach, kale, mustard greens, turnip greens, escarole, chard, arugula, beet greens, bok choy, dandelion green, mache, radicchio, rapini or broccoli de rabe, Swiss chard), oranges, lentils, pinto beans, garbanzo beans, asparagus, orange juice, broccoli, cauliflower, liver and brewer's yeast. The absorption efficiency of natural folates is approximately 50% that of folic acid (see Pharmacokinetics). Interestingly, folate was named because of its presence in green leafy vegetables (folium is Latin for leaf) and was originally isolated from four tons of spinach, such was the crudity of isolation techniques more than seven decades ago.

The principal biochemical function of folates is the mediation of one-carbon transfer reactions. 5-Methyltetrahydrofolate donates a methyl group to homocysteine, in the conversion of homocysteine to L-methionine. The enzyme that catalyzes the reaction is methionine synthase. Vitamin B_{12} is a cofactor in the reaction. This reaction is of great importance in the regulation of serum homocysteine levels and is the only reaction in the body in which folate and vitamin B_{12} are coparticipants. (See Vitamin B_{12}). The L-methione produced in the reaction can participate in protein synthesis and is also a major source for the synthesis of S-adenosyl-L-methionine (SAMe). The methyl group that was donated by 5-methyltetrahydrofolate to homocysteine in the formation of L-methionine is used by SAMe in a number of transmethylation reactions involving nucleic acids, phospholipids and proteins, as well as for the synthesis of epinephrine, melatonin, creatine and other molecules (see S-Adenosyl-L-Methionine). Tetrahydrofolate is the folate product of the methionine synthase reaction. 5-Methyltetrahydrofolate can be generated in only one way: conversion of 5,10-methylenetetrahydrofolate into 5-methyltetrahydrofolate via the enzyme methyleneterahydrofolate reductase (MTHFR). 5,10-Methylenetetrahydrofolate is regenerated from tetrahydrofolate via the enzyme serine hydroxymethyl-transferase, a reaction, which in addition to producing 5,10-methylenetetrahydrofolate, yields glycine.

5,10-Methylenetetrahydrofolate, in addition to its role in the metabolism of homocysteine, supplies the one-carbon group for the methylation of deoxyuridylic acid to form the DNA precursor thymidylic acid. This reaction is catalyzed by thymidylate synthase and the folate product of the reaction is dihydrofolate. Dihydrofolate is converted to tetrahydrofolate via the enzyme dihydrofolate reductase.

Folates are also involved in reactions leading to *de novo* purine nucleotide synthesis, interconversion of serine and glycine, generation and utilization of formate, the metabolism of L-histidine to L-glutamic acid, the metabolism of dimethylglycine to sarcosine and the metabolism of sarcosine to glycine.

One of the natural folates, folinic acid, is used as a pharmaceutical agent. Folinic acid, also known as leucovorin, citrovorum factor and 5-formyltetrahydrofolate, is used as rescue therapy following high-dose methotrexate in the treatment of osteosarcoma. It is also used to diminish the toxicity of methotrexate. It is used in the treatment of megaloblastic anemia due to folate deficiency and in the prevention or treatment of the toxic side effects of trimetrexate and pyrimethamine. The combination of folinic acid and 5-fluorouracil has until recently been standard therapy for metastatic colorectal cancer. Folinic acid increases the affinity of flurouracil for thymidylate synthase. Folinic acid is available as a calcium salt for parenteral or oral administration. See *Physicians' Desk Reference* for further discussion of folinic acid.

In addition to being known as pteroylglutamic acid or PGA, folic acid is known chemically as *N*-[4-[[(2-amino-1,4-di-hydro-4-oxo-6-pteridinyl)methyl]amino]benzoyl]-L-glutamic acid. Older names for folic acid are vitamin B_9, folicin, vitamin Bc and vitamin M. Its molecular formula is $C_{19}H_{19}N_7O_6$ and its molecular weight is 441.40 daltons. Folic acid forms yellowish-orange crystals. The color is imparted by the pteridine ring of folic acid. Pteridine also imparts color to butterfly wings.

ACTIONS AND PHARMACOLOGY
ACTIONS
Folic acid lowers the risk of neural tube defects and possibly other types of birth defects. It may also have antiatherogenic, anticarcinogenic, neuroprotective and antidepressant actions.

MECHANISM OF ACTION
Animal and epidemiologic studies have shown that folate deficiency is associated with defects of neural tube closure. Human studies have shown that folic acid, when taken by women planning to become pregnant, can greatly reduce the risk of bearing a child with spina bifida or other neural tube defects. The exact mechanism by which folic acid reduces the risk of neural tube defects and possibly other types of birth defects is not known. It is likely that this effect of folic acid is due to its role in nucleic acid synthesis and/or its role in the metabolism of homocysteine to methionine. Along a different line, it is hypothesized by some that folic acid may not prevent the occurrence of neural tube defects, but may instead selectively increase the abortion rate of affected fetuses.

A central feature of fetal development is widespread and sustained cell division. Folate plays a central role in the formation of nucleic acid precursors, such as thymidylic acid and purine nucleotides, which are essential for nucleic acid synthesis and cell division. The requirement for folate increases during times of rapid tissue growth. The teratogenic effect of folate deficiency may be a result of an insufficient supply of nucleic acid precursors in the rapidly dividing embryonic cells. Increasing folate tissue concentrations might overcome a metabolic deficiency of the vitamin in the production of nucleic acids, and possibly also proteins, at the time of neural tube closure, which typically occurs 24 to 28 days after conception. An insufficient supply of nucleic acid precursors, however, might be expected to cause more general birth defects than the highly specific and predictable nature of the congenital defects caused by folate deficiency. Although derivatives of the neural ectoderm are affected more than other tissues by folate deficiency, all of the embryonic tissues are dividing rapidly during the susceptible developmental period. An insufficient supply of nucleic acid precursors may play some role in the mechanism of folate deficiency-induced neural tube defects, but it is not a sufficient explanation for these congenital disorders.

Some studies have found that homocysteine levels in pregnant women who subsequently gave birth to children with neural tube defects, were significantly higher than those of pregnant women who gave birth to normal children. This would be expected to occur in pregnant women with low folate status. The enzyme that metabolizes homocysteine to methionine, methionine synthase, uses 5-methyltetrahydrofolate, as well as vitamin B_{12}, as a cofactor. There is some evidence that pregnant women with elevated homocysteine levels have a defect in the methionine synthase enzyme. A defect in the enzyme would lead to decreased production of methionine and S-adenosylmethione (SAMe). SAMe is involved in a number of transmethylation reactions, including reactions involved in the formation of myelin. Further, increased homocysteine levels could result in increased oxidative stress which might be contributory to a teratogenic effect. Homocysteine has been found to be teratogenic in avian embryos. Avian embryos treated directly with D,L-homocysteine or with L-homocysteine thiolactone showed neural tube defects which were prevented with folic acid, indicating that homocysteine *per se* can cause dysmorphogenesis of the neural tube.

Hyperhomocysteinemia is associated with cardiovascular disease, cerebrovascular disease and carotid artery stenosis in adults. Folic acid can lower homocysteine blood levels by converting homocysteine to methionine. A high intake of folate has been associated with a lower risk of coronary events. There is evidence that hyperhomocysteinemia is a risk factor for coronary heart disease independent of other known risk factors (hypercholesterolemia, hypertension, diabetes, smoking). Folic acid, as mentioned above, can lower homocysteine blood levels, but the mechanism by which hyperhomocysteinemia might increase the risk of vascular disease is unclear. A number of hypotheses have been proposed. Homocysteine may promote atherogenesis through endothelial dysfunction and oxidative stress. Elevated homocysteine levels may result in increased oxidation of low-density lipoprotein cholesterol (LDL-C). Oxidized LDL-C is thought to be a major etiological factor in atherogenesis. Homocysteine can promote the growth of smooth muscle cells and increase platelet adhesiveness and affect several factors in the coagulation cascade. Thus, homocysteine can be thrombogenic.

Approximately 10% of the population have a defective folate metabolizing enzyme called methylenetetrahydrofolate reductase (MTHFR). MTHFR catalyzes the reduction of 5,10-methylenetetrahydrofolate to 5-methyltetrahydrofolate. 5-Methyltetrahydrofolate transfers its methyl group to homocysteine in the formation of methionine, in a reaction catalyzed by methionine synthase. Flavin adenine dinucleotide (FAD), derived from riboflavin (vitamin B_2) and reduced nicotinamide adenine dinucleotide phosphate (NADPH), derived from niacin, are cofactors in the reaction. Deficiency of MTHFR is the most common inborn error of folate metabolism and is a major genetic cause of hyperhomocysteinemia. The polymorphism A222V (alanine to valine substitution at residue 222 of the enzyme), in which there is a base change at position 677 of its gene, of cytosine to thymine, is homozygous in about 10% of the population. Those homozygous for the T677 allele are found to have elevated homocysteine levels which appear to be associated with an increased risk of vascular disease. The mutant enzyme is thermolabile and does not bind as tightly to its cofactor FAD as does the normal enzyme. Addition of folate

to the mutant enzyme stabilizes its binding to FAD and also stabilizes the enzyme against heat inactivation.

Folic acid may have antiatherogenic mechanisms other than that of lowering homocysteine levels. Impaired availability of endothelium-derived nitric oxide (NO), produced by the enzyme endothelial nitric oxide synthase (eNOS), has been identified as a mediator of atherosclerosis. Folic acid and 5-methyltetrahydrofolate have been demonstrated to restore impaired NO status in hypercholesterolemic subjects. In cultured endothelial cells, 5-methyltetrahydrofolate was found to enhance the enzymatic activity of partially tetrahydrobiopterin (BH_4)-repleted eNOS, enhancing NO formation. BH_4 is the cofactor for eNOS. The enhancement of eNOS activity may be another mechanism for the possible antiatherogenic activity of folic acid.

5-Methyltetrahydrofolate has been found to directly scavenge superoxide radicals *in vitro*. Activated eNOS also decreases the production of superoxide. Uncoupling of eNOS, which occurs under conditions of hypercholesterolemia, results in decreased production of NO and increased production of superoxide. Folate appears to restore impaired NO availability by an ameliorative effect on eNOS uncoupling.

Epidemiologic studies have shown that diminished folate status is associated with colorectal, lung, esophageal, brain, cervical and breast cancers. Data supporting the effect of folate status on carcinogenesis are most compelling for colorectal cancer. The mechanism of the possible anticarcinogenic activity of folate is not well understood. Folate deficiency may induce DNA hypomethylation and gene ''unsilencing.'' Folate is critical for the synthesis of the transmethylating agent S-adenosylmethione (SAMe). SAMe methylates certain bases in DNA leading to gene silencing. Gene ''unsilencing'' alters gene expression and can disrupt the integrity of the genome. DNA hypomethylation appears to be an early, and consistent event in carcinogenesis, including that of colorectal cancer. Folate deficiency may lead to increased uracil incorporation in DNA. Folate is critical for the formation of thymidylic acid from deoxyuridylic acid. Increased uracil incorporation in DNA can lead to disruption of the integrity of DNA. Folate deficiency may also result in diminished DNA repair, impaired natural killer cell surveillance, secondary choline deficiency, decreased stimulation of T lymphocytes by phytohemagglutinin and activation of tumorigenic viruses. A recent report demonstrated that folate deficiency produced progressive DNA strand breaks in the highly conserved region of the p53 tumor-suppressor gene in rat colon.

Low concentrations of folate in the blood have been associated with poor cognitive function, dementia and

Alzheimer's disease-related neurodegeneration of the brain. A recent report from the "Nun Study "showed that low serum folate was strongly associated with atrophy of the cerebral cortex. The mechanism of the neuroprotective effect of folate is not well understood. It has been suggested that elevated homocysteine levels secondary to folate deficiency may account, in large part, for neurodegeneration via increased oxidative stress and endothelial dysfunction, among other things. Elevated serum homocysteine levels were associated with progressive atrophy of the medial temporal lobe in subjects with Alzheimer' s disease, in one study.

Folate deficiency has been associated with depression and other psychiatric symptoms. Consistent findings in major depression have been low plasma and low erythrocyte folate levels which have been linked to poor response to antidepressants. Subjects with low plasma folate levels responded less well to the antidepressant fluoxetine than did those with normal folate levels. A recent study reported that folic acid enhanced the antidepressant action of fluoxetine in subjects who did not appear to be folate deficient. The mechanism by which folate affects brain functions is unclear. It is thought that the most likely explanation is folate's role in the synthesis of S-adenosylmethione (SAMe). 5-Methyltetrahydrofolate is the methyl donor in the formation of methionine from homocysteine. It is thought that this reaction is important for the maintenance of the SAMe pool (SAMe is formed from methionine). SAMe is the methylating agent in the formation of the catecholamine neurotransmitters in the brain. These neurotransmitters are important in maintaining the affective state. SAMe itself has been found to have mood-modulating activity (see SAMe).

PHARMACOKINETICS

Folic acid or pteroylglutamic acid (PGA) is the form of folate used in food fortification and the principal form of folate found in nutritional supplements. Natural food folates are pteroylpolyglutamate derivatives. Pteroylpolyglutamate derivatives are hydrolyzed to pteroylmonoglutamate forms prior to absorption from the small intestine. The enzyme that catalyzes the cleavage is called folate conjugase or gamma-glutamylhydrolase. The monoglutamate forms of folate, including folic acid, are transported across the proximal small intestine via a saturable pH-dependent process. Higher doses of the pteroylmonoglutamates, including folic acid, are absorbed via a nonsaturable passive diffusion process. The efficiency of absorption of the pteroylmonoglutamates is greater than that of the pteroylpolyglutamates.

Because of the difference in absorption efficiency between natural food folate and folic acid, the concept of dietary folate equivalents (DFEs) has been introduced. Folic acid taken on an empty stomach is twice as available as food folate. Folic acid taken with food is 1.7 times as available as food folate. For example, 400 micrograms of folic acid taken on an empty stomach is equivalent to 470 micrograms of folic acid taken with food and is equivalent to 800 micrograms of food folate. DFEs can be calculated as follows:

1 microgram of DFEs = 1 microgram of food folate = 0.5 micrograms of folic acid taken on an empty stomach = 0.6 micrograms of folic acid taken with meals.

Following absorption of physiological amounts of folic acid into the enterocytes, a certain percentage undergoes reduction. Reduced folate is transported to the liver via the portal circulation. Much of a pharmacological dose of folic acid is transported to the liver as such, without first undergoing metabolism in the enterocytes. The various natural pteroylmonoglutamate forms undergo some metabolism in the enterocytes to pteroylpolyglutamate forms, but for the most part are also transported as their unmetabolized forms via the portal circulation to the liver. The folates are taken up by the liver and metabolized to polyglutamate derivatives (principally pteroylpentaglutamates), via the action of folylpolyglutamate synthase. Folates are stored in tissue in their polyglutamate forms. Folate is metabolized to its various metabolic forms in the liver. The various pteroylpolyglutamate forms are the active cellular cofactor forms of folate. Folate polyglutamates are released from the liver to the systemic circulation and to the bile. When released from the liver into the circulation, the polyglutamate forms are hydrolyzed by gamma-glutamylhydrolase and reconverted to the monoglutamate forms.

The principal folate in the plasma is 5-methyltetrahydrofolate in its monoglutate form. 5-Methyltetrahydrofolate circulates in erythrocytes in its polyglutamate form. Approximately two-thirds of folate in plasma is protein bound. All tissue forms of folate are polyglutamates, while circulating forms of folate are monoglutamates. When pharmacological doses of folic acid are administered, a significant amount of unchanged folic acid is found in the plasma. The liver contains approximately 50% of the body stores of folate, or about 6 to 14 milligrams. The total body store of folate is about 12 to 28 milligrams.

Folate is excreted in the urine as folate cleavage products. Intact folate enters the glomerulus and is reabsorbed into the proximal renal tubule. Very little intact folate is excreted in the urine. Folate is excreted in the bile and much of it is reabsorbed via the enterohepatic circulation.

INDICATIONS AND USAGE

Folic acid is indicated for the prevention of some birth defects and appears, as well, to confer significant protection against cardiovascular disease and some forms of cancer.

While available evidence suggests significant preventive/protective effects against various cancers, the use of folic acid as an interventive treatment for cancer is too premature to recommend due to some preliminary findings that it might promote growth of some established cancers. There is very preliminary evidence that folic acid might be helpful in reducing the symptoms of some psychiatric disorders. It has been hypothesized that folic acid supplementation might help prevent Alzheimer's disease and recurrent spontaneous early pregnancy loss, but the research that might confirm or refute these suggestions has not been performed.

RESEARCH SUMMARY

So strong are the data indicating that folic acid can protect against neural tube birth defects that the Food and Drug Administration issued a regulation that became effective in 1998 requiring fortification of all uncooked cereal grain products and all flour with folic acid.

Several studies have shown that women with low plasma folate and vitamin B_{12} concentrations are at significantly increased risk of giving birth to babies with neural tube defects, as well as some other birth defects. Moreover, several double-blind, placebo-controlled studies have demonstrated that neural tube defects can be significantly prevented when women take folic acid supplements during the periconceptional period. A dose of 400 micrograms of folic acid daily is now widely recommended for women of reproductive age.

Additional studies have shown that multivitamin supplements containing folic acid also significantly reduce the incidence of neural tube defects. There is some preliminary indication that periconceptional supplementation with these preparations may reduce the incidence of orofacial clefts, limb defects and cardiovascular anomalies.

In a recent, updated meta-analysis of studies of the relationship between folic acid intakes and plasma homocysteine levels and between the incidence of coronary heart disease, cerebrovascular and peripheral vascular disease and homocysteine levels, these conclusions were reached: The association between elevated homocysteine and these diseases is "consistent and very strong." Folic acid intakes up to 600 micrograms daily significantly reduce homocysteine levels in a dose-dependent fashion.

Based upon findings from this updated meta-analysis, it has been estimated that, for every 50 microgram daily increase in average food folate intake, 4,000 to 18,000 deaths due to cardiovascular disease could be prevented annually. It was further estimated that with population-wide consumption of 400 micrograms daily of supplemental folic acid, 3,000 to 23,000 deaths from cardiovascular disease could be prevented each year. Another group of researchers has estimated

that ten percent of all U.S. heart disease is attributable to elevated homocysteine levels.

Promising as all these observations are, it must be pointed out that the well-designed controlled clinical trials that could conclusively prove the efficacy of folic acid in the prevention and, possibly, the treatment of cardiovascular disease have yet to be conducted.

It has been demonstrated, however, in a prospective, randomized, placebo-controlled trial that folic acid can help prevent some of the deleterious effects of triglyceride-rich lipoproteins on endothelium-dependent vasodilation in healthy volunteers challenged with an acute oral fat load. These protective effects were achieved with oral doses of folic acid (10 milligrams daily for two weeks). These same researchers had previously demonstrated that parenteral administration of folic acid could restore endothelial function *in vivo* in subjects with elevated LDL-cholesterol levels.

In a study of 45 subjects with established cardiovascular disease, folic acid intake was significantly inversely correlated with multiple indices of oxidized LDL-cholesterol. This correlation remained significant even when adjusted for potential confounding variables, including consumption of other vitamins and nutrients.

Folic acid appears to protect against a number of cancers, particularly colorectal cancers. Some 20 epidemiologic studies suggest that those with the highest folate intake have an approximately 40% reduction in risk of this cancer. In the Nurses Health Study, involving 88,756 women, there was a 75% reduction in risk of colorectal cancer among those using multivitamin supplements containing 400 or more micrograms of folic acid for 15 or more years, compared with those not using these supplements. This benefit was calculated after controlling for all relevant potential confounding factors.

Long-term folate supplementation was found, in another study, to reduce the incidence of colorectal neoplasia by 62% in subjects with extensive chronic ulcerative colitis. Such subjects, without this supplementation, typically have a 10-fold to 40-fold increased risk of developing colorectal neoplasia.

In recent double-blind, placebo-controlled studies, administration of 5 to 10 milligrams of folic acid daily for six months to a year had several positive effects, as measured, for example, by a reduced biomarker of colorectal cancer development in patients with either colorectal cancer or adenomas. Another placebo-controlled study involved subjects who were given 1 milligram of folic acid daily following polypectomy. At two years post-surgery, the supplemented group had a recurrence rate half that of the placebo group. Larger multi-center, prospective studies are now in progress to test the effects of 1-5 milligrams of folic acid daily on recurrence of colorectal adenoma.

Effects of folic acid on uterine cervical cancer are in doubt. Earlier reports that folic acid supplementation can bring about reversal or regression of cervical dysplasia have not been confirmed in recent, well-controlled human trials using 5-10 milligrams of folic acid daily for three to six months.

Epidemiological studies hint at the possibility that folic acid might be helpful in preventing cancers of the brain, stomach and esophagus. Other such studies have recently shown considerably stronger evidence that, in both premenopausal and postmenopausal women who consume 15 grams of alcohol daily (the equivalent of one drink), total folate intake of at least 600 micrograms daily is significantly protective against breast cancer. The same protection is not evident in women who consume less than 15 grams of alcohol daily. Two of three case-control studies have also found evidence that folate might be protective against breast cancer in some women.

Another case-control study suggests that folate may be protective against pancreatic cancer in male smokers. Higher baseline serum folate concentrations were associated with a 55% reduction in pancreatic cancer risk, compared with those with lower baseline serum levels of folate.

There have been two studies showing that folic acid, in combination with vitamin B_{12}, can reverse a precursor of bronchial squamous cell cancer of the lung. In one of these randomized, placebo-controlled studies, both of which involved heavy smokers, 10 milligrams of folic acid daily, combined with 500 micrograms of vitamin B_{12} daily, resulted, after four months, in a significant reduction in the number of subjects exhibiting abnormal bronchial cells said to be cancer precursors.

One folate researcher, while observing that "folate appears to be an ideal candidate for chemoprevention given its proven safety and cost," nonetheless cautions that "the optimal dose, duration, and timing, as well as the appropriate target population, of folate chemoprevention need to be clearly defined." This researcher adds that "some animal studies have suggested that supraphysiologic levels of folate supplementation do not confer protection and, in some cases, may enhance carcinogenesis."

In a genetic murine model of colon cancer, for example, folate supplementation prevented development of tumors when administered prior to the presence of any microscopic neoplastic foci. But when supplementation began after the appearance of such foci, it promoted tumor development in this experiment. "Therefore," this researcher concluded, "it

appears that folate supplementation should be implemented before the development of precursor lesions in the target organ or in individuals free of any evidence of neoplastic foci."

Given that there are some reports, as noted above, in which supplemental folic acid appeared to confer benefit in subjects with pre-cancerous lesions, it is not possible to assess risk in this regard without further research, though caution, as expressed by the researcher quoted above, appears to be indicated.

Since there is a reported high incidence of folate deficiency in some psychiatric patients, including those with depression, dementia and schizophrenia, some have suggested that supplemental folic acid might be beneficial in some of these individuals. Some open studies have shown some benefit from folic acid supplementation. Placebo-controlled studies have generally shown no therapeutic effect. These have often used very high doses (15-20 milligrams a day) with what one reviewer has called effects toxic enough to cause, rather than ameliorate, mental symptoms. Two placebo-controlled studies using smaller doses produced benefits in patients with psychopathology associated with folate deficiency and in another group of patients on long-term lithium therapy. The latter were treated with 200 micrograms of folic acid daily.

It has been hypothesized that, since folic acid deficiency is associated with reduced brain levels of S-adenosylmethionine and 5-hydroxytryptamine, supplemental folic acid might be helpful in some with depression. Studies have, in fact, confirmed that serum folate levels are often deficient in those suffering from depression. Whether supplemental folic acid would be of benefit remains unknown.

Similarly, an association has been made recently between low serum folate levels and the severity of atrophy of the neocortex in Alzheimer's disease subjects. But whether supplemental folic acid can be of any help in this disease has not been determined.

Finally, there has recently been a report that elevated homocysteine and reduced serum folate concentrations are significantly associated with recurrent spontaneous early pregnancy losses in humans. The suggestion has thus been made that folic acid supplementation might help prevent these recurrent early pregnancy losses. Again, this hypothesis has not yet been tested.

CONTRAINDICATIONS, PRECAUTIONS, ADVERSE REACTIONS
CONTRAINDICATIONS
Folic acid is contraindicated in those who are hypersensitive to any component of a folic acid-containing product.

PRECAUTIONS

Women of childbearing age, pregnant women and nursing mothers should ensure that their intake of folic acid from nutritional supplements and/or fortified food is 400 micrograms/day. A number of pre- and postnatal supplements deliver 1 milligram (1,000 micrograms) daily of folic acid. Doses higher than 1 milligam/day should only be used by the above groups if prescribed by their physicians.

The use of folic acid for the treatment of folate deficiency or for the treatment of any medical condition requires medical supervision.

The use of folic acid doses above 1 milligram/day may precipitate or exacerbate the neurological damage of vitamin B_{12} deficiency. Those who use folic acid doses above 1 milligram/day should only do so under medical supervision.

Those with undiagnosed anemia, should exercise caution in the use of supplementary folic acid. Doses of folic acid greater than 100 micrograms daily may result in hematologic improvement in those with vitamin B_{12} deficiency.

ADVERSE REACTIONS

Folic acid doses of up to 1 milligram daily are well tolerated. There are more than 100 reported cases in which vitamin B_{12}-deficient subjects who were receiving oral doses of folic acid of 5 milligrams daily or more experienced progression of neurological symptoms and signs. There are very few such reports in those receiving doses of folic acid less than 5 milligrams daily. There are rare reports of hypersensitivity reactions to oral folic acid. There is one report of a trial using oral doses of folic acid of 15 milligrams daily for one month in which some subjects experienced sleep disturbances, mental changes and gastrointestinal effects. Studies using comparable or higher doses, longer duration, or both, failed to confirm these findings.

INTERACTIONS

DRUGS

Anticonvulsants (carbamazepine, fosphenytoin, phenytoin, phenobarbital, primidone valproic acid): These first-generation anticonvulsants may cause decreased serum folate levels and increased serum homocysteine levels. High doses of folic acid may result in decreased serum levels of these drugs.

Cholestyramine: Concomitant use of cholestyramine and folic acid may cause decreased absorption of folic acid.

Colestipol: Concomitant use of colestipol and folic acid may cause decreased absorption of folic acid.

Colchicine: Colchicine is reported to depress blood folate levels.

Fluoxetine: The use of folic acid at a dose of 500 micrograms/day was found to enhance the antidepressant action of fluoxetine given at a dose of 20 milligrams daily in one study.

Lithium: The use of folic acid at a dose of 200 micrograms daily was found to improve the efficacy of maintenance lithium in one study.

Lometrexol: ("T64") Folic acid supplementation in mice was found to augment the therapeutic activity and ameliorate the adverse reactions of the experimental antifolate cancer chemotherapeutic agent lometrexol.

Metformin: Long-term use of metformin has been associated with elevated homocysteine levels which are reduced with folic acid administration.

Methotrexate: The use of folic acid at a dose of 1 milligram daily may significantly reduce the toxic side effects with no reduction in drug efficacy in those undergoing chronic methotrexate therapy for rheumatoid arthritis.

Nonsteroidal antiinflammatory drugs (NSAIDS), including ibuprofen, indomethacin, naproxen, mefenamic acid, piroxicam, sulindac: When taken in large therapeutic doses, these NSAIDS may exert antifolate activity.

Phenytoin: Phenytoin may decrease serum folate levels and negatively affect folate status. High doses of folic acid may cause a decrease in serum phenytoin levels.

Pyrimethamine: The use of high doses of folic acid concomitantly with pyrimethamine to prevent bone marrow depression may cause a pharmacodynamic antagonism of the antiparasitic effect of pyrimethamine.

Sulfasalazine: Sulfasalazine may reduce the absorption of folic acid when used concomitantly.

NUTRITIONAL SUPPLEMENTS

Vitamin B_6: Vitamin B_6 may work synergistically with folic acid in lowering serum homocysteine levels.

Vitamin B_{12}: Vitamin B_{12} may work synergistically with folic acid in lowering homocysteine levels.

Zinc: Supplemental folic acid has been said to adversely affect the absorption of zinc. However, a review of the literature reveals no effect of folic acid supplementation on zinc nutriture.

FOODS

Administration of folic acid with food marginally decreases its availability.

OVERDOSAGE

There are no reports of folic acid overdosage in the literature.

DOSAGE AND ADMINISTRATION

The principal form of supplementary folate is folic acid. Folate triglutamate (pteroyltriglutamate) is also available. Folic acid is available in single ingredient and in combination products. A typical daily dose is 400 micrograms. Unit doses of one milligram or greater require a prescription.

The Food and Nutrition Board of the Institute of Medicine of the National Academy of Sciences has recommended the following Dietary Reference Intakes (RDI) for folate, expressed as dietary folate equivalents (1 microgram of dietary folate equivalents [DFEs]=1 microgram of food folate = 0.5 micrograms of folic acid taken on an empty stomach = 0.6 micrograms of folic acid with meals):

Infants   Adequate Intakes (AI)
0 through 6 months   65 micrograms/day ≈ 9.4 micrograms/Kg

7 through 12 months   80 micrograms/day ≈ 8.8 micrograms/Kg

                               Recommended Dietary
Children   Allowances (RDA)
1 through 3 years   150 micrograms/day
4 through 8 years   200 micrograms/day

Boys
9 through 13 years   300 micrograms/day
14 through 18 years   400 micrograms/day

Girls
9 through 13 years   300 micrograms/day
14 through 18 years   400 micrograms/day

Men
19 years and older   400 micrograms/day

Women
19 years and older   400 micrograms/day

RDA for Pregnancy
14 through 50 years   600 micrograms/day

Lactation
14 through 50 years   500 micrograms/day

The U.S. RDA for folic acid, the value used for nutritional supplement and food labeling purposes, is 400 micrograms/day.

A Lowest-Observed-Adverse-Effect Level (LOAEL) for folate is set by the Food and Nutrition Board at 5 milligrams/day. Based on this LOAEL and assuming an uncertainty factor (UF) of 5, the Food and Nutrition Board has recommended the following Tolerable Upper Intake Levels (UL) for folate from fortified foods or supplements (folic acid):

Adults   (UL)
19 years and older   1,000 micrograms/day

Infants
                               Not possible to establish
0 through 12 months   for supplemental folic acid

Children
1 through 3 years   300 micrograms/day
4 through 8 years   400 micrograms/day
9 through 13 years   600 micrograms/day
14 through 18 years   800 micrograms/day

Pregnancy
14 through 18 years   800 micrograms/day
19 years and older   1,000 micrograms/day

Lactation
14 through 18 years   800 micrograms/day
19 years and older   1,000 micrograms/day

HOW SUPPLIED

Folic Acid is available in the following forms and strengths for Rx use:

Injection — 5 mg/mL

Tablets — 1 mg

Folic Acid is available in the following forms and strengths for OTC use:

Tablets — 0.4 mg, 0.8 mg

LITERATURE

Aarsand AK, Carlsen SM. Folate administration reduces circulating homocysteine levels in NIDDM patients on long-term metformin treatment. *J Intern Med*. 1998; 244:169-174.

Alati T, Worzalla JF, Shih C, et al. Augmentation of the therapeutic activity of lometrexol [(6-*R*)5,10-dideazetetra-hydrofolate] by oral folic acid. *Cancer Res*. 1996; 56:2331-2335.

Alpert JE, Fava M. Nutrition and depression: the role of folate. *Nutr Rev*. 1997; 55:145-149.

Anon. How folate fights disease. *Nature Struct biol*. 1999; 6:293-294.

Anon. Recommendations for the use of folic acid to reduce the number of cases of spina bifida and other neural tube defects. *MMWR Morb Mortal Wkly Rep*. 1992; 42(RR-14):1-7.

Berry RJ, Li Z, Erickson JD, et al. Prevention of neural-tube defects with folic acid in China. *N Eng J Med*. 1999; 341:1485-1490.

Boushey CJ, Beresford SA, Omenn GS, Motulsky AG. A quantitative assessment of plasma homocysteine as a risk factor for vascular disease. Probable benefits of increasing folic acid intakes. *JAMA*. 1995; 274:1049-1057.

Branda RF, Moldow CF, MacArthur JR, et al. Folate-induced remission in aplastic anemia with familial defect of cellular folate uptake. *N Eng J Med.* 1978; 298:469-475.

Butterworth CE Jr, Bendich A. Folic acid and the prevention of birth defects. *Annu Rev Nutr.* 1996; 16:73-97.

Butterworth CE Jr, Hatch KD, Macaluso M, et al. Folate deficiency and cervical dysplasia. *JAMA.* 1992; 267:528-533.

Butterworth CE Jr, Hatch KD, Soong SJ, et al. Oral folic acid supplementation for cervical dysplasia: a clinical intervention trial. *Am J Obstet Gynecol.* 1992; 166:803-809.

Campbell NRC. How safe are folic acid supplements? *Arch Intern Med.* 1996; 156:1638-1644.

Choi S-W, Mason JB. Folate and carcinogenesis: An integrated scheme. *J Nutr.* 2000; 130:129-132.

Coppen A, Bailey J. Enhancement of the antidepressant action of fluoxetine by folic acid: a randomized, placebo controlled trial. *J Affect Disord.* 2000; 60:121-130.

Coppen A, Chaudhry S, Swade C. Folic acid enhances lithium prophylaxis. *J Affect Disord.* 1986; 10:9-13.

Czeizel AE, Dudás I. Prevention of the first occurrence of neural-tube defects by periconceptional vitamin supplementation. *N Eng J Med.* 1992; 327:1832-1835.

Dietary Reference Intakes for Thiamin, Riboflavin, Niacin, Vitamin B6, Folate, Vitamin B12, Pantothenic Acid, Biotin, and Choline. Washington, DC: National Academy Press; 1998.

Giovannucci E, Stampfer MJ, Colditz GA, et al. Multivitamin use, folate, and colon cancer in women in the Nurses' Health Study. *Ann Intern Med.* 1998; 129:517-524.

Glade MJ. Workshop on folate, B12, and choline. Sponsored by the Panel on Folate and other B Vitamins of the Standing Committee on the Scientific Evaluation of Dietary Reference Intakes, Food and Nutrition Board, Institute of Medicine, Washington, D.C., March 3-4, 1997. *Nutrition.* 1999; 15:92-96.

Guenther BD, Sheppard CA, Tran P, et al. The structure and properties of methylenetetrahydrofolate reductase from *Escherichia coli* suggest how folate ameliorates human hyperhomocysteinemia. *Nature Struct Biol.* 1999; 6:359-365.

Heimburger DC, Alexander CB, Birch R, et al. Improvement in bronchial squamous metaplasia in smokers treated with folate and vitamin B12. Report of a preliminary randomized, double-blind intervention trial. *JAMA.* 1988; 259:1525-1530.

Herbert V. Folic acid. In: Shils ME, Olson JA, Shike M, Ross AC, eds. *Modern Nutrition in Health and Disease.* 9th ed. Baltimore, MD: Williams and Wilkins; 1999:433-446.

Homocysteine Lowering Trialists' Collaboration. Lowering blood homocysteine with folic acid based supplements: meta-analysis of randomized trials. *Brit Med J.* 1998; 316:894-898.

Hopkins PN, Wu LL, Wu J, et al. Higher plasma homocysteine and increased susceptibility to adverse effects of low folate in early familial coronary artery disease. *Arterioscler Thromb Vasc Biol.* 1995; 15:1314-1320.

Jacques PF, Selhub J, Bostom AG, et al. The effect of folic acid fortification on plasma folate and total homocysteine concentrations. *N Engl J Med.* 1999; 340:1449-1454.

Jacob RA. Folate, DNA methylation, and gene expression: factors of nature and nurture. *Am J Clin Nutr.* 2000; 72:903-904.

Kim Y-I. Folate and Cancer Prevention: A new medical application of folate beyond hyperhomocysteinemia and neural tube defects. *Nutr Rev.* 1999; 57:314-321.

Kim Y-I. Folate and carcinogenesis: Evidence, mechanisms, and implications. *J Nut Biochem.* 1999; 10:66-88.

Kim Y-I. Methyletetrahydrofolate reductase polymorphisms, folate and cancer risk: a paradigm of gene-nutrient interactions in carcinogenesis. *Nutr Rev.* 2000; 58:205-209.

Kim Y-I, Shirwadkar S, Choi S-W, et al. Effects of dietary folate on DNA strand breaks within mutation-prone exons of the p53 gene in the rat colon. *Gastroenterol.* 2000; 119:151-161.

Lucock M. Folic acid: nutritional biochemistry, molecular biology, and role in disease processes. *Mol Genet Metab.* 2000; 71:121-138.

Malinow MR, Duell PB, Hess DL, et al. Reduction of plasma homocyst(e)ine levels by breakfast cereal fortified with folic acid in patients with heart disease. *N Eng J Med.* 1998; 338:1009-1015.

Mills JL. Fortification of foods with folic acid-how much is enough? *N Eng J Med.* 2000; 342:1442-1445.

Morgan SL, Baggott JE, Vaughn WH, et al. Supplementation with folic acid during methotrexate therapy for rheumatoid arthritis. A double-blind, placebo-controlled trial. *Ann Intern Med.* 1994; 121:833-841.

MRC Vitamin Study Research Group Prevention of neural tube defects: results of the Medical Council Vitamin Study. *Lancet.* 1991; 388:131-137.

Nelen WL, Blom HJ, Steegers EA, et al. Homocysteine and folate levels as risk factors for recurrent early pregnancy loss. *Obstet Gynecol.* 2000; 95:519-524.

Oakley GP Jr. Eat right *and* take a multivitamin. *N Eng J Med.* 1998; 338:1060-1061.

Rampersaud GC, Kauwell GPA, Hutson AD, Cerda JJ, Bailey LB. Genomic DNA methylation decreases in response to moderate folate depletion in elderly women. *Am J Clin Nutr.* 2000:72:998-1003.

Rimm EB, Willett WC, Hu FB, et al. Higher intake of folate and vitamin B6 is associated with low rates of coronary artery disease in women. *JAMA.* 1998; 279:359-364.

Rosenquist TH, Ratashak SA, Selhub J. Homocysteine induces congenital defects of the heart and neural tube: Effect of folic acid. *Proc Natl Acad Sci USA.* 1996; 93:15227-15232.

Scholl TO, Johnson WG. Folic acid: influence on the outcome of pregnancy. *Am J Clin Nutr.* 2000; 71:1295S-1303S.

Snowdon DA, Tully CL, Smith CD, et al. Serum folate and the severity of atrophy of the neocortex in Alzheimer disease: findings from the Nun Study. *Am J Clin Nutr.* 2000; 71:993-998.

Song J, Sohn KJ, Medline A, et al. Chemopreventive effects of dietary folate on intestinal polyps in Apc+/-Msh2-/-mice. *Cancer Res.* 2000; 60:3191-3199.

Stroes ESG, van Faassen EE, Yo M, et al. Folic acid reverts dysfunctional nitric oxide synthase. *Circ Res.* 2000; 86:1129-1134.

Title LM, Cummings PM, Giddens K, et al. Effect of folic acid and antioxidant vitamins on endothelial dysfunction in patients with coronary artery disease. *J Amer Coll Cardiol.* 2000; 36:758-765.

Voutilainen S, Lakka TA, Porkkala-Sarataho E, et al. Low serum folate concentrations are associated with an excess incidence of acute coronary events: the Kuopio Ischaemic Heart Disease Risk Factor Study. *Eur J Clin Nutr.* 2000; 54:424-428.

Wilmink HW, Stroes ESG, Erkelens WD, et al. Influence of folic acid on postprandial endothelial dysfunction. *Arterioscler Thromb Vasc Biol.* 2000; 20:185-188.

Woo KS, Chook P, Lolin YI, et al. Folic acid improves arterial endothelial function in adults with hyperhomocysteinemia. *J Am Coll Cardiol.* 1999; 34:2002-2006.

Zhang S, Hunter DJ, Hankinson SE, et al. A prospective study of folate intake and the risk of breast cancer. *JAMA.* 1999; 281:1632-1637.

Fructo-oligosaccharides

DESCRIPTION

Fructo-oligosaccharides (FOS) typically refer to short-chain oligosaccharides comprised of D-fructose and D-glucose, containing from 3 to 5 monosaccharide units. Similar molecules are obtained by partial enzymatic hydrolysis of inulins (see Inulins). Those are called oligofructose. FOS, also called neosugar and short-chain FOS (scFOS), are produced on a commercial scale from sucrose using a fungal fructosyltransferase enzyme.

FOS are comprised of one molecule of D-glucose in the terminal position and from 2 to 4 D-fructose units. FOS containing 2 fructose residues is abbreviated GF_2 (G is for glucose, F, for fructose). Those with 3 fructoses are abbreviated GF_3, and those with 4 fructoses, GF_4. GF_2 is also called 1-kestose and GF_3 is called nystose. The linkage between fructose units in FOS is a beta-(2-1) glycosidic link. The structural formula is represented below.

Fructo-oligosaccharides
(The top sugar is glucose. n = 2-4 fructose residues)

FOS are resistant to digestion in the stomach and small intestine. The reason for this is the presence of the beta configuration of the anomeric C_2 in the D-fructose residues. The human digestive enzymes sucrase, maltase-isomaltase and alpha-glucosidase are specific for alpha-glycosidic linkages. FOS are considered nondigestible oligosaccharides. They are, however, fermented by a limited number of colonic bacteria. This could lead to changes in the colonic ecosystem in favor of some bacteria, such as bifidobacteria, which appear to be beneficial in some respects. FOS and other nondigestible oligosaccharides are referred to as bifidogenic factors.

Substances such as FOS that may promote the growth of beneficial bacteria in the colon are called prebiotics. Prebiotics are typically nondigestible oligosaccharides.

ACTIONS AND PHARMACOLOGY

ACTIONS

FOS may have anticarcinogenic, antimicrobial, hypolipidemic and hypoglycemic actions in some. They may also help improve mineral absorption and balance, and may have anti-osteoporotic and anti-osteopenic activities.

MECHANISM OF ACTION

The possible anticarcinogenic activity of FOS might be accounted for, in part, by the possible anticarcinogenic action of butyrate. Butyrate, along with other short-chain fatty acids, is produced by bacterial fermentation of FOS in the colon. Some studies suggest that butyrate may induce growth arrest and cell differentiation, and may also upregulate apoptosis, three activities that could be significant for antitumor activity. FOS may also aid in increasing the concentrations of calcium and magnesium in the colon. High concentrations of these cations in the colon may help control the rate of cell turnover. High concentrations of calcium in the colon may also lead to the formation of insoluble bile or salts of fatty acids. This might reduce the potential damaging effects of bile or fatty acids on colonocytes.

FOS may promote the growth of favorable bacterial populations, such as bifidobacteria, in the colon. Bifidobacteria may inhibit the growth of pathogenic bacteria, such as *Clostridium perfringens* and diarrheogenic strains of *Escherichia coli*.

FOS may lower serum triglyceride levels in some. The mechanism of this possible effect is unclear. Decreased hepatocyte triglyceride synthesis is a hypothetical possibility. FOS may also lower total cholesterol and LDL-cholesterol levels in some. Again, the mechanism of this possible effect is unclear. Propionate, a product of FOS fermentation in the colon, may inhibit HMG-CoA reductase, the rate-limiting step in cholesterol synthesis.

The possible effects of FOS on blood glucose may be explained in a few ways. FOS may delay gastric emptying and/or shorten small-intestinal tract transit time. Propionate may inhibit gluconeogenesis by its metabolic conversion to methylmalonyl-CoA and succinyl-CoA. These metabolites could inhibit pyruvate carboxylase. Propionate may also reduce plasma levels of free fatty acids. High levels of free fatty acids lower glucose utilization and induce insulin resistance. Propionate may enhance glycolysis via depletion of citrate in hepatocytes. Citrate is an allosteric inhibitor of phosphofructokinase.

FOS may bind/sequester such minerals as calcium and magnesium in the small intestine. The short-chain fatty acids formed from the bacterial fermentation of FOS may facilitate the colonic absorption of calcium and, possibly, also magnesium ions. This could be beneficial in preventing osteoporosis and osteopenia.

PHARMACOKINETICS

Little digestion of FOS occurs in the stomach and small intestine following ingestion of FOS. FOS are fermented in the colon by bifidobacteria and some other bacteria to produce the short-chain fatty acids (SCFA) acetate, propionate and butyrate; the gases hydrogen, hydrogen sulfide, carbon dioxide and methane; and lactate, pyruvate and succinate. Some acetate, propionate and butyrate is absorbed from the colon and transported by the circulation to various tissues where these SCFA undergo further metabolism. Many SCFA are metabolized by the colonocyes. Butyrate is an important respiratory fuel for the colonocytes.

Those with ileostomies may have a microbial population colonizing their ileums. In those cases, FOS could be fermented by some of the bacteria, much as they are in the colon.

INDICATIONS AND USAGE

Fructo-oligosaccharides appear to be of benefit in modulating the microbial ecology of the gut, boosting gastrointestinal immunity. FOS may also protect against colon cancer, and may have favorable lipid effects in some. FOS may also aid in calcium absorption.

RESEARCH SUMMARY

There is evidence that FOS can improve the microbial ecology of the gut and protect against some bacterial pathogens, particularly in the large intestine. FOS selectively stimulate the growth of bifidobacteria and also have many of the actions and benefits of dietary fibers.

A fermented milk product containing FOS significantly lowered LDL-cholesterol levels in male subjects with borderline elevated levels of serum total cholesterol. This double-blind, placebo-controlled study extended for three weeks. Other studies have credited FOS with lowering both cholesterol and triglyceride levels. FOS have been shown to lower hepatic lipogenesis. In one recent study, however, 15 grams of FOS daily for 20 days failed to favorably affect either blood glucose levels or serum lipid concentrations in patients with type 2 diabetes. More research is needed.

There is experimental evidence that FOS might inhibit colon cancer. In an animal model for both familial adenomatous polyposis and sporadic colon cancers, FOS were said to "dramatically" reduce the incidence of colon tumors.

FOS have also been shown to increase calcium absorption in animal studies.

CONTRAINDICATIONS, PRECAUTIONS, ADVERSE REACTIONS

CONTRAINDICATIONS

FOS are contraindicated in those who are hypersensitive to these substances. They are also contraindicated in those who are hypersensitive to inulins.

PRECAUTIONS

Those who develop gastrointestinal symptoms with the use of dietary fiber should exercise some caution in the use of FOS. Those with irritable bowel syndrome should exercise caution in the use of FOS. Those receiving whole body radiation or radiation to the gastrointestinal tract should avoid FOS supplements.

Those with lactose intolerance should exercise caution in the use of doses of FOS greater than 10 grams daily.

ADVERSE REACTIONS

Doses up to 10 grams daily are well tolerated. Higher doses may cause gastrointestinal symptoms. Doses greater than 30 grams daily can cause flatus. Doses greater than 40 grams daily can cause borborygmi and bloating. Doses greater than 50 grams daily can cause cramps and diarrhea. Some are more sensitive to FOS and may develop gastrointestinal symptoms at lower doses. Those with lactose intolerance have been reported to experience gastrointestinal symptoms at a dose of 25 grams.

DOSAGE AND ADMINISTRATION

FOS are available as nutritional supplements and in functional foods. Dosing is variable and ranges from 4 to10 grams daily and sometimes higher. Those who use more than 10 grams daily should split the dosage throughout the day.

LITERATURE

Alles MS, de Roos NM, Bakx JC, et al. Consumption of fructo-oligosaccharides does not favorably affect blood glucose and serum lipid concentrations in patients with type 2 diabetes. *Am J Clin Nutr.* 1999; 69:64-69.

Bouhnik Y, Vahedi K, Achour L, et al. Short-chain fructo-oligosaccharide administration dose-dependently increases fecal bifidobacteria in healthy humans. *J Nutr.* 1999; 129:113-116.

Buddington RK, Williams CH, Chen SC, Witherly SA. Dietary supplement of neosugar alters the fecal flora and decreases activities of some reductive enzymes in human subjects. *Am J Clin Nutr.* 1996; 63:709-716.

Luo J, van Yperselle M, Rizkalla SW, et al. Chronic consumption of short-chain fructo-oligasaccharides does not affect basal hepatic glucose production or insulin resistance in type 2 diabetics. *J Nutr.* 2000; 130:1572-1577.

Ohta A, Baba S, Takizawa T, Adachi T. Effects of fructo-oligosaccharides on the absorption of magnesium in the magnesium-deficient rat model. *J Nutr Sci Vitaminol (Tokyo).* 1994; 40:171-180.

Ohta A, Motohashi Y, Sakai K, et al. Dietary fructo-oligosaccharides increase calcium absorption and levels of mucosal calbindin-D9K in the large intestine of gastrectomized rats. *Scand J Gastroenterol.* 1998; 33:1062-1068.

Ohta A, Ohtsuki M, Hosoro A, et al. Dietary fructo-oligosaccharides prevent osteopenia after gastrectomy. *J Nutr.* 1998; 128:106-110.

Oku T, Tokunaga T, Hosoya N. Nondigestibility of a new sweetener, ''Neosugar,'' in the rat. *J Nutr.* 1984; 114:1574-1581.

Pierre F, Perrin P, Champ M, et al. Short-chain fructo-oligosaccharides reduce the occurrence of colon tumors and develop gut-associated lymphoid tissue in Min mice. *Cancer Res.* 1997; 57: 225-228.

Roberfroid MB, Delzenne NM. Dietary fructans. *Annu Rev Nutr.* 1998; 18:117-143.

Sahaafsma G, Meuling WJ, van Dokkum W, Bouley C. Effects of a milk product, fermented by *Lactobaccilus acidophilus* and with fructo-oligosaccharides added, on blood lipids in male volunteers. *Eur J Clin Nutr.* 1998; 52:436-440.

Teuri U, Vapaatalo H, Korpela R. Fructo-oligosaccharides and lactulose cause more symptoms in lactose maldigesters and subjects with pseudohypolactasia than in control lactose digesters. *Am J Clin Nutr.* 1999; 69:973-979.

Gamma-Butyrolactone (GBL)

> Products containing gamma-butyrolactone (GBL) or 1, 4 butanediol (BD) should not be used by anyone for supplementation.

DESCRIPTION

Gamma-butyrolactone or GBL is an organic oily liquid that is used as an intermediate in the synthesis of such substances as polyvinypyrrolidone and is also used as a solvent for polyacrylonitrile and cellulose acetate, among others. GBL is a constituent of paint removers, textile oils and drilling oils.

The reason GBL was introduced into the dietary supplement marketplace is because it is easily converted into gamma-hydroxybutyrate (GHB) after ingestion and is used as a prodrug of GHB.

GBL is also known chemically as dihydro-2 (3H)-furanone; butyrolactone; 1,2-butanolide; 1,4-butanolide; gamma-hydroxybutyric acid lactone; 3-hydroxybutyric acid lactone and 4-hydroxybutanoic acid lactone. The chemical structure is as follows:

Gamma-Butyrolactone

GHB has been classified as a schedule I substance and is illegal to use except in certain FDA-allowed clinical trials.

FDA has asked all GBL dietary supplement producers to recall their products.

Another organic solvent, 1,4 butanediol or BD, also gets converted to gamma-hydroxybutyrate upon ingestion. FDA has issued a warning regarding products that contain BD.

For more information on this substance, refer to the Gamma-Hydroxybutyrate (GHB) monograph.

LITERATURE

FDA. Warning on dietary supplements. *JAMA.* 1999; 282:1218.

Lo Vecchio F, Curry SC, Bagnasco T. Butyrolactone-induced central nervous system depression after ingestion of RenewTrient, a "dietary supplement." *NEJM*. 1998; 339:847-848.

MMWR Morb Mortal Wkly Rep. Adverse events associated with ingestion of gamma-butyrolactone-Minnesota, New Mexico, and Texas, 1998-1999. 1999; 48:137-140.

Poldrugo F, Snead OC 3d. 1, 4 Butanediol gamma-hydroxybutyric acid and ethanol. *Neuropharmacology*. 1984; 23:109-113.

Ramburg-Schepens MO, Buffet M, Durak C, Mathieu-Nolf M. Gamma-butyrolactone poisoning and its similarities to gamma-hydroxybutyric acid: two cases. *Vet Hun Toxicol*. 1997; 39:234-235.

Gamma-Hydroxybutyrate (GHB)

It is illegal to use GHB except if enrolled in certain FDA-allowed clinical trials or for FDA-approved indications.

DESCRIPTION

Gamma-hydroxybutyrate or GHB was sold in the 1980s as a nutritional supplement. It was used mainly as a claimed aid to bodybuilding and sleep. In November, 1990, FDA banned the OTC sale of GHB following reports of severe illness, including seizures and coma associated with use of GHB. In February, 2000, the U.S. House of Representatives approved federal legislation making GHB illegal while allowing medical formulations to be available for clinical testing and potential medical use. Illicitly made GHB is now a schedule I substance in company with heroin, LSD and cocaine. Medically formulated GHB, such as that being developed for the treatment of narcolepsy, is classified as a schedule III substance.

Gamma-hydroxybutyrate is also known chemically as 4-hydroxybutyrate and oxybate and is represented by the following chemical formula:

$$HO-CH_2-CH_2-CH_2-COOH$$

Gamma-Hydroxybutyric acid (GHB)

It typically is in the form of sodium oxybate, sodium gamma-hydroxybutyrate or sodium 4-hydroxybutyrate. Other names used for GHB have been liquid ecstasy, liquid X, somatomax PM and Gamma-OH. Some of the effects of GHB are reported to be similar to the effects of 3,4-methylenedioxymethamphetamine or MDMA, more commonly known as ecstasy.

GHB is found naturally in animal tissues, including the brain, kidney, heart muscle and fat. It was synthesized in 1969 and used in Europe as an intravenous anesthetic agent. It was also found to be useful for narcolepsy and is being developed for that use in the U.S. Studies to date indicate that GHB may reduce EDS or excessive daytime sleepiness in these patients.

ACTIONS AND PHARMACOLOGY

ACTIONS

GHB has anesthetic and hypnotic actions.

MECHANISM OF ACTIONS

GHB is derived from the neurotransmitter gamma-aminobutyric acid (GABA) and is also converted to GABA. GHB is thought to function as an inhibitory chemical transmitter in the central nervous system. Further, it is thought that its central nervous system depressant effect is probably mediated through specific receptors for GHB as well as interaction with the GABA (B) receptor.

GHB is also thought to be a specific inhibitor of central dopamine release. And, under certain conditions, e.g. during sedation or anesthesia or in the presence of a high concentration of calcium, GHB may stimulate dopamine release.

GHB has been found to stimulate the release of growth hormone when administered intravenously in healthy male volunteers.

PHARMACOKINETICS

Following oral ingestion, GHB is rapidly absorbed from the gastrointestinal tract and transported by the portal circulation to the liver where most of it gets metabolized to carbon dioxide and water by first-pass metabolism pathways. A certain amount crosses the blood-brain barrier. Mean value for the terminal half life ranges from 20 to 23 minutes.

INDICATIONS AND USAGE

GHB is regarded as an experimental drug. There are no indications for its use as a supplement. It is illegal to use it as a supplement.

RESEARCH SUMMARY

GHB has been banned as a supplement by the Food and Drug Administration. It is regarded as an experimental drug and can be used only in approved clinical trials. There are, however, products being sold that contain gamma-butyrolactone (GBL) for which many claims are made. GBL is converted in the body to GHB. Claims for GBL include anti-depressive effects, sleep aid, growth-hormone releaser, sexual and athletic enhancers. None of these claims has been proved. Several cases of GBL toxicity have been reported, manifestations of which include bradycardia, hypothermia, central nervous system depression and uncontrolled movements. Use of any GBL/GHB products is inadvisable.

CONTRAINDICATIONS, PRECAUTIONS, ADVERSE REACTIONS

CONTRAINDICATIONS

GHB is contraindicated in those with seizure disorders, those with bradycardia and other conditions associated with defects of cardiac conduction, those with cardiovascular disease, Cushing's syndrome, severe hypertension, hyperprolactinemia and those with severe illness of any kind.

PRECAUTIONS

GHB is illegal to use except if enrolled in certain FDA-allowed clinical trials or for any FDA-approved indications. Gamma-butyrolactone (GBL) and 1,4 butanediol (BD) are chemicals that may be available. GBL and BD are metabolized to GHB in the body and should be avoided by all.

Under no conditions should GHB, GBL or BD be used with alcohol, benzodiazepines, skeletal muscle relaxants, opioids, antihistamines, barbiturates, anticonvulsants, major tranquilizers or protease inhibitors.

ADVERSE REACTIONS

The most common adverse events reported in patients participating in U.S. clinical trials of the effects of sodium oxybate (sodium gamma-hydroxybutyrate) for the treatment of narcolepsy are dizziness, nausea, headache and enuresis. In these trials, subjects were randomized to doses of 3, 6 or 9 grams daily, and the side effects appeared to be dose-related.

Other adverse effects reported in those taking GHB include vomiting, lightheadedness, confusion, abnormal muscle movements, bradycardia, drowsiness, incoordination, orthostatic hypotension, diarrhea, loss of bladder control, loss of consciousness, temporary amnesia, sleepwalking and seizure-like activity.

INTERACTIONS

GHB taken with any of the following drugs may lead to life-threatening situations: alcohol, anticonvulsants, benzodiazepines, antihistamines (particularly sedating antihistamines), skeletal muscle relaxants, major tranquilizers, opioids and protease inhibitors used for the treatment of HIV.

OVERDOSAGE

It is unclear whether GHB ingestion alone can be fatal (without co-ingesting other CNS depressant agents or other drugs). Symptoms of GHB overdosage include markedly decreased levels of consciousness, bradycardia, hypothermia, respiratory acidosis and emesis. Patients typically regain consciousness spontaneously within five hours of ingestion.

GHB ingestion in a patient taking the protease inhibitors ritonavir and saquinavir caused a near-fatal reaction. Co-ingestion of GHB and alcohol and other "recreational drugs" has been associated with low respiratory rates (at times requiring intubation), coma and death. Over 145 cases of GHB poisoning, including eight deaths, have been reported. Typically, those involved were using other CNS-depressant agents such as alcohol along with GHB. These reports include ingestions of substances such as gamma-butyrolactone (GB) and 1,4 butanediol, both of which are converted to GHB in the body.

DOSAGE AND ADMINISTRATION

It is illegal to use GHB except if enrolled in certain FDA-allowed clinical trials or for FDA-approved indications.

LITERATURE

CDC. Gamma-hydroxybutyrate use-New York and Texas, 1995-1996. *MMWR*. 1997; 46:281-283.

Centers for disease control and prevention. Multistate outbreak of poisonings associated with illicit use of gamma-hydroxybutyrate. *MMWR*. 1990; 39:861-863.

Chin RL, Spores KA, Cullison B. Clinical course of gamma-hydroxybutyrate overdose. *Ann Emerg Med*. 1998; 31:716-722.

FDA. Warning on dietary supplements. *JAMA*. 1999; 282, 1218.

Harrington RD, Woodward JA, Hooton TM, Horn JR. Life-threatening interactions between HIV-I protease inhibitors and the illicit drugs MDMA and gamma-hydroxybutyrate. *Arch Intern Med*. 1999; 159:2221-2224.

Lammers GL, Arends J, Declerck AC, et al. Gamma-hydroxybutyrate and narcolepsy: a double-blind, placebo-controlled study. *Sleep*. 1993; 16:216-220.

Mamclak M, Scharf MB, Woods M. Treatment of narcolepsy with gamma-hydroxybutyrate. A review of clinical and sleep laboratory findings. *Sleep*. 1986; 9(1 pt 2):285-289.

Takahara J, Yunoki S, Yakushiji W, et al. Stimulatory effects of gamma-hydroxybutyric acid on growth hormone and prolactin release in humans. *J Clin Endocrinol Metab*. 1977; 44:1014-1017.

Tunnicliff G. Sites of action of gamma-hydroxybutyrate(GHB)-a neuroactive drug with abuse potential. *J Toxicol Clin Toxicol*. 1997; 35:581-590.

Gamma-Linolenic Acid (GLA)

TRADE NAMES

Tona-lean 1000 CLA (Action Labs) and Star GLA (GNC).

DESCRIPTION

Gamma-linolenic acid or GLA is an n-6 (omega-6) polyunsaturated fatty acid. It is comprised of 18 carbon atoms and three double bonds. GLA is an a11-cis n-6 polyunsaturated fatty acid also known as GLA, 18: 3n-6; 6,9,12-octadecatrienoic acid; (Z, Z, Z)- 6,9,12-octadecatrienoic acid; cis-6, cis-9, cis-12-octadecatrienoic acid, and gamolenic acid. The structural formula of GLA is:

GLA (gamma-linolenic acid)

GLA is found naturally to varying extents in the fatty acid fraction of some plant seed oils. In evening primrose seed oil, it is present in concentrations of 7 to 14% of total fatty acids; in borage seed oil, 20 to 27%; and in blackcurrant seed oil, 15 to 20%. GLA is also found in some fungal sources. GLA is produced naturally in the body as the delta 6-desaturase metabolite of the essential fatty acid linoleic acid. Under certain conditions, e.g. decreased activity of the delta-6 desaturase enzyme, GLA may become a conditionally essential fatty acid. GLA is present naturally in the form of triacylglycerols (TAGs). The stereospecifity of GLA varies among different oil sources. GLA is concentrated in the sn-3 position of evening primrose seed oil and blackcurrant seed oil and in the sn-2 position in borage seed oil. GLA is concentrated evenly in both the sn-2 and sn-3 positions of fungal oil.

ACTIONS AND PHARMACOLOGY

ACTIONS
GLA may have anti-inflammatory and antithrombotic actions. It may also have lipid-lowering activity.

MECHANISM OF ACTION
The anti-inflammatory and anti-aggregatory actions can be accounted for by reviewing its role in eicosanoid biosyntheses. GLA is a precursor in the synthesis of prostaglandin E_1 (PGE_1) as well as the series-3 prostaglandins. It also serves as a precursor in the synthesis of eicosapentaenoic acid (EPA). EPA is a precursor of the series-3 prostaglandins, the series-5 leukotrienes and the series-3 thromboxanes. These eicosanoids have anti-thrombogenic, anti-inflammatory and anti-atherogenic properties. PGE_1 inhibits platelet aggregation and has a vasodilation action. The incorporation of GLA and it metabolites in cell membranes may also play a role in the possible anti-inflammatory and anti-proliferative actions of GLA.

PHARMACOKINETICS
GLA-laden triacylglycerols (TAGs) following ingestion undergo hydrolysis via lipases to form monoglycerides and free fatty acids. Once formed, the monoglycerides and free fatty acids are absorbed by the enterocytes. In the enterocytes, a reacylation takes place reforming TAGs that are then assembled with phospholipids, cholesterol and apoproteins into chylomicrons. The chylomicrons are released into the lymphatics from whence they are transported to the systemic circulation. In the circulation, the chylomicrons are degraded by lipoprotein lipase and the fatty acids including GLA are distributed to various tissues in the body.

GLA is metabolized to the 20 carbon polyunsaturated fatty acid, dihomo-gamma-linolenic acid (DHLA) or eicosatrienoic acid (ETA), which is converted to prostaglandin E_1 (PGE_1). It is also metabolized to eicosapentaenoic acid (EPA). GLA and DHLA are normally not found in the free state in the cell to any appreciable degree but occur as components of phospholipids, neutral lipids and cholesterol esters, mainly in cell membranes. PGE_1 is metabolized to smaller prostaglandin remnants, which are primarily polar dicarboxylic acids. Most of the metabolites are excreted in the urine.

INDICATIONS AND USAGE
GLA appears to be effective in some cases of rheumatoid arthritis and may be indicated in some other inflammatory disorders, such as Sjogren's syndrome and ulcerative colitis. Possible other indications include diabetic neuropathy, acute respiratory distress syndrome, hypertension and elevated serum lipids. GLA has been used with some success in some cancers, principally cerebral gliomas. It has not proved useful for tardive dyskinesia, premenstrual syndrome or menopausal flushing. It may be indicated in some cases for atopic eczema and atopic dermatitis, particularly to help with itching, as well as for uremic skin conditions in hemodialysis patients. It should probably not be used in efforts to enhance immunity as it may be immunosuppressive.

RESEARCH SUMMARY
GLA, supplied in the form of evening primrose oil or borage seed oil, has been studied for many years for its possible effects in arthritis and other inflammatory processes. This is not surprising given its ability to modulate the pathways toward an anti-inflammatory state. It has been shown to suppress inflammation and reduce joint tissue injury in many animal models. Since an early double-blind study demonstrated significant improvement in sufferers of rheumatoid arthritis (RA) who received 540 milligrams of GLA per day for a year (relapsing when switched to placebo for three months), several other clinical studies have followed. These have yielded some encouraging results.

In a randomized double-blind, placebo-controlled study of RA sufferers, those receiving 1.4 grams of GLA in borage seed oil daily experienced significant relief. GLA reduced the number of tender joints 36% and the swollen joint count by 28%. Those on placebo experienced no significant improvement or declined in condition. The dose used in this study was much higher than in most other studies. Other recent studies similarly suggest that GLA is an effective treatment option for some with RA, particularly given its safety profile.

There is preliminary evidence that GLA might also be useful in Sjogren's syndrome and perhaps some other rheumatological disorder. It may be helpful for various dry-eye conditions. Recent animal work suggests GLA may enhance calcium absorption, reduce calcium excretion and increase calcium deposition in bone and thus play a therapeutic role in managing and preventing osteoporosis. A clinical pilot study noted encouraging results in elderly women given supplements of GLA, eicosapentaenoic acid (EPA) along with calcium carbonate. Those treated experienced increased lumbar and femoral bone mineral density over 36 months.

There is some evidence that prolonged use of GLA may result in reduced blood pressure in some hypertensive individuals, as well as fewer coronary events. These effects warrant further investigation.

There is some evidence that higher doses of GLA than typically used may improve blood lipids. In a small study, 17 subjects were assigned to two groups. One group of eight received 2 grams daily of GLA for six weeks, the other group received 500 milligrams daily for the same length of time. At the end of six weeks, the group that received 2 grams of GLA had a 37% lowering of their triglycerides and a 13% lowering of cholesterol. The lower dose showed no triglyceride or cholesterol-lowering activity. Unfortunately, there are no followup studies.

With respect to cancer, GLA has been shown to selectively kill 40 different human cancer cell lines in tissue culture without harm to normal cells. GLA appears to induce apoptotic death of tumor cells or, in various other ways, to suppress oncogene expression, at least in tissue culture. While the clinical use of GLA in cancer is only beginning, there is early encouraging news that it can help regress cerebral gliomas by 1 to 2 years. Other preliminary studies indicate GLA, alone or in combination with other substances, may be of some benefit in the treatment of pancreatic cancer, a finding that certainly warrants followup.

GLA's role in treating some skin disorders has focused primarily on atopic eczema, where the results continue to be mixed after years of study. In one of the best double-blind, multicenter studies to date, 160 patients with eczema of moderate severity were randomized to receive 500 milligrams of borage oil or placebo daily for a 24-week period. Various improvements were noted using GLA, and these reached statistical significance in one of the studies' subgroups. GLA has also been shown to have some efficacy in treating atopic dermatitis in both infant and adults, though here, too, results are mixed. GLA seems to have a positive effect on itching. One recent study showed that oral GLA supplementation can significantly relieve multiple uremic skin symptoms in hemodialysis patients.

GLA is being used to help ameliorate diabetic neuropathy with some encouraging results. In one multi-center randomized, double-blind, placebo-controlled study, those patients given 480 milligrams of GLA per day improved by all test parameters (at a level of statistical significance for 13 of the 16 parameters) over a one-year period. However, not all studies have been positive. There may be subgroups with diabetic neuropathy who could benefit from GLA. In a recent meta-analysis of treatments for tardive dyskinesia, no support was found for the use of GLA in this disorder. It has been suggested that GLA may be helpful in ulcerative colitis, but more research is needed to determine its role.

Treatment with GLA and EPA in the form of borage seed oil and fish oil significantly reduced the need for ventilatory support in 150 patients with acute respiratory distress syndrome. Patients thus treated were confined to intensive care an average of 12.8 days versus 17.5 days for controls.

Claims that GLA is useful in treating premenstrual syndrome (PMS) have not been supported by research findings, and GLA was found to be no better than placebo in preventing/treating menopausal flushing.

As an immune-modulator, GLA may primarily be an immune dampener rather than enhancer. Its ability to dampen some immune functions may make it useful in fighting some auto-immune disorders.

CONTRAINDICATIONS, PRECAUTIONS, ADVERSE REACTIONS

CONTRAINDICATIONS
None known.

PRECAUTIONS
GLA should not be used by pregnant women and nursing mothers unless recommended by a physician. Because of possible antithrombotic activity, those who take warfarin and hemophiliacs should exercise caution in its use. GLA should not be used before surgery.

ADVERSE REACTIONS
There have been no reports of serious adverse events in those taking GLA supplements. GLA is usually tolerated very well with no significant adverse effects.

INTERACTIONS
No interactions between GLA and aspirin, other NSAIDs, or herbs, such as *Allium sativum* (garlic) or *Ginkgo biloba* (Ginkgo), have been reported. Such interactions, if they were to occur, might be manifested by nosebleeds and/or increased susceptibility to bruising. If this does occur, GLA intake should be lowered or stopped.

OVERDOSAGE

No overdosing has been reported.

DOSAGE AND ADMINISTRATION

There are several forms of GLA supplements. A concentrated form of GLA is available. GLA is also available as evening primrose oil, borage seed oil and blackcurrant seed oil. Doses tried for rheumatoid arthritis and other conditions range from about 360 milligrams to 2.8 grams daily in divided doses and usually with meals. Doses of up to 2 grams daily may be helpful in those with elevated triglycerides. The concentrations of GLA varies in the different oil preparations and, depending on the concentration, the number of capsules daily may be smaller or larger in order to make up the desired dose.

HOW SUPPLIED

Capsules — 200 mg, 300 mg, 1000 mg

LITERATURE

Belch JJ, Ansell D, Madhok R, et al. Effects of altering dietary essential fatty acids on requirements for non-steroidal anti-inflammatory drugs in patients with rheumatoid arthritis: a double-blind, placebo-controlled study. *Ann Rheum Dis.* 1988; 47:96-104.

Berth-Jones J, Graham-Brown RA. Placebo-controlled trial of essential fatty acid supplementation in atopic dermatitis. *Lancet.* 1993; 341:1557-1560.

Chaintreuil J, Monnier L, Colette C, et al. Effects of dietary gamma-linolenate supplementation on serum lipids and platelet function in insulin-dependent diabetic patients. *Hum Nutr: Clin Nutr.* 1984; 38C:121-130.

Das UN, Prasad VV, Reddy DR. Local application of gamma-linolenic acid in the treatment of human gliomas. *Cancer Lett.* 1995; 94:147-155.

Fan YY, Chapkin RS. Importance of dietary gamma-linolenic acid in human health and nutrition. *J Nutr.* 1998; 128:1411-1414.

Gadek JE, De Michele SJ, Karlstad MD, et al. Effect of enteral feeding with eicosapentaenoic acid, gamma-linolenic acid, and antioxidants in patients with acute respiratory distress syndrome. Enteral nutrition in ARDS Study Group. *Crit Care Med.* 1999; 27:1409-1420.

Galli E, Picardo M, Chine L, et al. Analysis of polyunsaturated fatty acids in newborn sera: a screening tool for atopic dermatitis? *Int Arch Allergy Appl.* 1994; 82:422-423.

Henz BM, Jablonska S, Van De Kerkhof PC, et al. Double-blind, multicentre analysis of the efficacy of borage oil in patients with atopic eczema. *Br J Dermatol.* 1999; 149:685-688.

Horrobin DF, Morse PF. Evening primrose oil and atopic eczema. *Lancet.* 1995; 345: 260-261.

Hrelia S, Bordoni A, Biagi P, et al. gamma-Linoleic supplementation can affect cancer cell proliferation via modification of fatty acid composition. *Biochem Biophys Res Commun.* 1996; 14:441-447.

Huang Y-S, Mills DEM, eds. *Gamma-Linolenic Acid. Metaolism and its Roles in Nutrition and Medicine.* Champaign, IL: AOCS Press; 1996.

Keen H, Payan J, Allawi J. Treatment of diabetic neuropathy with gamma-linolenic acid. The gamma-Linolenic Acid Multicenter Trial Group. *Diabetes Care.* 1993; 16:8-16.

Kernoff PBA, Willis AL, Stone KJ, et al. Antithrombotic potential of di-homo-gamma-linolenic in man. *Brit Med J.* 1977; 2:1441.

Kruger MC, Coetzer H, de Winter R, et al. Calcium, gamma-linolenic acid and eicosapentaenoic acid supplementation in senile osteoporosis. *Aging (Milano).* 1998; 10: 385-394.

Morse PF, Horrobin DF, Manku MS, et al. Meta-analysis of placebo-controlled studies of the efficacy of gamma-linolenic acid in the treatment of atopic eczema. *Br J Dermatol.* 1989; 121:75-90.

Sim AK, Mc Craw AP. The activity of gamma-linolenate and dihomo-gamma linolenate methyl esters in non-human primates and in man. *Throm Res.* 1977; 10: 385-397.

Zurier RB, Rossett RG, Jacobson EW, et al. gamma-Linolenic acid treatment of rheumatoid arthritis. A randomized, placebo-controlled trial. *Arthritis Rheum.* 1996; 39: 1808-1817.

Gamma-Tocopherol

DESCRIPTION

Gamma-tocopherol is one of the four natural tocopherol homologues or isoforms, the others being alpha-, beta- and delta-tocopherol. Tocopherols and tocotrienols comprise the vitamin E family (See Vitamin E). Gamma-tocopherol is the principal tocopherol found in the lipid fraction of many seeds and nuts, including soybeans, corn and walnuts, and is the major tocopherol in the American diet. Because of the wide use of oils derived from these sources, gamma-tocopherol makes up approximately 65 to 70% of the total dietary intake of tocopherols, the other major dietary tocopherol being alpha-tocopherol.

Although gamma-tocopherol is the principal dietary tocopherol, plasma levels of this tocopherol average five times lower than alpha-tocopherol. Apparently, alpha-tocopherol is the only tocopherol maintained in human plasma. This situation is believed to be accounted for by the presence in the liver of alpha-tocopherol transfer protein (alpha-TTP). Alpha-TTP preferentially secretes alpha-tocopherol from the liver into the blood. This protein binds most strongly to alpha-tocopherol. Because alpha-tocopherol is the only tocopherol maintained in human plasma, the Food and Nutrition Board in their most recent report, and for the purpose of establishing RDAs for vitamin E, included only certain alpha-tocopherol forms in their definition of vitamin E activity.

Gamma-tocopherol is also known as d-gamma-tocopherol, RRR-gamma-tocopherol, 2R, 4'R, 8'R-gamma-tocopherol and 2, 7, 8-trimethyl-2 (4', 8', 12'-trimethyldecyl)-6-chromanol. It is abbreviated as gamma-TOH, gamma-T and gamma-TH. Gamma-tocopherol is a slightly viscous, pale yellow oil which is practically insoluble in water. Alpha-tocopherol differs from gamma-tocopherol by the presence of a methyl group in the 5 position of the chromanol ring. Gamma-tocopherol lacks this methyl group. Practically all supplemental RRR-alpha-tocopherol, commonly known as d-alpha-tocopherol, is produced from soybean oil-derived gamma-tocopherol by a chemical methylation. The structure is identical to natural d-alpha-tocopherol, but, since it is a semi-synthetic product, it is called natural-source alpha-tocopherol. In contrast to alpha-tocopherol, synthetic forms of gamma-tocopherol, such as *all rac*-gamma-tocopherol or dl-gamma-tocopherol, are not sold as nutritional supplements. Supplemental gamma-tocopherol is marketed as the free or unesterified form.

ACTIONS AND PHARMACOLOGY

ACTIONS

Gamma-tocopherol has antioxidant activity. It may also have anti-atherogenic, anti-apoptotic, antithrombotic, anticoagulant, anticarcinogenic and immunomodulatory actions.

MECHANISM OF ACTION

Gamma-tocopherol is a lipid soluble, chain-breaking, peroxyl radical scavenger. It can protect polyunsaturated fatty acids (PUFAs) within membrane phopholipids, as well as PUFAs within such plasma lipoproteins as low density lipoproteins (LDL), from oxidation. In this regard, gamma-tocopherol is considered to be a less-efficient scavenger of reactive oxygen species (ROS), such as peroxyl radicals, than alpha-tocopherol. This belief is based mainly on *in vitro* studies comparing the various tocopherol homologues.

A recent rat study demonstrated that both alpha-and gamma-tocopherol decreased arterial peroxidation and LDL oxidation and also increased endogenous superoxide dismutase activity. Interestingly, the effects of gamma-tocopherol were found to be more potent than those of alpha-tocopherol. The relative antioxidant activity of the various tocopherol homologous against ROS needs clarification.

It is clear, however, that gamma-tocopherol is a more effective scavenger of reactive nitrogen species (RNS) than is alpha-tocopherol. Gamma-tocopherol is more effective than alpha-tocopherol in inhibiting the oxidation of phopholipids by the RNS peroxynitrite. Peroxynitrite is formed by the reaction of nitric oxide with superoxide and may cause

significant cellular damage by reacting with DNA and proteins, as well as with phospholipids. It is postulated by one group of investigators ''that gamma-tocopherol acts *in vivo* as a trap for membrane-soluble electrophilic nitrogen oxides and other electrophilic mutagens, forming stable carbon-centered adducts through the nucleophilic 5-position, which is blocked in alpha-tocopherol.'' The chemical difference between alpha-tocopherol and gamma-tocopherol is the presence in alpha-tocopherol of a methyl group in the 5-position of the chromanol ring.

Gamma-tocopherol may have antiatherogenic activity. One study reported that those with coronary artery disease (CAD) have lower serum levels of gamma-tocopherol but not alpha-tocopherol, when compared with those without CAD. A few mechanisms have been postulated to account for the possible antiatherogenic activity of gamma-tocopherol. These include inhibition of LDL oxidation, inhibition of platelet aggregation and inhibition of apoptosis of coronary artery endothelial cells. Oxidized (ox)-LDL induces apoptosis of human coronary artery endothelial cells in culture, in part by activation of the NF-Kappa B signal transduction pathway. Gamma-tocopherol has been found in cell culture to inhibit ox-LDL-induced apoptosis of human coronary artery endothelial cells by inhibiting the activation of NF-Kappa B. In another study in human coronary smooth muscle cells, ox-LDL was found to mediate apoptosis of these cells, and both gamma- and alpha-tocopherol were found to inhibit this process. Both of these tocopherol homologues —alpha more so than gamma — were found to inhibit two of the pathways leading to apoptosis in these cells, the mitogen-activated protein kinase (MAPK) and Jun kinase pathways. Peroxynitrite is a potent mutagenic oxidant. It is formed during activation of phagocytes (polymorphonuclear leukocytes, monocytes and macrophages). Chronic inflammation induced by these cells is thought to play a major role in the etiology of cancer and other degenerative disease. The possible anticarcinogenic activity of gamma-tocopherol may be accounted for, in part, by its peroxynitrite-scavenging activity.

Gamma-tocopherol, as well as the other tocopherol homologues, enhance both spontaneous and mitogen-stimulated lymphocyte proliferation. The mechanism of the possible immunomodulatory activity of gamma-tocopherol, as well as that of the other homologues, is unclear.

PHARMACOKINETICS

The efficiency of absorption of gamma-tocopherol, as is true for all the members of the vitamin E family, is low and variable. Absorption is lower on an empty stomach than with meals. Gamma-tocopherol is absorbed from the lumen of the small intestine into the enterocytes by passive diffusion. Prior to its absorption, gamma-tocopherol participates in micelle formation with dietary fats and products of lipid hydrolysis. This is aided by bile salts secreted by the liver. Gamma-tocopherol is secreted by the enterocytes into the lymphatics in the form of chylomicrons. Chylomicrons undergo metabolism in the circulation via lipoprotein lipase to form chylomicron remnants. During this process, some gamma-tocopherol is transferred to various tissues such as adipose tissue, muscle and possibly the brain. Chylomicron remnants can transfer it to LDL and very low density lipoproteins (VLDL). Chylomicron remnants can also acquire apolipoprotein E (apoE), which directs them to the liver for metabolism.

The chylomicron remnants are taken up by the liver. Gamma-tocopherol does not bind very well to hepatic alpha-tocopherol transfer protein (alpha-TTP). This is the protein that is involved in the secretion of alpha-tocopherol in VLDLs. It is for this reason, that even though gamma-tocopherol is the major dietary tocopherol in the American diet, (excluding alpha-tocopherol from nutritional supplements), alpha-tocopherol levels in plasma and most other tissues are about five-fold higher than gamma-tocopherol. Gamma-tocopherol is also more rapidly taken up and turned over in tissues, compared with alpha-tocopherol.

Reaction of gamma-tocopherol and peroxynitrite *in vitro* results in the formation of four major products: 2, 7, 8-trimethyl-2-(4, 8, 12-trimethyldecyl)-5-nitro-6-chromanol (NGT or tocoyellow), 2, 7, 8-trimethyl-2-(4, 8, 12-trimethyl-decyl)-5,6-chromaquinone (tocored) and two diastereomers of 8a-(hydroxy)-gamma-tocopherol.

About half of ingested and absorbed gamma-tocopherol is excreted in the urine, mainly as a glucuronide conjugate of 2, 7, 8-trimethyl-2-(2'-carboxyethyl)-6-hydroxychroman or gamma-CEHC. Fecal excretion is the main route of excretion of oral gamma-tocopherol. Fecal excretion substances includes non-absorbed gamma-tocopherol and gamma-tocopherol that may be excreted via the biliary route.

The gamma-tocopherol metabolite gamma-CEHC, also known as LLU (Loma Linda University)-alpha, is reported to have natriuretic activity. This is thought to be mediated by inhibition of a potassium channel in the apical membrane of the thick ascending limb of the kidney.

INDICATIONS AND USAGE

There is some evidence that both alpha- and gamma-tocopherol may have complementary antioxidant activities. There might thus be indications and uses of gamma-tocopherol that are distinct from those of alpha-tocopherol, or circumstances in which one works better than the other. In general, however, gamma-tocopherol is likely to have some or most of the same indications and uses as alpha-tocopherol (See Vitamin E), although it has not been as extensively studied as alpha-tocopherol. There is preliminary evidence that gamma-tocopherol may be more protective against cardiovascular disease than alpha-tocopherol. There is also some preliminary evidence that it could be more effective in preventing some cancers. On the other hand, there is one recent report that elevated blood levels of gamma-tocopherol may be associated with an increased incidence of knee osteoarthritis, especially in those who are black.

RESEARCH SUMMARY

Some studies have indicated that gamma-tocopherol is more potent than alpha-tocopherol in protecting against nitric-oxide initiated lipid peroxidation. This has been demonstrated in vitro and in animal experiments. Human data are more equivocal. Some studies have suggested that both tocopherols are required for optimal protection against reactive nitrogen species. Several researchers have thus suggested that gamma-tocopherol should be part of "standard" vitamin E supplements.

Recently, an *in vitro* study showed that gamma-tocopherol significantly reduced oxidized-LDL-induced apoptosis of human coronary artery endothelial cells. In a recent animal study, gamma-tocopherol, significantly more than alpha-tocopherol, was found to decrease platelet aggregation and to delay intra-arterial thrombus formation. Research continues.

There are some experimental data suggesting that gamma-tocopherol may, more effectively than alpha-tocopherol, prevent neoplastic transformation. Recently, gamma-tocopherol was shown to inhibit (more effectively than alpha-tocopherol) the growth of a human prostate cancer cell line.

There is one study in which an association has been made between high blood levels of gamma-tocopherol and increased incidence of knee osteoarthritis, especially in those who are black. More research will have to be done before causality can be determined. Research is continuing.

CONTRAINDICATIONS, PRECAUTIONS, ADVERSE REACTIONS

CONTRAINDICATIONS

Gamma-tocopherol is contraindicated in those with known hypersensitivity to the substance.

PRECAUTIONS

Those on warfarin should be cautious in using high doses of gamma-tocopherol (doses greater than 100 milligrams daily) and, if they do so, they should have their INRs carefully monitored and their warfarin doses appropriately adjusted if indicated. Likewise, those with vitamin K deficiencies, such as those with liver failure, should be cautious in using high doses of gamma-tocopherol. Gamma-tocopherol should be used with caution in those with lesions with a propensity to bleed (e.g., bleeding peptic ulcers), those with a history of hemorrhagic stroke and those with inherited bleeding disorders (e.g., hemophilia).

High dose gamma-tocopherol supplementation should be stopped about one month before surgical procedures and may be resumed following recovery from the procedure. Those taking iron supplements should not take gamma-tocopherol concomitantly with the iron.

ADVERSE REACTIONS.
Gamma-tocopherol has only recently been introduced into the nutritional supplement marketplace. No adverse reactions have been reported.

INTERACTIONS
DRUGS
Antiplatelet drugs, such as aspirin, dipyridamole, eptifibatide, clopidogrel, ticlopidine, tirofiban and abciximab: High doses of gamma-tocopherol may potentiate the effects of these antiplatelet drugs.

Cholestyramine: may decrease gamma-tocopherol absorption.

Colestipol: may decrease gamma-tocopherol absorption.

Isoniazid: may decrease gamma-tocopherol absorption.

Mineral oil: may decrease gamma-tocopherol absorption.

Neomycin: may impair utilization of gamma-tocopherol.

Orlistat: is likely to inhibit gamma-tocopherol absorption.

Sucralfate: may interfere with gamma-tocopherol absorption.

Warfarin: High dose (greater than 100 milligrams daily) gamma-tocopherol may enhance the anticoagulant response of warfarin. Monitor INRs and appropriately adjust dose of warfarin if necessary.

NUTRITIONAL SUPPLEMENTS
Alpha-tocopherol: Supplemental alpha-tocopherol may decrease plasma concentration of gamma-tocopherol.

Desiccated ox bile: may increase the absorption of gamma-tocopherol.

Iron: Most iron supplements contain the ferrous form of iron. This form can oxidize gamma-tocopherol, which is marketed in a free, unesterified form, to its pro-oxidant form, if taken concomitantly.

Medium-chain triglycerides: may enhance absorption of gamma-tocopherol if taken concomitantly.

Phytosterols and phytostanols, including beta-sitosterol and beta-sitostanol: may lower plasma gamma-tocopherol levels.

Plant phenolic compounds and flavonoids: may participate in redox cycling reactions and help maintain levels of reduced gamma-tocopherol.

Selenium: may function synergistically with gamma-tocopherol.

Vitamin C: may help maintain gamma-tocopherol in its reduced (antioxidant) form.

FOODS
Olestra: is likely to inhibit the absorptin of gamma-tocopherol. Although alpha-tocopherol is added to olestra, gamma-tocopherol is not.

HERBS
Some herbs, including garlic and ginkgo, possess antithrombotic activity. High doses of gamma-tocopherol used concomitantly with these herbs may enhance their antithrombotic activity.

OVERDOSAGE
There are no reports of gamma-tocopherol overdoses in the literature.

DOSAGE AND ADMINISTRATION
Presently marketed forms of gamma-tocopherol contain about 60% gamma-tocopherol along with smaller amounts of the other tocopherol homologues. The gamma-tocopherols, as well as the other tocopherols, are present in the free (unesterified) form. Typical doses are about 200 milligrams daily (as gamma-tocopherol).

LITERATURE
Brigelius-Flohe R, Traber MG. Vitamin E: function and metabolism. *FASEB J.* 1999; 13:1145-1155.

Christen S, Woodall AA, Shigenaga MK, et al. Gamma-tocopherol traps mutagenic electrophiles such as NOx and complements alpha-tocopherol: physiological implications. *Proc Natl Acad Sci USA.* 1997; 94:3217-3222.

Cooney RV, Harwood PJ, Franke AA, et al. Products of gamma-tocopherol reaction with NO2 their formation in rat insulinoma (RINm5f) cells. *Free Rad Biol Med.* 1995; 19:259-269.

Cooney RV, Franke AA Harwood PJ, et al. Gamma-tocopherol detoxification of nitrogen dioxide: superiority to alpha-tocopherol. *Proc Natl Acad Sci USA.*

1993; 90:1771-1775.

de Nigris F, Franconi F, Maida I, et al. Modulation by alpha- and gamma-tocopherol and oxidized low-density lipoprotein of apoptotic signaling in human coronary smooth muscle cells. *Biochem Pharmacol.* 2000; 59:1477-1487.

Handelman GJ, Machlin LJ, Fitch K, et al. Oral alpha-tocopherol supplements decrease plasma gamma-tocopherol levels in humans. *J Nutr.* 1985; 115:807-813.

Hoglen NC, Waller SC, Sipes IG, Liebler DC. Reactions of peroxynitrite with gamma-tocopherol. *Chem Res Toxicol*. 1997; 10:401-407.

Li D, Saldeen T, Mehta JL. Gamma-tocopherol decreases ox-LDL-mediated activation of nuclear factor-KappaB and apoptosis in human coronary artery endothelial cells. *Biochem Biophys Res Commun*. 1999; 259:157-161.

Li D, Saldeen T, Romero F, Mehta JL. Relative effects of alpha- and gamma-tocopherol on low-density lipoprotein oxidation and superoxide dismutase and nitric oxide synthase activity and protein expression in rats. *J Cardiovasc Pharmacol Ther*. 1999; 4:219-226.

Mc Intyre BS, Briski KP, Tirmenstein MA, et al. Antiproliferative and apoptotic effects of tocopherols and tocotrienols on normal mouse mammary epithelial cells. *Lipids*. 2000; 35:171-180.

Parker RS, Swanson JE. A novel 5^1-carboxychroman metabolite of gamma-tocopherol secreted by HepG2 cells and excreted in human urine. *Biochem Biophys Res Commun*. 2000; 269:580-583.

Saldeen T, Li D, Mehta JL. Differential effects of alpha- and gamma-tocopherol on low-density lipoprotein oxidation, superoxide activity, platelet aggregation and arterial thrombogenesis. *J Am Coll Cardiol* 1999; 34:1208-1215.

Stone WL, Papas AM. Tocopherols and the etiology of colon cancer. *J Natl Cancer Inst*. 1997; 89:1006-1014.

Wechter WJ, Kantoci D, Murray ED Jr., et al. A new natriuretic factor: LLU-alpha. *Proc Natl Acad Sci USA*. 1996; 93:6002-6007.

Wolf G. Gamma-tocopherol: an efficient protector of lipids against nitric oxide-isolated peroxidative damage. *Nutr Rev*. 1997; 55:376-378.

Wu D, Meydani M, Beharka AA, et al. In vitro supplementation with different tocopherol homologues can affect the function of immune cells in ol zd mice. *Free Rad Biol Med*. 2000; 28:643-651.

Yamashita K, Takeda N, Ikeda S. Effects of various tocopherol-containing diets on tocopherol secretion into bile. *Lipids*. 2000; 35:163-170.

Gelatin Hydrolysates

DESCRIPTION

Gelatin is a heterogeneous mixture of proteins derived from animal collagen by hydrolysis. It is not found naturally. It typically is obtained by boiling bovine, pig and ox skin and bones. Gelatin has many uses in the food and pharmaceutical industries. Nutritionally, it is an incomplete protein because it lacks L-tryptophan. It is used in foods as stabilizers, thickeners and texturizers. Pharmaceutically, it is used as an encapsulating agent. Gelatin capsules are widely used both in the pharmaceutical and nutritional supplement industries.

Recently, gelatin subjected to greater hydrolysis in order to produce water-soluble peptides of various molecular weights has entered the nutritional supplement marketplace for use in bone and joint health. The gelatin peptides are rich in the amino acids found in collagen, including L-proline, L-hydroxyproline and glycine. Gelatin and hydrolyzed collagen are similar (see Hydrolyzed Collagen).

ACTIONS AND PHARMACOLOGY

ACTIONS

Gelatin hydrolysates have putative activity against degenerative joint disease (DJD).

MECHANISM OF ACTION

The mechanism of the putative anti-arthritic activity of gelatin hydrolysates is a matter of speculation. Although the amino acids in gelatin hydrolysates are identical to those in collagen, it is unlikely that these amino acids would make a significant contribution to the synthesis of collagen in, for example, joint cartilage. L-hydroxyproline is not a genetic amino acid. Thus, it is not a precursor to protein synthesis but, rather, is formed post-translationally. Both glycine and L-proline are synthesized by the body, and it is unlikely that these amino acids in gelatin hydrolysates would play any role in the *de novo* synthesis of collagen. There is speculation that gelatin hydrolysates may contain certain oligopeptides, which may stimulate collagen synthesis. This is far from proven.

PHARMACOKINETICS

The digestion, absorption and metabolism of gelatin hydrolysates are similar to those that occur with dietary proteins and peptides.

INDICATIONS AND USAGE

Claims that gelatin can fight arthritis and help maintain healthy joint cartilage and bone are to date poorly supported.

RESEARCH SUMMARY

A mixture of gelatin, vitamin C and calcium has been promoted as an effective interventive in joint disease. Some preliminary studies supporting this claim need more rigorous follow-up.

CONTRAINDICATIONS, PRECAUTIONS, ADVERSE REACTIONS

CONTRAINDICATIONS

None known.

PRECAUTIONS

Pregnant women and nursing mothers should avoid supplemental gelatin hydrolysates.

Those with renal failure or liver failure should exercise caution in the use of supplemental gelatin hydrolysates.

Those who use gelatin hydrolysates produced from bovine sources should only use products derived from raw materials (bovine skin and bone) classified as carrying no detectable infectivity. Bovine nervous system parts may carry the bovine spongiform encephalopathy (BSE) agent, the etiological agent of mad cow disease.

ADVERSE REACTIONS
No reports.

INTERACTIONS
There is one report of a collagen hydrosylate enhancing the effect of calcitonin in the treatment of osteoporosis.

DOSAGE AND ADMINISTRATION
Gelatin hydrolysates are available in powder form, usually in combination with other nutritional supplements, such as vitamin C and calcium. A typical dose is 10 grams daily. Gelatin hydrolysates are also available in capsules, usually in combination with other supplements, such as glucosamine, curcumin, chondroitin sulfate and willow bark.

HOW SUPPLIED
Capsules— 10 grains

LITERATURE
Adam M, Spacek P, Hulejova H, et al. [Postmenopausal osteoporosis. Treatment with calcitonin and a diet rich in collagen proteins.] [Article in Czech.] *Cas Lek Cesk.* 1996; 135:44-78.

Genistein

TRADE NAMES
Genistein PhytoEstrogen (Solaray), Genistein Isoflavone Rich Soyfood Supplement (Source Naturals).

DESCRIPTION
Genistein belongs to the isoflavone class of flavonoids. It is also classified as a phytoestrogen. Phytoestrogens are plant-derived nonsteroidal compounds that possess estrogen-like biological activity. Genistein has been found to have both weak estrogenic and weak anti-estrogenic effects.

Genistein is the aglycone (aglucon) of genistin. The isoflavone is found naturally as the glycoside genistin and as the glycosides 6''-O-malonylgenistin and 6''-O-acetylgenistin. Genistein and its glycosides are mainly found in legumes, such as soybeans and chickpeas. Soybeans and soy foods are the major dietary sources of these substances. Nonfermented soy foods, such as tofu, contain higher levels of the genistein glycosides, while fermented soy foods, such as tempeh and miso, contain higher levels of the aglycone.

Genistein is a solid substance that is practically insoluble in water. Its molecular formula is $C_{15}H_{10}O_5$, and its molecular weight is 270.24 daltons. Genistein is also known as 5, 7-dihydroxy-3-   (4-hydroxyphenyl)-4*H*-1-benzopyran-4-one, and 4', 5, 7-trihydroxyisoflavone. Genistin, which is the 7-beta glucoside of genistein, has greater water solubility than genistein. Genistein has the following structural formula:

Genistein

Genistein, when marketed as a nutritional supplement, is mainly present in the form of its glycoside genistin.

ACTIONS AND PHARMACOLOGY
ACTIONS
Genistein has estrogenic and antioxidant activities. It may also have anticarcinogenic, anti-atherogenic and anti-osteoporotic activities.

MECHANISM OF ACTION
Genistein has weak estrogenic activity as measured in *in vivo* and *in vitro* assays. *In vivo*, its estrogenic activity is one-third that of glycitein and four times greater than that of daidzein.

Genistein has been found to have a number of antioxidant activities. It is a scavenger of reactive oxygen species and inhibits lipid peroxidation. It also inhibits superoxide anion generation by the enzyme xanthine oxidase. In addition, genistein, in animal experiments, has been found to increase the activities of the antioxidant enzymes superoxide dismutase, glutathione peroxidase, catalase and glutathione reductase.

Several mechanisms have been proposed for genistein's putative anticarcinogenic activity. These include upregulation of apoptosis, inhibition of angiogenesis, inhibition of DNA topoisomerase II and inhibition of protein tyrosine kinases. Genistein's weak estrogenic activity has been suggested as another mechanism for genistein's putative anti-prostate cancer activity. In addition to the above mechanisms, other mechanisms of genistein's putative anti-prostate cancer activity include inhibition of nuclear factor (NF)-Kappa B in prostate cancer cells, downregulation of TGF (transforming growth factor)-beta and inhibition of EGF (epidermal growth factor)-stimulated growth. Genistein's anti-estrogenic action may be another possible mechanism to explain its putative anti-breast cancer activity. In the final analysis, the mechanism of genistein's putative anticarcinogenic activity is unclear.

The possible anti-atherogenic activity of genistein may be attributed, in part, to its antioxidant activity. Genistein may have some lipid-lowering activity, but the mechanism of this is unclear. The weak estrogenic activity of genistein may also contribute to its possible anti-atherogenic action.

Genistein's weak estrogenic effect may help protect against osteoporosis by preventing bone resorption and promoting increased bone density. Genistein has been found to maintain trabecular bone tissue in rats. However, the mechanism of genistein's possible anti-osteoporotic effect is unclear.

PHARMACOKINETICS

The pharmacokinetics of genistein in humans is complex and not well understood. The major dietary and supplemental form of genistein is the glycoside genistin. Some genistin may be hydrolyzed by hydrochloric acid in the stomach to genistein and some may be hydrolyzed by beta-glucosidases in food to genistein. Most of ingested genistin, however, is delivered to the large intestine intact. In the large intestine, bacterial beta-glucosidases hydrolyze genistin to genistein. Genistein is either absorbed or further metabolized in the large intestine to dihydrogenistein and 6'-hydroxy-O-desmethylangolensin. Genistein, which is absorbed from the large intestine and small intestine, is eventually transported to the liver. There, it undergoes conjugation with glucuronate and sulfate via hepatic phase II enzymes (UDP-glucuronosyl-transferases and sulfotransferases). The glucuronate and sulfate conjugates of genistein are excreted in the urine and in the bile. The genistein conjugates may be deconjugated to release genistein, which may be reabsorbed via the enterohepatic circulation.

There is considerable individual variation in the absorption and metabolism of ingested genistin and genistein. There are some data suggesting that genistein may be more bioavailable than genistin. However, other data suggest that the extent of absorption of genistein is similar for the aglycone and the glucoside forms. There are little data available on the tissue distribution of genistein.

INDICATIONS AND USAGE

INDICATIONS

There is a growing body of *in vitro* and animal studies suggesting that genistein may be helpful in preventing and treating some cancers, principally breast and prostate cancers. The clinical studies that might support or refute claims that genistein has anti-atherogenic properties and that it can safely and effectively be used as "natural" estrogen-replacement therapy have not been conducted. There are, however, preliminary data suggesting that soy isoflavones, including genistein, may be helpful in some problems associated with menopause, including osteoporosis and "hot flashes." See Soy Isoflavones.

Epidemiological data have long suggested that dietary isoflavones may confer protection against various cancers, especially breast and prostate cancer. High dietary intake of soy products in parts of Asia significantly correlated with reduced incidence of both breast and prostate cancers. Epidemiological data have not been entirely consistent in this regard, but most studies suggest protective effects. Some studies have shown, moreover, that this protection is lost in the second generation of those Asians emigrating to the United States.

These data led to experimental animal studies demonstrating protective effects. In one study, genistein perinatally fed to rats significantly protected offspring from subsequent chemically induced mammary cancers. These researchers concluded that adequate perinatal exposure to genistein can confer permanent protective effects against breast cancer. They have further speculated that protective effects in humans, with respect to breast cancer specifically, may depend upon exposure to genistein early in life. More research is needed to clarify this issue.

A number of studies have shown that genistein can inhibit prostate cancer-cell growth *in vitro*. Some recent *in vitro* studies suggest that genistein may be both chemopreventive and therapeutic in prostate cancers regardless of androgen responsiveness. Clinical trials are needed.

Also see Soy Isoflavones.

CONTRAINDICATIONS, PRECAUTIONS, ADVERSE REACTIONS

CONTRAINDICATIONS

Genistein is contraindicated in those who are hypersensitive to any component of a genistin, or genistein-containing product.

PRECAUTIONS

Pregnant women and nursing mothers should avoid the use of genistein/genistin supplements pending long-term safety studies.

Men with prostate cancer should discuss the advisability of the use of genistein/genistin supplements with their physicians before deciding to use them.

Women with estrogen receptor-positive tumors should exercise caution in the use of genistein/genistin supplements and should only use them if they are recommended and monitored by a physician.

Genistein/genistin intake has been associated with hypothyroidism in some.

DOSAGE AND ADMINISTRATION

Genistein is available in a few different isoflavone formulas. A standard soy isoflavone formula contains genistein mainly in the form of genistin, as well as daidzin and glycitin. The percentages of the various isoflavones present in this soy formula reflect the percentages of these substances as found in soybeans and are: genistin, about 50%; daidzin, about 38%; and glycitin, about 12%. A 50 mg dose of soy isoflavones—a typical daily dose—provides 25 mg of genistin, 19 mg of daidzin and about 6 mg of glycitin. Usually, 40% of the formula is comprised of soy isoflavones. Therefore, to get a dose of 50 mg of soy isoflavones, one needs 125 mg of the soy preparation.

Smaller amounts of genistein as the aglycone are available in some red clover preparations (see Biochanin A).

HOW SUPPLIED
Capsules
Powder
Tablets — Products labeled as 1000 mg relates to soybean content. Some tablets contain up to 20 mg genistein.

LITERATURE
Barnes S. Effect of genistein on in vitro and in vivo models of cancer. *J Nutr.* 1995; 125:777S-783S.

Barnes S, Peterson TG. Biochemical targets of the isoflavone genistein in tumor cell lines. *Proc Soc Exp Biol Med.* 1995; 208:103-108.

Constantinou A, Huberman E. Genistein as an inducer of tumor cell differentiation: possible mechanisms of action. *Proc Soc Exp Biol Med.* 1995; 208:109-115.

Dalu A, Haskell JF, Coward L, Lamartiniere CA. Genistein, a component of soy, inhibits the expression of the EGF and Erb B2/Neu receptors in the rat dorsolateral prostate. *The Prostate.* 1998; 37:36-48.

Davis JN, Kucuk O, Sarkar FH. Genistein inhibits NF-Kappa B activation in prostate cancer cells. *Nutr Biochem.* 1999; 35:167-174.

Davis JN, Muqim N, Bhuiyan M, et al. Inhibition of prostate specific antigen expression by genistein in prostate cancer cells. *Int J Oncol.* 2000; 16:1091-1097.

Fotsis T, Pepper M, Adlercreutz H, et al. Genistein, a dietary-derived inhibitor of *in vitro* angiogenesis. *Proc Natl Acad Sci USA.* 1993; 90:2690-2694.

Geller J, Sionit L, Partido C, et al. Genistein inhibits the growth of human-patient BPH and prostate cancer in histoculture. *The Prostate.* 1998; 34:75-79.

Lamartiniere CA. Protection against breast cancer with genistein: a component of soy. *Amer J Clin Nutr.* 2000; 71:1705S-1707S.

Wang TT, Sathyamoorthy N, Phang JM. Molecular effects of genistein on estrogen receptor mediated pathways. *Carcinogenesis.* 1996; 17:271-275.

Wei H, Bowen R, Cai Q, et al. Antioxidant and antipromotional effects of the soybean isoflavone genistein. *Proc Soc Exp Biol Med.* 1995; 208:124-130.

Germanium

TRADE NAMES
Germanium Forte (The Key Company), GE-132 (Douglas Lab/Amni) and GE-150 (Bio-Tech Pharmacal).

DESCRIPTION
Germanium is a metalloid element with atomic number 32 and atomic symbol Ge. Germanium is found in the earth's crust, in certain minerals and in living matter such as plants and the human body. Germanium is not an essential nutrient for humans.

A germanium-deficient diet fed to rats has been found to alter the mineral composition of bone and liver and decrease DNA in the tibia. Little more is known about the biologic role of this element.

Typical daily dietary intakes of germanium range from about 0.4 to 1.5 milligrams. Plant foods, such as wheat, vegetables, bran and leguminous seeds, are rich sources of germanium. Animal foods are low in germanium.

Some organic complexes of germanium are reported to inhibit tumor growth in animals. Some humans who consumed high amounts of these organic germanium supplements, which were contaminated with germanium dioxide (which is nephrotoxic), died from renal failure.

The main nutritional supplement form of germanium is known as Ge-132, Germanium-132, germanium sesquioxide or bis-carboxyethyl germanium sesquioxide. This is a synthetic organic product. It has not been found naturally. Noteworthy is that many of the clinical trials studying the effect of germanium on subjects with various cancers used another synthetic germanium compound, spirogermanium or 8,8-diethyl-N,N-dimethyl-2-aza-8-germaspiro (4,5) decane-2-propranamine dihydrochloride. Spirogermanium has great toxicity, especially neurotoxicity. Spirogermanium is not sold as a nutritional supplement.

Topical products containing inorganic germanium are marketed in Japan for relief of pain and swelling.

ACTIONS AND PHARMACOLOGY
ACTIONS
Bis-carboxyethyl germanium sesquioxide, Ge-132, may have antiproliferative activity. Ge-132 may also have antioxidant activity.

MECHANISM OF ACTION
The mechanism of the possible antiproliferative activity is unknown. Ge-132 is not effective in cell culture. It is speculated that Ge-132's possible antiproliferative activity is due to immune enhancement. There are reports that Ge-132

stimulates natural killer (NK) cell and cytotoxic T lymphocyte activity, as well as increased production of interferon.

Ge-132 was reported to prevent paraquat-induced hepatic oxidant injury in mice. The mechanism of this possible antioxidant effect is unknown.

PHARMACOKINETICS
Reported studies indicate that about 30% of an ingested dose of Ge-132 is absorbed from the small intestine. Little metabolism of Ge-132 appears to occur, and the substance is mainly excreted by the kidneys.

INDICATIONS AND USAGE
There are no indications for the use of supplemental germanium. Some inorganic forms of germanium, such as germanium dioxide, have been shown to be severely toxic to the liver and kidneys, resulting in some fatalities. Some organic forms of germanium, notably germanium lactate citrate, have also been shown to be severely toxic. The risk of contamination in putatively non-toxic forms of supplemental germanium outweighs any possible benefits, none of which, in any case, is yet well established.

RESEARCH SUMMARY
The Food and Drug Administration reported in 1997 that at least 31 human cases linked intake of germanium products with renal failure and, in some cases, death. Other adverse effects noted included anemia, muscle weakness and peripheral neuropathy. The total dose (not the daily dose) ingested in the cases reported on varied from 15 to more than 300 grams. Exposure varied from two to 36 months.

The Center For Food Safety and Applied Nutrition concluded: "Based on the evidence of persistent renal toxicity associated with germanium dioxide, the lack of conclusive findings of differential nephrotoxicity of organic germanium compounds, and the possibility of contamination of the organic germanium products with inorganic germanium, it is clear that germanium products present a potential human health hazard."

Some case histories are instructive. Based upon claims that germanium is an "anti-cancer" and "immunostimulatory" agent, a 25-year-old woman with stage II HIV disease consumed a total of 47 grams of germanium-lactate-citrate 18%. She developed severe renal insufficiency and hepatomegaly. A 55-year-old woman who consumed a similar amount of germanium compounds over a 19-month period was admitted to a hospital with general malaise, muscular weakness, anorexia and weight loss. She was found to have renal failure and muscular and nerve damage. Her decline soon ended in death. Other deaths have been reported in those who used germanium compounds as a general elixir, as well as in attempts to treat specific disorders.

A recent report described complete remission of pulmonary spindle cell carcinoma in a patient taking large doses of germanium sesquioxide. However, this would be considered pharmaceutical, not nutritional usage of this substance.

CONTRAINDICATIONS, PRECAUTIONS, ADVERSE REACTIONS
CONTRAINDICATIONS
Those with renal failure or those who are at risk for renal problems (for example, those with diabetes and those on potentially nephrotoxic drugs).

PRECAUTIONS
Because of the possibility of contamination of Ge-132 with germanium-containing compounds known to be toxic, including germanium dioxide and germanium lactate citrate, use of Ge-132 supplements requires extreme caution and is not recommended. Although pure Ge-132 has not yet been associated with renal failure, this possibility has not been ruled out.

Children, pregnant women, nursing mothers, those with renal failure and those with diabetes should absolutely avoid Ge-132 supplements. Also, those taking potentially nephrotoxic drugs should avoid Ge-132.

ADVERSE REACTIONS
Adverse reactions reported for those taking Ge-132—supposedly 100% pure—include nausea, diarrhea and skin eruptions. Germanium dioxide and germanium lactate citrate are nephrotoxic. Spirogermanium causes neurotoxicity and pulmonary toxicity.

Adverse effects reported for germanium dioxide and germanium lactate citrate, in addition to nephrotoxicity, include anemia, muscle weakness and peripheral neuropathy.

INTERACTIONS
There are no known interactions with Ge-132. There is always the possibility that Ge-132 might potentiate the nephrotoxicity of potentially nephrotoxic drugs.

OVERDOSAGE
Overdosage with pure Ge-132 has not been reported. However, overdosage with other forms of germanium has; in at least one case, multiple organ dysfunction, shock and death occurred.

DOSAGE AND ADMINISTRATION
No recommended dose. Germanium, in the form of Ge-132, also known as Germanium-132, germanium sesquioxide and bis-carboxyethyl germanium sesquioxide, is available as a nutritional supplement in capsules containing 30 to 150 milligrams. It is also available as a powder. Those who decide to use these supplements are cautioned to dose only under strict medical supervision and to be certain that the supplement (Ge-132) they are taking is 100% pure. Germani-

um may also be present in colloidal or liquid mineral preparations.

HOW SUPPLIED
Capsules — 25 mg, 150 mg
Powder
Sublingual Tablets — 25 mg, 150 mg

LITERATURE

Hess B, Raisin J, Zimmermann A, et al. Tubulointerstitial nephropathy persisting 20 months after discontinuation of chronic intake of germanium lactate citrate. *Am J Kidney Dis.* 1993; 21:548-552.

Kuebler JP, Tormey DC, Harper GR, et al. Phase II study of spirogermanium in advanced breast cancer. *Canc Treat Report.* 1984; 68:1515-1516.

Mainwaring MG, Poor C, Zander DS, Harman E. Complete remission of pulmonary spindle cell carcinoma after treatment with oral germanium sesquioxide. *Chest.* 2000; 117:591-593.

Nielsen FH. Ultratrace minerals. In: Shils ME, Olson JA, Shike M, Ross AC, eds. *Modern Nutrition in Health and Disease*, 9th ed. Baltimore MD: Williams and Wilkins; 1999:283-303.

Raisin J, Hess B, Blatter M, et al. [Toxicity of an organic germanium compound: deleterious consequences of a "natural remedy."] [Article in German.] *Schweiz Med Wochenschr.* 1992; 122:11-13.

Sanai T, Okuda S, Onoyama K, et al. Chronic tubulointerstitial changes induced by germanium dioxide in comparison with carboxyethylgermanium sesquioxide. *Kidney Int.* 1991; 40:882-890.

Schauss AG. Nephrotoxicity in humans by the ultratrace element germanium. *Ren Fail.* 1991; 13:1-4.

Shamir M, Sprung CL. [Fatal multiple organic system dysfunction associated with germanium metal used in complementary therapy.] [Article in Hebrew.] *Harefuah.* 1997; 133; 446-447, 502.

Takeuchi A, Yoshizawa N, Oshima S, et al. Nephrotoxicity of germanium compounds: report of a case and review of the literature. *Nephron.* 1992; 60:436-442.

Glandulars

DESCRIPTION
The term glandulars as used in the nutritional supplement marketplace refers to dried and ground-up raw animal glandular and nonglandular tissues or extracts of these tissues. The tissues include those from the following glands and organs: adrenal, thyroid, thymus, testis, ovary, pituitary, liver, pancreas, spleen, kidney, lung, heart, brain, uterus and prostate. Glandulars are believed by some to improve the function of the gland or organ from which the extract was produced. Most of these substances are derived from bovine sources; some are derived from ovine sources and some from porcine sources.

Glandulars and other tissue extracts have had roles in traditional medicine. At one time, extract of bone marrow was used as a hematinic agent for the treatment of iron-deficiency anemia. Desiccated thyroid is still used by many physicians in the management of hypothyroidism. Desiccated thyroid is the cleaned, dried and powdered thyroid gland, purified of fat and connective tissue; it is derived principally from hogs, but also from cows and sheep. Thymus extracts are being studied for their possible immunomodulatory activity.

ACTIONS AND PHARMACOLOGY
ACTIONS
The different glandulars and glandular extracts have various putative activities. Thymus and spleen extracts have putative immunomodulatory activities. Thyroid extracts have putative activity in managing hypothyroidism. Adrenal extracts have putative antiallergic and anti-inflammatory activities. Testis extracts have putative androgenic activity, and ovary extracts have putative estrogenic activity.

MECHANISM OF ACTION
For the most part, the various putative actions of the glandulars may be explained by the hormones and other factors that these tissue extracts contain. However, most of the glandulars marketed as nutritional supplements are unlikely to have physiologically meaningful levels of these bioactive substances. Some immune-modulatory substances have been isolated from thymus extracts as well as spleen extracts. Desiccated natural thyroid is available as a prescription drug for the management of hypothyroidism. The pharmaceutical preparation is standardized and contains both thyroxine and triiodothyronine. Thyroid extracts marketed as nutritional supplements are not allowed to have these hormones in them. Adrenal extracts may contain some cortisol. Cortisol does have anti-inflammatory and anti-allergic activities, but the amount of cortisol in the supplements is likely to be too low to have meaningful physiological activity. Testis extracts and ovary extracts contain testosterone and estrogen, respectively, but again, the amount of these hormones in the glandular supplements are unlikely to be physiologically significant.

PHARMACOKINETICS
The components of the various glandular supplements are digested, absorbed and metabolized by normal physiological processes.

INDICATIONS AND USAGE
Glandulars are said to have gland-restorative activity, immunomodulatory effects, androgenic and estrogenic properties and various rejuvenating qualities. A pharmaceutical

thyroid preparation is used to treat hypothyroidism, but supplemental thyroid products are not useful for this purpose and should not be substituted for pharmaceutical therapy. Testis and ovary supplements, similarly, should not be substituted for androgen and estrogen therapies recommended by physicians. Claims, including antiallergy and anti-inflammatory claims, made for glandular supplements are not supported by credible evidence.

RESEARCH SUMMARY

There is no credible evidence showing that supplemental glandulars rejuvenate glands.

Most clinical trials, which have been few in number, have produced non-significant results using glandulars. Some have shown immunomodulatory effects, but these findings are inconclusive.

CONTRAINDICATIONS, PRECAUTIONS, ADVERSE REACTIONS

CONTRAINDICATIONS

Glandulars are contraindicated in those who are hypersensitive to any component of a glandular-containing supplement.

Supplemental testis extracts are contraindicated in those with cancer of the prostate or benign prostatic hypertrophy (BPH).

Supplemental ovary extracts are contraindicated in those with breast cancer, ovarian cancer and uterine cancer and in those at risk for these cancers.

PRECAUTIONS

Glandulars should be avoided by pregnant women, nursing mothers and children.

Glandulars marketed as nutritional supplements should never be used for estrogen replacement, androgen replacement, thyroid replacement or cortisol replacement.

DOSAGE AND ADMINISTRATION

No recommended doses.

LITERATURE

Kouttab NM, Prada M, Cazzola P. Thymodulin: biological properties and clinical applications. *Med Oncol Tumor Pharmacother.* 1989; 6:5-9.

Valesini G, Barnaba V, Benvenuto R, et al. A calf thymus acid lysate improves clinical symptoms and T-cell defects in the early stages of HIV inflection. Second report. *Eur J Cancer Clin Oncol.* 1987; 23:1915-1919.

Wysocki J, Wicrusz-Wysocka B, Wykratowicz A, Wysocki H. The influence of thymus extracts on the chemotaxis of polymorphonuclear neutrophils (PMN) from patients with insulin-dependent diabetes mellitus (IDD). *Thymus.* 1992; 20:63-67.

Also, see Liver Hydrolysate/Desiccated Liver.

Glucomannan

DESCRIPTION

Glucomannan is a hydrocolloidal polysaccharide comprised of D-glucose and D-mannose residues (hence, the name) bonded together in beta-1,4 linkages. Approximately 60% of the polysaccharide is made up of D-mannose and approximately 40%, of D-glucose. Some of the sugar residues in glucomannan are acetylated. The molecular weight of this slightly branched polysaccharide ranges from 200 kilodaltons to 2,000 kilodaltons.

Glucomannan, which is also classified as a soluble dietary fiber, is derived from konjac flour. Konjac flour itself is derived from the *Amorphophallus* species, plants which are related to the common philodendron house plant and which grow in only certain parts of the world, including some regions in China and Japan. One member of the *Amorphophallus* genus called *Amorphophallus konjac*, is also known as voodoo lilly, devil's tongue and konjac. Konjac flour, however is derived from the tubers of various species of *Amorphophallus*, and the term konjac is used generically for the various species, as well as for the flour from their tubers. In addition to being known as konjac, the plant is called ju ruo (pronounced in Chinese) by the Chinese people, and called konjaku or konnyaku by the Japanese.

Konjac flour has a long history of use in both China and Japan as a food substance and as a folk remedy. Glucomannan products are widely used in Japan and China as general health aids, topically, for skin care and as a thickening agent for foods, among other things. Glucomannan, sometimes called konjac mannan, is marketed in the United States as a dietary supplement. Polysaccharides containing D-mannose and D-glucose in similar proportions to that found in konjac flour are found in other organisms, such as certain yeasts. Yeast glucomannan is not marketed as a dietary supplement.

ACTIONS AND PHARMACOLOGY

ACTIONS

Glucomannan may have laxative activity. It may also have activity in the control of serum glucose and lipid levels. Glucomannan has putative bariatric activity.

MECHANISM OF ACTION

The laxative effect of glucomannan is thought to be due to the swelling of glucomannan with consequent increase in stool bulk.

Some studies indicate that glucomannan may improve glycemic control in Type 2 diabetics. The mechanism of this effect is unclear. Glucomannan may delay the absorption of carbohydrates by increasing gastric-emptying time and/or decreasing small intestinal transit time.

The mechanism of glucomannan's possible hypocholesterolemic activity is likewise, unclear. The polysaccharide may stimulate the conversion of cholesterol to bile acids, as well as the fecal excretion of bile acids. Glucomannan may also decrease the intestinal absorption of cholesterol.

The putative bariatric (weight reduction) effect of glucomannan is not well understood. The swelling of glucomannan that occurs when it absorbs water in the gastrointestinal tract, may confer a feeling of satiety in some.

PHARMACOKINETICS

Following ingestion of glucomannan, very little of it is digested in the small intestine. Glucomannan is resistant to hydrolysis by the digestive enzymes. Significant degradation occurs in the large intestine via the action of colonic bacteria. Products of degradation in the large intestine, include formic acid, acetic acid, butyric acid, propionic acid, beta-1,4-D-mannobiose (4-O-beta-D-mannopyranosyl-D-mannopyranose), cellobiose(4-O-beta-D-glucopyranosyl-D-glucopyranose), 4-O-beta-D-glucopyr-anosyl-D-mannopyranose, glucose and mannose. There may be some absorption of these degradation products from the large intestine. Most of them are excreted in the feces, along with unchanged glucomannan. Butyrate is used as a respiratory fuel by the colonocytes.

INDICATIONS AND USAGE

INDICATIONS

Glucomannan has demonstrated some usefulness in the management of obesity, diabetes and constipation. It has some favorable effects on lipids.

RESEARCH SUMMARY

Some studies have demonstrated that glucomannan has some efficacy in the management of obesity. In an eight-week, double-blind study, 20 obese subjects received 1 gram of glucomannan or placebo daily. Subjects were instructed not to change eating or exercise habits. Glucomannan-supplemented subjects had a significant mean weight loss of 5.5 pounds. Serum cholesterol and LDL cholesterol were significantly reduced, as well, in the treated group.

In a double-blind trial, this one involving 60 children under age 15 with childhood obesity, there was a significant reduction in weight in both treated and placebo groups. Further, there was a concommitant significant reduction in alpha-lipoprotein and an increase in triglycerides in the treated group but not in the placebo group. However, in another controlled study of childhood obesity, excess weight and triglycerides were significantly decreased in treated subjects but not in controls.

In a 3-month study of severely obese patients, a hypocaloric diet therapy by itself was tested against the same hypocaloric diet in combination with 4 grams of glucomannan (in three doses) daily. The combination therapy resulted in more significant weight loss in relation to fatty mass alone, in an overall improvement in lipid status and carbohydrate tolerance and a greater adherence to the diet. The researchers concluded: "Due to the marked ability to satiate patients and the positive metabolic effects, glucomannan diet supplements have been found to be particularly efficacious and well tolerated even in the long-term treatment of severe obesity."

Glucomannan, given in a long-term feeding program to baboons, showed beneficial effects on glucose homeostasis. Subsequently, it was shown that 2.6-grams and 5.2-grams daily doses of glucomannan, added to a carbohydrate rich breakfast in eight patients with previous gastric surgery, improved their reactive hypoglycemia and decreased the postprandial rise in plasma insulin. Benefits were achieved without unpalatability and carbohydrate malabsorption.

In a recent randomized, placebo-controlled metabolic trial, glucomannan was found to improve metabolic control in high-risk Type 2 diabetic patients, as measured by glucose and lipid levels and blood pressure. More research is warranted.

Several studies have demonstrated that glucomannan is an effective treatment for many with chronic constipation. This has been demonstrated in double-blind, placebo-controlled and multicenter studies. One to 4 grams daily, in divided doses, are typically used in these studies of constipation.

CONTRAINDICATIONS, PRECAUTIONS, ADVERSE REACTIONS

CONTRAINDICATIONS

Glucomannan is contraindicated in those hypersensitive to any component of a glucomannan-containing product. It is also contraindicated in those with intestinal obstruction, difficulty in swallowing and esophageal narrowing.

PRECAUTIONS

Pregnant women and nursing mothers should avoid glucomannan supplements.

Glucomannan must be taken with adequate amounts of fluids. Inadequate fluid intake may cause glucomannan to swell and block the throat, esophagus or intestines.

Tablet forms of glucomannan should be avoided.

Glucomannan should not be taken before going to bed.

Type 2 diabetics who use glucomannan, may require adjustment of their antidiabetic medications.

ADVERSE REACTIONS

A few cases of esophageal obstruction have been reported with the use of glucomannan tablets. The most common adverse reactions are flatulence and abdominal distension. Diarrhea is occasionally reported.

INTERACTIONS

NUTRITIONAL SUPPLEMENTS

Fat-soluble vitamins (A, D, E, K): Concomitant intake of fat soluble vitamins and glucomannan may decrease the absorption of the fat-soluble vitamins.

FOODS

Glucomannan may decrease the absorption of fat-soluble vitamins found in foods.

OVERDOSAGE

Glucomannan overdosage has not been reported.

DOSAGE AND ADMINISTRATION

Glucomannan supplements are mainly available in capsules. Glucomannan powder is also available and there are glucomannan combination products.

Doses used range from one to four grams daily, taken in divided doses and with plenty of liquids.

LITERATURE

Arvill A, Bodin L. Effect of short-term ingestion of konjac glucomannan on serum cholesterol in healthy men. *Am J Clin Nutr.* 1995; 61:585-589.

Doi K, Matsuura M, Kawara A, et al. Influence of dietary fiber (konjac mannan) on absorption of vitamin B_{12} and vitamin E. *Tohoku J Exp Med.* 1983; 141 Suppl:677-681.

Henry DA, Mitchell AS, Aylward J, et al. Glucomannan and risk of oesophageal obstruction. *Br Med J.* 1986; 292:591-592.

Hopman WP, Houben PG, Speth PA, Lamers CB. Glucomannan prevents postprandial hypoglycemia in patients with previous gastric surgery. *Gut.* 188; 29:930-934.

Hou YH, Zhang LS, Zhou HM, et al. Influences of refined konjac meal on the levels of tissue lipids and the absorption of four minerals in rats. *Biomed Environ Sci.* 1990; 3:306-314.

Livieri C, Novazi F, Lorini R. [The use of highly purified glucomannan-based fibers in childhood obesity]. [Article in Italian]. *Pediatr Med Chir.* 1992; 14:195-198.

Matsuura Y. Degradation of konjac glucomannan by enzymes in human feces and formation of short-chain fatty acids by intestinal anaerobic bacteria. *J Nutr Sci Vitaminol (Tokyo).* 1998; 44:423-436.

Melga P, Giusto M, Ciuchi E, et al. [Dietary fiber in the dietetic therapy of diabetes mellitus. Experimental data with purified glucomannans]. [Article in Italian]. *Riv Eur Sci Med Farmacol.* 1992; 14:367-373.

Passaretti S, Franzoni M, Comin U, et al. Action of glucomannans on complaints in patients affected with chronic constipation: a multicentric clinical evaluaion. *Ital J Gastroenterol.* 1991; 23:421-425.

Staiano A, Simeone D, Del Giudice E, et al. Effect of the dietary fiber glucomannan on chronic constipation in neurologically impaired children. *J Pediatr.* 2000; 136:41-45.

Venter CS, Vorster HH, Van der Nest DG. Comparison between physiological effects of konjac-glucomannan can

propionate in baboons fed "Western" diets. *J Nutr.* 1990; 120:1046-1053.

Vido L, Facchin P, Antonello I, et al. Childhood obesity treatment: double blinded trial on dietary fibres (glucomannan) versus placebo. *Padiatr Padol.* 1993; 28:133-136.

Vita PM, Restelli A, Caspani P, Klinger R. [Chronic use of glucomannan in the dietary treatment of severe obesity]. [Article in Italian]. *Minerva Med.* 1992; 83:135-139.

Vorster HH, De Jager J. The effect of the long-term ingestion of konjac-glucomannan on glucose tolerance and immunoreactive insulin values of baboons. *S Afr Med J.* 1984; 65:805-808.

Vuksan V, Jenkins DJ, Spadofora P, et al. Konjac-mannan (glucomminan) improves glycemia and other associated risk factors for coronary heart disease in Type 2 diabetes. A randomized controlled metabolic trial. *Diabetes Care.* 1999; 22:913-919.

Vuksan V, Sievenpiper JL, Owen R, et al. Beneficial effects of viscous Konjac-mannan in subjects with the insulin resistance syndrome. *Diabetes Care.* 2000; 23:9-14.

Walsh DE, Yaghoubian V, Behforooz A. Effect of glucomannan on obese patients: a clinical study. *Int J Obesity.* 1984; 8:289-293.

Glucosamine

TRADE NAMES

Glucosamine is available from numerous manufacturers generically. Branded products include Aflexa (Mcneil Consumer), Natures Blend Glucosamine (National Vitamin Co.), GS-500 (Enzymatic Therapy), Glucosamine Complex (Schiff), Maxi GS (Maxi-Health Research), NAG (Twinlab).

DESCRIPTION

Glucosamine is an amino monosaccharide found in chitin, glycoproteins and glycosaminoglycans (formerly known as mucopolysaccharides) such as hyaluronic acid and heparan sulfate. Glucosamine is also known as 2-amino-2-deoxyglucose, 2-amino-2-deoxy-beta-D-glucopyranose and chitosamine. Glucosamine has the following chemical structure:

Glucosamine

Glucosamine is available commercially as a nutritional supplement in three forms: glucosamine hydrochloride or glucosamine HCl, glucosamine sulfate and N-acetyl-glucosamine.

At neutral as well as physiologic pH, the amino group in glucosamine is protonated, resulting in its having a positive charge. Salt forms of glucosamine contain negative anions to neutralize the charge. In the case of glucosamine hydrochloride, the anion is chloride, and in glucosamine sulfate the anion is sulfate. N-acetylglucosamine is a delivery form of glucosamine in which the amino group is acetylated, thus neutralizing its charge. To date, most of the clinical studies examining the effect of glucosamine on osteoarthritis have been performed with either the sulfate or the chloride salts of glucosamine. All three forms are water soluble.

The glucosamine used in supplements is typically derived from marine exoskeletons. Synthetic glucosamine is also available.

ACTIONS AND PHARMACOLOGY

ACTIONS

The actions of supplemental glucosamine have yet to be clarified. It may play a role in the promotion and maintenance of the structure and function of cartilage in the joints of the body. Glucosamine may also have anti-inflammatory properties.

MECHANISM OF ACTION

Until the specific actions of supplemental glucosamine are determined, the mechanism of action in relieving arthritic pain and in repair of cartilage is a matter of speculation. However, we do know a great deal about the biochemistry of the molecules in which glucosamine is found. Biochemically, glucosamine is involved in glycoprotein metabolism. Glycoproteins, known as proteoglycans, form the ground substance in the extra-cellular matrix of connective tissue. Proteoglycans are polyanionic substances of high-molecular weight and contain many different types of heteropolysaccharide side-chains covalently linked to a polypeptide-chain backbone. These polysaccharides make up to 95% of the proteoglycan structure. In fact, chemically, proteoglycans resemble polysaccharides more than they do proteins.

The polysaccharide groups in proteoglycans are called glycosaminoglycans or GAGs. GAGs include hyaluronic acid, chondroitin sulfate, dermatan sulfate, keratan sulfate, heparin and heparan sulfate. All of the GAGs contain derivatives of glucosamine or galactosamine.

Glucosamine derivatives are found in hyaluronic acid, keratan sulfate and heparan sulfate. Chondroitin sulfate contains derivatives of galactosamine.

The glucosamine-containing glycosaminoglycan hyaluronic acid is vital for the function of articular cartilage. GAG chains are fundamental components of aggrecan found in articular cartilage. Aggrecan confers upon articular cartilage shock-absorbing properties. It does this by providing cartilage with a swelling pressure that is restrained by the tensile forces of collagen fibers. This balance confers upon articular cartilage the deformable resilience vital to its function.

In the early stages of degenerative joint disease, aggrecan biosynthesis is increased. However, in later stages, aggrecan synthesis is decreased, leading eventually to the loss of cartilage resiliency and to most of the symptoms that accompany osteoarthritis.

During the progression of osteoarthritis, exogenous glucosamine may have a beneficial role. It is known that, *in vitro*, chondrocytes do synthesize more aggregan when the culture medium is supplemented with glucosamine. N-acetylglucosamine is found to be less effective in these *in vitro* studies. Glucosamine has also been found to have antioxidant activity and to be beneficial in animal models of experimental arthritis.

The counter anion of the glucosamine salt (i.e. chloride or sulfate) is unlikely to play any role in the action or pharmacokinetics of glucosamine. Further, the sulfate in glucosamine sulfate supplements should not be confused with the glucosamine sulfate found in such GAGs as keratan sulfate and heparan sulfate. In the case of the supplement, sulfate is the anion of the salt. In the case of the above GAGs, sulfate is present as an ester. Also, there is no glucosamine sulfate in chondroitin sulfate.

PHARMACOKINETICS

Pharmacokinetics of glucosamine are derived primarily from animal studies. About 90% of glucosamine administered orally as a glucosamine salt gets absorbed from the small intestine, and from there it is transported via the portal circulation to the liver. It appears that a significant fraction of the ingested glucosamine is catabolized by first-pass metabolism in the liver. Free glucosamine is not detected in the serum after oral intake, and it is not presently known how much of an ingested dose is taken up in the joints in humans. Some uptake in the articular cartilage is seen in animal studies.

INDICATIONS

Glucosamine may be indicated for the treatment and prevention of osteoarthritis, either by itself or in combination with chondroitin sulfate (see Chondroitin Sulfate).

RESEARCH SUMMARY

Two recent meta-analyses have confirmed that glucosamine is useful in the treatment of osteoarthritis. One of these meta-analyses included all double-blind, placebo-controlled trials that lasted four weeks or longer. This meta-analysis also included trials that studied the effects of chondroitin sulfate (see Chondroitin Sulfate). In all, there were 13 of these studies (six involving glucosamine and seven involving chondroitin sulfate).

All 13 studies found positive results in hip or knee osteoarthritis. The authors of the meta-analysis judged a trial positive if there was 25% or more improvement in the treatment group compared with placebo. The Levesque Index and global pain scores were used to assess improvement. Very significant improvement was associated with both glucosamine (39.5%) and chondroitin sulfate (40.2%), compared with placebo.

In another recent meta-analysis of nine randomized, controlled trials of glucosamine, glucosamine was significantly superior to placebo in seven of the studies and was superior to ibuprofen and equal to ibuprofen in the other two studies.

Recently, a long-term, randomized placebo-controlled trial of glucosamine sulfate's effects on osteoarthritis ended with the conclusion that the supplement halts progression of structural joint damage and reduces symptoms of those with osteoarthritis of the knee. The study involved 212 patients 50 years or older who received 1500 milligrams of glucosamine sulfate daily or placebo.

Radiographic evidence, at a three-year followup, showed joint space narrowing—the prime indicator of arthritic joint damage—in the placebo group consistent with what has been documented to be typical in untreated osteoarthritis. The glucosamine-supplemented subjects, on the other hand, showed only a non-significant increase in joint space at the same three-year followup.

There has been one study demonstrating an apparent synergistic effect using glucosamine and chondroitin together. The combination was more effective than either substance alone in inhibiting progression of degenerative cartilage lesions in an experimental study.

Clinical research is needed to determine if this effect is truly synergistic, additive or non-existent. The National Institutes of Health has started a large, multi-center study that may shed further light on this issue.

It is probably not surprising that glucosamine may be helpful in osteoarthritis. Glucosamine is crucial for the construction of glycosaminoglycans (GAGs) in articular cartilage. Reduced GAG content in osteoarthritic cartilage matrix corresponds with the severity of osteoarthritis. Oral glucosamine appears to be capable of prompting the chondrocytes to secrete more GAGs. This knowledge, derived from animal

and *in vitro* studies, has prompted clinical trials of glucosamine in osteoarthritis.

CONTRAINDICATIONS, PRECAUTIONS, ADVERSE REACTIONS

CONTRAINDICATIONS

There are no known contraindications to glucosamine supplementation.

WARNINGS AND PRECAUTIONS

Glucosamine may increase insulin resistance. Glucosamine increases insulin resistance in normal and experimentally diabetic animals. In these animals, intravenous glucosamine significantly decreases the rate of glucose uptake in skeletal muscle. In animals given oral glucosamine, this is not observed.

Those with type 2 diabetes and those who are overweight and have problems with glucose tolerance should have their blood sugars carefully monitored if they use glucosamine supplements. Because of insufficient safety data, children, pregnant women and nursing mothers should avoid using glucosamine.

ADVERSE REACTIONS

Side effects that have been reported are mainly mild gastrointestinal complaints such as heartburn, epigastric distress and diarrhea. No allergic reactions have been reported including sulfa-allergic reactions to glucosamine sulfate.

INTERACTIONS

Glucosamine may increase insulin resistance and consequently affect glucose tolerance. Diabetics who, under medical advisement, decide to use glucosamine supplements will need to monitor their blood glucose and may need to adjust the doses of the medications they take to control blood glucose. This needs to be done under medical supervision. No other drug, nutritional supplement, food or herb interaction is known.

OVERDOSAGE

None known.

DOSAGE AND ADMINISTRATION

The three forms of glucosamine available commercially are glucosamine hydrochloride, glucosamine sulfate and N-acetyl glucosamine. The usual dose used by those with osteoarthritis is 1,500 milligrams daily in divided doses. These three forms of glucosamine are available in 500 milligram capsules.

The amount of glucosamine base varies with the supplemental form. Pure glucosamine hydrochloride is about 83% in glucosamine base, pure glucosamine sulfate is about 65% in glucosamine base, and pure N-acetyl glucosamine, about 75% in glucosamine base. It is important that all clinical studies standardize the glucosamine dose of the form used to glucosamine base.

Supplements are available containing glucosamine and low-molecular-weight chondroitin sulfate. (See Chondroitin Sulfate.)

It usually takes several weeks of supplementation before effects, if any, are noted.

HOW SUPPLIED

Capsules — 500 mg, 550 mg, 750 mg, 1000 mg
Powder
Liquid — 500 mg/5 mL
Tablets — 340 mg, 500 mg, 1000 mg

LITERATURE

Deal CL, Moskowitz RW. Nutraceuticals as therapeutic agents in osteoarthritis. The role of glucosamine, chondroitin sulfate, and collagen hydrolysate. *Rheum Dis Clin North Am.* 1999; 25:379-395.

Drovanti A, Bignamini AA, Rovati AL. Therapeutic activity of oral glucosamine sulfate in osteoarthritis, a placebo-controlled double-blind investigation. *Clin Ther.* 1980; 3:260-272.

Houpt JB, McMillan R, Wein C, Paget-Dello SD. Effect of glucosamine hydrochloride in the treatment of pain of osteoarthritis of the knee. *J Rheumatol.* 1999; 26:2423-2430.

Leffler CT, Philippi AF, Leffler SG, et al. Glucosamine, chondroitin, and manganese ascorbate for degenerative joint disease of the knee or low back: a randomized double-blind, placebo-controlled pilot study. *Mil Med.* 1999; 64:85-91.

McClain DA, Crook, ED. Hexosamines and insulin resistance. *Diabetes.* 1996; 45:l003-l006.

Noack W, Fischer, M., Forster, KK, et al. Glucosamine sulfate in osteoarthritis of the knee. *Osteoarthritis Cartilage.* 1994; 2:51-59.

Pujalte JM, Llavore EP, Ylescupidez FR. Double-blind evaluation of oral glucosamine sulfate in the basic treatment of osteoarthritis. *Curr Med Res Opin.* 1980; 7:110-114.

Reichelt A, Forster K, Fisher M, et al. Efficacy and safety of intramuscular glucosamine sulfate in osteoarthritis of the knee. A randomized, placebo-controlled, double-blind study. *Arzneimittelforschung.* 1999; 44:75-80.

Setnikar I, Giacchetti C, Zanolo G. Pharmacokinetics of glucosamine in the dog and in man. *Arzneimittelfors.* 1986; 36*chung*:729-735.

Setnikar I, Palumbo R, Canali S, Zanolo G. Pharmacokinetics of glucosamine in man. *Arzneimittelforschung.*1993; 43:1109-1113.

Towheed TE, Anastassiades TP. Glucosamine and chondroitin for treating symptoms of osteoarthritis. Evidence is widely touted but incomplete. JAMA. 2000; 283:1483-1484.

Towheed TE, Anastassiades TP. Glucosamine therapy for osteoarthritis. Editorial. *J Rheumatol* 1999; 26:2294-2297.

Glutamine Peptides

DESCRIPTION

Glutamine peptides refer to certain dipeptides used in total parenteral nutrition (TPN) as delivery forms of L-glutamine. The term also refers to peptides containing L-glutamine, which are found in some nutritional supplements, particularly those marketed as sports and fitness products.

L-glutamine depletion is a typical feature of such metabolic stress conditions as trauma (including surgical trauma), infection, sepsis, cancer and severe burns. The metabolic response to these conditions is characterized by catabolism and negative nitrogen balance. Under these conditions, L-glutamine, which is normally manufactured by the body (mainly in skeletal muscles) in sufficient quantities to satisfy physiological demands, is required exogenously. Under these conditions, L-glutamine becomes an essential amino acid and must be supplied to the body in order to prevent breakdown of muscle tissue, immune dysfunction and compromise of the gut mucosal barrier function with consequent bacterial translocation into the body. L-glutamine is arguably the most needed amino acid and, indeed, one of the most needed nutrients under these circumstances.

Until recently, L-glutamine was lacking from TPN. The reason for this is because L-glutamine is not very soluble in water—one gram dissolves in 20.8 ml of water at 30 degrees Celsius—and L-glutamine is unstable in solution. The problem has been solved by the synthesis of glutamine-containing dipeptides, which are very soluble in water and stable in solution.

Two synthetic glutamine-containing dipeptides that may be used in TPN are L-alanyl-L-glutamine (Ala-Gln) and glycyl-L-glutamine (Gly-Gln). The molecular weight of Ala-Gln is 217.24 daltons, and L-glutamine comprises 67% of the dipeptide. L-glutamine comprises 72% of Gly-Gln, and its molecular weight is 203.22 daltons.

ACTIONS AND PHARMACOLOGY

ACTIONS

Glutamine peptides may have immunomodulatory, anticatabolic/anabolic, gut mucosal barrier-protective and antioxidant actions.

MECHANISM OF ACTION

The glutamine dipeptides, Ala-Gln and Gly-Gln, have demonstrated immunomodulatory, anticatabolic/anabolic, gastrointestinal mucosal protective and antioxidant activities when used in TPN. These activities have not yet been demonstrated with glutamine peptides marketed as nutritional supplements for fitness purposes. The mechanism of the immunomodulatory action of the glutamine dipeptides is unclear. The mechanism may in part be due to the ability of

L-glutamine to ameliorate the negative effects of TPN on the immune system. Also, L-glutamine is the preferred respiratory fuel for lymphocytes and appears to be required to support the proliferation of mitogen-stimulated lymphocytes, as well as the production of interleukin-2 (IL-2) and interferon-gamma (IFN-gamma). It also appears to be required for the maintenance of lymphokine-activated killer cells (LAK). It can also enhance phagocytosis by neutrophils and monocytes.

The anticatabolic/anabolic action of the glutamine dipeptides can be explained by their effect in sparing skeletal muscle L-glutamine stores. Most of the L-glutamine in the body is synthesized in skeletal muscle, where it is also stored. Under conditions of metabolic stress, skeletal muscle can be depleted of its L-glutamine, which is used for metabolic activities of other tissue/cells, such as enterocytes and lymphocytes.

The gastrointestinal mucosal-protective effect of the glutamine dipeptides can be explained in a few ways. L-glutamine is the preferred respiratory fuel for enterocytes and colonocytes. Maintaining the bioenergetics of these cells is fundamental to maintaining the integrity of the intestine. In addition, L-glutamine helps maintain secretory IgA, which functions primarily by preventing the attachment of bacteria to mucosal cells. L-glutamine may inhibit translocation of Gram-negative bacteria from the intestine into the body.

Metabolic stress goes hand in hand with oxidative stress. L-glutamine can help in ameliorating oxidative stress by serving as precursor to glutathione.

PHARMACOKINETICS
Glutamine dipeptides in TPN are transported via the circulation to the various tissues of the body, where they are taken up by cells and metabolized. Ala-Gln is first metabolized to L-alanine and L-glutamine, while Gly-Gln is metabolized to glycine and L-glutamine. L-glutamine participates in various metabolic activities, including the production of L-glutamate and other amino acids, glutathione, energy, proteins, pyrimidine and purine nucleotides and amino sugars. L-glutamine is eliminated by glomerular filtration and is almost completely reabsorbed by the renal tubules.

Most of the glutamine dipeptides administered orally or enterally are absorbed intact from the lumen of the small intestine into the enterocytes. A portion of the glutamine dipeptides gets metabolized within the enterocytes. That which is not metabolized enters the portal circulation from whence it is transported to the liver. Again, some metabolism takes place in the liver, and that portion not metabolized enters the systemic circulation and is distributed to various tissues of the body.

INDICATIONS AND USAGE
Like glutamine itself (see Glutamine), the dipeptide forms added to TPN are credited with helping in the recovery of trauma, surgical and other critically ill patients. There is as yet no credible evidence that oral use of glutamine peptide supplements has anabolic or ergogenic effects in those who are not metabolically compromised.

RESEARCH SUMMARY
Studies have shown that glutamine and glutamine dipeptides exert similar metabolic effects. The dipeptides themselves are now being used in clinical nutrition.

In one recent, double-blind, randomized, controlled study, duration of hospital stay was significantly reduced in patients who had undergone major abdominal surgery and who had received glutamine dipeptides via TPN over a five-day period. Mean cumulative nitrogen balance was significantly better in these patients, as was immune function, as measured by lymphocyte counts and generation of cysteinyl leukotrienes by polymorphonuclear neutrophils, a measure of neutrophil function.

CONTRAINDICATIONS, PRECAUTIONS, ADVERSE REACTIONS
CONTRAINDICATIONS
Glutamine peptides are contraindicated in those hypersensitive to any component of a glutamine peptide-containing product.

PRECAUTIONS
The use of glutamine dipeptides in TPN must be done under medical supervision.

Those with renal and liver failure should exercise caution in the use of glutamine peptide supplements.

Pregnant women and nursing mothers should avoid the use of oral glutamine peptide supplements unless prescribed by their physicians.

ADVERSE REACTIONS
There are rare reports of constipation and bloating with high dose glutamine peptides in TPN.

INTERACTIONS
DRUGS
See L-Glutamine.

OVERDOSAGE
No reports of overdosage.

DOSAGE AND ADMINISTRATION
The use of glutamine dipeptides in TPN is relatively recent. The two synthetic dipeptides used are L-alanyl -L-glutamine and glycyl-L-glutamine. Doses suggested (given as L-glutamine) are 12 grams daily for surgical trauma and about 25 grams daily for severe trauma and infections.

Those who use oral glutamine peptide supplements for fitness or sports purposes use 1.5 to 4.5 grams (as L-glutamine) daily.

LITERATURE

Decker-Baumann C, Buhl K, Frohmuller S, et al. Reduction of chemotherapy-induced side-effects by parenteral glutamine supplementation in patients with metastatic colorectal cancer. *Eur J Cancer.* 1999; 35:202-207.

Furst P, Pogan K, Stehle P. Glutamine dipeptides in clinical nutrition. *Nutrition.* 1997; 13:731-737.

Khan J, Iiboshi Y, Cui L, et al. Alanyl-glutamine-supplemented parenteral nutrition increases luminal mucus gel and decreases permeability in the rat small intestine. *J Parenter Enteral Nutr.* 1999; 23:24-31.

Li YS, L. JS, Jiang JW, et al. Glycyl-glutamine-enriched long-term total parenteral nutrition attenuates bacterial translocation following small bowel transplantation in the pig. *J Surg Res.* 1999; 82:106-111.

Minami H, Morse EL, Adibi SA. Characteristics and mechanism of glutamine-dipeptide absorption in human intestine. *Gastroenterology.* 1992; 103:3-11.

Morlion BJ, Stehle P, Wachtler P, et al. Total parenteral nutrition with glutamine dipeptide after major abdominal surgery: a randomized, double-blind, controlled-study. *Ann Surg.* 1998; 227:302-308.

Schroder J, Kahlke V, Fandrich F, et al. Glutamine dipeptide-supplemented parenteral nutrition reverses gut mucosal structure and interleukin-6 release of rat intestinal mononuclear cells after hemorrhagic shock. *Shock.* 1998; 10:26-31.

Glutathione

DESCRIPTION

The term glutathione is typically used as a collective term to refer to the tripeptide L-gamma-glutamyl-L-cysteinylglycine in both its reduced and dimeric forms. Monomeric glutathione is also known as reduced glutathione and its dimer is also known as oxidized glutathione, glutathione disulfide and diglutathione. In this monograph, reduced glutathione will be called glutathione— this is its common usage by biochemists—and the glutathione dimer will be referred to as glutathione disulfide.

Glutathione is widely found in all forms of life and plays an essential role in the health of organisms, particularly aerobic organisms. In animals, including humans, and in plants, glutathione is the predominant non-protein thiol and functions as a redox buffer, keeping with its own SH groups those of proteins in a reduced condition, among other antioxidant activities. Glutathione has the following structural formula:

Glutathione

Glutathione is present in tissues in concentrations as high as one millimolar. Cysteine, the business residue of glutathione, neither has the solubility nor activity of glutathione at physiological pH. It appears that nature has built the cysteine molecule into the glutathione tripeptide to make the amino acid more soluble and allow it to have redox buffering activity in a living tissue environment. Glutathione also plays roles in catalysis, metabolism, signal transduction, gene expression and apoptosis. It is a cofactor for glutathione S-transferases, enzymes which are involved in the detoxification of xenobiotics, including carcinogenic genotoxicants, and for the glutathione peroxidases, crucial selenium-containing antioxidant enzymes (see Selenium). It is also involved in the regeneration of ascorbate from its oxidized form, dehydroascorbate (see Vitamin C). There are undoubtedly roles of glutathione that are still to be discovered.

Glutathione is present in the diet in amounts usually less than 100 milligrams daily, and it does not appear that much of the oral intake is absorbed from the intestine into the blood (see Pharmacokinetics). Glutathione is not an essential nutrient since it can be synthesized from the amino acids L-cysteine, L-glutamate and glycine. It is synthesized in two ATP-dependent steps: first, gamma-glutamylcysteine is synthesized from L-glutamate and cysteine via the enzyme gamma-glutamylcysteine synthetase—the rate limiting step— and second, glycine is added to the C-terminal of gamma-glutamylcysteine via the enzyme glutathione synthetase. The liver is the principal site of glutathione synthesis. In healthy tissue, more than 90% of the total glutathione pool is in the reduced form and less than 10% exists in the disulfide form. The enzyme glutathione disulfide reductase is the principal enzyme that maintains glutathione in its reduced form. This latter enzyme uses as its cofactor NADPH (reduced nicotinamide adenine dinucleotide phosphate). NADPH is generated by the oxidative reaction in the pentose phosphate pathway.

The consequences of a functional glutathione deficiency, which results in tissue oxidative stress, can be seen in some pathological conditions. For example, those with glucose 6-phosphate dehydrogenase deficiency produce lower amounts of NADPH and hence, lower amounts of reduced glutathione. This condition is characterized by a hemolytic anemia. Conditions causing chronic glutathione deficiency all result in hemolytic anemia, among other pathological consequences. Oxidative stress caused by glutathione deficiency results in fragile erythrocyte membranes. Malaria-causing organisms (*Plasmodia* species) do not like to feed on these sick erythrocytes. That is about the only good news regarding this situation. Chronic functional glutathione deficiency is also associated with immune disorders, an increased incidence of malignancies, and in the case of HIV disease, probably accelerated pathogenesis of the disease. Acute manifestations of functional glutathione deficiency can be seen in those who have taken an overdosage of acetaminophen. This results in depletion of glutathione in the hepatocytes, leading to liver failure and death, if not promptly treated.

Glutathione is an orphan drug for the treatment of AIDS-associated cachexia. It is thought that this disorder is due, in part, to oxidatively-stressed and damaged enterocytes. There is some evidence that although orally administered glutathione may not be absorbed into the blood from the small intestine to any significant extent, that it may be absorbed into the enterocytes where it may help repair damaged cells. Glutathione in one form or another is the subject of some medicinal chemistry research and some clinical trials. For example, an aerosolized form of glutathione is being studied in AIDS and cystic fibrosis patients. Glutathione, the principal antioxidant of the deep lung, appears to be diminished in those with AIDS. Prodrugs of gamma-L-glutamyl-L-cysteine are being evaluated as anticataract agents.

Glutathione (reduced) is known chemically as *N*-(*N*-L-gamma-glutamyl-L-cysteinyl)glycine and is abbreviated as GSH. Its molecular formula is $C_{10}H_{17}N_3O_6S$ and its molecular weight is 307.33 daltons. Glutathione disulfide is also known as L-gamma-glutamyl-L-cysteinyl-glycine disulfide and is abbreviated as GSSG. Its molecular formula is $C_{20}H_{32}N_6O_{12}S_2$.

The marketed glutathione dietary supplement products are obtained from yeast fermentation, as is the orphan drug. L-Cysteine and N-acetylcysteine are precursors of glutathione and are also available as dietary supplements (see L-Cysteine and N-Acetylcysteine).

ACTIONS AND PHARMACOLOGY
ACTIONS
Glutathione has antioxidant activity. It may have detoxification, and immunomodulatory activities, and may have beneficial effects on sperm motility and in the protection against noise-induced hearing loss.

MECHANISM OF ACTION
Glutathione is the principal intracellular non protein thiol and plays a major role in the maintenance of the intracellular redox state. It may be thought of as an intracellular redox buffer. Glutathione is a nucleophilic scavenger and an electron donor via the sulfhydryl group of its business residue, cysteine. Its reducing ability maintains molecules such as ascorbate and proteins in their reduced state. Glutathione is also the cofactor for the selenium-containing glutathione peroxidases (see Selenium), which are major antioxidant enzymes. These enzymes detoxify peroxides, such as hydrogen peroxide and other peroxides. Another antioxidant activity of glutathione is the maintenance of the antioxidant/reducing agent ascorbate in its reduced state. This is accomplished via glutathione-dependent dehydroascorbate reductase which is comprised of glutaredoxin and protein isomerase reductase. Glutathione may also react with the reactive nitrogen species peroxynitrite to form *S*-nitrosoglutathione.

Glutathione S-transferases (GSTs) consist of a family of multifunctional enzymes that metabolize a wide variety of electrophilic compounds via glutathione conjunction. GSTs are involved in the detoxification of xenobiotic compounds and in the protection against such degenerative diseases as cancer. The mechanism of these enzymes involves a nucleophilic attack by glutathione on an electrophilic substrate. The resulting glutathione conjugates that form are more soluble than the original substrates and thus more easily exported from the cell. The release of glutathione-S-conjugates from cells is an ATP-dependent process mediated by membrane glycoproteins belonging to the multidrug-resistance protein (MRP) family. Proteins of the MRP family are essential for the transport of glutathione S-conjugates into the extracellular space. They are also known as glutathionine-S-conjugate pumps.

Absorption of orally administered glutathione has been observed in some animals (mice, rats, guinea pigs). Oral glutathione has been demonstrated to reverse age-associated decline in immune responsiveness in mice. In one study, glutathione was found to enhance T-cell mediated responsiveness, including delayed-type hypersensitivity (DTH). The mechanism of this effect was ascribed to the antioxidant activity of glutathione.

Parenterally administered glutathione was found to improve sperm motility in a small human trial. Again, the effect was thought to be due to the antioxidant activity of this substance.

Noise-induced hearing loss is thought to be due to oxidative stress. Intraperitoneal administration of glutathione to guinea pigs was found to protect against noise-induced hearing loss and once more, the antioxidant activity of glutathione was thought to account for this effect.

PHARMACOKINETICS

The pharmacokinetics of oral glutathionine in humans are not well understood. It appears that in some animals (mice, rats, guinea pigs), serum glutathione levels do increase following its oral administration. Most human studies of glutathione have not found this to be the case. It appears that oral glutathione is hydrolyzed in the intestine via the intestinal gamma-glutamyl transferase enzyme. A small amount of orally administered glutathione may reach the portal circulation, but apparently this is also rapidly metabolized by hepatic gamma-glutamyltransferase. Thus, most studies have not observed a significant increase in circulating glutathione following its oral administration. However, there is an occasional study that does show an increase in circulating glutathione after oral administration. Further, there is some evidence that glutathione may be absorbed into the enterocytes following ingestion, but may not be released by these cells into the circulation. Research is needed to resolve the issue of glutathione absorption.

INDICATIONS AND USAGE

Though glutathione is undoubtedly a potent antioxidant, indications for its use as a supplement are not yet well established. There is preliminary evidence that it might eventually prove to be useful in the management of some cancers, atherosclerosis, diabetes, lung disorders, noise-induced hearing loss, male infertility and to help prevent or ameliorate various toxicities. It may also have some antiviral activity. Glutathione is an orphan drug for the treatment of AIDS-associated cachexia.

RESEARCH SUMMARY

The use of glutathione in cancer treatment has been two-fold. It has been investigated as an antitumor agent in its own right and as a chemoprotectant used to diminish the toxicities of some cancer drugs. In one animal study, glutathione produced significant regression of aflatoxin-induced liver cancers and significantly enhanced survival. All rats exposed to aflatoxin but not given glutathione died within 24 months of exposure to the carcinogen, but 81% of the glutathione-treated animals were still alive at the end of the 24 months. The researchers concluded that the glutathione-effect noted in this study ''strongly suggests that this antioxidant merits further investigation as a potential antitumor agent in humans.''

Human cancer studies, so far, have utilized glutathione in a secondary role—principally to protect against the toxicity of cisplatin. Its role in this regard has been found effective in several studies wherein it has been demonstrated to diminish cisplatin-induced nephrotoxicity and neurotoxicity.

Early research indicates that exogenous glutathione may significantly inhibit platelet aggregation and improve other hemostatic and hemorheological factors in atherosclerotic patients. In other preliminary clinical work, glutathione has been found to help preserve renal function in patients who had coronary artery bypass operations.

A glutathione aerosol preparation has been helpful in reversing the oxidant-antioxidant imbalance in idiopathic pulmonary fibrosis, and it has helped suppress lung epithelial surface inflammatory cell-derived oxidants in patients with cystic fibrosis. Similar aerosol treatment has been given to HIV patients to augment deficient glutathione levels of the lower respiratory tract with the idea of improving host defense in these immuno-compromised individuals. More research is needed.

Glutathione has also been shown to enhance insulin secretion in elderly subjects with impaired glucose tolerance. There are some further preliminary indications that glutathione might be helpful in some with diabetes, but more research is needed before any meaningful conclusions can be made.

In a double-blind, placebo-controlled study, injected glutathione demonstrated a significant positive effects on sperm motility and morphology in infertile men. And, finally, in another study that needs followup, glutathione exhibited significant *in vitro* inhibition of herpes simplex virus type 1 replication. It appears that the mechanism of this effect is due to glutathione's redox-modulating active. Some viral infections, including HIV infection, result in oxidative stress which may be a major mechanism of their pathogenesis, Modulating oxidative stress could be an antiviral maneuver.

CONTRAINDICATIONS, PRECAUTIONS, ADVERSE REACTIONS

CONTRAINDICATIONS

Glutathione is contraindicated in those hypersensitive to any component of a glutathione-containing product.

PRECAUTIONS

Pregnant women and nursing mothers should avoid the use of supplementary glutathione.

Glutathione is an orphan drug for the treatment of AIDS-associated cachexia. Its use for this indication must be medically supervised.

ADVERSE REACTIONS

Oral doses of up to 600 milligrams daily are well tolerated. There are no reports of adverse reactions.

INTERACTIONS

DRUGS

Cisplatin: Glutathione, administered parenterally, may ameliorate some of the adverse reactions of cisplatin.

OVERDOSAGE

There have been no reports of glutathione overdosage in the literature.

DOSAGE AND ADMINISTRATION

Glutathione is available as a single ingredient dietary supplement or in combination products. Dosage ranges from 50 to 600 milligrams daily.

HOW SUPPLIED

Capsules—50 mg, 250 mg

Powder

Tablets

LITERATURE

Anderson ME, Luo JL. Glutathione therapy: from prodrugs to genes. *Semin Liver Dis.* 1998; 18:415-424.

Aw TW, Wierzbicka G, Jones DP. Oral glutathione increases tissue glutathione in vivo. *Chem Biol Interact.* 1991; 80:89-97.

Bains JS, Shaw CA. Neurodegenerative disorders in humans: the role of glutathione in oxidative stress-mediated neuronal death. *Brain Res Brain Res Rev.* 1997; 25:335-358.

Borok Z, Buhl R, Grimes GJ, et al. Effect of glutathione aerosol on oxidant-antioxidant imbalance in ideopathic pulmonary fibrosis. *Lancet.* 1991; 338:215-216.

Broquist HP. Buthionine sulfoximine, an experimental tool to induce glutathionine deficiency: elucidation of glutathionine and ascorbate in their role as antioxidants. *Nutr Rev.* 1992; 50:110-111.

Brown LA, Bai C, Jones DP. Glutathione protection in aveolar type II cells from fetal and neonatal rabbits. *Am J Physiol.* 1992; 262:L305-L312.

Cascinu S, Cordella L, Del Ferro E, et al. Neuroprotective effect of reduced glutathione on cisplatin-based chemotherapy in advanced gastric cancer: a randomized double-blind placebo-controlled study. *J Clin Oncol.* 1995; 13:26-32.

Cheung P-Y, Wang W, Schulz R. Glutathione protects against ischemia-perfusion injury by detoxifying peroxynitrite. *J Mol Cell Cardiol.* 2000; 32:1669-1678.

De Mattia G, Bravi MC, Laurenti O, et al. Influence of reduced glutathione infusion on glucose metabolism in patients with non-insulin-dependent diabetes mellitus. *Metabolism.* 1998; 47:993-997.

Exner R, Wessner B, Manhart N, Roth E. Therapeutic potential of glutathione. *Wien Klin Wochenschr.* 2000; 112:610-616.

Favilli F, Marraccini P, Iantomasi T, Vincenzini MT. Effect of orally administered glutathione levels in osme organs of rats: role of specific transporters. *Br J Nutr.* 1997; 78:293-300.

Flagg EW, Coates RJ, Eley JW, et al. Dietary glutathione intake in humans and the relationship between intake and plasma total glutathionine level. *Nutr Canc.* 1994; 21:33-46.

Furukawa T, Meydani SN, Blumberg JB. Reversal of age-associated decline in immune responsiveness by dietary glutathione supplementation in mice. *Mech Ageing Dev.* 1987; 38:107-117.

Griffith OW. Biologic and pharmacologic regulation of mammalian glutathione synthesis. *Free Rad Biol Med.* 1999; 27:922-935.

Hagen TM, Jones DP. Transepithelial transport of glutathione in vascularly perfused small intestine of rat. *Am J Physiol.* 1987; 252(5 Pt 1):G607-G613.

Hagen TM, Wierzbicka GT, Sillau AH, et al. Bioavailability of dietary glutathione: effect on plasma concentration. *Am J Physiol.* 1990; 259(4 Pt 1):G524-G529.

Hayes JD, McLellan LI. Glutathione and glutathione-dependent enzymes represent a co-ordinately regulated defence against oxidative stress. *Free Rad Res.* 1999; 31:273-300.

Hayes JD, Strange RC. Glutathione S-transferase polymorphisms and their biological consequences. *Pharmacology.* 2000; 61:154-166.

Hercbergs A, Brok-Simoni F, Holtzman F, et al. Erythrocyte glutathione and tumor response to chemotherapy. *Lancet.* 1992; 339:1074-1076.

Holroyd KJ, Buhl R, Borok Z, et al. Correction of glutathione deficiency in the lower respiratory tract of HIV seropositive individuals by glutathione aerosol treatment. *Thorax.* 1993; 48:985-989.

Hwang C, Sinskey AJ, Lodish HF. Oxidized redox state of glutathione in the endoplasmic reticulum. *Science.* 1992; 257:1496-1502.

Janaky R, Ogita K, Pasqualotta BA, et al. Glutathione and signal transduction in the mammalian CNS. *J Neurochem.* 1999; 73:889-902.

Lash LH, Hagen TM, Jones DP. Exogenous glutathione protects intestinal epithelial cells from oxidative injury. *Proc Natl Acad Sci USA.* 1986; 83:4641-4645.

Lenzi A, Culasso F, Gandini L, et al. Placebo-controlled, double-blind, cross-over trial of glutathione therapy in male infertility. *Hum Reprod.* 1993; 8:1657-1662.

Lenzi A, Picardo M, Gandini L, et al. Glutathione treatment of dyspermia: effect on the lipoperoxidation process. *Hum Reprod.* 1994; 9:2044-2050.

Loguercio C, Di Pierro M. The role of glutathione in the gastrointestinal tract: a review. *Ital J Gastroenterol Hepatol.* 1999; 31:401-407.

Lyons J, Rauh-Pfeiffer A, Yu YM, et al. Blood glutathione synthesis rates in healthy adults receiving a sulfur amino acid-free diet. *Proc Natl Acad Sci USA.* 2000; 97:5071-5076.

Martensson J, Jain A, Meister A. Glutathione is required for intestinal function. *Proc Natl Acad Sci USA.* 1990; 87:1715-1719.

Meister A. On the antioxidant effects of ascorbic acid and glutathionine. *Biochem Pharmacol.* 1992; 44:1905-1915.

Murphy ME, Scholich H, Sies H. Protection by glutathione and other thiol compounds against the loss of protein thiols and tocopherol homologs during microsomal lipid peroxidation. *Eur J Biochem.* 1992; 210:139-146.

Nagasawa HT, Cohen JF, Holleschau AM, Rathbun WB. Augmentation of human and rat lenticular glutathione in vitro by prodrugs of gamma-L-glutamyl-L-cysteine. *J Med Chem.* 1996; 39:1676-1681.

Novi AM. Regression of aflatoxin B₁-induced hepatocellular carcinomas by reduced glutathione. *Science.* 1981; 212:541-542.

Ohinataab Y, Yamasobac T, Schachta J, Millera JM. Glutathione limits noise-induced hearing loss. *Hear Res.* 2000; 146:28-34.

Palamara AT, Perno C-F, Ciriolo MR, et al. Evidence for antiviral activity of glutathione: in vitro inhibition of herpes simplex virus type 1 replication. *Antiviral Res.* 1995; 27:237-253.

Paolisso G, Giugliano D, Pizza G, et al. Glutathione infusion potentiates glucose-induced insulin secretion in aged patients with impaired glucose tolerance. *Diabetes Care.* 1992; 15:1-7.

Roum JH, Borok Z, McElvaney NG, et al. Glutathione aerosol suppresses lung epithelial surface inflammatory cell-derived oxidants in cystic fibrosis. *J Appl Physiol.* 1999; 87:438-443.

Samiec PS, Drews-Botsch C, Flagg EW, et al. Glutathione in human plasma: decline in association with aging, age-related macular degeneration, and diabetes. *Free Radic Biol Med.* 1998; 24:699-704.

Schmidinger M, Budinsky AC, Wenzel C, et al. Glutathione in the prevention of cisplatin induced toxicities. A prospectively randomized pilot trial in patients with head and neck cancer and non small cell lung cancer. *Wien Klin Wochenschr.* 2000; 112:617-623.

Shaw CA, ed. *Glutathione in the Nervous System.* London: Taylor and Francis; 1998.

Sies H. Glutathione and its role in cellular functions. *Free Rad Biol Med.* 1999; 27:916-921.

Smyth JF, Bowman A, Perren T, et al. Glutathione reduces the toxicity and improves quality of life of women diagnosed with ovarian cancer treated with cisplatin: results of a double-blind, randomized trial. *Ann Oncol.* 1997; 8:569-573.

Sternberg P Jr, Davidson PC, Jones DP, et al. Protection of retinal pigment epithelium from oxidative injury by glutathione and precursors. *Invest Opthalmol Vis Sci.* 1993; 34:3661-3668.

Witschi A, Reddy S, Stofer B, Lauterburg BH. The systemic availability of oral glutathione. *Eur J Clin Pharmacol.* 1992; 43:667-669.

Glycerol

TRADE NAMES

Glycerol Fuel (Twinlab)

DESCRIPTION

Glycerol is one of the most common alcohols found in human metabolism. It is a 3-carbon molecule containing three hydroxyl groups. Its molecular formula is $C_3H_8O_3$, and its molecular weight is 92.09 daltons. A syrupy liquid with a sweet taste, glycerol is about 0.6 times as sweet as cane sugar. Glycerol is also known as glycerin, glycerine, 1,2,3-propanetriol and trihydroxypropane. The structural formula for glycerol is:

Glycerol

Glycerol is the backbone of triacylglycerols (triglycerides or neutral fats) and phospholipids. These substances are present in most life forms, and dietary intake of glycerol comes mainly from these molecules in animal and plant products. Glycerol is also used as a sweetner in syrup, liquor and some foods.

Glycerol has had diverse uses in medicine. It has moisturizing and lubricating properties and can increase serum osmolality. It is given orally to reduce intraocular pressure and vitreous volume in eye surgery and is used as an adjunct in the management of acute glaucoma. Glycerol may also be used topically to reduce corneal edema, which may be of use in eye examinations. Glycerol has also been used (intravenously or orally) for the management of cerebral edema secondary to acute stroke, to lower intracranial pressure and to improve rehydration during acute gastrointestinal disease. It is a hyperosmotic laxative and may be used rectally in suppositories. It is used as a cerumenolytic and as a demulcent in cough preparations.

Oral glycerol by itself may have dehydrating activity. However, if ingested with added fluid, it may increase total body water. This is known as glycerol hyperhydration, and glycerol is used by some athletes to improve thermoregulation and endurance during exercise or exposure to hot environments.

ACTIONS AND PHARMACOLOGY

ACTIONS

Supplemental glycerol has putative hyperhydration and athletic performance-enhancing activities.

MECHANISM OF ACTION

The main effect of glycerol itself results from its dehydrating activity. For example, oral glycerol can increase serum osmalility, thus drawing fluid from other parts of the body. This is the mechanism, at least in part, for its ocular hypotensive effect in the treatment of acute glaucoma.

Therefore, it seems paradoxical to talk about glycerol's hyperhydration effect. However, in combination with ample water, it may be more hydrating than water alone, at least for some. The mechanism of this effect and how it may relate to enhanced athletic performance is still highly unclear.

PHARMACOKINETICS

Following ingestion, glycerol is efficiently absorbed and rapidly metabolized. It is absorbed from the lumen of the small intestine into the enterocytes and from those cells into the portal circulation, from whence it is transported to the liver. In the hepatocytes, much of glycerol is phosphorylated via the enzyme glycerol kinase to produce L-glycerol 3-phophate. ATP is necessary for this reaction.

Some L-glycerol 3-phosphate reacts with fatty acyl CoA molecules to ultimately form triglycerides (triacylglycerols) and phospholipids. Most L-glycerol 3-phosphate undergoes oxidation to dihydroxyacetone phosphate, catalyzed either by cytosolic glycerol 3-phosphate dehydrogenase, an enzyme that requires NAD^+ as electron receptor, or by mitochondrial glycerol 3-phosphate dehydrogenase. The coupling of the two glycerol 3-phosphate dehydrogenases leads to the passage of electrons from NADH to enter the mitochondrial electron transfer chain for the production of ATP. This transfer of electrons from cytosolic NADH to the mitochondrial electron transport chain is known as the glycerol phosphate shuttle. Dihydroxyacetone phosphate can either move in the direction of further oxidation to finally yield carbon dioxide, water and ATP or be converted to glyceraldehyde 3-phosphate and move in the direction of glucose and glycogen synthesis.

Glycerol not metabolized in the liver is transported to various tissues and undergoes metabolism. Similar reactions to those discussed above occur in the kidney.

Glycerol is eliminated in the kidney by filtration and, in concentrations up to 0.15 mg/ml, undergoes complete tubular reabsorption. In higher concentration, glycerol begins to appear in the urine and induces an osmotic diuresis.

The elimination half-life of glycerol is from 30 to 45 minutes.

INDICATIONS AND USAGE

Glycerol may be useful for improving hydration and, thus, exercise endurance in some, but research results related to this putative benefit are mixed. There is no evidence that glycerol helps with weight loss. Intravenous glycerol is helpful in some with acute ischemic cerebral infarct. Oral glycerol has been useful in preventing some of the neurologic and audiologic sequellae of childhood bacterial meningitis.

RESEARCH SUMMARY

Pre-exercise administration of glycerol significantly improved cycling endurance time in two double-blind, randomized, cross-over trials. Mean heart rate was also reduced in glycerol-supplemented subjects.

Pre-exercise administration of glycerol in another study, however, failed to affect exercise performance in a group of triathletes. Results of animal work have been similarly mixed, and more research is needed.

Glycerol did not increase weight loss in a placebo-controlled trial.

Intravenous administration of glycerol in subjects with acute ischemic cerebral infarct has resulted in significantly fewer neurological deficits in one study. Several other trials demonstrating similar benefits have been double-blind, randomized trials, but some of these benefits have been transient.

Glycerol-treated infants and children with bacterial meningitis had less severe hearing impairment and fewer neurologic deficits than did controls. Oral administration of glycerol was utilized.

CONTRAINDICATIONS, PRECAUTIONS, ADVERSE REACTIONS

CONTRAINDICATIONS

Supplemental glycerol is contraindicated in those with severe dehydration, anuria, congestive heart failure and pulmonary edema. It is also contraindicated in those who are hypersensitive to glycerol.

PRECAUTIONS

Glycerol supplementation should be avoided by pregnant women and nursing mothers.

Those with cardiac, renal or hepatic problems should avoid supplemental glycerol, as should those with diabetes and those with hemolytic anemia.

Anyone using oral glycerol for supplementation must drink plenty of fluid concomitantly. See Dosing and Administration.

Those using glycerol need to be aware that contact of glycerol with strong oxidizing agents, such as potassium permanganate, potassium chlorate or chromium trioxide, may produce an explosion.

ADVERSE REACTIONS

There are rare reports of cardiac dysrhythmias occurring with oral glycerol use and one report of hypertension occurring. Other adverse reactions include headache, dizziness, confusion and amnesia (in elderly subjects) and hyperglycemia. Hyperosmolarity, which occurs with oral glycerol, is usually clinically significant only in those with type 2 diabetes. Those with type 2 diabetes may develop nonketotic hyperosmolar hyperglycemia.

The most frequent adverse reactions are gastrointestinal and include nausea and vomiting, bloating and diarrhea.

DOSAGE AND ADMINISTRATION
The doses are variable in those who use glycerol for hydration purposes and for possible exercise performance enhancement. Some use 2 to 4 tablespoons of glycerol in water, orange juice or a sports drink. The ratio of fluids to glycerol is about 20 to 1. This is taken approximately 2.5 hours prior to exercise. The volume of a tablespoon is 15 ml, and one ml of glycerol weighs 1.25 grams. The energy value of glycerol is about 4 kcal or 4 Cal per gram. Pharmaceutical grade glycerol is used.

HOW SUPPLIED
Liquid

LITERATURE
Inder WJ, Swanney MP, Donald RA, et al. The effect of glycerol and desmopressin on exercise performance and hydration in triathletes. *Med Sci Sports Exerc.* 1998; 30:1263-1269.

Montner P, Stark DM, Riedesel ML, et al. Pre-exercise glycerol hydration improves cycling endurance time. *Int J Sports Med.* 1996; 17:27-33.

Robergs RA, Griffin SE. Glycerol. Biochemistry, pharmacokinetics and clinical and practical applications. *Sports Med.* 1998; 26:145-167.

Wagner DR. Hyperhydrating with glycerol: implications for athletic performance. *J Am Diet Assoc.* 1999; 99:207-212.

Glycine

DESCRIPTION
Glycine is a protein amino acid found in the protein of all life forms. It is the simplest amino acid in the body and the only protein amino acid that does not have chirality. Although most glycine is found in proteins, free glycine is found in body fluids as well as in plants. The normal diet contributes approximately 2 grams of glycine daily.

Glycine is not considered an essential amino acid, i. e., the cells in the body can synthesize sufficient amounts of glycine to meet physiological requirements. However, glycine is of major importance in the synthesis of proteins, peptides, purines, adenosine triphosphate (ATP), nucleic acids, porphyrins, hemoglobin, glutathione, creatine, bile salts, one-carbon fragments, glucose, glycogen, and L-serine and other amino acids. Glycine is also a neurotransmitter in the central nervous system (CNS). Glycine and gamma-aminobutyric acid (GABA) are the major inhibitory neurotransmitters in

the CNS. Recently, a glycine-gated chloride channel has been identified in neurophils that can attenuate increases in intracellular calcium ions and diminish oxidant damage mediated by these white blood cells. Thus, glycine may be a novel antioxidant.

Glycine is also known as amino acetic acid, aminoethanolic acid, glycocoll, glycinium and sucre de gelatine. Its IUPAC abbreviation is Gly and its one-letter abbreviation, used when spelling out protein structures, is G. It is a neutral amino acid. Glycine is a solid water-soluble substance that has a sweetish taste. Its structural formula is:

Glycine

ACTIONS AND PHARMACOLOGY
ACTIONS
Supplemental glycine may have antispastic activity. Very early findings suggest it may also have antipsychotic activity as well as antioxidant and anti-inflammatory activities.

MECHANISM OF ACTION
In the CNS, there exist strychnine-sensitive glycine binding sites as well as strychnine-insensitive glycine binding sites. The strychnine-insensitive glycine-binding site is located on the NMDA receptor complex. The strychnine-sensitive glycine receptor complex is comprised of a chloride channel and is a member of the ligand-gated ion channel superfamily. The putative antispastic activity of supplemental glycine could be mediated by glycine's binding to strychnine-sensitive binding sites in the spinal cord. This would result in increased chloride conductance and consequent enhancement of inhibitory neurotransmission.

The ability of glycine to potentiate NMDA receptor-mediated neurotransmission raised the possibility of its use in the management of neuroleptic-resistant negative symptoms in schizophrenia.

Animal studies indicate that supplemental glycine protects against endotoxin-induced lethality, hypoxia-reperfusion injury after liver transplantation, and D-galactosamine-mediated liver injury. Neutrophils are thought to participate in these pathologic processes via invasion of tissue and releasing such reactive oxygen species as superoxide. *In vitro* studies have shown that neutrophils contain a glycine-gated chloride channel that can attenuate increases in intracellular calcium and diminsh neutrophil oxidant production. This research is ealy-stage, but suggests that supplementary glycine may turn out to be useful in processes where neutrophil infiltration contributes to toxicity, such as ARDS.

PHARMACOKINETICS

Following ingestion of glycine, the amino acid is absorbed from the small intestine via an active transport mechanism. From the small intestine, glycine is transported to the liver by means of the portal circulation where a portion enters into one of several metabolic pathways. Glycine not metabolized in the liver enters the systemic circulation and is distributed to various tissues in the body. Glycine readily crosses the blood-brain barrier.

INDICATIONS AND USAGE

Glycine may be indicated to help alleviate the symptoms of spasticity. An indication for potentiating some anti-convulsant drugs and preventing some seizures could emerge, as could an indication for its use in managing schizophrenia. Research in progress also suggests usefulness in some cancers. There is no evidence to support use of glycine as an ergogenic aid, and it is too early to say whether it can play any useful role in lipid metabolism. There are no well-designed clinical trials to support its use in benign prostate hypertrophy.

RESEARCH SUMMARY

Glycine first attracted interest in the medical research community for its reputed ability to dampen reflex excitability in the CNS. A pilot study of its effects on severe chronic leg spasticity (most of the subjects were suffering from chronic multiple sclerosis) yielded improvement in spasticity and mobility of the lower limbs, rated at about 25% overall. The dose used was 1 gram daily for six months to a year. All patients noted some benefits, and no adverse events were recorded. Other researchers have since reported that glycine can potentiate some but not all anticonvulsant drugs in some animal models. It has also been shown to prevent some experimentally produced seizures.

The effects of oral glycine (200 mg/kg/day) were tested in two siblings suffering from 3-phosphoglycerate dehydrogenase deficiency, an inborn error of L-serine biosynthesis. A significant amount of glycine is made from L-serine. Among the features of this disorder are intractable seizures. L-serine in doses up to 500 mg/kg/day failed to control the seizures, but oral glycine completely stopped them, and electroencephalographic abnormalities resolved after six months of treatment.

High-dose glycine may be beneficial in the management of enduring negative symptoms of schizophrenia. Twenty-two treatment-resistant schizophrenic patients participated in a double-blind, placebo-controlled, six-week, crossover treatment trial with 0.8 grams per kilogram daily of glycine added to their ongoing antipsychotic medication. Glycine

intake ranged from 40 to 90 grams daily. Only mild gastrointestinal side effects (nausea and vomiting) were reported in one patient taking glycine. Patients taking glycine experienced significantly diminished negative symptoms. Followup studies are planned.

Recent animal studies suggest that glycine may have some anti-cancer properties. In one recent study, 51 weeks of glycine supplementation did not stop early foci formation of cancer but reduced formation of small liver tumors by 23%, medium-sized tumors by 64% and large tumors by nearly 80% in rats given an agent that is a peroxisome proliferator and liver carcinogen.

In another recent study, dietary glycine inhibited B16 melanoma tumors in mice. Glycine-supplemented mice had tumors that were 50 to 70% smaller in size than those in controls. The protective mechanism in this case appeared to be inhibition of angiogenesis effected by suppressed endothelial-cell proliferation. Tumors in mice fed glycine had 70% fewer arteries than were present in the tumors of controls.

Whether very preliminary data suggesting some positive effects of glycine on lipid metabolism will be mirrored in human research remains to be seen.

Partly because glycine is a precursor of creatine, some have assumed that it might have some of the same ergogenic potential that has been claimed for creatine. This, so far, has not been demonstrated. Glycine is claimed to be beneficial for benign prostatic hypertrophy based on a dated clinical study that has never been confirmed.

CONTRAINDICATIONS, PRECAUTIONS, ADVERSE REACTIONS

CONTRAINDICATIONS

Glycine supplementation is contraindicated in those hypersensitive to any component of the preparation. It is also contraindicated in those who are anuric (some glycine gets converted to ammonia).

PRECAUTIONS

Glycine supplementation should be avoided by pregnant women and nursing mothers. Because of some conversion of glycine to ammonia, those with hepatic impairment should avoid glycine supplementation unless prescribed.

ADVERSE REACTIONS

Doses of 1 gram daily are very well tolerated. Mild gastrointestinal symptoms are infrequently noted. In one study doses of 90 grams daily were also well tolerated.

INTERACTIONS

Antispastic drugs. Theoretically, supplemental glycine might have additive effects when used in conjunction with baclofen, diazepam, dantrolene sodium and tizanidine.

No other drug, nutritional supplement, food or herb interactions are known.

OVERDOSAGE

There are no reports of overdosage in humans. The majority of mice receiving 3 to 4.5 grams per kilogram by intravenous infusion experienced bradycardia, prolongation of the PQ interval, QRS duration and death.

DOSAGE AND ADMINISTRATION

Glycine is available in 500 milligram tablets and capsules. Those who supplement use up to 1 gram daily in divided doses. Doses used for management of schizophrenia have ranged from 40 to 90 grams daily.

HOW SUPPLIED

Capsules — 500 mg, 600 mg

Irrigation Solution — 1.5%

Powder

Tablets — 500 mg, 600 mg

LITERATURE

Barbeau A. Preliminary study of glycine administration in patients with spasticity. *Neurol.* 1974; 24:392.

de Kooning JT, Duran M, Dorling L, et al. Beneficial effects of L-serine and glycine in the management of seizures in 3-phosphoglycerate dehydrogenase deficiency. *Ann Neurol.* 1998; 44:261-265.

Heresco-Levy U, Javitt DC, Ermilov M, et al. Efficacy of high-dose glycine in the treatment of enduring negative symptoms of schizophrenia. *Arch Gen Psychiatry.* 1999; 56:29-36.

Olsson J, Hahn RG. Glycine toxicity after high-dose i.v. infusion of 1.59 % glycine in the mouse. *Br J Anaest.* 1999; 82:250-254.

Rose ML, Cattley RC, Dunn C, et al. Dietary glycine prevents the development of liver tumors caused by the peroxisome proliferator WY-14, 643. *Carcinogenesis.* 1999; 20:2075-2081.

Rose ML, Madren J, Bunzendahl H, Thurman RG. Dietary glycine inhibits the growth of B16 melanoma tumors in mice. *Carcinogenesis.* 1999; 20:793-798

Simpson RK Jr, Gondo M, Robertson CS, Goodman JC. The influence of glycine and related compounds on spinal cord injury-related spasticity. *Neurochem Res.* 1995; 20:1203-1210.

Simpson RK Jr, Robertson CS, Goodman JC. The role of glycine in spinal shock. 1996; 19:215-224.

Smith JE, Hall PV, Galvin MR, et al. Effects of glycine administration on canine experimental spinal spasticity and the levels of glycine, glutamate, and aspartate in the lumbar spinal cord. *Neurosurg.* 1979; 4:153-156.

Toth E, Lajtha A. Glycine potentiates the action of some anticonvulsant drugs in some seizure models. *Neurochem Res.* 1984; 9:1711-1718.

Wheeler M, Stachlewitz RT, Yamashina S, et al. Glycine-gated channels in neutrophils attenuate calcium influx and superoxide production. FASEB J. 2000; 14:476-484.

Wheeler MD, Ikejema K, Mol Life Sci. Enomoto N, et al. Glycine: a new anti-inflammatory immunonutrient. *Cell Mol Life Sci.*1999; 56:843-856.

Yagasaki K, Funabiki R. Effects of dietary supplemented amino acids on endogenous hypercholesterolemia in rats. *J Nutr Sci Vitaminol.* 1990; 36 Suppl 12:S165-S168.

Glycitein

DESCRIPTION

Glycitein belongs to the isoflavone class of flavonoids. It is also classified as a phytoestrogen since it is a plant-derived nonsteroidal compound that possesses estrogen-like biological activity. Glycitein has been found to have weak estrogenic activity.

Glycitein is the aglycone of glycitin. The isoflavone is found naturally as the glycoside (glucoside) glycitin and as the glycosides 6''-0-malonylglycitin and 6''-0-acetylglycitin. Glycitein and its glycosides are mainly found in legumes, such as soybeans and chickpeas. Soybeans and soy foods are the major dietary sources of these substances. Glycitein glycosides are the least abundant of the isoflavones in soybeans and soy foods, where they comprise about 5 to 10% of the total isoflavones. However, in soy germ, glycitein glycosides comprise about 40% of the isoflavones.

Glycitein is a solid substance that is virtually insoluble in water. Glycitein is also known as 7-hydroxy-6-methoxy-3-(4-hydroxyphenyl)- 4*H*-1-benzopyran-4-one and 4', 7-dihydroxy-6-methoxyisoflavone.

Glycitein, when marketed as a nutritional supplement, is mainly present in the form of its beta-glucoside, glycitin.

ACTIONS AND PHARMACOLOGY

ACTIONS

Glycitein has estrogenic activity. It may also have antioxidant, anticarcinogenic, anti-atherogenic and anti-osteoporotic activities.

MECHANISM OF ACTION

Of all the soy isoflavones, glycitein has been the least studied. The chemical structure of glycitein is similar to that of genistein and daidzein, and it would be expected to have similar possible activities. However, except for its probable antioxidant activity, this cannot be certainly stated, since small differences in chemical structure often produce great differences in biological activities. What is known is that glycitein has weak estrogenic activity as measured in *in vivo* and *in vitro* assays. *In vivo*, its estrogenic activity is the highest of the soy isoflavones: three times greater than that of genistein and 12 times greater than that of daidzein. Any further discussion of the mechanism of glycitein's possible actions would be entirely speculative.

PHARMACOKINETICS

Little is known about the pharmacokinetics of glycitein in humans. Studies show that, following ingestion of soy isoflavones, glycitein is found in the plasma, indicating that it is absorbed to some extent. It is likely that the pharmacokinetics of glycitein are similar to that of genistein and daidzein.

See Genistein and Daidzein.

INDICATIONS AND USAGE

Though not as studied as genistein and daidzein, two other soy isoflavones, glycitein presumably has some of the same anticancer effects. It may also have some of the benefits observed in the use of soy isoflavones, with respect to atherogenesis and problems associated with menopause, including "hot flashes" and osteoporosis.

See Soy Isoflavones, Genistein and Daidzein.

RESEARCH SUMMARY

Because glycitein is found only in small amounts in soybeans, glycitein research has lagged far behind research on genistein and daidzein, two other soy isoflavones. Recently, however, research has shown that 40% of the plant estrogens in soy germ is glycitein. Its estrogenicity, which is higher than that of daidzein and genistein, coupled with another recent finding that glycitein may be more readily absorbed in the body, has resulted in increased interest in this isoflavone. More research is underway.

CONTRAINDICATIONS, PRECAUTIONS, ADVERSE REACTIONS

CONTRAINDICATIONS

Glycitein is contraindicated in those who are hypersensitive to any component of a glycitein or glycitin-containing product.

PRECAUTIONS

Pregnant women and nursing mothers should avoid the use of glycitein/glycitin-containing supplements pending long-term safety studies.

Men with prostate cancer should discuss the advisability of the use of glycitein/glycitin-containing supplements with their physicians before deciding to use them.

Women with estrogen receptor-positive tumors should exercise caution in the use of glycitein/glycitin-containing supplements and should use them only if they are recommended and monitored by a physician.

DOSAGE AND ADMINISTRATION

Glycitein is available in a few different formulations. A standard soy isoflavone formula contains glycitein principally in the form of glycitin, as well as genistin and daidzin with much smaller amounts of the aglycones glycitein, genistein and daidzein. The percentage of the soy isoflavones present in such a supplement reflect the percentages of these substances in soybeans and are: glycitin, about 12%; genistin, about 50%; and daidzin, about 38%. A 50-milligram dose of the soy isoflavone supplement—a typical daily dose—delivers about 6 mg of glycitin, 25 mg of genistin and 19 mg of daidzin. Usually 40% of the supplement is comprised of soy isoflavones. Therefore, to get a dose of 50 mg of soy isoflavones, which includes 6 mg of glycitin, 125 mg of the soy supplement are required.

Soy isoflavone supplements derived from soy germ are richer in glycitin. Typically, about 40% of a soy germ isoflavone supplement is comprised of glycitin, about 50% of daidzin and about 10% of genistin.

LITERATURE
Song TT, Hendrich S, Murphy PA. Estrogenic activity of glycitein, a soy isoflavone. *J Agric Food Chem.* 1999; 47:1607-1610.

Zhang Y, Wang G-J, Song TT, et al. Urinary disposition of the soybean isoflavones daidzein, genistein and glycitein differs among humans with moderate fecal isoflavone degradation activity. *J Nutr.* 1999; 129:957-962.

For additional references, see Soy Isoflavones.

Grape Seed Proanthocyanidins

TRADE NAMES

Proanthodyn Grape Seed Extract (Source Naturals), Activin Grape Seed Extract (Natrol), Grape Seed Power (Nature's Herbs), Grape Pips (Nutricology), Grape Seed Phytosome (Enzymatic Therapy), Grapenol (Solaray).

DESCRIPTION

Grape seed proanthocyanidins refer to procyanidin mixtures extracted from grape (*Vitis vinifera*) seeds. Procyanidins are derivatives of the flavan-3-ol class of flavonoids. This class includes (+)-catechin, commonly referred to as catechin, and (-)-epicatechin, commonly referred to as epicatechin. Procyanidins are dimers and oligomers of catechin and epicatechin and their gallic acid esters. Procyanidins are widely distributed in the plant kingdom and, in addition to being found in grape seeds, are found in cocoa and chocolate, apples, peanuts, almonds, cranberries, blueberries and in the bark of pines, among other plant sources.

Grape seed proanthocyanidins are mainly comprised of dimers, trimers and tetramers of catechin and epicatechin and their gallates. They also contain smaller amounts of pentamers, hexamers and heptamers of these flavan-3-ols and their gallates. The procyanidin dimers and oligomers are also known as oligomeric procyanidins (OPCs) and procyanidolic oligomers or PCOs. Grape seed proanthocyanidins comprise approximately 60 to 70% of the polyphenol content of grapes. The procyanidins are colorless in their pure state.

See also Cocoa Flavonoids and Pycnogenol.

ACTIONS AND PHARMACOLOGY

ACTIONS

Grape seed proanthocyanidins have antioxidant activity. They may also have anti-inflammatory, anticarcinogenic and anti-atherogenic activities.

MECHANISM OF ACTION

Grape seed proanthocyanidins have been found to have a number of antioxidant activities in the laboratory. These include scavenging of hydroxyl and peroxyl radicals, and inhibition of the oxidation of low-density lipoprotein (LDL). The inhibitory potential related to lipid peroxidation appears to increase with the degree of polymerization of the molecules. That is, grape seed proanthocyanidins with a greater number of catechin and epicatechin units appear to have more potent inhibitory activity than those with fewer catechin and epicatechin units. Further, the position of linkage between inter-flavan units also appears to influence lipid peroxidation inhibitory activity. Procyanidin isomers with a 4-6 inter-flavan linkage appear to show stronger inhibitory activity than those with a 4-8 linkage. Finally, the presence of a gallate group also appears to affect the inhibitory activity of the procyanidins with respect to lipid peroxidation. A procyanidin dimer with a gallate group linked at the 3-hydroxy position appears to show much greater inhibition of lipid peroxidation than a dimer without such a group.

Grape seed proanthocyanidins have shown anti-inflammatory, anticarcinogenic and anti-atherogenic activities, again in the laboratory. These activities are thought to be due, in large part, to the antioxidant activities of these molecules. These proanthocyanidins have been found to be cytotoxic for some human cancer lines in culture. Upregulation of apoptosis by the proanthocyanidins in these cancer lines is another possible mechanism for their possible anticarcinogenic activity.

PHARMACOKINETICS

Little is known about the pharmacokinetics of grape seed proanthocyanidins in humans. It appears that they do, at least in part, get absorbed. However, the extent of absorption appears to vary widely, not only among the various components of the grape seed proanthocyanidins, but also among subjects.

INDICATIONS AND USAGE

Experimental data suggest that grape seed proanthocyanidins may have anticancer activity, that they protect against some forms of lipid peroxidation and that they may be cardioprotective, hepatoprotective and capillary protective. They appear to have anti-inflammatory activity. Claims that they are useful in the treatment of arthritis, varicose veins, diabetic retinopathy and some allergies are largely based upon anecdotal testimony; clinical trials are lacking.

RESEARCH SUMMARY

Antitumor-promoting activity, described as highly significant, has been observed in animals treated with topical grape seed proanthocyanidins. Skin tumor incidence, multiplicity and volume were all significantly inhibited. These effects were attributed to inhibition of epidermal lipid peroxidation. Higher doses resulted in greater degrees of cancer inhibition.

An extract of grape seed proanthocyanidins has significantly inhibited human breast cancer, lung cancer and gastric adenocarcinoma cells in vitro. The extract did not inhibit neoplastic K562 myelogenous leukemic cells. In the same experiment, the extract enhanced growth and viability of normal human gastric mucosal cells and J774A.1 murine macrophage cells. These promising preliminary findings warrant more research.

Grape seed proanthocyanidins have been shown to significantly inhibit the peroxidation of polyunsaturated fatty acids and some other lipids in animal and in vitro studies. Some experimental data suggest that these effects might help protect capillaries, heart, brain and liver tissues in some circumstances. In one study, a grape seed proanthocyanidin extract more potently protected brain and hepatic tissues from the damage of experimentally induced reactive oxygen species damage than did other antioxidants (vitamin C, vitamin E succinate and beta-carotene). In other in vitro experiments, grape seed proanthocyanidins have strongly inhibited reactive oxygen species activities implicated in microvascular injury.

Acetaminophen-induced programmed and unprogrammed liver-cell death was dramatically prevented and reduced in mice treated with a grape seed proanthocyanidin extract. Exposure to the extract for seven days prior to acetaminophen administration was notably more effective than pretreatment for three days. The extract significantly counteracted acetaminophen-promoted apoptotic DNA fragmentation.

In another animal model, grape seed proanthocyanidins were shown to increase resistance to myocardial ischemia reperfusion injury. And in a recent experiment utilizing cholesterol-fed rabbits, an extract of grape seed proanthocyanidins significantly attenuated the development of aortic atherosclerosis compared with controls that did not receive the extract.

CONTRAINDICATIONS, PRECAUTIONS, ADVERSE REACTIONS

CONTRAINDICATIONS

Grape seed proanthocyanidins are contraindicated in those with a known hypersensitivity to any of the ingredients in a grape seed proanthocyanidin-containing product.

PRECAUTIONS

Grape seed proanthocyanidin supplementation should be avoided by pregnant women and nursing mothers.

DOSAGE AND ADMINISTRATION

Grape seed proanthocyanidins are available in products called grape seed extracts. These products contain grape seed procyanidins as well as catechin and epicatechin. Typical doses are 50 to 100 mg daily. Products called OPCs or PCOs (procyanidolic oligomers) are typically grape seed extracts.

HOW SUPPLIED

Capsules — 40 mg, 50 mg, 100 mg, 150 mg, 200 mg

Tablets — 40 mg, 50 mg, 100 mg, 200 mg

LITERATURE

Bagchi D, Garg A, Krohn RL, et al. Protective effects of grape seed proanthocyanidins and selected antioxidants against TPA-induced hepatic and brain lipid peroxidation and DNA fragmentation, and peritoneal macrophage activation in mice. *Gen Pharmacol.* 1998; 30:771-776.

Gabetta B, Fuzzati N, Griffini A, et al. Characterization of proanthocyanidins from grape seeds. *Fitoterapia.* 2000; 71:162-175.

Sato M, Maulik G, Ray PS, et al. Cardioprotective effects of grape seed proanthocyanidins against ischemic reperfusion injury. *J Mol Cell Cardiol.* 1999; 31:1289-1297.

Yamakoshi J, Kataoka S, Koga T, Ariga T. Proanthocyanidin-rich extract from grape seed attenuates the development of aortic atherosclerosis in cholesterol-fed rabbis. *Atherosclerosis.* 1999; 142:139-149.

Ye X, Krohn RL, Liu W, et al. The cytotoxic effects of a novel IH636 grape seed proanthocyanidin extract on cultured human cancer cells. *Mol Cell Biochem.* 1999; 196:99-108.

Zhao J, Wang J, Chen Y, Agarwal R. Anti-tumor-promoting activity of a polyphenolic fraction isolated from grape seed in the mouse skin two-stage initiation-promotion protocol and identification of procyanidin B5-3' -gallate as the most effective antioxidant constituent. *Carcinogenesis.* 1999; 20:1737-1745.

Green Tea Catechins

TRADE NAMES

Dexatrim Green Tea (Ginsana), Earl Green Tea (Traditional Medicinal Teas), Green Tea Gold (Prince of Peace), Green Tea Power (Nature's Herbs), Ambootia Green Tea (Nature's Essence), Emerald Gardens Green Tea (Celestial Seasoning) Arkopharma Exolise (Health From the Sun).

DESCRIPTION

Catechins belong to the flavan-3-ol class of flavonoids. Green tea catechins are the flavan-3-ols found in green tea leaves (*Camellia sinensis*). The major four catechins in green tea leaves are (-)-epigallocatechin gallate (EGCG), (-)-epicatechin gallate (ECG), (-)-epigallocatechin (EGC) and (-)-epicatechin (EC). They are all polyphenolic substances. Black tea leaves have a much lower content of these catechins. That's because black tea leaves undergo extensive fermentation, during which the majority of the catechins are enzymatically oxidized to the major pigments of black tea leaves, theaflavin and thearubigen.

The green tea catechins make up approximately 30% of the dry weight of green tea leaves. Of the catechins, EGCG is the most abundant one in green tea leaves. Green tea, an aqueous infusion of green tea leaves, has been a popular beverage in China and Japan for centuries. In these countries, it is thought that green tea has a number of health-promoting benefits, and it is used in the management of various disorders. Epidemiological studies suggest that green tea may have cancer chemopreventive, as well as anti-atherogenic, properties.

The possible health benefits of green tea are attributed to the catechins. These polyphenolic substances are antioxidants. EGCG appears to be the most potent antioxidant of all the green tea catechins.

ACTIONS AND PHARMACOLOGY

ACTIONS

Green tea catechins have antioxidant activity. They may also have anticarcinogenic, anti-inflammatory, anti-atherogenic, thermogenic and antimicrobial activities.

MECHANISM OF ACTION

Green tea catechins have been found to have a number of antioxidant activities, including scavenging of such reactive oxygen species as superoxide, hydroxyl and peroxyl radicals, inhibition of lipid peroxidation, inhibition of 2'-deoxyguanosine oxidation in DNA to 8-hydroxy-2'-deoxyguanosine and inhibition of the oxidation of low-density lipoproteins. EGCG appears to have the greatest antioxidant activity of all the green tea catechins and, in some studies, it has been found to be a more potent antioxidant than ascorbate and reduced glutathione.

The possible anticarcinogenic activity of the green tea catechins may be accounted for by a number of different mechanisms. Much of the research has been done with EGCG, and it appears that, just as EGCG appears to be the most potent antioxidant of the green tea catechins, it also may have the greatest possible anticarcinogenic activity. EGCG and also EGC and ECG have been found to induce apoptosis in some tumor cell lines. EGCG has been shown to inhibit angiogenesis. EGCG and ECG have been demonstrated to inhibit tyrosine phosphorylation of the receptor tyrosine kinase PDGF-Rbeta (platelet-derived growth factor receptor-beta) and its downstream signaling pathway and, consequently, to inhibit transformation of human glioblastoma cells. Interestingly, only the green tea catechins possessing the gallate group in their structure had this activity. Green tea catechins have also been found to upregulate the synthesis of some hepatic phase II enzymes that are involved in the detoxication (detoxification) of some xenobiotics, including chemical carcinogens.

In addition to their possible activity in preventing malignant transformation and inhibiting tumor growth, the green tea catechins may have antimetastatic potential. In this regard, EGCG has been found to inhibit the proteolytic enzyme urokinase. Urokinase is an enzyme that cancer cells may use in order to invade normal tissue and form metastases. EGCG and ECG have been demonstrated to inhibit metalloproteinase- -2(MMP-2) (also known as gelatinase A) and metalloproteinase-9(MMP-9) (also known as gelatinase B). These enzymes also appear to play an important role in tumor invasion and metastases. Finally, EGCG has been found to downregulate the expression of the androgen receptor in human prostate cancer cells in culture, consequently inhibiting androgen action. This and its inhibition of 5-alpha reductase may account for EGCG's antiproliferative effect on cultured human prostate cancer cells.

The possible anti-inflammatory activity of the green tea catechins may, in large part, be accounted for by their antioxidant actions. EGCG has been found to inhibit the activity of the transcription factors AP-1 and NF-kappa B, both of which may mediate many inflammatory processes and both of which may be activated by reactive oxygen species. EGCG's antioxidant activity may itself mediate this inhibition.

Again, a few different mechanisms may come into play in the possible anti-atherogenic activity of the green tea catechins. PDGF-R beta, which was discussed above, may also be involved in smooth muscle proliferation. Smooth muscle proliferation is involved in the pathogenic process of atherosclerosis. EGCG and ECG have been shown to inhibit tyrosine phosphorylation of PDGF-Rbeta and its downstream signaling pathway and, consequently, the proliferation of smooth muscle.

The inhibition of the oxidation of low-density lipoproteins is another possible anti-atherogenic mechanism. The green tea catechins may also have antithrombotic activity and may aid in lowering total cholesterol and LDL-cholesterol levels. The antithrombotic effect appears to be at the platelet level. These catechins have been found to inhibit ADP- and collagen-induced platelet aggregation in rats. Coagulation parameters were not affected. The mechanism of the possible cholesterol-lowering effect is unclear. It is thought that the green tea catechins may stimulate the secretion of bile salts and the fecal excretion of cholesterol.

The green tea catechins have been found to promote thermogenesis. The proposed mechanism for this is inhibition of the enzyme catechol-O-methyl-transferase. This enzyme inactivates norepinephrine.

The mechanism of the possible antimicrobial activity of the green tea catechins is unclear.

PHARMACOKINETICS
The pharmacokinetics of the green tea catechins in humans remain incompletely understood. They are absorbed from the gastrointestinal tract following ingestion, and blood levels of the various catechins have been measured. However, the extent of their absorption, as well as of their distribution, metabolism and excretion, is unclear. A recent human study indicates that the green tea catechins are mainly found in blood in the protein-rich fraction of plasma and in high-density lipoproteins. They are also found in low-density lipoproteins (LDL), but it is unclear if they are present in sufficient amounts in LDL to enhance its resistance to oxidation. Another recent human study has detected two catechin metabolites in the urine following ingestion of green tea. These metabolites are (-)-5(3', 4', 5' -trihydroxyphenyl)-gamma-valerolactone and (-)-5-(3', 4' -dihydroxyphenyl)-gamma-valerolactone. They appear to be produced by intestinal microorganisms with EGC and EC as the precursors of the above metabolites, respectively. These metabolites were also detected in the plasma and the feces. Human pharmacokinetic studies of the green tea catechins are needed in order to better understand their possible beneficial health effects.

INDICATIONS AND USAGE
Green tea catechins may have anticarcinogenic, anti-atherosclerotic, anti-inflammatory and antimicrobial activities. It has been suggested that their reported thermogenic effects might be helpful in controlling body weight.

RESEARCH SUMMARY
Though epidemiological data are mixed with respect to the effects of green tea consumption on the incidence of cancer,

the predominant data suggest that green tea confers protective effects against many cancers. The incidence of prostate cancer, for example, is the lowest in the world in China, a country with high green tea consumption. Esophageal cancer risk has been found to be reduced by 60% in those who consume two to three cups of green tea daily in China. And smokers in Japan are reportedly less likely to develop lung cancer if they regularly consume green tea.

A prospective cohort study of 8,552 Japanese found a significant inverse relationship between green tea consumption and cancer incidence. Females consuming more than 10 cups of green tea daily had the most notable protection, compared with those consuming less than three cups per day.

Green tea consumption has also been associated with a better outcome in some with breast cancer. Higher intakes of green tea (mean: 8 cups/day), compared with lower intakes (mean: 2 cups/day), are associated with a significantly reduced recurrence rate and a longer disease-free period, particularly among premenopausal women with histologically classified stage I and II breast cancer. Stage III cancer patients did not appear to benefit from green tea consumption. Among the specific green tea-related benefits noted in the stage I and II patients were decreased numbers of axillary lymph node metastases.

Preliminary associations have now been made between higher green tea consumption and reduced levels of breast, prostate, stomach, pancreas, colon and lung cancers.

Additionally, both green tea generally, and green tea catechins specifically, have shown efficacy in combating several cancers in animal models of carcinogenesis and *in vitro* tests. Epigallocatechin-3-gallate (EGCG) especially has shown marked anti-cancer effects against breast, colon, prostate, pancreatic, skin, bladder, lung, stomach, ovarian, leukemic and liver cancer, among others. EGCG has been shown to induce apoptosis in several of these cancer types while leaving normal cells unaffected. EGCG has also been shown to inhibit urokinase, a proteolytic enzyme often required for cancer growth. Further, angiogenesis has been shown to be significantly inhibited by EGCG. Recently, EGCG demonstrated an ability to inhibit androgen activity in an androgen-responsive prostate cell line.

Green tea and its catechins have protected against a broad range of chemically induced cancers in *in vitro* and animal studies. Those effects have been reported in all stages of some cancers. Additionally, green tea has been reported to enhance the activity of some anti-cancer drugs. It has increased concentrations of doxorubicin, for example, in some cancer cells without also increasing doxorubicin concentrations in normal cells.

The incidence of cardiovascular disease in China is about 80% lower than in developed countries. High consumption of green tea in China has been associated with this notable decreased risk of cardiovascular disease. Numerous epidemiological studies have associated higher intakes of green tea with decreased risk of atherogenesis in Japan and elsewhere. *In vitro* and animal studies have shown that green tea and its catechins, especially EGCG, can help prevent oxidation of LDL-cholesterol. Recently, a human study demonstrated that EGCG inhibits phospholipid hydroperoxidation in plasma. Mixed results have been reported on the ability of green tea to significantly reduce LDL-cholesterol oxidation in humans. One recent study produced results suggesting that daily consumption of seven to eight cups of green tea might reduce LDL-cholesterol oxidation to an extent possibly sufficient to reduce the risk of cardiovascular disease. In *in vitro* and animal studies green tea and its catechins have reduced total cholesterol and LDL-cholesterol levels, have exhibited anti-thrombotic effects and have inhibited the proliferation of smooth muscle, activities that further suggest anti-atherogenic properties.

Green tea and its constituents have exhibited a variety of anti-inflammatory effects, raising hopes that they might be helpful in treating some forms of arthritis, dermatosis, gout and other inflammatory conditions. In an animal model of inflammatory polyarthritis with similarities to human rheumatoid arthritis, green tea polyphenols, in three experiments, significantly reduced the incidence of arthritis (33 to 50%), compared with controls (84 to 100%). Inflammatory cytokines, tumor necrosis factor and interferon-gamma and RA-specific immunoglobulin-G were all reduced in the animals given the green tea polyphenols.

These polyphenols, administered orally and topically, have also protected against chemical- and solar-induced skin inflammations in animal experiments. Significant protection against UVB-radiation was reported in one experiment utilizing hairless mice. Oral feeding was more effective than topical application in this case.

Recently, a green tea extract was tested to see if it could help reduce the risk of cutaneous squamous cell carcinoma and melanoma in subjects whose psoriasis and some other skin diseases were being treated with a combination of psoralens and exposure to ultraviolet A radiation. While this combination treatment has been shown to be very effective, it has also been shown to significantly increase skin cancer risk. In the recent study alluded to above, a green tea extract, given pre- and post-treatment, significantly prevented the DNA damage and inflammatory processes associated with the combination treatment in animals and in human subjects.

Anther recent study reached the conclusion that green tea extracts increase energy expenditure and fat oxidation in humans. These thermogenic effects were said to go beyond green tea's thermogenic caffeine effects and to be synergistic with them. Compared with placebo, 90 mg of EGCG and 50 mg of caffeine produced a significant 4% increase in 24-hour energy expenditure and a significant decrease in 24-hour respiratory quotient in healthy men. Supplementation with 50 mg of caffeine alone did not have significant thermogenic effects.

The researchers concluded that ''green tea has thermogenic properties and promotes fat oxidation beyond that explained by its caffeine content per se. The green tea extract may play a role in the control of body composition via sympathetic activation of thermogenesis, fat oxidation, or both.''

Finally, there is *in vitro* evidence that green tea and its catechins have some antiviral and other antimicrobial activities. Recently, various green tea catechins were shown to inhibit extracellular release of vero toxin from enterohemorrhagic *Escherichia coli*.

CONTRAINDICATIONS, PRECAUTIONS, ADVERSE REACTIONS

CONTRAINDICATIONS

Green tea catechin supplementation is contraindicated in those who are hypersensitive to any component of a green tea catechin-containing preparation.

PRECAUTIONS

Pregnant women and nursing mothers should avoid green tea catechin supplementation pending long-term safety studies. Catechins may decrease platelet aggregation. Those taking drugs affecting platelet aggregation, such as aspirin, those taking warfarin and those with either genetic or acquired bleeding tendencies should exercise caution in the use of green tea catechin supplements.

Green tea catechin supplementation should be stopped before any surgical procedure.

ADVERSE REACTIONS

None known.

INTERACTIONS

DRUGS

Platelet active drugs: Green tea catechins may enhance the effect of these drugs.

Caffeine: Green tea catechins and caffeine may have a synergistic effect in enhancing thermogenesis. Green tea catechins may inhibit catechol-O-methyl-transferase, an enzyme that metabolizes norepinephrine. Caffeine may inhibit cyclic AMP phosphodiesterase, an enzyme that metabolizes norepinephrine-induced cyclic AMP.

Chemotherapeutic agents: Animal studies suggest that green tea catechins may enhance the effects of chemotherapeutic agents such as doxorubicin and that they may ameliorate some of their toxiocity. There is no human data on this.

OVERDOSAGE

There are no reports of overdosage.

DOSAGE AND ADMINISTRATION

Green tea catechin supplements in a number of green tea extract formulas are available. EGCG is the principal catechin in these supplements. Typical doses are 125 mg to 250 mg daily (of the catechins). There are a number of green tea food products available.

HOW SUPPLIED

Bags

Bulk Powder

Capsules — 175 mg, 250 mg, 500 mg

Liquid

Tablets — 100 mg

LITERATURE

Ahmad N, Mukhtar H. Green tea polyphenols and cancer: biologic mechanisms and practical implications. *Nutr Rev.* 1999; 57:78-83.

Cao Y, Cao R. Angiogenesis inhibited by drinking tea. *Nature.* 1999; 398:381.

Demeule M, Brossard M, Pagé, M, et al. Matrix metalloproteinase inhibition by green tea catechins. *Biochim Biophys Acta.* 2000; 1478:51-60.

Dulloo AG, Duret C, Rohrer D, et al. Efficacy of a green tea extract rich in catechin polyphenols and caffeine in increasing 24-h energy expenditure and fat oxidation in humans. *Am J Clin Nutr.* 1999; 70:1040-1045.

Dulloo AG, Seydoux J, Girardier L, et al. Green tea and thermogenesis: interactions between catechin-polyphenols, caffeine and sympathetic activity. *Int J Obes Relat Metab Disord.* 2000; 24:252-258.

Gupta S, Ahmad N, Mukhtar H. Prostate cancer chemoprevention by green tea. *Semin Urol Oncol.* 1999; 17:70-76.

Haqqi TM, Anthony DD, Gupta S, et al. Prevention of collagen-induced arthritis in mice by a polyphenolic fraction from green tea. *Proc Natl Acad Sci USA.* 1999; 96:4524-4529.

Jankun J, Selman SH, Swiercz R, Skrzypczak-Jankun E. Why drinking green tea could prevent cancer. *Nature.* 1997; 387:561.

Kang WS, Lim IH, Yuk DY, et al. Antithrombotic activities of green tea catechins and (-)-epigallocatechin gallate. *Throm Res.* 1999; 96:229-237.

L'Allemain G. [Multiple actions of EGCG, the main component of green tea]. [Article in French]. *Bull Cancer.* 1999; 86:721-724.

Li C, Lee M-J, Sheng S, et al. Structural identification of two metabolites of catechins and their kinetics in human urine and blood after tea ingestion. *Chem Res Toxicol*. 2000; 13:177-184.

Miura Y, Chiba T, Miura S, et al. Green tea polyphenols (flavan 3-ols) prevent oxidative modification of low density lipoproteins: an ex vivo study in humans. *J Nutr Biochem*. 2000; 11:216-222.

Mukhtar H, Katiyar SK, Agarwal R. Green tea and skin — anticarcinogenic effects. *J Invest Dermatol*. 1994; 102:3-7.

Nakagawa K, Ninomiya M, Okubo T, et al. Tea catechin supplementation increases antioxidant capacity and prevents phospholipid hydroperoxidation in plasma of humans. *J Agric Food Chem*. 1999; 47:3967-3973.

Okushio K, Suzuki M, Matsumoto N, et al. Identification of (-)-epicatechin metabolites and their metabolic fate in the rat. *Drug Metab Disp*. 1999; 27:309-316.

Sachinidis A, Seul C, Seewald S, et al. Green tea compounds inhibit tyrosine phosphorylation of PDGF beta-receptor and transformation of A172 human glioblastoma. *FEBS Lett*. 2000; 471:51-55.

Shi X, Ye J, Leonard SS, et al. Antioxidant properties of (-)-epicatechin-3-gallate and its inhibition of Cr (VI)-induced DNA damage and Cr (IV)- or TPA-stimulated NF-Kappa B activation. *Mol Cell Biochem*. 2000; 206:125-132.

Suganuma M, Okabe S, Sueoka N, et al. Green tea and cancer chemoprevention. *Mutation Res*. 1999; 428:339-344.

Sugita-Konishi Y, Hara-Kudo Y, Amano F, et al. Epigallocatechin gallate and gallocatechin gallate in green tea catechins inhibit extracellular release of Vero toxin from enterohemorrhagic Escherichia coli. O157:H7. *Biochem Biophys Acta*. 1999; 1472:42-50.

Yang TTC, Koo MWL. Inhibitory effect of Chinese green tea on endothelial cell-induced LDL oxidation. *Atherosclerosis*. 2000; 148:67-73.

Hemp Seed Oil

DESCRIPTION

Hemp seed oil is derived from the seeds of the plant *Cannabis sativa*. Hemp seed oil is a relatively rich source of alpha-linolenic acid (ALA) and is one of the few plant seed oils containing more than small amounts of gamma-linolenic acid (GLA). ALA concentrations in hemp seed oil range from approximately 15% to 25%. GLA concentration ranges from approximately 1% to 6%. The most abundant fatty acid in hemp seed oil is linoleic acid, which comprises approximately 50% to 70% of the fatty acid content.

Hemp seed and hemp seed oil normally do not contain significant quantities of tetrahydrocannabinol or any of the other psychoactive substances produced by *Cannabis sativa*. However, trace amounts of these substances have been reported in some batches of the oil. This is most likely due to contamination of the seed by adherent resin or other plant residues.

ALA, GLA, linoleic acid and all fatty acids in hemp seed oil are present in the form of triglycerides or neutral fats.

ACTIONS AND PHARMACOLOGY

ACTIONS

Hemp seed oil has putative antithrombotic and anti-inflammatory activities.

MECHANISM OF ACTION

Antithrombotic and anti-inflammatory activities have not been demonstrated with hemp seed oil. Therefore, any proposed mechanism of actions is entirely speculative. Hemp seed oil is relatively rich in ALA, which may be metabolized to eicosapentaenoic acid (EPA). EPA is a precursor of the anti-inflammatory and antithrombotic eicosanoids. ALA metabolites may also inhibit the production of some pro-inflammatory eicosanoids, as well as some of the pro-inflammatory cytokines.

GLA is a precursor in the synthesis of prostaglandin E_1 (PGE$_1$), which inhibits platelet aggregation and has vasodilatory activity.

PHARMACOKINETICS

There are no reported pharmacokinetic studies of hemp seed oil. However, much is known about the physiology and biochemistry of edible oils, and certain assumptions can be made. ALA- and GLA-laden triglycerides in hemp seed oil are probably absorbed from the small intestine, aided by bile salts. During the process, there is some deacylation of the fatty acids of the triglycerides. Reacylation takes place within the mucosal cells of the small intestine, and the ALA- and GLA-laden triglycerides enter the lymph system in the form of chylomicrons. ALA- and GLA-laden chylomicrons are transported from the lymph into the blood, where ALA and GLA are then carried in lipid particles to the various cells of the body. They then get metabolized to EPA, PGE$_1$ and various eicosanoids.

INDICATIONS AND USAGE

It has been claimed that hemp seed oil inhibits platelet aggregation, favorably affects lipids and reduces the risk of heart attack. Other claims include usefulness in arthritis, autoimmune disorders and inflammation, in general. There is no research that supports any of these claims.

RESEARCH SUMMARY

There is no published research showing benefit (or lack of benefit) from the use of hemp seed oil. To the extent that it is a source of alpha-linolenic acid, as well as gamma-linolenic acid, it may have some of the benefits of those substances.

CONTRAINDICATIONS, PRECAUTIONS, ADVERSE REACTIONS

CONTRAINDICATIONS

None known.

PRECAUTIONS

Pregnant women and nursing mothers should avoid supplemental hemp seed oil. Because of possible antithrombotic activity of hemp seed oil, those with hemophilia and those taking warfarin should be cautious. Likewise, hemp seed oil should be halted in those having surgical procedures. Hemp seed oil is abundant in linoleic acid. Some laboratory studies suggest linoleic acid may stimulate the growth of prostate cancer and breast cancer cells. It is unclear if this has relevance to those with prostate or breast cancer. However, to be on the safe side, those with prostate or breast cancer should be cautious about using this substance. Cannabinoids have been found in certain batches of hemp seed oil.

ADVERSE REACTIONS

Hemp seed oil may cause mild gastrointestinal symptoms, such as nausea and diarrhea.

INTERACTIONS

DRUGS

Interactions may occur between hemp seed oil, ALA and its metabolites, and aspirin and other NSAIDs. Such interactions, if they were to occur, might be manifested by nosebleeds and increased susceptibility to bruising. If this occurs, consideration should be given to lowering or stopping intake. Such interaction may also occur between hemp seed oil and warfarin.

NUTRITIONAL SUPPLEMENTS

Interactions may occur if hemp seed oil is used with such nutritional supplements as fish oils, which have possible antithrombotic activity.

HERBS

Interactions may occur between hemp seed oil, ALA and its metabolites, and such herbs as garlic (*Allium sativum*) and ginkgo (*Ginkgo biloba*). Such interactions might be manifested by nosebleeds and easy bruising.

OVERDOSAGE

There are no reports of hemp seed overdosage.

DOSAGE AND ADMINISTRATION

Hemp seed oil comes in capsules and bottles of oil. The ALA content ranges from 15 to 25%. Three to 4 grams of ALA is approximately equivalent to the 0.3 grams, which one would derive from a fish-rich diet. Since hemp seed oil is easily oxidized, it is important that it contain an antioxidant, such as vitamin E.

HOW SUPPLIED

Lip Balm

LITERATURE

Costantino A, Schwartz RH, Kaplan P. Hemp oil ingestion causes positive urine tests for delta 9-tetrahydrocannabinol carboxylic acid. *J Anal Toxicol.* 1997; 21:482-485.

Deferne J-D, Pate DW. Hemp seed oil: a source of valuable essential fatty acids. *J Int Hemp Assoc.* 1996; 3:4-7.

Lehman T, Sager F, Brenneisen R. Excretion of cannabinoids in urine after ingestion of cannabis seed oil. *J Anal Toxicol.* 1997; 21:373-375.

Rose DP. Effects of dietary fatty acids on breast and prostate cancers: evidence from *in vitro* experiments and animal studies. *Am J Clin Nutr.* 1997; 66:1513S-1522S.

Rose DP, Connolly JM. Effects of fatty acids and eicosanoid synthesis inhibitors in the growth of two human prostate cancer cell lines. *Prostate.* 1991; 18:243-254.

Rose DP, Connolly JM. Stimulation of growth of human breast cancer cell lines in culture by linoleic acid. *Biochem Biophys Res Commun.* 1989; 164:277-283.

Struempler RE, Nelson G, Urry FM. A positive cannabinoids workplace drug test following the ingestion of commercially available hemp seed oil. *J Anal Toxicol.* 1997; 21:283-285.

Hesperetin

DESCRIPTION

Hesperetin belongs to the flavanone class of flavonoids. Hesperetin, in the form of its glycoside hesperidin, is the predominant flavonoid in lemons and oranges.

Hesperetin is a solid substance that is poorly soluble in water. Its molecular formula is $C_{16}H_{14}O_6$, and its molecular weight is 302.28 daltons. It is also known as 3',5,7-trihydroxy-4'-methoxyflavanone and (S)-2,3- dihydro-5,7-dihydroxy-2-(3-hydroxy-4-methoxyphenyl)-4-*H*-1-benzopyran-4-one. Hesperetin is the aglycone (aglucon) of hesperedin. Hesperetin has the following structural formula:

Hesperetin

ACTIONS AND PHARMACOLOGY

ACTIONS

Hesperetin may have antioxidant, anti-inflammatory, anti-allergic, hypolipidemic, vasoprotective and anticarcinogenic actions.

MECHANISM OF ACTION

Hesperetin is a phenolic antioxidant. It may scavenge such reactive oxygen species as superoxide anions and may protect against peroxidation.

Hesperetin's possible anti-inflammatory activity may be accounted for by its interference with the metabolism of arachidonic acid and histamine release. There is evidence that hesperetin inhibits phospholipase A_2, lipoxygenase and cyclo-oxygenase. Hesperetin may inhibit histamine release from mast cells.

Hesperetin may reduce plasma cholesterol levels by inhibition of 3-hydroxy-3-methylglutaryl coenzyme A (HMG-CoA) reductase as well as acylcoenzyme A: cholesterol acyltransferase (ACAT). Inhibition of these enzymes has been demonstrated in rats fed a high-cholesterol diet.

The mechanism of hesperetin's possible vasoprotective action is unclear. Hesperetin has been shown to decrease microvascular permeability. It may protect endothelial cells from hypoxia by stimulating certain mitochondrial enzymes such as succinate dehydrogenase.

The mechanism of hesperetin's possible anticarcinogenic action is also unclear. It may be accounted for, in part, by hesperetin's possible antioxidant activity. Other possibilities include inhibition of polyamine biosynthesis and inhibition of lipoxygenase and cyclo-oxygenase.

PHAMACOKINETICS

Hesperetin is typically administered as hesperidin. See Hesperidin.

INDICATIONS AND USAGE

Hesperetin may be helpful in lowering cholesterol and, possibly, otherwise favorably affecting lipids. *In vitro* and animal research also suggests the possibility that hesperetin might have some anticancer effects and that it might have some anti-aromatase activity, as well as activity against *Helicobacter pylori*. More research will be required before hesperetin is indicated for any of these situations.

RESEARCH SUMMARY

Like hesperidin, hesperetin has shown some favorable effects on lipids, but, unlike hesperidin, this research has so far been confined to *in vitro* and animal studies. In the best-designed of the animal studies to date, hesperetin significantly lowered plasma cholesterol levels (but not triglyceride levels) in rats fed a high-cholesterol diet.

No conclusions can yet be drawn from early animal work that suggests hesperetin-induced anticancer effects. Similarly, isolated studies showing anti-aromatase and anti-*Helicobacter pylori* activity *in vitro* need follow-up.

CONTRAINDICATIONS, PRECAUTIONS, ADVERSE REACTIONS

See Hesperidin.

DOSAGE AND ADMINISTRATION

Hesperetin is typically administered as hesperidin. See Hesperidin.

LITERATURE

Ameer B, Weitraub RA, Johnson JV, et al. Flavanone absorption after naringinin, hesperidin and citrus administration. *Clin Pharmacol Ther.* 1996; 60:34-40.

Bae EA, Han MJ, Kim DH. In vitro anti-Helicobacter pylori activity of some flavonoids and their metabolites. *Planta Med.* 1999; 65:442-443.

Borradaile NM, Carroll KK, Kurowaska EM. Regulation of HepG2 cell apolipoprotein B metabolism by the citrus flavanones hesperetin and naringenin. *Lipids.* 1999; 34:591-598.

Choi JS, Park KV, Moon SH, et al. Antimutagenic effect of plant flavonoids in the Salmonella assay system. *Arch Pharm Res.* 1994; 17:71-75.

Franke AA, Cooney RV, Custer LJ, et al. Inhibition of neoplastic transformation and bioavailability of dietary flavonoid agents. *Adv Exp Med Biol.* 1998; 439:237-248.

Jeong HJ, Shin YG, Kim IH, Pezzuto JM. Inhibition of aromatase activity by flavonoids. *Arch Pharm Res.* 1999; 22:309-312.

Lee S-H, Jeong T-S, Park YB, et al. Hypocholesterolemic effect of hesperetin mediated by inhibition of 3-hydroxy-3-methylglutaryl coenzyme A reductase and acyl coenzyme A: cholesterol acyltransferase in rats fed high-cholesterol diet. *Nutr Res.* 1999; 19:1245-1258.

Hesperidin

DESCRIPTION

The flavonoid hesperidin is a flavanone glycoside (glucoside) comprised of the flavanone (a class of flavonoids) hesperitin and the disaccharide rutinose. Hesperidin is the predominant flavonoid in lemons and oranges. The peel and membranous parts of these fruits have the highest hesperidin concentrations. Therefore, orange juice containing pulp is richer in the flavonoid than that without pulp. Sweet oranges *(Citrus sinensis)* and tangelos are the richest dietary sources of hesperidin. Hesperidin is classified as a citrus bioflavonoid.

Hesperidin, in combination with a flavone glycoside called diosmin, is used in Europe for the treatment of venous insufficiency and hemorrhoids. Hesperidin, rutin and other flavonoids thought to reduce capillary permeability and to have anti-inflammatory action were collectively known as vitamin P. These substances, however, are not vitamins and are no longer referred to, except in older literature, as vitamin P.

Hesperidin is a solid substance with low solubility in water. It is, however, much more soluble in water than its aglycone hesperetin. Hesperidin's molecular formula is $C_{28}H_{34}O_{15}$, and its molecular weight is 610.57 daltons.

The disaccharide of hesperidin, rutinose, is comprised of the sugars rhamnose (6-deoxy-L-mannose) and glucose. Hesperidin is also known as hesperetin 7-rhamnoglucoside, hesperetin-7-rutinoside and (S)-7-[[6-0-(6-deoxy-alpha-L-mannopyranosyl)-beta-D-glucopyranosyl] oxy]-2, 3-dihydro-5-hydroxy-2-(3-hydroxy-4-methoxyphenyl)-4*H*-1-benzopyran-4-one. Hesperidin is represented by the following chemical structure:

Hesperidin

ACTIONS AND PHARMACOLOGY
ACTIONS
Hesperidin may have antioxidant, anti-inflammatory, anti-allergic, hypolipidemic, vasoprotective and anticarcinogenic actions.

MECHANISM OF ACTION
Although some studies indicate that hesperidin has antioxidant activity *in vivo*, others do not demonstrate antioxidant activity *in vitro*.

The possible anti-inflammatory action of hesperidin is probably due to the possible anti-inflammatory action of its aglycone hesperetin. Hesperetin appears to interfere with the metabolism of arachidonic acid as well as with histamine release. Hesperetin appears to inhibit phospholipase A2, lipoxygenase and cyclo-oxygenase. There is evidence that hesperetin inhibits histamine release from mast cells, which would account for the possible anti-allergic activity of hesperidin.

Again, the possible hypolipidemic effect of hesperidin is probably due to hesperetin's possible action in lipid lowering. Hesperetin may reduce plasma cholesterol levels by inhibition of 3-hydroxy-3-methylglutaryl coenzyme A

(HMG CoA) reductase, as well as acyl coenzyme A: cholesterol acytransferase (ACAT). Inhibition of these enzymes by hesperetin has been demonstrated in rats fed a high cholesterol diet.

The mechanism of hesperidin's possible vasoprotective action is unclear. Animal studies have shown that hesperidin decreases microvascular permeability. Hesperidin, itself or via hesperetin, may protect endothelial cells from hypoxia by stimulating certain mitochondrial enzymes, such as succinate dehydrogenase.

The mechanism of hesperidin's possible anticarcinogenic action is also unclear. One explanation may be the inhibition of polyamine synthesis. Inhibition of lipoxygenase and cyclo-oxygenase is another possibility.

PHARMACOKINETICS
There is not much known about the pharmacokinetics of hesperidin in humans. It is unclear if hesperidin itself is absorbed from the intestine intact as a glycoside. The aglycone hesperetin is detected in the serum following ingestion and may be formed prior to or following absorption. Hesperetin may undergo glucuronidation in the wall of the intestine, as well as in the liver. Hesperetin is detected in the urine within three hours after ingestion of hesperidin. Urinary excretion appears to be the major route of excretion of the aglycone. Not much more is known about the metabolism of hesperidin.

INDICATIONS AND USAGE
Hesperidin has demonstrated some ability to favorably affect lipids and to treat some vascular disorders in humans. Other claims made for hesperidin are based on *in vitro* and animal studies. These include claims that hesperidin is useful in cancer and immune disorders. There are also claims that hesperidin is an anti-allergen and anti-inflammatory agent based on results from animal experiments.

RESEARCH SUMMARY
In several animal studies, hesperidin has significantly increased HDL-cholesterol while lowering total lipid and triglyceride plasma levels. A recent clinical trial tested the effects of hesperidin-rich orange juice in 25 subjects with elevated cholesterol levels. Subjects drank one glass of orange juice daily for four weeks, two glasses daily for four weeks and three glasses daily for four weeks. By the third phase of the study, HDL levels in these subjects increased 21% and the LDL/HDL ratio dropped 16%. Folate levels significantly increased. This was interpreted as a positive result, as well, since folate has been shown to cause declines in levels of homocysteine which, at high levels, is believed to increase the risk of heart disease.

These positive effects, attributed by the researchers to the hesperidin content of orange juice, persisted throughout a five-week washout period that followed the conclusion of testing. During that period, subjects were asked not to drink any juice.

Hesperidin has demonstrated antihypertensive and diuretic effects in both normotensive rats and spontaneously hypertensive rats. It has also shown some ability to protect against ischemia-reperfusion tissue damage in some animal models.

In combination with micronized diosmin, hesperidin has significantly improved acute internal hemorrhoids of pregnancy in a clinical open trial.

Anticancer, antimutagenic and immune-modulating effects have been seen with the use of hesperidin in numerous *in vitro* and animal studies. Among the cancers investigated in these studies are esophageal, colon, urinary bladder and skin cancers. In one study that compared the cancer-inhibiting effects of a number of dietary flavonoids and bioflavonoids, hesperidin, hesperetin and catechin were said to be the most potent. More research is needed.

Similarly, more research is warranted to see whether preliminary animal studies suggesting that hesperidin may have significant antiallergenic and antiinflammatory effects will have clinical relevance.

CONTRAINDICATIONS, PRECAUTIONS, ADVERSE REACTIONS

CONTRAINDICATIONS

Hesperidin is contraindicated in those who are hypersensitive to hesperidin or any component of an hesperidin-containing product.

PRECAUTIONS

Pregnant women and nursing mothers should avoid use of supplemental hesperidin at doses higher than may be found in some multivitamin preparations (about 20 mg) unless such use is recommended by a physician.

ADVERSE REACTIONS

Supplemental hesperidin is usually well tolerated. Adverse reactions include gastrointestinal ones, such as nausea.

INTERACTIONS

NUTRITIONAL SUPPLEMENTS

Vitamin C: The interaction between flavonoids, such as hesperidin and hesperetin, and vitamin C is unclear. It has been believed for some time that flavonoids work synergistically with vitamin C, enhancing the absorption of the vitamin and preventing its oxidation. However, recent research indicates that flavonoids, such as hesperetin, may actually inhibit the uptake of vitamin C into cells. More research is needed to clarify this issue.

OVERDOSAGE

There are no reports of overdosage.

DOSAGE AND ADMINISTRATION

Hesperidin is present in such nutritional supplements as vitamin C with bioflavonoids. Typical dose in these products is about 20 mg. Hesperidin is available in hesperidin-complex supplements. Doses for this type of supplement are usually 500 mg to 2 grams daily. In Europe, hesperidin is available for the management of venous insufficiency and hemorrhoids in a combination product with diosmin. A 500-mg dose of this combination product is comprised of 50 mg of hesperidin and 450 mg of diosmin. Dose for this mixed flavonoid product, for the above conditions, is 1 to 3 grams daily. Another flavonoid, hesperidin methyl chalcone, is often marketed in formulations with hesperidin. This is a different flavonoid, and very few studies have been performed using it. A good source of hesperidin is orange juice containing pulp.

LITERATURE

Ameer B, Weintraub RA, Johnson JV, et al. Flavanone absorption after naringin, hesperidin, and citrus administration. *Clin Pharmacol Ther.* 1996; 60:34-40.

Berkarda B, Koyuncu H, Soybir GT, Baykut F. Inhibitory effect of hesperidin on tumor initiation and promotion in mouse skin. *Res Exp Med. (Berl).* 1998; 198:93-99.

Bok SH, Lee SH, Park YB, et al. Plasma and hepatic cholesterol and hepatic activities of 3-hydroxy-3-methyl-glutaryl-CoA reductase and acyl CoA: cholesterol transferase are lower in rats fed citrus peel extract or a mixture of citrus bioflavonoids. *J Nutr.* 1999; 129:1182-1185.

Emin JA, Oliveira AB, Lapa AJ. Pharmacological evaluation of the anti-inflammatory activity of a citrus bioflavonoid, hesperidin, and the isoflavonoids duartin and claussequinone in rats and mice. *J Pharm Pharmacol.* 1994; 46:118-122.

Galati EM, Monforte MT, Kirjavainen S, et al. Biological effects of hesperidin, a citrus flavonoid (Note I): anti-inflammatory and analgesic activity. *Farmaco.* 1994; 40:709-712.

Galati EM, Trovato A, Kirjavainen S, et al. Biological effects of hesperidin, a citrus flavonoid. (Note III): antihypertensive and diuretic activity in rat. *Farmaco.* 1996; 51:219-221.

Koyuncu H, Berkarda B, Baykut F, et al. Preventive effect of hesperidin against inflammation in CD-1 mouse skin caused by tumor promoter. *Anticancer Res.* 1999; 19(4B):3237-3241.

Matsuda H, Yano M, Kubo M, et al. [Pharmacological study on citrus fruits. II. Anti-allergic effect of fruit of Citrus unshiu MARKOVICH (2). On flavonoid components.] [Article in Japanese.] *Yakugaku Zasshi.* 1991; 111:193-198.

Miyake Y, Yamamoto K, Tsujihara N, Osawa T. Protective effects of lemon bioflavonoids on oxidative stress in diabetic rats. *Lipids.* 1998; 33:689-695.

Montforte MT, Trovato A, Kirjavainen S, et al. Biological effects of hesperidin, a citrus flavonoid. (Note II): hypolipidemic activity on experimental hypercholesterolemia in rat. *Farmaco.* 1995; 50:595-599.

Tanaka T, Makita H, Kawabata K, et al. Chemoprevention of azoxymethane-induced rat colon carcinogenesis by the naturally occurring flavonoids, diosmin and hesperidin. *Carcinogenesis.* 1997; 18:957-965.

Hexacosanol

DESCRIPTION

Hexacosanol is a 26-carbon, long-chain, saturated primary alcohol. Along with other long-chain alcohols, such as docosanol, octacosanol and triacontanol, it belongs to a family of organic compounds called fatty alcohols. It is a component of vegetable waxes and is found in wheat germ oil, rice bran oil and wool wax, among other things. Hexacosanol has also been isolated from the plant *Hygrophilia erecta*, a medicinal herb that grows in India and Vietnam.

Hexacosanol is also known as 1-hexacosanol, n-hexacosanol and ceryl alcohol.

ACTIONS AND PHARMACOLOGY

ACTIONS

Hexacosanol may have neuroprotective activity and neurotrophic activity, and it may increase phagocytic activity of macrophages.

MECHANISM OF ACTION

Hexacosanol has been shown to attenuate the degeneration of cholinergic neurons after injury, to possess neurotrophic activities on cultured neurons and to increase the phagocytic activity of mice macrophages. It has also been found to increase the regeneration of both sensory and motor axons in the sciatic nerve of the mouse *in vivo*. The mechanism of these actions is unknown.

PHARMACOKINETICS

Little is known about the pharmacokinetics of hexacosanol in humans. It is likely, as in the case of its close relative, octacosanol, that absorption of this fatty alcohol is variable and poor. There are no published reports regarding its distribution, metabolism and excretion. Again, in comparison with octacosanol, it is likely that bile is the main route of excretion.

INDICATIONS AND USAGE

Hexacosanol has demonstrated significant neuroprotective effects in preliminary *in vitro* and *in vivo* studies. *In vitro* and *in vivo* animal studies have demonstrated that hexacosanol can inhibit glucose-stimulated insulin secretion. It has also been shown to stimulate phagocytosis in cultured macrophages.

RESEARCH SUMMARY

Hexacosanol has shown an ability to promote the maturation of central neurons in culture. It significantly increased both neurite outgrowth and the number of collaterals. It was said to strikingly enhance biochemical differentiation of cultured neurons.

In a subsequent *in vitro* study, hexacosanol strongly attenuated degeneration of cholinergic neurons. The researchers described this as the first report of an *in vivo* neurotrophic influence exerted by an exogenously administered long-chain fatty alcohol and concluded that ''the low dosage needed and the peripheral administration of this compound may be of great advantage in the reduction of cell loss in some neurodegenerative disorders like Alzheimer's disease or stroke.''

Still more recent studies have further confirmed the neurotrophic properties of hexacosanol. In one of these studies conducted in an animal model, injected hexacosanol significantly protected the pyramidal neurons of the hippocampus from the neurotoxic substance kainic acid. It was estimated that hexacosanol spared 72% of the toxin-exposed neurons.

Hexacosanol also significantly inhibited the increased locomotor activity normally associated with exposure to kainic acid. Some researchers have stated: ''The peripheral administration of hexacosanol may lead to a significant breakthrough in the treatment of excitotoxin-related human diseases.''

In yet another *in vivo* study, hexacosanol was tested to see whether it has nerve-regeneration effects. Mice with crushed sciatic nerves, given injected hexacosanol, exhibited a 40% increase in the regeneration rate of sensory fibers compared with controls. There was significant recovery of neuromuscular function, as measured by quantitative electromyography and sensorimotor tests, in the hexacosanol-treated animals. Research is ongoing.

Hexacosanol has also shown an ability to inhibit glucose-stimulated insulin secretion, in both *in vitro* and *in vivo* animal studies. These studies have suggested a direct hexacosanol effect on islets of Langerhans. This activity may prevent insulin resistance.

And, finally, a preliminary study has demonstrated that hexacosanol can increase the phagocytosis activity of cultured macrophages. More research is warranted.

CONTRAINDICATIONS, PRECAUTIONS, ADVERSE REACTIONS

CONTRAINDICATIONS

None known.

PRECAUTIONS

Because of lack of long-term safety studies, children, pregnant women and nursing mothers should avoid supplemental hexacosanol.

ADVERSE REACTIONS

None known.

OVERDOSAGE

No reports of overdosage.

DOSAGE AND ADMINISTRATION

Hexacosanol is available as a nutritional supplement, typically in combination with other long-chain fatty alcohols, such as octacosanol. Doses used are 500 to 1250 micrograms daily.

LITERATURE

Azzouz M, Kenel PF, Warter J-M, et al. Enhancement of mouse sciatic nerve regeneration by the long-chain fatty acid, n-hexacosanol. *Exp Neurol.* 1996; 138:189-197.

Borg J. The neurotrophic factor, n-hexacosanol, reduces the neuronal damage induced by the neurotoxin, kainic acid. *J Neurosci Res.* 1991; 29:62-67.

Borg J, Kesslak PJ, Cotman CW. Peripheral administration of a long-chain fatty alcohol promotes septal cholinergic neurons survival after fimbria-fornix transection. *Brain Res.* 1990; 518:295-298.

Borg J, Toazara J, Hietter H, et al. Neurotrophic effect of naturally occurring long-chain fatty alcohols on cultured CNS neurons. *FEBS Lett.* 1987; 213:406-410.

Damge C, Hillaire-Buys D, Koenig M, et al. Effect of n-hexacosanol on insulin secretion in the rat. *Eur J Pharmacol.* 1995; 274:133-139.

Moosbrugger I, Bischoff P, Beck JP, et al. Studies on the immunological effects of fatty alcohols—I. Effects of n-hexacosanol on murine macrophages in culture. *Int J Immunopharmacol.* 1992; 14:292-302.

Human Growth Hormone and Secretagogues

TRADE NAMES

Recapture HGH (Transcend Marketing International), HGH 2000 (Global Nutrition), Eden GH1 (Nutribolics), Biogevity (Neways), Bioregenics GH (Oasis Wellness Network).

DESCRIPTION

Human growth hormone (HGH) is a heterogenous mixture of polypeptides secreted by the anterior pituitary gland. The principal form of HGH is a polypeptide containing 191 amino acids with a molecular weight of 215,000 daltons. This form of HGH is produced by recombinant DNA technology and is marketed for the treatment of short stature in growth hormone(GH)-deficient children and adolescents. Recombinant HGH or somatropin is also used for the treatment of GH deficiency in adults, short stature in association with renal insufficiency, AIDS-related wasting and short stature associated with Turner's Syndrome. In all of these cases, GH must be administered parenterally since it has very poor oral bioavailability.

GH is the primary hormone responsible for growth in humans, as well as other mammals, and it helps regulate such metabolic processes as anabolism and lipolysis. Normal human aging is associated with decreased GH secretion. Mean GH level in those over the age of 60 is about half of that in young adults. The reduction in GH levels with aging is believed to contribute to age-related decreases in muscle mass and strength and decreased lipolysis.

The effects of GH are largely mediated via IGF-1 (insulin-like growth factor 1). IGF-1 is a mitogen and may promote some cancers, including prostate, breast and colorectal cancers. Clearly, long-term safety studies, as well as efficacy studies, are essential to evaluate the role, if any, of GH replacement in the aging population.

The release of GH from somatotroph cells of the anterior pituitary gland is a complex process involving multiple regulators. The hypothalamic peptide GHRH (growth hormone-releasing hormone) acts on the somatotrophs to release GH, while the inhibitory peptide somatostatin blocks GH release. In addition, GH release appears to be influenced by a third, separate mechanism, as well—a growth hormone secretagogue pathway. GH secretagogues, abbreviated GHSs, can be amino acids, such as L-arginine, small peptides and nonpeptides. Further, neurotransmitters, such as acetylcholine, dopamine and norepinephrine, and neuropeptides, such as opioid peptides, are also involved in the control of GH secretion.

Recently, HGH has entered the dietary supplement marketplace, as have IGF-1 (see Insulin-Growth Factor 1) and several so-called GH secretagogues or releasers. The substances being marketed as GH secretagogues or releasers include the amino acids L-arginine, L-glutamine, L-ornithine, glycine, L-dopa, as well as such substances as ornithine alpha-ketoglutarate (see Ornithine Alpha-Ketoglutarate) and the herbs *Macuna pruriens* and *Tribulus terrestris*.

ACTIONS AND PHARMACOLOGY

ACTIONS

Supplemental HGH and secretagogues or releasers have putative anabolic and lipolytic activities, as well as putative "anti-aging" activity.

MECHANISM OF ACTION

The mechanism of the putative actions of supplemental HGH and secretagogues or releasers is unknown. The actions of endogenous GH and parenteral GH are thought to be mediated via the anabolic hormone IGF-1 and by interaction with specific GH receptors that are widely distributed in body tissues.

PHARMACOKINETICS

Orally administered GH has very poor bioavailability. It is claimed that GH is significantly absorbed from the oral mucosa if delivered by a spray. There is no substantiation for this. It is likely that orally administered GH is digested in the small intestine to the amino acids thah comprise the molecule.

INDICATIONS AND USAGE

There are no indications for the non-pharmaceutical use of HGH in any form. Claims that it is an anti-aging substance, that it enhances athletic and sexual performance, that it promotes joint health, is a sleep aid and an immune enhancer, that it has antidiabetic and antiatherosclerotic effects, and is a neuroprotector, are unsupported by credible evidence. Injected HGH may reduce fat and increase lean body mass in some, but serious side effects may attend the use of HGH for this purpose. There is preliminary evidence that injected HGH may be of benefit in some with Crohn's disease and that it might be helpful in treating dilated cardiomyopathy. There is some fear that high doses of HGH might promote some cancers.

RESEARCH SUMMARY

Recombinant human growth hormone, given parenterally to men aged 61 to 81, reportedly resulted in significant improvements in lean body mass, muscle tone, skin thickness and density of lumbar vertebrae. Significant loss of adipose tissue was also reported. The researchers concluded that "the effects of six months of human growth hormone treatment on lean body mass and adipose tissue were equivalent in magnitude to the changes incurred during 10 to 20 years of aging."

Subsequent studies also demonstrated some positive effects of HGH replacement therapy on body composition in those over 60. Some serious side effects were also noted, however, including arthralgias of both small and large joints, insulin resistance leading to higher serum fasting glucose levels, fluid retention in the lower extremities, carpal tunnel syndrome, gynecomastia and headaches. Due to the prevalence of some of these side effects, the researchers who conducted the first human trial reduced the dosage of HGH they had been using by half.

In a preliminary study, recombinant human growth hormone, given parenterally for three months to patients with idiopath-

ic dilated cardiomyopathy, was reported to increase myocardial mass and reduce the size of the left ventricular chamber. These changes were associated with improved clinical status.

Recently, in another preliminary study, injected HGH was said to be beneficial in some with Crohn's disease. Improvement was measured by scores on the Crohn's Disease Activity Index over a four-month period.

There is no credible evidence that oral HGH has any health benefit.

CONTRAINDICATIONS, PRECAUTIONS, ADVERSE REACTIONS

(For information on the pharmaceutical use of somatropin, see *Physicians' Desk Reference*.)

CONTRAINDICATIONS

Supplemental human growth hormone is contraindicated in those with any evidence of active malignancy. It is also contraindicated in those who are hypersensitive to any component of an HGH-containing product.

PRECAUTIONS

Pregnant women and nursing mothers should avoid the use of HGH-containing supplements.

Adolescents should avoid the use of supplemental HGH.

Those with diabetes should avoid the use of supplemental HGH.

Oral forms of HGH are not meant to be used parenterally and should never be used in such a manner.

ADVERSE REACTIONS

None known for HGH-containing supplements.

INTERACTIONS

None known for HGH-containing supplements.

DOSAGE AND ADMINISTRATION

Oral recombinant human growth hormone is available and marketed as a dietary supplement, typically in the form of an oral spray. There are no recommended doses.

HOW SUPPLIED

Sublingual spray

LITERATURE

Bengtsson B-Å, Eden S, Lonn L, et al. Treatment of adults with growth hormone deficiency with recombinant human GH. *J Clin Endocrinol Metab.* 1993; 76:309-317.

Cohn L, Feller AG, Draper MW, Rudman IW, Rudman D. Carpal tunnel syndrome and gynaecomastia during growth hormone treatment of elderly men with low circulating IGF-1 concentrations. *Clin Endocrinol.* 1993; 39:417-425.

Fazio S, Sabatini D, Capaldo B, et al. A preliminary study of growth hormone in the treatment of dilated cardiomyopathy. 1996; 334:809-814.

Marcus R, Hoffman AR. Growth hormone as therapy for older men and women. *Annu Rev Pharmacol Toxicol.* 1998; 38:45-61.

Rudman D, Feller AG, Nagraj HS, et al. Effects of human growth hormone in men over 60 years old. *N Engl J Med.* 1990; 323:1-6.

Huperzine A

TRADE NAMES

Huperzine A is available from numerous manufacturers generically. Branded products include Memorall (PharmAssure), Huperzine Rx-Brain (Nature's Plus).

DESCRIPTION

Huperzine A is a plant alkaloid derived from the Chinese club moss plant, *Huperzia serrata*, which is a member of the *Lycopodium* species. *Huperzia serrata* has been used in Chinese folk medicine for the treatment of fevers and inflammation.

Huperzine A has been found to have acetylcholinesterase activity. Huperzine B, also derived from *Huperzia serrata*, is a much less potent acetylcholinesterase inhibitor. Natural huperzine A is a chiral molecule also called L-huperzine A or (-)-huperzine A. Synthetic huperzine A is a racemic mixture called (±)-huperzine A. Huperzine A is also known as HUP, hup A and selagine. In Chinese medicine, the extract of *Huperzia serrata* is known as Chien Tseng Ta and shuangyiping. Huperzine A derivatives are being developed for pharmaceutical application.

ACTIONS AND PHARMACOLOGY

ACTIONS

Huperzine A may have cognition-enhancing activity in some.

MECHANISM OF ACTION

Alzheimer's disease is a neurodegenerative disorder associated with neuritic plaques that affect the cerebral cortex, amygdala and hippocampus. There is also neurotransmission damage in the brain. One of the major functional deficits in Alzheimer's disease is a hypofunction of cholinergic neurons. This leads to the cholinergic hypothesis of Alzheimer's disease and the rationale for strategies to increase acetylcholine in the brains of Alzheimer's disease patients. Two FDA-approved drugs for the treatment of Alzheimer's disease, tacrine and donepezil, are acetylcholinesterase inhibitors.

Huperzine A is also an acetylcholinesterase inhibitor and has been found to increase acetylcholine levels in the rat brain following its administration. It also increases norepinephrine and dopamine, but not serotonin levels. The natural L or (-)-huperzine A is approximately three times more potent than the racemic or (±)-huperzine A *in vitro*.

PHARMACOKINETICS

There are limited pharmacokinetic studies with huperzine A. It appears that huperzine A is rapidly absorbed from the gastrointestinal tract and transported to the liver via the portal circulation. Some first-pass metabolism takes place in the liver, and huperzine A and its metabolites are distributed widely in the body, including to the brain. Following ingestion, the time to reach peak blood level is approximately 80 minutes.

INDICATIONS AND USAGE

Huperzine A has potent pharmacological effects and, particularly since long-term safety has not been determined, it should only be used with medical supervision. It may have some effectiveness in Alzheimer's disease and age-related memory impairment. It has been used to treat fever and some inflammatory disorders, but there is no credible scientific evidence to support these uses.

RESEARCH SUMMARY

Numerous studies, most of them from China, suggest that huperzine A may be as effective as the drugs tacrine and donepezil in Alzheimer's disease. This is not so surprising since *in vitro* and animal model tests have demonstrated that huperzine A effectively inhibits acetylcholinesterase, an enzyme that catalyzes acetylcholine breakdown. Tacrine and donepezil work in the same way to conserve acetylcholine in the brain—the mode by which they presumptively improve memory and cognition in those with Alzheimer's and age-related cognitive impairment. Huperzine A may prove superior to tacrine (dose-limited due to its hepatotoxicity) if long-range studies, yet to be conducted, demonstrate its safety.

In one double-blind, randomized study, huperzine A, in injectable form, was tested against a saline control in 56 patients with multi-infarct dementia or senile dementia and in 104 patients with senile and pre-senile simple memory disorders. Huperzine A produced significant positive effects as measured by the Wechsler Memory Scale. Dizziness was experienced by a few of the huperzine A-treated patients.

In another study, this one multicenter, double-blind, placebo-controlled and randomized, 50 subjects with Alzheimer's disease were given huperzine A or placebo for eight weeks. Significant improvement was noted in 58 percent of the patients in terms of memory, cognitive and behavioral functions. Research is ongoing.

CONTRAINDICATIONS, PRECAUTIONS, ADVERSE REACTIONS

CONTRAINDICATIONS

None known.

PRECAUTIONS

Huperzine A should be avoided by children, pregnant women and nursing mothers.

Because of possible adverse effects in those with seizure disorders, cardiac arrhythmias and asthma, those with these disorders should avoid huperzine A. Those with irritable bowel disease, inflammatory bowel disease and malabsorption syndromes should avoid huperzine A.

ADVERSE REACTIONS

Adverse effects reported with huperzine A include gastrointestinal effects, such as nausea and diarrhea, sweating, blurred vision, fasciculations and dizziness. Possible adverse effects include vomiting, cramping, bronchospasm, bradycardia, arrhythmias, seizures, urinary incontinence, increased urination and hypersalivation.

INTERACTIONS

DRUGS

Acetylcholinesterase Inhibitors: Use of huperzine A along with the acetylcholinesterase inhibitors donepezil or tacrine may produce additive effects, including additive adverse effects. Other acetylcholinesterase inhibitors include neostigmine, physostigmine and pyridostigmine, and use of these agents along with huperzine A may produce additive effects, including additive adverse effects.

Cholinergic Drugs: Use of huperzine A along with cholinergic drugs, such as bethanechol, may produce additive effects, including additive adverse effects.

NUTRITIONAL SUPPLEMENTS

Use of huperzine A with choline, phosphatidylcholine, CDP-choline and L-alpha-glycerylphosphorylcholine hypothetically might produce additive effects, including additive adverse effects.

OVERDOSAGE

There are no reports of overdosage with huperzine A.

DOSAGE AND ADMINISTRATION

There are various forms of huperzine A available, including extracts of *Huperzia serrata*, natural (-)-huperzine A and synthetic racemic (±)-huperzine A. Natural (-)-huperzine A is approximately three times more potent than the synthetic racemic mixture. The doses of natural (-)-huperzine A used in clinical studies ranged from 60 micrograms to 200 micrograms daily. Huperzine A should only be used with a physician's recommendation and monitoring.

HOW SUPPLIED

Capsules — 50 mcg
Tablets — 50 mcg

LITERATURE

Cheng DH, Tang XC. Comparative studies of huperzine A, E-2020 and tacrine on behavior and cholinesterase activities. *Pharmacol Biochem Behav.* 1998; 60:377-386.

Cheng DH, Ren H, Tang XC. Huperzine A, a novel promising acetylcholinesterase inhibitor. *Neuroreport.* 1996; 8:97-101.

Quian BC, Wang M, Zhou ZF, et al. Pharmacokinetics of tablet huperzine A in six volunteers. *Chung Kuo Yao Li Hsueh Pao.* 1995; 16:396-398.

Tang XC, Kindel GH, Kozikowski AP, Hanin I. Comparison of the effects of natural and synethetic huperzine A on rat brain cholinergic function in vitro and in vivo. *J Ethnopharmacol.* 1994; 44:147-155.

Xiong ZQ, Tang XC. Effect of huperzine A, a novel acetylcholinesterase inhibitor, on radial maze performance in rats. *Pharmacol Biochem Behav.* 1995; 51:415-419.

Xu SS, Gao ZX, Weng Z, et al. Efficacy of tablet huperzine-A on memory, cognition and behavior in Alzheimer's disease. *Chung Kuo Yao Li Hsueh Pao.* 1995; 16:391-395.

Ye JW, Cai JX, Wang LM, Tang XC. Improving effects of huperzine A on spatial working memory in aged monkeys and young adult monkeys with experimental cognitive impairment. *J Pharmacol Exp Ther.* 1999; 288:814-819.

Zhang RW, Tang XC, Han YY, et al. Drug evaluation of huperzine A in the treatment of senile memory disorders. [Article in Chinese] *Chung Kuo Yao Li Hsueh Pao.* 1991; 12:250-252.

Hydrolyzed Collagen

DESCRIPTION

Hydrolyzed collagen refers to enzymatically or chemically processed collagen, which is mainly derived from bovine, ox and pig skin and bone. Hydrolyzed collagen consists of water-soluble peptides of various molecular weights. These peptides are rich in the amino acids found in collagen, including glycine, L-proline and L-hydroxyproline. Nutritional supplements containing hydrolyzed collagen are marketed for bone and joint health purposes. Hydrolyzed collagen and gelatin hydrolysates are similar. See Gelatin.

ACTIONS AND PHARMACOLOGY

ACTIONS

Hydrolyzed collagen has putative activity against degenerative joint disease (DJD).

MECHANISM OF ACTION

The mechanism of the putative anti-arthritic activity of hydrolyzed collagen is a matter of speculation. It is claimed that the amino acids of hydrolyzed collagen contribute to the synthesis of new collagen and new cartilage in joints. If this were the case, then hydrolyzed cartilage would be a disease-modifying substance. The amino acids in hydrolyzed collagen may contribute to joint collagen synthesis. However, if they did, it is unlikely that this contribution would be significant. L-hydroxyproline is not a genetic amino acid. It is formed in collagen post-translationaly. Therefore, L-hydroxyproline in hydrolyzed collagen would not contribute to collagen synthesis. Further, both glycine and L-proline are synthesized by the body, and it is entirely unclear how any glycine or L-proline in hydrolyzed collagen would make any significant contribution to collagen synthesis in joints. There is speculation that some oligopeptides that may be found in hydrolyzed collagen might have a stimulatory effect on collagen synthesis.

PHARMACOKINETICS

The digestion, absorption and metabolism of hydrolyzed collagen are similar to those of dietary proteins and peptides.

INDICATIONS AND USAGE

It is claimed that hydrolyzed collagen is useful in counteracting degenerative joint diseases. There is little convincing evidence to support this claim.

RESEARCH SUMMARY

Some preliminary research suggests that hydrolyzed collagen may have effects that could be beneficial in some with degenerative joint diseases. Well-designed clinical studies, however, are lacking.

CONTRAINDICATIONS, PRECAUTIONS, ADVERSE REACTIONS

CONTRAINDICATIONS

Hydolyzed collagen is contraindicated in those who are hypersensitive to any component of a hydrolyzed collagen-containing product.

PRECAUTIONS

Pregnant women and nursing mothers should avoid the use of supplemental hydrolyzed collagen.

Those with renal failure or liver failure should exercise caution in the use of hydrolyzed collagen.

Those who use hydrolyzed collagen produced from bovine sources should be sure that the products are derived from raw materials (bovine skin and bone) classified as carrying no detectable infectivity. Bovine nervous system parts may carry the bovine spongiform encephalopathy (BSE) organism, the etiological agent of mad cow disease.

INTERACTIONS

There is one report of hydrolyzed collagen enhancing the effect of calcitonin in the treatment of osteoporosis.

DOSAGE AND ADMINISTRATION

Hydrolyzed collagen is available in powder form by itself or in combination with other nutritional supplements, including glucosamine and chondroitin sulfate. A typical dose is 10 grams daily.

LITERATURE

Adam M, Spacek P, Hulejova H, et al. [Postmenopausal osteoporosis. Treatment with calcitonin and a diet rich in collagen proteins]. [Article in Czech]. *Cas Lek Cesk.* 1996; 135: 74-78.

Koepff P, Muller A, Scheiber R, Turowski A, Braumer K. Agents for the treatment of arthroses. United States Patent Number 4,804,745. Feb. 14, 1989.

Hydroxycitric Acid

DESCRIPTION

(-) - Hydroxycitric acid, commonly called hydroxycitric acid, is found in the fruits of the genus *Garcinia*. Supplemental hydroxycitric acid is typically an extract of the rinds of *Garcinia cambogia* fruit, also called Brindle berry. Fruit of this plant has long been used in India as a condiment, and the dried rind is used as a flavoring agent. The dried fruit rind is also used in Indian folk medicine for gastrointestinal complaints and rheumatism. Hydroxycitric acid is the principal acid in the fruits of *Garcinia cambogia* and makes up to 16% of the content of the dried fruit.

Hydroxycitric acid, in addition to being called (-)- hydroxycitric acid, is also known as hydroxycitrate, (-) — threo-hydroxycitric acid and 4S-hydroxycitric acid. It is abbreviated as (-)-HCA and sometimes as HCA. It is a different substance than either citric acid or isocitric acid, which are key intermediates in the tricarboxylic acid or Krebs cycle. The terms for the acid and anion forms, hydroxycitric acid and hydroxycitrate, respectively, are used interchangeably. However, the anion form is the form that occurs under biological conditions.

ACTIONS AND PHARMACOLOGY

ACTIONS

Hydroxycitric acid is a putative antiobesity agent.

MECHANISM OF ACTION

Hydroxycitric acid is a competitive inhibitor of the enzyme adenosine triphosphate-citrate (*pro-3S*) — lyase or ATP citrate lyase. In the cytosol, ATP citrate lyase catalyzes the conversion of citrate and coenzyme A to oxaloacetate and acetyl coenzyme A (acetyl CoA). Acetyl CoA is used in the synthesis of fatty acids, cholesterol and triglycerides and also in the synthesis of acetylcholine in the central nervous system.

Oxaloacetate may enter the gluconeogenic pathway, which can lead to the production of glucose and glycogen. It is believed that the putative antiobesity effect of hydroxycitric acid is due to suppression of fatty acid and fat synthesis. In addition, hydroxycitric acid is thought to suppress food intake via an anorectic effect. This is believed to be accounted for by hydroxycitric acid's stimulation of liver gluconeogenesis.

PHARMACOKINETICS

There is little reported on the pharmacokinetics of hydroxycitric acid in humans. Animal studies indicate that it is absorbed via the gastrointestinal tract and transported to the liver and other body tissues. There are no reports indicating if the marketed hydroxycitric acid is transported into liver cells in humans.

INDICATIONS AND USAGE

Claims are made that hydroxycitric acid is an effective weight-loss agent. These claims are not presently supported by well-controlled studies.

RESEARCH SUMMARY

A suggestion from animal work that hydroxycitric acid might be an effective antiobesity agent has not been confirmed in human studies. A recent well-controlled trial of hydroxycitric acid failed to produce any significant weight loss compared with placebo. This was a 12-week double-blind study in which overweight subjects were randomized to receive 1500 milligrams of hydroxycitric acid daily or placebo.

In another recent study, also conducted double-blind, placebo-controlled and randomized, researchers sought to see whether hydroxycitric acid supplementation could increase fat oxidation in human subject. The researchers found no significant effect.

CONTRAINDICATIONS, PRECAUTIONS, ADVERSE REACTIONS

CONTRAINDICATIONS
None known.

PRECAUTIONS
Pregnant women and nursing mothers should avoid hydroxycitric acid supplements. Because of the theoretical possibility that hydroxycitric acid might affect the formation of acetylcholine in the brain, those with dementia syndromes, including Alzheimer's disease, should avoid hydroxycitric acid. Those with diabetes should be cautious about using hydroxycitric acid.

ADVERSE REACTIONS
In a 12-week weight loss study comparing hydroxycitric acid, 1500 milligrams daily, against a placebo, the number of reported adverse reactions was not significantly different between the placebo group and hydroxycitric acid groups.

OVERDOSAGE

There are no reports of overdosage.

DOSAGE AND ADMINISTRATION

Hydroxycitric acid is available in *Garcinia cambogia* extracts. Some products contain hydroxycitric acid in the lactone form, which has not shown activity in animal models. There are products available that are free of the lactone form. Typical doses are about 1500 milligrams (as hydroxycitric acid) daily.

LITERATURE

Conte AA. A non-prescription alternative in weight reduction therapy. *Am J Bariatr Med.* 1993; Summer:17-19.

Greenwood MR, Cleary MP, Gruen R, et al. Effect of (-)-hydroxycitrate on development of obesity in the Zucker obese rat. *Am J Physiol.* 1981; 240:E72-E78.

Heymsfield SB, Allison DB, Vasseli JR, et al. *Garcinia cambogia* (hydroxycitric acid) as a potential antiobesity agent: a randomized controlled trial. *JAMA.* 1998; 280:1596-1600.

Kriketos AD, Thompson HR, Greene H, Hill JO. (-)-Hydroxycitric acid does not affect energy expenditure and substrate oxidation in adult males in a post-absorptive state. *Int J Obes Relat Metab Disord.* 1999; 23:867-873.

Hydroxyethylrutosides

DESCRIPTION

Hydroxyethylrutosides (HR) refer to a mixture of semi-synthetic derivatives of the flavonoid rutin. Rutin is a naturally occurring flavonol glycoside comprised of the flavonol quercetin and the disaccharide rutinose (see Rutin). Hydroxyethylrutosides are comprised of the mono-, di-, tri- and tetrahydroxyethyl derivatives of rutin and are prepared by the hydroxyethylation of the phenolic groups of rutin.

Formulations, mainly consisting of the trihydroxyethyl derivative of rutin, are used in Europe, Mexico and other Latin American countries for the treatment of such venous disorders as varicose veins and hemorrhoids. The generic name for these formulations is troxerutin.

Trihydroxyethylrutoside, the principal flavonoid in troxerutin, is also known as 7, 3', 4'-tris [O- (2-hydroxyethyl)]rutin, trioxyethylrutin and 2- [3, 4-bis (2-hydroxyethoxy) phenyl]-3 [[6-O-(6-deoxy-alpha-L-mannopyranosyl)-beta-D-glucopyranosyl]oxy] -5-hydroxy-7- (2-hydroxyethoxy) -4*H*-1-benzopyran-4-one. It is a solid, yellow substance that is soluble in water. Its molecular formula is $C_{33}H_{42}O_{19}$, and its molecular weight is 742.69 daltons.

ACTIONS AND PHARMACOLOGY

ACTIONS
Hydroxyethylrutosides may have venoprotective, vasoprotective and antioxidant actions.

MECHANISM OF ACTION
The mechanisms of the possible veno- and vasoprotective actions of HR are not clear. During blood stasis, such as occurs during venous insufficiency, hypoxic conditions can activate endothelial cells. The activation of endothelial cells may result in phospholipase A2 activation, leading to the

release of inflammatory mediators, neutrophil adhesiveness to the endothelium with subsequent release of superoxide anions and leukotriene B4, and depletion of ATP. At least *in vitro*, HR appear to inhibit some of these processes, such as the activation of phospholipase A2 and the recruitment and activation of neutrophils. HR may have reactive oxygen and nitrogen species scavenging activity, which could also contribute to the possible protective effects. It is unclear, however, what the active forms of HR are *in vivo*.

PHARMACOKINETICS

There is little known about the pharmacokinetics of HR in humans. Radioactive labeling studies indicate that HR are absorbed from the intestine following absorption and that the major route of HR excretion is via the biliary-enteric route. However, it is unclear how much HR are absorbed intact—that is, as the glycosides—and it is also unclear what the metabolic fate of HR is following absorption.

INDICATIONS AND USAGE

Hydroxyethylrutosides have demonstrated significant efficacy in the treatment of venous insufficiency and related disorders. There is preliminary evidence that HR might be useful in some with Meniere's disease.

RESEARCH SUMMARY

A meta-analysis of randomized, placebo-controlled trials using HR in the treatment of chronic venous insufficiency found improvement in HR-treated subjects, compared with placebo, as measured by significant disappearance of the following symptoms: pain, cramps, tired legs, swelling and restless legs.

In another review of the therapeutic efficacy of HR, the substance was found to show ''promise as a useful additional option for the management of edema and other symptoms of chronic venous insufficiency.'' Positive effects were confirmed in venous insufficiency associated with pregnancy and lymphoedema. Reductions in retinal vascular permeability have been seen in HR-treated patients with diabetic retinopathy, and HR have been shown, in other studies, to be efficacious in treating some women with hemorrhoids of pregnancy.

Finally, there is a double-blind, placebo-controlled, crossover study showing significant, positive HR effects in the treatment of subjects with well-defined Meniere's disease. Dose in this trial was 2 grams of HR daily for three months. Side effects were few.

CONTRAINDICATIONS, PRECAUTIONS, ADVERSE REACTIONS

CONTRAINDICATIONS

Hydroxyethylrutosides are contraindicated in those hypersensitive to any component of an HR-containing product.

PRECAUTIONS

HR should be avoided by pregnant women and nursing mothers unless they are prescribed by physicians.

ADVERSE REACTIONS

HR are generally well tolerated. Gastrointestinal side effects, such as nausea, are occasionally reported.

DOSAGE AND ADMINISTRATIONS

Troxerutin (trihydroxyethylrutoside) is available is some combination products. It is used in Europe and Latin American countries in the management of varicose veins and hemorrhoids. Doses used for these conditions range from 500 mg to 2 grams daily.

LITERATURE

Janssens D, Michiels C, Arnould T, Remacle J. Effects of hydroxyethylrutosides on hypoxia-induced activation of human endothelial cells *in vitro*. *Br J Pharmacol*. 1996; 118:599-604.

MacLennan WJ, Wilson J, Rattenhuber V, et al. Hydroxyethylrutosides in elderly patients with chronic venous insufficiency: its efficacy and tolerability. *Gerontology*. 1994; 40:45-52.

Moses M, Ranacher G, Wilmot TJ, Golden GJ. A double-blind clinical trial of hydroxyethylrutosides in Meniere's disease. *J Laryngol Otol*. 1984; 98:265-272.

Poynard T, Valterio C. Meta-analysis of hydroxyethylrutosides in the treatment of chronic venous insufficiency. *Vasa*. 1994; 23:244-250.

Wadworth AN, Faulds D. Hydroxyethylrutosides. A review of its pharmacology, and therapeutic efficacy in venous insufficiency and related disorders. *Drugs*. 1992; 44: 1013-1032.

Indole-3-Carbinol

DESCRIPTION

Indole-3-carbinol or I3C is a breakdown product of the glucosinolate glucobrassicin, also known as indole-3-glucosinolate. Glucosinolates are beta-thioglucoside N-hydroxysulfates, which are primarily found in cruciferous vegetables (cabbage, broccoli sprouts, brussels sprouts, cauliflower, bok choy and kale).

Indole-3-carbinol may have cancer chemopreventive activity. Glucosinolates themselves have minimal anticancer activity. Indole-3-carbinol is produced from indole-3-glucosinolate via the action of the enzyme myrosinase (thioglucoside glucohydrolase), an enzyme which is present in cruciferous vegetables and activated upon maceration of the vegetables.

The possible anticancer activity of substances such as I3C was recognized by the Roman statesman, Cato the Elder (234-149 BC), who in his treatise on medicine wrote: ''If a cancerous ulcer appears upon the breasts, apply a crushed cabbage leaf and it will make it well.'' Crushing a cabbage leaf would convert indole-3-glucosinolate to I3C, among other reactions.

ACTIONS AND PHARMACOLOGY

ACTIONS
Indole-3-carbinol may modulate estrogen metabolism. It may also have anticarcinogenic, antioxidant and anti-atherogenic activities.

MECHANISM OF ACTION
The estrogen metabolites 16 alpha-hydroxyestrone and 4-hydroxyestrone have been demonstrated to be carcinogens and are thought to be responsible for the possible carcinogenic effects of estrogen. On the other hand, the estrogen metabolite 2-hydroxyestrone has been found to be protective against several types of cancer, including breast cancer. Indole-3-carbinol has been shown to increase the ratio of 2-hydroxyestrone to 16 alpha-hydroxyestrone and also to inhibit the 4-hydroxylation of estradiol. Indole-3-carbinol increases 2-hydroxylation of estrogens via induction of cytochrome P4501A1 (CYP1A1). Indole-3-carbinol is converted by stomach acid to diindolymethane (DIM) and indole (3,2,b) carbazole (ICZ). DIM and ICZ have similar activities regarding estrogen metabolism.

Regarding its possible anticarcinogenic effects, indole-3-carbinol has been shown to modulate the activities of both Phase I enzymes, such as cytochrome P4501A1, -1A2, -2B1, -2B2, -3A1 and -3A2, and Phase II enzymes, such as glutathione S-transferase (GST), quinone reductase and uridine glucuronide transferase. Indole-3-carbinol modulates the metabolism of carcinogens, such as benzo(a)pyrene, aflatoxin B_1 and 4-(methylnitrosoamino)-1-(3-pyridyl)-1-butanone (NNK). Indole-3-carbinol has also been shown to upregulate apoptosis in some cancer cell lines.

As mentioned above, indole-3-carbinol induces the synthesis of 2-hydroxyestrone. 2-hydroxyestrone has been found to inhibit the oxidation of low-density lipoprotein. This indicates that indole-3-carbinol has indirect antioxidant activity. 2-hydroxyestrone also appears to inhibit smooth muscle proliferation. Inhibition of smooth muscle proliferation and inhibition of the oxidation of LDL could account for the possible anti-atherogenic activity of indole-3-carbinol.

PHARMACOKINETICS
There is much unknown about the pharmacokinetics of indole-3-carbinol in humans. It is converted to DIM and ICZ by stomach acid, and DIM and ICZ are absorbed from the gastrointestinal tract. The extent of absorption of I3C, DIM and ICZ, as well as their distribution, metabolism and excretion, are currently being studied.

INDICATIONS AND USAGE
I3C may have anticarcinogenic effects and, possibly, some anti-atherogenic activity. It may be useful in inhibiting the formation of papillomatosis cysts caused by the human papilloma virus (HPV). Claims that it helps build muscle are unsubstantiated.

RESEARCH SUMMARY
I3C has significantly reduced the number of tumor-bearing animals and the number of tumors per animal, compared with controls, in an animal model of spontaneous mammary tumorogenesis. I3C, administered after carcinogen initiation, also significantly inhibited chemically induced mammary tumors.

Aflatoxin-induced tumors in fish were inhibited by I3C when given before exposure to aflatoxin. On the other hand, I3C appeared to promote aflatoxin-induced tumor activity when given after initiation with aflatoxin in these animals. In a rat study, however, I3C had inhibitory effects on aflatoxin-induced tumor formation when given both before and after aflatoxin exposure. More research on this issue is needed. Still other animal studies have demonstrated that I3C exerted protective effects of various types against cancers of the endometrium, lung, tongue, colon and liver.

Cell culture work has shown that HPV proliferation was inhibited by the action of I3C. Subsequently, it was shown that feeding I3C to nude mice significantly inhibited the formation of papillomatous cysts. This, in turn, led to a human study in which I3C again significantly inhibited the formation of these lesions—this time in children.

There is preliminary evidence from *in vitro* studies that I3C-induced metabolites can inhibit oxidation of LDL-cholesterol and that they can also inhibit smooth muscle cell proliferation.

CONTRAINDICATIONS, PRECAUTIONS, ADVERSE REACTIONS.

CONTRAINDICATIONS
Indole-3-carbinol is contraindicated in those hypersensitive to this substance or to any component of an indole-3-carbinol-containing product.

PRECAUTIONS
Pregnant women and nursing mothers should avoid indole-3-carbinol supplements pending long-term safety studies. Those with cancer should confer with their physician before deciding to use indole-3-carbinol.

INTERACTIONS

DRUGS
Antacids, H2 blockers, proton-pump inhibitors: The conversion of indole-3-carbinol to DIM and ICZ requires stomach acid. It is unclear if indole-3-carbinol itself would have all

the possible activities mentioned above if it were not converted to DIM and ICZ.

Tamoxifen: Indole-3-carbinol may be synergistic with tamoxifen in protecting against breast cancer.

DOSAGE AND ADMINISTRATION

Indole-3-carbinol is available as a stand-alone supplement and in combination products. Dosage ranges from 200 mg to 800 mg daily.

Indole-3-carbinol, as well as diindolylmethane, are available in combination formulas used by some body builders.

LITERATURE

Albert-Puleo M. Physiological effects of cabbage with reference to its potential as a dietary cancer-inhibitor and its use in ancient medicine. *J Ethnopharm.* 1983; 9:261-272.

Bailey GS, Hendricks JD, Shelton DW, et al. Enhancement of carcinogenesis by the natural anti-carcinogen indole-3-carbinol. *J Natl Cancer Inst.*1987; 78:931-934.

Bradlow HL, Michnovicz JJ, Wong GYC, et al. Long term responses of women to indole-3-carbinol or a high fiber diet. *Cancer Epidemiol Biomarkers Prev.* 1994; 3:591-595.

Bradlow HL, Sepkovic DW, Telang NT, Osborne MP. Multifunctional aspects of the action of indole-3-carbinol as an antitumor agent. *Ann NY Acad Sci.*1999; 889:204-213.

Cover CM, Hsieh SJ, Cram EJ, et al. Indole-3-carbinol and tamoxifen cooperate to arrest the cell cycle of MCF-7 human breast cancer cells. *Cancer Res.* 1999; 59:1244-1251.

Grubbs CJ, Steele VE, Casebolt T, et al. Chemoprevention of chemically-induced mammary carcinogenesis by indole-3-carbinol. *Anticancer Res.* 1995; 15:709-716.

He Y-H, Freisen MD, Ruch RJ, Schut HAJ. Indole-3-carbinol as a chemopreventive agent in 2-amino-1-methyl-6-phenylimidazo [4,5-*b*] pyridine (PhIP) carcinogenesis: inhibition of PhIP-DNA adduct formation, acceleration of PhIP metabolism, and induction of cytochrome P450 in female F344 rats. *Food Chem Toxicol.* 2000; 38:15-23.

Kim DJ, Han BS, Ahn B, et al. Enhancement by indole-3-carbinol of liver and thyroid gland neoplastic development in a rat medium-term multiorgan carcinogenesis model. *Carcinogenesis.* 1997; 18:377-381.

Michnovicz JJ, Bradlow HL. Induction of estradiol metabolism by dietary indole-3-carbinol in humans. *J Natl Cancer Inst.* 1990; 50:947-950.

Niwa T, Swaneck G, Bradlow HL. Alterations in estradiol metabolism in MCF-7 cells induced by treatment with indole-3-carbinol and related compounds. *Steroids.* 1994; 59:523-527.

Wong GYC, Bradlow HL, Sepkovic DW, et al. A dose-ranging study of indole-3-carbinol for breast cancer prevention. *J Cell Biol.*1988; 28:111-116.

Zeligs MA. Diet and estrogen status: the cruciferous connection. *J Med Food.* 1998; 1:67-82.

Inosine

TRADE NAMES

Inosine is available generically from numerous manufacturers. Branded products include Inosine Mega (Twinlab).

DESCRIPTION

Inosine is a purine ribonucleoside widely found in plants, animals and other forms of living matter. It is comprised of the purine base hypoxanthine and the sugar D-ribose. The structural formula is:

Inosine

Inosine, in the form of its nucleotide, inosine 5'-monophosphate (inosinate), is the precursor of adenosine monophosphate (AMP) and guanosine monophosphate (GMP) in the *de novo* biosynthesis of purine nucleotides. It is also an intermediate in the so-called salvage pathway of purine nucleotide synthesis, and it is an intermediate in the degradation of purines and purine nucleosides to the purine end-product, uric acid. Inosine is also found as a minor nucleoside in transfer RNA.

Disodium inosinate is commonly used in foods for flavor enhancement and comprises a significant proportion of the dietary intake of inosine. Inosine itself has been used as a pharmaceutical agent. Some time ago, Trophicardyl was used in France for the treatment of cardiovascular conditions, including ischemia, cardiomyopathy and arrythmias. The active drug was inosine. In Russia, Riboxin, again inosine, was and is still used for the treatment of similar disorders. Inosine pranobex (Isoprinosine), a delivery form of inosine, is an orphan drug indicated for the treatment of subacute sclerosing panencephalitis. This drug is also thought to have immunomodulatory activity.

Inosine is also known as hypoxanthine riboside, 9-beta-D-ribofuranosylhypoxanthine and hypoxanthosine. It is abbreviated I.

ACTIONS AND PHARMACOLOGY

ACTIONS

Inosine may have neuroprotective, cardioprotective, anti-inflammatory and immunomodulatory activities.

MECHANISM OF ACTION

Inosine has been found to have potent axon-promoting effects *in vivo* following unilateral transection of the corticospinal tract of rats. The mechanism of this action is unclear. Possibilities include serving as an agonist of a nerve growth factor-activated protein kinase (N-Kinase), conversion to cyclic nucleotides that enable advancing nerve endings to overcome the inhibitory effects of myelin, stimulation of differentiation in rat sympathetic neurons, augmentation of nerve growth factor-induced neuritogenesis and promotion of the survival of astrocytes, among others.

The mechanism of inosine's possible cardioprotective effect is similarly unclear. Inosine has been reported to have a positive inotropic effect and also to have mild coronary vasodilation activity. Exogenous inosine may contribute to the high-energy phosphate pool of cardiac muscle cells and favorably affect bioenergetics generally. Inosine has also been reported to enhance the myocardial uptake of carbohydrates relative to free fatty acids as well as glycolysis.

In cell culture studies, inosine has been found to inhibit the production, in immunostimulated macrophages and spleen cells, of the proinflammatory cytokines, tumor necrosis factor (TNF)-alpha, interleukin (IL)-1, interleukin (IL)-12, macrophage-inflammatory protein-1 alpha and interferon (IFN)-gamma. It also suppressed proinflammatory cytokine production and mortality in a mouse endotoxemic model. These actions might account for the possible immunomodulatory, anti-inflammatory and anti-ischemic actions of inosine.

PHARMACOKINETICS

Ingested inosine is absorbed from the small intestine, from whence it is transported via the portal circulation to the liver. In the liver, inosine may be catabolized by a series of reactions culminating in the production of uric acid and also may be metabolized to adenine- and guanine-containing nucleotides. Inosine not metabolized in the liver is transported via the systemic circulation and distributed to various tissues of the body, where it is metabolized in similar fashion as in the liver. Uric acid, the purine end-product of inosine catabolism, is excreted in the urine.

INDICATIONS AND USAGE

The primary popular claim made for inosine, that it enhances exercise and athletic performance, is refuted by the available research data. There is some preliminary evidence that inosine may have some neurorestorative, anti-inflammatory, immunomodulatory and cardioprotective effects.

RESEARCH SUMMARY

In a double-blind, placebo-controlled, cross-over study of nine highly trained endurance runners, 6 grams daily of inosine failed to demonstrate any benefit in various exercise tests, including a three-mile treadmill run. By one of the measures used, placebo was significantly superior to inosine.

In another placebo-controlled study, inosine again failed to confer any advantage over placebo in 10 competitive male cyclists, as measured by tests of aerobic and anaerobic cycling performance. Here too, inosine was actually inferior to placebo under some test conditions, suggesting, the researchers concluded, that it might have an ergolytic effect.

Preliminary research has suggested that inosine can suppress proinflammatory cytokine production and mortality in a mouse endotoxemic model and that it has some cardioprotective effects in an animal model of ischemic heart. This was associated with an observed inosine-linked increase in glycolytic activity and improved energy production.

Inosine has also recently shown neurorestorative effects in the rat corticospinal tract after injury. It had previously been shown to induce axon outgrowth from primary neurons in culture. The more recent *in vivo* study encouraged the researchers to hope that inosine "might help to restore essential circuitry after injury to the central nervous system." More research is needed.

CONTRAINDICATIONS, PRECAUTIONS, ADVERSE REACTIONS

CONTRAINDICATIONS

Supplemental inosine is contraindicated in those with a history of gouty arthritis with acute attacks.

PRECAUTIONS

Pregnant women and nursing mothers should avoid supplemental inosine.

Those with a history of hyperuricemia should be extremely cautious about use of inosine.

ADVERSE REACTIONS

Mild gastrointestinal symptoms, such as abdominal discomfort and nausea, have occasionally been reported.

OVERDOSAGE

No reports of overdosage.

DOSAGE AND ADMINISTRATION

No typical doses. Doses of 5 to 10 grams daily were used in the above-reported studies of the effects of inosine on athletic performance.

HOW SUPPLIED

Capsules — 100 mg, 500 mg

Tablets — 500 mg

LITERATURE

Benowitz LI, Goldberg DE, Madsen JR, et al. Inosine stimulates extensive axon collateral growth in the rat corticospinal tract after injury. *Proc Natl Acad Sci.* 1999; 96:13486-13490.

Hasko G, Kuhel DG, Nemeth ZH, et al. Inosine inhibits inflammatory cytokine production by a posttranscriptional mechanism and protects against endotoxin-induced shock. *J Immunol*. 2000; 164:1013-1019.

Korotkov AA, Zhorzholiani TD, Chkheidze LG, Shalamberidze DN. [Effect of inosine after early infusion of contrykal and heparin in various hemodynamic types of acute myocardial ischemia.] [Article in Russian.] *Kardiologiia*. 1998; 28:91-94.

Lewandowski ED, Johnston DL, Roberts R. Effects of inosine on glycolysis and contracture during myocardial ischemia. *Cir Res*. 1991; 68:578-587.

Mc Naughton L, Dalton B, Tarr J. Inosine supplementation has no effect on aerobic or anaerobic cycling performance. *Int J Sports Nutr*. 1999; 9:333-334.

Milano S, Dieli M, Millott S, et al. Effect of isoprinosine on IL-3, IFN-gamma and IL-4 production *in vivo* and *in vitro*. *Int J Immunopharmacol*. 1991; 13:1013-1018

Renoux G, Renoux M, Guillaumin J-M. Isoprinosine as an immunopotentiator. *J Immunopharmacol*. 1979; 1:337-356.

Starling RD, Trappe TA, Short KR, et al. Effect of inosine supplementation on aerobic and anaerobic cycling performance. *Med Sci Sports Exerc*. 1996; 28:1193-1198.

Williams MH, Kreider RB, Hunter DW, et al. Effect of inosine supplementation on 3-mile treadmill run performance and VO_2 peak. *Med Sci Sports Exec*. 1990; 22:517-522.

Zimmer HG. Effect of inosine on cardiac adenine nucleotide metabolism in rats. *Adv Myocardiol*. 1985; 6:173-183.

Inositol Hexaphosphate

DESCRIPTION

Inositol hexaphosphate, also known as phytate, is a component of most cereal grains and seeds, occurring in conjunction with plant fiber, and is a source of *myo*-inositol in the diet. Inositol hexaphosphate is responsible for storing more than 80 percent of the total phosphate in cereals and legumes. Phytate has strong chelating power for doubly charged metal ions, such as magnesium, calcium and zinc. Some studies suggest that phytate may slow tumor growth rates.

Inositol hexaphosphate, in addition to being known as phytate, is known as *myo*-inositol hexaphosphate, and *myo*-inositol 1,2,3,4,5,6-hexakisphosphate. Inositol hexaphosphate is abbreviated as $InsP_6$ and sometimes as IP-6. The structural formula is:

Inositol hexaphosphate

ACTIONS AND PHARMACOLOGY

ACTIONS

Inositol hexaphosphate is a putative antiproliferative agent and may have antioxidant activity.

MECHANISM OF ACTIONS

Some speculate that inositol hexaphosphate's possible antiproliferative activity is due to its chelating divalent cations which may be important for tumor growth. Others speculate that inositol hexaphosphate, along with inositol, are metabolized to inositol triphosphates, which are believed to be involved in cell signaling and regulating cell growth, and that this may underlie its possible effects. Chelation by inositol hexaphosphate of ferrous cations could inhibit the Fenton reaction, a reaction which generates reactive oxygen species. Enhancement of natural killer cell activity is offered as still another speculative mechanism.

PHARMACOKINETICS

It is unclear how much inositol hexaphosphate is absorbed in humans following ingestion. Inositol hexaphosphate may, in part, be hydrolyzed to *myo*-inositol. (See *myo*-inositol.)

INDICATIONS AND USAGE

There is preliminary evidence that inositol hexaphosphate may eventually find some use in the treatment of some cancers.

RESEARCH SUMMARY

A few studies performed *in vitro* and in animal models suggest that inositol hexaphosphate inhibits some cancers, specifically epithelial cancers, including breast and colon cancers. It has also significantly inhibited human rhabdomyosarcoma in an animal model. More research is needed to see whether this substance can play a role in the clinical treatment of some cancers. There is some epidemiologic data suggesting that dietary phytate may have chemopreventive activity.

CONTRAINDICATIONS, PRECAUTIONS, ADVERSE REACTIONS

CONTRAINDICATIONS

None known.

PRECAUTIONS
Supplemental inositol hexaphosphate should be avoided by pregnant women and nursing mothers, due to lack of long-term safety studies.

ADVERSE REACTIONS
No significant adverse effects were noted in one report on the use of a daily dose of 8.8 grams of inositol hexaphosphate taken for several months.

INTERACTIONS
Inositol hexaphosphate may form chelates with divalent cations such as calcium, magnesium, manganese, zinc, copper and iron found in foods, if taken with foods or nutritional supplements containing these elements. It may also interact with food proteins.

OVERDOSAGE
No reports of overdosage.

DOSAGE AND ADMINISTRATION
None recommended.

LITERATURE
Graf E, Eaton JW. Antioxidant function of phytic acid. *Free Rad Biol Med.* 1990; 8:61-69.

Jariwalla RJ, Sabin R, Lawson S, Herman ZS. Lowering of serum cholesterol and triglycerides and modulation by dietary phytates. *J Appl Nutr.* 1990; 42:18-28.

Jariwalla RJ, Sabin R, Lawson S, et al. Effect of dietary phytic acid (phytate) on the incidence and growth rate of tumors promoted in Fisher rats by magnesium supplement. *Nutr Res.* 1988; 8:813-827.

Porres JM, Stahl CH, Cheng W-H, et al. Dietary intrinsic phytate protects colon from lipid peroxidation in pigs with a moderately high dietary iron intake. *Proc Soc Exp Biol Med.* 1999; 221:80-86.

Shamsuddin AM. Inositol phosphates have novel anticancer function. *J Nutr.* 1995; 125:725S-732S.

Shamsuddin AM. Reduction of cell proliferation and enhancement of NK-cell activity. 1992. United States Patent Number 5,082,833.

Vucenik I, Kalebic T, Tantivejkulk, Shamsuddin A. Novel anticancer function of inositol hexaphosphate. Inhibition of human rhabdomyosarcoma *in vitro* and *in vivo. Anticanc Res.* 1998; 18:1377-1384.

Inositol Nicotinate

TRADE NAMES
No Flush Niacin (Twinlab, Nature's Life and others), No Flush Niacin Vegicaps (Solgar)

DESCRIPTION
Inositol nicotinate is a delivery form of nicotinic acid that has been used in Europe and Japan for the treatment of hyperlipidemias, peripheral vascular disorders, including Raynaud's disease, intermittent claudication, Buerger's disease (thromboangiitis obliterans), and necrobiosis lipoidica, a disorder marked by shiny leg lesions due to atrophy of the skin. Inositol nicotinate is marketed in the United States as a nutritional supplement. The flushing reaction ("niacin flush") which occurs in those taking immediate-release or crystalline nicotinic acid, is usually not as severe with inositol nicotinate.

Inositol nicotinate is also known as inositol niacinate, *myo*-inositol hexa-3-pyridinecarboxylic acid, hexanicotinoyl inositol, *meso*-inositol hexanicotinate, inositol hexanicotinate, inositol hexaniacinate and hexanicotinyl *cis*-1,2,3,5-*trans*-4,6-cyclohexane. Its molecular formula is $C_{42}H_{30}N_6O_{12}$ and its molecular weight is 810.73 daltons. Each molecule of inositol nicotinate contains six molecules of nicotinic acid esterified to one molecule of *myo*-inositol. By weight, approximately 80% of inositol nicotinate is nicotinic acid and 20% is *myo*-inositol. The chemical structure of inositol nicotinate is represented as follows:

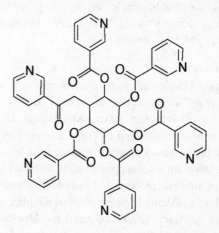

Inositol Nicotinate

ACTIONS AND PHARMACOLOGY
ACTIONS
Inositol nicotinate may have antihyperlipidemic activity. It may also have activity in the management of certain peripheral vascular diseases, such Raynaud's disease and intermittent claudication.

MECHANISM OF ACTION
The possible antihyperlipidemic activity of inositol nicotinate is accounted for by its metabolic conversion to nicotinic acid. See monograph on Niacin (Nicotinic Acid) for a discussion of the possible mechanisms of the antihyperlipidemic activity of nicotinic acid.

Inositol nicotinate has shown some activity in some with Raynaud's disease and intermittent claudication. Features of Raynaud's disease include intense vasoconstriction or vasospasm and platelet aggregation. The mechanism of inositol nicotinate's possible activity in Raynaud's disease is unknown. Nicotinic acid, the principal metabolite of inositol nicotinate, can cause vasodilation of cutaneous vessels. This results in increased blood flow principally to the face, neck and chest and is responsible for the so called niacin-flush. The vasodilatory activity of nicotinic acid is thought to be prostaglandin-mediated. However, the vasodilatory effect of nicotinic acid is transitory and unlikely to play a significant role in the possible activity of inositol nicotinate in Raynaud's disease.

Intermittent claudication results from occlusive arterial disease of the lower limbs and is characterized by pain, which develops during exercise and which disappears at rest. The pain is due to ischemia resulting from the obstruction or vasoconstriction of peripheral arteries. Inositol nicotinate may help some with this disorder. Again, the possible activity of inositol nicotinate is most likely mediated via its metabolite nicotinic acid. The mechanism of this possible effect is not understood. Hypothetical possibilities include nicotinic acid's hypolipidemic activity, its possible fibrinogen-lowering activity and, less likely, nicotinic acid's transient vasodilatory activity.

PHARMACOKINETICS

The pharmacokinetics of inositol nicotinate are not completely known. The molecule, at least in part, is absorbed from the small intestine intact. Metabolism of inositol nicotinate to *myo*-inositol and nicotinic acid appears to occur principally in the blood. Serum nicotinic acid levels appear to reach peak serum levels approximately 10 hours following ingestion of inositol nicotinate. Inositol nicotinate may be considered as a sustained-release form of nicotinic acid. See monographs on Niacin (Nicotinic Acid) and *Myo*-Inositol for discussions of the pharmacokinetics of these substances.

INDICATIONS AND USAGE

Inositol nicotinate has uses similar to those of nicotinic acid (see monograph on Niacin [Nicotinic Acid]). It has shown some promise in the treatment of hyperlipidemia, Raynaud's disease, intermittent claudication and other peripheral vascular diseases. Its use in dermatological conditions is too preliminary to support conclusions.

RESEARCH SUMMARY

Much of the research that applies to nicotinic acid applies to inositol nicotinate (see monograph on Niacin [Nicotinic Acid]). Inositol nicotinate is sometimes used for the treatment of Raynaud's disease. In one double-blind, placebo-controlled trial, 23 patients with primary Raynaud's disease were randomized to receive placebo or 4 grams of inositol hexanicotinate daily during cold weather. The treated subjects had significantly fewer and shorter vasospasm attacks than did the controls.

CONTRAINDICATIONS, PRECAUTIONS, ADVERSE REACTIONS

CONTRAINDICATIONS

Inositol nicotinate is contraindicated in those hypersensitive to any component of an inositol nicotinate-containing product. It is also contraindicated in those with hepatic dysfunction, unexplained elevations of serum aminotransferases (transaminases), active peptic ulcer disease and arterial bleeding.

PRECAUTIONS

Pregnant women and nursing mothers should avoid the use of inositol nicotinate.

The use of inositol nicotinate as an antihyperlipidemic agent or for the management of peripheral vascular disorders such as Raynaud's disease and intermittent claudication, or for any medical condition requires medical supervision.

Those with diabetes, gout, renal dysfunction and cardiovascular disease (especially acute myocardial infarction and unstable angina) should exercise caution in the use of inositol nicotinate, as should those with a past history of hepatobiliary disease, jaundice, peptic ulcer disease or gastritis.

Inositol nicotinate should not be substituted for equivalent doses of immediate-release (regular crystalline) nicotinic acid. Cases of severe hepatic toxicity, including fulminant hepatic necrosis, have occurred in those who have substituted sustained-release nicotinic acid products for immediate-release nicotinic acid at equivalent doses. Even though this has not been reported for inositol nicotinate, since inositol nicotinate behaves as a sustained-release form of nicotinic acid, this situation is theoretically possible. Those who switch from immediate-release nicotinic acid to inositol nicotinate, should start off, under medical supervision, with low doses of inositol nicotinate and the dose should be slowly increased to obtain the desired therapeutic response.

Inositol nicotinate, at high doses, may adversely affect glucose tolerance. Diabetics who use inositol nicotinate for lipid lowering, should have their serum glucose levels carefully monitored and the dose of their antidiabetic medications adjusted as necessary.

ADVERSE REACTIONS

Adverse reactions of high-dose nicotinic acid include flushing, pruritis, dizziness, palpitations, impaired glucose tolerance, elevated uric acid levels and liver dysfunction. Inositol nicotinate appears to be a well-tolerated delivery form of nicotinic acid. It has only recently been introduced into the

United States marketplace. However, few adverse reactions have been reported in Europe where the product has been in use for about three decades.

INTERACTIONS

See Niacin (Nicotinic Acid).

OVERDOSAGE

There have been no reported overdoses involving inositol nicotinate reported in the literature.

DOSAGE AND ADMINISTRATION

Inositol nicotinamide is available as a single ingredient product or in combination with other nutritional supplements. Dosage used has ranged from 500 milligrams to 4 grams daily taken with meals. Doses higher than 4 grams are rarely used.

HOW SUPPLIED

Capsules — 500 mg

Tablets — 500 mg

LITERATURE

Head KA. Inositol hexanicotinate: a safer alternative to niacin. *Alt Med Rev.* 1996; 1:176-184.

Holti G. An experimentally controlled evaluation of the effect of inositol nicotinate upon the digital blood flow of patients with Raynaud's phenomenon. *J Int Med Res.* 1979; 7:473-483.

O'Hara J, Jolly PN, Nicol CG. The therapeutic efficacy of inositol nicotinate (Hexopal) in intermittent claudication: a controlled trial. *Br J Clin Pract.* 1988; 42:377-383.

Ring EF, Bacon PA. Quantitative thermographic assessment of inositol nicotinate therapy in Reynaud's phenomena. *J Int Med Res.* 1977; 5:217-222.

Sunderland GT, Belch JJ, Sturrock RD, et al. A double blind randomized placebo controlled trial of hexopal in primary Reynaud's disease. *Clin Rheumatol.* 1988; 7:46-49.

Insulin-Like Growth Factor 1 (IGF-1)

DESCRIPTION

Insulin-like growth factor-1 (IGF-1) is a single-chain polypeptide of 70 amino acids. It is a trophic factor that circulates at high levels in the blood-stream and mediates many, if not most, of the effects of growth hormone. Although the main source of IGF-1 in the serum is the liver, many other tissues synthesize it and are sensitive to its trophic action. IGF-1 was called somatomedin in the older literature. IGF-1 and insulin have similar three-dimensional structures.

IGF-1 appears to influence neuronal structure and functions throughout the life span. It has been shown to have the ability to preserve nerve cell function and promote nerve

growth in experimental studies. Because of these properties, recombinant human IGF-1 is in clinical trials for the treatment of amyotrophic lateral sclerosis (ALS).

Recently, recombinant human IGF-1 has entered the dietary supplement marketplace, as have recombinant human growth hormone and several so-called growth hormone secretagogues or releasers.

ACTIONS AND PHARMACOLOGY

ACTIONS

Supplemental IGF-1 has putative anabolic and lipolytic activities.

MECHANISM OF ACTION

The mechanism of the putative actions of supplemental IGF-1 is unknown.

PHARMACOKINETICS

Orally administered IGF-1 has very poor bioavailability. There is no credible evidence that IGF-1 is absorbed from the oral mucosa if administered as a spray. It is likely that orally administered IGF-1 is digested in the small intestine to the amino acids that comprise the molecule.

INDICATIONS AND USAGE

Claims for supplemental IGF-1 are sweeping and include antiaging, promotion of lean muscle mass, enhanced athletic and sexual performance, joint protection, antidiabetic and antiatherosclerotic effects, sleep aid, immune enhancer, neuroprotector and much more. There is no credible evidence to support these claims for oral IGF-1. High levels of IGF-1 have been associated with elevated risk of several cancers, especially prostate cancer.

RESEARCH SUMMARY

There is no research to support the use of IGF-1 as a nutritional supplement, whether in oral or injected form. There is research showing associations between high levels of circulating IGF-1 and several cancers.

Claims that IGF-1 supplements significantly increase lean muscle mass are unsubstantiated. Use of IGF-1 in doses far higher than those used by most bodybuilders failed to produce more than very modest anabolic effects in AIDS patients. It is possible that some clinical indications, but not supplemental indications, will emerge from experimental work currently underway with IGF-1. There is a hint in some of this work that IGF-1 might, for example, have some neuroprotective and neurorestorative effects in some conditions.

CONTRAINDICATIONS, PRECAUTIONS, ADVERSE REACTIONS

CONTRAINDICATIONS

Supplemental IGF-1 is contraindicated in those with any evidence of active malignancy. It is also contraindicated in those who are hypersensitive to any component of an IGF-1-containing product.

PRECAUTIONS
Pregnant women and nursing mothers should avoid the use of supplemental IGF-1-containing products.

Adolescents should avoid the use of supplemental IGF-1-containing products.

Supplemental IGF-1 is not meant to be used parenterally and should never be used in such a manner.

ADVERSE REACTIONS
None known for supplemental IGF-1-containing supplements.

INTERACTIONS
There are no known interactions for supplemental IGF-1-containing supplements.

OVERDOSAGE
No reports for supplemental IGF-1-containing supplements.

DOSAGE AND ADMINISTRATION
Supplemental IGF-1 is available and marketed as a dietary supplement, typically in the form of an oral spray. There are no recommended doses.

LITERATURE
Carro E, Nuñez A, Busiguina S, Torres-Aleman I. Circulating insulin-like growth factor 1 mediates effects of exercise on the brain. *J Neurosci.* 2000; 20:2926-2933.

Chan JM, Stampfer MJ, Giovanucci E, et al. Plasma insulin-like growth factor 1 and prostate cancer risk: a prospective study. *Science.* 1998; 279:563-566.

Giovannucci E, Pollak MN, Platz EA, et al. A prospective study of plasma insulin-like growth factor-1 and binding protein-3 and risk of colorectal neoplasia in women. *Cancer Epidemiol Biomarkers Prev.* 2000; 9:345-349.

Hankinson SE, Willett WC, Colditz GA, et al. Circulating concentrations of insulin-like growth factor-1 and risk of breast cancer. *Lancet.* 1998; 351:1393-1396.

Le Roith D. Insulin-like growth factors. *N Engl J Med.* 1997; 336:633-640.

Lewis ME, Neff NT, Contreras PC, et al. Insulin-like growth factor-1: potential for treatment of motor neuronal disorders. *Exp Neurol.* 1993; 124:73-88.

Magee BA, Shooter GK, Wallace JC, Francis GL. Insulin-like growth factor 1 and its binding proteins: a study of the binding interface using B-domain analogues. *Biochem.* 1999; 38:15863-15870.

Mantzoros CS, Tzonou A, Signorello LB, et al. Insulin-like growth factor 1 in relation to prostate cancer and benign prostate hyperplasia. *Brit J Cancer.* 1997; 76:1115-1118.

Niblock MM, Brunso-Bechtold J, Riddle DR. Insulin-like growth factor 1 stimulates dendritic growth in primary somatosensory cortex. *J Neurosci.* 2000; 20:4165-4176.

Inulins

DESCRIPTION
Inulins refer to a group of naturally occurring fructose-containing oligosaccharides. They belong to a class of carbohydrates known as fructans. Fructans, in addition to inulins, include another group of naturally occurring fructose-containing oligosaccharides called levans. Inulins are usually of plant origin, while levans are found in fungi and bacteria. Inulins are mainly comprised of fructose units and typically have a terminal glucose. The bond between fructose units in inulins is a beta-(2-1) glycosidic linkage. Plant inulins contain 2 to 150 fructose units. The smallest inulin is called 1-kestose and is composed of two residues of fructose and one of glucose. Inulins are naturally synthesized from sucrose.

Chemically, inulins with a terminal glucose are known as alpha-D-glucopyranosyl-[beta-D-fructofuranosyl](n-1)-D-fructofuranosides, which is abbreviated GpyFn. Inulins without glucose are beta-D-fructopyranosyl-[D-fructofuranosyl](n-1)-D-fructofuranosides, abbreviated as FpyFn. Lower case n refers to the number of fructose residues in inulin; py is the abbreviation for pyranosyl. The basic structural formula follows:

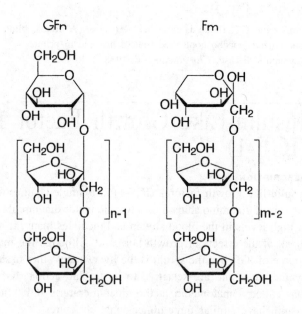

Inulin
n or m equal the number of fructose units
G = glucose, F = fructose

Inulins are present in onions, leeks, garlic, bananas, asparagus and artichokes, among other vegetables and fruits. Because of their sweet taste and their texture, inulins are added to various foods. Inulin intake in the U.S. ranges from 1 to 4 grams daily. It is higher in the European diet.

Inulins are only slightly digested in the small intestine. They are, however, fermented by a limited number of colonic bacteria. This could lead to changes in the colonic ecosystem in favor of some bacteria, such as bifidobacteria, which may have health benefits. Inulins are considered to be bifidogenic factors. Their energy content is about half that of digestible carbohydrates or about 1 to 2 kcal/grams.

Substances such as inulins that promote the growth of beneficial bacteria in the colon are called prebiotics. Prebiotics are typically nondigestible oligosaccharides.

Inulins are marketed as nutritional supplements and functional foods. The sources of these inulins are roots of chicory (*Cichorium intybus*) and Jerusalem artichokes (*Helianthus tuberosus*). Oligofructose refers to the partial enzymatic hydrolysate of inulins. Fructooligosaccharrides usually refer to synthetic short-chain fructans. The average chain length in inulins is 10.

ACTIONS AND PHARMACOLOGY

ACTIONS
Inulins may have antitumor, antimicrobial, hypolipidemic and hypoglycemic actions. They may also help to improve mineral absorption and balance and may have antiosteoporotic activity.

MECHANISM OF ACTION
The possible antitumor activity of inulins, particularly with respect to colon cancer, might be accounted for, in part, by the possible antitumor action of butyrate. Butyrate, the anion of the short-chain fatty acid butyric acid, is produced by bacterial fermentation of inulins in the colon. Some studies suggest that butyrate may induce growth arrest and cell differentiation and upregulate apoptosis, three activities that could be significant for antitumor activity. Inulins may also aid in increasing the concentrations of calcium and magnesium in the colon. High concentrations of these cations in the colon may help control the rate of cell turnover. High concentrations of calcium may also lead to the formation of insoluble bile or salts of fatty acids. This might reduce the potential damaging effects of bile or fatty acids on colonocytes.

Inulins may promote the growth of favorable bacterial populations, such as bifidobacteria, in the colon. Bifidobacteria may inhibit the growth of pathogenic bacteria, such as *Clostridium perfringens* and diarrheogenic strains of *Escherichia coli*.

Inulins have been found to lower serum triglycerides in rats, and there is some indication that they may lower serum triglycerides in some humans, as well. The mechanism of this possible effect is unclear. It is speculated that the possible triglyceride-lowering effect is due to decreased triglyceride synthesis in the liver. Inulins may lower cholesterol levels in some type 2 diabetics. There is less evidence that inulins lower cholesterol in those with hypercholesterolemia who do not have diabetes. Propionate, a product of inulin fermentation in the colon, may inhibit hydroxymethylglutaryl-CoA (HMG-CoA) reductase, the rate-limiting step in cholesterol biosynthesis.

The possible beneficial effects of inulins on blood glucose—there is some evidence that inulins may lower fasting blood sugar in type 2 diabetics—may be explained as follows: Inulins may delay gastric emptying and/or shorten small-intestinal transit time. Propionate may inhibit gluconeogenesis. It may do this by its metabolic conversion to methylmalonyl-CoA and succinyl CoA, metabolites that may inhibit pyruvate carboxylase. Propionate may reduce plasma levels of free fatty acids. High levels of plasma free fatty acids lower glucose utilization and induce insulin resistance. Propionate may also enhance glycolysis via depletion of citrate in hepatocytes. Citrate is an allosteric inhibitor of phosphfructokinase.

Inulins, similar to dietary fiber, may bind/sequester such minerals as calcium and magnesium in the small intestine. The short-chain fatty acids (acetate, propionate, butyrate) formed from the bacterial fermentation of inulins in the intestinal tract may facilitate the colonic absorption of calcium and possibly also magnesium ions. This could be beneficial in preventing osteoporosis and osteopenia.

PHARMACOKINETICS
Little digestion of inulins takes place in the stomach and small intestine following ingestion of inulins. Inulins are fermented in the colon by bifidobacteria and some other bacteria to produce the short-chain fatty acids acetate, propionate and butyrate; the gases hydrogen, hydrogen sulfide, carbon dioxide and methane; and lactate, pyruvate and succinate. Acetate, propionate and butyrate that are not metabolized in colonocytes are absorbed from the colon and transported via the portal circulation to the liver. These short-chain fatty acids are extensively metabolized in hepatocytes. Acetate, propionate and butyrate that are not metabolized in hepatocyes are transported by the circulation to various tissues, where they undergo further metabolism. Butyrate is an important respiratory fuel for the colonocytes and is metabolized in them to carbon dioxide and water. Energy, in the form of ATP, is produced from the catabolism of butyrate.

Those with ileostomies may have a microbial population colonizing their ileums. In those cases, inulins could be fermented by some of the bacteria in similar fashion to the way they are fermented in the colon.

INDICATIONS AND USAGE

Inulins, like some other prebiotic substances, may help protect against colorectal cancer and some infectious bowel diseases. They may also have lipid-lowering effects. Animal research is suggestive of these benefits, but human research is in short supply.

RESEARCH SUMMARY

There is the suggestion from animal research that inulins may help prevent colon carcinogenesis by stimulating growth of bifidobacteria. In experiments with rats, dietary administration of inulins inhibited the development of colonic aberrant crypt foci, putative preneoplastic lesions that are believed to give rise to colonic adenomas and carcinomas. Oligofructose, a partial enzymatic hydrolysate of inulins, also inhibited these crypt foci but not as effectively as inulins.

Recently, 12 healthy male volunteers ate a breakfast cereal containing 18% inulin for several weeks. At the end of the trial, plasma total cholesterol and triacylglycerol levels were significantly decreased.

CONTRAINDICATIONS, PRECAUTIONS, ADVERSE REACTIONS

CONTRAINDICATIONS

Inulins are contraindicated in those who are hypersensitive to these substances.

PRECAUTIONS

Those who develop gastrointestinal symptoms with the use of dietary fiber should exercise caution in the use of inulins. Those with irritable bowel syndrome should exercise caution in the use of inulins. Those receiving whole body-radiation or radiation to the gastrointestinal tract should avoid supplementation with inulins.

ADVERSE REACTIONS

Doses up to 10 grams daily are well tolerated. Higher doses may cause such gastrointestinal symptoms as flatulence, bloating and diarrhea.

Occasional allergic reactions have been reported.

INTERACTIONS

NUTRITIONAL SUPPLEMENTS

Inulins may enhance the colonic absorption of calcium and magnesium supplements if used concomitantly with them.

Probiotics: The possible beneficial effects of inulins may be enhanced if used in combination with probiotics.

FOODS

Inulins may enhance the colonic absorption of calcium and magnesium in foods.

OVERDOSAGE

No reports of overdosage.

DOSAGE AND ADMINISTRATION

Inulins are available in tablets, powder and functional foods. Dosing is variable and ranges from 4 to 10 grams daily. Those who use more than 10 grams daily should split the dosage throughout the day. Doses higher than 30 grams daily may cause significant gastrointestinal discomfort.

LITERATURE

Brighenti F, Casiraghi MC, Canzi E, Ferrari A. Effect of consumption of a ready-to-eat breakfast cereal containing inulin on the intestinal milieu and blood lipids in healthy male volunteers. *Eur J Clin Nutr.* 1999; 53:726-733.

Menne E, Guggenbuhl N, Roberfroid M. Fn-type chicory inulin hydrolysate has a prebiotic effect in humans. *J Nutr.* 2000; 130:1197-1199.

Reddy BS, Hamid R, Rao CV. Effect of dietary oligofructose and inulin on colonic preneoplastic aberrant crypt foci inhibition. *Carcinogenesis.* 1997; 18:1371-1374.

Roberfroid MB, Delzenne NM. Dietary fructans. *Annu Rev Nutr.* 1998; 18:117-143.

Roberfroid MB, Van Loo JA, Gibson GR. The bifidogenic nature of chicory inulin and its hydrolysis products. *J Nutr.* 1998; 128:11-19.

Williams CM. Effects of inulin on lipid parameters in humans. *J Nutr.* 1999; 129(7 Suppl):1471S-1473S.

Iodine

TRADE NAMES

Kelp-Tabs (The Key Company), Kelp Natural Iodine (Apothecary Products)

DESCRIPTION

Iodine, consumed principally as its iodide salts, is an essential trace element which is vital to the function of the thyroid gland. It is an essential component of thyroid hormones, which are required for normal development and metabolism. The fact that trace element composition of foods is very much dependent on geography was first recognized with respect to iodine. Iodine is present in low amounts in the earth's crust and thus in its soil. It is plentiful in the oceans and is found in sea animals and sea plants, such as seaweeds. Iodine is a non-metallic element belonging to the halogen group. Its atomic number is 53, and its atomic mass is 126.90 daltons. Its atomic symbol is I. The terms iodine and iodide are frequently used interchangeably.

The thyroid hormones are iodine-containing substances and they do not function without iodine. Approximately 80% of the body's iodine pool, or about 15 milligrams in adults, is present in the thyroid gland. Moderate deficiency of iodine may result in a goiter. Severe iodine deficiency may result in endemic myxedema among adults and in endemic cretinism among infants. Iodine deficiency results in decreased production of the thyroid hormones thyroxine or T_4 and triiodothyronine or T_3. The fall in the level of T_4 leads to increased thyroid stimulating hormone (TSH) output from the pituitary gland, resulting in an increase in the size of the thyroid gland which can lead to the formation of a goiter. In addition to causing goiters, iodine deficiency may result in a wide spectrum of effects on growth and development, particularly on brain development. Iodine deficiency is the most common cause of preventable mental deficit in the world.

In the early 1900s and prior to that, iodine deficiency and endemic goiter were very common in the United States. In the early 1920s, it was demonstrated in school children in Ohio that endemic goiter could be prevented and reduced by administration of small amounts of iodine in the form of iodide. Shortly afterwards, mass prophylaxis of endemic goiter with iodized salt was introduced in the United States and Switzerland, leading to a sharp fall in the incidence of goiter, as well as cretinism. Goiter, myxedema and other iodine deficiency disorders (IDD), including cretinism, still continue to be major public health problems on the global level. Approximately 20% of the world's population is iodine-deficient and at risk for IDD.

In addition to iodized salt, rich sources of iodine include fish and sea vegetables (seaweeds). Iodine is also available in animal products, such as eggs, milk, meat and poultry. In industrialized countries, most animal feeds are enriched with iodine.

ACTIONS AND PHARMACOLOGY

ACTIONS

Iodine's major action is its precursor role in the formation of thyroid hormones. Iodine may also be protective against radioactive iodine and consequent thyroid cancer. Iodine is used therapeutically for the treatment of certain hyperthyroid conditions and thyroid storm. The radionuclide ^{123}I is used for thyroid imaging and ^{131}I is used therapeutically for radioactive ablation of benign overactive thyroid and of locally invasive or metastatic thyroid cancer.

MECHANISM OF ACTION

Iodine in the form of iodide is preferentially taken up by the thyroid gland. Iodide is accumulated in the thyroid by means of an active iodide transport mechanism which is catalyzed by a sodium/iodide symporter, which mediates the sodium/potassium ATPase-dependent coupling of inward iodide and sodium fluxes. The thyroid gland is not the only organ capable of iodide uptake. However, the thyroid is the only organ known to organify iodide. Iodide is released by the thyroid cells into the colloid follicle phase, and there it is oxidized by hydrogen peroxide formed from the thyroid peroxidase system. Iodine reacts with tyrosine residues in thyroglobulin to form thyroxine (T_4) and triiodothyronine (T_3). The formation of T_4 and T_3 takes place post-translationally. The iodinated thyroglobulin is absorbed back into the thyroid cells where proteolytic enzymes break it down. The thyroid hormones T_4 and T_3 are released into the circulation and distributed to the various tissues of the body.

Potassium iodide may be used following radiation exposure from a nuclear reactor accident. Pharmacological doses of iodide block uptake by the thyroid of radioactive isotopes, particularly ^{131}I, thus minimizing the risk of radiation-induced thyroid cancer.

PHARMACOKINETICS

Iodine in the form of iodide is rapidly and efficiently absorbed from the small intestine following ingestion. A large fraction of absorbed iodine is taken up by the thyroid gland via the sodium/iodide symporter. In addition to the thyroid gland, active iodide occurs in the salivary glands, the gastric mucosa and in the lactating mammary gland. The nonlactating mammary gland does not accumulate iodide. Recently, it has been reported that accumulation of iodide via a sodium/iodide symporter appears to occur in human breast cancer tissue The major route of excretion of excess iodine is by the kidneys.

INDICATIONS AND USAGE

Apart from its use in iodine-deficiency disorders and for certain hyperthyroid conditions and thyroid storm, iodine is used as an expectorant and has demonstrated some ability to protect against the toxic effects of radioactive materials. It has also shown some preliminary efficacy in the treatment of sarcoidosis and has ameliorated some of the symptoms of fibrocystic disease of the breast. There are some preliminary reports that iodine is helpful in the treatment of erythematous dermatoses. Recently, some researchers have expressed concern that those on vegetarian diets may be at increased risk of iodine deficiency. Similarly, those on salt-restricted diets in general may be at the same or greater increased risk.

RESEARCH SUMMARY

There are reports that potassium iodide is a useful expectorant in chronic obstructive pulmonary disease including bronchitis, emphysema and asthma. It has been used in some studies of these conditions at doses of 300 to 1,000 milligrams two or three times daily. While somewhat effective, potassium iodide is not often used in this context due to the availability of more effective and safer expectorants.

Potassium iodide can effectively reduce thyroid uptake of radioiodine by 90% to 99% when administered immediately after exposure. Dosage used for this purpose has been reported at 130 milligrams per day. A 50% reduction in uptake of radioiodine has been achieved when potassium iodide was administered three to four hours after exposure to radiation. Limited benefit was seen when therapy began between four and twelve hours post-exposure. Potassium iodide has not protected against other radioactive substances.

The World Health Organization (WHO) has recommended that communities near nuclear reactors stockpile potassium iodides. Some credit Poland's prompt and widespread use of potassium iodide after the 1986 Chernobyl nuclear reactor disaster with the fact that Poland did not experience a significant increase in the incidence of childhood thyroid cancers, while fallout areas in Ukraine, Belarus and Russia (where potassium iodide was not widely used) have experienced large increases in these cancers.

Treatment with elemental iodine for four months has reportedly produced significant relief from symptoms of fibrocystic breast disease in one study. Upon discontinuing iodine, women in this study suffered a recurrence of pain and soreness. Some subsequent studies have also reported significant benefit from supplementation with other iodine-containing compounds used to treat this condition. Sodium iodide exhibited marked efficacy but was accompanied by a high rate of side effects. In one analysis of three clinical studies, molecular iodine was found to be the most beneficial in the treatment of fibrocystic breast disease.

There is one case report in which 300 milligrams of potassium iodide three times daily was of significant benefit in subjects with sarcoidosis. Pain and swelling in the arthritic ankle largely disappeared within 48 hours after initiation of treatment, and there was rapid regression of erythema nodosum on the leg.

Some others have reported benefit from 200 milligrams of potassium iodide three times daily in subjects with erythema nodosum. Best response has been seen when given soon after onset in patients with positive C-reactive protein reactions. There is also very preliminary evidence that the same doses of potassium iodide may be helpful in some with erythema multiforme and nodular vasculitis. More research is needed to confirm these findings.

Recently, some researchers have concluded that vegetarians, especially "strict" vegetarians who exclude all animal products from their diets, may be at increased risk of iodine deficiency. Both strict vegan diets and lactovegetarian diets that exclude seaweed and iodized salt provide very low iodine, according to the findings of one recent study. Non-vegetarian diets that exclude iodized salt and naturally rich sources of iodine, especially fish and seafood, also deliver very little iodine.

Urinary excretion studies have suggested that there has been a decline in iodide intake in several populations tested, e.g., school children in Switzerland and blood donors in New Zealand. Some have attributed this to the growing popularity of salt-restriction in diet generally. Some European populations have also recently been reported to exhibit overt and borderline iodine deficiencies.

One researcher has concluded that "the subclinical effects of low iodine intake and the physiological significance of low iodine excretion need to be studied further."

CONTRAINDICATIONS, PRECAUTIONS, ADVERSE REACTIONS

CONTRAINDICATIONS

Iodide and iodine are contraindicated in those hypersensitive to iodide- and iodine-containing products.

PRECAUTIONS

Pregnant women and nursing mothers should avoid intakes of iodine (iodide) greater than RDA amounts. These amounts are 175 micrograms daily for pregnant women and 200 micrograms daily for nursing mothers. Use of iodide doses much higher than 175 micrograms daily by pregnant women may cause fetal damage. Use by nursing mothers of iodide doses much greater than 200 micrograms daily may cause rash and thyroid suppression in the infant.

Older people with nodular goiters are at risk of developing hyperthyroidism from use of potassium iodide and iodized salt.

Potassium iodide and iodized salt may exacerbate symptoms in some with autoimmune thyroiditis.

Children with cystic fibrosis appear to have an exaggerated susceptibility to the goitrogenic effect of high doses of iodide.

ADVERSE REACTIONS

Doses of iodide up to 1,000 micrograms daily are generally well tolerated. Pharmacological doses of iodide have caused a number of adverse reactions. The adverse reactions include hypersensitivity reactions, flare-up of adolescent acne, rashes, arrhythmias, central nervous system effects (confusion, numbness, tingling, weakness in the hands or feet), hypothyroidism, hyperthyroidism (Jod-Basedow phenomenon), parotitis (iodide mumps), thyroid adenoma and small bowel lesions.

Manifestations of hypersensitivity reactions include angioedema, symptoms resembling serum sickness (fever, arthralgia, eosinophilia, lymphadenopathy), cutaneous and mucosal hemorrhages, urticaria, thrombotic thrombocytopenia purpura (TTP) and fatal periarteritis. Nonspecific small bowel lesions manifested by stenosis with or without ulcerations have been associated with the use of enteric-coated potassium iodide. These lesions may cause hemorrhage, obstruction, perforation and death.

Chronic intake of pharmacological doses of iodides can lead to iodism. Iodism is characterized by frontal headache, pulmonary edema, coryza, eye irritation, skin eruptions, gastric disturbances and inflammation of the tonsils, larynx, pharynx and submaxillary and parotid glands.

The most common adverse effect of salt iodization is the development of iodine-induced hyperthyroidism (IIH). IIH affects mainly older people with nodular goiter. Another possibility is the exacerbation of autoimmune thyroiditis. Theoretically, salt iodization can induce hypothyroidism by acute blockage of the synthesis and secretion of thyroid hormones. Hypothyroidism, however, has not been reported with salt iodization. Also, allergic responses to salt iodization are rare. IIH may develop when iodine deficiency increases thyrocyte proliferation and mutation rates. This can lead to the development of hyperfunctioning autonomous nodules in the thyroid gland and hyperthyroidism following iodine supplementation. A recent study reported transient hyperthyroidism in one out of 32 young adults with goiter and hypothyroidism after receiving 200 micrograms daily of iodine.

INTERACTIONS

DRUGS
Antithyroid Drugs: Concomitant use of antithyroid drugs and iodide may potentiate the hypothyroid effect of iodides.

Lithium: Concomitant use of pharmacological doses of potassium iodide and lithium may result in hypothyroidism.

Warfarin: Concomitant use of pharmacological doses of potassium iodide (for hyperthyroidism) and warfarin may decrease the anticoagulant effectiveness of warfarin.

NUTRITIONAL SUPPLEMENTS
Selenium: Intake of selenium and iodide may have synergistic activity in the treatment of Kashin-Beck disease, an osteoarthropathy (see Selenium).

FOODS
Certain foods contain substances which are metabolized to 5-vinyloxazolidine-2-thione and thiocyanate. 5-Vinyloxazolidine-2-thione and thiocyanate may compete with iodide and negatively affect the iodine status of the thyroid gland and may cause hypothyroidism. These food substances are called goitrogens and are found in foods such as cassava and such cruciferous foods as cabbage, Brussels sprouts, broccoli, cauliflower and rutabaga. Certain flavonoids may have goitrogenic activity. C-gluosylflavones such as vitexin, which are found in millet, have been found to inhibit thyroid peroxidase activity. The soybean isoflavones genistein and daidzein have also been found to inhibit thyroid peroxidase.

OVERDOSAGE
The administration of pharmacological doses of potassium iodide to those with impaired renal function may lead to serious hyperkalemia.

DOSAGE AND ADMINISTRATION
Potassium iodide is available as a nutritional supplement, typically in combination products. Doses are usually 150 micrograms daily for adults.

Approximately 77% of potassium iodide is comprised of iodide.

Iodine is commonly available in iodized salt. Iodine content in iodized salt ranges from 20 to 40 milligrams per kilogram or 20 to 40 micrograms per gram.

Iodized oil is used in some countries as a dietary iodine source.

The Food and Nutrition Board of the U.S. National Academy of Sciences has recommended the following daily dietary intakes of iodine (iodide):

Age (years) or status	Intake (micrograms/day)
0 to 0.5	40
0.5 to 1	50
1 through 10	70 to 120
Greater than 11	120 to 150
Pregnancy	175
Lactation	200

The World Health Organization's (WHO) recommendations are slightly different and are:

Age (years) or status	Intake (micrograms/day)
0 to 1	50
1 to 6	90
7 to 12	120
Greater than 12	150
Pregnancy	200
Lactation	200

HOW SUPPLIED
Tablets — 0.15 mg

LITERATURE
Carrasco N. Iodide transport in the thyroid gland. *Biochim Biophys Acta.* 1993; 1154:65-82.

Caserio RJ, Eaglstein WH, Allen CM. Treatment of granuloma annulare with potassium iodide. (letter). *J Am Acad Dermatol.* 1984; 10:294.

Crocker DG. Nuclear reactor accidents-the use of KI as a blocking agent against radioiodine uptake in the thyroid-a review. *Health Physics.* 1984; 46:1265-1279.

Davidsson L. Are vegetarians an 'at risk group' for iodine deficiency? *Br J Nutr.* 1999; 81:3-4.

Delange F. Risks and benefits of iodine supplementation. *Lancet.* 1998; 351:923-924.

Ghent WR, Eskin BA, Low DA, Hill LP. Iodine replacement in fibrocystic disease of the breast. *Can J Surg.* 1993; 36:453-460.

Graham N, Hogan DB, Simpson D. Potassium iodide in the treatment of sarcoidosis (letter). *Can Med Assoc J.* 1981; 124:124-127.

Hetzel BS. Iodine and neuropsychological development. *J Nutr.* 2000; 130:493S-495S.

Hetzel BS, Clugston GA. Iodine. In: Shils ME, Olson JA, Shike M, Ross CA. *Modern Nutrition in Health and Disease,* 9th ed. Baltimore, MD: Williams and Wilkens; 1999:253-264.

Horio T, Danno K, Okamoto H, et al. Potassium iodide in erythema nodosum and other erythematous dermatoses. *J Am Acad Dermatol.* 1983; 9:77-81.

Horio T, Imamura S, Danno K, et al. Potassium iodide in the treatment of erythema nodosum and nodular vasculitis. *Arch Dermatol.* 1981; 117:29-31.

Kahaly G, Dienes HP, Beyer J, Hommel G. Randomized, double-blind, placebo-controlled trial of low dose iodide in endemic goiter. *J Clin Endocrinol Metab.* 1997; 82:4049-4053.

La Rosa GL, Lupo L, Giuffrida D, et al. Levothyroxine and potassium iodide are both effective in treating benign solitary solid cold nodules of the thyroid. *Ann Int Med.* 1995; 122:1-8.

Moreno-Reyes R, Suetens C, Mathieu F, et al. Kashin-Beck osteoarthropathy in rural Tibet in relation to selenium and iodide status. *N Eng J Med.* 1998; 339:1112-1120.

Nauman J, Wolff J. Iodide prophylaxis in Poland after the Chernobyl reactor accident: benefits and risks. *Am J Med.* 1993; 94:524-532.

Remer T, Neubert A, Manz F. Increased risk of iodine deficiency with vegetarian's nutrition. *Br J Nutr.* 1999; 81:45-49.

Tazebay UH, Wapnir IL, Levy O, et al. The mammary gland iodide transporter is expressed during lactation and in breast cancer. *Nature Med.* 2000; 6:871-878.

Tonglet R, Bourdoux P, Minga T, Ermans A-M. Efficacy of low oral doses of iodized oil in the control of iodine deficiency in Zaire. *N Eng J Med.* 1992; 326:236-241.

Ipriflavone

TRADE NAMES

Ipriflavone is available from numerous manufacturers generically. Branded products include Ostivone (Natrol).

DESCRIPTION

Ipriflavone is a synthetic derivative of the plant isoflavone, genistein. Genistein is mainly found in soya in the form of genistin but also found in other plant sources, as well, in lower amounts. Ipriflavone occurs in trace amounts in some soy sauces. Although ipriflavone is sometimes classified as a phytoestrogen, it has no direct estrogenic activity. Ipriflavone does not activate any of the estrogen receptors. It does appear to have a favorable impact on bone density, and ipriflavone has been approved for the treatment of involutional osteoporosis in some European countries and in Japan.

The structural formula of ipriflavone is:

Ipriflavone

Ipriflavone is also known as 7-isopropoxy-3-phenyl-4H-1-benzopyran-4-one; 7-(1-methylethoxy)-3-phenyl-4H-1-benzopyran-4-one; 7-isopropoxy-3-phenylchromone and 7-isopropoxyisoflavone. Ipriflavone is abbreviated as IP. It is a solid substance that has poor solubility in water.

ACTIONS AND PHARMACOLOGY

ACTIONS

Ipriflavone may have a beneficial action on bone density.

MECHANISM OF ACTION

Osteoporosis is the consequence of an imbalance between osteoclastic and osteoblastic activity, coupled with an increased rate of bone turnover that occurs with menopause. Osteoclasts are the bone-resorbing cells, and osteoblasts are the bone-forming cells. In osteoporosis, a net loss of bone mass occurs due to either excessive-bone-resorbing activity of osteoclasts or impaired bone-forming activity of osteoblasts.

In vitro and animal studies suggest ipriflavone inhibits osteoclastic bone resorption and that it may also stimulate bone formation. Ipriflavone does not possess any estrogenic activity. The mechanism of action of ipriflavone on osteocasts and their precursor cells is not well understood. There is some evidence that ipriflavone may stimulate osteoblast activity by down-regulation of endothelin receptors. Ipriflavone may also reduce the ability of endothelin-1 to inhibit mineralization. Ipriflavone was found to be effective in preventing bone loss in ovariectomized rats. Ipriflavone, in contrast to estradiol, did not lower ovariectomized-induced rise in serum alkaline phosphatase or insulin-like growth factor-1 (IGF-1) and IGF-1 binding protein (IGFBP-3) concentrations.

PHARMACOKINETICS

Ipriflavone is absorbed from the small intestine; from there it enters the portal circulation. Greater absorption is obtained with food, and lipid-containing foods especially enhance its absorption. Ipriflavone is metabolized in the liver. The two major metabolites are 7-hydroxy-ipriflavone and 7-(1-carboxy-ethoxy)-isoflavone. Ipriflavone and its metabolites are distributed to the various tissues of the body via the systemic circulation.

In the blood, ipriflavone and its metabolites are bound to albumin. Elimination of ipriflavone and its metabolites is mainly by the urinary route. A smaller fraction of ingested ipriflavone is eliminated in the feces.

INDICATIONS AND USAGE

Ipriflavone may be indicated to help prevent and reduce bone resorption in osteoporosis. It may also help relieve bone pain associated with osteoporosis. There is some evidence that it can help correct some lipid disturbances associated with estrogen deficiency. Because ipriflavone does not have direct estrogenic effects, it may be suitable for use in aging men with bone loss, as well as in women. It has been suggested that ipriflavone might help prevent or reduce bone loss in men who have prostate cancer and are receiving androgen-reducing therapies.

RESEARCH SUMMARY

Ipriflavone is a currently approved drug indicated for the treatment and prevention of osteoporosis in Japan, Italy, Hungary and some other countries. It is available as a supplement in the United States. Its efficacy is increased when it is combined with calcium and other supplements that help diminish bone loss associated with menopause and aging. It is also sometimes combined with low-dose estrogen preparations.

Ipriflavone's efficacy in osteoporosis is well established by the results of numerous clinical studies, as well as studies involving many animal models. Many carefully controlled studies demonstrate that oral doses of 200 milligrams of ipriflavone three times a day (often combined with one gram of oral calcium daily) can have significant effects, increasing bone mineral density, reducing bone pain and diminishing the incidence of bone fractures—usually in post-menopausal women. Significant improvements in mobility have also been observed. Some studies have continued for as long as two years without incidence of significant side-effects.

Ipriflavone may exert its beneficial effects by inhibiting formation of the osteoclasts that are involved in bone resorption and by promoting the activity of the osteoblasts involved in building new bone. Its lack of direct estrogenic effects may make it a useful alternative in some cases to standard therapies and may, in particular, make it a useful therapy in men with bone loss associated with aging or androgen-limiting therapies (such as those sometimes used in the treatment of prostate cancer). More study is needed to determine ipriflavone's efficacy in this context.

CONTRAINDICATIONS, PRECAUTIONS, ADVERSE REACTIONS

CONTRAINDICATIONS

PRECAUTIONS

Because of lack of long-term safety studies, ipriflavone should be avoided by pregnant women and nursing mothers. Those taking theaphylline should be aware of an interaction with ipriflavone causing higher theophylline levels.

ADVERSE REACTIONS

Mild gastrointestinal side effects such as nausea have been reported.

INTERACTIONS

DRUGS

Theophylline: Ipriflavone is reported to inhibit the metabolism and elimination of theophylline. Both ipriflavone and its metabolite 7-hydroxy-isoflavone inhibit CYP (cytochrome P450) 1A2 and also CYP2C9. Inhibition of cytochrome P450 metabolism of theophylline produces higher serum levels of theophylline per given theophylline dose and, therefore, those on theophylline who also take ipriflavone must have their serum theophylline levels carefully monitored in order to avoid any toxic effects of elevated theophylline levels.

Tolbutamide: Ipriflavone and 7-hydroxy-ipriflavone inhibit tolbutamide hydroxylase activity. Consequently, use of ipriflavone may be expected to give higher levels of tolbutamide when the two are administered concurrently.

Nifedipine: 7-hydroxy-ipriflavone inhibits nifedipine oxidase activity. Consequently, use of ipriflavone may be expected to give higher levels of nifedipine in those using these products together.

Estrogen: Ipriflavone may add to the effects of estrogen.

SERM's: Ipriflavone may add to the effects of selective estrogen receptor modulators (SERMs).

Calcitonin: Ipriflavone may add to the effects of calcitonin.

Biphosphonates: Ipriflavone may add to the effects of and biphosphonates in the management of osteoporosis.

NUTRITIONAL SUPPLEMENTS

Ipriflavone may add to the effects of vitamins D and K, calcium, fluoride and boron in the management of osteoporosis.

OVERDOSAGE

There are no reports of ipriflavone overdosage.

DOSAGE AND ADMINISTRATION

The typical dose for use in the management of osteoporosis is 200 milligrams taken twice or three times daily.

HOW SUPPLIED

Capsules — 100 mg, 200 mg, 300 mg

LITERATURE

Agnusedi D, Crepaldi G. Isaia G, et al. A double blind, placebo-controlled trial of ipriflavone for prevention of postmenopausal spinal bone loss. *Calcif Tissue Int.* 1997; 61:142-147.

Agnusdei D, Bufalino L. Efficacy of ipriflavone in established osteoporosis and long-term safety. *Calif Tissue Int.* 1997; 61 Suppl 1:S23-S27.

Albanese CV, Cudd A, Argentino L, et al. Ipriflavone directly inhibits osteoclastic activity. *Biochem Biophys Res Communi.* 1994; 199:930-936.

Arjmandi BH, Birnbaum RS, Barengolts E, Kakreja SC. The synthetic phytoestrogen, ipriflavone, and estrogen prevent bone loss by different mechanisms. *Calcif Tissue Int.* 2000; 66:61-65.

Ferene L, Istvan S. Pharmacokinetics of ipriflavone. *Acta Pharm Hung.* 1995; 66:219-222.

Gennari C, Agnusdei D, Crepaldi G, et al. Effect of ipriflavone-a synthetic derivative of natural isoflavones-on bone mass loss in the early years after menopause. *Menopause.* 1998; 5:9-15.

Hagiwara H, Naruse M, Adachi C, et al. Ipriflavone down-regulates endothelin receptor levels during differentiation of rat calvarial osteoblast-like cells. *J Biochem.* 1999; 126:168-173.

Head, KA. Ipriflavone: an important bone-building isoflavone. *Altern Med Rev.* 1999; 4:10-22.

Kitatani K, Morii H. Ipriflavone. *Nippon Rinsho.* 1998; 56:1537-1543.

Melis GB, Paoletti AM, Cagnacci A, et al. Lack of any estrogenic effect of ipriflavone in postmenopausal women. *J Endocrinol Invest.* 1992; 15:755-761.

Monostory K, Vereczkey L, Levai F, Szatmari I. Ipriflavone as an inhibitor of human P450 enzymes. *Br J Pharmacol.* 1998; 123:605-610.

Reginster JY. Ipriflavone: pharmacological properties and usefulness in postmenopausal osteoporosis. *Bone Miner.* 1993; 23:223-232.

Sato M, Grese TA, Dodge JA, et al. Emerging therapies for the prevention or treatment of postmenopausal osteoporosis. *J Med Chem.* 1999; 42:1-24.

Schreiber MD, Rebar RW. Isoflavones and postmenopausal bone health: a viable alternative to estrogen therapy? *Menopause.* 1999; 6:233-241.

Iron

TRADE NAMES

Feostat (Forest Pharmaceuticals), Ircon (Kenwood Therapeutics), Ferretts (Pharmics), Hemocyte (U.S. Pharmaceutical Corp.), Nephro-Fer (R & D Labs), Fergon (Bayer Consumer), Feronate (Prime Marketing), Fe-40 (Bio-Tech Pharmacal), Ferro-Caps (Nature's Bounty), Ferro-Time (Time-Cap Labs), Vitedyn-Slo (Edyn Corp.), Feosol (SmithKline Beecham Consumer), Yieronia (R.I.D. Inc.), Fer-In-Sol (Mead Johnson), Ed-In-Sol (Edwards Pharmaceutical), Siderol (A.G. Marin Pharmaceutical), Mol-Iron (Schering Plough Heathcare), Feratab (Upsher-Smith Labs), Ferrousal (Prime Marketing), Slow Fe (Novartis Consumer).

DESCRIPTION

Iron is an essential trace mineral in human nutrition. It is involved in the entire process of respiration, including oxygen transport and electron transport. The principal goal of respiration is the production of biologic energy. Iron-deficiency, which can lead to a microcytic, hypochromic anemia, is the most common nutritional disorder in the world. Approximately 25% of the world's population is iron-deficient. Even iron-deficiency states which do not lead to anemia may have global effects on human health. On the other hand, iron overload disorders, which can lead to cirrhosis, coronary heart disease and congestive heart failure, among other things, is also a public health concern.

Iron is a transition metal with atomic number 26 and an atomic mass of 55.85 daltons. Its chemical symbol is Fe. Physiologically, iron exists in one of two oxidation states: ferrous (II) iron or ferric (III) iron.

The function and synthesis of hemoglobin, which carries most of the oxygen in the blood, is dependent on iron. Basic to the electron transport reactions that produce energy in the mitochondria of cells is the combining of oxygen with hydrogen to form water. The reaction occurs by means of a flow of electrons, derived from the oxidation of foodstuffs, across electron-carrier proteins called cytochromes, and via the final combination of these electrons with oxygen to produce water. The final enzyme in the electron transport chain is cytochrome oxidase. The cytochromes and cytochrome oxidase rely on iron for their production and function. Iron is also involved in the production of myoglobin, L-carnitine and aconitase, all of which are involved in energy production in the body. In addition to its fundamental roles in energy production, iron is involved in DNA synthesis and iron may also play roles in normal brain development and in immune function. Iron is also involved in the synthesis of collagen and in the synthesis of serotonin, dopamine and norepinephrine.

Although iron is clearly essential for a wide range of vital biological processes, it is also a potentially toxic substance. The shift back and forth between its two oxidation states—ferrous (II) and ferric (III)—via single electron-transfer reactions is the property that makes iron such an essential component of the cytochromes in the electron transport chain. However, this redox property also contributes to its potential toxicity. Redox cycling between ferrous (II) and ferric (III) can generate the highly reactive oxygen species hydroxyl radicals, which can damage lipids, DNA and proteins. The symptoms of the iron overload disorder hereditary hemochromatosis are due to iron toxicity.

The best dietary sources of iron are green vegetables, legumes and meat. Milk products, snack foods and soft drinks are not good sources of iron. Much of the iron ingested in the American diet in the form of bread and cereals is not well absorbed. The average dietary intake of iron in the United States ranges from 10 to 20 milligrams daily. Many, including adolescents and pregnant and lactating women, may be at risk for iron deficiency.

ACTIONS AND PHARMACOLOGY

ACTIONS

The major activity of supplemental iron is in the prevention and treatment of iron deficiency anemia. Iron has putative immune-enhancing, anticarcinogenic and cognition-enhancing activities.

MECHANISM OF ACTION

Iron is necessary for the production of hemoglobin. Iron-deficiency can lead to decreased production of hemoglobin and a microcytic, hypochromic anemia.

Under experimental conditions, iron-deficient subjects were found to have certain abnormalities in cell-mediated immunity and in the ability of neutrophils to kill different bacteria. The mechanism of those possible immune effects of iron is unknown. On the other hand, free iron may stimulate the growth of pathogenic bacteria.

Iron-deficiency has been associated with the Plummer-Vinson syndrome. In this condition, there is difficulty swallowing solid food because of a thin, web-like membrane that grows across the upper passageway of the esophagus. Those with Plummer-Vinson syndrome are at increased risk of cancer of the esophagus and stomach. Iron supplementation can prevent this syndrome. There is no other human evidence that iron has anticarcinogenic activity. The mechanism of iron's action in the Plummer-Vinson syndrome is unknown.

Some studies have suggested that children and adolescents with iron-deficiency may also have learning problems and that iron supplementation may increase cognitive skills in some children and adolescents with iron deficiency. The possible role of iron in these cases may be accounted for, in part, by iron's role in neurotransmitter synthesis, particularly in the synthesis of dopamine. Iron deficient rats have been reported to have phenylketonuria and disturbed brain function. It has been suggested that iron-deficiency in the rats resulted in altered phenylalanine metabolism producing phenylketonuria. Phenylketonuria has not been reported in iron-deficient humans.

PHARMACOKINETICS

The absorption of iron from the gastrointestinal tract is highly regulated. In fact, iron homeostasis is maintained by regulating its absorption, since the body does not have a regulated mechanism to excrete excess iron. Much remains unknown about its absorption, as well as the pharmacokinetics of iron in humans, in general. Dietary iron sources include heme iron, elemental iron which is used in food fortification, dietary ferric iron and iron salts used for supplementation. The discussion will begin with the iron salts.

The efficiency of absorption depends on the salt form, the amount administered, the dosing regimen and the size of iron stores. Subjects with normal iron stores absorb 10% to 35% of an iron dose. Those who are iron deficient may absorb up to 95% of an iron dose. Ingested inorganic iron is solubilized and ionized by the acid gastric juice. Iron supplements are mainly in the ferrous form (Fe II). Iron supplements that may be in the ferric form (Fe III) are reduced to the ferrous form. Absorption of iron may occur at any level of the small intestine but is most efficient in the duodenum. Iron is taken up by one of a few proteins on the luminal surface of the mucosal epithelium of the small intestine. Possible iron-binding proteins include a beta$_3$-integrin, the Hfe protein which functions together with beta-microglobulin and Nramp2 or divalent metal ion transporter1 (DMT1). Each of these proteins are transmembrane proteins. It is unclear how they operate in the transport of iron into the enterocytes. Nramp2 (DMT1) is a member of a class of proteins called natural resistance-associated macrophage proteins.

Within the enterocyte, iron—still in the ferrous form—is transferred to the cytosolic proteins mobilferrin and paraferritin. Paraferritin transports iron to the serosal surface of the enterocyte from whence it enters the portal circulation. As it enters the portal circulation, ferrous (Fe II) iron is oxidized to ferric (Fe III) iron by the copper-containing protein ceruloplasmin. Ferric iron bound to transferrin is carried in the portal circulation to the liver and then to all of the tissues of the body.

Transferrin, the principal iron transporter in the blood and other body fluids, distributes ferric (Fe III) iron throughout the body, principally to the red blood cell precursors in the bone marrow for hemoglobin synthesis. Approximately 70% to 90% of transferrin-bound iron is taken up by the erythropoietic cells of bone marrow for hemoglobin synthesis. Smaller amounts are delivered to other cells for the formation of cytochromes, cytochrome oxidase, myoglobin, or for other iron-requiring enzymes. Transferrin binds to a transferrin receptor located on the cell membrane forming an iron-transferrin-transferrin receptor complex which enters the cell by endocytosis. Within the cell, iron is released into the cytosol. Within the cytosol of the erythroblast, iron is transported by an unknown mechanism to mitochondria where it is inserted into protoporphyrin to form heme.

Iron in excess of need is stored principally as ferritin in the reticuloendothelial system of liver, spleen, bone marrow and other organs. Iron is released from ferritin in the form of ferrous (Fe II) iron and enters the plasma where it is oxidized by ceruloplasmin to ferric (Fe III) iron and taken up and transported in the plasma by transferrin.

Iron loss occurs principally through nonspecific mechanisms, including exfoliation of intestinal cells, urinary and biliary secretions and menstruation. Pre-menopausal women normally lose iron via menstrual bleeding. Iron losses can occur from gastrointestinal bleeding, bleeding from trauma, including surgical procedures, and from uterine bleeding in post-menopausal women on hormone replacement therapy. The body has a limited capacity to excrete iron. Very little iron is excreted by the kidneys or via the biliary route. Some iron losses occur through sloughing of skin and mucosal cells.

The absorption of heme iron is not well understood. To be absorbed, iron contained in heme proteins must first be freed by digestion of the protein to yield heme. Heme is absorbed from the small intestine by an unknown mechanism. Within the enterocytes, iron is freed from protoporphyrin by the enzyme heme oxygenase which converts the porphyrin ring to bilirubin and also yields ferric (III) iron and carbon monoxide. Ferric (III) iron binds to paraferritin which releases ferric iron from the serosal side of the cell into the circulation where it binds to transferrin. The remaining pharmacokinetics are as described above.

Dietary ferric (III) iron is solubilized and ionized by acid gastric juice. Some fraction of dietary ferric iron is reduced in the stomach. Some binds to mucin and is transported to the small intestine. Mucin protects ferric (III) iron against precipitation at the alkaline pH of the small intestine. The enzyme ferric reductase, which resides in the brush border of the duodenum, is capable of converting ferric iron to the ferrous form, which may be transported into the enterocytes by such iron-transport proteins as Nramp2, also known as divalent metal ion transporter1 (DMT1). The remaining pharmacokinetics of dietary ferric iron are as described above.

Iron-fortified cereals contain so-called reduced iron. This is finely powdered metallic iron and is generally poorly assimilated. It must first be oxidized to ferric (III) iron and then reduced to ferrous (II) iron in the stomach and small intestine before it can be absorbed.

Carbonyl iron or iron pentacarbonyl (diiron enneacarbonyl) is another nutritional supplement form of iron. Carbonyl iron requires stomach acid for its absorption.

In the treatment of iron deficiency anemia, an increase in the reticulocyte count is seen in three to four days and peaks in seven to ten days. The hemoglobin values may increase at a rate of 1.5 to 2.2 grams per deciliter per week for the first two weeks, followed by 0.7 to 1.6 grams per deciliter per week until normal values are achieved.

INDICATIONS AND USAGE

Apart from its use in preventing and treating iron-deficiency anemia, iron has been used with some success in reducing the frequency of breath-holding spells (BHS) in children. It is helpful in Plummer-Vinson syndrome and, in that context, may help prevent cancer of the esophagus and stomach in those with this syndrome. There is the suggestion in some research that iron might diminish learning problems and enhance cognition in some children and adolescents with iron deficiency. It may have some favorable effects on immunity and exercise performance—but, again, these benefits are most likely largely limited to those with frank or borderline iron deficiency. Iron's efficacy in malaria appears to be limited to improving iron status; it has no apparent effect on parasite rate or density. There is very preliminary evidence that it may have some modest, indirect beneficial effects in promotion of weight loss. Unrecognized iron deficiency may be significant in patients with critical illnesses, generally, according to findings of one recent study. In recent years, several research efforts have suggested that excess iron levels pose health risks for some groups.

RESEARCH SUMMARY

The frequency of breath-holding spells (BHS) diminished significantly in children with this disorder given iron 5 mg/kg/day for 16 weeks, compared with controls. Some 88% of those given iron had complete or partial responses compared with 6% in the placebo group. In a more recent study, 63 of 91 children with BHS had concomitant iron deficiency anemia. Complete or partial remission from BHS was achieved in children receiving 6 mg/kg/day for three months. Controls had a 21% partial or complete rate of remission.

Iron supplementation has been useful in preventing Plummer-Vinson syndrome characterized by difficulty in swallowing due to a membrane that grows across the upper esophagus. This condition is associated with an increased incidence of esophageal and gastric cancers. There is no other credible evidence that supplemental iron has other anticarcinogenic effects.

Iron deficiency anemia is associated, in some instances, with emotional, social and learning disorders in children and adolescents. Iron supplementation has improved these conditions in some studies. Iron deficiency in the absence of anemia can also cause some of these same problems and can be helped with iron supplementation, another study suggests.

Some researchers have reported that up to 25% of adolescent girls in the United States are iron deficient. In one study, the effects of iron supplements were tested in adolescent girls with non-anemia iron deficiency to see if they might improve cognition. This was a double-blind, placebo-controlled trial. Subjects were randomized to receive 650 milligrams of iron twice daily or placebo for eight weeks. Those with iron supplementation were reported to perform significantly better than those in the placebo group on tests related to verbal learning and memory.

Iron deficiency is known to diminish various aspects of immune function. Adequate levels help maintain cellular immunity and help to protect against some infections. Cell-mediated immune response may be impaired when iron deficiency negatively impacts the iron-requiring enzyme called ribonucleotide reductase, an enzyme that appears to be essential for the proper function of the T-lymphocyte arm of immunity. Resistance to candida, herpes simplex virus and some other pathogens appears to be reduced in those with poor iron status. On the other hand, excess iron may predispose individuals to some infections.

Claims that iron boosts energy and enhances exercise performance may be true—provided the claim is limited to those who are iron deficient. Muscle weakness and decreased exercise tolerance can occur in those who are iron deficient but not necessarily suffering from iron-deficiency anemia. Iron deficiency without anemia is not uncommon among some endurance athletes (e.g., long-distance runners), more among women than men.

Supplemental iron has been reported to be of some benefit in women on very-low calorie weight reduction diets. In one study, obese women on these diets lost more (but not significantly greater) weight when given supplemental iron.

The researchers concluded: "The greater recovery of thyroid hormone levels may have maintained metabolic rates to allow for greater weight loss." Some follow-up may be warranted.

Iron deficiency may be more widespread than generally believed. One recent study reported the presence of functional iron deficiency in 35% of 51 consecutive adult patients presenting to the general intensive care unit of a teaching hospital over a six-week period. Patients with massive hemorrhage or exchange transfusion in the two weeks before admission, those who were pregnant or lactating, those older than 80 years, those with hematological malignant disorders and those with bone marrow depression were excluded. Patients with functional iron deficiency had longer stays in intensive care than did those without iron deficiency (mean length of stay 7.6 days versus 3.3 days, respectively).

On the other hand, there is also evidence that some population subsets may be getting too much iron, some of it through supplementation. One group has estimated that up to one million people in the United States may have hemochromatosis, a hereditary disorder characterized by excess intestinal absorption of iron. Early symptoms include fatigue and joint pain. Fatal complications can include diabetes, cancer, heart disease and cirrhosis of the liver. One recent study found that stroke victims who have elevated levels of iron are significantly more likely to experience more severe neurological damage than are those with normel iron levels. Research is ongoing.

CONTRAINDICATIONS, PRECAUTIONS, ADVERSE REACTIONS

CONTRAINDICATIONS

Iron supplements are contraindicated in those with hemochromatosis and hemosiderosis.

Iron supplements are contraindicated in those who are hypersensitive to any component of an iron-containing supplement.

PRECAUTIONS

Iron supplements should not be used for the treatment of anemias other than iron deficiency anemia.

Treatment of iron deficiency anemia must only be undertaken under medical supervision.

Those with elevated serum ferritin levels should be extremely cautious in the use of iron supplements.

Pregnant women and nursing mothers should not use supplemental doses of iron higher than RDA amounts (30 and 15 milligrams daily, respectively) unless higher doses are recommended by their physicians.

Iron supplements can be highly toxic or lethal to small children. Those who use iron supplements should use childproof bottles and keep the bottles away from children.

Iron supplements should be used with extreme caution in those with chronic liver failure, alcoholic cirrhosis, chronic alcoholism and pancreatic insufficiency.

Carbonyl iron requires adequate stomach acid for absorption. Therefore, carbonyl iron should be taken with food and should not be used with antacids.

Iron should be used with caution in those with a history of gastritis, peptic ulcer disease or gastrointestinal bleeding.

ADVERSE REACTIONS

The most common side effects are gastrointestinal ones and include nausea, vomiting, bloating and other abdominal discomfort, black stools, diarrhea, constipation and anorexia.

Temporary staining of teeth occurs from iron-containing liquids.

INTERACTIONS

DRUGS

Acid Pump Inhibitors: (lansoprazole, omeprazole, pantoprazole, rabeprazole): Use of acid pump inhibitors may suppress the absorption of carbonyl iron.

Antacids: Aluminum-or magnesium-containing antacids may decrease the absorption of iron if used concomitantly.

Bisphosphonates (alendronate, etidronate, risedronate): Concomitant use of a bisphosphonate and a ferrous (II) iron supplement may decrease the absorption of the bisphosphonate.

H₂ Blockers (cimetidine, famotidine, nizatidine, ranitidine): Use of H₂ blockers may suppress the absorption of carbonyl iron.

Levodopa: Concomitant intake of levodopa and iron may reduce absorption of levodopa.

Levothyroxine: Concomitant intake of levothyroxine and iron may decrease the absorption of levothyroxine.

Penicillamine: Concomitant intake of iron and penicillamine may decrease the absorption of penicillamine.

Quinolones (ciprofloxacin, gatifloxacin, levofloxacin, lomefloxacin, moxifloxacin, norfloxacin, ofloxacin, sparfloxacin, trovafloxacin): Concomitant use of a quinolone and iron may decrease the absorption of the quinolone and iron.

Tetracyclines (doxycycline, minocycline, tetracycline): Concomitant intake of a tetracycline and iron may decrease the absorption of both the tetracycline and iron.

NUTRITIONAL SUPPLEMENTS

Beta-carotene: Beta-carotene may enhance the absorption of iron if they are taken concomitantly.

Calcium: Calcium carbonate may decrease absorption of iron if used concomitantly.

Copper: Intake of iron supplements may decrease the copper status of tissues.

Inositol Hexaphosphate: Concomitant intake of inositol hexaphosphate and iron may depress the absorption of iron.

L-Cysteine: Concomitant intake of L-cysteine and iron may increase the absorption of iron.

Magnesium: Concomitant intake of magnesium and iron may decrease the absorption of iron.

N-Acetyl-L-Cysteine: Concomitant intake of N-acetyl-L-cysteine and iron may increase the absorption of iron.

Tocotrienols: Concomitant intake of tocotrienols—which are typically used in their nonesterified forms—and iron may cause oxidation of the tocotrienols.

Vanadium: Concomitant intake of vanadium and iron may decrease the absorption of iron.

Vitamin C: Concomitant intake of vitamin C and iron may enhance the absorption of iron.

Vitamin E (alpha-tocopherol, gamma-tocopherol, mixed tocopherols): Concomitant intake of non-esterified tocopherols and iron may cause oxidation of the tocopherols.

Zinc: Concomitant intake of zinc and iron may decrease the absorption of iron.

FOODS

Cysteine-containing Proteins: Foods rich in cysteine-containing proteins (e.g. animal muscle tissue) may increase the absorption of iron if ingested concomitantly.

Oxalic Acid: Concomitant intake of iron with foods rich in oxalic acid (spinach, sweet potatoes, rhubarb and beans) may decrease the absorption of iron.

Phytic Acid: Concomitant intake of iron with foods rich in phytic acid (unleavened bread, raw beans, seeds, nuts and grains and soy isolates) may decrease the absorption of iron.

Teas: Concomitant intake of tea and iron may cause decreased absorption of iron. This is attributed to the tannins in tea.

LABORATORY TESTS

Guaic assay: Earlier studies reported a high false positive rate for guaic assay for occult blood in those receiving iron supplements. However, more recent data indicate that iron supplementation has no significant effect on guaic or other tests for occult blood.

OVERDOSAGE

Acute iron overdosage can be divided into four stages. In the first stage, which occurs up to six hours after ingestion, the principal symptoms are vomiting and diarrhea. Other symptoms include hypotension, tachycardia and CNS depression ranging from lethargy to coma. The second phase may occur at 6-24 hours after ingestion and is characterized by a temporary remission. In the third phase, gastrointestinal symptoms recur accompanied by shock, metabolic acidosis, coma, hepatic necrosis and jaundice, hypoglycemia, renal failure and pulmonary edema. The fourth phase may occur several weeks after ingestion and is characterized by gastrointestinal obstruction and liver damage.

In a young child, 75 milligrams per kilogram is considered extremely dangerous. A dose of 30 milligrams per kilogram can lead to symptoms of toxicity. Estimates of a lethal dosage range from 180 milligrams per kilogram and upwards. A peak serum iron concentration of five micrograms or more per ml is associated with moderate to severe poisoning in many.

DOSAGE AND ADMINISTRATION

There are several forms used for iron supplementation. They include ferrous sulphate, ferrous fumarate, ferrous gluconate, ferrous ascorbate and carbonyl iron.

The approximate amount of the above forms required to supply 60 milligrams of elemental iron are:

ferrous ascorbate	437 mg
ferrous fumarate	183 mg
ferrous gluconate	518 mg
ferrous sulphate	186 mg
carbonyl iron	300 mg

Iron replacement therapy for adults is 2-3 mg/kg daily in three divided doses. This must be done under a physician's supervision.

Iron is present in some combination supplements at doses of 10 to 18 milligrams daily.

The Food and Nutrition Board of the National Academy of Sciences has recommended the following daily dietary intakes for iron:

Age (years) or status	RDA milligrams/day
0.0 to 0.5	6
0.5 to 1.0	10
1 to 3	10
4 to 6	10
7 to 10	10
Males	
11 to 14	12
15 to 18	12
19 to 24	10
25 to 50	10
51 and over	10
Females	
11 to 14	15
15 to 18	15
19 to 24	15
25 to 50	15
51 and over	10
Pregnant	30
Lactating	15

HOW SUPPLIED

Ferrous fumarate is available in the following forms and strengths:

Chewable Tablets — 100 mg

Suspension — 100 mg/5 mL

Tablets — 200 mg, 300 mg, 325 mg, 350 mg

Ferrous gluconate is available in the following forms and strengths

Enteric Coated Tablets — 325 mg

Tablets — 300 mg, 320 mg, 324 mg, 325 mg

Ferrous sulfate is available in the following forms and strengths:

Capsules, Extended Release — 250 mg

Enteric Coated Tablets — 324 mg, 325 mg

Elixir — 220 mg/5 mL

Liquid — 75 mg/0.6 mL

Tablets — 195 mg, 300 mg, 324 mg, 325 mg

Exsiccated ferrous sulfate is available in the following forms and strengths:

Capsules — 150 mg, 159 mg

Enteric Coated Tablets — 200 mg

Tablets — 200 mg

Tablet, Extended Release — 160 mg

LITERATURE

Adish AA, Esrey SA, Gyorkos TW, et al. Effect of consumption of food cooked in iron pots on iron status and growth of young children: a randomised trial. *Lancet*. 1999; 353:712-716.

Anderson GJ. Control of iron absorption. *J Gastroenterol Hepatol*. 1996; 11:1030-1032.

Andrews NC. Disorders of iron metabolism. *N Eng J Med.* 1999; 341:1986-1995.

Andrews NC, Fleming MD, Gunshin H. Iron transport across biological membranes. *Nutr Rev.* 1999; 57:114-123.

Baer D. Hereditary iron overload and African Americans (editorial). *Am J Med.* 1996; 101:5-8.

Beard JL. Iron requirements in adolescent females. *J Nutr.* 2000; 130(2S Suppl):440S-442S.

Beguin Y, Huebers HA, Josephson B, Finch CA. Transferrin receptors in rat plasma. *Proc Natl Acad Sci USA.* 1988; 85:637-640.

Bellamy MC, Gedney JA. Unrecognized iron deficiency in critical illness. *Lancet.* 1998; 352:1903.

Beutler E, Larsh SE, Gurney CW. Iron therapy in chronically fatigued nonanemic women: a double-blind study. *Ann Intern Med.* 1960; 52:378-394.

Bruner AB, Joffe A, Duggan A, et al. Randomised study of cognitive effects of iron supplementation in non-anaemic iron-deficient adolescent girls. *Lancet.* 1996; 348:992-997.

Dallman PR. Iron deficiency and the immune response. *Am J Clin Nutr.* 1987; 46:329-334.

de Valk B, Marx JJM. Iron, atherosclerosis, and ischemic heart disease. *Arch Int Med.* 1999; 159:1542-1548.

Fairbanks VF. Iron in medicine and nutrition. In: Shils ME, Olson JA, Shike M, Ross AC, eds. *Modern Nutrition in Health and Disease.* Baltimore, MD: Williams and Wilkins; 1999:193-221.

Feder JN, Gnirke A, Thomas W, et al. A novel MHC class I like gene is mutated in patients with hereditary hemochromatosis. *Nat Genet.* 1996; 13:399-408.

Finch CA, Huebers H. Perspectives in iron metabolism. *N Engl J Med.* 1982; 306:1520-1528.

Garcia-Casal MN, Leets I, Layrisse M. Beta-carotene and inhibitors of iron absorption modify iron uptake by Caco-2 cells. *J Nutr.* 2000; 130:5-9.

Harris ED. The iron-copper connection: the link to ceruloplasmin grows stronger. *Nutr Rev.* 1995; 53:170-173.

Huebers HA, Beguin Y, Pootrakul P, et al. Intact transferrin receptors in human plasma and their relation to erythropoiesis. *Blood.* 1990; 75:102-107.

Kurz KM, Galloway R. Improving adolescent iron status before childbearing. *J Nutr.* 2000; 130:(2S Suppl):437S-439S.

Lehto P, Kivisto KT, Neuvonen PJ. The effect of ferrous sulfate on the absorption of norfloxacin, ciprofloxacin and ofloxacin. *B J Clin Pharmacol.* 1994; 37:82-85.

Mendler MH, Turlin B, Moirand R, et al. Insulin resistance-associated hepatic iron overload. *Gastroenterology.* 1999; 117:1155-1163.

Moirand R, Mortaji AM, Loréal O, et al. A new syndrome of liver iron overload with normal transferrin saturation. *Lancet.* 1997; 349:95-97.

Morse AC, Beard JL, Jones BC. A genetic development model of iron deficiency: biological aspects. *Proc Soc Exp Biol Med.* 1999; 220:147-152.

Neuvonen PJ, Turakka H. Inhibitory effect of various iron salts on the absorption of tetracycline in man. *Eur J Clin Pharmacol.* 1974; 7:357-360.

Oski FA. Iron deficiency in infancy and childhood. *N Engl J Med.* 1993; 329:190-193.

Pigeon C, Turlin B, Iancu TC, et al. Carbonyl-iron supplementation induces hepatocyte nuclear changes in BALB/CJ male mice. *J Hepatol.* 1999; 30:926-934.

Salonen JT, Nyyssönen K, Korpela H, et al. High stored iron levels are associated with excess risk of myocardial infarction in Eastern Finnish men. *Circulation.* 1992; 86:803-811.

Scrimshaw NS, San Giovanni JP. Synergism of nutrition, infection, and immunity: an overview. *Am J Clin N.* 1997; 66:464S-477S.

Smith MA, Harris PLR, Sayre LM, Perry G. Iron accumulation in Alzheimer disease is a source of redox-generated free radicals. *Proc Acad Sci USA.* 1997; 94:9866-9868.

Wessling-Resnick M. Iron transport. *Annu Rev Nutr.* 2000; 20:120-151.

Wienk KJH, Marx JJM, Beynen AC. The concept of iron bioavailability and its assessment (review). *Eur J Nutr.* 1999; 38:51-75.

Wurapa RK, Gordeuk VR, Brittenham GM, et al. Primary iron overload in African Americans. *Am J Med.* 1996; 101:9-18.

Kombucha

DESCRIPTION

Kombucha, also known as the Manchurian or Kargasok mushroom, is not a mushroom but a symbiotic mixture of bacteria, including *Acetobacter xylinum*, *Acetobacter ketogenum* and *Pichia fermentans*, and various yeasts. The yeasts are usually of the genera *Saccharomyces*, *Brettanomyces* and *Zygosaccharomyces*. Kombucha is used as a tea and is prepared by incubating it in sugared black or green tea. The tea is mildly effervescent and has a cider-like acid taste.

Anecdotes abound regarding Kombucha's ability to treat a wide spectrum of disorders, including AIDS and baldness. A few years ago, a media stir was created when it was reported that a patient with far-advanced AIDS made a "miraculous" recovery after drinking Kombucha tea. What wasn't reported was that the patient had begun a new FDA-allowed experimental therapy at the same time.

Kombucha tea is prepared by the user, and it is possible for the home-brewed version to become contaminated with pathogenic bacteria or fungi.

ACTIONS AND PHARMACOLOGY

ACTIONS

Kombucha has putative "cure-all" activity.

MECHANISM OF ACTION

Kombucha tea may have some antibiotic activity.

PHARMACOKINETICS

There are no reports on the pharmacokinetics of kombucha, and it is unlikely that any pharmacokinetic studies have been performed.

INDICATIONS AND USAGE

Claims have been made that kombucha tea cures everything from AIDS to baldness, flatulence and cancer. There is no credible evidence that it is effective in preventing or treating any disorder, and its use has been associated with significant toxicity in some cases. Its use in immuno-compromised individuals is particularly inadvisable.

RESEARCH SUMMARY

There is no credible research that supports the use of kombucha for any purpose. Its use has been associated with occasional allergic reactions, jaundice, nausea, vomiting, and head and neck pain. The Iowa Department of Public Health recommended against its use when two cases of severe unexplained illness (one of which ended in death) were reported in two individuals who had been consuming kombucha tea daily for two months. Two cases of symptomatic lead poisoning were reported in individuals who drank kombucha tea brewed in a ceramic pot. It was hypothesized that the tea elucted lead from the glaze pigment of the pot.

CONTRAINDICATIONS, PRECAUTIONS, ADVERSE REACTIONS

CONTRAINDICATIONS

Kombucha is contraindicated in those who are hypersensitive to any component of the preparation.

PRECAUTIONS

Children, pregnant women, nursing mothers, the elderly and those with compromised immune systems should avoid the use of kombucha.

Kombucha may contain antibiotic substances and, theoretically, could cause antibiotic resistance.

Those who use kombucha should be extremely careful in its preparation in order to avoid contamination with pathogenic bacteria and or fungi. The tea should not be prepared or stored in ceramic or lead containers, as lead can leach into the tea.

ADVERSE REACTIONS

Those who drink more than 4 ounces daily of Kombucha tea frequently experience nausea, vomiting and headaches. There have been reports of allergic reactions, jaundice, and head and neck pain. There are reports of two women with unexplained metabolic acidosis following use of kombucha tea. One died. However, it was unclear whether the kombucha tea had any role in causing the metabolic acidosis. Another 115 people who made tea from the same batch of kombucha had no adverse reactions. There are a few reports of elevated serum liver tests and a report of lead poisoning from drinking kombucha tea prepared in a ceramic pot. A case of cutaneous anthrax associated with kombucha has been reported, possibly secondary to contamination of the tea during its preparation.

OVERDOSAGE

There are no reported cases of overdosage with kombucha.

DOSAGE AND ADMINISTRATION

There is no typical dosage and no recommended dosage.

HOW SUPPLIED

Capsules — 450 mg

Liquid

Tea

LITERATURE

Currier RW, Goddard J, Buehler K, et al. Unexplained severe illness possibly associated with consumption of Kombucha tea-Iowa, 1995. *MMWR Morb Mort Wkly Rep.* 1995; 44:892-893,899-900.

Hauser SP, [Dr. Sklenar's Kombucha mushroom infusion—a biological cancer therapy. Documentation No. 18.] [Article in German.] *Schweiz Rundsch Med Prax.* 1990; 79:243-246.

Mayser P, Fromme S, Leitzmann C, Grunder K. The yeast spectrum of the 'tea fungus Kombucha.' *Mycoses.* 1995; 38:289-295.

Phan TG, Estell J, Duggin G, et al. Lead poisoning from drinking Kombucha tea brewed in a ceramic pot. *Med J Aust.* 1998; 169:644-646.

Sadjadi J. Cutaneous anthrax associated with the Kombucha "mushroom" in Iran. *JAMA.* 1998; 280:1567-1568.

Srinivasan R, Smolinske S, Greenbaum D. Probable gastrointestinal toxicity of Kombucha tea: is this beverage healthy or harmful? *J Gen Int Med.* 1997; 12:643-644.

Lactoferrin

DESCRIPTION

Lactoferrin is a glycoprotein that belongs to the iron transporter or transferrin family. It was originally isolated from bovine milk, where it is found as a minor protein component of whey proteins (see Whey Proteins). Lactoferrin contains 703 amino acids and has a molecular weight of 80 kilodaltons. In addition to its presence in milk, it is also found in exocrine secretions of mammals and is released from neutrophil granules during inflammation.

Lactoferrin is considered a multifunctional or multi-tasking protein. It appears to play several biological roles. Owing to its iron-binding properties, lactoferrin is thought to play a role in iron uptake by the intestinal mucosa of the suckling neonate. That is, it appears to be the source of iron for breast-fed infants. It also appears to have antibacterial, antiviral, antifungal, anti-inflammatory, antioxidant and immunomodulatory activities.

Three isoforms of lactoferrin have been isolated: lactoferrin-alpha, lactoferrin-beta and lactoferrin-gamma. Lactoferrin-beta and lactoferrin-gamma have RNase activity, whereas lactoferrin-alpha does not. Receptors for lactoferrin are found in monocytes, lymphocytes, neutrophils, intestinal tissue and on certain bacteria. Lactoferrin is abbreviated LF and Lf. Bovine lactoferrin is abbreviated bLF.

Bovine lactoferrin, derived from whey proteins, is marketed as a nutritional supplement. Supplemental lactoferrin typically contains low amounts of iron.

ACTIONS AND PHARMACOLOGY

ACTIONS

Supplemental lactoferrin may have antimicrobial, immunomodulatory, antioxidant and anti-inflammatory actions.

MECHANISM OF ACTION

The possible antibacterial activity of supplemental lactoferrin might be accounted for, in part, by its ability to strongly bind iron. Iron is essential to support the growth of pathogenic bacteria. Lactoferrin may also inhibit the attachment of bacteria to the intestinal wall. A breakdown product of lactoferrin is the peptide lactoferricin. Lactoferricin, classified as a bioactive peptide, may also have antibacterial, as well as antiviral, activity. The possible antiviral activity of supplemental lactoferrin may be due to its inhibition of virus-cell fusion and viral entry into cells.

A few mechanisms are proposed for lactoferrin's possible immunomodulatory activity. Lactoferrin may promote the growth and differentiation of T lymphocytes. Lactoferrin appears to bind uniquely in the region of major histocompatability (MHC) proteins and the CD4 and CD8 determinants on T4 (helper) and T8 (suppressor) lymphocytes; it bears sequence homologies with the MHC Class II determinant. Lactoferrin also appears to play a role in the regulation of cytokines and lymphokines, such as tumor necrosis (TNF)-alpha and interleukin (IL)-6. Lactoferrin's possible antioxidant activity may also contribute to its possible immunomodulatory activity.

Lactoferrin's possible antioxidant activity can also be accounted for by its ability to strongly bind iron. Free iron is a major contributor to the generation of reactive oxygen species via the Fenton reaction.

Lactoferrin's possible anti-inflammatory action may be accounted for by its possible antioxidant and immunomodulatory activities.

PHARMACOKINETICS

Little is known of the pharmacokinetics of oral lactoferrin. Lactoferrin appears much more resistant to proteolytic action than most dietary proteins. Lactoferrin is digested in the intestine to the bioactive peptide lactoferricin. Most of the possible actions of oral lactoferrin may be confined to the gut. There is some preliminary evidence that lactoferrin and lactoferricin may be absorbed, in part, from the lumen of the small intestine into enterocytes and that these molecules enter other cells as well. However, this is unclear.

INDICATIONS AND USAGE

There is some preliminary evidence from *in vitro* and animal research that supplemental lactoferrin may have some immune-enhancing effects. There is no evidence that it is effective as a treatment or preventive in any form of cancer. Neither is there any credible evidence to support claims that it helps those with fatigue or allergy.

RESEARCH SUMMARY

A number of *in vitro* and animal studies have shown that lactoferrin has various bactericidal and fungicidal effects. It has exhibited significant activity against *Escherichia coli*, *Proteus mirabilis*, *Staphyloccocus aureus*, *Candida albicans* and other pathogens in these studies. *In vitro*, lactoferrin has similarly shown some significant activity against HIV, herpes simplex virus type 1, hepatitis C virus, cytomegalovirus and some other viruses.

Human studies, however, are almost entirely lacking. One small, recent study showed that oral lactoferrin reduced the duration and severity of bacterial infection in five neutropenic patients receiving chemotherapy for acute myelogenous leukemia, compared with nine matched controls. More research is needed.

CONTRAINDICATIONS, PRECAUTIONS, ADVERSE REACTIONS

CONTRAINDICATIONS

Supplemental lactoferrin is contraindicated in those with hypersensitivity to any component of a lactoferrin-containing product.

PRECAUTIONS

Pregnant women and nursing mothers should avoid using lactoferrin supplements.

INTERACTIONS

Some in vitro studies suggest that lactoferrin acts synergistically with antifungal agents.

DOSAGE AND ADMINISTRATION

Oral lactoferrin dosed at 40 mg daily has been used in a couple of clinical trials of the substance. Those who supplement with lactoferrin typically take 250 mg daily. Lactoferrin is also found in whey protein supplements.

LITERATURE

Adamik B, Zimecki M, Wlaszczyk A, et al. Lactoferrin effects on the *in vitro* immune response in critically ill patients. *Arch Immunol Ther Exp (Warcz)*. 1998; 46:169-176.

Baveye S, Elass E, Mazurier J, et al. Lactoferrin: a multifunctional glycoprotein involved in the modulation of the inflammatory process. *Clin Chem Lab Med*. 1999; 37:281-286.

Britigan BE, Serody JS, Cohen MS. The role of lactoferrin as an anti-inflammatory molecule. *Adv Exp Med Biol*. 1994; 357:143-156.

Ikeda M, Nozak A, Sugiyama K, et al. Characterization of antiviral activity of lactoferrin against hepatitis C virus infection in human cultured cells. *Virus Res*. 2000; 66:51-63.

Levay PF, Viljoen M. Lactoferrin: a general review. *Haemtologica*. 1995; 80:252-267.

Lonnerdal B, Iyer S. Lactoferrin: molecular structure and biological function. *Annu Rev Nutr*. 1995; 15:93-110.

Swart PJ, Kuipers EM, Smit C, et al. Lactoferrin. Antiviral activity of lactoferrin. *Adv Exp Med Biol*. 1998; 443:205-213.

Trumpler U, Straub PW, Rosenmund A. Antibacterial prophylaxis with lactoferrin in neutropenic patients. *Eur J Clin Microbiol Infect Dis*. 1989; 8:310-313.

Vorland LH. Lactoferrin: a multifunctional glycoprotein. *APMIS*. 1999; 107:971-981.

Vorland LH, Ulvatne H, Andersen J, et al. Antibacterial effects of lactoferricin B. *Scand J Infect Dis*. 1999; 31:179-184.

Zimecki M, Wlaszczyk A, Cheneau P, et al. Immunoregulatory effects of a nutritional preparation containing bovine lactoferrin taken orally by healthy individuals. *Arch Immunol Ther Exp (Warcz)*. 1998; 46:231-240.

Lactulose

TRADE NAMES

Duphalac (Solvay), Chronulac (Aventis), Constilac (Alra), Cephulac (Aventis), Generlac (Morton Grove), Constulose (Alpharma), Enulose (Alpharma), Cholac (Alra), Kristalose (Bertek).

DESCRIPTION

Lactulose is a semisynthetic disaccharide comprised of the sugars D-lactose and D-fructose. It is not found naturally. The sugars are joined by a beta glycosidic linkage making it resistant to hydrolysis by human digestive enzymes. There is no disaccharidase in the microvillus membrane of small intestine enterocytes that can hydrolyze lactulose; nor is the disaccharide absorbed from the small intestine. Lactulose is, however, fermented by a limited number of colonic bacteria. This can lead to changes in the colonic ecosystem in favor of

some bacteria, such as lactobacilli and bifidobacteria, which may confer some health benefits.

Lactulose is used in the treatment of constipation and hepatic encephalopathy. The efficacy of lactulose in these conditions is based on its fermentation in the colon by certain bacteria and the increase of the biomass of these bacteria in the colon. The products of fermentation are mainly organic acids, such as lactic acid and small-chain fatty acids, which, by exerting a local osmotic effect in the colon, result in increased fecal bulk and stimulation of peristalsis. The higher doses used for hepatic encephalopathy lower the colonic pH, and ammonia, in the form of ammonium ions, is used by the bacteria for amino acid and protein synthesis. This lowers the serum ammonia levels and improves mental function.

The stimulation of the growth of bacteria, such as bifido-bacteria, may have other health benefits, such as protection against cancer of the colon. Lactulose is referred to as a bifidogenic factor. Substances such as lactulose that promote the growth of beneficial bacteria in the colon are called prebiotics. Prebiotics are typically nondigestible oligosac-charides. In addition to its uses in treatment of hepatic encephalopathy and constipation, lactulose is used in Japan in functional foods and as a nutritional supplement. These uses of lactulose are being explored in the United States, as well.

Lactulose is a solid substance that is very soluble in water and has a sweet taste. It is sweeter than lactose but not as sweet as fructose. Lactulose is also known as 4-O-beta-D-galactopyranosyl-D-fructofuranose. Its molecular formula is $C_{12}H_{22}O_{11}$, and its molecular weight is 342.30 daltons. The structural formula is:

Lactulose

ACTIONS AND PHARMACOLOGY

ACTIONS

Therapeutically, lactulose has laxative and ammonia-detoxifying actions.

Supplemental lactulose may have antitumor, antimicrobial, hypolipidemic and hypoglycemic actions in some. It may also help improve mineral absorption and balance, and may have antiosteoporotic activity.

MECHANISM OF ACTION

The possible antitumor activity of lactulose might be accounted for, in part, by the possible antitumor action of butyrate. Butyrate, along with other short-chain fatty acids, is produced by bacterial fermentation of lactulose in the colon. Some studies suggest that butyrate may induce growth arrest and cell differentiation and may also upregulate apoptosis, three activities that could be significant for possible antitumor activity. Lactulose may also aid in increasing the concentrations of calcium and magnesium in the colon. High concentrations of these cations in the colon may help control the rate of cell turnover. High concentrations of calcium in the colon may also lead to the formation of insoluble bile or salts of fatty acids. This might reduce the potential damaging effects of bile or fatty acids on colonocytes.

Lactulose may promote the growth of favorable bacterial populations, such as bifidobacteria, in the colon. Bifidobacteria may inhibit the growth of pathogenic bacteria, such as *Clostridium perfringens* and diarrheogenic *Escherichia coli*.

Lactulose may aid in lowering serum triglycerides in some. The mechanism of this possible effect is unclear. Decreased hepatocyte *de novo* synthesis of triglycerides is one hypothetical possibility. Lactulose may also lower total cholesterol and LDL-cholesterol levels in some. Again, the mechanism of this possible effect is unclear. Propionate, a product of lactulose fermentation in the colon, may inhibit HMG-CoA reductase, the rate-limiting step in cholesterol synthesis.

The possible effects of lactulose on blood glucose may be explained in a few ways. Lactulose may delay gastric emptying and/or shorten small-intestinal tract transit time. This may be via the short-chain fatty acids produced from lactulose in the colon. Short-chain fatty acids may be involved in the so-called "ileocolonic brake," which refers to the inhibition of gastric emptying by nutrients reaching the ileo-colonic junction. Short-chain fatty acids may also stimulate contractions of the ileum and shorten ileal emptying. In addition, propionate may inhibit gluconeogenesis by its metabolic conversion to methylmalonyl-CoA and succinyl-CoA. These metabolites could inhibit pyruvate carboxylase. Propionate may also reduce plasma levels of free fatty acids. High levels of free fatty acids lower glucose utilization and induce insulin resistance. Finally, propionate may enhance glycolysis via depletion of citrate in hepatocytes. Citrate is an allosteric inhibitor of phosphofructokinase.

Lactulose may bind/sequester such minerals as calcium and magnesium in the small intestine. The short-chain fatty acids formed from the bacterial fermentation of lactulose may facilitate the colonic absorption of calcium and, possibly, also magnesium ions. This could be beneficial in preventing osteoporosis and osteopenia.

PHARMACOKINETICS

Following ingestion, lactulose reaches the colon with very little digestion or absorption taking place in the stomach or small intestine. Lactulose is fermented by bifidobacteria, lactobacilli and some other bacteria in the colon to produce the short-chain fatty acids acetate, propionate and butyrate; the gases hydrogen, hydrogen sulfide, carbon dioxide and methane; and lactate, pyruvate, succinate and formate. Acetate, propionate and butyrate that are not metabolized in colonocyes are absorbed from the colon and transported via the portal circulation to the liver. These short-chain fatty acids are extensively metabolized in hepatocytes. Acetate, propionate and butyrate that are not metabolized in hepatocytes are transported by the circulation to various tissues, where they undergo further metabolism. Butyrate is an important respiratory fuel for the colonocytes. Lactulose is completely metabolized in the colon, and no lactulose is excreted in the feces.

Those with ileostomies may have a microbial flora colonizing their ileums. In those cases, lactulose could be fermented by some of the bacteria in a fashion similar to their fermentation in the colon.

INDICATIONS AND USAGE

Lactulose is used to treat constipation and hepatic encephalopathy. Preliminary research suggests that it might protect against a number of intestinal pathogens, that it might be helpful in the treatment of some inflammatory bowel diseases and that it could help prevent colorectal cancers. There is additional preliminary evidence suggesting that it could be of benefit in osteoporosis, diabetes mellitus and renal failure.

RESEARCH SUMMARY

Lactulose has proved effective in the treatment of some with chronic constipation, helping to restore normal peristalsis and defecation rhythm, softening stools and diminishing pain and other symptoms of dyspeptic disorders.

Lactulose is used with good results in some with compensated liver disease; lactulose has been shown in various studies to increase protein tolerance and help prevent hepatic encephalopathy.

Lactulose has helped protect against *Salmonella* infection and has shown activity against a number of other intestinal pathogens. It has reduced the incidence of bacterial translocation from the gut to mesenteric lymph nodes in rats with obstructive jaundice. It has also prevented bacterial translocation in animal models of surgical trauma. Other experiments suggest that lactulose might be helpful in idiopathic, as well as infectious inflammatory bowel diseases.

Lactulose has suppressed experimentally induced colonic aberrant crypt foci in rats and has helped protect colonic mucosa against a known colon carcinogen.

There is some early but promising clinical work. In one controlled study, patients who had undergone endoscopic removal of colorectal polyps were given antioxidant vitamins or lactulose to see if these substances could reduce the recurrence rate of adenomatous polyps. Over the course of this five-year study, polyps recurred in 5.7% of those taking the vitamins (A, C and E) and in 14.7% of those taking lactulose, compared with a recurrence rate of 35.9% in untreated controls. There were 209 subjects in the study.

Lactulose has also been shown to significantly stimulate calcium absorption in postmenopausal women, though the research has not yet been done to see whether it slows the rate of bone loss in aging subjects. There is, in addition, preliminary research suggesting that lactulose might improve glucose tolerance and have other effects on carbohydrate metabolism that could be of benefit in those with diabetes mellitus.

Finally, there is the suggestion in other preliminary research that lactulose might be helpful in the treatment of chronic renal failure. Lactulose has been shown to promote fecal excretion of water, sodium, potassium, amonium, urea, creatine and hydronium ions.

CONTRAINDICATIONS, PRECAUTIONS, ADVERSE REACTIONS

CONTRAINDICATIONS

Some lactulose preparations contain galactose. Therefore, lactulose is contraindicated in those who require a low galactose diet. Lactulose is also contraindicated in those who are hypersensitive to any component of a lactulose-containing preparation.

PRECAUTIONS

In the United States, lactulose is a prescription drug. Its use requires medical supervision. Its use as a dietary supplement is considered experimental.

Those who develop gastrointestinal symptoms (flatus, bloating, diarrhea) with the use of dietary fiber should exercise caution in the use of lactulose.

Those with lactose intolerance should exercise caution in the use of lactulose.

One of the metabolites of lactulose is hydrogen gas. Hypothetically, this represents a potential hazard for those using lactulose who may be required to undergo electrocautery procedures during proctoscopy or colonoscopy. Accumulation of hydrogen gas in significant amounts in the presence of an electric spark may result in an explosion. Therefore, those undergoing these procedures should stop lactulose intake at least a week before the procedure.

Pregnant women and nursing mothers should avoid lactulose.

ADVERSE REACTIONS

Laxative doses are typically 20 to 40 grams daily. Doses up to 10 grams daily are usually well tolerated. Some may be more sensitive to the possible gastrointestinal side effects of lactulose. The adverse reactions are mainly gastrointestinal and include flatus and abdominal cramps. Doses of greater than 13 grams daily can cause diarrhea. Also, nausea and vomiting have been reported following the higher doses. Some find the taste of lactulose to be disagreeable.

INTERACTIONS

DRUGS

Concomitant use of nonabsorbable antacids with lactulose may inhibit the desired lactulose-induced drop in colonic pH which might affect laxative activity and activity in the treatment of hepatic encephalopathy.

NUTRITIONAL SUPPLEMENTS

The concomitant use of such probiotics as *Bifidobacterium longum* and lactulose may enhance the possible health benefits of lactulose.

Lactulose may enhance the colonic absorption of calcium and magnesium supplements if used concomitantly.

FOODS

Lactulose may enhance the colonic absorption of calcium and magnesium in foods.

OVERDOSAGE

There have been no reports of overdosage.

DOSAGE AND ADMINISTRATION

Lactulose is available in some functional foods and nutritional supplements in Japan. Its use in the U.S. for supplemental purposes is still experimental. Supplemental doses used in Japan are about 2 to 5 grams daily. Doses higher than 10 grams daily are likely to cause gastrointestinal side effects (flatus, abdominal cramping, diarrhea). Doses of 10 to 20 grams daily and up to 40 grams daily are used to treat constipation. Doses from 60 to 120 grams daily are used to treat hepatic encephalopathy. Pharmaceutical lactulose is available in solutions and in the form of a crystalline powder. Lactulose is a prescription drug in the U.S. for pharmaceutical uses.

HOW SUPPLIED

Powder — 10 g/packet
Solution — 10 g/15 ml
Syrup — 10 g/15 ml

LITERATURE

Bianchi G, Ronchi M, Marchesini G. Effects of lactulose on carbohydrate metabolism and diabetes mellitus. *Scand J Gastroenterol Suppl.* 1997; 222:62-64.

Challa A, Rao JR, Chawan CB, Shackelford L. *Bifidobacterium longum* and lactulose suppress azoxymethane-induced colonic aberrant crypt foci in rats. *Carcinogenesis.* 1997; 18:517-521.

Clausen MR, Mortensen PB. Lactulose, disaccharides and colonic flora. Clinical consequences. *Drugs.* 1997; 53:930-942.

Gardiner KR, Erwin PJ, Anderson NH, et al. Lactulose as an antiendotoxin in experimental colitis. *Br J Surg.* 1995; 82:469-472.

Horsmans Y, Solbreux PM, Daenens C, et al. Lactulose improves psychomotor testing in cirrhotic patients with subclinical encephalopathy. *Aliment Pharmacol Ther.* 1997; 11:165-170.

Huchzermeyer H, Schumann C. Lactulose — a multifaceted substance. *Z Gastroenterol.* 1997; 35:945-955.

Ozcelik MF, Eroglu C, Pekmezci S, et al. The role of lactulose in the prevention of bacterial translocation in surgical trauma. *Acta Chir Belg.* 1996; 96:44-48.

Physicians' Desk Reference. 54th ed. Montvale, NJ: Medical Economics Company; 2000.

Ponz de Leon M, Roncucci L. Chemoprevention of colorectal tumors: role of lactulose and of other agents. *Scan J Gastroenterol Suppl.* 1997; 222:72-75.

Rowland IR, Bearne CA, Fischer R, Pool-Zobel BL. The effect of lactulose on DNA damage induced by DMH in the colon of human flora-associated rats. *Nutr Cancer.* 1996; 26:37-47.

Salminen S, Salminen E. Lactulose, lactic acid bacteria, intestinal microecology and mucosal protection. *Scand J Gastroenterol Suppl.* 1997; 222:45-48.

Teuri U, Vapaatalo H, Korpela R. Fructooligosaccharides and lactulose cause more symptoms in lactose maldigesters and subjects with pseudohypolactasia than in control lactose digesters. *Am J Clin Nutr.* 1999; 69:973-979.

Van den Heuvel EG, Muijs T, Van Dokkum W, Schaafsma G. Lactulose stimulates calcium absorption in postmenopausal women. *J Bone Miner Res.* 1999; 14:1211-1216.

L-Alpha-Glycerylphosphorylcholine (Alpha-GPC)

DESCRIPTION

L-alpha-glycerylphosphorylcholine is a substance derived from soy lecithin. It is phosphatidylcholine without the two fatty acid chains contained within the phosphatidylcholine structure. Although it is popularly referred to as a phospholipid, it is not. It is a phospholipid-derived substance.

Alpha-GPC has the following structural formula:

L-alpha-glycerylphosphorylcholine

L-alpha-glycerylphosphorylcholine is either abbreviated as alpha-GPC or GPC. It is also known as choline alfoscerate; choline-glycerophosphate, and choline-hydroxide, (R)-2,3-dihydroxypropyl hydrogen phosphate, inner salt. Alpha-GPC is believed to be a delivery form of choline (see Choline).

ACTIONS AND PHARMACOLOGY

ACTIONS

Alpha-GPC is a putative cognition enhancer and a putative growth hormone secretagogue.

MECHANISM OF ACTION

The actions of supplemental alpha-GPC are speculative and, therefore, any proposed mechanism of action is likewise speculative. Alpha-GPC is a delivery form of choline, and choline can be metabolized to acetylcholine. Some with Alzheimer's disease may suffer from a cholinergic defect, and, theoretically, a delivery form of choline may positively affect some with cognition disorders in which there exists a cholinergic deficit. In a similar speculative vein, it is known that cholinergic potentiation may modulate the growth hormone (GH) response to the hypothalamic hormone GHRH or growth hormone releasing hormone. Again, if alpha-GPC is a significant precursor of acetylcholine, it may have a GH secretagogue effect.

PHARMACOKINETICS

Some pharmacokinetic data are available from animal studies. Human pharmacokinetic data are lacking. It is unclear as to how much of an ingested dose of alpha-GPC gets into the brain or, for that matter, how much choline from a dose of ingested alpha-GPC gets to the brain.

INDICATIONS AND USAGE

It has been claimed that alpha-GPC is indicated for situations in which increased human growth hormone secretion is desirable and for the treatment of cognitive disorders. Evidence is insufficient to warrant support for either of these claimed indications at this time.

RESEARCH SUMMARY

The claim has been made that this putative acetylcholine precursor encourages the body to secrete increased levels of human growth hormone. There is some preliminary evidence that this is so, but whether this has any therapeutic significance remains to be seen. Safety data are also lacking. Claims that alpha-GPC is helpful in the treatment of cognitive disorders in the elderly are based upon scant and preliminary findings which, nonetheless, may warrant further investigation.

CONTRAINDICATIONS, PRECAUTIONS, ADVERSE REACTIONS

CONTRAINDICATIONS

Alpha-GPC is contraindicated in those who are hypersensitive to any component of the preparation.

PRECAUTIONS

Because of lack of long-term safety data, children, pregnant women and nursing mothers should avoid use of alpha-GPC.

ADVERSE REACTIONS

To date, no adverse reactions have been reported.

INTERACTIONS

There are no known drug, nutritional supplement, food or herb interactions.

OVERDOSAGE

There are no reports of overdosing.

DOSAGE AND ADMINISTRATION

Those who use alpha-GPC take 500 milligrams to 1 gram daily. About 40% of alpha-GPC is choline.

LITERATURE

Amenta F, Del Valle M, Vega JA, Zaccheo D. Age-related structural changes in the rat cerebellar cortex: effect of choline alfoscerate treatment. *Mech Ageing Dev.* 1991; 61: 173-186.

Amenta F, Ferrante F, Vega JA, Zaccheo D. Long term choline alfoscerate treatment counters age-dependent microanatomical changes in rat brain. *Prog Neuropsychopharmacol Biol Psychiatry.* 1994; 18:915-924.

Ceda GP. Ceresini. G. Denti L, et al. Alpha-glycerylphosphorylcholine administration increases the GH responses to GHRH of young and elderly subjects. *Horm Metab Res.* 1992; 24:119-121.

Ricci A, Bronzetti E, Vega JA, Amenta F. Oral choline alfoscerate counteracts age-dependent loss of mossy fibres in the rat hippocampus. *Mech Ageing Dev.* 1992; 66: 81-91.

Larch Arabinogalactan

DESCRIPTION

Larch arabinogalactan refers to a polysaccharide derived from wood of the Western larch or *Larix occidentalis.*

Arabinogalactans occur in other types of larch, but that which is marketed for supplemental usage comes from the Western larch. Larch arabinogalactan is not one substance but a mixture of several different arabinogalactans with molecular weights as low as 3,000 daltons and as high as 100,000 daltons.

Arabinogalactans are water-soluble polysaccharides widely found in plants, fungi and bacteria. They are comprised of D-galactose and L-arabinose residues in the form of a beta-D-(1-3)-galactan main chain with side chains made up of galactose and arabinose units of various lengths. Galactan itself is a polymer of galactose.

In plants, arabinogalactans occur as arabinogalactan proteins. These proteins are proteoglycans involved in plant growth and development; they may also be involved in signal transduction in plants.

Dietary intake of arabinogalactans comes from carrots, radishes, tomatoes, pears and wheat, among other plant foods. Gum arabic, a commonly used food additive, is composed of highly branched arabinogalactan. Arabinogalactans are also found in such herbs as *Echinacea* spp. and such edible mushrooms as *Ganoderma lucidum.* Arabinogalactans are thought to contribute to the possible immune-enhancing activities of echinacea and ganoderma.

Larch arabinogalactan is considered a nondigestible soluble dietary fiber. It is also thought to stimulate the colonic growth of such bacteria as bifidobacteria and lactobacilli. These bacteria may confer certain health benefits. Substances that stimulate the growth of bifidobacteria are called bifidogenic factors. Substances that promote the colonic growth of beneficial bacteria are called prebiotics.

ACTIONS AND PHARMACOLOGY

ACTIONS

Larch arabinogalactan may have immune-enhancing activity.

MECHANISM OF ACTION

Larch arabinogalactan has shown some immune-enhancing activity in the laboratory, particularly with regard to the stimulation of human natural killer cell cytotoxicity.

The mechanism of the possible immune-enhancing activity is not known.

PHARMACOKINETICS

Little is reported on the pharmacokinetics of larch arabinogalactan in humans. It appears that there is little digestion of the polysaccharide in the stomach and small intestine. Like similar substances, it is most likely fermented in the colon to produce the short-chain fatty acids acetate, propionate and butyrate; the gases hydrogen, hydrogen sulfide, carbon dioxide and methane; and lactate, pyruvate and succinate. This requires corroboration by human studies.

INDICATIONS AND USAGE

Larch arabinogalactan exhibits immune-enhancing properties in animal and *in vitro* studies.

RESEARCH SUMMARY

Larch arabinogalactan has enhanced natural killer (NK) cell cytotoxicity and has also enhanced the function of some other immune-system components in experimental studies. It has inhibited the metastasis of tumor cells to the liver in the laboratory. Human trials are needed.

CONTRAINDICATIONS, PRECAUTIONS, ADVERSE REACTIONS

CONTRAINDICATIONS

Larch arabinogalactan is contraindicated in those hypersensitive to any component of a larch arabinogalactan-containing preparation.

PRECAUTIONS

Since larch arabinogalactan contains galactose and since the pharmacokinetics of the polysaccharide in humans has not been clarified, those who require a low galactose diet should avoid the substance.

Pregnant women and nursing mothers should avoid larch arabinogalactan supplements, pending long-term safety studies.

Those with lactose intolerance should exercise caution in the use of supplemental larch arabinogalactan.

ADVERSE REACTIONS

Doses of up to 10 grams daily appear to be well tolerated. There are no reports of adverse reactions. However, as with similar products, it would be expected that at higher doses (e.g., greater than 30 grams daily) gastrointestinal side effects, such as flatus, abdominal cramps and diarrhea, would be likely to occur in some.

INTERACTIONS

No known interactions with drugs, nutritional supplements, foods or herbs.

OVERDOSAGE

There are no reports of overdosage.

DOSAGE AND ADMINISTRATION

Larch arabinogalactan is available in capsules, powder and combination products marketed as nutritional supplements. Dosage is variable and ranges from 1 to 3 grams daily and sometimes higher.

LITERATURE

Hauer J, Anderer FA. Mechanism of stimulation of human natural killer cytotoxicity by arabinogalactan from *Larix occidentalis. Cancer Immunol Immunother.* 1993; 36:237-244.

He Y,Li.R, Chen Q, et al. [Chemical studies of immunologically active polysaccharides of Ganoderma lucidum (Leyss.ex Fr.) Karst.] [Article in Chinese.] *Chung Kuo Chung Yao Tsa Chih.* 1992; 17:226-228,256.

Kelly GS. Larch arabinogalactan: clinical relevance of a novel immune—enhancing polysaccharide. *Altern Med Rev.* 1999; 4:96-103.

Odonmazig P, Ebringerova A, Machova E, Alfodi J. Structural and molecular properties of the arabinogalactan isolated from Mongolian larchwood (*Larix dahurica* L). *Carbohydr Res.* 1994; 252:317-324.

Ponder GR, Richards GN. Arabinogalactan from Western larch. Part III: alkaline degredation revisited, with novel conclusions on molecular structure. *Carbohydrate Polymers.* 1997; 34:251-261.

L-Arginine

TRADE NAMES

R-Gene 10 (Pharmacia Corp.)

DESCRIPTION

L-arginine is a protein amino acid present in the proteins of all life forms. It is classified as a semi-essential or conditionally essential amino acid. This means that under normal circumstances the body can synthesize sufficient L-arginine to meet physiological demands. There are, however, conditions where the body cannot. L-arginine is essential for young children and for those with certain rare genetic disorders in which synthesis of the amino acid is impaired. Some stress conditions that put an increased demand on the body for the synthesis of L-arginine include trauma (including surgical trauma), sepsis and burns. Under these conditions, L-arginine becomes essential, and it is then very important to ensure adequate dietary intake of the amino acid to meet the increased physiological demands created by these situations.

L-arginine, even when it is not an essential amino acid as defined above, is a vital one. In addition to participating in protein synthesis, it plays a number of other roles in the body. These include the detoxification of ammonia formed during the nitrogen catabolism of amino acids via the formation of urea. In addition, L-arginine is a precursor in the formation of nitric oxide, creatine, polyamines, L-glutamate, L-proline, agmatin (a possible neurotransmitter in the brain) and the arginine-containing tetrapeptide tuftsin, believed to be an immunomodulator. L-arginine is a glycogenic amino acid; it can be converted to D-glucose and glycogen if needed by the body or it can be catabolized to produce biological energy.

L-arginine, when administered in high doses, stimulates pituitary release of growth hormone and prolactin and pancreatic release of glucagon and insulin. Intravenous L-arginine may be used as an aid in the evaluation of problems with growth and stature that may be due to growth hormone deficiency. Intravenous arginine hydrochloride may be used as a fourth-line agent in the treatment of severe metabolic alkalosis. L-arginine is also used as an immunonutrient in enteral and parenteral nutrition to help improve the immune status in those suffering from sepsis, burns and trauma.

L-arginine is predominately synthesized in the kidney. It is a key intermediate in the Krebs-Henseleit urea cycle. L-ornithine and L-citrulline are precursors in the synthesis of L-arginine, and L-arginine is converted to urea and L-ornithine via the enzyme arginase. The portion of L-arginine that is not converted to urea enters the circulation, and is distributed to the various tissues and metabolized as discussed above. A much smaller amount of L-arginine is produced in the liver.

The typical dietary intake of L-arginine is 3.5 to 5 grams daily. Most dietary L-arginine comes from plant and animal proteins. Small amounts of free L-arginine are found in vegetable juices and fermented foods, such as miso and yogurt. Soy protein and other plant proteins are richer in L-arginine than are animal proteins, which are richer in lysine. It is thought that the possible hypocholesterolemic effect of soy protein is due, at least in part, to the higher L-arginine content in this protein.

L-arginine is a basic amino acid with the molecular formula $C_6H_{14}N_4O_2$ and with a molecular weight of 174.20 daltons. It has 3 pKs: $pK_1=2.18$, $pK_2=9.09$ and $pK_3=13.2$. Therefore, it carries a positive charge at physiological pH. The stereoisomer of L-arginine, D-arginine, does not have any biological activity, as far as we know. L-arginine is also known as 2-amino-5-guanidinovaleric acid and (S)-2-amino-5-[(aminoiminomethyl)amino] pentaenoic acid. Its one-letter abbreviation is R. It is also abbreviated as Arg. The terms L-arginine and arginine are frequently used interchangeably. The structural formula of L-arginine is as follows:

L-arginine

ACTIONS AND PHARMACOLOGY
ACTIONS
Supplemental L-arginine may have anti-atherogenic, antioxidant and immunomodulatory actions. It may also have wound-repair activity.

MECHANISM OF ACTION
Many of supplemental L-arginine's activities, including its possible anti-atherogenic actions, may be accounted for by its role as the precursor to nitric oxide or NO. NO is produced by all tissues of the body and plays very important roles in the cardiovascular system, immune system and nervous system. NO is formed from L-arginine via the enzyme nitric oxide synthase or synthetase (NOS), and the effects of NO are mainly mediated by 3,'5' -cyclic guanylate or cyclic GMP. NO activates the enzyme guanylate cyclase, which catalyzes the synthesis of cyclic GMP from guanosine triphosphate or GTP. Cyclic GMP is converted to guanylic acid via the enzyme cyclic GMP phosphodiesterase.

NOS is a heme-containing enzyme with some sequences similar to cytochrome P-450 reductase. Several isoforms of NOS exist, two of which are constitutive and one of which is inducible by immunological stimuli. The constitutive NOS found in the vascular endothelium is designated eNOS and that present in the brain, spinal cord and peripheral nervous system is designated nNOS. The form of NOS induced by immunological or inflammatory stimuli is known as iNOS. iNOS may be expressed constitutively in select tissues such as lung epithelium.

All the nitric oxide synthases use NADPH (reduced nicotinamide adenine dinucleotide phosphate) and oxygen (O_2) as cosubstrates, as well as the cofactors FAD (flavin adenine dinucleotide), FMN (flavin mononucleotide), tetrahydrobiopterin and heme. Interestingly, ascorbic acid appears to enhance NOS activity by increasing intracellular tetrahydrobiopterin. eNOS and nNOS synthesize NO in response to an increased concentration of calcium ions or in some cases in response to calcium-independent stimuli, such as shear stress.

In vitro studies of NOS indicate that the Km of the enzyme for L-arginine is in the micromolar range. The concentration of L-arginine in endothelial cells, as well as in other cells, and in plasma is in the millimolar range. What this means is that, under physiological conditions, NOS is saturated with its L-arginine substrate. In other words, L-arginine would not be expected to be rate-limiting for the enzyme, and it would not appear that supraphysiological levels of L-arginine—which could occur with oral supplementation of the amino acid—would make any difference with regard to NO production. The reaction would appear to have reached its maximum level. However, *in vivo* studies have demonstrated that, under certain conditions, e.g. hypercholesterolemia, supplemental L-arginine could enhance endothelial-dependent vasodilation and NO production.

The discordance between the *in vivo* results—increased NO production under certain conditions—and the *in vitro* enzyme studies described above is known as the "arginine paradox." There are a few explanations for the "arginine paradox." NOS may be inhibited by asymmetric dimethylarginine or ADMA, which is known to be elevated in hypercholesterolemia and which increases mononuclear cell (monocyte and T-lymphocyte) adhesiveness in hypercholesterolemics. ADMA is formed by post-translational methylation of L-arginine residues in proteins and is released from the proteins following their hydrolysis. The "arginine paradox" may be explained in part by increasing levels of L-arginine overcoming the inhibition of NOS by ADMA. In addition to hypercholesterolemia, elevated levels of ADMA are associated with hypertension, diabetes, preeclampsia, smoking and aging. Elevation of ADMA may be due to altered metabolism of this substance by dimethylarginine dimethylaminohydrolase or DDAH. DDAH is the major enzyme involved in ADMA catabolism. Decreased levels of DDAH have been found in diabetic and hypercholesterolemic animal models.

Other explanations of the "arginine paradox" include the presence of other inhibitors of NOS yet to be discovered, impaired transport of L-arginine into or within endothelial cells and impaired regeneration of L-arginine from L-citrulline. There is another interesting possibility. A non-enzymatic pathway by which NO may be produced has recently been described. Endothelial dysfunction is associated with increased oxidative stress resulting in increased formation of such reactive oxygen species as hydrogen peroxide and superoxide anions. Further, during conditions of oxidative stress, enzymatic synthesis of NO may decrease, and NO reacts with superoxide anions to form the reactive nitrogen species peroxynitrite. Under these conditions, L-arginine can essentially scavenge hydrogen peroxide and superoxide to form NO non-enzymatically. Interestingly, in this non-enzymatic reaction, L-arginine, as well as the non-biological D-arginine, can both form NO.

NO formed from supplemental L-arginine can play a major role in the possible anti-atherogenic activity of L-arginine. NO inhibits mononuclear cell adhesion, platelet aggregation, proliferation of vascular smooth muscle, production of some reactive oxygen species, such as superoxide anions, and promotion of endothelium-dependent dilation. Leukocyte adhesion, platelet aggregation, smooth muscle proliferation, endothelial dysfunction and oxidative stress are all part of the process of atherogenesis. L-arginine may also have anti-atherogenic activity independent of its role in the enzymatic formation of NO.

L-arginine may itself have antioxidant activity. L-arginine has been found to inhibit the oxidation of low-density lipoproteins (LDL) to oxidized LDL (oxLDL). The oxidation of LDL to oxLDL is believed to be a pivotal early step in atherogenesis. L-arginine may also scavenge superoxide anions and hydrogen peroxide (see above), as well as inhibit lipid peroxidation.

L-arginine has been shown to have immunomodulatory activity. For example, in human breast cancer, supplementation with this amino acid has been reported to increase the quantity and cytotoxic activity of natural killer (NK) cells and lymphokine-activated-killer (LAK) cells. L-arginine is considered an immunonutrient and is added to enteral and parenteral feedings for burn, sepsis and trauma patients. The mechanism of L-arginine's possible immunomodulating activity is not entirely clear. It may, at least in part, be again due to L-arginine's role in the production of NO. Production of NO, with consequent decrease of the cyclic AMP/cyclic GMP ratio in NK cells, would favor the production of interleukin-1, which is known to activate NK cells and may directly enhance NK cell cytotoxicity. L-arginine is also a precursor in the synthesis of the tetrapeptide tuftsin, which itself appears to have immunomodulatory activity. Tuftsin's activity appears to depend on two of the four amino acids present in its structure, L-arginine and L-proline. L-arginine also participates in the synthesis of L-proline.

L-arginine's possible activity in wound repair may be due to its precursor role in the formation of L-ornithine and, ultimately, L-proline. L-proline is a key element in collagen biosynthesis.

PHARMACOKINETICS

Following ingestion, L-arginine is absorbed from the lumen of the small intestine into the enterocytes. Absorption is efficient and occurs by an active transport mechanism. Some metabolism of L-arginine takes place in the enterocytes. L-arginine not metabolized in the enterocytes enters the portal circulation from whence it is transported to the liver, where again some portion of the amino acid is metabolized. L-arginine not metabolized in the liver enters the systemic circulation, where it is distributed to the various tissues of the body. L-arginine participates in various metabolic activities, including the production of proteins, D-glucose, glycogen, L-ornithine, urea, nitric oxide, L-glutamate, creatine, polyamines, L-proline, agmatin and tuftsin. L-arginine is eliminated by glomerular filtration and is almost completely reabsorbed by the renal tubules. L-arginine produces peak plasma levels approximately one to two hours after oral administration.

INDICATIONS AND USAGE

L-arginine shows promise in the treatment and prevention of cardiovascular disease (including atherosclerosis, hypertension, hyperlipidemia and angina pectoris), in the treatment of some forms of male infertility and some kidney disorders and it is helpful in accelerating wound healing in some circumstances. It has demonstrated some positive immune-modulating and anticancer effects. There is preliminary evidence that it could be helpful in some men with erectile dysfunction and in some others with migraine, liver disease and primary ciliary dyskinesia. There is conflicting but mostly negative evidence related to claims that it can improve exercise performance and promote lean muscle mass.

RESEARCH SUMMARY

Numerous *in vitro* experiments have shown that L-arginine has effects on endothelial cells that could be expected to inhibit cardiovascular disease. Inferences have been drawn from these studies suggesting that L-arginine, through its nitric oxide activity, especially in the endothelial cells of the blood vessels, inhibits vasoconstriction, thrombolytic activity, cell proliferation, inflammation and other activities that promote cardiovascular disease.

Some of the promise of these *in vitro* studies has been realized in animal and clinical studies. In hypercholesterolemic animal models, L-arginine helps normalize lipids and vasodilatory response, inhibits platelet aggregation and formation of intimal lesions. Further, it has been seen in some of these animal studies to cause pre-existing lesions to regress.

Similarly, L-arginine has had significant positive effects in hypercholesterolemic and hypertensive humans. It has also been helpful in those with angina pectoris. In a recent long-term study, supplemental L-arginine, given for six months, resulted in significant improvement in coronary small-vessel endothelial function associated with a decrease in plasma endothelin concentrations.

In a double-blind, placebo-controlled study of 22 subjects with stable angina, supplemental L-arginine (1 gram twice daily) significantly improved exercise capacity. L-arginine supplementation resulted in a 70% reduction in angina attacks in another study.

In other studies, L-arginine was credited with significantly reducing lipid peroxidation in patients with diabetes mellitus. Conflicting results were produced by two studies related to L-arginine's effects on vasomotor response in smokers. In one of these studies, L-arginine significantly reversed abnormal myocardial blood flow response to a cold pressor test; in the other small study, no significant positive effect was seen.

The treatment of oligospermia with L-arginine was first reported many years ago. In one of these early studies, 178 men with oligospermia were given 4 grams of L-arginine daily. Severe oligospermia was diagnosed in 93 of these subjects. Treatment ceased in subjects who showed no

improvement after two months. A 100% increase in sperm count was achieved in 42 cases, resulting in 15 pregnancies. There was marked increase in sperm number and motility in an additional 69 patients, resulting in another 13 pregnancies.

Subsequent studies have shown that L-arginine improves sperm count and motility. A recent small study credited L-arginine with producing pregnancies, but larger clinical trials are needed to confirm the efficacy seen in the early work.

L-arginine is of benefit in some kidney diseases and shows some promise in interstitial cystitis. It helps improve kidney function in some diabetic animal models and prevents chronic renal failure in others. A recent study indicated that L-arginine facilitates renal vasodilatation and natriuresis in renal transplant patients. There was also the suggestion in this study that L-arginine counteracts the antinatriuretic effect of cyclosporin.

Several studies have found that L-arginine benefits some with interstitial cystitis. Other studies, however, have not reported benefit. It appears that L-arginine can decrease pain and urgency in some subsets of interstial cystitis patients, but more research is needed to confirm this.

L-arginine has long been used following trauma and during sepsis. Studies have shown that L-arginine improves nitrogen balance and thus reduces protein catabolism. Animal studies have shown that L-arginine can be of significant benefit after severe burn injury, increasing survival, improving cardiac function and preventing bacterial translocation. Intravenous L-arginine has been helpful in some human traumas, helping to speed healing while inhibiting post-injury wasting and weight loss.

L-arginine shows many effects on immune function both *in vitro* and *in vivo*. In various animal studies, L-arginine has, reportedly, improved host immunity in a variety of conditions through its effects on the thymus and T-lymphocytes. It has also been reported to reduce the incidence of chemically induced tumors and to reduce the size of pre-existing tumors. It has significantly inhibited metastatic spread of some cancers in animal work.

In human work, oral L-arginine has increased the responsiveness of some immune components and has decreased the number and percent of T suppressor/cytotoxic cells (CD8) in healthy human volunteers. In a clinical trial involving patients undergoing abdominal surgery, intravenous L-arginine diminished postoperative reduction in the mitogenic responses of peripheral blood lymphocytes to ConA and PHA. Enhancement of these same responses was reported in a study in which L-arginine was given to HIV patients. L-arginine supplementation in this study, did not, however, alter T-lymphocyte subsets or ratios.

In a more recent study of L-arginine's effects in HIV-infected subjects, supplementation for six months (7.4 grams daily) failed to produce any improvement in immunological parameters measured, but body weight increased in L-arginine-supplemented subjects.

In healthy human volunteers, administering 30 grams of L-arginine daily for three days resulted in enhanced natural-killer (NK) and lymphokine-activated-killer (LAK) cell activity. A mean rise of 91% in NK cell activity and a mean rise of 58% in LAK cell activity were observed. The researchers concluded: ''The substantial enhancement of human NK and LAK cell activity by large doses of L-arginine could be useful in many immunosuppressed states, including malignant disease, AIDS and HIV infection, in which depressed NK cell activity is an important component of the disease process.''

Supplementation with L-arginine has significantly increased the quantity and cytotoxic activity of NK cells and lympho-kine-activated cells in patients with breast cancer in one study. Research is ongoing.

There is recent, preliminary evidence that oral L-arginine can help some men with erectile dysfunction. In a double-blind, placebo-controlled study, 50 men with this disorder were randomized to receive 5 grams of L-arginine daily or placebo for six weeks. Nine of 29 L-arginine-supplemented subjects and two of 17 controls reported significant subjective improvement in erectile function. All nine of the L-arginine responders had low urinary levels of stable metabolites of nitric oxide at baseline. These levels doubled by the end of the study. More research is needed.

In another recent study, L-arginine was found to be helpful in subjects suffering from primary ciliary dyskinesia, a genetic disorder characterized by impaired cilia motility and abnormally low levels of nasal nitric oxide. L-arginine, in combination with ibuprofen, also proved helpful in significantly reducing migraine pain intensity compared with placebo in another recent, preliminary, multi-center study of 40 migraine patients.

Research related to L-arginine's claimed hepatoprotective effects is dated. The data, however, looked promising and deserve follow-up.

Claims that L-arginine enhances exercise performance and promotes development of lean body mass while burning fat in healthy individuals are poorly supported. Weight gain was decreased in obese mice fed L-arginine, but there are no human data to support anti-obesity claims for L-arginine.

There are hypothetical reasons to believe that L-arginine, popular with some body builders, might have ergogenic/anabolic effects but, so far, these effects have not been demonstrated. High dose oral L-arginine has, however, been shown to induce release of growth hormone and prolactin but, again, no studies have been conducted to see whether this could have any meaningful ergogenic or anabolic effect.

CONTRAINDICATIONS, PRECAUTIONS, ADVERSE REACTIONS
CONTRAINDICATIONS
Supplemental L-arginine is contraindicated in those with the rare genetic disorder argininemia. It is also contraindicated in those hypersensitive to any component of an arginine-containing preparation.

PRECAUTIONS
Because of absence of long-term safety studies, and because of the possibility of growth hormone stimulation, pregnant women and nursing mothers should avoid L-arginine supplementation.

Those with renal or hepatic failure should exercise caution in the use of supplemental L-arginine.

Proteins of the herpes simplex virus are rich in L-arginine, and there are a few reports (mainly anecdotal) of those taking supplemental L-arginine who have had recurrences of oral herpes lesions. Although it is unlikely that those with a history of herpes simplex virus infection will have recurrences if they use L-arginine supplements, they should nevertheless be aware of this possibility.

ADVERSE REACTIONS
Oral supplementation with L-arginine at doses up to 15 grams daily are generally well tolerated. The most common adverse reactions of higher doses — from 15 to 30 grams daily — are nausea, abdominal cramps and diarrhea. Some may experience these symptoms at lower doses.

INTERACTIONS
DRUGS

Cyclosporine: L-arginine may counteract the antinaturetic effect of cyclosporin.

Ibuprofen: L-arginine may increase the absorption of ibuprofen if taken concomitantly.

Organic nitrates: L-arginine supplements theoretically may potentiate the effects of organic nitrates if taken concomitantly.

Sildenafil citrate: Theoretically, L-arginine supplements taken concomitantly with sildenafil citrate, may potentiate the effects of the drug.

HERBS

Yohimbe: L-Arginine, if used concomitantly, may enhance the effect of yohimbe.

DOSAGE AND ADMINISTRATION

L-arginine is available in tablet, capsule and powder form and as L-arginine hydrochloride and free base L-arginine. It is also available in medical foods as an aid in the enhancement of immune function.

Various doses are used. For cardiovascular health reasons, doses from 8 to 21 grams daily have been used in divided doses. To help aid with sperm quantity and quality, doses of 10 to 20 grams daily have been used in divided doses. Doses of 5 grams daily have been used for erectile dysfunction. Doses of 1.5 to 2.4 grams daily have been used for interstitial cystitis.

HOW SUPPLIED

Capsules — 500 mg, 700 mg

Injection — 10%

Powder

Tablets — 500 mg, 1000 mg

LITERATURE

Adams MR, McCredie R, Jessup W, et al. Oral L-arginine improves endothelium-dependent dilatation and reduces monocyte adhesion to endothelial cells in young men with coronary artery disease. *Atherosclerosis.* 1997; 129:261-269.

Andres A, Morales JM, Praga M, et al. L-arginine reverses the antinatriuretic effect of cyclosporin in renal transplant patients. *Nephrol Dial Transplant.* 1997; 12:1437-1440.

Barbul A. Arginine: biochemistry, physiology, and therapeutic implications. *JPEN.* 1986; 10:227-238.

Barbul A, Sisto DA, Wasserkrug HL, Efron G. Arginine stimulates lymphocyte immune response in healthy human beings. *Surgery.* 1981; 90:244-251.

Bode-Boger SM, Boger RH, Galland A, et al. L-arginine-induced vasodilation in healthy humans: pharmacokinetic-pharmacodynamic relationship. *Br J Clin Pharmacol.* 1998; 46:489-497.

Brandes RP, Brandes S, Boger RH, et al. L-Arginine supplementation in hypercholesterolemic rabbits normalizes leukocyte adhesion to non-endothelial matrix. *Life Sci.* 2000; 66:1519-1524.

Cartledge JJ, Davies A-M, Eardley I. A randomized double-blind placebo-controlled crossover trial of the efficacy of L-arginine in the treatment of interstitial cystitis. *BJU Int.* 2000; 85:421-426.

Chan JS, Boger RH, Bode-Boger SM. Et al. Asymmetric dimethylarginine increases mononuclear cell adhesiveness in hypercholesterolemic humans. *Arterioscler Thromb Vasc Biol.* 2000; 20:1040-1046.

Chen J, Wollman Y, Chernichovsky T, et al. Effect of oral administration of high-dose nitric oxide donor L-arginine in men with organic erectile dysfunction: results of a double-blind, randomized, placebo-controlled study. *BJU Int.* 1999; 83:269-273.

Clarkson P, Adams MR, Powe AJ, et al. Oral L-arginine improves endothelium-dependent dilation in hypercholesterolemic young adults. *J Clin Invest.* 1996; 97:1989-1994.

Cooke JP. Singer AH, Tsao P, et al. Antiatherogenic effects of L-arginine in the hypercholesterolemic rabbit. *J Clin Invest.* 1992; 90:1168-1172.

Griffith RS, DeLong DC, Nelson JD. Relation of arginine-lysine antagonism to herpes simplex growth in tissue culture. *Chemotherapy.* 1981; 27:209-213.

Hambrecht R, Hilbrich L, Erbs S, et al. Correction of endothelial dysfunction in chronic heart failure: additional effects of exercise training and oral L-arginine supplementation. *J Am Coll Cardiol.* 2000; 35:701-713.

Horton JW, White J, Maass D, Sanders B. Arginine in burn injury improves cardiac performance and prevents bacterial translocation. *J Appl Physiol.* 1998; 84:695-702.

Isidori A, Lo Monaco A, Cappa M. A study of growth hormone release in man after oral administration of amino acids. *Current Med Res Opinion.* 1981; 7:475-481.

Kapuler AM, Gurusiddiah S. The amino acids precursory to proteins are primary human food: proline, glutamine, and arginine found free in the juices of common vegetables and herbs. *J Med Food.* 1998; 1:97-115.

Korting GE, Smith SD, Wheeler MA, et al. A randomized double-blind trial of oral L-arginine for treatment of interstitial cystitis. *J Urol.* 1999; 161:558-565.

Lerman A, Burnett JC Jr, Higano ST, et al. Long-term L-arginine supplementation improves small-vessel coronary endothelial function in humans. *Circulation.* 1998; 97:2123-2128.

Loukides S, Kharitonov S, Wodehouse T, et al. Effect of arginine on mucocilliary function in primary ciliary dyskinesia. *Lancet.* 1998; 352:371-372.

Lubec B, Hayn M, Kitzmü ller E, et al. L-arginine reduces lipid peroxidation in patients with diabetes mellitus. *Free Rad Biol Med.* 1997; 22:355-357.

Mantha SV. Mediation of L-arginine-induced retardation of hypercholesterolemic atherosclerosis in rabbits by antioxidant mechanisms. *Nutr Res.* 1999; 10:1529-1539.

Nagase S, Takemura K, Ueda A, et al. A novel nonenzymatic pathway for the generation of nitric oxide by the reaction of hydrogen peroxide and D- or L-arginine. *Biochem Biophys Res Commun.* 1997; 233:150-153.

Narita I, Border WA, Ketteler M, et al. L-arginine may mediate the therapeutic effects of low protein diets. *Proc Natl Acad Sci USA.* 1995; 92:4552-4556.

Park KGM, Hayes PD, Garlick PJ et al. Stimulation of lymphocyte natural cytotoxicity by L-arginine. *Lancet.* 1991; 337:645-646.

Reis DJ, Regunathan S. Is agmatine a novel neurotransmitter in brain? *Trends Pharmacol Sci.* 2000; 21:187-193.

Sandrini G, Franchini S, Lanfranchi S, et al. Effectiveness of ibuprofen-arginine in the treatment of acute migraine headaches. *Int J Clin Pharmacol Res.* 1998; 18:145-150.

Schachter A, Goldman JA, Zuckerman Z. Treatment of oligospermia with the amino acid arginine. *J Urology.* 1973; 110:311-313.

Scibona M, Meschini P, Capparelli S, et al. [L-arginine and male infertility]. [Article in Italian]. *Minerva Urol Nefrol.* 1994; 46:251-253.

Tangphao O, Grossman M, Chalon S, et al. Pharmacokinetics of intravenous and oral L-arginine in normal volunteers. *Br J Clin Pharmacol.* 1999; 47:261-266.

Tentolouris C, Tousoulis D, Davies GJ, et al. Serum cholesterol level, cigarette smoking, and vasomotor responses to L-arginine in narrowed epicardial coronary arteries. *Amer J Cardiol.* 2000; 85:500-503.

Wascher TC, Posch K, Wallner S, et al. Vascular effects of L-arginine: anything beyond a substrate for the NO-synthase? *Biochem Biophys Res Commun.* 1997; 234:35-38.

L-Aspartate

TRADE NAMES

L-Aspartate is available as magnesium, potassium, calcium and zinc salts from numerous manufacturers. It is available in the base form as L-aspartic acid (Tyson).

DESCRIPTION

L-aspartate is a protein amino acid naturally found in all life forms. L-aspartate is a dicarboxylic amino acid. Although most L-aspartate is in proteins, small amounts of free L-aspartate are found in body fluids and in plants. The normal diet contains about 2 grams of L-aspartate daily. L-aspartate is also in the alternative dipeptide sweetener aspartame; the amount of L-aspartate from the sweetener is a small fraction of total L-aspartate consumed.

L-aspartate is considered a non-essential amino acid, meaning that, under normal physiological conditions, sufficient amounts of the amino acid are synthesized in the body to meet the body's requirements. L-aspartate is formed by the transamination of the Krebs cycle intermediate oxaloacetate. The amino acid serves as a precursor for synthesis of proteins, oligopeptides, purines, pyrimidines, nucleic acids and L-arginine. L-aspartate is a glycogenic amino acid, and it can also promote energy production via its metabolism in the Krebs cycle. These latter activities were the rationale for the

claim that supplemental aspartate has an anti-fatigue effect on skeletal muscle, a claim that was never confirmed.

L-aspartate is also known as L-amino succinate. Its IUPAC abbreviation is Asp. Its one-letter abbreviation, used when spelling out protein structures, is D. It is a solid, with an acid form that is slightly soluble in water, and with salt forms that are more water-soluble. Available salts include magnesium, calcium, potassium, zinc and combinations thereof. L-aspartate is used interchangeably with the term aspartic acid. The biological form of this substance, however, is the anion of aspartic acid, L-aspartate. Aspartic acid has the following chemical structure:

Aspartic acid

ACTIONS AND PHARMACOLOGY

ACTIONS

L-aspartate salts are delivery forms for cations such as magnesium, potassium, calcium and zinc.

MECHANISM OF ACTION

L-aspartates can form salts with cations such as magnesium, potassium, calcium and zinc.

PHARMACOKINETICS

Following ingestion, L-aspartate is absorbed from the small intestine by an active transport process. Following absorption, L-aspartate enters the portal circulation and from there is transported to the liver, where much of it is metabolized to protein, purines, pyrimidines and L-arginine, and is catabolized as well. L-aspartate is not metabolized in the liver; it enters the systemic circulation, which distributes it to various tissues of the body. The cations associated with L-aspartate independently interact with various substances in the body and participate in various physiological processes.

INDICATIONS AND USAGE

There is no support for the claim that aspartates are exercise performance enhancers, i.e. ergogenic aids.

RESEARCH SUMMARY

There are claims that L-aspartate is a special type of mineral transporter for cations, such as magnesium, into cells. Magnesium aspartate has not been found to be more biologically effective when compared with other magnesium salts.

There are also claims that L-aspartate has ergogenic effects, that it enhances performance in both prolonged exercise and short intensive exercise. It is hypothesized that L-aspartate, especially the potassium magnesium aspartate salt, spares stores of muscle glycogen and/or promotes a faster rate of glycogen resynthesis during exercise. It has also been hypothesized that L-aspartate can enhance short intensive exercise by serving as a substrate for energy production in the Krebs cycle and for stimulating the purine nucleotide cycle.

An animal study using injected aspartate failed to find any evidence of a glycogen-sparing effect or any ergogenic effects whatsoever. A more recent double-blind human study of male weight trainers similarly found aspartate supplementation to have no effect, and another study of the effect of aspartate on short intensive exercise again found no effect.

CONTRAINDICATIONS, PRECAUTIONS, ADVERSE REACTIONS

CONTRAINDICATIONS

L-aspartate supplementation is contraindicated in those hypersensitive to any component of the preparation.

PRECAUTIONS

Because of lack of long-term safety studies, L-aspartate salts should be avoided by children, pregnant women and lactating women.

ADVERSE REACTIONS

Mild gastrointestinal side effects including diarrhea have been reported.

INTERACTIONS

No drug, nutritional supplement, food or herb interactions are known.

OVERDOSAGE

Overdosage has not been reported.

DOSAGE AND ADMINISTRATION

L-aspartate salts of potassium, magnesium, calcium and zinc are available, as well as mixed salts of magnesium potassium aspartate and calcium magnesium aspartate. See Calcium, Magnesium, Potassium and Zinc for dose recommendations of these minerals.

HOW SUPPLIED

Capsules — 600 mg
Powder

LITERATURE

Bac P, Pages N, Herrenknecht CLA, Teste JF. Inhibition of mouse-killing behavior in magnesium-deficient rats: effect of pharmacological doses of magnesium pidolate, magnesium aspartate, magnesium lactate, magnesium gluconate and magnesium chloride. *Magnes Res.* 1995; 8:37-45.

de Haan A, van Doorn JE, Westra HG. Effects of potassium + magnesium aspartate on muscle metabolism and force development during short static exercise. *Int J Sports Med.* 1985; 6:44-49.

Hagan RD, Upton SJ, Duncan JJ, et al. Absence of effect of potassium- magnesium aspartate on physiologic responses to prolonged work in aerobically trained men. *Int J Sports Med.* 1982; 3:177-181.

Hicks JT. Treatment of fatigue in general practice: a double-blind study. *Clinical Medicine.* 1964; 71:85-90.

Maughan RJ, Sadler DJ. The effects of oral administration of salts of aspartic acid on the metabolic response to prolonged exhausting exercise in man. *Int J Sports Med.* 1983; 4:119-123.

Trudeau F, Murphy R. Effects of potassium-aspartate salt administration on glycogen use in the rat during a swimming stress. *Physiol Behav.* 1993; 54:7-12.

Tuttle JL, Potteiger JA, Evans BW, Ozmun JC. Effects of acute potassium-magnesium aspartate supplementation on ammonia concentrations during and after resistance training. *Int J Sport Nutr.* 1995; 5:102-109.

L-Carnitine

TRADE NAMES

Carnitine and L-carnitine are available generically from numerous manufacturers. Branded products include Carnitor (Sigma-Tau), Carnitine-300 (Key Company), Carni Fuel (Twinlab), Mega L-Carnitine (Twinlab) and Maximal Burner Carnitine (Bricker Labs), Proxeed (Sigma-Tau).

DESCRIPTION

L-carnitine, an amino acid derivative, is found in nearly all cells of the body. L-carnitine transports long-chain fatty acids across the inner mitochondrial membranes in the mitochondria, where they are processed by beta-oxidation to produce biological energy in the form of adenosine triphosphate or ATP.

L-carnitine is known chemically as (R)-3-carboxy-2-hydroxy-N,N,N-trimethyl-1-propanaminium hydroxide, inner salt; beta-hydroxy-gamma-N,N,N-trimethylaminobutyrate; gamma-amino-beta-hydroxybutyric acid trimethylbetaine; (3-carboxy-2-hydroxypropyl) trimethylammonium hydroxide, inner salt; gamma-trimethyl-beta-hydroxybutyrobetaine, and 3-hydroxy-4-(trimethylammonio) butanoate. L-carnitine is also known as levocarnitine and was formerly called vitamin BT. L-carnitine is a quarternary amine and belongs to the same chemical family as choline and is soluble in water. L-carnitine is represented by the following chemical structure:

$$CH_3 \quad HO \quad H \quad\quad O$$
$$CH_3 - N^+ - CH_2 - C - CH_2 - C - O^-$$
$$CH_3$$

L-Carnitine

L-carnitine occurs naturally in animal products. Generally, only very small amounts of it are found in plants, with few exceptions, such as avocado and some fermented soy products, e.g. tempeh. L-carnitine is a chiral molecule. Its stereoisomer D-carnitine does not have the biological activity of L-carnitine and may even antagonize L-carnitine in its biological roles.

L-carnitine is synthesized in the human body, chiefly in the liver and kidneys, from the essential amino acids L-lysine and L-methionine. Niacin, vitamins B$_6$ and C, and iron are involved in its biosynthesis. L-carnitine is described as a conditionally essential nutrient. This refers to certain conditions where exogenous L-carnitine may be required, such as in long-term parenteral nutrition, those on valproic acid therapy and possibly for the elderly.

L-carnitine is available in a few forms. Oral L-carnitine is available as a nutritional supplement and as a prescribed orphan drug treatment for primary and secondary L-carnitine deficiencies. Intravenous L-carnitine (levocarnitine) is available as a prescription orphan drug for the treatment of primary and secondary L-carnitine deficiencies. Acetyl-L-carnitine, another delivery form of both L-carnitine and acetyl groups, is available as a nutritional supplement. Another delivery form of L-carnitine, proprionyl-L-carnitine, is available in Europe but not at present in the U.S.

ACTIONS AND PHARMACOLOGY

ACTIONS
Supplemental L-carnitine may have cardioprotective activity in addition to beneficially affecting cardiac function. It may have a triglyceride-lowering effect in some as well as help to elevate HDL-cholesterol levels. L-carnitine may also have antioxidant properties.

Acetyl-L-carnitine may have neuroprotective activity. It may also aid in the treatment of age-related cholinergic deficits, such as those found in dementia disorder, including Alzheimer's disease (see Acetyl-L-carnitine).

MECHANISM OF ACTION
There are at least two major functions of L-carnitine. All tissues except the brain use long-chain fatty acids for bioenergy production. In cardiac and skeletal muscle, a major contribution of bioenergy comes from the beta-oxida-tion of long-chain fatty acids. Long-chain fatty acids require L-carnitine to transport them across the inner membranes of the mitochondria, wherein their metabolism produces bioenergy. Following the delivery of long-chain fatty acids into other mitochondria, L-carnitine, either by itself or esterified to an acyl group, recrosses the mitochondrial membrane to allow for continual use in this shuttle process.

Another function of L-carnitine is to remove short-chain and medium-chain fatty acids from the mitochondria in order to maintain coenzyme A levels in these organelles. These fatty acids accumulate as a result of normal and abnormal metabolism. This mechanism prevents the build-up in the mitochondria of short-chain and medium-chain fatty acids that may interfere with the bioenergy-producing process vital to the normal function of the cell.

Two types of L-carnitine deficiency states exist: primary systemic carnitine deficiency (SCD) and secondary carnitine deficiency syndromes. SCD is an autosomal recessive disorder characterized by progressive cardiomyopathy, skeletal myopathy, hypoglycemia and hyperammonemia. SCD appears to be due, in part, to loss of function of the transporter protein called OCT N2, which helps carry L-carnitine into cells. Patients with SCD have low L-carnitine levels in liver and skeletal muscle and variable concentrations of L-carnitine in the serum. Treatment with large doses of L-carnitine either orally or intravenously is sometimes beneficial in this rare genetic disorder.

Secondary L-carnitine deficiency disorders include a large number of entities. Some of these are genetic defects of metabolism such as methylmalonic aciduria, cytochrome C oxidase deficiency, fatty acyl-coenzyme A dehydrogenase deficiency, including long-chain and medium-chain deficiency, isovaleric acidemia, glutaric aciduria and propionic acidemia.

The mechanism of L-carnitine deficiency in these disorders is unclear. Some hypothesize that an accumulation of short-chain and medium-chain fatty acyl CoA molecules occurs in the mitochondria because insufficient L-carnitine is available to expel them. This accumulation would disturb the bioenergy-producing processes of the mitochondria. Symptoms of secondary muscle L-carnitine deficiency, not surprisingly, include muscle weakness and fatigue.

Secondary L-carnitine deficiency may also be found secondary to other conditions such as chronic renal failure treated by hemodialysis, cirrhosis with cachexia, chronic severe myopathies, myxedema, hypopituitarism, adrenal insufficiency, hyperammonemia associated with valproic acid therapy, valproate-induced Reye's syndrome, advanced AIDS and pregnancy. It may also be seen in those with HIV who are being treated with the nucleoside analogues didanosine (ddI), zalcitabine (ddC) and stavudine (d4T). In addition, it may occur in premature infants receiving parenteral nutrition. There is some preliminary evidence that secondary L-carnitine deficiency may also be associated with aging.

L-carnitine may possess antioxidant properties. A disturbance in long-chain fatty acid oxidation in mitochondria and/ or the accumulation of small-chain and medium-chain fatty acyl CoA molecules in the mitochondria might be expected to increase oxidative stress. There is some evidence that proprionyl-L-carnitine, a delivery form of L-carnitine, might protect the ischemic heart from reperfusion injury via an antioxidant effect.

PHARMACOKINETICS
About 60 to 75% of L-carnitine from food is absorbed. The percentage absorbed from supplements appears to be lower. In one study only 20% of a 2-gram dose of L-carnitine was found to be absorbed following ingestion. Most of an ingested dose of L-carnitine is absorbed by the small intestine, apparently by facilitative diffusion and active transport. Following the administration of a dose of L-carnitine of 1,980 milligrams twice daily, the maximum plasma concentration level (C_{max}) was 80 nanomoles per milliliter, and the time to maximum concentration (T_{max}) occurred at 3.3 hours. The bioavailability of oral L-carnitine is about 15%. L-carnitine is not bound to plasma protein or albumin.

Five normal adult male volunteers, administered a dose of [^{3}H-methyl]-L-carnitine following 15 days of a high-carnitine diet and additional L-carnitine supplement, excreted 58 to 65% of administered radioactive dose in 5 to 11 days in the urine and feces. Maximum concentration of [^{3}H-methyl]-L-carnitine in serum occurred from 2.0 to 4.5 hours after radioactive L-carnitine administration. Major metabolites found were trimethyl N-oxide, primarily in urine (8% to 49% of the administered dose) and [^{3}H]-gamma-butyrobetaine, primarily in feces (0.44% to 45% of the administered dose). Fecal excretion of total L-carnitine was less then 1% of total L-carnitine excretion. After attainment of steady state following four days of oral administration of about 2,000 milligrams twice a day of L-carnitine, urinary excretion of L-carnitine was about 9% of the orally administered dose. Approximately 95% of filtered L-carnitine is reabsorbed in healthy humans. Hypothyroidism decreases the urinary excretion of L-carnitine, while hyperthyroidism increases it.

Following absorption from the intestine, about 25% of L-carnitine may be acylated in the intestinal mucosa. Orally administered L-carnitine and its acylated metabolite are distributed to most tissues of the body. Uptake of L-carnitine into cells is thought to occur by facilitative diffusion and, in some cases, by active transport. Most of the body's stores of L-carnitine are found in cardiac and skeletal muscle.

INDICATIONS AND USAGE
The strongest evidence for the use of supplemental L-carnitine may be in the management of cardiac ischemia and peripheral arterial disease. It may also more generally be indicated for cardioprotection. It lowers triglyceride levels and increases levels of HDL-cholesterol in some. It is used with some benefit in those with primary and secondary carnitine deficiency syndromes. There is less evidence to support arguments that carnitine is indicated in liver, kidney and immune disorders or in diabetes and Alzheimer's disease. There is little evidence that supplemental L-carnitine boosts energy, increases athletic performance or inhibits obesity. There is no support for the claim that healthy vegetarians require L-carnitine supplementation.

RESEARCH SUMMARY
Favorable results have been reported for many years with regard to the use of L-carnitine in the treatment of various forms of cardiovascular disease. The walking capacity of patients with intermittent claudication was significantly improved in one double-blind, cross-over study of patients receiving oral L-carnitine. The data in this study suggests that L-carnitine enhances pyruvate utilization and oxidative phosphorylation efficiency in the skeletal muscle of the ischemic leg.

In a more recent, multicenter study, propionyl-L-carnitine was compared with placebo in the treatment of those with peripheral arterial disease of the legs. The study of 162 patients receiving propionyl-L-carnitine and 166 patients receiving placebo continued for one year. Walking ability and quality of life were evaluated at regular intervals. Those initially presenting with the most severe disability (able to walk no more than 250 meters) exhibited significant improvement, increasing walking distance by 98 meters compared with 54 meters in the placebo group. Those able to walk more than 250 meters at baseline also improved, versus placebo, but not at a level of statistical significance.

Supplemental L-carnitine has been helpful in some rare primary genetic L-carnitine deficiency syndromes, as well as in more common secondary L-carnitine deficiency syndromes (see pharmacology). It has been estimated that about 40% of those with the myopathies associated with the secondary deficiency syndromes respond to dietary L-carnitine, evidenced by enhanced muscle strength and reduced myoglobinuria.

An indirect role for supplemental L-carnitine in some forms of liver disease is suggested, because hepatic disease impairs the last stage of L-carnitine synthesis resulting in L-carnitine deficiencies in heart and skeletal muscle. Preliminary work suggests that L-carnitine can reduce fat deposits in some fatty livers. Research is ongoing.

The kidney is also an important locus of carnitine synthesis. Chronic kidney disease may eventually be an indication for L-carnitine supplementation, but more research is needed to demonstrate this. There is some evidence that dialysis patients can benefit from L-carnitine supplementation since dialysis removes the low-molecular-weight L-carnitine.

There is no evidence that L-carnitine will prevent diabetes, although abnormal carnitine metabolism is associated with diabetes. Ongoing research may demonstrate some benefit from L-carnitine supplementation. Animal model work in diabetes has shown improved myocardial function with administration of parenteral L-carnitine.

The claim that L-carnitine may have beneficial effects in Alzheimer's disease is unproved. Acetyl-L-carnitine, a derivative of L-carnitine and a delivery form of the substance, on the other hand, has shown some very preliminary benefit in this regard (see Acetyl-L-Carnitine). Investigation of L-carnitine may have some positive impact on some immune disorders, including AIDS. In a study of 20 patients with advanced AIDS, subjects were randomly assigned to receive either placebo or 6 grams of L-carnitine daily. At baseline, L-carnitine concentrations in the peripheral blood mononuclear cells (PBMC) of the AIDS patients were found to be lower than in healthy controls, even though the AIDS patients had normal serum concentrations of L-carnitine.

The study continued for two weeks. It demonstrated a significant trend toward restoration of normal intracellular L-carnitine levels. This increase in cellular L-carnitine was strongly associated with improved lymphocyte proliferative responsiveness to mitogens. The researchers suggested that "L-carnitine supplementation could have a role as a complementary therapy for HIV-infected individuals." The study also noted a significant decrease in the triglyceride levels of those patients receiving L-carnitine supplements. More research is clearly warranted.

L-carnitine effects on immunity are suggested, as well, from animal model work. Reductions in circulating cytokines and tumor necrosis factor have been observed.

There is little convincing evidence that L-carnitine supplements have any significant impact on physical performance or obesity. There is no support for the claim that vegetarians, including strict vegetarians, require L-carnitine supplementation. There is no evidence of carnitine deficiency in this population. Plasma carnitine concentrations in strict vegetarians are only an insignificant 10% lower than in omnivores.

CONTRAINDICATIONS, PRECAUTIONS, ADVERSE REACTIONS

CONTRAINDICATIONS
None known.

PRECAUTIONS
Standard assays for mutagenicity indicate that L-carnitine is not mutagenic.

Reproductive studies have been performed in rats and rabbits at doses up to 3.8 times the human doses used for the treatment of primary and secondary L-carnitine deficiency on the basis of surface area and have revealed no evidence of impaired fertility or harm to the fetus due to L-carnitine. However, there are no adequate and well-controlled studies in pregnant women. Because animal reproduction studies are not always predictive of human response, supplemental L-carnitine should be used by pregnant women only if clearly indicated and only under medical supervision. It is not known whether L-carnitine is excreted in human milk. Supplemental L-carnitine is not advised for nursing mothers. Those with seizure disorders should only use L-carnitine under medical advisement and supervision.

ADVERSE REACTIONS
Mild gastrointestinal symptoms have been reported in those taking oral L-carnitine, including transient nausea and vomiting, abdominal cramps and diarrhea. Mild myasthenia has been reported in uremic patients taking the racemic mixture D,L-carnitine. There are no reports of mild myasthenia in uremic patients receiving L-carnitine. Supplemental L-carnitine is generally well tolerated.

Although the incidence is low, seizures have been reported to occur in those with or without pre-existing seizure disorders receiving either oral or intravenous L-carnitine. In those with pre-existing seizure activity, an increase in seizure frequency and/or severity has been reported.

INTERACTIONS
Therapy with valproic acid, the nucleoside analogues didanosine (ddI), zalcitabine (ddC) and stavudine (d4T) may produce secondary L-carnitine deficiencies. So might the pivalic acid-containing antibiotics, pivampicillin, pivmecillinam and pivcephalexin. These antibiotics are used in Europe.

Choline supplementation may lead to increased L-carnitine retention. Vitamin C deficiency may lead to secondary L-carnitine deficiency.

OVERDOSAGE
There have been no reports of toxicity from L-carnitine overdosage. The oral LD_{50} of L-carnitine in mice is 19.2 grams per kilogram.

DOSAGE AND ADMINISTRATION
L-carnitine is available in a few forms. Oral L-carnitine is available as a nutritional supplement and as a prescribed

treatment for primary and secondary L-carnitine deficiencies. Intravenous L-carnitine is available as a prescription drug for the treatment of primary and secondary L-carnitine deficiencies. Acetyl-L-carnitine is available as a nutritional supplement. Propionyl-L-carnitine is available in Europe but not currently in the United States. DL-carnitine should be avoided. The available salts of L-carnitine are L-carnitine HC1, L-carnitine tartrate and L-carnitine fumarate.

Those who take supplemental L-carnitine for cardiovascular health (and most other possible indications) take 500 milligrams to 2 grams daily. The higher amounts are taken in divided doses. The doses are taken with or without food.

See Physician's Desk Reference for dosage and administration of levocarnitine in the treatment of primary and secondary L-carnitine deficiencies. See Acetyl-L-carnitine for dosage of this supplement.

HOW SUPPLIED

Capsules — 250 mg, 300 mg, 500 mg

Injection — 200 mg/mL

Liquid

Solution — 100 mg/mL

Tablets — 250 mg, 330 mg, 500 mg, 1000 mg

Wafer — 500 mg

LITERATURE

Bohles H, Richter K, Wagner-Thiesson E, Schafer H. Decreased serum carnitine in valproate induced Reye syndrome. *Eur J Pediatr.* 1982; 139:185-186.

Bohmer T, Rynding A, Solberg HE. Carnitine levels in human serum in health and disease. *Clin Chim Acta.* 1974; 57:55-61.

Borum PR. Carnitine. An*n Rev Nutr.* 1983; 3:233-259.

Brevetti G, Diehm C, Lambert D. European multicenter study on propionyl-L-carnitine in intermittent claudication. *J Am Coll Cardiol.* 1999; 35:1618-1624.

Brevetti G, Chiarello M, Ferulano G, et al. Increases in walking distance in patients with peripheral vascular disease: a double-blind, cross-over study. *Circul.* 1988; 77:767-773.

Brooks H, Goldberg L, Holland R, et al. Carnitine-induced effects on cardiac and peripheral hemodynamics. *J Clin Pharmacol.* 1977; 17:561-578.

Christiansen R, Bremer J. Active transport of butyrobetaine and carnitine into isolated liver cells. *Biochem Biophys Acta.* 1977; 448:562-577.

de Simone C, Famularo G, Tzantzoglov S, et al. Carnitine depletion in peripheral blood mononuclear cells from patients with AIDS: effect of L-carnitine. *AIDS.* 1994; 8:655-660.

Famularo G, Moretti S, Marcellini S, et al. Acetyl-carnitine deficiency in AIDS patients with neurotoxicity on treatment with antiretroviral nucleoside analogues. *AIDS.* 1997; 11:185-190.

Lindstedt S, Lindstedt G. Distribution and excretion of carnitine $^{14}CO_2$ in the rat. *Acta Chim Scand.* 1961; 15:701-702.

Maebashi M, Kawamura N, Sato M, et al. Lipid-lowering effects of carnitine in patients with type-IV hypolipoproteinaemia. *Lancet.* 1978; 2:805-807.

Marzo A, Arrigoni Martelli E, Mancinelli A, et al. Protein binding of L-carnitine family components. *Eur J Drug Met Pharmacokin* Special Issue III. 1992; 364-368.

Nezu J, Tamai I, Oku A, et al. Primary systemic carnitine deficiency is caused by mutations in a gene encoding sodium ion-dependent carnitine transporter. *Nat Gen.* 1999; 21:91-94.

Opie LH. Role of carnitine in fatty acid metabolism of normal and ischemic myocardium. *Am Heart J.* 1979; 97:375-388.

Levocarnitine. *Physicians' Desk Reference.* 54 ed. Montvale, NJ; Medical Economics Company. 2000:2957-2959.

Pola P, Savi L Grilli M, et al. Carnitine in the therapy of dyslipidemic patients. *Curr Therapeu Res.* 1980; 27:208-216.

Prockup LD, Engel WK, Shug AL. Nearly fatal muscle carnitine deficiency with full recovery after replacement therapy. Neur*ol.* 1983; 33:1629-1631.

Rebouche CJ. Carnitine. In: Shils ME, Olson JA, Shike M, Ross AC, eds. Modern Nutrition in Health and Disease. 9th ed. Baltimore, MD: Williams & Wilkins; 1999:505-512.

Rebouche CJ. Carnitine function and requirements during the life cycle. FAS*EB J.* 1992; 6:3379-3386.

Rebouche CJ, Engel AG. Carnitine metabolism and deficiency syndromes. *Mayo Clin* Proc. 1983; 58:533-540.

Rebouche CJ, Paulson DJ. Carnitine metabolism and function in humans. *Ann Rev Nutr.* 1986; 6:41-68.

Rossi CS, Siliprandi N. Effects of carnitine on serum HDL-cholesterol: report of two cases. *Johns Hopkins Medical J.* 1982; 150:51-54.

Sachan DS, Rhew TH, Ruark RA. Ameliorating effects of carnitine on alcohol-induced fatty liver. *Am J Clin Nutr.* 1984; 39:738-744.

Triggs WJ, Bohan TP, Shen-Nan L, Wilmore J. Valproate-induced coma with ketosis and carnitine insufficiency. *Arch Neurol.* 1990; 47 006031-1133.

Vacha GM, Giorcelli G, Siliprandi N, Corsi G. Favorable effects of L-carnitine treatment on hypertriglyceridemia in hemodialysis patients: decisive role of low levels of high-density lipoprotein-cholesterol. *Am J Clin Nutr.* 1983; 38:532-540.

L-Cysteine

TRADE NAMES

L-cysteine is available generically from numerous manufacturers. Branded products include Cysteine-500 (Key Company) and Cystech (Bio-tech Pharmacal).

DESCRIPTION

L-cysteine is a protein amino acid naturally present in the proteins of life forms. L-cysteine is a sulfur amino acid and contains a sulfhydryl group. Although most cysteine is found in proteins, small amounts of free cysteine are found in body fluids and in plants. The normal diet contributes approximately 1 gram of L-cysteine daily.

L-cysteine is considered a nonessential amino acid, meaning that, under normal physiologic conditions, sufficient amounts of this amino acid are formed from the dietary essential amino acid L-methionine and the nonessential amino acid L-serine via a transsulfuration reaction. L-cysteine is a conditionally essential amino acid under certain circumstances, for example, for preterm infants.

L-cysteine serves as a precursor for synthesis of proteins, glutathione, taurine, coenzyme A and inorganic sulfate. Glutathionine itself has a number of biochemical functions, including maintenance of normal cellular redox state. Certain conditions, e.g. an acetaminophen overdose, can deplete hepatic glutathione, and this can be life-threatening. The antidote to an acetaminophen overdose is L-cysteine, in the delivery form of N-acetylcysteine. The L-cysteine derived from N-acetylcysteine helps to restore hepatic glutathione.

L-cysteine is also known as L-2-amino-3-mercaptopropanoic acid, 2-amino-3-mercaptopropanoic acid, beta-mercaptoalanine, 2-amino-3 mercaptopropionic acid and alpha-amino-beta-thiolpropionic acid. L-cysteine is represented by the following chemical structure:

L-cysteine

Its IUPAC abbreviation is Cys, and its one-letter abbreviation, used when spelling out protein structures, is C. L-cysteine is a white, solid substance that is soluble in water. It is hygroscopic and slowly decomposes and oxidizes. In solution, it undergoes oxidation to L-cystine, which is a dimer of L-cysteine. N-acetylcysteine is a preferred delivery form of L-cysteine because of greater stability and possible higher absorbability. (See N-Acetylcysteine).

ACTIONS AND PHARMACOLOGY

ACTIONS

The most significant action of supplemental L-cysteine is as a redox modulator.

MECHANISM OF ACTION

Certain conditions, e.g. an acetaminophen overdose, deplete hepatic glutathione and subject the tissues to oxidative stress resulting in loss of cellular integrity. L-cysteine serves as a major precursor for synthesis of glutathione.

PHARMACOKINETICS

Following ingestion, some L-cysteine is oxidized to L-cystine, and both L-cysteine and L-cystine are absorbed from the small intestine by active-transport processes. L-cysteine absorption is largely sodium-dependent, while L-cystine is absorbed by a sodium-independent transport system. Following absorption, L-cysteine enters the portal circulation, which distributes it to the liver. There, much of it is metabolized to protein, glutathione, taurine and sulfate. L-cysteine, which does not get metabolized by the liver, enters the systemic circulation which distributes it to various tissues of the body.

INDICATIONS AND USAGE

It has been claimed that L-cysteine has anti-inflammatory properties, that it can protect against various toxins, and that it might be helpful in osteoarthritis and rheumatoid arthritis. More research will have to be done before L-cysteine can be indicated for any of these conditions. Research to date has mostly been in animal models.

RESEARCH SUMMARY

There is some evidence from animal studies that cysteine can help ensure adequate glutathione synthesis during and after inflammatory challenge, thus helping to "ameliorate," in the words of one research group, "adverse effects of oxidative damage induced by disease or drugs."

Cysteine-supplemented mice and guinea pigs have enjoyed significantly extended life spans, and other animals, challenged with various toxins, have, when pre-supplemented with cysteine, survived considerably longer than non-supplemented controls. In one of these studies, 90% of control rats given large doses of acetaldehyde died. But other rats first given a combination of vitamins C and B, along with cysteine, and then exposed to the same dose of acetaldehyde, all survived. Cysteine's protective mechanisms could relate to its own antioxidant properties, its promotion of glutathione (a major antioxidant) or even, it has been hypothesized, to some ability to participate in DNA repair.

There is inconclusive evidence that cysteine could play a positive role in the treatment of osteoarthritis and rheumatoid arthritis.

CONTRAINDICATIONS, PRECAUTIONS, ADVERSE REACTIONS

CONTRAINDICATIONS

L-cysteine supplementation is contraindicated in those hypersensitive to any component of the preparation.

PRECAUTIONS

Because of lack of long-term safety studies, L-cysteine supplementation should be avoided by children, pregnant women and nursing mothers.

Although the incidence of cystine renal stones is low, they do occur. Those who form renal stones, particularly cystine stones, should avoid L-cysteine supplements.

L-cysteine, like other sulfhydryl-containing substances, could produce a false-positive result in the nitroprusside test for ketone bodies used in diabetes.

ADVERSE REACTIONS

With typical doses of 1 to 1.5 grams daily, the most commonly reported side effects have been gastrointestinal, such as nausea. There are rare reports of cystine renal stone formation.

INTERACTIONS

NUTRITIONAL SUPPLEMENTS

Zinc: L-cysteine complexes with zinc and may increase the absorption of zinc.

Vitamin C: Ascorbic acid may inhibit the oxidation of L-cysteine to L-cystine.

OVERDOSAGE

There are no reports of overdosage in those taking L-cysteine supplements. However, large doses of L-cysteine are neuroexcitotoxic in several species. Single injections of L-cysteine (0.6-1.5 g/kg) into 4-day-old pups resulted in massive damage to cortical neurons, permanent retinal dystrophy, atrophy of the brain and hyperactivity.

DOSAGE AND ADMINISTRATION

The usual supplemental dosage of L-cysteine is 500 milligrams to 1.5 grams daily. Those who supplement with L-cysteine should drink at least six to eight glasses of water daily in order to prevent cystine renal stones. Some studies indicate that an intake of 3 to 5 grams daily of vitamin C may prevent cystine stones. However, high-dose vitamin C itself may contribute to renal stones in some (see Vitamin C).

Another delivery form of L-cysteine is N-acetylcysteine (see N-Acetylcysteine).

HOW SUPPLIED

Capsules — 500 mg, 750 mg
Injection — 50 mg/mL
Powder
Tablets — 500 mg

LITERATURE

Anderson R, Lukey PT, Theron AJ, Dippenaar U. Ascorbate and cysteine-mediated selective neutralization of extracellular oxidants during N-formyl peptide activation of human phagocytes. *Agents Actions.*1987;20:77-86.

Anderson R, Theron AJ, Ras GJ. Regulation by the antioxidants ascorbate, cysteine, and dapsone of the increased extracellular and intracellular generation of reactive oxidants by activated phagocytes from cigarette smokers. *Am Rev Respir Dis.* 1987; 135:1027-1032

Asper R, Schmucki O. Cystinuric therapy by ascorbic acid. *Urol Int.*1982;37:91-109.

Campbell NR, Reade PC, Radden BG. Effect of cysteine on the survival of mice with transplanted malignant lymphoma. *Nature.* 1974;251:158-159.

Csako G. False-positive results for ketone with the drug mensa and other free-sulfhydryl compounds. *Clin Chem.* 1987;33(2 pt 1):289-292.

Fettman MJ, Valerius KD, Ogilvie GK. Effects of dietary cysteine on blood sulfur amino acid, glutathione, and malondialdehyde concentrations in cats. *Am J Vet Res.* 1999;60:328-333.

Oeriu S, Vachitu E. The effect of the administration of compounds which contain sulfhydryl groups on the survival rate of mice, rats and guinea pigs. *Journ Geront.* 1965;20;47.

Stipanuk MH. Homocysteine, cysteine and taurine. In: Shils ME, Olson JA, Shike M, Ross AC, eds. *Modern Nutrition in Health and Disease.* Ninth edition. Baltimore, MD: Williams & Wilkins; 1999:543-558.

L-Glutamine

TRADE NAMES

Glutamine Fuel Powder (Twinlab), Glutamine Fuel Mega (Twinlab), Glutamine Express (Genetic Evolutionary Nutrition), L-Glutamine Power (Champion Nutrition), Earthlink Science Glutamine Chews Chocolate (Amerifit).

DESCRIPTION

L-glutamine is a protein amino acid found in proteins of all life forms. It is classified as a semi-essential or conditionally essential amino acid. This means that under normal circumstances the body can synthesize sufficient L-glutamine to meet physiological demands. However, there are conditions where the body cannot do so. Recently, L-glutamine has come to be regarded as one of the most important of the amino acids when the body is subjected to such metabolic stress situations as trauma (including surgical trauma), cancer, sepsis and burns. Under such conditions, L-glutamine becomes an essential amino acid, and it is therefore very important to ensure adequate intakes of the amino acid in order to meet the increased physiological demands created by these situations.

L-glutamine is the most abundant amino acid in the body, and plasma glutamine levels are the highest of any amino acid. L-glutamine is predominantly synthesized and stored in skeletal muscle. The amino acid L-glutamate is metabolized to L-glutamine in a reaction catalyzed by the enzyme glutamine synthase, a reaction which, in addition to L-glutamate, requires ammonia, ATP and magnesium.

L-glutamine is a very versatile amino acid and participates in many reactions in the body. It is important in the regulation of acid-base balance. L-glutamine allows the kidneys to excrete an acid load, protecting the body against acidosis. This is accomplished by the production of ammonia, which binds hydrogen ions, to produce ammonium cations that are excreted in the urine along with chloride anions. Bicarbonate ions are simultaneously released into the bloodstream. L-glutamine helps protect the body against ammonia toxicity by transporting ammonia, in the form of L-glutamine's amide group, from peripheral tissues to visceral organs, where it can be excreted as ammonium by the kidneys or converted to urea by the liver.

The amide group can also participate in other metabolic activities, as can the amino group of L-glutamine. L-glutamine serves as the most important nitrogen shuttle, supplying nitrogen for metabolic purposes (from glutamine-producing tissues, such as skeletal muscle) to glutamine-consuming tissues.

L-glutamine participates in the formation of purine and pyrimidine nucleotides, amino sugars (such as glucosamine), L-glutamate and other amino acids, nicotinamide adenine dinucleotide and glutathione. It also participates in protein synthesis, energy production and, if necessary, the production of D-glucose and glycogen. Importantly, L-glutamine can serve as the primary respiratory substrate for the production of energy in enterocytes and lymphocytes. L-glutamine is considered an immunonutrient, and supplemental L-glutamine is used in medical foods for such stress situations as trauma, cancer, infections and burns.

The typical dietary intake of L-glutamine is 5 to 10 grams daily. Most dietary L-glutamine comes from animal and plant proteins. Small amounts of free L-glutamine are found in vegetable juices and fermented foods, such as miso and yogurt. L-glutamine is the amide of L-glutamic acid. Its molecular formula is $C_5H_{10}N_2O_3$, and its molecular weight is 146.15 daltons. The structural formula is:

L-glutamine

L-glutamine is also known as 2-aminoglutaramic acid, levoglutamide, (S)-2, 5-diamino-5-oxopentaenoic acid and glutamic acid 5-amide. Its one-letter abbreviation is Q, and it is also abbreviated as Gln. The terms L-glutamine and glutamine are used interchangeably. D-glutamine, the stereo-isomer of L-glutamine, does not have, as far as is known, biological activity. L-glutamine is not very soluble in water, and aqueous solutions are unstable at temperatures of 22 to 24 degrees Celsius. For these reasons, the more soluble and more stable glutamine dipeptides are used as delivery forms of L-glutamine in total parenteral nutrition (TPN) solutions. See Glutamine Peptides.

ACTIONS AND PHARMACOLOGY
ACTIONS
Supplemental L-glutamine may have immunomodulatory, anticatabolic/anabolic and gastrointestinal mucosal-protective actions. It may also have antioxidant activity.

MECHANISM OF ACTION
Supplemental L-glutamine's possible immunomodulatory role may be accounted for in a number of ways. L-glutamine appears to play a major role in protecting the integrity of the gastrointestinal tract and, in particular, the large intestine. During catabolic states, the integrity of the intestinal mucosa may be compromised with consequent increased intestinal permeability and translocation of Gram-negative bacteria from the large intestine into the body. The demand for L-glutamine by the intestine, as well as by cells such as lymphocytes, appears to be much greater than that supplied by skeletal muscle, the major storage tissue for L-glutamine. L-glutamine is the preferred respiratory fuel for enterocytes, colonocytes and lymphocytes. Therefore, supplying supplemental L-glutamine under these conditions may do a number of things. For one, it may reverse the catabolic state by sparing skeletal muscle L-glutamine. It also may inhibit translocation of Gram-negative bacteria from the large intestine. L-glutamine helps maintain secretory IgA, which functions primarily by preventing the attachment of bacteria to mucosal cells.

L-glutamine appears to be required to support the proliferation of mitogen-stimulated lymphocytes, as well as the production of interleukin-2 (IL-2) and interferon-gamma (IFN-gamma). It is also required for the maintenance of lymphokine-activated killer cells (LAK). L-glutamine can enhance phagocytosis by neutrophils and monocytes. It can lead to an increased synthesis of glutathione in the intestine, which may also play a role in maintaining the integrity of the intestinal mucosa by ameliorating oxidative stress.

The exact mechanism of the possible immunomodulatory action of supplemental L-glutamine, however, remains unclear. It is conceivable that the major effect of L-glutamine occurs at the level of the intestine. Perhaps enteral L-glutamine acts directly on intestine-associated lymphoid tissue and stimulates overall immune function by that mechanism, without passing beyond the splanchnic bed.

The anticatabolic/anabolic activity of supplemental L-glutamine can be explained by its effect in sparing skeletal muscle L-glutamine stores.

PHARMACOKINETICS

Following ingestion, L-glutamine is absorbed from the lumen of the small intestine into the enterocytes. Absorption is efficient and occurs by an active transport mechanism. Some metabolism of the amino acid takes place in the enterocytes. L-glutamine that is not metabolized in the enterocytes enters the portal circulation from whence it is transported to the liver, where again some portion of the amino acid is metabolized. L-glutamine not metabolized in the liver enters the systemic circulation, where it is distributed to the various tissues of the body. L-glutamine participates in various metabolic activities, including the formation of L-glutamate catalyzed by the enzyme glutaminase. It also participates in the synthesis of proteins, glutathione, pyrimidine and purine nucleotides and amino sugars. The transport of L-glutamine into cells is via an active process. L-glutamine is eliminated by glomerular filtration and is almost completely reabsorbed by the renal tables.

INDICATIONS AND USAGE

Glutamine has been shown to be beneficial when administered in the form of glutamine peptides via TPN in some patients with varying forms of catabolic stress, e.g., some cancer, transplantation, intensive-care, surgical and immune-suppressed patients. Benefits from enteral glutamine supplementation are generally less pronounced, but preliminary significant results have been reported with the use of oral glutamine in very-low-birth-weight infants and in some major trauma patients in whom glutamine seems to strengthen immunity, particularly in the gastrointestinal tract. Glutamine may help protect against some of the side effects of cancer chemotherapy and radiotherapy.

There is little concurring evidence that glutamine is an effective ergogenic aid, but there is some suggestion that it might help protect against exercise-induced immune impairment. Some dated research suggesting that glutamine might help curb alcohol craving has not been followed up. Claims that it helps prevent neurodegenerative disorders or that it modulates mood have not been substantiated.

RESEARCH SUMMARY

Several well-designed studies have demonstrated that the addition of glutamine to TPN helps decrease intestinal permeability and mucosal and villous atrophy in the small intestine. Inhibition of intestinal permeability is believed to decrease microbial translocation and thus reduce infective opportunities in the gut. Increased intestinal permeability has been associated with a number of traumas, illnesses and some surgeries.

Studies have shown worthwhile reductions in length of hospital stay attributed to glutamine-supplemented TPN in bone-marrow transplantation patients and in those who had resection for colon or rectal cancer. In another study, mortality was significantly better in intensive-care patients who received TPN supplemented with glutamine than in those whose TPN did not include glutamine.

In addition, glutamine in TPN has been credited with improving nutritional status in some critically ill patients, including cancer patients. And it appears to allow for more aggressive radiotherapy and chemotherapy by protecting against some of the side effects of those treatments.

Enteral glutamine has also demonstrated positive results. In a recent placebo-controlled study, oral glutamine significantly decreased the severity and duration of painful oral mucositis (stomatitis) in autologous bone-marrow transplantation patients. It was similarly helpful in alleviating radiation-induced oral mucositis in a recent randomized pilot trial. Very-low-birth-weight infants orally supplemented with glutamine between days 3 and 30 of life had far less hospital-acquired sepsis than controls (11% versus 30%) and had better tolerance to enteral feedings.

In a placebo-controlled study examining infectious morbidity in multiple trauma patients, oral glutamine was credited with significantly reducing the incidence of pneumonia, sepsis and bacteremia. In another recent randomized study of critically ill patients, supplementation with oral glutamine was said to have significant hospital cost benefits, reducing cost per survivor by 30%.

While claims that glutamine is an effective ergogenic aid are poorly supported, there is some evidence that the substance can help protect against some of the immune impairment that is sometimes seen in exercise "overtraining." Lower resting levels of plasma glutamine have been observed in some athletes suffering from overtraining syndrome, characterized, in part, by transient immunosuppression. In a few preliminary studies, oral glutamine supplementation appears to improve some measures of immunity and to decrease post-exercise infection. Results are not consistent, however, and more research is needed.

Some dated research suggesting that oral glutamine might help curb alcohol craving has not been followed up. One study demonstrated a significant decrease in voluntary alcohol consumption in rats supplemented with glutamine. A subsequent small, uncontrolled study focused on a group of subjects with extensive history of alcoholism. Considerable improvement was noted. More research is needed.

CONTRAINDICATIONS, PRECAUTIONS, ADVERSE REACTIONS
CONTRAINDICATIONS
Supplemental L-glutamine is contraindicated in those hypersensitive to any component of a glutamine-containing product.

PRECAUTIONS
Pregnant women and nursing mothers should avoid supplemental L-glutamine unless prescribed by a physician.

Those with renal or hepatic failure should exercise caution in the use of supplemental L-glutamine.

ADVERSE REACTIONS
Doses of L-glutamine up to 21 grams daily appear to be well tolerated. Reported adverse reactions are mainly gastrointestinal and not common. They include constipation and bloating. There is one older report of two hypomanic patients whose manic symptoms were exacerbated following the use of 2 to 4 grams daily of L-glutamine. The symptoms resolved when the L-glutamine was stopped. These patients were not rechallenged, nor are there any other reports of this nature.

INTERACTIONS
DRUGS
Human growth hormone: Concomitant use of L-glutamine and human growth hormone may enhance nutrient absorption in those with severe short bowel syndrome. L-glutamine has orphan drug status for this indication.

Indomethacin: Concomitant use of L-glutamine and indomethacin may ameliorate increased intestinal permeability caused by indomethacin. The reported dose used for L-glutamine was 21 grams daily taken in divided doses three times a day. Further, misoprostol is reported to have a synergistic effect with this combination in ameliorating intestinal permeability.

Methotrexate: There is one report that methotrexate may decrease the possible effectiveness of supplemental L-glutamine for chemotherapy-induced mucositis. In another report, nine patients with breast cancer were reported to have decreased symptoms of methotrexate-related toxicity when given supplemental L-glutamine at a dose of 0.5 gram/kilogram/day.

Paclitaxel: In one report, L-glutamine at a dose of 10 grams three times daily, given 24 hours after receiving paclitaxel, appeared to prevent the development of myalgia and arthralgia, adverse reactions of paclitaxel.

DOSAGE AND ADMINISTRATION
L-glutamine is available in capsules, tablets and powder form. It is also available in medical foods for oral and enteral nutrition use and in a dipeptide form for parenteral nutrition use. (See Glutamine Peptides.) Typical doses for those with cancer, AIDS, trauma, burns, infections and other stress-related conditions range from 4 to 21 grams daily. Those who take L-glutamine for these indications must be under medical supervision.

Those with chemotherapy- or radiation-induced stomatitis have taken doses of 2 to 4 grams twice daily or 2 grams four times daily. This was done by dissolving a given amount of L-glutamine in water or normal saline — one gram dissolves in 20.8 ml of water at 30 degrees Celsius — and using it as a swish and swallow. Again, this must be performed under medical supervision. Since L-glutamine is unstable in water, fresh solutions should be prepared daily.

Those who use supplemental L-glutamine as a possible ergogenic aid use between 1.5 to 4.5 grams daily, taken between meals.

HOW SUPPLIED
Capsules — 500 mg, 750 mg
Powder
Tablets — 500 mg, 750 mg, 1000 mg

LITERATURE
Abcouwer SF, Souba WW. Glutamine and arginine. In: Shils ME, Olson JA, Shike M, Ross AC, eds. *Modern Nutrition in Health and Disease.* 9th ed. Baltimore, MD: Williams and Wilkins. 1999:559-569.

Anderson PM, Ramsay NK, Shu XO, et al. Effect of low-dose oral glutamine on painful stomatitis during bone marrow transplantation. *Bone Marrow Transplant.* 1998;22:339-344.

Anderson PM, Schroeder G, Skubitz KM. Oral glutamine reduces the duration and severity of stomatitis after cytotoxic cancer chemotherapy. *Cancer.* 1998;83:1433-1439.

Antonio J, Street C. Glutamine: a potentially useful supplement for athletes. *Can J Appl Physiol.* 1999;24:1-14.

Bulus N, Cersosimo E, Ghishan F, Abumrad NN. Physiologic importance of glutamine. *Metabolism.* 1989;38(Suppl1):1-5.

Byrne TA, Morrissey TB, Nattakom TV, et al. Growth hormone, glutamine, and a modified diet enhance nutrient absorption in patients with severe short bowel syndrome. *J Parenter Enteral Nutr.* 1995;19:296-302.

Cao Y, Feng Z, Hoos A, Klimberg VS. Glutamine enhances gut glutathione production. *J Parenter Enteral Nutr.* 1998;22:224-247.

Furukawa S, Saito H, Inoue T, et al. Supplemental glutamine augments phagocytosis and reactive oxygen intermediate production by neutrophils and monocytes from postoperative patients *in vitro. Nutrition.* 2000;16:323-329.

Furukawa S, Saito H, Ming-Tsan L, et al. Enteral administration of glutamine in purulent peritonitis. *Nutrition.* 1999;15:29-31.

Haub MD, Potteiger JA, Nau KL, et al. Acute L-glutamine ingestion does not improve maximal effort exercise. *J Sports Med Phys Fitness.* 1998;38:240-244.

Hond ED, Peeters M, Hiele M, et al. Effect of glutamine on the intestinal permeability changes induced by indomethacin in humans. *Aliment Pharmacol Ther.* 1999;13:679-685.

Houdijk, APJ, Rijnsburger ER, Jansen J, et al. Randomized trial of glutamine-enriched enteral nutrition on infectious morbidity in patients with multiple trauma. *Lancet.* 1998;352:772-776.

Huang EY, Leung SW, Wang CJ, et al. Oral glutamine to alleviate radiation-induced oral mucositis: a pilot randomized trial. *Int J Rad Oncol Biol Phys.* 2000;46:535-539.

Ito A, Higashiguchi T. Effects of glutamine administration on liver regeneration following hepatectomy. *Nutrition.* 1999;15:23-28.

Lacey JM, Wilmore DW. Is glutamine a conditionally essential amino acid? *Nutr Rev.* 1990;48:297-309.

Mebane AH. L-Glutamine and mania. *Am J Psychiatry.* 1984;141:1302-1303.

Neu J, Roig JC, Meetze WH, et al. Enteral glutamine supplementation for very low birth weight infants decreases mortality. *J Pediatr.* 1997;131:691-699.

Noyer CM, Simon D, Borczuk A, et al. A double-blind placebo-controlled pilot study of glutamine therapy for abnormal intestinal permeability in patients with AIDS. *Am J Gastroenterol.* 1998;93:972-975.

Rogers LL, Pelton RB, Williams RJ. Voluntary alcohol consumption of rats following administration of glutamine. *J Biol Chem.* 1955;214:503-506.

Rohde T, MacLean DA, Klarlund Pedersen B. Glutamine, lymphocyte proliferation and cytokine production. *Scan J Immunol.* 1996;44:648-650.

Rohde T, MacLean DA, Pedersen BK. Effect of glutamine supplementation on changes in the immune system induced by repeated exercise. *Med Sci Sports Exerc.* 1998;30:856-862.

Sacks GS. Glutamine supplementation in catabolic patients. *Ann Pharmacother.* 1999;33:348-354.

Wilmore DW, Schloerb PR, Ziegler TR. Glutamine in the support of patients following bone marrow transplantation. *Curr Opin Clin Nutr Metab Care.* 1999;2:323-327.

Windmueller HG, Spaeth AF. Identification of ketone bodies and glutamine as the major respiratory fuels *in vivo* for postabsorptive rat small intestine. *J Biol Chem.* 1978;253:69-76.

Ziegler TR, Benfell K, Smith RJ, et al. Safety and metabolic effects of L-glutamine administration in humans. *J Parenter Enteral Nutr.* 1990;14:137S-146S.

L-Histidine

DESCRIPTION

L-histidine is a protein amino acid that is found in the proteins of all life forms. Although most L-histidine is found in proteins, a small amount of free L-histidine does exist in plants and fermented foods. The naturally occurring dipeptides found in muscle, carnosine and anserine are both comprised of L-histidine and beta-alanine.

L-histidine is one of the 10 essential amino acids for infants. It has never been clear if L-histidine is an essential amino acid for adults. At the very least, it is a conditional essential amino acid for adults. That is, even though L-histidine is synthesized in adult human tissues, sufficient quantities may not be made to meet the physiological requirements imposed by certain stress or disease situations.

L-histidine is a solid water-soluble substance. Chemically, it is called (S)-alpha-amino-1H-imidazole-4-propanoic acid; alpha-amino-4 (or 5)-imidazolepropionic acid; L-2-amino-3-(1H-imidazol-4yl) propionic acid, and glyoxaline-5-alanine. Its IUPAC abbreviation is His, and its one-letter abbreviation is H. L-histidine is classified as a basic amino acid. L-histidine has the following structural formula:

L-Histidine

ACTIONS AND PHARMACOLOGY

ACTIONS

The actions of supplemental L-histidine are entirely unclear. It may have some immunomodulatory as well as antioxidant activity.

MECHANISM OF ACTION

Since the actions of supplemental L-histidine are unclear, any postulated mechanism is entirely speculative. However, some facts are known about L-histidine and some of its metabolites, such as histamine and trans-urocanic acid, which suggest that supplemental L-histidine may one day be shown to have immunomodulatory and/or antioxidant activities. Low free histidine has been found in the serum of some rheumatoid arthritis patients. Serum concentrations of other amino acids have been found to be normal in these patients. L-histidine is an excellent chelating agent for such metals as copper, iron and zinc. Copper and iron participate in a reaction (Fenton reaction) that generates potent reactive oxygen species that could be destructive to tissues, including joints.

L-histidine is the obligate precursor of histamine, which is produced via the decarboxylation of the amino acid. In experimental animals, tissue histamine levels increase as the amount of dietary L-histidine increases. It is likely that this would be the case in humans as well. Histamine is known to possess immunomodulatory and antioxidant activity. Suppressor T cells have H_2 receptors, and histamine activates them. Promotion of suppressor T cell activity could be beneficial in rheumatoid arthritis. Further, histamine has been shown to down-regulate the production of reactive oxygen species in phagocytic cells, such as monocytes, by binding to the H_2 receptors on these cells. Decreased reactive oxygen species production by phagocytes could play antioxidant, anti-inflammatory and immunomodulatory roles in such diseases as rheumatoid arthritis.

This latter mechanism is the rationale for the use of histamine itself in several clinical trials studying histamine for the treatment of certain types of cancer and viral diseases. In these trials, down-regulation by histamine of reactive oxygen species formation appears to inhibit the suppression of natural killer (NK) cells and cytotoxic T lymphocytes, allowing these cells to be more effective in attacking cancer cells and virally infected cells.

PHARMACOKINETICS

L-histidine is absorbed from the small intestine via an active transport mechanism requiring the presence of sodium. From the small intestine, L-histidine is transported to the liver by means of the portal circulation, where some is metabolized and from whence some enters the systemic circulation to be distributed to various tissues in the body.

L-histidine is metabolized in several different ways. It is a substrate for protein synthesis; decarboxylation produces histamine; it is converted to trans-urocanate in the skin; it forms the dipeptides carnosine and anserine in muscle; it is a precursor of the thiol antioxidant, L-ergothioneine; and it forms alpha-ketoglutarate.

INDICATIONS AND USAGE

L-histidine may be indicated for use in some with rheumatoid arthritis. It is not indicated for treatment of anemia or uremia or for lowering serum cholesterol.

RESEARCH SUMMARY

It has been reported that rheumatoid arthritis (RA) sufferers have abnormally low blood levels of this amino acid. In a pilot study, RA patients received up to 6 grams of supplemental histidine daily and were said to benefit with as little as 1 gram daily. A subsequent study with 4.5 grams daily in some with more active and prolonged disease found much less benefit—but still enough to warrant further research.

CONTRAINDICATIONS, PRECAUTIONS, ADVERSE REACTIONS

CONTRAINDICATIONS

L-histidine supplementation is contraindicated in anyone hypersensitive to any component of the preparation.

PRECAUTIONS

L-histidine supplements should be avoided by children, pregnant women and nursing mothers. Those with allergies or peptic ulcer disease should only use L-histidine supplements under strict medical supervision. Although there are no reports of adverse events in these groups, increased histamine production from L-histidine might negatively affect those with these conditions.

ADVERSE REACTIONS

Mild gastrointestinal side effects have been reported. L-histidine is generally well tolerated.

INTERACTIONS

Medroxyprogesterone Acetate: L-histidine was observed to enhance (in tissue culture) the effect of medroxyprogesterone acetate in reducing the number of human breast cancer cells that were in the S phase.

H_1 and H_2 Blockers: Although not reported, L-histidine, via its metabolism to histamine, might decrease the efficacy of H_1 and H_2 blockers.

No other drug, nutritional supplement, food or herb interaction are known.

OVERDOSAGE

None reported.

DOSAGE AND ADMINISTRATION

Tablets and capsules typically are available in 500 milligram to 1000 milligram dosages. Dosages have ranged from 500 milligrams to 4.5 grams daily.

HOW SUPPLIED

Capsules — 600 mg
Powder
Tablets — 500 mg, 600 mg

LITERATURE

Blumenkrantz MJ, Shapiro DJ, Swendseid ME, Kopple JD. Histidine supplementation for treatment of anaemia of uraemia. *Br Med J.* 1975; 2(5970):530-533.

Gerber DA. Decreased concentration of free histidine in serum in rheumatoid arthritis, an isolated amino acid abnormality not associated with generalized hypoaminoacidemia. *J Rheumatol.* 1975; 2:384-392.

Gerber DA. Low free serum histidine concentration in rheumatoid arthritis. A measure of disease activity. *J Clin Invest.* 1975; 55:1124-1173.

Gerber DA, Sklar JE, Niedwiadowiez J. Lack of effect of oral L-histidine on the serum cholesterol in human subjects. *Am J Clin Nutr.* 1971; 24:1382-1383.

Gerber DA, Tanenbaum L, Ahrens M. Free serum histidine levels in patients with rheumatoid arthritis and control subjects following an oral load of free L-histidine. *Metabolism.* 1976; 25:655-657.

Ghezzo F, Racca S, Conti G, et al. L-histidine medroxyprogesterone acetate interaction modulates human breast cancer cell growth and progestin receptor expression in vitro. *Pharmacy Res.* 1997; 35:119-122.

Griswold DE, Alessi S, Badger AM, et al. Inhibitions of T suppressor cell expression by histamine type 2 (H₂) receptor antagonists. *J Immunol.* 1984; 132:3054-3057.

Hellstrand K, Dalgren C, Hermodsson S. Histaminergic regulation of NK cells. Role of monocyte-derived reactive oxygen metabolites. *J Immunol.* 1994; 153:4940-4947.

Lee NS, Fitzpatrick D, Meier E, Fisher H. Influence of dietary histidine on tissue histamine concentration, histidine decorboxylase and histamine methyltransferase activity in the rat. *Agents Actions.* 1981; 11:307-311.

Pinals RS, Harris ED, Burnett JB, Gerber DA. Treatment of rheumatoid arthritis with L-histidine: a randomized, placebo-controlled, double-blind trial. *J Rheumatol.* 1977; 4:414-419.

Lithium

TRADE NAMES

Trade names of prescription-only products include Eskalith and Eskalith-CR (SmithKline Beecham), and Lithobid (Solvay).

DESCRIPTION

Lithium is the lightest element of the alkali-metal group and the lightest metal. Its atomic number is 3 and its symbol Li. Lithium is a very reactive metal and is found naturally as lithium salts. Lithium is best known for its pharmaceutical use in the treatment of bipolar disorder or manic-depressive illness. Lithium is not currently considered an essential nutrient for humans. However, certain lithium deficiency states have been reported in some animals. Rats fed diets low in lithium were found to have depressed fertility, birth weight, litter size and weaning weight. Goats fed diets deficient in lithium were reported to have depressed fertility, birth weight and life span, as well as altered activity of several liver and blood enzymes. At least for rats and goats, lithium may serve an essential nutrient role.

Lithium is present in the human diet in ultratrace quantities and is found in some natural mineral waters. The typical daily dietary intake of lithium is approximately 200 to 600 micrograms. Fish, processed meat, milk, milk products, eggs,

potatoes and vegetables are rich sources of this mineral. It has been suggested that lithium, at low-dosage levels, has a generally beneficial effect on human behavior. This suggestion was based on a report that associated higher incidence of violent crimes with low-lithium drinking water.

Lithium carbonate and lithium citrate are the pharmaceutical forms used for the treatment of bipolar affective disorder. Lithium gamma-linolenic acid is in clinical studies for the treatment of certain types of cancer. Lithium succinate is used in the United Kingdom as a topical treatment for seborrheic dermatitis.

For information on the pharmaceutical use of lithium for the treatment of manic-depressive illness, refer to the *Physicians' Desk Reference*. For information on lithium interactions, refer to the *Physicians' Desk Reference Companion Guide*.

ACTIONS AND PHARMACOLOGY

ACTIONS

None known for dietary lithium.

INDICATIONS

There are no indications for the supplemental use of lithium. Suggestions that it might be useful in treating alcoholism, cancer or immune disorders are unfounded. Its use in treating manic-depressive illness requires strict medical supervision. There is very little safety margin between therapeutic and toxic doses.

RESEARCH SUMMARY

There is no credible research to support the supplemental or medically unsupervised use of lithium for any purpose.

CONTRAINDICATIONS, PRECAUTIONS, ADVERSE REACTIONS

CONTRAINDICATIONS

None known for dietary lithium. See *Physicians' Desk Reference* for pharmaceutical use of lithium.

OVERDOSAGE

None known for dietary lithium. See *Physicians' Desk Reference* for pharmaceutical lithium.

DOSAGE AND ADMINISTRATION

No recommended dosage. Lithium may be found in colloidal minerals and some mineral waters.

HOW SUPPLIED

OTC Forms and strengths include:

Tablets — 50 mcg

Prescription-only forms and strengths include:

Capsules — 150 mg, 300 mg, 600 mg

Extended Release Tablets — 300 mg, 450 mg

Syrup — 300 mg/5 ml

LITERATURE

Nielsen FH. Ultratrace minerals. In: Shils ME, Olson JA, Shike M, Ross AC, eds. *Modern Nutrition in Health and Disease.* 9th ed. Baltimore, MD: Williams and Wilkins; 1999: 283-303.

Pickett EE, O'Dell BL. Evidence for dietary essentiality of lithium in the rat. *Biol Trace Elem Res.* 1992; 34:299-319.

Schrauzer GN, Shrestha KP. Lithium in drinking water and the incidence of crimes, suicides and arrests related to drug addictions. *Biol Trace Elem Res.* 1990; 25:105-113.

Lithium Gamma-Linolenic Acid (Li-GLA)

DESCRIPTION

Lithium gamma-linolenic acid is the lithium salt of the 18-carbon, n-6 polyunsaturated fatty acid gamma-linolenic acid or GLA. (See GLA.) Lithium gamma-linolenic acid, abbreviated Li-GLA, was developed to enhance the water solubility of GLA.

Lithium gamma-linolenic acid, in addition to being known as Li-GLA, is known as lithium gammalinolenate.

ACTIONS AND PHARMACOLOGY

ACTIONS

Li-GLA has putative cytotoxic activity against cells chronically infected with HIV-1 and putative antiproliferative activity in tumor cells.

MECHANISM OF ACTION

The mechanism of the putative actions of Li-GLA are speculative. It is hypothesized that the antiproliferative activity in tumor cells is due to the generation, from Li-GLA, of reactive oxygen species, which damage the tumor cells. Likewise, it is speculated that such reactive oxygen species are cytotoxic to cells chronically infected with HIV-1.

PHARMACOKINETICS

Studies of Li-GLA on pancreatic cancer patients have used intravenous infusions of the substance. Little information is available on the pharmacokinetics of oral Li-GLA.

INDICATIONS AND USAGE

Li-GLA has shown activity against HIV infected T-cells. It also has shown antiproliferative activity in tumor cells.

RESEARCH SUMMARY

Li-GLA has been reported, in preliminary research, to have selective cell-killing effects in human T-lymphoblastoid cells chronically infected with HIV. This *in vitro* work needs follow-up.

Li-GLA inhibits the growth of pancreatic cancer cells *in vitro*. It has also been reported to prolong the survival of those with pancreatic cancer. Follow-up with randomized prospective studies is needed to determine if Li-GLA might have any role to play in the management of pancreatic cancer or any other type of cancer.

CONTRAINDICATIONS, PRECAUTIONS, ADVERSE REACTIONS

CONTRAINDICATIONS

None known.

PRECAUTIONS

Li-GLA should not be used by pregnant women or nursing mothers unless recommended by a physician. Li-GLA should not be used before surgery.

ADVERSE REACTIONS

Li-GLA has mainly been used in clinical studies administered intravenously. There is little experience with oral Li-GLA.

INTERACTIONS

No interactions between Li-GLA and warfarin, aspirin, other NSAIDs or herbs, such as *Allium sativum* (garlic) or *Ginkgo biloba,* have been reported. Such interactions, if they were to occur, might be manifested by nosebleeds and/or increased susceptibility to bruising. If this does occur, Li-GLA intake should be lowered or stopped.

OVERDOSAGE

There have been no reports of overdosage in the literature.

DOSAGE AND ADMINISTRATION

Oral Li-GLA is presently not available.

LITERATURE

Botha JH, Robinson KM, Leary WP. The response of human carcinoma cell lines to gamma-linolenic acid with special reference to the effects of agents which influence prostaglandin and thromboxane syntheses. *Prostaglandins Leukot Med.* 1985; 19:63-77.

de Antueno R, Elliot M, Ells G, et al. *In vivo* and *in vitro* biotransformation of the lithium salt of gamma-linolenic acid by three human carcinomas. *Br J Cancer.* 1997; 75:1812-1818.

Fearon KC, Falconer JS, Ross JA, et al. An open-label phase I/II dose escalation study of the treatment of pancreatic cancer using lithium gammalinolenate. *Anticancer Res.* 1996; 16; 867-874.

Ferguson PJ. Synergistic cytotoxicity between gamma-linolenic acid and the flavonoid naringenin against a human oral squamous carcinoma cell line (Meeting abstract). *Proc Annu Meet Am Assoc Cancer Res.* 1997; 38:A2148.

Ilc K, Ferrero JM, Fischel JL, et al. Cytotoxic effects of two gamma linolenic salts (lithium gammalinolenate or meglumine gammalinolenate) alone or associated with a nitrosourea: an experimental study on human glioblastoma cell lines. *Anticancer Drugs.* 1999; 10:413-417.

Kairemo KJ, Jekunen AP, Korppi-Tommola ET, Pyrhonen SO. The effect of lithium gamma-linolenate therapy of pancreatic cancer on perfusion in liver and pancreatic tissues. *Pancreas.* 1998; 16:105-106.

Kinchington D, Randall S, Winther M, Horrobin D. Lithium gamma-linolenate-induced cytotoxicity against cells chronically infected with HIV-1. *FEBS Lett.* 1993; 330:219-221.

Ravichandran D, Cooper A, Johnson CD. Effect of lithium gamma-linoenate on the growth of experimental human pancreatic carcinoma. *Br J Surg.* 1998; 85:1201-1205.

Ravichandran D, Cooper A, Johnson CD. Growth inhibitory effect of lithium gammalinolenate on pancreatic cancer cell lines: the influence of albumin and iron. *Eur J Cancer.* 1998; 34:188-192.

Seegers JC, Lotterling ML, Panzer A, et al. Comparative antimitotic effects of lithium gamma-linolenate, gamma-linolenic acid and arachidonic acid, on transformed and embryonic dells. *Prostaglandins Leukot Essent Fatty Acids.* 1998; 59:285-291.

Liver Hydrolysate/ Desiccated Liver

TRADE NAMES
L.I.B. (Merit Pharmaceuticals), Beef Liver Argentine (Ultimate Nutrition), Uni-Liver (Universal Nutrition), Livitrate (Progressive Laboratories), Argentine Liver Concentrate (Kal), Raw Liver (Premier Labs).

DESCRIPTION
Liver hydrolysate and desiccated liver have been marketed as nutritional supplements for over a century. They are principally used as a source of heme iron (see Iron).

Liver hydrolysate is typically prepared from bovine liver by partial enzymatic hydrolysis and processed to remove most of the fat and cholesterol. Desiccated liver is typically prepared by a freeze-drying process and retains fat and cholesterol. Liver hydrolysate is also known as liver extract and liquid liver extract.

ACTIONS AND PHARMACOLOGY
ACTIONS
Liver hydrolysate and desiccated liver may have hematinic activity. Liver hydrolysate has putative hepatoprotective activity.

MECHANISM OF ACTION
Hematinic activity refers to the ability of a substance to improve the quality of the blood, including the hemoglobin level and the number of erythrocytes. Liver hydrolysate and desiccated liver contain heme iron, an absorbable form of iron, which may promote the production of hemoglobin.

The putative hepatoprotective activity of liver hydrolysate is unknown.

PHARMACOKINETICS
The components of liver hydrolysate and desiccated liver are digested, absorbed and metabolized by normal physiological processes.

INDICATIONS AND USAGE
Claims are made that liver supplements improve fat metabolism, impart energy, help damaged tissues regenerate and protect the liver. There is no credible evidence to support any of these claims.

RESEARCH SUMMARY
There are no credible studies supporting the use of liver supplements.

CONTRAINDICATIONS, PRECAUTIONS, ADVERSE REACTIONS
CONTRAINDICATIONS
Liver hydrolysate and desiccated liver are contraindicated in those who are hypersensitive to any component of a liver hydrolysate- or desiccated liver-containing supplement.

PRECAUTIONS
Liver hydrolysate and desiccated liver supplements should be avoided by pregnant women, nursing mothers and children.

Those with hemochromatosis, sickle cell anemia, sideoblastic anemia and thalassemia should be extremely cautious in the use of liver hydrolysate and desiccated liver supplements.

Those who receive frequent blood transfusions and those with chronic liver failure should be extremely cautious in the use of liver hydrolysate and desiccated liver supplements.

The treatment of iron-deficiency anemia should be under the advice and supervision of a physician. Liver hydrolysate and desiccated liver are not standard treatments for iron-deficiency anemia.

ADVERSE REACTIONS
No reports.

INTERACTIONS
DRUGS
Heme iron is unlikely to have the types of drug interactions that iron salts do (see Iron).

NUTRITIONAL SUPPLEMENTS
Heme iron in liver hydrolysate and desiccated liver may be additive to the effects of iron supplements.

DOSAGE AND ADMINISTRATION
There are several forms of liver hydrolysate and desiccated liver that are marketed as nutritional supplements. There are no typical doses of these supplements.

HOW SUPPLIED
Capsules — 475 mg, 500 mg, 550 mg, 1000 mg, 2000 mg
Injection

Tablets — 10.5 gr, 30 gr

LITERATURE

Fujisawa K. Therapeutic effects of liver hydrolysate preparation on chronic hepatitis: a double-blind, controlled study. *Asian Med J*. 1984; 26:497-526.

Ohbayashi A, Akioka T, Tasaki H. A study of effects of liver hydrolysate on hepatic circulation. *J Therapy*. 1972; 54:1582-1585.

Washizuka M, Hiraga Y, Furuichi H, et al. [Effect of liver hydrolysate on ethanol- and acetaldehyde- induced deficiencies]. [Article in Japanese]. *Nippon Yakurigaku Zasshi*. 1998; 111:117-125.

L-Lysine

TRADE NAMES

Free Form L-Lysine (Thompson), L-Lysine Premium (Ultimate Nutrition).

DESCRIPTION

L-lysine is protein amino acid. It is classified as an essential amino acid for humans and therefore must be supplied in the diet. Certain proteins, such as those found in meat, poultry and milk are rich in L-lysine. Proteins found in grains, cereals and their products are typically low in L-lysine. For example, wheat is low in L-lysine; wheat germ, however, is rich in L-lysine. Small amounts of free L-lysine are found in vegetables, vegetable juices and in such fermented foods as miso and yogurt.

L-lysine's popularity as a nutritional supplement arose as a result of some studies suggesting that the amino acid may decrease the recurrence rate of some infected with herpes simplex virus.

L-lysine is a basic amino acid and carries a positive charge at physiological pH. It is a solid substance that is very soluble in water. L-lysine has three pKa's: $pKa_1=2.20$, $pKa_2=8.90$ and $pKa_3=10.28$. L-lysine is marketed as a nutritional substance, either as L-lysine monohydrochloride or as the free base, L-lysine. The molecular weight of L-lysine is 146.19 daltons, its molecular formula is $C_6H_{14}N_2O_2$, and its structural formula is:

L-lysine

L-lysine is also known as (S)- 2, 6, -diaminohexanoic acid and alpha, epsilon-diaminocaproic acid It is abbreviated as Lys or by its one letter abbreviation, K. L-lysine and lysine are frequently used interchangeably. The D-stereoisomer (D-lysine) is not biologically active.

ACTIONS AND PHARMACOLOGY

ACTIONS

Supplemental L-lysine has putative anti-herpes simplex virus activity. There is preliminary research suggesting that it may have some anti-osteoporotic activity.

MECHANISM OF ACTION

Proteins of the herpes simplex virus are rich in L-arginine, and tissue culture studies indicate an enhancing effect on viral replication when the amino acid ratio of L-arginine to L-lysine is high in the tissue culture media. When the ratio of L-lysine to L-arginine is high, viral replication and the cytopathogenicity of herpes simplex virus have been found to be inhibited.

L-lysine may facilitate the absorption of calcium from the small intestine.

PHARMACOKINETICS

Following ingestion, L-lysine is absorbed from the lumen of the small intestine into the enterocytes by an active transport process. Some metabolism of L-lysine takes place within the enterocytes. That which is not metabolized is transported to the liver via the portal circulation. In the liver, L-lysine, along with other amino acids, participates in protein biosynthesis. Some is metabolized to L-alpha-aminoadipic acid semialdehyde, which is further metabolized to acetoacetyl-CoA. The intermediate in this pathway is saccharopine. L-lysine does not participate in transamination. It is the exception to the general rule that the first step in catabolism of an amino acid is the removal of its alpha-amino group by transamination to form the respective alpha-keto acid. L-lysine is both a glycogenic and a ketogenic amino acid. It can participate in the formation of D-glucose and glycogen, as well as lipids. It can also participate in the production of energy.

L-lysine that is not metabolized in the liver is transported to the various tissues of the body, where it is involved in reactions similar to those described above. L-hydroxylysine, found in collagen and elastin, is formed post-translationally.

INDICATIONS AND USAGE

Lysine may reduce the recurrence rate of herpes simplex virus (HSV) infections and/or reduce their severity in some, though research results have been mixed with respect to this putative benefit. Very preliminary research indicates a possible role for lysine in the prevention and treatment of osteoporosis.

RESEARCH SUMMARY

A number of clinical studies have found that lysine is useful in preventing and sometimes shortening outbreaks of herpes simplex infections. A few studies have found no effect. *In vitro* and animal studies have also found evidence of lysine's anti-herpetic effects.

In a double-blind, placebo-controlled, multicenter trial of oral lysine, the treatment group received 1000 mg of lysine three times daily (3000 mg daily) for six months. During that period, the treated subjects had an average of 2.4 fewer HSV infections, and their symptoms were significantly less severe and healing times significantly reduced.

In another randomized, double-blind, cross-over study, a daily dose of 1248 mg (but not 624 mg) of lysine was found to decrease the recurrence rate of HSV in non-immunocompromised subjects. In this study, the 1248 mg dosage did not shorten healing time.

There is one study suggesting that supplemental lysine can both enhance intestinal absorption and improve renal conservation of absorbed calcium and that it might thus be helpful in osteoporosis. Further research is needed.

CONTRAINDICATIONS, PRECAUTIONS, ADVERSE REACTIONS

CONTRAINDICATIONS

L-lysine supplementation is contraindicated in those with the rare genetic disorder hyperlysinemia/hyperlysinuria.

PRECAUTIONS

Pregnant women and nursing mothers should only consider using supplemental L-lysine if their diets are low in this amino acid. They should avoid supplemental L-lysine for other reasons.

Proteins such as casein, which are high in L-lysine relative to L-arginine, are associated with elevated cholesterol levels. Those with hypercholesterolemia who are interested in taking supplemental L-lysine should be aware of this.

Those with hepatic or renal failure should exercise caution in the use of supplemental L-lysine.

ADVERSE REACTIONS

Doses up to 3 grams daily are generally well tolerated. Very high doses—greater than 10 to 15 grams daily—may cause gastrointestinal symptoms, such as nausea, abdominal cramps and diarrhea.

There is one report of Fanconi's syndrome and tubulointestinal nephritis in a 44-year old woman associated with the use of supplemental L-lysine.

INTERACTIONS

NUTRITIONAL SUPPLEMENTS

Concomitant use of calcium supplements and L-lysine may increase calcium absorption. This is based on a very preliminary study that needs follow-up.

OVERDOSAGE

There are no reports of overdosage with L-lysine.

DOSAGE AND ADMINISTRATION

Typical dosage used for possible prevention of herpes simplex virus recurrence is 500 mg to 3 grams daily. The average dose is 1 gram daily. Higher doses are split throughout the day.

HOW SUPPLIED

Capsules — 500 mg
Powder
Tablets — 333 mg, 500 mg, 1000 mg

LITERATURE

Civitelli R, Villareal DT, Agnusedei D, et al. Dietary L-lysine and calcium metabolism in humans. *Nutrition.* 1992; 8:400-405.

Di Giovanna JJ, Blank H. Failure of lysine in frequently recurrent herpes simplex infection. Treatment and prophylaxis. *Arch Dermatol.* 1984; 120:48-51.

Flondin NW. The metabolic roles, pharmacology, and toxicology of lysine. *J Am Coll Nutr.* 1997; 16:7-21.

Griffith RS, De Long DC, Nelson JD. Relation of L-arginine—lysine antagonism to herpes simplex growth in tissue culture. *Chemotherapy.* 1981; 27:209-213.

Griffith RS, Walsh DE, Myrmel KH, et al. Success of L-lysine therapy in frequently recurrent herpes simplex infection. Treatment and prophylaxis. *Dermatologica.* 1987; 175:183-190.

Lo JC, Chertow GM, Rennke H, Seifter JL. Fanconi's syndrome and tubulointestinal nephritis in association with L-lysine ingestion. *Am J Kidney Dis.* 1996; 28:614-617.

McCune MA, Perry HO, Muller SA, O'Fallon WM. Treatment of recurrent herpes simplex infections with L-lysine monohydrochloride. *Cutis.* 1984; 34:366-373.

Rajamohan T, Kurup PA. Lysine: arginine ratio of a protein influences cholesterol metabolism: Part 1—studies on sesame protein having low lysine: arginine ratio. *Indian J Exp Biol.* 1997; 35:1218-1223.

Thein DJ, Hurt WC. Lysine as a prophylactic agent in the treatment of recurrent herpes simplex labialis. *Oral Surg Oral Med Oral Pathol.* 1984; 58:659-666.

L-Methionine

DESCRIPTION

L-methionine is a protein amino acid. It is classified as an essential amino acid for humans and therefore must be supplied in the diet. According to the Food and Agriculture Organization of the United Nations (FAO) and World Health Organization (WHO), recommended daily L-methionine intake is 13 mg per kg or about one gram daily for adults. Actual intake is higher. This is principally derived from dietary proteins. Rich sources of L-methionine include cheeses, eggs, fish, meat and poultry. L-methionine is also found in fruits and vegetables, but not as abundantly. Small amounts of free L-methionine occur in vegetables, vegetable juices and fermented foods.

In addition to its role as a precursor in protein synthesis, L-methionine participates in a wide range of biochemical reactions, including the production of S-adenosylmethionine (SAM or SAMe), L-cysteine, glutathione, taurine and sulfate. SAM itself, as a methyl donor (see SAMe), is involved in the synthesis of creatine, epinephrine, melatonin and the polyamines spermine and spermidine, among several other substances.

L-methionine is also a glycogenic amino acid and may participate in the formation of D-glucose and glycogen. The ability of L-methionine to reduce the liver-toxic effects of such hepatotoxins as acetaminophen and methotrexate has led to the suggestion that methionine should be added to acetaminophen products. However, there is some recent research suggesting that elevated L-methionine intake may promote intestinal carcinogenesis. This is unclear. Further, one of the metabolites of L-methionine, L-homocysteine, has been implicated as a significant factor in coronary heart disease and other vascular diseases.

L-methionine is a sulfur-containing amino acid that is minimally soluble in water. Its molecular formula is $C_5H_{11}NO_2S$, and its molecular weight is 149.21 daltons. L-methionine is also known as 2-amino-4-(methylthio)butyric acid, alpha-amino-gamma-methylmercaptobutyric acid, (S)-2-amino-4-(methylthio)butanoic acid and gamma-methyl-thio-alpha-aminobutyric acid. It is abbreviated as Met and its one-letter abbreviation is M. The terms L-methionine and methionine are used interchangeably. The D-stereoisomer, D-methionine, does not possess biological activity with regard to protein synthesis and the biochemical reactions mentioned above. However, D-methionine, as well as L-methionine, may possess antioxidant activity. L-methionine is represented by the following chemical structure:

L-methionine

ACTIONS AND PHARMACOLOGY

ACTIONS

L-methionine may protect against the toxic effects of hepatotoxins, such as acetaminophen. Methionine may have antioxidant activity.

MECHANISM OF ACTION

The mechanism of the possible anti-hepatotoxic activity of L-methionine is not entirely clear. It is thought that metabolism of high doses of acetaminophen in the liver lead to decreased levels of hepatic glutathione and increased oxidative stress. L-methionine is a precursor to L-cysteine. L-cysteine itself may have antioxidant activity. L-cysteine is also a precursor to the antioxidant glutathione. Antioxidant activity of L-methionine and metabolites of L-methionine appear to account for its possible anti-hepatotoxic activity. Recent research suggests that methionine itself has free-radical scavenging activity by virtue of its sulfur, as well as its chelating ability.

PHARMACOKINETICS

Following ingestion, L-methionine is absorbed from the lumen of the small intestine into the enterocytes by an active transport process. Some metabolism of L-methionine takes place within the enterocytes. That which is not metabolized is transported to the liver via the portal circulation. In the liver, L-methionine, along with other amino acids, participates in protein biosynthesis. It may also participate in a wide variety of metabolic reactions, including the formation of SAMe, L-homocysteine, L-cysteine, taurine and sulfate. It can also be metabolized to produce D-glucose and glycogen. L-methionine not metabolized in the liver is transported to the various tissues of the body where it is involved in reactions similar to those described above.

INDICATIONS AND USAGE

There are no indications for the use of supplemental methionine unless specifically recommended by a physician. It is effective as an antidote in some cases of acetaminophen poisoning. But, because some research suggests that it may promote some cancers, its use as a supplement is inadvisable.

RESEARCH SUMMARY

When given within 10 hours of acetaminophen poisoning, oral methionine has been found to be as effective as N-acetylcysteine in preventing severe liver damage and death. There is preliminary evidence that methionine might also help protect against some of the adverse side effects of methotrexate and gentamicin, among others.

On the other hand, high intake of methionine can lead to increased levels of the oxidant homocysteine. There is some fear that high intake of dietary methionine can promote some cancers, and there is some very preliminary experimental data to support that fear. There is also some epidemiological data suggesting a link between increased dietary methionine and increased risk of gastric cancer. More research is needed.

CONTRAINDICATIONS, PRECAUTIONS, ADVERSE REACTIONS

CONTRAINDICATIONS

L-methionine is contraindicated in those with the genetic disorder homocystinuria. It is also contraindicated in those who are hypersensitive to any component of a methionine-containing product.

PRECAUTIONS

L-methionine supplements should be avoided by pregnant women and nursing mothers unless they are prescribed by a physician.

L-methionine supplementation should be avoided by those with neoplastic disease. It should also be avoided by those with elevated homocysteine levels and used with caution in those with coronary heart disease.

Supplemental L-methionine should be used with great caution in those with schizophrenia and those with hepatic and renal failure. In any case, L-methionine supplements should only be used if recommended and monitored by a physician.

ADVERSE REACTIONS

Doses of L-methionine of up to 250 mg daily are generally well tolerated. Higher doses may cause nausea, vomiting and headache. Healthy adults taking 8 grams of L-methionine daily for four days were found to have reduced serum folate levels and leucocytosis. Healthy adults taking 13.9 grams of L-methionine daily for five days were found to have changes in serum pH and potassium and increased urinary calcium excretion. Schizophrenic patients given 10 to 20 grams of L-methionine daily for two weeks developed functional psychoses. Single doses of 8 grams precipitated encephalopathy in patients with cirrhosis.

INTERACTIONS

DRUGS

Acetaminophen and methotrexate: L-methionine may decrease hepatic toxicity in those with acetaminophen overdosage or in those taking methotrexate. Theoretically, it may decrease hepatic toxicity in the case of other potential hepatotoxic drugs, as well.

Gentamicin: Methionine may protect against the ototoxic effects of gentamicin.

NUTRITIONAL SUPPLEMENTS

Dietary supplementation with L-methionine was found to decrease glycine levels when given to healthy women on a low-protein diet.

High L-methionine intake in a diet high in salt and nitrites/nitrates may increase the risk of stomach cancer.

OVERDOSAGE

There are no reports of overdosage.

DOSAGE AND ADMINISTRATION

L-methionine supplements should only be taken with a physician's recommendation.

HOW SUPPLIED

Capsules — 500 mg

Powder

Tablets — 200 mg, 500 mg

LITERATURE

Bellone J, Farello G, Bartoletta E, et al. Methionine potentiates both basal and GHRH-induced GH secretion in children. *Clin Endocrinol (Oxf).* 1997; 47:61-64.

Breillot F, Hadida F, Echinard-Darin P, et al. Decreased rat rhabdomyosarcoma pulmonary metastases in response to low methionine diet. *Anticanc Res.* 1986; 76:6299-639.

Duranton B, Freund JN, Galluser M, et al. Promotion of intestinal carcinogenesis by dietary methionine. *Carcinogenesis.* 1999; 20:493-497.

Hladovec J, Sommerova Z, Pisarikova A. Homocysteinemia and endothelial damage after methionine load. *Thrombo Res.* 1997; 88:361-364.

Jones AL, Hayes PC, Proudfoot AT, Vale JA, Prescott LF, Krenzelok EP. Should methionine be added to every paracetamol tablet? *BMJ.* 1997; 315:301-304.

Kroger H, Hauschild A, Ohde M, et al. Nicotinamide and methionine reduce the liver toxic effects of methotrexate. *Gen Pharmacol.* 1999; 33:203-206.

La Vecchia C, Negri E, Franceschi S, Decarli A. Case-control study on influence of methionine, nitrite, and salt on gastric carcinogenesis in northern Italy. *Nutr Canc.* 1997; 27:65-68.

Meakins TS, Persaud C, Jackson AA. Dietary supplementation with L-methionine impairs the utilization of urea-nitrogen and increases 5-L-oxoprolinuria in normal women consuming a low protein diet. *J Nutr* 1998; 128:720-727.

Sha S-H, Schacht J. Antioxidants attenuate gentamicin-induced free radical formation *in vitro* and ototoxicity *in vivo*: D-methionine is a potential protectant. *Hearing Res.* 2000; 142:34-40.

Vale JA, Meredith TJ, Goulding R. Treatment of acetaminophen poisoning. The use of oral methionine. *Arch Int Med.* 1981; 141(3 Spec No):394-396.

L-Ornithine

TRADE NAMES

L-Ornithine is available from numerous manufacturers generically; branded products include OKG (Nature's Bounty).

DESCRIPTION

L-Ornithine is a nonprotein amino acid. It is used in the body in the biosynthesis of L-arginine, L-proline and polyamines. L-Ornithine is a basic amino acid, positively charged at physiological pH. It is also known as alpha,delta-diaminovaleric acid and 2,5-diaminopentanoic acid. The molecular formula of L-ornithine is $C_5H_{12}N_2O_2$, and its molecular weight is 132.16 daltons. The structural formula is:

L-Ornithine

L-Ornithine is used as a nutritional supplement principally for its putative anabolic activity. There is little evidence to support this use. However, a derivative of L-ornithine called ornithine alpha-ketoglutarate or OKG (see Ornithine Alpha-Ketoglutarate) may, under certain conditions, have immunomodulatory and anticatabolic and/or anabolic actions.

ACTIONS AND PHARMACOLOGY

ACTIONS

L-Ornithine has putative anabolic, immunomodulatory and wound-healing activities.

MECHANISM OF ACTION

L-Ornithine may at very high doses—around 30 grams—stimulate the pituitary release of growth hormone by virtue of its metabolism to L-arginine (see L-Arginine).

Burn injury and other traumas affect the status of L-arginine in the various tissues of the body. *De novo* synthesis of L-arginine during these conditions is probably not sufficient for normal immune function, nor for normal protein synthesis. Under these conditions, L-ornithine may have immunomodulatory and wound-healing activities, again, by virtue of its metabolism to L-arginine.

PHARMACOKINETICS

Following ingestion, L-ornithine is absorbed from the small intestine via a sodium-dependent active transport process. The transport system for L-ornithine is shared with L-arginine, L-lysine and L-cystine. L-ornithine is transported via the portal circulation to the liver where it undergoes extensive metabolism to L-arginine, polyamines and proline, among other metabolites. L-Ornithine that is not metabolized in the liver is distributed by the systemic circulation to the various cells of the body.

INDICATIONS AND USAGE

It is claimed that ornithine has anabolic effects and improves athletic performance, that it has wound-healing effects and is immuno-enhancing. There is little support for these claims. There is at least preliminary evidence, however, that the better-studied ornithine alpha-ketoglutarate may have some of these activities. Inasmuch as ornithine is metabolized to arginine, which also demonstrates some of these effects, it is possible that ornithine, when more thoroughly studied, might exhibit some similar effects. See Arginine and Ornithine Alpha-Ketoglutarate.

RESEARCH SUMMARY

In one double-blind, placebo-controlled study, a combination of 1 gram of arginine and 1 gram of ornithine daily, used in conjunction with a high-intensity strength-training program over a five-week period, increased total strength and lean body mass in adult males, compared with controls. Most trials using ornithine alone, however, have reported no significant anabolic effects. Most of these studies have failed to show that ornithine supplementation has any significant effect on insulin secretion or human growth hormone levels in bodybuilders. There is apparently only one study reporting that ornithine increased growth hormone levels in bodybuilders, and this study used a very high dose of the supplement (13 grams daily). Numerous gastrointestinal side effects were associated with this dosage.

CONTRAINDICATIONS, PRECAUTIONS, ADVERSE REACTIONS

CONTRAINDICATIONS

L-Ornithine is contraindicated in those with a deficiency of ornithine-delta-aminotransferase. This is a genetic disorder resulting in gyrate atrophy of the choroid and retina and progressive blinding chorioretinal degeneration. It is rare.

L-Ornithine is also contraindicated in those hypersensitive to any component of an ornithine-containing supplement.

PRECAUTIONS

Pregnant women and nursing mothers should avoid L-ornithine supplementation.

ADVERSE REACTIONS

Doses higher than 10 grams daily may cause such gastrointestinal symptoms as nausea, abdominal cramps and diarrhea.

DOSAGE AND ADMINISTRATION

Those who use L-ornithine take doses of 500 milligrams to 2 grams, usually before bedtime and on an empty stomach. Some combine L-ornithine with similar doses of L-arginine.

HOW SUPPLIED

Capsules — 500 mg, 650 mg, 750 mg, 1000 mg

Powder

LITERATURE

Barbul A. Arginine: biochemistry, physiology, and therapeutic implications. *J Parenter Enteral Nutr.* 1986; 10:227-238.

Bucci L, Hickson JF Jr, et al. Ornithine ingestion and growth hormone release in bodybuilders. *Nutr Res.* 1990; 10:239-245.

Bucci LR, Hickson JF Jr, Wolinsky I, Pivarnik JM. Ornithine supplementation and insulin release in bodybuilders. *Int J Sport Nut.* 1992; 2:289-291.

DeBandt J-P, Coudray-Lucas C, Lioret N, et al. A randomized controlled trial of the influence of the mode of enteral ornithine alpha-ketoglutarate administration in burn patients. *J Nutr.* 1998; 128:563-569.

Elam RP, Hardin DH, Sutton RA, Hagen L. Effects of arginine and ornithine on strength, lean body mass and urinary hydroxyproline in adult males. *J Sports Med Phys Fitness.* 1989; 29:52-56.

Fogelholm GM, Naveri HK, Kiilavuori KT, Harkoner MH. Low-dose amino acid supplementation: no effects on serum human growth hormone and insulin in male weightlifters. *Int J Sport Nutr.* 1993; 3:290-297.

Iwasaki K, Mano K, Ishihara M, et al. Effects of ornithine or arginine administration on serum amino acid levels. *Biochem Int.* 1987; 14:971-976.

Jeevanandam M, Holaday NJ, Petersen SR. Ornithine alpha-ketoglutarate (OKG) supplementation is more effective than its component salts in traumatized rats. *J Nutr.* 1996; 126:2141-2150.

Lambert MI, Hefer JA, Millar RP, Macfarlane PW. Failure of commercial oral amino acid supplements to increase serum growth hormone concentrations in male body builders. *Int J Sport Med.* 1993; 3:298-305.

Torre PM, Ronnenberg AG, Hartman WJ, Prior RL. Supplemental arginine and ornithine do not affect splenocyte proliferation in surgically treated rats. *J Parenter Enteral Nut.* 1993; 17:532-536.

L-Phenylalanine

DESCRIPTION

L-phenylalanine is a protein amino acid. It is classified as an essential amino acid because the body requires a dietary source of the amino acid to meet its physiological demands. L-phenylalanine is found in proteins of all life forms. Dietary sources of the amino acid are principally derived from animal and vegetable proteins. Vegetables and juices contain small amounts of the free amino acid. The free amino acid is also found in fermented foods such as yogurt and miso. The alternative sweetener aspartame is a dipeptide of L-phenylalanine, as is the methyl ester, and L-aspartic acid.

In addition to being involved in protein synthesis, L-phenylalanine is the precursor of L-tyrosine. The conversion of L-phenylalanine to L-tyrosine is via the enzyme L-phenylalanine hydroxylase. It is this enzyme that is virtually absent in those with the inborn error of metabolism phenylketonuria (PKU). L-tyrosine produced from L-phenylalanine is a precursor in the synthesis of the neurotransmitters norepinephrine and dopamine, among other reactions. L-phenylalanine is marketed as a nutritional supplement and used by some for its putative antidepressant activity.

L-phenylalanine is also known as beta-phenylalanine, alpha-aminohydrocinnamic acid, (S)-2-amino-3- phenylpropanoic acid and alpha-amino-beta-phenylpropionic acid. It is abbreviated as either Phe or by its one-letter abbreviation F. The molecular formula of L-phenylalanine is $C_9H_{11}NO_2$, and its molecular weight is 165.19 daltons. L-phenylalanine is an aromatic amino acid with the following structural formula:

L-phenylalanine

ACTIONS AND PHARMACOLOGY

ACTIONS

L-phenylalanine has putative antidepressant activity. It may also, when used in conjunction with UVA irradiation, have antivitiligo activity.

MECHANISM OF ACTION

The mechanism of L-phenylalanine's putative antidepressant activity may be accounted for by its precursor role in the synthesis of the neurotransmitters norepinephrine and dopamine. Elevated brain norepinephrine and dopamine levels are thought to be associated with antidepressant effects.

The mechanism of L-phenylalanine's possible antivitiligo activity is not well understood. It is thought that L-phenylalanine may stimulate the production of melanin in the affected skin.

PHARMACOKINETICS

Following ingestion, L-phenylalanine is absorbed from the small intestine by a sodium dependent active transport process. L-phenylalanine is transported from the small intestine to the liver via the portal circulation. In the liver, L-phenylalanine is involved in a number of biochemical reactions, including protein synthesis, the formation of L-tyrosine and oxidative catabolic reactions. L-phenylalanine that is not metabolized in the liver is distributed via the systemic circulation to the various tissues of the body, where it undergoes metabolic reactions similar to those that take place in the liver.

INDICATIONS AND USAGE

L-phenylalanine may be helpful in some with depression. It may also be useful in the treatment of vitiligo. There is some evidence that L-phenylalanine may exacerbate tardive dyskinesia in some schizophrenic patients and in some who have used neuroleptic drugs.

RESEARCH SUMMARY

Both oral and intravenous administration of L-deprenyl and L-phenylalanine in doses of 5 to 10 milligrams and 250 milligrams per day, respectively, demonstrated significant antidepressant effects in 155 unipolar depressed patients. In another preliminary study, L-phenylalanine was said to have mood-elevating effects in 31 of 40 depressed subjects. Followup is needed.

Several clinical studies have shown that L-phenylalanine may be helpful in the treatment of vitiligo in both children and adults. L-phenylalanine, in doses up to 100 mg/kg/day significantly improved vitiligo in 200 subjects when combined with UVA/sunlight. Best results were achieved in early-stage disease, but significant repigmentation occurred in some with later-stage disease who used the supplement/sunlight combination for prolonged periods. Another study confirmed these effects but found that no added benefit was derived from doses exceeding 50 mg/kg/day.

Recently, other researchers have reported on their six-year experience in treating vitiligo with L-phenylalanine in combination with daily sun exposure. Subjects treated by these researchers received oral L-phenylalanine 50 or 100 mg/kg/day plus topical 10% phenylalanine gel daily. The total average improvement rate was rated at 83.1%, but the improvement rate limited to those judged to have good response was 56.7%, with a 90.3% rate for the face, 42.8% for the trunk and 37.1% for the limbs. This uncontrolled, retrospective study involved 193 patients, male and female, children and adults, with evolving vitiligo of various types. There was no statistically significant difference in response rates between those who received 50 mg/kg/day versus those receiving 100 mg/kg/day or between children and adults.

On the negative side, there is a report that a loading dose of 100 mg/kg of L-phenylalanine exacerbated symptoms of tardive dyskinesia in some neuroleptic-treated depressives. In another study, the same L-phenylalanine challenge exacerbated tardive dyskinesia symptoms in schizophrenic subjects.

CONTRAINDICATIONS, PRECAUTIONS, ADVERSE REACTIONS

CONTRAINDICATIONS

L-phenylalanine is contraindicated in those with phenylketonuria. It is also contraindicated in those taking non-selective monoamine oxidase (MAO) inhibitors. L-phenylalanine is contraindicated in those hypersensitive to any component of an L-phenylalanine-containing supplement.

PRECAUTIONS

Pregnant women and nursing mothers should avoid supplementation with L-phenylalanine.

Tardive dyskinesia has been reported to be exacerbated after ingestion of L-phenylalanine by schizophrenics. Therefore, those with schizophrenia should exercise extreme caution in the use of supplemental L-phenylalanine.

Use of L-phenylalanine for vitiligo must be done under medical supervision.

Those with hypertension should exercise caution in the use of L-phenylalanine.

ADVERSE REACTIONS

L-phenylalanine will exacerbate symptoms of phenylketonuria if used by phenylketonurics. L-phenylalanine was reported to exacerbate tardive dyskinesia when used by some with schizophrenia.

INTERACTIONS

DRUGS

Non-selective monoamine oxidase (MAO) inhibitors: including phenelzine sulfate, tranylcypromine sulfate and pargyline HC1 — Concomitant use of L-phenylalanine and non-selective MAO inhibitors may cause hypertension.

Selegiline: L-phenylalanine and the selective MAO inhibitor selegiline may have synergistic antidepressant activity if used concomitantly.

Neuroleptic Drugs: L-phenylalanine may potentiate the tardive dyskinesia side reactions of neuroleptic drugs if used concomitantly with them.

OVERDOSAGE

There are no reports of Phenylalanine overdosage in the literature.

DOSAGE AND ADMINISTRATION.

L-phenylalanine supplements as well as DL-phenylalanine (see DL-Phenylalanine) supplements are available in the nutritional supplement marketplace. Those who use L-phenylalanine supplements typically use 500 milligrams to 1.5 grams daily.

HOW SUPPLIED

Capsules — 200 mg, 500 mg, 600 mg
Powder
Tablets — 500 mg

LITERATURE

Birkmayer W, Riederer P, Linauer W, Knoll J. L-deprenyl plus L-phenylalanine in the treatment of depression. *J Neural Transm.* 1984; 59:81-87.

Camacho F, Mazuecos J. Treatment of vitiligo with oral and topical phenylalanine: 6 years of experience. *Arch Dermatol.* 1999; 135:216-217.

Gardos G, Cole JO, Matthews JD, et al. The acute effects of a loading dose of phenylalanine in unipolar depressed patients with and without tardive dyskinesia. *Neuropsychopharmacology.* 1992; 6:241-247.

Gibbs J, Falasco JD, McHugh PR. Cholecystokinin-decreased food intake in rhesus monkeys. *Am J Physiol.* 1976; 230:15-18.

Kostiuk PG, Martyniuk AE. [Possible molecular mechanisms of brain dysfunction in phenylketonuria.] [Article in Russian.] *Patol Fiziol Eksp Ter.* 1992; Jul-Aug(4):34-36.

Kuiters GR, Hup JM, Siddiqui AH, Cormane RH. Oral phenylalanine loading and sunlight as source of UVA irradiation in vitiligo on the Caribbean island of Curacao. *J Trop Med Hyg.* 1986; 89:149-155.

Mosnik DM, Spring B, Rogers K, Baruah S. Tardive dyskinesia exacerbated after ingestion of phenylalanine by schizophrenic patients. *Neuropsycopharmacology.* 1997; 16:136-146.

Sabelli HC, Fawcett J, Gusovsky F, et al. Clinical studies on the phenylalanine hypothesis of affective disorder: urine and blood phenylacetic acid and phenylalanine dietary supplements. *J Clin Psychiatry.* 1986; 47:66-70.

Schulpis CH, Antoniou C, Michas T, Starigos J. Phenylalanine plus ultraviolet light: preliminary report of a promising treatment for childhood vitiligo. *Pediatr Dermatol.* 1989; 6:332-335.

Siddiqui AH, Stolk LM, Bhaggoe R, et al. L-phenylalanine and UVA irradiation in the treatment of vitiligo. *Dermatology.* 1994; 188:215-218.

Zhao G. [Inherited metabolic aberration of phenylalanine in the family members of patients with essential hypertension and stroke]. [Article in Chinese]. *Chung Hua I Hsueh Tsa Chih.* 1991; 71:388-390.

L-Theanine

DESCRIPTION

L-theanine is a non-protein amino acid mainly found naturally in the green tea plant *(Camellia sinensis)*. L-theanine is the predominant amino acid in green tea and makes up 50% of the total free amino acids in the plant. The amino acid constitutes between 1% and 2% of the dry weight of green tea leaves. L-theanine is considered the main component responsible for the taste of green tea, which in Japanese is called umami. L-theanine is marketed in Japan as a nutritional supplement for mood modulation.

L-theanine is a derivative of L-glutamic acid. It is a water-soluble solid substance with the molecular formula $C_7H_{14}O_3N$ and a molecular weight of 160.19 daltons. L-theanine is also known as gamma-ethylamino-L-glutamic acid, gamma-glutamylethylamide, r-glutamylethylamide, L-glutamic acid gamma-ethylamide and L-N-ethylglutamine. The chemical structure is:

L-theanine

ACTIONS AND PHARMACOLOGY

ACTIONS

L-theanine may have activity in modulating the metabolism of cancer chemotherapeutic agents and ameliorating their side effects. It may also have mood-modulating activity.

MECHANISM OF ACTION

In animal tumor models, L-theanine has been found to increase the antitumor activity of some anthracyline agents (doxorubicin, idarubicin) and to ameliorate some of the side effects of these agents. It appears that L-theanine inhibits the efflux of these agents from tumor cells, increasing the inhibitory concentration of the drugs in the target cells. At the same time, L-theanine appears to decrease the oxidative stress caused by these agents on normal cells. Most of the side effects of these agents are due to oxidative stress. The mechanism by which L-theanine inhibits the efflux of such cancer chemotherapeutic agents as doxorubicin is unclear. L-theanine appears to have modest antioxidant activity, and this may explain, in part, L-theanine's ability to ameliorate some of the side effects of the chemotherapeutic agents. Further, L-theanine, by an unclear mechanism, appears to inhibit the influx of chemotherapeutic normal cells.

The mechanism of L-theanine's possible mood-modulating activity is also unclear. The amino acid might affect the metabolism and the release of some neurotransmitters in the brain, such as dopamine.

PHARMACOKINETICS.

Little is known about the pharmacokinetics of L-theanine in humans. From animal studies, it appears that L-theanine is absorbed from the small intestine via a sodium-coupled active transport process and appears to cross the blood-brain barrier. Not much is known beyond that. However, research is ongoing.

INDICATIONS AND USAGE

L-theanine has exhibited anticancer effects and an ability to favorably modulate the activity of some anticancer drugs in *in vitro* and animal experiments. It has also demonstrated hypotensive effects in animal work. It has inhibited LDL-cholesterol oxidation in preliminary *in vitro* tests. It was recently reported to enhance learning ability in animals and to induce relaxation in human subjects, possibly through its effects on serotonin, dopamine and other neurotransmitters. It has also been shown to inhibit caffeine stimulation in another preliminary animal study.

RESEARCH SUMMARY

L-theanine has been shown to enhance the anticancer activity of doxorubicin and idarubicin in *in vitro* and animal studies. In an *in vitro* study, L-theanine increased doxorubicin's inhibition of Ehrlich ascites carcinoma more than two-fold and increased nearly three-fold the concentration of doxorubicin in the tumor compared with treatment with doxorubicin alone.

Subsequently, L-theanine, in combination with doxorubicin, was shown to significantly reduce tumor weight (to 62% of the control level) in M5076 ovarian sarcoma-bearing mice. The doxorubicin dose used in this combination was ineffective by itself in inhibiting tumor growth. L-theanine was reported to increase doxorubicin concentration in the tumor by two- to seven-fold while simultaneously decreasing doxorubicin concentrations in normal tissues.

A combination of L-theanine and doxorubicin significantly inhibited both primary ovarian sarcoma and hepatic metastasis of the tumor. L-theanine was credited in this study with enhancing the activity of doxorubicin.

In another study, L-theanine was used in conjunction with idarubicin, a recently synthesized anthracyline derivative being used clinically in some parts of the world to treat acute myelocytic leukemia. The use of idarubicin had been limited due to the frequency with which it produces severe leukopenia. Combined with idarubicin in the treatment of P388 leukemia-bearing mice, L-theanine significantly inhibited suppression of bone marrow cells and leukopenia, while simultaneously enhancing the antitumor activity of idarubicin.

Very recently, L-theanine, in combination with doxorubicin, was further shown to have the ability to significantly inhibit even doxorubicin-resistant leukemia in mice.

In an *in vitro* test, L-theanine showed some ability to inhibit LDL peroxidation. The polyphenol component of a green-tea extract was more potent in this regard than the L-theanine component. The caffeine component, on the other hand, was less effective than L-theanine.

L-theanine has also exhibited hypotensive effects in spontaneously hypertensive rats but not in Wistar kyoto rats. Recently, L-theanine, at certain doses, was shown to inhibit caffeine stimulation, measured by electroencephalography in rats.

Recently, L-theanine, previously shown to penetrate the blood-brain barrier through the leucine-preferring transport system, has been demonstrated to produce significant increases in serotonin and/or dopamine concentrations in the brain, principally in the striatum, hypothalamus and hippocampus.

These findings led to recent studies investigating the possibility that L-theanine might enhance learning ability, induce relaxation and relieve emotional stress. Memory and learning ability were said to be improved in young male Wistar rats given 180 mg of L-theanine daily for four months. Performance was assessed using a test for learning ability and passive and active avoidance tests for memory.

The mental effects of L-theanine were tested in a small group of volunteers divided into two groups defined as "high-anxiety" and "low-anxiety" groups. The volunteers were females aged 18 to 22. Their level of anxiety was assessed by a manifest anxiety scale. Subjects received water, 50 mg of L-theanine or 200 mg of L-theanine solution once a week. Brain waves were measured 60 minutes after administration. The 200 mg dose (dissolved in 100 ml of water) resulted in significantly greater production of alpha waves than was observed in subjects receiving water. Greatest production was consistently seen about 40 minutes after L-theanine intake. The effect was dose-dependent. The researchers regarded the significantly increased production of alpha-brain wave activity as an index of increased relaxation. More rigorous followup is needed.

CONTRAINDICATIONS, PRECAUTIONS, ADVERSE REACTIONS

CONTRAINDICATIONS

L-theanine is contraindicated in those who are hypersensitive to any component of an L-theanine-containing product.

PRECAUTIONS

Pregnant women and nursing mothers should avoid L-theanine supplements. Use of L-theanine supplements concomitantly with cancer chemotherapeutic agents must be done under medical supervision.

ADVERSE REACTIONS

There are no known adverse reactions.

INTERACTIONS

DRUGS

Doxorubicin and Idarubicin: L-theanine may enhance the antitumor effects of these drugs and may ameliorate some of their side effects.

DOSAGE AND ADMINISTRATION

L-theanine supplements are available in Japan for promotion of relaxation and modulation of mood. Doses used are between 50 and 200 mg, as necessary.

L-theanine is available in some green tea preparations. The amino acid constitutes between 1% and 2% of the dry weight of green tea leaves.

LITERATURE

Juneja LR, Chu D-C, Okubo T, et al. L-Theanine — a unique amino acid of green tea and its relaxation effect in humans. *Trends Food Sci Tech.* 1999; 10:199-204.

Kaduka T, Nozawa A, Unno T, et al. Inhibiting effects of theanine on caffeine stimulation evaluated by EEG in the rat. *Biosci Biotechnol Biochem.* 2000; 64:287-293.

Kitaoka S, Hayashi H, Yokogoshi H, Suzuki Y. Transmural potential changes associated with the in vitro absorption of theanine in the guinea pig intestine. *Biosci Biotechnol Biochem.* 1996; 60:1768-1771.

Sadzuka Y, Sugiyama T, Miyagishima A, et al. The effects of theanine, as a novel biochemical modulator, on the antitumor activity of adriamycin. *Cancer Lett.* 1996; 105; 203-209.

Sadzuka Y, Sugiyama T, Sonobe T. Efficacies of tea components on doxorubicin induced antitumor activity and reversal of multidrug resistance. *Toxicology Lett.* 2000; 113:155-162.

Sugiyama T, Sadzuka Y. Enhancing effects of green tea components on the antitumor activity of adriamycin against M5076 ovarian carcinoma. *Cancer Lett.* 1998; 133:19-26.

Sugiyama T, Sadzuka Y. Combination of theanine with doxorubicin inhibits hepatic metastasis of M5076 ovarian sarcoma. *Clin Cancer Res.* 1999; 5:413-416.

Sugiyama T, Sadzuka Y, Sonobe T. Theanine, a major amino acid in green tea, inhibits leukopenia and enhances antitumor activity induce by idarubicin. *Proc Am Assoc Cancer Res.* 1999; 40:10(Abstract 63).

Yokogoshi H, Kato Y, Sagesaka YM, et al. Reduction effect of theanine on blood pressure and brain 5-hydroxyindoles in spontaneous hypertensive rats. *Biosci Biotechnol Biochem.* 1995; 59:615-618.

Yokogoshi H, Kobayashi M. Hypotensive effect of gamma-glutamylmethylamide in spontaneously hypertensive rats. *Life Sci.* 1998; 62:1065-1068.

Yokogoshi H, Kobayashi M, Mochizuki M, Terashima T. Effect of theanine, r-glutamylethylamide on brain monoamines and striatal dopamine release in conscious rats. *Neurochem Res.* 1998; 23:667-673.

L-Tyrosine

TRADE NAMES
Rxosine (Tyson Neutraceuticals), Free-Form L-Tyrosine (Solaray), Tyrosine Power (Nature's Herbs).

DESCRIPTION
L-tyrosine is a protein amino acid. It is classified as a conditionally essential amino acid.

Under most circumstances, the body can synthesize sufficient L-tyrosine, principally from L-phenylalanine, to meet its physiological demands. However, there are conditions where the body requires a dietary source of the amino acid for its physiological demands. For example, L-tyrosine is an essential amino acid for those with phenylketonuria. L-tyrosine is found in proteins of all life forms. Dietary sources of L-tyrosine are principally derived from animal and vegetable proteins. Vegetables and juices contain small amounts of the free amino acid. The free amino acid is also found in fermented foods such as yogurt and miso.

In addition to being involved in protein synthesis, L-tyrosine is a precursor for the synthesis of the catecholamines epinephrine, norepinephrine and dopamine, the thyroid hormones thyroxine and triiodothyronine, and the pigment melanin.

L-tyrosine is also known as beta- (para-hydroxyphenyl) alanine, alpha-amino-para-hydroxyhydrocinnamic acid and *(S)*- alpha-amino-4-hydroxybenzenepropanoic acid. It is abbreviated as either Tyr of by its one-letter abbreviation Y. The molecular formula of L-tyrosine is $C_9H_{10}NO_3$, and its molecular weight is 181.19 daltons. L-tyrosine is an aromatic amino acid with the following structural formula:

L-tyrosine

ACTIONS AND PHARMACOLOGY
ACTIONS
L-tyrosine has putative antidepressant activity.

MECHANISM OF ACTION
The mechanism of L-tyrosine's putative antidepressant activity may be accounted for by the precursor role of L-tyrosine in the synthesis of the neurotransmitters norepinephrine and dopamine. Elevated brain norepinephrine and dopamine levels are thought to be associated with antidepressant effects.

PHARMACOKINETICS
Following ingestion, L-tyrosine is absorbed from the small intestine by a sodium-dependent active transport process. L-tyrosine is transported from the small intestine to the liver via the portal circulation. In the liver, L-tyrosine is involved in a number of biochemical reactions, including protein

synthesis and oxidative catabolic reactions. L-tyrosine that is not metabolized in the liver is distributed via the systemic circulation to the various tissues of the body.

INDICATIONS AND USAGE

Results are mixed, but largely negative, with respect to claims that tyrosine is an effective antidepressant. Claims that it can alleviate some of the mental and physical symptoms of environmental stress are based on preliminary evidence. Further claims that tyrosine is useful in narcolepsy and attention deficit disorder have been refuted by some studies. Another study found that tyrosine supplementation did not improve neuropsychological performance in subjects with phenylketonuria. Claims that tyrosine is helpful in alleviating symptoms of premenstrual syndrome (PMS) and drug withdrawal are largely anecdotal and unconfirmed. There is no evidence tyrosine has any effect on dementia, Alzheimer's disease or Parkinson's disease.

RESEARCH SUMMARY

Two small, early studies suggested that tyrosine might have useful antidepressant effects. A subsequent follow-up with more subjects and conducted in a randomized, double-blind fashion failed to find any significant antidepressant activity, compared with placebo, in subjects with major depression. The dose used was 100 mg/kg/day of tyrosine for four weeks.

One study has concluded that tyrosine can protect against some forms of environmental stress. Subjects were given a 100 mg/kg dose of tyrosine and then exposed for 4.5 hours to cold and hypoxia in this double-blind, placebo-controlled crossover study. Tyrosine was reported to significantly decrease adverse symptoms, including mood and performance impairment. Follow-up is needed.

In another double-blind, placebo-controlled trial, tyrosine had no significant effect on subjects with narcolepsy and associated cataplexy. Dose used was 9 grams daily for four weeks. Similarly, tyrosine failed to produce lasting, significant improvement in subjects with attention deficit disorder. In this small, open study, tyrosine seemed to improve this condition after two weeks of supplementation, but this improvement was not sustained.

Recently, tyrosine was tested to see if it could improve the neuropsychological test performances of individuals with phenylketonuria. This was a randomized, double-blind, placebo-controlled crossover study. Maximum dosage used was 100 to 150 mg/kg/day. The supplementation increased plasma tyrosine concentrations. Higher tyrosine levels correlated at baseline with improved performance on the neuropsychological tests, yet higher concentrations achieved through supplementation in this trial did not enhance test scores.

CONTRAINDICATIONS, PRECAUTIONS, ADVERSE REACTION

CONTRAINDICATIONS

L-tyrosine is contraindicated in those with the inborn errors of metabolism alkaptonuria and tyrosinemia type I and type II. It is also contraindicated in those taking non-selective monoamine oxidase (MAO) inhibitors. L-tyrosine is contraindicated in those hypersensitive to any component of an L-tyrosine-containing supplement.

PRECAUTIONS

Pregnant women and nursing mothers should avoid supplementation with L-tyrosine.

Those with hypertension should exercise caution in the use of L-tyrosine.

Those with melanoma should avoid L-tyrosine supplements.

ADVERSE REACTIONS

L-tyrosine is generally well tolerated. There are some reports of those taking supplemental L-tyrosine experiencing insomnia and nervousness.

INTERACTIONS

DRUGS

Non-selective MAO inhibitors: including phenelzine sulfate, tranylcypromine sulfate and pargyline HC1 —Concomitant use of L-tyrosine and non-selective MAO inhibitors may cause hypertension.

DOSAGE AND ADMINISTRATION

Those who use supplemental L-tyrosine typically take 500 to 1500 mg daily.

HOW SUPPLIED

Capsules — 300 mg, 500 mg
Powder
Tablets — 300 mg, 500 mg, 1000 mg

LITERATURE

Banderet LE, Lieberman HR. Treatment with tyrosine, a neurotransmitter precursor, reduces environmental stress in humans. *Brain Res Bull.* 1989; 22:759-762.

Elwes RD, Crewes H, Chesterman LP, et al. Treatment of narcolepsy with L-tyrosine: double-blind, placebo-controlled trial. *Lancet.* 1989; 2(8671):1067-1069.

Gelenberg AJ, Gibson CJ. Tyrosine for the treatment of depression. *Nutr Health.* 1984; 3:163-173.

Gelenberg AJ, Wojcik JD, Falk WE, et al. Tyrosine for depression: a double-blind trial. *J Affect Disord.* 1990; 19:125-132.

Gelenberg AJ, Wojcik JD, Gibson CJ, Wurtman RJ. Tyrosine for depression. *J Psychiatr Res.* 1982-83; 17:175-180.

Reimherr FW, Wender PH, Wood DR, Ward M. An open trial of L-tyrosine in the treatment of attention deficit disorder, residual type. *Am J Psychiatry.* 1987; 144:1071-1073.

Smith ML, Hanley WB, Clarke JTR, et al. Randomised controlled trial of tyrosine supplementation on neuropsychological performance in phenylketonuria. *Arch Dis Child.* 1998; 78:116-121.

Young SN. Behavioral effects of dietary neurotransmitter precursors: basic and clinical aspects. *Neurosci Biobehav Rev.* 1996; 20:313-323.

Lutein and Zeaxanthin

DESCRIPTION

Lutein and zeaxanthin are members of the carotenoid family, a family best known for another one of its members, beta-carotene (see Beta-Carotene). They are natural fat-soluble yellowish pigments found in some plants, algae and photosynthetic bacteria. They serve as accessory light-gathering pigments and to protect these organisms against the toxic effects of ultra-violet radiation and oxygen. They also appear to protect humans against phototoxic damage. Lutein and zeaxanthin are found in the macula of the human retina, as well as the human crystalline lens. They are thought to play a role in protection against age-related macular degeneration (ARMD) and age-related cataract formation. They may also be protective against some forms of cancer. These two carotenoids are sometimes referred to as macular yellow, retinal carotenoids or macular pigment.

Food sources of lutein and zeaxanthin, include corn, egg yolks and green vegetables and fruits, such as broccoli, green beans, green peas, brussel sprouts, cabbage, kale, collard greens, spinach, lettuce, kiwi and honeydew. Lutein and zeaxanthin are also found in nettles, algae and the petals of many yellow flowers. In green vegetables, fruits and egg yolk, lutein and zeaxanthin exist in non-esterified forms. They also occur in plants in the form of mono-or diesters of fatty acids. For example, lutein and zeaxanthin dipalmitates, dimyristates and monomyristates are found in the petals of the marigold flower (*Tagetes erecta*). Many of the marketed lutein nutritional supplements contain lutein esters, with much smaller amounts of zeaxanthin esters, which are derived from the dried petals of marigold flowers.

Lutein dipalmitate is found in the plant *Helenium autumnale* L. Compositae. It is also known as helenien and it is used in France for the treatment of visual disorders. Zeaxanthin in its fatty acid ester forms, is the principal carotenoid found in the plant *Lycium chinese* Mill. *Lycium chinese* Mill, also known as Chinese boxthorn, is used in traditional Chinese medicine for the treatment of a number of disorders, including visual problems.

Lutein and zeaxanthin belong to the xanthophyll class of carotenoids, also known as oxycarotenoids. The xantho-phylls, which in addition to lutein and zeaxanthin, include alpha-and beta-cryptoxanthin, contain hydroxyl groups. This makes them more polar than carotenoids, such as beta-carotene and lycopene, which do not contain oxygen. Although lutein and zeaxanthin have identical chemical formulas and are isomers, they are not stereoisomers, as is sometimes believed. They are both polyisoprenoids containing 40 carbon atoms and cyclic structures at each end of their conjugated chains. Also, they both occur naturally as *all-trans* (*all-E*) geometric isomers. The principal difference between them is in the location of a double bond in one of the end rings. This difference gives lutein three chiral centers rather than the two that are found in zeaxanthin. The chemical structures are illustrated below.

Lutein

Zeaxanthin

Owing to its three chiral centers, there are 2^3 or 8 stereoisomers of lutein. The principal natural stereoisomer of lutein is (3R,3'R,6'R)-lutein. Lutein is also known as xanthophyll (also, the group name of the oxygen-containing carotenoids), vegetable lutein, vegetable luteol and beta, epsilon-carotene-3,3'diol. The molecular formula of lutein is $C_{40}H_{56}O_2$ and its molecular weight is 568.88 daltons. The chemical name of the principal natural stereoisomer of lutein is (3R,3'R,6'R)-beta,epsilon-carotene-3,3'-diol.

Zeaxanthin has two chiral centers and therefore, 2^2 or 4 stereoisomeric forms. One chiral center is the number 3 atom in the left end ring, while the other chiral center is the number 3' carbon in the right end ring. One stereoisomer is (3R,3'R)-zeaxanthin; another is (3S-3'S)-zeaxanthin. The third stereoisomer is (3R,3'S)-zeaxanthin, and the fourth, (3S,3'R)-zeaxanthin. However, since zeaxanthin, in contrast to lutein, is a symmetric molecule, the (3R,3'S)-and (3S,3'R)-stereoisomers are identical. Therefore, zeaxanthin has only three stereoisomeric forms. The (3R,3'S)-or (3S,3'R)-stereoisomer is called *meso*-zeaxanthin.

The principal natural form of zeaxanthin is (3R,3'R)-zeaxanthin. (3R,3'R)-and *meso*-zeaxanthin are found in the macula of the retina, with much smaller amounts of the (3S,3'S)-stereoisomer. It is thought that *meso*-zeaxanthin in the macula is formed from (3R,3'R,6'R)-lutein. Zeaxanthin is also known as beta, beta-carotene-3,3'-diol, *all-trans*-beta-carotene-3,3'-diol, (3R,3'R)-dihydroxy-beta-carotene (the principal natural stereoisomer), zeaxanthol and anchovyxanthin. Its molecular formula is $C_{40}H_{56}O_2$ and its molecular weight is 568.88 daltons. Zeaxanthin is the principal pigment of yellow corn *zea mays* L, from which its name is derived. It is also produced by certain bacteria, such as *Flavobacterium multivorum*, which are yellow in color.

Chicken egg yolks are a rich food source of lutein and zeaxanthin. The average amount of lutein in chicken egg yolk is approximately 290 micrograms per yolk, and the average amount of zeaxanthin, approximately 210 micrograms per yolk. Lutein-containing plant extracts, which are mainly derived from marigolds, are widely fed to chickens in order to give their egg yolks and skin a deeper yellow color. However, the downside of obtaining lutein and zeaxanthin via consuming egg yolks, is a possible elevation of LDL-cholesterol.

ACTIONS AND PHARMACOLOGY

ACTIONS
Lutein and zeaxanthin may be ophthalmoprotective.

MECHANISM OF ACTION
Lutein and zeaxanthin, which are naturally present in the macula of the human retina, filter out potentially phototoxic blue light and near-ultraviolet radiation from the macula. The protective effect is due in part, to the reactive oxygen species quenching ability of these carotenoids. Further, lutein and zeaxanthin are more stable to decomposition by pro-oxidants than are other carotenoids such as beta-carotene and lycopene. Zeaxanthin is the predominant pigment in the fovea, the region at the center of the macula. The quantity of zeaxanthin gradually decreases and the quantity of lutein increases in the region surrounding the fovea, and lutein is the predominant pigment at the outermost periphery of the macula. Zeaxanthin, which is fully conjugated (lutein is not), may offer somewhat better protection than lutein against phototoxic damage caused by blue and near-ultraviolet light radiation.

Lutein and Zeaxanthin, which are the only two carotenoids that have been identified in the human lens, may be protective against age-related increases in lens density and cataract formation. Again, the possible protection afforded by these carotenoids may be accounted for, in part, by their reactive oxygen species scavenging abilities.

PHARMACOKINETICS
Lutein and zeaxanthin exist in several forms. Nutritional supplement forms are comprised of these carotenoids either in their free (non-esterified) forms or in the form of fatty acid esters. Lutein and zeaxanthin exist in a matrix in foods. In the case of the chicken egg yolk, the matrix is comprised of lipids (cholesterol, phospholipid, triglycerides). The carotenoids are dispersed in the matrix along with fat-soluble nutrients, including vitamins A, D and E. In the case of plants, lutein and zeaxanthin are associated with chloroplasts or chromoplasts.

The efficiency of absorption of lutein and zeaxanthin is variable, but overall appears to be greater than that of beta-carotene. Esterified forms of these carotenoids may be more efficiently absorbed when administered with high-fat meals (about 36 grams), than with low-fat meals (about 3 grams). Lutein and zeaxanthin esters are hydrolyzed in the small intestine via esterases and lipases. Lutein and zeaxanthin that are derived from supplements or released from the matrices of foods, are either solubilized in the lipid core of micelles (formed from bile salts and dietary lipids) in the lumen of the small intestine, or form clathrate complexes with conjugated bile salts. Micelles and possibly clathrate complexes deliver lutein and zeaxanthin to the enterocytes.

Lutein and zeaxanthin are released from the enterocytes into the lymphatics in the form of chylomicrons. They are transported by the lymphatics to the general circulation via the thoracic duct. In the circulation, lipoprotein lipase hydrolyzes much of the triglycerides in the chylomicrons, resulting in the formation of chylomicron remnants. Chylomicron remnants retain apolipoproteins E and B48 on their surfaces and are mainly taken up by the hepatocytes and to a smaller degree by other tissues. Within hepatocytes, lutein and zeaxanthin are incorporated into lipoproteins. Lutein and zeaxanthin appear to be released into the blood mainly in the form of high-density lipoproteins (HDL) and, to a lesser extent, in the form of very-low density lipoprotein (VLDL). Lutein and zeaxanthin are transported in the plasma predominantly in the form of HDL.

Lutein and zeaxanthin are mainly accumulated in the macula of the retina, where they bind to the retinal protein tuberlin. Zeaxanthin is specifically concentrated in the macula, especially in the fovea. Lutein is distributed throughout the retina.

The form of lutein in the plasma is (3R,3'R,6'R)-lutein. Zeaxanthin found in plasma is predominantly (3R,3'R)-zeaxanthin. Lutein appears to undergo some metabolism in the retina to *meso*-zeaxanthin.

INDICATIONS AND USAGE
Lutein and zeaxanthin show some promise of protecting against macular degeneration and may reduce the risk of cataracts in some.

RESEARCH SUMMARY
Epidemiological data have found a relationship between low plasma concentrations of the carotenoids, lutein and zeaxan-

thin, and risk of developing age-related macular degeneration (AMD). Laboratory evidence has suggested that supplemental lutein and/or zeaxanthin might help protect against AMD.

In a multi-center study of 356 subjects aged 55 to 80 years, all diagnosed with advanced stage AMD, a high dietary intake of carotenoids was associated with a 43% lower risk for AMD compared with those consuming low quantities of these carotenoids. Lutein and zeaxanthin were most strongly associated with reduced AMD risk.

Lutein esters, equivalent to 30 milligrams of free lutein per day, given over a period of 140 days, significantly increased macular pigment density in two subjects. A low density of this pigment is believed to be a risk factor for AMD. Controlled clinical trials are needed.

There is also epidemiological evidence that increased lutein and zeaxanthin intake are associated with lower risk of cataract development. In one epidemiological study, those found to have the highest intake of lutein and zeaxanthin had a 22% decreased risk of cataract extraction compared with those who consumed the least amounts of these carotenoids. These findings are consistent with those of similar studies. Again, clinical studies are needed.

CONTRAINDICATIONS, PRECAUTIONS, ADVERSE REACTIONS

CONTRAINDICATIONS

Lutein and zeaxanthin are contraindicated in those hypersensitive to any component of lutein-and zeaxanthin-containing products.

PRECAUTIONS

Pregnant women and nursing mothers should try to obtain lutein and zeaxanthin from the consumption of five or more servings daily of fruits and vegetables. Chicken egg yolk is also rich in lutein and zeaxanthin, and pregnant women and nursing mothers who do not have problems with elevated cholesterol levels, should try to include this item in their diets, as well.

Lutein and zeaxanthin supplements should not be used for the treatment of vitamin A deficiency, since these carotenoids are not converted to vitamin A.

ADVERSE REACTIONS

Adverse reactions involving lutein and zeaxanthin have not been reported.

INTERACTIONS

DRUGS

Cholestyramine: Concomitant intake of lutein/zeaxanthin and cholestyramine may decrease the absorption of these carotenoids.

Colestipol: Concomitant intake of lutein/zeaxanthin and colestipol may decrease the absorption of these carotenoids.

Mineral oil: Concomitant intake of mineral oil and lutein/zeaxanthin may reduce the absorption of these carotenoids.

Orlistat: Orlistat may decrease the absorption of lutein/zeaxanthin.

NUTRITIONAL SUPPLEMENTS

Beta-carotene: Concomitant intake of beta-carotene and lutein may decrease the absorption of these carotenoids.

Medium-chain triglycerides: Concomitant intake of medium-chain triglycerides and lutein/zeaxanthin may enhance the absorption of these carotenoids.

Pectin: Concomitant intake of pectin and lutein/zeaxanthin may decrease the absorption of these carotenoids.

FOODS

Oils: Some dietary oil, such as corn oil, may increase the absorption of lutein/zeaxanthin, especially the ester forms of these carotenoids.

Olestra: Concomitant intake of olestra and lutein/zeaxanthin may decrease the absorption of these carotenoids.

OVERDOSAGE

Overdosage of lutein and zeaxanthin have not been reported in the literature.

DOSAGE AND ADMINISTRATION

Lutein/zeaxanthin supplements are available in free (non-esterified) and esterified (with fatty acids) forms, and as single ingredient or combination products. The amount of zeaxanthin in these products is considerably lower than that of zeaxanthin. Products that deliver higher amounts of zeaxanthin are being developed. Dosage is variable, and optimal dosage for ophthalmological health is not known. Dietary intake of lutein of 6.9-11.7 milligrams daily has been associated with a decreased risk of age-related macular degeneration. Nutritional supplements containing lutein deliver from 250 micrograms (0.25 milligrams) to 20 milligrams daily.

Green leafy vegetables are good dietary sources of lutein, but poor sources of zeaxanthin. Good dietary sources of zeaxanthin, include yellow corn, orange pepper, orange juice, honeydew, mango and chicken egg yolk.

HOW SUPPLIED

Lutein is available in the following forms and strengths:

Capsules — 6 mg, 20 mg

LITERATURE

Berendschot TT, Goldbohm RA, Klö pping WA, et al. Influence of lutein supplementation on macular pigment, assessed with two objective techniques. *Invest Opthalmol Vis Sci.* 2000; 41:3322-3326.

Bone RA, Landrum JT, Dixon Z, et al. Lutein and zeaxanthin in the eyes, serum and diet of human subjects. *Exp Eye Res.* 2000; 71:239-245.

Bone RA, Landrum JT, Friedes LM, et al. Distribution of lutein and zeaxanthin stereoisomers in the human retinal. *Exp Eye Res.* 1997; 64:211-218.

Bone RA, Landrum JT, Tarsis SL. Preliminary identification of the human macular pigment. *Vision Res.* 1985; 25:1531-1535.

Bowen PE, Clark JP. *Lutein esters having high bioavailability.* International patent publication number: WO 98/45241. International publication date: 15 October 1998.

Brown L, Rimm EB, Seddon JM, et al. A prospective study of carotenoid intake and risk of cataract extraction in U.S. men. *Am J Clin Nutr.* 1999; 70:517-524.

Chasan-Taber L, Willett WC, Seddon JM, et al. A prospective study of carotenoid and vitamin A intakes and risk of cataract extraction in U.S. women. *Am J Clin Nutr.* 1999; 70:509-516.

Dietary Reference Intakes for Vitamin C, Vitamin E, Selenium, and Carotenoids. Washington, DC: National Academy Press; 2000:325-382.

Erdman JW Jr. Variable bioavailability of carotenoids from vegetables (editorial). *Am J Clin Nutr.* 1999; 70:179-180.

Garnett KM, Glerhart DL, Guerra-Santos LH. *Method of making pure 3R-3' R stereoisomer of zeaxanthin for human ingestion.* United States Patent Number: 5,854,015. Date of Patent: Dec. 29, 1998.

Hammond BR Jr, Wooten BR, Snodderly DM. Density of the human crystalline lens is related to the macular pigment carotenoids, lutein and zeaxanthin. *Optom Vis Sci.* 1997; 74:499-504.

Handelman GJ, Nightingale ZD, Lichtenstein AH, et al. Lutein and zeaxanthin concentrations in plasma after dietary supplementation with egg yolk. *Am J Clin Nutr.* 1999; 70:247-251.

Khachik F. *Process for extraction and purification of lutein, zeaxanthin and rare carotenoids from marigold flowers and plants.* International patent publication number: WO 99/20587. International publication date: 29 April 1999.

Koonsvitsky BP, Berry DA, Jones MB, et al. Olestra affects serum concentrations of alpha-tocopherol and carotenoids but not vitamin D or vitamin K status in free-living subjects. *J Nutr.* 1997; 127(8 Suppl):1636S-1645S.

Kostic D, White WS, Olson JA. Intestinal absorption, serum clearance, and interactions between lutein and beta-carotene when administered to human adults in separate or combined oral doses. *Am J Clin Nutr.* 1995; 62:604-610.

Landrum JT, Bone RA, Joa H, et al. A one year study of the macular pigment: the effect of 140 days of a lutein supplement. *Exp Eye Res.* 1997; 65:57-62.

Mares-Perlman JA. Too soon for lutein supplements (editorial). *Am J Clin Nutr.* 1999; 70:431-432.

Nussbaum JJ, Pruett RC, Delori FC. Historic perspectives. Macular yellow pigment. The first 200 years. *Retina.* 1981; 1:296-310.

Olson JA. Carotenoids. In: Shils ME, Olson JA, Shike M, Ross AC. *Modern Nutrition in Health and Disease.* Baltimore, MD: Williams and Wilkins; 1999:525-541.

Roodenburg AJ, Leenen R, van het Hof KH, et al. Amount of fat in the diet affects bioavailability of lutein esters but not of alpha-carotene, beta-carotene, and vitamin E in humans. *Am J Clin Nutr.* 2000; 71:1187-1193.

Siems WG, Sommerburg O, van Kuijk FJ. Lycopene and beta-carotene decompose more rapidly than lutein and zeaxanthin upon exposure to various pro-oxidants in vitro. *Biofactors.* 1999; 10:105-113.

Sommerburg O, Keunen JE, Bird AC, et al. Fruits and vegetables that are sources for lutein and zeaxanthin: the macular pigment in human eyes. *B J Opthalmol.* 1998; 82:907-910.

Sommerburg OG, Siems WG, Hurst JS, et al. Lutein and zeaxanthin are associated with photoreceptors in the human retina. *Curr Eye Res.* 1999; 19:491-495.

van den Berg H. Effect of lutein on beta-carotene absorption and cleavage. *Int J Vitam Nutr Res.* 1998; 68:360-365.

van het Hof KH, Brouwer IA, West CE, et al. Bioavailability of lutein from vegetables is 5 times higher than that of beta-carotene. *Am J Clin Nutr.* 1999; 70:261-268.

Lycopene

TRADE NAMES

Lycopene (Nature's Answer)

DESCRIPTION

Lycopene is a member of the carotenoid family of chemical substances. Lycopene, similar to other carotenoids, is a natural fat-soluble pigment (red, in the case of lycopene) found in certain plants and microorganisms, where it serves as an accessory light-gathering pigment and to protect these organisms against the toxic effects of oxygen and light. Lycopene may also protect humans against certain disorders, such as prostate cancer and perhaps some other cancers, and coronary heart disease.

Carotenoids are the principal pigments responsible for the colors of vegetables and fruits (see Beta-Carotene and Lutein and Zeaxanthin). Lycopene is responsible for the red color of red tomatoes. In addition to tomatoes (*Lycopersicon esculentum*) and tomato-based products, such as ketchup, pizza sauce, tomato juice and tomato paste, lycopene is also found in watermelon, papaya, pink grapefruit and pink guava.

Processed tomato products are more available dietary sources of lycopene than fresh tomatoes. The average daily intake of lycopene is approximately 25 milligrams, with 50% of this in the form of processed tomato products.

Lycopene is an acyclic isomer of beta-carotene. Beta-carotene, which contains beta-ionone rings at each end of the molecule, is formed in plants, including tomatoes, via the action of the enzyme lycopene beta-cyclase. Lycopene is a 40 carbon atom, open chain polyisoprenoid with 11 conjugated double bonds. The structural formula of lycopene is represented as follows:

Lycopene

All-trans lycopene is the predominant geometric isomer found in plants. *Cis* isomers of lycopene are also found in nature, including 5-*cis*, 9-*cis*, 13-*cis* and 15-*cis* isomers. Lycopene found in human plasma is a mixture of approximately 50% *cis* lycopene and 50% all-*trans* lycopene. Lycopene in processed foods, is mainly in the form of the *cis*-isomer.

Lycopene is a lipophilic compound and is insoluble in water. Lycopene is also known as psi-carotene. Its molecular formula is $C_{40}H_{56}$ and its molecular weight is 536.88 daltons. In contrast to beta-carotene, lycopene has no vitamin A activity and thus is a nonprovitamin A carotenoid.

ACTIONS AND PHARMACOLOGY

ACTIONS

Lycopene may have anticarcinogenic and antiatherogenic activities.

The intake of tomato-based foods, especially processed tomato products, is associated with a significantly lower risk for prostate cancer, and also appears to be associated with a lower risk for lung cancer. The mechanism of the possible anticarcinogenic activity of lycopene is not well understood, but there are a few hypotheses. Cancer, as well as several other chronic diseases, is linked to oxidative stress. *In vitro* studies have demonstrated that lycopene has the highest antioxidant activity of all the carotenoids. It has the ability to quench singlet oxygen (more so than beta-carotene), to trap peroxyl radicals, to inhibit the oxidation of DNA, to inhibit lipid peroxidation, and in some studies, to inhibit the oxidation of low-density lipoprotein (LDL).

MECHANISM OF ACTION

Non-antioxidant mechanisms have also been proposed. Failure of cell signaling may be a cause of cell overgrowth and eventually cancer. Lycopene may stimulate gap junction communication between cells. It is speculated that lycopene may suppress carcinogen-induced phosphorylation of regulatory proteins such as p53 and Rb antioncogenes and stop cell division at the G_0-G_1 cell cycle phase. One researcher has hypothesized that lycopene-induced modulation of the liver metabolizing enzyme cytochrome P450 2E1 may be the underlying mechanism of protection against carcinogen-induced preneoplastic lesions in the rat liver. Lycopene may also reduce cellular proliferation induced by insulin-like growth factors. There is some preliminary *in vitro* evidence for the latter proposal.

The mechanism of the possible antiatherogenic activity of lycopene is likewise unclear. Lycopene's antioxidant activity is a possibility. Lycopene has also been found to inhibit cholesterol synthesis, to inhibit HMG-CoA (hydroxymethylglutaryl coenzyme A) reductase activity and to upregulate LDL receptor activity in macrophages. A small preliminary study in humans, reported an LDL-cholesterol-lowering effect of lycopene.

PHARMACOKINETICS

Lycopene is available in nutritional supplements in the form of an oleoresin, in phospholipid complexes and in oils. In foods, lycopene exists as part of a matrix (in chloroplasts or chromoplasts) within the vegetables or fruit. The efficiency of absorption of lycopene from supplements and foods is variable. The efficiency of absorption of lycopene from tomatoes, in which lycopene is tightly bound within the matrix, is low. It is much higher in processed tomato products. The improved availability of lycopene from processed foods is due to its release from the ruptured plant cells following the mechanical and thermal processing, as well as heat induced-*trans* to *cis* isomerization. *Cis*-lycopene is reported to be more bioavailable than *trans*-lycopene. Lipids increase the absorption of lycopene. For example, the combination of tomato sauce and olive oil delivers more absorbable lycopene than tomato sauce without oil.

Lycopene from supplements or from the matrices of foods is either solubilized in the lipid core of micelles (formed from bile salts and dietary fat) in the lumen of the small intestine or forms clathrate complexes with conjugated bile salts. Micelles and clathrate complexes deliver lycopene to the enterocytes.

Lycopene is released from the enterocytes into the lymphatics in the form of chylomicrons. Lycopene is transported by the lymphatics to the general circulation via the thoracic duct. In the circulation, lipoprotein lipase hydrolyzes much of the triglycerides in the chylomicrons, resulting in the formation of chylomicron remnants. Chylomicron remnants retain apolipoproteins E and B48 on their surfaces and are mainly taken up by hepatocytes and to lesser degrees by other tissues. Within hepatocytes, lycopene is incorporated into lipoproteins. Lycopene is released into the blood from the hepatocytes in the form of very-low density lipoproteins (VLDL) and low-density lipoproteins (LDL). In the plasma, VLDL is converted by lipoprotein lipase to LDL. Lycopene is transported in the plasma predominantly in the form of LDL.

There is much unknown about the pharmacokinetics of lycopene, in particular its distribution and its metabolism.

INDICATIONS AND USAGE

Lycopene may be helpful in preventing and possibly also managing some cancers, particularly prostate cancer, and may confer some protection against cardiovascular disease. Research, though suggestive of these positive effects, is far from conclusive. And there is far too little evidence of efficacy from very preliminary studies to support any indication for lycopene in the management of HIV disease or other immune dysfunction or in the management of neurodegenerative disorders.

RESEARCH SUMMARY

In a prospective study that followed the eating habits of 47,000 men for six years, a positive correlation was found between tomato-based food consumption and apparent resistance to development of prostate cancer. There was a 35% reduction in risk of developing prostate cancer among those who consumed more than 10 servings of tomato products weekly, compared with those who consumed fewer than 1.5 servings weekly. Most of these servings (82%) were in the form of tomatoes, tomato sauce and pizza. Tomato sauce appeared to be the most protective.

This study reinforced the findings of an earlier prospective study that examined the eating habits of Seventh Day Adventist men over a six-year period. This study found that the relative risk of prostate cancer was 0.60 among Adventist men who ate tomatoes more than five times weekly, compared with those who consumed them less than once weekly.

A recent review of 72 studies found 57 reports of inverse associations between tomato consumption or blood lycopene levels and risk of various types of cancer; 35 of these associations were significant. Evidence of lycopene protective effects were highest for cancers of the prostate, lung and stomach.

While cautioning that these associations do not establish a cause-and-effect relationship, the reviewer observed that

"the consistency of the results across numerous studies in diverse populations, for case-control and prospective studies, and for dietary-based and blood-based investigations argues against bias or confounding as the explanation for these findings."

Recently, more direct, though still preliminary, evidence emerged suggestive of lycopene protective and, perhaps, interventive effects in prostate cancer. In this study, 33 men scheduled for surgery to remove cancerous prostate glands, were randomized to receive 30 milligrams of lycopene (in two 15-milligram capsules) daily or nothing. Dosing commenced 30 days prior to surgery.

Examination of the prostate glands post-surgery revealed that cancer had spread to the very edge of the glands in seven of the 21 lycopene-treated subjects compared with the same extent of spread in 9 of the 12 subjects who did not receive lycopene. Pre-cancerous tissue in the lycopene group was judged to be less abnormal than pre-cancerous tissue in the group that did not receive lycopene. Prostate specific antigen (PSA) fell 20% in the lycopene group between initial dosing and surgery. PSA levels were unchanged in the group not receiving lycopene. Research is ongoing.

Recent epidemiological studies have reported an inverse relationship between higher tissue and serum levels of lycopene and the risk of coronary artery disease. And a recent study in which 19 healthy subjects consumed a variety of tomato products for three weeks reported no change in serum cholesterol levels but significant decrease in lipid peroxidation and LDL-cholesterol oxidation. Numerous *in vitro* and animal studies have also reported results suggestive of lycopene effects that might help prevent or ameliorate cardiovascular disease. Research continues.

CONTRINDICATIONS, PRECAUTIONS, ADVERSE REACTIONS

CONTRAINDICATIONS

Lycopene is contraindicated in those hypersensitive to any component of a lycopene-containing product.

PRECAUTIONS

Pregnant women and nursing mothers should obtain their lycopene intake from food sources rather than supplements.

INTERACTIONS

DRUGS

Cholestyramine: Concomitant intake of cholestyramine and lycopene may decrease the absorption of lycopene.

Colestipol: Concomitant intake of colestipol and lycopene may decrease the absorption of lycopene.

Mineral oil: Concomitant intake of mineral oil and lycopene may reduce the absorption of lycopene.

Orlistat: Orlistat may decrease the absorption of lycopene.

NUTRITIONAL SUPPLEMENTS

Beta-carotene: Concomitant intake of beta-carotene and lycopene may increase the absorption of lycopene.

Medium-chain triglycerides: Concomitant intake of medium-chain triglycerides and lycopene may enhance the absorption of lycopene.

Pectin: Concomitant intake of pectin and lycopene may decrease the absorption of lycopene.

FOODS

Oils: Dietary oils, such as olive oil, may enhance the absorption of lycopene.

Olestra: Olestra may reduce the absorption of lycopene.

DOSAGE AND ADMINISTRATION

Lycopene supplements are available as oleoresin preparations, phospholipid preparations and in oils, such as medium chain triglycerides. Doses range from 5 to 15 milligrams daily.

The optimal dose of lycopene is not known.

The following lists the lycopene contents of some foods:

Food	Lycopene content (micrograms/gram wet weight)
Fresh tomatoes	8.8-42.0
Cooked tomatoes	37
Tomato sauce	62
Tomato paste	54-1,500
Tomato powder	1,126-1,265
Tomato soup (condensed)	80
Tomato juice	50-116
Pizza sauce	127
Ketchup	99-134
Watermelon	23-72
Pink guava	54
Pink grapefruit	34
Papaya	20-53

HOW SUPPLIED

Capsules — 5 mg, 6 mg, 10 mg

Tablets — 10 mg

LITERATURE

Agarwal S, Rao AV. Tomato lycopene and its role in human health and chronic diseases. *CMAJ.* 2000; 163:739-744.

Agarwal S, Rao AV. Tomato lycopene and low density lipiprotein oxidation: a human dietary intervention study. *Lipids.* 1998; 33:981-984.

Arab L, Steck S. Lycopene and cardiovascular disease. *Am J Clin Nutr.* 2000; 71(suppl); 1691S-1695S.

Bohm Y, Bitsch R. Intestinal absorption of lycopene from different matrices and interactions to other carotenoids, the lipid status, and the antioxidant capacity of human plasma. *Eur J Nutr.* 1999; 38:118-125.

Boileau AC, Merchen NR, Wasson K, et al. Cis-lycopene is more bioavailable than trans-lycopene in vitro and in vivo in lymph-cannulated ferrets. *J Nutr.* 1999; 129:1176-1181.

Bramley PM. Is lycopene beneficial to human health? *Phytochem.* 2000; 54:233-236.

Clinton SK. Lycopene: chemistry, biology, and implications for human health and disease. *Nutr Rev.* 1998; 56:35-51.

Clinton SK, Emenhiser C, Schwartz SJ, et al. Cis-trans lycopene isomers, carotenoids, and retinol in the human prostate. *Cancer Epidemiol Biomarkers Prev.* 1996; 5:823-833.

Gann PH, Ma J, Giovannucci E, et al. Lower prostate cancer risk in men with elevated plasma lycopene levels: results of a prospective analysis. *Cancer Res.* 1999; 59:1225-1230.

Gartner C, Stahl W, Sies H. Lycopene is more bioavailable from tomato paste than from fresh tomatoes. *Am J Clin Nutr.* 1997; 66:116-122.

Giovannucci E. Tomatoes, tomato-based products, lycopene, and cancer: Review of the epidemiologic literature. *J Natl Cancer Inst.* 1999; 91:317-331.

Giovannucci E, Ascherio A, Rimm EB, et al. Intake of carotenoids and retinol in relation to risk of prostate cancer. *J Natl Cancer Inst.* 1995; 87:1767-1976.

Johnson EJ. The role of lycopene in health and disease. *Nutr Clin Care.* 2000; 3:35-43.

Johnson EJ, Qin J, Krinsky NI, Russell RM. Ingestion by men of a combined dose of beta-carotene and lycopene does not affect the absorption of beta-carotene but improves that of lycopene. *J Nutr.* 1997; 127:1833-1837.

Leal M, Shimada S, Ruiz F, et al. Effect of lycopene on lipid peroxidation and glutathione-dependent enzymes induced by T-2 toxin in vivo. *Toxicol Lett.* 1999; 109:1-10.

Michaud DS, Feskanich D, Rimm EB, et al. Intake of specific carotenoids and risk of lung cancer in 2 prospective U.S. cohorts. *Am J Clin Nutr.* 2000; 72:990-997.

Paetau I, Rao D, Wiley ER, et al. Carotenoids in human buccal mucosa cells after 4 wk of supplementation with tomato juice or lycopene supplements. *Am J Clin Nutr.* 1999; 70:490-494.

Rao AV, Agarwal S. Bioavailability and in vivo antioxidant properties of lycopene from tomato products and their possible role in the prevention of cancer. *Nutr Cancer.* 1998; 31:199-203.

Rao AV, Agarwal S. Role of lycopene as antioxidant carotenoid in the prevention of chronic diseases: a review. *Nutr Res.* 1999; 19:305-323.

Rao AV, Fleshner N, Agarwal S. Serum and tissue lycopene and biomarkers of oxidation in prostate cancer patients: a case-control study. *Nutr Cancer.* 1999; 33:159-164.

Riso P, Pinder A, Santangelo A, Porrini M. Does tomato consumption effectively increase the resistance of lymphocyte DNA to oxidative damage? *Am J Clin Nutr.* 1999; 69:712-718.

Sengupta A, Das S. The anti-carcinogenic role of lycopene, abundantly present in tomato. *Eur J Cancer Prev.* 1999; 8:325-330.

Sies H, Stahl W. Lycopene: antioxidant and biological effects and its bioavailability in the human. *Proc Soc Exp Biol Med.* 1998; 218:121-124.

Sutherland WH, Walker RJ, De Jong SA, Upritchard JE. Supplementation with tomato juice increases plasma lycopene but does not alter susceptibility to oxidation of low-density lipoproteins from renal transplant patients. *Clin Nephrol.* 1999; 52:30-36.

Magnesium

TRADE NAMES

Magnacaps (The Key Company), M2 Magnesium (Miller Pharmacal), Magimin-Forte (The Key Company), Elite Magnesium (Miller Pharmacal), Mag Delay (Major Pharmaceuticals), Slow-Mag (Roberts Laboratories), Mag-SR (Cypress Pharmaceuticals), Magonate (Fleming and Company), Magtrate (Mission Pharmacal), Almora (Forest Pharmaceuticals), Mag-G (Cypress Pharmaceuticals), Mag-Tab SR (Niche Pharmaceuticals), Uro-Mag (Blaine Pharmaceuticals), Mag-Ox 400 (Blaine Pharmaceuticals)

DESCRIPTION

Magnesium is an essential mineral in human nutrition with a wide range of biological functions. Magnesium is involved in over 300 metabolic reactions. It is necessary for every major biological process, including the production of cellular energy and the synthesis of nucleic acids and proteins. It is also important for the electrical stability of cells, the maintenance of membrane integrity, muscle contraction, nerve conduction and the regulation of vascular tone, among other things.

Magnesium is an alkaline earth metal with atomic number 12 and an atomic weight of 24.31 daltons. Its chemical symbol is Mg. Magnesium exists under physiological conditions in its divalent (+2 or II) state. The total body magnesium content of an adult is about 25 grams. About 50%-60% exists in bone. Magnesium is the second most abundant intracellular cation; potassium is the most abundant. Approximately 1% of the body's magnesium is found extracellularly.

Magnesium is intimately interlocked, biologically with calcium. In some reactions, such as the synthesis of nucleic acids and protein, calcium and magnesium are antagonistic. Magnesium is necessary for these processes, while calcium can inhibit them. Magnesium and calcium cooperate, however, in the production of adenosine triphosphate or ATP. Magnesium has been called ''nature's physiological calcium

channel blocker'' since it appears to regulate the intracellular flow of calcium ions.

Symptoms and signs of magnesium deficiency include anorexia, nausea and vomiting, diarrhea, generalized muscle spasticity, paresthesias, confusion, tremor, focal and generalized seizures, confusion, loss of coordination, cardiac arrhythmias, laboratory abnormalities, such as hypokalemia and hypocalcemia, muscle cramps, hypertension and coronary and cerebral vasospasms. Magnesium deficiency may be found in diabetes mellitus, malabsorption syndromes, alcoholism and hyperthyroidism, among other disorders. Use of certain drugs may also lead to magnesium deficiency. These drugs include thiazide diuretics (when used for long periods of time), loop diuretics, cisplatin, amphotericin, pentamidine (when used intravenously), aminoglycosides and cyclosporine. Magnesium deficiency itself is an important cause of hypokalemia.

In addition to its use for the treatment of hypomagnesemia, magnesium is used for the treatment of certain cardiac arrhythmias, in particular torsade de pointes, and eclampsia. It is also used as a laxative and antacid. Magnesium may also have value for the prevention of osteoporosis and for the management of migraine headaches in some. There is preliminary evidence that magnesium may help some with premenstrual syndrome, type 2 diabetes mellitus and hypertension. The role of magnesium, if any, in the management of acute myocardial infarction remains controversial.

Foods rich in magnesium include unpolished grains, nuts and green vegetables. Green leafy vegetables are particularly good sources of magnesium because of their chlorophyll content. Chlorophyll is the magnesium chelate of porphyrin. Meats, starches and milk are less rich sources of magnesium. Refined and processed foods are generally magnesium-poor. The mean daily magnesium intake in the U.S. in males nine years and older is estimated to be about 323 milligrams; for females nine years and older, it is estimated to be 228 milligrams. Some surveys report lower intakes, and some believe that the dietary intake for many may be sub-optimal.

ACTIONS AND PHARMACOLOGY

ACTIONS

Magnesium may have anti-osteoporotic activity. Magnesium has anti-arrhythmic activity. Magnesium has activity in the management of preeclampsia. Magnesium may have anti-hypertensive, glucose-regulatory and bronchodilatory activities. Magnesium has putative myocardial protective activity during an acute myocardial infarction and putative anti-migraine activity.

MECHANISM OF ACTION

Significant reductions in bone mineral content and serum magnesium have been reported in women with postmenopausal osteoporosis compared to age-matched controls. Bone mineral content and bone mineral density have been positively correlated with dietary magnesium in a few, but not all, studies of postmenopausal women. A couple of studies have demonstrated increased bone mineral density in postmenopausal women which was associated with intake of supplemental magnesium. Magnesium influences both matrix and mineral metabolism in bone. Magnesium depletion can cause cessation of bone growth, decrease dosteoblastic and osteoclastic activity, osteopenia and increased bone fragility. Bone mineral with decreased magnesium content results in larger and more perfect bone mineral crystals, which may be more brittle than amorphous crystals.

Magnesium depletion is associated with a number of cardiac arrhythmias, including atrial fibrillation, premature atrial and ventricular beats, ventricular tachycardia and ventricular fibrillation. Magnesium is effective in treating these arrhythmias in those who are magnesium deficient. Magnesium may also be effective in treating cardiac arrhythmias in those who are not magnesium deficient. This is especially true for the treatment, by magnesium, of torsade de pointes. The mechanism of the anti-arrhythmic action of magnesium is not fully understood. The anti-arrhythmic effect of magnesium may be related to its role in maintaining intracellular potassium. It may also be related to its role as a natural calcium channel blocker.

Magnesium sulfate is widely used to prevent eclamptic seizures in pregnant women with hypertension. Vasospasm in preeclampsia is thought to be a consequence of endothelial dysfunction. Magnesium has been found, both *in vitro* and *in vivo*, to increase production of the vasodilator prostacyclin. Magnesium may also protect against damage to the endothelium by reactive oxygen species. The action of magnesium sulfate in the treatment of eclampsia can be accounted for by the release of endothelial prostaglandin by magnesium, its protection against reactive oxygen species damage to the endothelium and by its possible inhibition of platelet aggregation. It may act as an anticonvulsant via neuronal calcium-channel blockade and antagonism of the glutamate N-methyl-D-aspartate (NMDA) receptor.

Some studies have reported that some populations with low dietary intake of magnesium have increased incidence of hypertension. Another study reported dietary intake of magnesium in normotensives to be significantly greater than intake in untreated hypertensive subjects. Intervention studies with magnesium therapy for hypertensives have led to conflicting results. The mechanism of the possible anti-hypertensive activity of magnesium is unclear. A possibility is that magnesium, acting in a calcium channel blocking capacity, may have a vasodilatory action.

A few studies have reported that magnesium depletion results in insulin resistance as well as impaired secretion of insulin. Insulin resistance and abnormal glucose tolerance may be accounted for, in part, by inadequate magnesium. Some studies have reported improved insulin response in elderly type 2 diabetics who received magnesium. The mechanism of the possible role of magnesium in improving glycemic control is unclear. Magnesium is a cofactor for phosphorylation reactions. Magnesium may affect insulin signal transduction. Magnesium may also alter insulin receptor binding. These are some speculative possibilities.

Intravenous magnesium has been demonstrated to have bronchodilatory activity in some with asthma. The mechanism of this activity is unclear.

The mechanism of the putative myocardial protective activity of magnesium during an acute myocardial infarction is also unclear. Speculative possibilities include magnesium's anti-arrhythmic activity, as well as its possible activity in inhibiting platelet aggregation. Magnesium's possible vasodilatory activity—via its acting as a calcium channel blocker—and possible reduction of reperfusion dysfunction are two additional speculative mechanisms for this putative activity. The mechanism of the possible anti-migraine activity is unknown.

PHARMACOKINETICS

The efficiency of absorption of magnesium is inversely proportional to the amount of magnesium ingested. The fractional absorption of magnesium from 7 to 36 milligrams was found to be 65% to 70% in one study. The same study reported a fractional absorption of 11% to 14% with a magnesium intake of 960 to 1,000 milligrams. One study of magnesium absorption from food sources reported a fractional absorption of 40% to 60% of a daily intake of 380 milligrams of magnesium in healthy older men.

Magnesium appears to be absorbed from both the small intestine and the colon. The sites of maximal magnesium absorption appear to be the distal jejunum and ileum. The efficiency of absorption (fractional absorption) of a magnesium salt appears to principally depend on its solubility in intestinal fluids, as well as on the amount digested. Enteric-coated magnesium salts are less efficiently absorbed than non enteric-coated preparations. Salts with high solubility, e.g., magnesium citrate, appear to be more efficiently absorbed than salts with poor solubility, e.g., magnesium oxide. There are a few reports that suggest that the counter anion of the magnesium salt may influence its absorption. Magnesium aspartate and magnesium orotate are reported by some to be more available forms of magnesium than other magnesium salts. However, there are no compelling data that indicate that the nature of the counter anion makes any significant difference on the availability of magnesium salt, independent of its possible effect on the solubility of the salt.

Magnesium appears to be absorbed by both a saturable active transport mechanism and an unsaturable passive mechanism. The saturable active transport mechanism may account for the higher absorption efficiency at lower magnesium intakes. There is no good evidence that vitamin D and its active metabolite, 1, 25-dihydroxyvitamin D (1, 25(OH)$_2$D) play a significant role in the absorption of magnesium, as some have suggested.

Magnesium is transported to the liver via the portal circulation and to the rest of the body via the systemic circulation. A large fraction of ingested magnesium is taken up by bone. Magnesium transport into cells appears to require the presence of carrier-mediated transport systems. Magnesium is excreted by the kidneys, and the kidney is the principal organ involved in magnesium homeostasis. There is no tubular secretion of magnesium. Magnesium is filtered and reabsorbed. About 65% of filtered magnesium is reabsorbed in the loop of Henle and 20% to 30% in the proximal convoluted tubule.

About 3% to 5% of filtered magnesium is excreted in the urine. The regulatory mechanisms of the kidney in maintaining magnesium homeostasis are unclear.

There is much about the pharmacokinetics of magnesium that is not known. Research is ongoing.

INDICATIONS AND USAGE

Magnesium deficiency is associated with the pathogenesis of numerous serious disorders, notably ischemic heart disease, congestive heart failure, sudden cardiac death, cardiac arrhythmias, diabetes mellitus, pre-eclampsia/eclampsia and hypertension, among others. Treatment with supplemental magnesium is often helpful in these conditions. There is also evidence that it can be of benefit in some with osteoporosis, alcoholism, migraine, asthma, pre-menstrual syndromes, kidney stones and strokes. It may help prevent or reduce the incidence of cerebral palsy and mental retardation in early pre-term infants. There is little or no evidence to support claims that magnesium enhances athletic/exercise performance, that it is an effective antidepressant or that it is helpful in bipolar disorder.

RESEARCH SUMMARY

There is considerable epidemiological data associating low magnesium intake with an increased incidence of cardiovascular disease. Some recent data have suggested the presence of serum magnesium abnormality in sick inpatient and outpatient populations ranging from 12% to 40%. Hypomagnesemia has frequently been associated with those suffering from various forms of cardiovascular disease.

Magnesium's role as a cofactor in various crucial intracellular enzymatic reactions related to myocardial metabolism and contractility is well established. It is not surprising, then, that magnesium deficiencies, perhaps even borderline deficiencies, can negatively impact cardiovascular health. At the same time, due to lack of an accurate assay of intracellular magnesium, it has been difficult to assess the efficacy of supplemental magnesium in some of these conditions. ''Also uncertain,'' two reviewers of the data have stated in an editorial, ''is whether magnesium administration merely corrects an underlying deficiency state or exerts specific beneficial pharmacologic effects.'' That caveat can be applied equally not only to the possible cardiologic indications for the use of supplemental magnesium but to all other possible indications, as well.

In addition to the epidemiological data, there are also some experimental and clinical data supporting the use of magnesium in some with cardiovascular disease. Frank magnesium deficiency has clearly been shown to induce vascular damage in the heart and kidneys and to promote atherosclerosis. In pharmacological concentrations, infusion of magnesium inhibits platelet aggregation, exerts anti-arrhythmic effects and induces vasodilatation of blood vessels. In animals it has protected against ischemia-reperfusion injury.

In some randomized, double-blind, placebo-controlled studies, intravenous magnesium has significantly improved outcome in subjects with acute myocardial infarction. However, in a recent prospective study assessing the effects of early captopril, oral mononitrate and intravenous magnesium in 58,050 patients with suspected acute myocardial infarction, no beneficial effects were observed with magnesium. Some have argued that because the magnesium was administered after iatrogenic or spontaneous reperfusion this difference in timing might explain, at least in part, its poor performance. Reviewers of these data have concluded that there is, as yet, insufficient evidence of magnesium efficacy to recommend it for routine use in patients with suspected myocardial infarction. They have recommended further study. It should also be pointed out that, as of yet, there are no randomized studies showing a magnesium mortality benefit in congestive heart failure.

Epidemiological data indicate that low dietary magnesium intake is associated with a higher incidence of hypertension. Magnesium supplementation has significantly reduced blood pressure in some, but not all, studies. Some of these positive studies have been criticized as being methodologically flawed. Larger, better designed studies are needed.

Intravenous administration of magnesium has been effective in suppressing some, but not all, cardiac arrhythmias. It is the treatment of choice for controlling torsade de pointes and is an option for treating refractory or recurrent ventricular fibrillation or tachycardia.

There is also an inverse association between dietary magnesium intake and risk of total stroke in men. In some animal experiments, magnesium has demonstrated significant neuroprotective effects. A large multicenter trial of intravenous magnesium's possible efficacy post-acute stroke is now underway.

Magnesium's possible usefulness in protecting against atherosclerosis was suggested by findings in experimental animals that magnesium deficiency promotes vascular damage and other atherosclerotic processes. In addition, supplemental magnesium has lowered serum cholesterol and triglyceride levels and has inhibited atherosclerotic lesions in other animal studies. More research is needed.

Magnesium was first used in 1906 to help prevent eclamptic seizures. It is now routinely used for this purpose in hypertensive pregnant women. It showed marked benefit in this condition and significant superiority over diazepam and phenytoin in the Collaborative Eclampsia Trial. There is also good evidence that treating pregnant women with magnesium pre-delivery may reduce the incidence of mental retardation and cerebral palsy in early preterm infants. Intravenous magnesium has also been used to inhibit premature labor with some success in one study.

Magnesium deficiency has been implicated in increased insulin resistance and a higher incidence of cardiovascular disease among those with diabetes mellitus. Hypomagnesemia has been reported in 25% to 38% of diabetic patients; its incidence is highest in those with the poorest metabolic control. In a small early study of eight elderly subjects with NIDDM, supplementation with two grams of magnesium daily significantly improved insulin response and action, compared with placebo. Some other small studies have suggested benefits with daily doses as low as 100 milligrams of magnesium daily. Recently, however, the large, well-designed prospective Atherosclerosis Risk in Communities (ARIC) study found no relationship between low dietary magnesium intake and increased risk of type 2 diabetes in a middle-aged population. On the other hand, there was a significant inverse correlation between serum total magnesium levels and incidence in the caucasian subset of this study. The same correlation was not seen in the black subset. More study is needed.

Magnesium has been used with some success in a few studies to promote bronchodilation and improve lung function in some asthmatic patients. In one recent meta-analysis, intravenous magnesium was found to significantly reduce the rate of hospital admissions and to improve pulmonary function in patients treated in emergency departments for severe acute asthma. The same benefit was not reported for those with mild to moderate asthma. Epidemiological data have also shown that higher dietary intakes of magnesium are associated with a lower incidence of airway reactivity and respiratory symptoms. More research is needed to further determine the relative value of supplemental magnesium in the prevention and treatment of asthma and related conditions.

Alcoholics have a high incidence of magnesium deficiency. This deficiency contributes, some research indicates, to an increased incidence of osteoporosis and cardiovascular disease among chronic alcoholics. Alcohol is known to be a potent magnesium diuretic. Supplemental magnesium has shown benefit in some alcoholics. In one randomized study, supplemental magnesium improved a number of metabolic variables and muscle strength, compared with placebo, in chronic alcoholics. Alcohol consumption was the same before and during the trial. The favorable metabolic changes suggested that supplemental magnesium might improve liver cell function and electrolyte status, as well as muscle strength, in chronic alcoholics.

Magnesium and phenobarbital have been reported to be effective in easing the symptoms of alcohol withdrawal. A double-blind, placebo-controlled trial of magnesium in the ethanol withdrawal syndrome, however, found no benefit from intramuscular injections of magnesium, compared with saline control. The researchers concluded that magnesium is not indicated for alcohol withdrawal unless withdrawal is characterized by cardiac arrhythmias.

Other researchers, reviewing the literature on the use of magnesium in delirium tremens between 1954 and 1987, have similarly concluded that there is most likely no causal relationship between hypomagnesemia and delirium tremens. They cite more recent research findings showing that hypomagnesemia is not universal among chronic alcoholics and that magnesium concentrations return to normal in some alcoholics without use of magnesium supplements. They have recommended against the routine use of parenteral magnesium in patients with delirium tremens.

Magnesium supplements may significantly protect post menopausal women from osteoporosis according to researchers who tested the supplement in a group of these women for two years. Magnesium's role in regulating active calcium transport has made its importance in bone metabolism manifest. Women in the two-year study received varying doses of magnesium, from 250 milligrams to 750 milligrams, and were compared with unsupplemented age-matched controls. The magnesium-treated women also had significantly increased bone density by the end of the study while the controls did not. Follow-up is needed.

Magnesium levels have been found to be diminished in some with premenstrual syndrome (PMS). In one double-blind, randomized study, women with PMS received placebo or 360 milligrams of magnesium three times a day from day 15 of the menstrual cycle to the onset of menstrual flow. Magnesium performed better than placebo in some measures related to premenstrual mood changes. Both placebo and magnesium seemed to reduce pain associated with PMS. More rigorous studies are needed before any conclusion can be drawn with respect to magnesium's possible efficacy in alleviating symptoms of PMS. Finally, two double-blind, studies have suggested that chronic oral magnesium supplementation may reduce the frequency of migraine headaches. Refractory patients have, reportedly, been helped with intravenous magnesium. Magnesium concentrations have been shown to affect serotonin receptors, nitric oxide synthesis and release and NMDA receptors, all believed to play some role in migraine. In a multi-center, placebo-controlled, double-blind, randomized study, 81 patients, aged 18-65 years, with a mean migraine frequency attack of 3-6 per month, were given 600 milligrams of magnesium or placebo orally each day for 12 weeks. In weeks 9-12, attack frequency was reduced by 41.6% in the magnesium group and by 15.8% in the placebo group, compared with baseline. More research is warranted.

CONTRAINDICATIONS, PRECAUTIONS, ADVERSE REACTIONS

CONTRAINDICATIONS

Magnesium is contraindicated in those with renal failure. It is also contraindicated in those with high-grade atrioventricular (AV) blocks unless those with high-grade AV blocks have artificial pacemakers.

Magnesium is contraindicated in those who are hypersensitive to any component of a magnesium-containing supplement.

PRECAUTIONS

Pregnant women and nursing mothers should avoid magnesium doses greater than 350 milligrams daily (in supplementary form) unless higher doses are prescribed by their physicians.

Those with myasthenia gravis should avoid the use of magnesium supplements. Magnesium supplements may exacerbate weakness and trigger a myasthenic crisis.

ADVERSE REACTIONS

The most common adverse reaction from the use of magnesium supplements is diarrhea. Other gastrointestinal symptoms that may occur with the use of magnesium supplements are nausea and abdominal cramping. If magnesium supplements are taken with food, diarrhea and other gastrointestinal symptoms are less likely to occur. Diarrhea and other gastrointestinal symptoms typically occur with magnesium doses greater than 350 milligrams daily. Doses of 350 milligrams or lower are generally well tolerated.

Those with renal failure may develop hypermagnesemia with use of magnesium supplements (see Contraindications). Serious adverse reactions with the use of oral magnesium supplements in those with normal renal function are rare but they have been reported. An eight week-old infant developed metabolic alkalosis, diarrhea and dehydration after receiving large amounts of magnesium oxide powder on each of two successive days. An adult woman developed metabolic alkalosis and hypokalemia from the repeated daily ingestion of 30 grams of magnesium oxide. Paralytic ileus has been reported in adults taking large, cathartic doses of magnesium. One suicide patient given 465 grams of magnesium sulfate as a cathartic to counteract an intentional drug overdose had a cardiopulmonary arrest. A few deaths have been reported in patients with renal failure who took very large doses of magnesium as magnesium sulfate or magnesium oxide.

INTERACTIONS

DRUGS

Bisphosphonates (alendronate, etidronate, risedronate): Concomitant intake of a bisphosphonate and magnesium may decrease the absorption of the bisphosphonate.

Quinolones (ciprofloxacin, gatifloxacin, levofloxacin, lomefloxacin, moxifloxacin, norfloxacin, ofloxacin, sparfloxacin, trovafloxacin): Concomitant use of a quinolone and magnesium may decrease the absorption of the quinolone.

Tetracyclines (doxycyline, monocycline, tetracycline): Concomitant intake of a tetracycline and magnesium may decrease the absorption of the tetracycline.

NUTRITIONAL SUPPLEMENTS

Boron: Boron may increase magnesium levels.

Calcium: Concomitant intake of high doses of calcium—greater than 2 grams—may decrease the absorption of magnesium. Most studies have shown that concomitant intakes of typical doses of calcium and magnesium do not decrease the absorption of magnesium.

Inositol Hexaphosphate: Concomitant intake of inositol hexaphosphate and magnesium may depress the absorption of magnesium.

Iron: Concomitant intake of magnesium and iron may decrease the absorption of iron.

Manganese: Concomitant intake of magnesium and manganese may decrease the absorption of manganese.

Non-digestible oligosaccharides (fructo-oligosaccharides, inulin): Concomitant use of non-digestible oligosaccharides and magnesium may increase the colonic absorption of magnesium.

Phosphate: Concomitant intake of phosphate and magnesium may decrease the absorption of both phosphate and magnesium.

Sodium Alginate: Concomitant intake of sodium alginate and magnesium may decrease the absorption of magnesium.

FOODS
Concomitant intake of a magnesium supplement with foods rich in oxalic acid (spinach, sweet potatoes, rhubarb and beans) or phytic acid (unleavened bread, raw beans, seeds, nuts and grains and soy isolates) may decrease the absorption of magnesium.

OVERDOSAGE
See Adverse Reactions.

There is a report of a patient having a cardiopulmonary arrest after ingesting 465 grams of magnesium sulfate, and there are a few reports of deaths in those with renal failure who took very large doses of magnesium.

DOSAGE AND ADMINISTRATION
There are several forms of magnesium used for nutritional supplementation. These include: magnesium oxide, magnesium gluconate, magnesium chloride, magnesium citrate, magnesium hydroxide, magnesium aspartate, magnesium orotate, magnesium arginate, magnesium pidolate and other amino acid and oligopeptide chelates of magnesium. Magnesium supplements are available as stand-alone supplements or in combination products. Some products contain mixtures of a few magnesium forms, e.g., magnesium oxide, magnesium chloride and magnesium gluconate. Many combination products are available.

Typical doses of magnesium (expressed as elemental magnesium) range from 100 to 350 milligrams daily.

Taking magnesium supplements with food is less likely to cause diarrhea.

The Food and Nutrition Board of the Institute of Medicine of the United States National Academy of Sciences has recommended the following Adequate Intake (AI) and Recommended Dietary Allowance (RDA) values for magnesium:

Infants	(AI)
0 through 6 months	30 mg/day
7 through 12 months	75 mg/day

Children	(RDA)
1 through 3 years	80 mg/day
4 through 8 years	130 mg/day

Boys	
9 through 13 years	240 mg/day
4 through 18 years	410 mg/day

Girls	
9 through 13 years	240 mg/day
4 through 18 years	360 mg/day

Men	
19 through 30 years	400 mg/day
31 through 50 years	420 mg/day
51 through 70 years	420 mg/day
Greater than 70 years	420 mg/day

Women	
19 through 30 years	310 mg/day
31 through 50 years	320 mg/day
51 through 76 years	320 mg/day
Greater than 70 years	320 mg/day

Pregnancy	
14 through 18 years	400 mg/day
19 through 30 years	350 mg/day
31 through 50 years	380 mg/day

Lactation	
14 through 18 years	360 mg/day
19 through 30 years	310 mg/day
31 through 50 years	320 mg/day

The Food and Nutrition Board has recommended the following upper limits (UL) for supplementary magnesium (i.e., nonfood source magnesium).

Infants	(UL)
0 through 12 months	Not possible to establish for supplementary magnesium

Children	
1 through 3 years	65 mg of supplementary magnesium
4 through 8 years	110 mg of supplementary magnesium

Pregnancy	
14 through 50 years	350 mg of supplementary magnesium

Lactation	
14 through 50 years	350 mg of supplementary magnesium

Adolescents and Adults	350 mg of supplementary magnesium

The Food and Nutrition Board recognizes that those with certain clinical conditions, such as neonatal tetany, hyperuricemia, hyperlipidemia, lithium toxicity, hyperthyroidism, cardiac arrhythmias and digitalis intoxication, may benefit from the prescribed use of magnesium supplements exceeding the above ULs.

HOW SUPPLIED

Magnesium chloride is available in the following forms and strengths for Rx use:

Injection — 200 mg/mL

Magnesium chloride is available in the following forms and strengths for OTC use:

Tablet, Extended Release — 535 mg

Magnesium gluconate is available in the following forms and strengths for OTC use:

Liquid — 3.25 mg/mL, 1000 mg/5 mL
Tablet — 500 mg

Magnesium Lactate is available in the following forms and strengths for OTC use:

Tablet, Extended Release — 84 mg

Magnesium Oxide is available in the following forms and strengths for OTC use:

Capsules — 140 mg, 600 mg
Powder
Tablets — 200 mg, 250 mg, 400 mg, 420 mg, 500 mg

Magnesium Sulfate is available in the following forms and strengths for Rx use:

Injection — 40 mg/mL, 80 mg/mL, 125 mg/mL, 500 mg/mL

LITERATURE

Abbott L, Nadler J, Rude RK. Magnesium deficiency in alcoholism: possible contribution to osteoporosis and cardiovascular disease in alcoholics. *Alcohol Clin Exp Res.* 1994; 18:1076-1082.

Altura BM, Altura BT. Role of magnesium and calcium in alcohol-induced hypertension and strokes as probed by in vivo television microscopy, digital image microscopy, optical spectroscopy, 31P-NMR, spectroscopy and a unique magnesium ion-selective electrode. *Alcohol Clin Exp Res.* 1994; 18:1057-1068.

Baxter GF, Sumeray MS, Walker JM. Infant size and magnesium: insights into LIMIT-2 and ISIS-4 from experimental studies. *Lancet.* 1996; 348:1424-1426.

Britton J, Pavord I, Richards K, et al. Dietary magnesium, lung function, wheezing, and airway hyper-reactivity in a random adult population sample. *Lancet.* 1994; 344:357-362.

Casscells W. Magnesium and myocardial infarction. *Lancet.* 1994; 343:807-809.

Christiansen CW, Rieder MA, Silverstein EL, Gencheff NE. Magnesium sulfate reduces myocardial infarct size when administered before but not after coronary reperfusion in a canine model. *Circulation.* 1995; 92:2617-2621.

de Lourdes Lima M, Cruz T, Carreiro Pousada J, et al. The effect of magnesium supplementation in increasing doses on the control of type 2 diabetes. *Diabetes Care.* 1998; 21:682-686.

Dietary Reference Intakes for Calcium, Phosphorous, Magnesium, Vitamin D, and Fluoride. Washington, DC: National Academy Press; 1997.

Durlach J, Durlach V, Bac P, et al. Magnesium and therapeutics. *Magnes Res.* 1994; 7:313-328.

Elisaf M, Merkouropoulos M, Tsianos EV. Siamopoulos KC. Pathogenetic mechanisms of hypomagnesemia in alcoholic patients. *J Trace Elem Med Biol.* 1995; 9:210-214.

Facchinetti F, Borella P, Sances G, et al. Oral magnesium successfully relieves premenstrual mood changes. *Obstet Gynecol.* 1991; 78:177-181.

Gullestad L, Dolva LO, Soyland E, et al. Oral magnesium supplementation improves metabolic variables and muscle strength in alcoholics. *Alcohol Clin Exp Res.* 1992; 16:986-990.

Herzog WR, Schlossberg ML, MacMurdy KS, et al. Timing of magnesium therapy affects experimental infarct size. *Circulation.* 1995; 92:2622-2626.

Iseri LT, French JH. Magnesium: nature's physiologic calcium blocker. *Am Heart J.* 1984; 108:188-193.

ISIS-4 (Fourth International Study of Infarct Survival) Collaborative Group. ISIS-4: a randomised factorial trial assessing early oral captopril, oral mononitrate, and intravenous magnesium sulfate in 58,050 patients with suspected acute myocardial infarction. *Lancet.* 1995; 345:669-685.

Jermain DM, Crisman ML, Nisbet RB. Controversies over the use of magnesium sulfate in delirium tremens. *Ann Pharmacother.* 1992; 26:650-652.

Kao WHL, Folsom AR, Nieto J, et al. Serum and dietary magnesium and the risk for type 2 diabetes mellitus (editorial). *Arch. Int Med.* 1999; 159:2151-2159.

Lim R, Herzog WR. Magnesium for cardiac patients: is it a valuable treatment supplement? *Contemp Int Med.* 1998; 10:6-9.

Lucas MJ, Leveno KJ, Cunningham FG. A comparison of magnesium sulfate with phenytoin for the prevention of eclampsia. *N Engl J Med.* 1995; 333:201-205.

Martini LA. Magnesium supplementation and bone turnover. *Nutr Rev.* 1999; 57:227-229.

Mauskop A, Altura BM. Role of magnesium in the pathogenesis and treatment of migraines. *Clin Neurosci.* 1998; 5:24-27.

Orchard TJ. Magnesium and type 2 diabetes mellitus (editorial). *Arch Int Med.* 1999; 159:2119-2120.

Peikert A, Wilimzig C, Kohne-Volland R. Prophylaxis of migraine with oral magnesium: results from a prospective, multi-center, placebo-controlled and double-blind randomized study. *Cephalalgia*. 1996; 16:257-263.

Paolisso G, Sgamabato S, Pizza G, et al. Improved insulin response and action by chronic magnesium administration in aged NIDDM. *Diabetes Care*. 1989; 12:265-269.

Rivlin RS. Magnesium deficiency and alcohol intake: mechanisms, clinical significance and possible relation to cancer development (a review). *J Am Coll Nutr*. 1994; 13:416-423.

Roberts JM. Magnesium for preeclampsia and eclampsia. *N Engl J Med*. 1995; 333:250-251.

Roffe C, Fletcher S, Woods KL. Investigation of the effects of intravenous magnesium sulphate on cardiac rhythm in acute myocardial infarction. *Br Heart J*. 1994; 71:141-145.

Saris N-EL, Mervaala E, Karppanen H, et al. Magnesium. An update on physiological, clinical and analytical aspects (review). *Clinica Chimica Acta*. 2000; 294:1-26.

Schendel DE, Berg CJ, Yeargin-Allsopp M, et al. Prenatal magnesium sulfate exposure and the risk for cerebral palsy or mental retardation among very low-birth-weight children aged 3 to 5 years. *JAMA*. 1996; 276:1805-1810.

Shils ME. Magnesium. In: Shils M, Olson JA, Shike M, Ross AC, eds. *Modern Nutrition in Health and Disease*. 9th ed. Baltimore, MD: Williams and Wilkins; 1999:169-192.

Sojka JE. Magnesium supplementation and osteoporosis. *Nutr Rev*. 1995; 53:71-80.

Terblanche S, Noakes TD, Dennis SC, et al. Failure of magnesium supplementation to influence marathon running performance or recovery in magnesium-replete subjects. *Int J Sports Nutr*. 1992; 2:154-164.

Toba Y, Kajita Y, Masuyama R, et al. Dietary magnesium supplementation affects bone metabolism and dynamic strength of bone in ovariectomized rats. *J Nutr*. 2000; 130:216-220.

Tosiello L. Hypomagnesemia and diabetes mellitus. A review of clinical implications. *Arch Intern Med*. 1998; 156:1143-1148.

Woods KL, Fletcher S. Long-term outcome after intravenous magnesium sulphate in suspected acute myocardial infarction: the second Leicester Intravenous Magnesium Intervention Trial (LIMIT-2). *Lancet*. 1994; 343:816-819.

Malic Acid

TRADE NAMES
Fibralgia (Nature's Sunshine)

DESCRIPTION
Malic acid, an alpha-hydroxy organic acid, is sometimes referred to as a fruit acid. This is because malic acid is found in apples and other fruits. It is also found in plants and animals, including humans. In fact, malic acid, in the form of its anion malate, is a key intermediate in the major biochemical energy-producing cycle in cells known as the citric acid or Krebs cycle located in the cells' mitochondria.

Malic acid, also known as apple acid, hydroxybutanedioic acid and hydroxysuccinic acid, is a chiral molecule. The naturally occurring stereoisomer is the L-form. The L-form is also the biologically active one. There is some preliminary evidence that malic acid, in combination with magnesium, may be helpful for some with fibromyalgia. Malic acid sold as a supplement is mainly derived from apples and, therefore, is the L-form. L-malic acid has the following chemical structure:

L-malic Acid

ACTIONS AND PHARMACOLOGY

ACTIONS
Malic acid, in combination with magnesium, has putative antifibromyalgic activity.

MECHANISM OF ACTION
The mechanism of malic acid's putative antifibromyalgic activity is unknown.

PHARMACOKINETICS
Malic acid is absorbed from the gastrointestinal tract from whence it is transported via the portal circulation to the liver. There are a few enzymes that metabolize malic acid. Malic enzyme catalyzes the oxidative decarboxylation of L-malate to pyruvate with concomitant reduction of the cofactor NAD+ (oxidized form of nicotinamide adenine dinucleotide) or NADP+ (oxidized form of nicotinamide adenine dinucleotide phosphate). These reactions require the divalent cations magnesium or manganese. Three isoforms of malic enzyme have been identified in mammals: a cytosolic NADP+-dependent malic enzyme, a mitochondrial NADP+-dependent malic enzyme and a mitochondrial NAD(P)+-dependent malic enzyme. The latter can use either NAD+ or NADP+ as the cofactor but prefers NAD+. Pyruvate formed from malate can itself be metabolized in a number of ways, including metabolism via a number of metabolic steps to glucose. Malate can also be metabolized to oxaloacetate via the citric acid cycle. The mitochondrial malic enzyme, particularly in brain cells, may play a key role in the pyruvate recycling pathway, which utilizes dicarboxylic acids and substrates, such as glutamine, to provide pyruvate to maintain the citric acid cycle activity when glucose and lactate are low.

Clearly, the metabolism of malic acid is complex and what any of the above has to do, if anything, with malic acids' putative activity in those with fibromyalgia is entirely unclear.

INDICATIONS AND USAGE

Malic acid may help some with fibromyalgia.

RESEARCH SUMMARY

Results have been mixed in studies of malic acid's possible effects in those with fibromyalgia. In a double-blind, placebo-controlled crossover study, subjects with primary fibromyalgia syndrome were randomized to receive a combination of 200 milligrams of malic acid and 50 milligrams of magnesium per tablet (three tablets twice a day) or placebo for four weeks. This was followed by a six-month, open-label trial with dose escalating up to six tablets twice a day. Outcome variables were measures of pain and tenderness, as well as functional and psychological measures.

No clear benefit was observed for the malic acid/magnesium combination in the lower-dose blinded trial. But in the open-label trial, at higher doses, there were significant reductions in the severity of all three primary pain/tenderness measures. Follow-up is needed.

CONTRAINDICATIONS, PRECAUTIONS, ADVERSE REACTIONS

CONTRAINDICATIONS

None known for malic acid. See Magnesium.

PRECAUTIONS

Because of lack of long-term safety studies, supplementary malic acid should be avoided by pregnant women and lactating mothers. See Magnesium.

INTERACTIONS

None reported for malic acid. See Magnesium.

DOSAGE AND ADMINISTRATION

The doses used in the fibromyalgia studies were L-malic acid, 1200 to 2400 milligrams daily, and magnesium, 300 to 600 milligrams daily.

HOW SUPPLIED

Tablets — 350 mg

LITERATURE

Russell IJ, Michalek JE, Flechas JD, Abraham GE. Treatment of fibromyalgia syndrome with Super Malic: a randomized, double-blind, placebo-controlled pilot study. *J Rheumatol*. 1995; 22:953-958.

Young Z, Floyd DL, Loeber G, Tong L. Structure of a closed form of human malic enzyme and implications for catalytic mechanism. *Nature Struct Biol*. 2000; 7:251-257.

Manganese

DESCRIPTION

Manganese is an essential trace mineral in animal nutrition and is believed to be an essential trace mineral in human nutrition, as well. Manganese is a metallic element with atomic number 25 and an atomic weight of 54.94 daltons. Its chemical symbol is Mn. Manganese exists in the oxidation states Mn^{2+} or Mn(II) and Mn^{3+} or Mn(III) under physiological conditions.

Dietary manganese-deficiency in animals results in a wide variety of structural and physiological defects, including growth retardation, skeletal and cartilage malformations, impaired reproductive function, congenital ataxia due to abnormal inner ear development, optic nerve abnormalities, impaired insulin metabolism and abnormal glucose tolerance, alterations in lipoprotein metabolism and an impaired oxidant defense system.

Manganese deficiency states have not been well documented in humans. There is one report of a man maintained for four months on a manganese-deficient diet and also given magnesium-containing antacids. The symptoms which occurred included a decrease in serum cholesterol, depressed growth of hair and nails, scaly dermatitis, weight loss, reddening of his black hair and beard and impaired blood clotting. He responded to a diet containing manganese. In another report, men fed a low-manganese diet manifested low serum cholesterol levels and dermatitis. Short-term manganese supplementation did not reverse these symptoms.

In still another report, young women fed a manganese-poor diet were found to have mildly abnormal glucose tolerance and increased menstrual losses of manganese, calcium, iron and total hemoglobin. Finally a child on long-term total parenteral nutrition (TPN) lacking manganese manifested bone demineralization and impaired growth that were corrected by supplementation with manganese.

Manganese is the preferred metal cofactor for glycosyltransferases. Glycosyltransferases are important in the synthesis of glycoproteins and glycosaminoglycans (GAGs or mucopolysaccharides). Glycoproteins are involved in the synthesis of myelin and the clotting factors, among other things. Manganese-containing metalloenzymes include manganese superoxide dismutase, the principal antioxidant enzyme of mitochondria, arginase, pyruvate carboxylase and glutamine synthetase.

The richest dietary sources of manganese include whole grains, nuts, leafy vegetables and teas. Manganese is concentrated in the bran of grains which is removed during processing. Mean intakes of manganese worldwide range from 0.52 to 10.8 milligrams daily.

ACTIONS AND PHARMACOLOGY
ACTIONS
Manganese may have antioxidant activity. Manganese has putative anti-osteoporotic and anti-arthritic activities.

MECHANISM OF ACTION
Manganese ions have been found to scavenge hydroxyl and superoxide radicals. The mechanism of binding of manganese ions to these reactive oxygen species is not known. Manganese is a crucial component of the metalloenzyme manganese superoxide dismutase (MnSOD). MnSOD is found in mitochondria and is the principal constituent of the mitochondrial oxidant defense system. Rats and mice fed manganese-deficient diets are found to have reduced MnSOD activity in heart muscle and nervous tissue. They also have mitochondrial abnormalities and pathological changes in these tissues. The pathological changes are thought to result from oxidative damage due to the decreased activity of MnSOD which normally would protect against this damage.

Dietary manganese deficiency results in skeletal and cartilage malformations in animals and in one human report. It is thought that this is due to decreased activity of the manganese-dependent glycosyltransferases which, among other things, are involved in the synthesis of glycosaminoglycans or GAGs. GAGs are crucial for healthy cartilage and bone. However, there is as yet only very preliminary evidence that supplemental manganese has any effect on the promotion of bone or cartilage formation in humans who are not manganese-deficient. One study reported that manganese when taken in combination with calcium, copper and zinc may improve bone mineral density in postmenopausal women with osteoporosis.

PHARMACOKINETICS
There is scant information on the pharmacokinetics of manganese in humans. The efficiency of absorption (fractional absorption) of ingested manganese appears to be low, about 5%. Absorption efficiency appears to decrease as dietary intake of manganese increases. It increases with low dietary intake of manganese. Absorption appears to occur throughout the small intestine and appears to occur by both active-transport and passive diffusion mechanisms. Manganese ions are transported via the portal circulation to the liver. In what forms manganese is transported to the liver—bound to albumin, alpha$_2$-macroglobulin, hydrated manganese complexes, etc.—is also unclear. A fraction of manganese is taken up by hepatocytes and a fraction is transported by the systemic circulation to the various tissues of the body. Some manganese is bound to the plasma protein transferrin, but there also appear to be other carriers that transport manganese in the systemic circulation. Manganese is found principally in the mitochondria of cells. Absorbed manganese is excreted primarily via the biliary route. Very little manganese is excreted in the urine.

INDICATIONS AND USAGE
Apart from its uses in rare overt deficiency disorders, manganese might have some efficacy in osteoporosis and osteoarthritis as well as in some with premenstrual syndrome (PMS). Evidence for these benefits is preliminary.

RESEARCH SUMMARY
Manganese supplementation, in combination with calcium, zinc and copper, showed some efficacy in postmenopausal osteoporosis. Manganese ascorbate, in combination with glucosamine hydrochloride and chondroitin sulfate, was helpful in treating knee osteoarthritis pain in a recent randomized, double-blind, placebo-controlled pilot study. Followup on these studies is needed. Similarly, there is an isolated study needing followup that suggested some possible benefit from manganese in alleviating some PMS symptoms, including anxiety, depression, irritability and mood swings.

CONTRAINDICATIONS, PRECAUTIONS, ADVERSE REACTIONS
CONTRAINDICATIONS
Manganese supplements are contraindicated in those with liver failure. Some patients with end-stage liver disease have been found to accumulate manganese in their basal ganglia. It is thought that manganese may play a role in the hepatic encephalopathy in those with liver failure. Manganese is eliminated primarily through the bile, and hepatic dysfunction leads to depressed manganese excretion.

Manganese supplements are contraindicated in those hypersensitive to any component of a manganese-containing supplement.

PRECAUTIONS
Pregnant women and nursing mothers should avoid intakes of manganese above the upper limit of the estimated safe and adequate daily dietary intake (ESSADI). The ESSADI for those 11 years and older is 2.0 to 5.0 milligrams daily.

ADVERSE REACTIONS
Oral manganese supplements are generally well tolerated. Oral manganese, however, may be neurotoxic in those with liver failure. Manganese is primarily eliminated via the biliary route, and hepatic dysfunction leads to depressed manganese excretion. Manganese may accumulate in the basal ganglia of those with liver failure and may exacerbate hepatic encephalopathy and/or cause Parkinson's disease-like symptoms.

Manganese is toxic under certain conditions. Hepatic failure was discussed above. Mine workers exposed to high concentrations of manganese dust develop what is known in the mining villages of northern Chile, where this disorder has been found, as ''locura manganica'' or manganese madness. In later stages of this disease, symptoms similar to those of Parkinson's disease are observed. Levodopa is the treatment of the later stages of manganese madness.

There are a few reports of manganese intoxication occurring in those on long-term total parenteral nutrition (TPN) who developed parkinsonism which was treated with levodopa.

INTERACTIONS

DRUGS

Antacids: Magnesium-containing antacids, such as aluminum hydroxide/magnesium hydroxide, aluminum hydroxide/magnesium carbonate and aluminum hydroxide/magnesium trisilicate, may decrease the absorption of manganese if taken concomitantly.

Laxatives: Magnesium-containing laxatives may decrease the absorption of manganese if taken concomitantly.

Tetracycline: Tetracycline may reduce the absorption of manganese if taken concomitantly.

NUTRITIONAL SUPPLEMENTS

Calcium: Calcium supplements may decrease the absorption of manganese if taken concomitantly.

Iron: Non-heme iron supplements may reduce the absorption of manganese if taken concomitantly.

Magnesium: Magnesium supplements may decrease the absorption of manganese if taken concomitantly.

FOODS

Concomitant intake of manganese with foods rich in phytic acid (unleavened bread, raw beans, seeds, nuts and grains and soy isolates) or oxalic acid (spinach, sweet potatoes, rhubarb and beans) may depress the absorption of manganese.

DOSAGE AND ADMINISTRATION

There are several forms of supplementary manganese, including manganese gluconate, manganese sulfate, manganese ascorbate and manganese amino acid chelates. Manganese is available as a stand-alone supplement and also in combination products. One combination product used for bone/joint health contains chondroitin sulfate, glucosamine hydrochloride and manganese ascorbate.

Typical supplemental intake of manganese ranges from 2 to 5 milligrams daily.

The Food and Nutrition Board of the U.S. National Academy of Sciences has recommended the following estimated safe and adequate daily dietary intake (ESADDI) values for manganese:

Age (years)	ESADDI (milligrams)
0 to 0.5	0.3 to 0.6
0.5 to 1	0.6 to 1.0
1 to 3	1.0 to 1.5
4 to 6	1.5 to 2.0
7 to 10	2.0 to 3.0
11 to 18	2.0 to 5.0
Adults	2.0 to 5.0

Up to 10 milligrams daily of manganese is considered safe.

LITERATURE.

Baly DL, Schneiderman JS, Garcia-Welsh AL. Effect of manganese deficiency on insulin binding, glucose transport and metabolism in rat adipocytes. *J Nutr.* 1990; 120:1075-1079.

Fell JME, Reynolds AP, Meadows N, et al. Manganese toxicity in children receiving long-term parenteral nutrition. *Lancet.* 1996; 347:1218-1221.

Gong H, Amemiya T. Optic nerve changes in manganese-deficient rats. *Exp Eye Res.* 1999; 68:313-320.

Hussain S, Ali SF. Manganese scavenges superoxide and hydroxyl radicals: an in vitro study in rats. *Neuroscience Letters.* 1999; 261:21-24.

Keen CL, Ensunsa JL, Watson MH, et al. Nutritional aspects of manganese from experimental studies. *Neurotoxicol.* 1999; 20:213-223.

Krieger D, Krieger S, Jansen O, et al. Manganese and chronic hepatic encephalopathy. *Lancet.* 1995; 346:270-274.

Nagatomo S, Umehara F, Hanada K, et al. Manganese intoxication during total parenteral nutrition: report of two cases and review of the literature. *J Neurol Sci.* 1999; 162:102-105.

Nielsen FH. Ultratrace minerals. In: Shils ME, Olson JA, Shike M, Ross AC, eds. *Modern Nutrition in Health and Disease,* 9th ed. Baltimore, MD: Williams and Wilkins; 1999:283-303.

Strause L, Saltman P, Glowacki J. The effect of deficiencies of manganese and copper on osteo-induction and on resorption of bone particles in rats. *Calcif Tissue Int.* 1987; 41:145-150

Strause L, Saltman P, Smith KT, et al. Spinal bone loss in postmenopausal women supplemented with calcium and trace minerals. *J Nutr.* 1994; 124:1060-1064.

Strause LG, Hegenauer J, Saltman P, et al. Effects of long-term dietary manganese and copper deficiency on rat skeleton. *J Nutr.* 1986; 116:135-141.

Medium-Chain Triglycerides

TRADE NAMES

MCT Oil (Mead Johnson)

DESCRIPTION

Medium-chain triglycerides, commonly abbreviated MCT or MCTs, are medium-chain fatty acid esters of glycerol.

Medium-chain fatty acids are fatty acids containing from six to 12 carbon atoms. These fatty acids are constituents of coconut and palm kernel oils and are also found in camphor tree drupes. Coconut and palm kernel oils are also called lauric oils because of their high content of the 12 carbon fatty acid, lauric or dodecanoic acid.

Medium-chain triglycerides used for nutritional and other commercial purposes are derived from lauric oils. In the process of producing MCTs, lauric oils are hydrolyzed to medium-chain fatty acids and glycerol. The glycerol is drawn off from the resultant mixture, and the medium-chain fatty acids are fractionally distilled. The medium-chain fatty acid fraction used commercially is mainly comprised of the eight carbon caprylic or octanoic acid and the 10 carbon capric or decanoic acid. There are much smaller amounts of the six carbon caproic or hexanoic acid and the 12 carbon lauric acid in the commercial products. The caprylic- and capric-rich mixture is finally re-esterified to glycerol to produce medium-chain triglycerides that are mainly glyceral esters of caproic (C_6) caprylic (C_8), capric (C_{10}) and lauric acid (C_{12}) in a ratio of approximately 2:55:42:1. MCTs are represented by the following chemical structures:

Medium-chain triglycerides

R represents the alkyl moieties primarily of C_8, caprylic (octanoic) and C_{10}, capric (decanoic) acids.

$$CH_3(CH_2)_5CH_2 \text{---} C(\text{=}O) \text{---} OH$$

Caprylic Acid

$$CH_3(CH_2)_7CH_2 \text{---} C(\text{=}O) \text{---} OH$$

Capric acid

MCT is also known as fractionated coconut oil. In a process called interesterification, long-chain fatty acids, such as oleic and linoleic acid, are introduced into the final product. MCT derivatives produced by the interesterification process are referred to as structural lipids or structural triglycerides. Unlike most natural oils of animal or vegetable origin, MCT is stable and resistant to oxidation owing mainly to the saturation of the medium-chain fatty acids.

ACTIONS AND PHARMACOLOGY

ACTIONS

MCT's major action is as an energy-yielding substrate, particularly beneficial for those with malabsorption syndromes. MCT is also ketogenic.

MECHANISM OF ACTION

The physiology and biochemistry of medium-chain triglycerides are very different from those of long-chain triglycerides. MCT is rapidly absorbed from the small intestine, intact or following hydrolysis, into the portal circulation. From there, it is transported to the liver. Long-chain triglycerides are first hydrolyzed in the small intestine to long-chain fatty acids. They are in turn re-esterified in the mucosal cells of the small intestine to long-chain triglyerides, which are then carried by chylomicrons and transported via the lymphatic system to the systemic circulation. The systemic circulation in turn distributes the long-chain triglycerides to various tissues of the body, including adipose tissue and the liver.

Since MCT, in contrast with long-chain fatty acids, does not require pancreatic enzymes or bile salts for digestion and absorption, MCT is better handled in those with malabsorption syndromes than are the long-chain fatty acids. These syndromes include pancreatic disorders, hepatic disorders, gastrointestinal disorders and disorders of the lymph system.

Medium-chain fatty acids are taken up by hepatocytes and converted to medium-chain fatty acyl CoA which enters mitochondria without requiring the aid of carnitine. On the other hand, long-chain fatty acids, which are also converted to their coenzyme A esters in cells, including hepatocytes, require that they be converted from coenzyme A esters to carnitine esters in order to be transported across the mitochondrial membrane. Within the hepatocyte mitochondria, medium-chain fatty acyl CoA is converted to acetoacetate and beta-hydroxybutyrate and subsequently to carbon dioxide, water and energy. The oxidation of MCT produces 8.3 kilocalories of energy per gram ingested.

MCTs are therefore easier to metabolize, which could be advantageous to those who are critically ill and those with carnitine deficiencies.

MCT is ketogenic. The metabolism of MCT in hepatocytes produces two so-called ketone bodies, acetoacetate and beta-hydroxybutyrate. These ketone bodies are carried by the bloodstream to other tissues of the body, where they are used for energy production, as well as for other biochemical processes. It is believed that ketosis may raise the seizure threshold and reduce seizure severity. This is still hypothetical but is the rationale for the use of ketogenic diets in the treatment of seizure disorders.

PHARMACOKINETICS

MCT is rapidly absorbed from the small intestine, intact or hydrolyzed, after ingestion and is transported to the liver via the portal circulation. Medium-chain fatty acids are transported into hepatocytes and converted to medium-chain fatty acyl CoA esters. Medium-chain fatty acyl CoAs (mainly of caprylic and capric acids) are transported into mitochondria, where they are metabolized to acetoacetate and beta-hydroxybutyrate. The first mitochondrial enzyme in this process is medium-chain acyl CoA dehydrogenase. Acetoacetate and beta-hydroxybutyrate may be further metabolized in the liver to carbon dioxide, water and energy, and may enter some other metabolic pathways in the liver or be transported by the systemic circulation to other tissues, where they undergo metabolism mainly to CO_2, H_2O and energy. Very little ingested MCT is deposited in the body as fat.

INDICATIONS AND USAGE

Though MCT's are being promoted in the supplement marketplace for weight loss and to increase athletic performance, numerous studies have shown that MCT's are ineffective for achieving these goals. On the other hand, MCT does appear to be helpful for nutritional support in a number of conditions, including enteral and total parenteral nutrition in some infants and surgical patients, as well as in some of those who are critically ill with immunosuppression, pulmonary disease, liver disease, neurologic injury and various malabsorption syndromes. MCT may also be useful in some with epilepsy and other disorders characterized by seizures. There is preliminary evidence that MCT may be helpful in some cancers and may have some positive effects on immunity.

RESEARCH SUMMARY

A large number of studies have sought to determine whether MCT can promote long-chain fatty acid oxidation, inhibit the rate of muscle glycogen depletion, and enhance exercise and athletic performance. Many of these studies have tested subjects, some of them elite athletes, on bicycle ergometers. Some of these trials have been randomized, double-blind, placebo-controlled. Almost all have found no effect of MCT on rates of long-chain fatty acid oxidation, muscle glycogen utilization or performance. "At present," one research group concluded, "there is insufficient scientific evidence to recommend that athletes either ingest fat, in the form of MCTs, during exercise, or 'fat adapt' in the weeks prior to a major endurance event to improve athletic performance."

It should be noted that some have reported that exercise performance is actually impaired in some taking high doses of MCT. This diminished performance was associated with increased gastrointestinal complaints, primarily intestinal cramping.

Research on weight loss associated with MCT intake is not as abundant but presents a mixed and mostly negative conclusion. MCT diets have been compared with LCT (long-chain triglyceride) diets and show no superiority. There are no convincing data that diets high in MCT are effective for weight loss.

MCT shows considerable promise, on the other hand, for the nutritional support of some premature infants, surgical patients and the critically ill, particularly those needing total parenteral nutrition (TPN). Lipid emulsions containing significant quantities of MCT as part of TPN have demonstrated significant benefits in some with pulmonary diseases, AIDS, liver disease, neurologic injury and several other illnesses.

AIDS patients, for example, who were suffering from fat malabsorption and chronic diarrhea with weight loss, were significantly benefited by a 12-week regimen of MCT. There was a significant decrease in stool number, stool fat and stool weight compared with baseline, regardless of the etiology of the diarrhea.

Surgical patients have shown more improvement in some studies, using MCT, compared with LCT. The same is true in some patients with some forms of liver disease. MCT is more readily utilized than LCT and is not deposited in the liver. MCT combined with LCT was found to be superior to LCT alone in septic patients with ARDS. Nutritional support with MCT has also helped prevent gestational hyperlipidemic pancreatitis, with resulting successful childbirth.

MCT's usefulness in drug-resistant epilepsy was demonstrated in a trial with 50 children, eight of whom achieved complete control of seizures (four without further use of anticonvulsant drugs). In another trial, five of 17 MCT-treated subjects with previously intractable drug-resistant seizures achieved complete control of seizures with diminished or discontinued use of drugs. Five others had some improvement. Other types of intractable seizures have also yielded to MCT supplementation. Seven girls with Rett syndrome who suffered from drug-resistant seizures were given MCT therapy; five showed clinical benefit.

There is very preliminary evidence that MCT may have some positive effects on immunity and may exert some anti-cancer effects. Compared with LCT, MCT enhanced macrophage response in an animal model and suppressed Malassezia infection *in vitro*. This is significant, in particular, since lipophilic Malassezia species frequently grow on standard lipid infusions and can induce catheter-associated sepsis in newborns and immunocompromised patients receiving parenteral lipids.

In an animal model of cachexia-inducing colon adenocarcinoma, an MCT regimen reduced weight loss and was associated with a marked reduction in tumor size. LCT, on the other hand, did not have these effects. *In vitro* studies have indicated that MCT is significantly cytotoxic against some human tumor cells. More research is underway.

CONTRAINDICATIONS, PRECAUTIONS, ADVERSE REACTIONS

CONTRAINDICATIONS
MCT is contraindicated in those with hepatic encephalopathy.

PRECAUTIONS
Great caution should be exercised in the use of MCT in those with diabetes, acidosis, ketosis, cirrhosis and the inborn error of metabolism, medium-chain acyl CoA dehydrogenase deficiency. Those with cirrhosis may accumulate free fatty acids and glycerol if given MCT.

ADVERSE REACTIONS
Adverse effects reported include diarrhea, nausea, vomiting, irritability and, with high doses (over 80 grams taken at one time), intestinal cramping.

INTERACTIONS

DRUGS
Theoretically, MCT may facilitate the uptake of some lipophilic drugs.

NUTRITIONAL SUPPLEMENTS
MCT may facilitate the absorption of vitamin E, magnesium and calcium. Theoretically, MCT may facilitate the absorption of the fat-soluble vitamins A, D and K, carotenoids, lipophilic polyphenols and supplemental long-chain fatty acids (ALA, EPA, DHA, GLA).

FOODS
MCT may facilitate the absorption of magnesium, calcium, fat-soluble vitamins and other lipophilic nutrients (carotenoids, flavonoids) and long-chain fatty acids in foods.

HERBS
Theoretically, MCT may facilitate the absorption of lipophilic substances in herbs.

OVERDOSAGE
There are no reports of overdosage with MCT.

DOSAGE AND ADMINISTRATION
Medium-chain triglycerides are available in several medical food products, many for use in a hospital setting. Doses of these medical food products are as prescribed by a physician.

MCT (100 percent) is available as a nutritional supplement. Those with malabsorption syndromes typically use one tablespoon up to three times a day with food or as directed by a physician. One tablespoon is equivalent to approximately 15 grams of MCT.

Those who use MCT as a supplement for any other reason typically use one tablespoon once to three times daily taken with food.

Doses greater than 80 grams (over five tablespoons) taken at one time may cause intense intestinal cramping.

HOW SUPPLIED
Oil

LITERATURE

Babayan VK. Medium chain length fatty acid esters and their medical and nutritional applications. *J Am Oil Chem Soc.* 1981; 58:49A-51A.

Bach AC, Ingenbleek Y, Frey A. The usefulness of dietary medium-chain triglycerides in body weight control: fact or fancy? *J Lipid Res.* 1996; 37:708-726.

Bach AC, Babayan VK. Medium-chain triglycerides: an update. *Am J Clin Nutr.* 1982; 36:950-962.

Craig GB, Darnell BE, Weinsier RL, et al. Decreased fat and nitrogen losses in patients with AIDS receiving medium-chain-triglyceride-enriched formula vs. those receiving long-chain-triglyceride-containing formula. *J Am Diet Assoc.* 1997; 97:605-611.

Fan, ST. Review: nutritional support for patients with cirrhosis. *Gastroenterol Hepatol.* 1997; 12:282-286.

Greenberger NJ, Skillman TG. Medium-chain triglycerides. Physiologic consideration and clinical implications. *N Engl J Med.* 1969; 280:1045-1058.

Haas RH, Rice MA, Trauner DA, Merritt TA. Therapeutic effects of a ketogenic diet in Rett syndrome. *Am J Med Genet Suppl.* 1986; 1:225-246.

Hawley JA, Brouns F, Jeukendrup A. Strategies to enhance fat utilization during exercise. *Sports Med.* 1998; 25:241-257.

Hinton PS, Peterson CA, McCarthy DO, Ney DM. Medium-chain compared with long-chain triacylglycerol emulsions enhance macrophage response and increase mucosal mass in parenterally fed rats. *Am J Clin Nutr.* 1998; 67:1265-1272.

Jeukendrup AE, Thielen JJ, Wagenmakers AJ, et al. Effect of medium-chain triacylglycerol and carbohydrate ingestion during exercise on substrate utilization and subsequent cycling performance. *Am J Clin Nutr.* 1998; 67:397-404.

Jiang ZM, Zhang SY, Wang XR, et al. A comparison of medium-chain and long-chain triglycerides in surgical patients. *Ann Surg.* 1993; 217:175-184.

Kimoto Y, Tanji Y, Taguchi T, et al. Antitumor effect of medium-chain triglyceride and its influence on the self-defense system of the body. *Cancer Detect Prev.* 1998; 22:219-224.

Kimura T, Fukui E, Kageyu A, et al. Enhancement of oral bioavailability of d-alpha-tocopherol acetate by lecithin-dispersed aqueous preparation containing medium-chain triglycerides in rats. *Chem Pharm Sci.* 1989; 37:439-441.

Mizushima T, Ochi K, Matsumura N, et al. Prevention of hyperlipidemic acute pancreatitis during pregnancy with medium-chain triglyceride nutritional support. *Int J Pancreatol.* 1998; 23:187-192.

Papamandjaris AA, MacDougall DE, Jones PJ. Medium chain fatty and metabolism and energy expenditure: obesity treatment implications. *Life Sci.* 1998; 62:1203-1215.

Papavassilis C, Mach KK, Mayser PA. Medium-chain triglycerides inhibit growth of Malassezia: implications for prevention of systemic infection. *Crit Care Med.* 1999; 27:1781-1786.

Ruppin DC, Middleton WRJ. Clinical use of medium chain triglycerides. *Drugs.* 1980; 20:216-224.

Sanchez R, Hendler S. Delivery formulation for probucol. 1996; U.S. Patent No. 5, 494, 936

Sills MA, Forsythe WI, Haidukewych D, et al. The medium chain triglyceride diet and intractable epilepsy. *Arch Dis Child.* 1986; 61:1168-1172.

Smirniotis V, Kostopanagiotou G, Vassiliou J, et al. Long chain versus medium chain lipids in patients with ARDS: effects on pulmonary haemodynamics and gas exchange. *Intensive Care Med.* 1998; 24:1029-1033.

Tisdale MJ, Brennan RA. A comparison of long-chain triglycerides and medium-chain triglycerides on weight loss and tumour size in a cachexia model. *Br J Cancer.* 1988; 58:580-583.

Trauner DA. Medium-chain triglyceride (MCT) diet in intractable seizure disorder. *Neurology.* 1985; 35:237-238.

Wanke CA, Pleskow D, Degirolami PC, et al. A medium chain triglyceride-based diet in patients with HIV and chronic diarrhea reduces diarrhea and malabsorption: a prospective, controlled trial. *Nutrition.* 1996; 12:766-771.

Melatonin

TRADE NAMES

Melatonin is available from numerous manufacturers generically. Branded products include Melatonex (Sun Source), Mela-T (Alacer), Night Rest (Source Naturals).

DESCRIPTION

Melatonin is the principal hormone of the vertebrate pineal gland, and it is also produced by extra-pineal tissues in amphibians. It is found in plants as well, but at much lower concentrations than in animals. This hormone is involved in setting the timing (entrainment) of mammalian circadian rhythms, as well as regulating seasonal responses to changes in day length in seasonally breeding mammals—so called photoperiodic responses. Photoperiodic responses include changes in reproductive status, behavior and body weight. Seasonal effects on reproduction in humans are subtle, and the role of melatonin here, if any, is unclear. Recently, melatonin supplementation has become popular as a possible aid for sleep disorders among other things.

Melatonin is synthesized endogenously by the pinealocytes of the pineal gland. The essential amino acid L-tryptophan is a precursor in the synthesis of melatonin. In this synthesis, L-tryptophan first gets metabolized to 5-hydroxytryptophan from which 5-hydroxytryptamine, also known as serotonin, is made. 5-hydroxytryptamine is converted to melatonin in a two-step process, occurring mainly in the pineal gland.

Melatonin is also known as N-acetyl-5-methoxytryptamine and N-[2-(5-Methoxy-1H-indol-3-yl) ethyl] acetamide. The structural formula is:

Melatonin

Melatonin is a solid, lipophilic, hydrophobic substance, which is available as a supplement in synthetic form. Melatonin derived from the pineal glands of beef cattle is also marketed.

ACTIONS AND PHARMACOLOGY

ACTIONS

Supplemental melatonin may have a hypnotic action. It may also have antioxidant and anti-apoptotic activity.

MECHANISM OF ACTION

Melatonin is derived in pinealocytes from L-tryptophan. 5-hydroxytryptamine or serotonin is an intermediate in the biosynthetic process. The rate limiting step in the synthesis of melatonin is the n-acetylation of the 5-hydroxytryptamine by the enzyme arylalkylamine N-acetyltransferase (AA-NAT). Melatonin synthesis displays a circadian rhythm that is reflected in serum melatonin levels. The rhythm is generated by a circadian clock located in the suprachiasmatic nucleus (SCN) of the hypothalamus. The SCN clock is set to the 24 hour day by the natural light-dark cycle. Light signals through a direct retinal pathway to the SCN. The SCN clock sends circadian signals over a neural pathway to the pineal gland. This drives rhythmic melatonin synthesis. The neural input to the gland is norepinephrine, and the output is melatonin. Specifically, the rhythm of the enzyme AA-NAT is under SCN control, with the resulting melatonin rhythm characterized by high levels at night. Thus, the synthesis and release of melatonin are stimulated by darkness and inhibited by light.

The effects of hormones are typically mediated through receptors. Two forms of high-affinity melatonin receptors and one form of a low-affinity receptor have been identified. The high-affinity ML1 receptors are designated Mel1a and Mel1b. The low-affinity receptor is designated ML2.

The Mel1a receptor is expressed in the SCN and in the hypophyseal pars tuberalis. The SCN is the putative site of circadian action of melatonin, and the hypophyseal pars tuberalis is the putative site of its reproductive effects. The Mel1b receptor is expressed mainly in the retina. The ML1 melatonin receptors belong to the family of guanadine triphosphate-binding proteins or G protein-coupled receptors. Activation of the ML1 receptors results in inhibition of adenylate cyclase activity in target cells.

The distribution of the ML2 receptors has not yet been determined. These receptors are coupled to the stimulation of phosphoinositide hydrolysis.

In summary, melatonin is a hormone that has biological effects and that signals through a family of G protein-coupled receptors.

Melatonin has antioxidant activity. However, this activity is found only with very high pharmaceutical doses of this substance. The most significant antioxidant activity of melatonin appears to be its ability to inhibit metal ion-catalyzed oxidation processes, specifically the Fenton reaction.

Melatonin has been found to have anti-apoptotic activity in the thymus. Melatonin inhibits apoptosis in the thymus as well as in cultured dexamethasone-treated thymocytes (a standard model for the study of apoptosis). It is thought to do so by down-regulating the glucocorticoid receptor.

The mechanism of action of supplemental melatonin is speculative. The putative effect of melatonin as a hypnotic may be accounted for by receptor-mediated action on the limbic system. Pharmacologic doses of melatonin may produce a hypothermic effect, which may also play a role in its hypnotic effect.

PHARMACOKINETICS

The absorption and bioavailability of melatonin varies widely. Melatonin is absorbed from the small intestine and is transported by the portal circulation to the liver. Variable amounts of ingested melatonin are metabolized in the liver to 6-hydroxymelatonin. After conjugation with sulfuric or glucuronic acid, it is excreted by the kidneys. Nonmetabolized melatonin is transported via the systemic circulation to various tissues in the body. Serum half-life of ingested melatonin is approximately 35 to 50 minutes.

If melatonin causes drowsiness, this effect occurs about 30 minutes after ingestion and lasts for at least an hour. Melatonin given in the early evening appears to advance the nighttime peak of melatonin secretion by about three hours. Ingested melatonin that did not undergo first-pass metabolism in the liver is eventually metabolized, mainly in the liver, by hydroxylation to 6-hydroxymelatonin. After conjugation with sulfuric or glucuronic acid, it is excreted by the kidneys. A single nighttime dose is cleared by the following morning. With chronic dosing, however, some lipid storage occurs.

INDICATIONS AND USAGE

Melatonin may be indicated for some forms of insomnia and other sleep disturbances. Research results are mixed with respect to claims that melatonin can abolish some of the symptoms of jet lag. Use of the supplement in cancer and immune disorders is unsupported by current research; there are some promising findings, but they are very preliminary. There is no evidence to substantiate claims that melatonin can delay aging, be useful in cardiovascular disease, depression, seasonal affective disorder or sexual dysfunction.

RESEARCH SUMMARY

Numerous studies, many of them well-designed, suggest that supplemental melatonin can be effective in some sleep disorders, principally insomnia. These studies show that, in doses that raise serum melatonin levels to those that approximate normal nocturnal levels, sleep can be induced and sustained in some. Through its effects on circadian rhythms and possibly through an induced hypothermic effect, melatonin, in doses administered at carefully timed intervals, may be able to normalize various sleep disorders, such as those sometimes experienced by shift workers, and thus diminish fatigue.

The complexity of appropriate timing and dosage, however, has prompted some researchers to caution against melatonin use for sleep disturbance outside of laboratory settings or without medical supervision—at least until more research sheds further light on these issues. Even marginal drowsiness or lack of mental alertness could prove hazardous for some shift workers, for example.

In addition, a cautionary note has recently been issued with respect to the use of melatonin to treat sleep disturbances in children with neurologic disorders. Six such children, aged nine months to 18 years, were given 5 milligrams of melatonin at bedtime in as effort to treat their sleep disorder. Quality and quantity of sleep quickly increased in five of the six children. But in four of the subjects, all of whom had a prior history of seizures, incidence of seizures increased while taking melatonin. Discontinuance of the supplements led to seizure-incidence returning to pre-supplementation levels. But resumption of melatonin supplementation, this time at a reduced level of 1 milligram doses, again caused an increase in seizures, and the study was halted.

Some criticized these researchers for using inappropriately high doses, but the typical dose range in studies of melatonin's effects on sleep disturbance has been 0.3 milligrams to 5 milligrams, with 2 to 3 milligrams commonly being used. Clearly, more research is needed before melatonin can safely be recommended for use in individuals, whether children or adults, with seizure history. In addition, safety data, in general, is lacking for use of this supplement, particularly for long-term use. Certainly, if more research better defines the proper use of melatonin in sleep disturbances, the supplement might make a significant contribution considering that many sleep-deprived individuals become dependent upon benzodiazepine and other sedating drugs with potentially serious adverse effects in search of insomnia relief.

This point was made in a recent well-designed study that tested the effects of melatonin (2 milligrams daily) in a controlled release formula against placebo. During the course of the study, 34 long-term users of benzodiazepine were encouraged to reduce their benzodiazepine dosage incrementally. The goal was complete discontinuance during weeks five and six. The study proceeded double-blind through the six weeks of period one and then single-blind through the six weeks of period two, during which all subjects received melatonin and efforts to discontinue benzodiazepine resumed.

At the end of the study, 14 of 18 subjects who received melatonin in period one had completely discontinued benzodiazepine use; only four of 16 in the placebo group achieved this goal. An additional six subjects in the placebo group achieved complete discontinuance of benzodiazepine in period two. Sleep quality scores were significantly higher for the melatonin group than for the placebo group. A six-month post-study followup showed that 19 of the 24 subjects who discontinued benzodiazepine therapy continued to maintain good sleep quality. These subjects continued to use melatonin after the study ended and they did not resume use of benzodiazepine.

The use of melatonin to help alleviate some of the symptoms of jet lag has produced mixed results in trials to date. Often some benefit has been noted, but many studies have been criticized for being small and poorly designed. In the largest controlled trial to date, researchers recently reported that melatonin exerts no beneficial physiological effect on jet lag. Melatonin was tested against placebo in two doses and with different administration times. No melatonin regimen was superior to placebo.

Claims that melatonin can be used to prevent or treat cancer or immune dysfunction are unsupported by current research. There is some very preliminary data suggesting some beneficial effects in animal models and in *in vitro* studies. A small amount of clinical work has been done, and more seems warranted.

Claims that melatonin can favorably influence lipids, lower blood pressure and help prevent heart attacks are entirely baseless, as are claims that it can correct sexual dysfunction or otherwise enhance sexual performance. It has demonstrated no effect in seasonal affective disorder and, rather than help dispel depression it has been reported to cause or worsen it in some cases.

The sensational claim that melatonin dramatically delays aging is similarly without foundation. The claim was based, generally, on the long-held belief that endogenous melatonin secretion diminishes with age and, specifically, upon a single mouse study that has been criticized as seriously flawed by several researchers.

The idea that levels of serotonin fall with age was refuted in a recent study of 34 healthy subjects aged 65 to 81 in whom plasma melatonin concentrations were compared with those of a younger subject group (98 healthy individuals aged 18 to 30). No significant difference was noted between the two groups. The researchers have cautioned against the use of melatonin by the elderly, particularly since many of them may be using a variety of prescription drugs for which interactions with melatonin are unknown and could be potentially hazardous.

CONTRAINDICATIONS, PRECAUTIONS, ADVERSE REACTIONS
CONTRAINDICATIONS
None known.

PRECAUTIONS
Use of melatonin in children, pregnant women and nursing mothers is not advised.

Adverse reactions of supplemental melatonin include depression. Those who suffer from depression are advised against taking melatonin.

Because melatonin may cause both nighttime and daytime drowsiness, those who operate hazardous machinery are advised against taking melatonin.

Large doses of melatonin (not recommended) have been shown to inhibit ovulation. Women who are trying to conceive should avoid melatonin.

Melatonin use in some children with seizure disorders leads to increased seizure activity. Those with seizure disorders, both children and adults, should avoid melatonin supplements.

Those over 65 years old who take any sedating medications or herbs, or who use alcohol, should exercise caution in the use of melatonin.

ADVERSE REACTIONS

Adverse reactions associated with melatonin include stomach discomfort, morning grogginess, daytime "hangover," feeling of a "heavy head," depression, psychotic episodes (in combination with fluoxetine), headache, lethargy, fragmented disorientation, amnesia, inhibition of fertility, increased seizure activity, suppression of male sexual drive, hypothermia, retinal damage, gynecomastia and low sperm count. Typically, these reports are related to high doses. However, adverse effects have been reported and can occur with low doses as well.

INTERACTIONS

DRUGS

Aspirin and other NSAIDs may lead to decreased melatonin levels.

The bioavailability of oral melatonin is increased by coadministration of fluvoxamine. This is believed due to inhibition of the elimination of melatonin.

Beta blockers may lead to decreased melatonin levels.

A psychotic episode has been reported associated with the use of melatonin in a subject taking the antidepressant fluoxetine.

There is a report of melatonin augmenting the antitumor effect of interleukin-2.

There is a report of melatonin enhancing the activity of the anti-*Mycobacterium tuberculosis* drug, isoniazid.

Melatonin and progestin combinations can be additive in inhibiting ovarian function in women.

Use of melatonin with benzodiazepenes, sedating antihistamines, sedating antidepressants and other sedating drugs may cause additive sedation and increase incidence of adverse effects.

Use of melatonin with corticosteroids may interfere with the efficacy of the corticosteroids.

HERBS

Use of melatonin with valerian or kava kava may lead to additive sedation.

NUTRITIONAL SUPPLEMENTS

Use of melatonin with 5-hydroxytryptophan may lead to additive sedation.

ALCOHOL

Use of melatonin with alcohol may lead to additive sedation.

FOOD

No interactions are known.

OVERDOSAGE

None known. No apparent serious consequences have been reported in those taking up to 24 grams daily of melatonin for one month, though such doses are not recommended.

DOSAGE AND ADMINISTRATION

Those who use melatonin supplements for sleep disturbance or jet lag usually take no more than 0.3 milligrams to 3 milligrams at bedtime for short periods of time (no longer than two weeks). Higher doses and dosing for longer periods of time requires medical supervision. As with all nutritional supplements, the physician must know if his or her patient is taking melatonin. Melatonin supplements derived from animals should be avoided.

HOW SUPPLIED

Capsules — 1 mg, 2.5 mg, 3 mg, 5 mg

Liquid — 1 mg/mL, 1 mg/4 mL

Lozenges — 0.5 mg, 3 mg

Sublingual Tablets — 2.5 mg

Tablets — 0.2 mg, 0.3 mg, 0.5 mg, 1 mg, 3 mg, 5 mg

Tea

Timed Release Tablets — 1 mg, 2 mg, 3 mg

LITERATURE

Antunes F, Barclay LRC, Ingold KU. On the antioxidant activity of melatonin. *Free Rad Bio Med.* 1999; 26:117-128.

Barni S, Lissoni P, Cazzaniga M, et al. A randomized study of low-dose subcutaneous interleukin-2 plus melatonin versus supportive care alone in metastatic colorectal cancer patients progressing under 5-fluorouracil and folates. *Oncology.* 1995; 52:243-245.

Brzezinski A. Melatonin in humans. *N Engl J Med.* 1997; 336:186-195.

Bursztajn HJ. Melatonin therapy: from benzodiazepine-dependent insomnia to authenticity and autonomy. *Arch Intern Med.* 1999; 159:2393-2395.

Cupp MJ. Melatonin. *Am Fam Physician.* 1997; 56:1421-1425.

Dolberg OT, Hirschmann S, Grunhaus L. Melatonin for the treatment of sleep disturbances in major depressive disorder. *Am J Psychiat.* 1998; 155:1119-1121.

Force RW, Hansen L, Bedell M. Psychotic episode after melatonin [letter]. *Ann Pharmacother.* 1997; 31:1408.

Garfinkel D, Zisapel N, Wainstein J, Laudon M. Facilitation of benzodiazepine discontinuation by melatonin. *Arch Intern Med.* 1999; 159:2456-2460.

Hartter S, Grozinger M, Weigmann H, et al. Increased bioavailability of oral melatonin after fluvoxamine administration. *Clin Pharmacol Therap.* 2000; 67:1-6.

Middleton BA, Stone BM, Arendt J. Melatonin and fragmented sleep patterns. *Lancet.* 1996; 348:551-552.

Murphy PJ, Myers BL, Badia P. Nonsteroidal anti-inflammatory drugs alter body temperature and suppress melatonin in humans. *Physiol Behav.* 1996; 59:133-139.

Reiter RJ. Melatonin, active oxygen species and neurological damage. *Drug News Perspect.* 1998; 11:291-296.

Reppert SM, Weaver DR. Melatonin madness. Cell. 1995; 83:1059-1062.

Sainz RM, Mayo JC, Reiter RJ, et al. Melatonin regulates glucocorticoid receptor: an answer to its antiapoptotic action in thymus. *FASEB J.* 1999; 13:1547-1556.

Turjanski AG, Rosenstein RE, Estrin DA. Reactions of melatonin and related indoles with free radicals: a computational study. *J Med Chem.* 1998; 44:3684-3689.

Voorduow BC, Euser R, Verdonk RE, et al. Melatonin and melatonin-progestin combinations alter pituitary-ovarian function in women and can inhibit ovulation. *J Clin Encocrinol Metab.* 1992; 74:108-117.

Wiid I, Hoal-van Helden E, Hon D. et al. Potentiation of isoniazid activity against *Myobacterium tuberculosis* by melatonin. *Antimicrob Agents Chemother.* 1999; 43:975-977.

Methylsulfonylmethane (MSM)

DESCRIPTION

Methylsulfonylmethane, abbreviated MSM, is an organic sulfur-containing compound that occurs naturally in a variety of fruits, vegetables, grains and in animals, including humans in at least trace amounts. MSM has also been found in such plants as *Equisetem arvense*, also known as horsetail. The biological role of MSM, if any, is not known. MSM is a metabolite of dimethyl sulfoxide or DMSO (see Dimethyl Sulfoxide). It is believed that some of the possible effects of DMSO could be attributed to MSM.

MSM is a water-soluble, solid compound. It is also known as dimethyl sulfone, DMSO2, sulfonylbismethane and methyl sulfone.

ACTIONS AND PHARMACOLOGY

ACTIONS
None known.

PHARMACOKINETICS

Little is known about the pharmacokinetics of MSM in humans. Sulfur from MSM was found to be incorporated into protein methionine and cysteine when fed to guinea pigs. MSM was also detected in the brain of a normal 62-year old male, following its ingestion, using *in vivo* proton magnetic resonance spectroscopy. Thus, it appears that MSM gets absorbed and can cross the blood-brain barrier.

INDICATIONS AND USAGE

Claims for MSM include pain relief, particularly in arthritis, immune modulation in autoimmune disorders, muscle repair, sleep aid and diabetes therapy. There is no credible evidence to support any of these claims. There is very preliminary research suggesting some possible MSM anti-cancer effects.

RESEARCH SUMMARY

Two animal studies showed that MSM and other bipolar solvents can prolong latency period to time of tumor appearance in chemically induced animal model cancers. In one of these studies, there was no effect on tumor incidence; in the other, MSM seemed to reduce the incidence of poorly differentiated tumors. More research is indicated.

There is no research to support other claims made for MSM.

CONTRAINDICATIONS, PRECAUTIONS ADVERSE REACTIONS

CONTRAINDICATIONS
None known.

PRECAUTIONS
MSM should be avoided by pregnant women and nursing mothers.

ADVERSE REACTIONS
Reported adverse reactions include nausea, diarrhea and headache.

OVERDOSAGE
There are no reports of overdosage.

DOSAGE AND ADMINISTRATION
Doses used are typically 1 to 3 grams daily.

HOW SUPPLIED
Powder — 2600 mg/0.5 teaspoonful
Tablets — 750 mg

LITERATURE

Childs SJ. Dimethyl sulfone (DMSO2) in the treatment of interstitial cystitis. *Urol Clin North Am.* 1994; 21:85-98.

Kandorf H, Chirra AR, De Gruccio A, Girman DJ. Dimethyl sulfoxide modulation of diabetes onset in NOD mice. *Diabetes.* 1989; 38:194-197.

Kocsis JJ, Harkaway S, Snyder R. Biological effects of the metabolites of dimethyl sulfoxide. *Ann NY Acad Sci.* 1975; 243:104-109.

Layman DL. Growth inhibitory effects of dimethyl sulfoxide and dimethyl sulfone on vascular smooth muscle and endothelial cells in vitro. *In Vitro Cell Dev Biol.* 1987; 23:422-428.

Morton JI, Siegel BV. Effects of oral dimethyl sulfoxide and dimethyl sulfone on murine autoimmune lymphoproliferative disease. *Proc Soc Exp Biol Med.* 1986; 183; 227-230.

O'Dwyer PJ, McCabe DP, Sickle-Santanello BJ, et al. Use of polar solvents in chemoprevention of 1, 2-dimethylhydrazine-induced colon cancer. *Cancer.* 1988; 62:944-948.

Pearson TW, Dawson HJ, Lackey HB. Natural occurring levels of dimethyl sulfoxide in selected fruits, vegetables, grains and beverages. *J Agric Food Chem.* 1989; 29:1089-1091.

Richmond VL, Incorporation of methylsulfonylmethane sulfur into guinea pig serum proteins. *Life Sci.* 1986; 39:263-268.

Rose SE, Chalk JB, Galloway GJ, Doddrell DM. Detection of dimethyl sulfone in the human brain by in vivo proton magnetic resonance spectroscopy. *Magn Reson Imaging.* 2000; 18:95-98.

Modified Citrus Pectin

DESCRIPTION

Modified citrus pectin refers to citrus pectin which has been hydrolyzed to yield smaller molecular weight molecules which appears to render it more absorbable. Unmodified citrus pectin is not absorbable. Pectin (see Pectin) is a soluble fiber that is found in citrus fruits (oranges, lemons, grapefruits) and apples. Pectin obtained from orange or lemon rinds, both rich sources of pectin, is referred to as citrus pectin. Citrus pectin is a linear polysaccharide containing from about 300 to 1,000 monosaccharide units. D-galacturonic acid, an acid form of the sugar D-galactose, is the principal monosaccharide unit of citrus pectin. The D-galacturonic acid residues are bonded together by alpha-1,4 glycosidic linkages in linear chains. Neutral sugars, present in side chains on the pectin molecule, include D-galactose, L-arabinose, D-xylose and L-frucose. L-Rhamnose is also found in pectin. Some of the galacturonic acid residues in pectin are in the form of methyl esters. The molecular weight of citrus pectin ranges from 20,000 to 400,000 daltons, with the majority of the molecules having molecular weights ranging from 50,000 to 150,000 daltons.

Modified citrus pectin is formed from citrus pectin via a depolymerization process in which citrus pectin is first treated with sodium hydroxide at a pH of 10 for a short time, and then hydrochloric acid at a pH of 3 for a much longer period of time. The pectin fragments that are formed are principally comprised of D-polygalacturonates, absent the methoxyl groups. The molecular weight of modified citrus pectin ranges from 1,000 to 15,000 daltons, with an average weight of about 10,000 daltons. Modified citrus pectin is comprised of linear polygalacturonate chains containing from 5 to 90 galacturonic acid residues, with an average of approximately 55 residues. Also present, are D-galactose residues in side chains. Modified citrus pectin is also known as modified pectin, depolymerized pectin and pH-modified pectin. It is abbreviated as MCP. It is water soluble.

ACTIONS AND PHARMACOLOGY

ACTIONS

Modified citrus pectin has putative anticarcinogenic activity.

MECHANISM OF ACTION

Modified citrus pectin, when administered orally to rats, was found to inhibit spontaneous prostate carcinoma metastasis. It had no effect on the growth of the primary tumor. Injected modified citrus pectin was found to inhibit metastasis of melanoma cells in mice. The mechanism of these anticarcinogenic effects is not clear.

Galectins comprise a family of galactoside-binding mammalian lectins. Lectins themselves comprise a group of hemagglutinating proteins found in plant seeds, which bind the branching carbohydrate molecules of glycoproteins and glycolipids on cell surfaces, resulting in agglutination or proliferation, among other things. Galectins are proteins that can bind to carbohydrates via carbohydrate recognition domains (CRDs). At present, the galactin family includes 10 members. Apparently, galectins are secreted from cells via nonclassical secretory pathways. Galectin-3, one of the members of the family, is thought to be involved in mitosis and proliferation. On the cell surface, galectin-3 mediates cell-cell adhesion and cell-matrix interaction via binding to its complementary glycoconjugates, such as laminin and fibronectin, and thereby is thought to play an important role in the pathogenesis of cancer metastasis.

Some metastic events may involve cellular interactions that are mediated by cell surface components, including galectins. The galactose-containing carbohydrate side chains of modified citrus pectin may interfere with these cellular interactions by competing with the natural ligands of the galectins and by doing so, inhibit the metastatic process. It is thought that galectins may play a role in human prostate cancer, and in particular, human prostate cancer metastasis.

PHARMACOKINETICS

There is little on the pharmacokinetics of modified citrus pectin in humans. Based on rat studies, modified citrus pectin is probably absorbed to some degree following ingestion. However, research is necessary to determine its absorption efficiency, as well as its distribution, metabolism and excretion.

INDICATIONS AND USAGE

Modified citrus pectin has shown some ability to inhibit metastasis of prostate cancer in a rat study. It has also shown some activity against melanoma cells in culture and in mice. More research is needed before there can be any indication for the use of modified citrus pectin in cancer.

RESEARCH SUMMARY

There was the suggestion in one *in vitro* study of modified citrus pectin that it might have some ability to inhibit melanoma metastasis. Stronger, but still preliminary evidence emerged from a rat study that modified citrus pectin might similarly inhibit the spread of prostate cancer. The lungs of rats treated with this substance had significantly fewer metastatic colonies than controls. There was no effect on the primary tumor. Follow-up is needed.

CONTRAINDICATIONS, PRECAUTIONS, ADVERSE REACTIONS

CONTRAINDICATIONS

Modified citrus pectin is contraindicated in those hypersensitive to any component of a modified citrus pectin-containing product.

PRECAUTIONS

The use of modified citrus pectin for the management of prostate cancer or any type of cancer is considered experimental. Those who wish to use modified citrus pectin for the management of prostate cancer or any type of cancer must be under medical supervision.

Modified citrus pectin should be avoided by pregnant women and nursing mothers.

DOSAGE AND ADMINISTRATION

Modified citrus pectin is available as a dietary supplement both as a powder and in capsule form. Dosage is variable. See precautions regarding its use.

LITERATURE

Gopalkrishnan RV, Roberts T, Tuli S, et al. Molecular characterization of prostate carcinoma tumor antigen-1, PCTA-1, a human galectin-8 related gene. *Oncogene*. 2000; 19:4405-4416.

Hsieh TC, Wu JM. Changes in cell growth, cyclin/kinase, endogenous phosphoproteins and nm23 gene expression in human prostatic JCA-1 cells treated with modified citrus pectin. *Biochem Mol Biol Int*. 1995; 37:833-841.

Inohara H, Raz A. Effects of natural complex carbohydrate (citrus pectin) on murine melanoma cell properties related to galectin-3 functions. *Glycoconj J*. 1994; 11:527-532.

Pienta KJ, Naik H, Akhtar A, et al. Inhibition of spontaneous metastasis in a rat prostate cancer model by oral administration of modified citrus pectin. *J Natl Cancer Inst*. 1995; 87:348-353.

Platt D, Raz A. Modulation of the lung colonization of B16-F1 melanoma cells by citrus pectin. *J Natl Cancer Inst*. 1992; 84:438-442.

Rabinovich GA, Riera CM, Landa CA, Sotomayor CE. Galectins: a key intersection between glycobiology and immunology. *Braz J Med Biol Res*. 1999; 32:383-393.

Raz A, Pienta KJ. Method for treatment of cancer by oral administration of modified citrus pectin. United States Patent Number 5,895,784. Date of Patent: Apr. 20, 1999.

Molybdenum

TRADE NAMES

Moly-B (Carlson)

DESCRIPTION

Molybdenum is an essential trace mineral in animal and human nutrition. It is found in several tissues of the human body and is required for the activity of some enzymes that are involved in catabolism, including the catabolism of purines and the sulfur amino acids. Molybdenum is a transition metal with atomic number 42 and an atomic weight of 95.94 daltons. Its symbol is Mo. Compounds of molybdenum are among the scarcer constituents of the earth's crust. In fact, molybdenum is only about three times more abundant than gold. The principal ore of molybdenum is molybdenite (molybdenum disulfide). Organic forms of molybdenum are found in living matter, from bacteria to animals, including humans.

In spite of its low abundance, molybdenum deficiency in humans is rare but it has been described. A patient on long-term total parenteral nutrition (TPN) developed a syndrome characterized by hypouricemia, hypermethioninemia, low urinary sulfate excretion, tachycardia, tachypnea and mental and visual disturbances. The syndrome worsened with the administration of L-methionine and the patient eventually became comatose. The patient improved when molybdenum, in the form of ammonium molybdate, was added to the TPN. The deleterious effects of molybdenum deficiency were primarily due to the accumulation of sulfite coming from the catabolism of L-cysteine. Sulfite is toxic to the nervous system and molybdenum is necessary for its metabolism to a nontoxic form.

Animals can be made molybdenum deficient by feeding them diets containing high amounts of tungsten or copper. Both tungsten and copper are molybdenum antagonists. Molybdenum deficiency has also been produced experimentally in goats by feeding them purified diets, very low in molybdenum. Molybdenum deficiency in animals results in retarded weight gain, decreased food consumption, impaired reproduction and a shortened life expectancy.

High intake of molybdenum is antagonistic to copper and can produce a condition in animals known as molybdenosis.

Molybdenum-containing compounds, such as tetrathiomolybdate are currently in clinical trials for the treatment of metastatic cancer and Wilson disease. The use of copper antagonistic substances in these disorders, is known as copper depletion therapy.

ACTIONS AND PHARMACOLOGY

ACTIONS

Molybdenum prevents and treats molybdenum deficiency. Molybdenum has putative anticarcinogenic activity.

MECHANISM OF ACTION

The active biological form of molybdenum is known as the molybdenum cofactor or Moco. Moco is comprised of a molybdenum atom coordinated by the dithiolene moiety of a family of tricyclic pyranopterin structures, the simplest of which is known as molybdopterin. Moco is the cofactor for four human enzymes: xanthine dehydrogenase (xanthine: NAD$^+$ oxidoreductase), xanthine oxidase (a form of xanthine dehydrogenase), sulfite oxidase (sulfite dehydrogenase; sulfite: ferricytochrome c oxidoreductase), and aldehyde oxidase (aldehyde: oxygen oxidoreductase). Xanthine dehydrogenase catalyzes the conversion of hypoxanthine to xanthine, and xanthine to uric acid. In addition to uric acid, the end product of purine catabolism, NADH is formed from NAD$^+$ in the reaction. Xanthine oxidase also catalyzes the reactions of purine end metabolism. However, in the case of xanthine oxidase, which is formed from xanthine dehydrogenase, NAD$^+$ is not a participant in the reaction, and a reactive oxygen species, the superoxide anion, is a product of the reaction.

Sulfite oxidase is involved in the degradative metabolism of the sulfur amino acids methionine and cysteine. Sulfite oxidase, which is located in mitochondria, converts sulfite to sulfate. Sulfite is derived from the metabolism of cysteine. It also enters the body in the form of free sulfites which are used as food additives. Aldehyde oxidase is involved in a number of reactions, including the catabolism of pyrimidines and the biotransformation of xenobiotics.

Deficiency of the molybdenum cofactor (Moco) causes a severe disease in humans that usually results in premature death in early childhood and is inherited as an autosomal recessive trait. All of the Moco-dependent enzymes—xanthine dehydrogenase, sulfite oxidase and aldehyde oxidase—are affected. Moco deficiency is rare. Additional signs of this combined enzyme deficiency, are severe neurological abnormalities, dislocated ocular lenses, mental retardation, increased urinary excretion of sulfite, thiosulfate, S-sulfocysteine, taurine, hypoxanthine and xanthine, and reduced serum and urine levels of sulfate and urate. Isolated sulfite oxidase deficiency is also known. This is a rare autosomal-recessive disorder presenting at birth with seizures, severe neurologic disease and lens subluxation.

Lin Xian is a small region in Honan Province in north China which has had one of the highest incidences of esophageal cancer in the world. It was determined that the soil in this area was markedly low in molybdenum. In order for nitrates in the soil to be reduced to nitrogenous substances necessary for plant nutrition, a molybdenum-dependent enzyme, nitrate reductase (found in nitrogen-fixing bacteria), is required. When the molybdenum level in the soil is low, instead of being converted to amines, the nitrates get converted to nitrosamines, known carcinogenic substances. By enriching the soil with molybdenum, as ammonium molybdate, those living in this region are exposed to lower amounts of nitrosamines in their diets, and the incidence of esophageal cancer may be declining.

The possible anticarcinogenic activity in the above example is due to feeding the soil to produce lower amounts of carcinogens. When the inhabitants in the region were administered molybdenum as a supplement, this action did not appear to affect the incidence of esophageal or any other type of cancer. However, molybdenum may have anticarcinogenic activity for a few hypothetical reasons. Aldehyde oxidase may play a role in the detoxification of some carcinogenic xenobiotics. This needs to be studied. Molybdenum is involved in cofactors that are required for enzyme activity by some of the inhabitants of the microflora of the large intestine. Some of these molybdenum-dependent enzymes may also be involved in detoxifying carcinogenic xenobiotics. This too needs study. Finally, it has been shown that copper depletion suppresses tumor growth in an animal model. There is some evidence that copper is an important cofactor for angiogenesis, and therefore, copper deficiency may suppress angiogenesis. Tetrathiomolybdate, a molybdenum compound which antagonizes copper, is now in clinical trial to determine if copper depletion therapy via molybdenum is a viable approach for the treatment of cancer.

PHARMACOKINETICS

Molybdenum in nutritional supplements is in the form of either sodium molybdate or ammonium molybdate. Molybdenum in food is principally in the form of the organic molybdenum cofactors. The efficiency of absorption of nutritional supplement forms of molybdenum ranges from 88% to 93%, and the efficiency of absorption of molybdenum from foods ranges from about 57% to 88%. Absorption of molybdenum occurs rapidly from the stomach as well as the small intestine. The mechanism of absorption—passive, active or both—is unclear. Following absorption, molybdenum is transported via the portal circulation to the liver and via the systemic circulation to the other tissues of the body. Molybdate is carried in the blood bound to alpha-macroglobulin and by adsorption to erythrocytes. The liver and kidney retain the highest amounts of molybdenum. Within cells, molybdenum participates in the formation of the molybdenum cofactor. Molybdenum is excreted in the urine as molybdate. Some molybdenum is excreted in the bile. Excretion, rather than absorption, is the principal homeostatic mechanism for molybdenum.

INDICATIONS AND USAGE

Molybdenum is indicated in cases of molybdenum deficiency due to prolonged use of total parenteral nutrition. Despite some epidemiological evidence showing a higher incidence of esophageal carcinoma in those who live in areas where the soil is low in molybdenum, there is as yet no indication for the use of supplemental molybdenum in the prevention of cancer. Claims that molybdenum may help prevent anemia, that it protects against dental caries and helps in cases of sexual impotence have no credible support.

RESEARCH SUMMARY

Except for evidence of supplemental molybdenum's usefulness in some individuals made deficient due to prolonged total parenteral nutrition, research to date has revealed no further indications for the supplemental use of molybdenum.

An epidemiologic association has been made between the high incidence of esophageal cancer and the low intake of molybdenum in an area of China. In one study, supplementing some of those who live in this area with molybdenum for prolonged periods did not lower the incidence of cancer, although supplementation with beta carotene, vitamin E and selenium did reduce the incidence of some cancers in this study group.

Non-dietary forms of molybdenum, however, are being developed as experimental drugs for the treatment of cancer via their ability to deplete copper (see Actions and Pharmacology).

CONTRAINDICATIONS, PRECAUTIONS, ADVERSE REACTIONS

CONTRAINDICATIONS

Molybdenum is contraindicated in those who are hypersensitive to any component of a molybdenum-containing product.

PRECAUTIONS

Pregnant women and nursing mothers should avoid the use of supplemental molybdenum greater than U.S. RDA amounts (75 micrograms daily). Dietary intake of molybdenum in the United States ranges from about 120 to 240 micrograms daily, with an average intake of 180 micrograms daily. A supplementary intake of molybdenum of 75 micrograms daily brings the intake up to the upper limits of the estimated safe and adequate daily dietary intake for molybdenum.

Those with hyperuricemia and/or gout should exercise caution in the use of supplementation with doses of molybdenum greater than U.S. RDA amounts.

The use of molybdenum, specifically tetrathiomolybdate, for the treatment of cancer or Wilson disease is experimental.

ADVERSE REACTIONS

Doses of molybdenum of 10 to 15 milligrams daily have been associated with a gout-like syndrome and hyperuricemia. Supplementary doses of molybdenum of up to 500 micrograms are generally well tolerated. However, there is one report of a male who suffered acute toxicity with a molybdenum dose ranging from 300-800 micrograms daily for 18 days (see Overdosage).

INTERACTIONS

DRUGS

Acetaminophen: High doses of molybdate may inhibit the metabolism of acetaminophen.

NUTRITIONAL SUPPLEMENTS

Copper: High doses of molybdate may antagonize the absorption of copper. Likewise, high doses of copper may antagonize the absorption of molybdenum and overall decrease molybdenum status.

FOODS

High doses of molybdenum may antagonize absorption of copper from foods.

OVERDOSAGE

There is one report of acute clinical poisoning with molybdenum from a dietary molybdenum supplement. The subject, a male in his late thirties, consumed a cumulative dose of 13.5 milligrams of molybdenum over a period of 18 days, at an intake rate of 300-800 micrograms daily. This was followed by the development of acute psychosis (visual and auditory hallucinations), several petit mal seizures and one grand mal seizure. The subject was treated with chelation therapy and his symptoms and signs remitted after several hours. Neuropsychological tests and Spectral Emission Computer Tomography revealed frontal lobe damage of the brain. Major depression and learning disability persisted one year following the molybdenum incident. There are no other reports of overdosage. Further, other reports of those taking doses of molybdenum up to 500 micrograms daily or greater for extended periods of time, have not shown any adverse reactions.

DOSAGE AND ADMINISTRATION

Molybdenum supplements are usually available in the form of sodium molybdate and sometimes in the form of ammonium molybdate. Molybdenum is found in combination products, including multivitamin/multimineral formulas. A typical supplementary dose is 75 micrograms daily. The amounts of molybdenum on nutritional supplement labels, are expressed as elemental molybdenum.

The Food and Nutrition Board of the U.S. National Academy of Sciences has recommended the following estimated safe and adequate daily dietary intake (ESSADI) values for molybdenum:

Category	Age (years)	ESSADI (micrograms/day)
Infants	0-0.5	15-30
	0.5-1	20-40
Children	1 through 3	25-50
	4 through 6	30-75
	7 through 10	50-150
	11 through 18	75-250
Adults	19 years and older	75-250

The U.S. RDA for molybdenum, which is the value used for nutritional supplement and food labeling purposes, is 75 micrograms daily.

The richest dietary sources of molybdenum, include legumes, cereal grains, leafy vegetables, milk, beans, liver and kidney.

HOW SUPPLIED

Tablets — 150 mcg, 500 mcg

LITERATURE

Anon. Molybdenum deficiency in TPN. *Nutr Rev.* 1987; 45:337-341.

Barceloux DG. Molybdenum. *J Toxicol Clin Toxicol.* 1999; 37:231-237.

Barch DH. Esophageal cancer and microelements. *J Am Coll Nutr.* 1989; 8:99-107.

Beedham C. Molybdenum hydroxylases as drug-metabolizing enzymes. *Drug Metab Rev.* 1985; 16:119-156.

Blot WJ, Li JY, Taylor PR, et al. Nutrition intervention trials in Linxian, China: supplementation with specific vitamin/mineral combinations, cancer incidence, and disease-specific mortality in the general population. *J Natl Cancer Inst.* 1993; 85:1483-1492.

Boles JW, Klaassen CD. Effects of molybdate and pentachlorophenol on the sulfation of acetaminophen. *Toxicology.* 2000; 146:23-35.

Brewer GJ, Dick RD, Grover DK, et al. Treatment of metastatic cancer with tetrathiomolybdate, an anticopper, antiangiogenic agent: Phase I study. *Clin Cancer Res.* 2000; 6:1-10.

Brewer GJ, Johnson V, Dick RD, et al. Treatment of Wilson disease with ammonium tetrathiomolybdate. II. Initial therapy in 33 neurologically affected patients and follow-up with zinc therapy. *Arch Neurol.* 1996; 53:1017-1025.

Edwards MC, Johnson JL, Marriage B, et al. Isolated sulfite oxidase deficiency: review of two cases in one family. *Ophthalmology.* 1999; 106:1957-1961.

Hille R. Molybdenum enzymes. *Essays Biochem.* 1999; 34:125-137.

Johnson JL, Cohen HJ, Rajagopalan KV. Molecular basis of the biological function of molybdenum. *J Biol Chem.* 1974; 249:5046-5055.

Johnson JL, Waud WR, Rajagopalan KV, et al. Inborn errors of molybdenum metabolism: Combined deficiencies of sulfite oxidase and xanthine dehydrogenase in a patient lacking the molybdenum cofactor. *Proc Natl Acad Sci USA.* 1980; 77:3715-3719.

Luo XM, Wei HJ, Hu GG, et al. Molybdenum and esophageal cancer in China. *Federation Proceedings.* 1981; 46:928(Abstract#3962).

Mendel RR. The role of the molybdenum cofactor in humans. *Biofactors.* 2000; 11:147-148.

Momcilovic B. a case of acute human molybdenum toxicity from a dietary molybdenum supplement—a new member of the "Lucor metallicum" family. *Arh Hig Rada Toksikol.* 1999; 50:289-297.

Nielsen FH. Ultratrace minerals. In: Shils ME, Olson JA, Shike M, Ross AC, eds. *Modern Nutrition in Health and Disease.* 9th ed. Baltimore, MD: Williams and Wilkins; 1999:283-303.

Rajagopalan KV. Molybdenum—an essential trace element. *Nutr Rev.* 1987; 45:321-328.

Recommended Dietary Allowances. 10th Edition. Washington, DC: National Academy Press; 1989.

Thompson KH, Scott KC, Turnlund JR. Molybdenum metabolism in men with increasing molybdenum intakes: changes in kinetic parameters. *J Appl Physiol.* 1996; 81:1404-1409.

Turnland JR, Keyes WR, Peiffer GL. Molybdenum absorption, excretion, and retention studied with stable isotopes in young men at five intakes of dietary molybdenum. *Am J Clin Nutr.* 1995; 62:790-796.

Vyskocil A, Viau C. Assessment of molybdenum toxicity in humans. *J Appl Toxicol.* 1999; 19:185-192.

Wuebbens MW, Liu MTW, Rajagopalan KV, Schlindelin H. Insights into molybdenum cofactor deficiency provided by the crystal structure of the molybdenum cofactor biosynthesis protein MoaC. *Strucutre.* 2000; 8:709-718.

Myco-Polysaccharides

DESCRIPTION

Some mushrooms and other fungal entities have possible immunomodulatory activities and possible other health benefits. It is thought these health benefits are mainly due to polysaccharides and polysaccharide-protein complexes, which comprise the cell walls of these organisms. The principal bioactive substances are believed to be the beta-D-glucans. Beta-D-glucans, usually called beta-glucans, are nondigestible polysaccharides found in nature in such sources as cereal grains, including oats and barley, as well as in yeast, bacteria, algae and mushrooms.

It is likely that the activities of the various myco-beta-D-glucans depend on such chemical characteristics as their molecular weight, their branching patterns, their solubility in water and their tertiary structure. The most studied mushroom beta-glucans, all of which are available in Japan for use as biological response modifiers, are lentinan from *Lentinus edodes*; grifolan (also called GRN and grifolan LE) from *Grifola frondosa*; schizophyllan (also called SPG, sonifilan, sizofiran and sizofilan) from *Schizophyllum commune*; SSG from *Sclerotinia sclerotiorum*; PSK (also called krestin) from *Coriolus versicolor*; and PSP (polysaccharide peptide), also from *Coriolus versicolor*.

The beta-glucan lentinan is comprised of a beta-(1→3)-D-glucan backbone with beta-(1→ 6)-glucan side chains. The molecular weight of lentinan is approximately 5×10^5 daltons, the degree of branching is 2/5, and the tertiary structure of lentinan is a triple helix. Grifolan is also comprised of a beta-(1→3)-D-glucan backbone with beta-(1→6)-glucan side chains. The molecular weight of grifolan is approximately 5×10^5 daltons, the degree of branching is 1/3, and its tertiary structure is a triple helix. Both schizophyllan and SSG also contain beta-(1→3)-D-glucan backbones and beta-(1→6)-glucan side chains; they have triple helix tertiary structures. The degree of branching in schizophyllan is 1/3; in SSG, it is 1/3. PSK and PSP are glycoproteins containing beta-glucans.

ACTIONS AND PHARMACOLOGY

ACTIONS
Myco-polysaccharides may have immunomodulatory, antitumor, antimicrobial, lipid-lowering and glucose-regulating activities.

MECHANISM OF ACTION
The best studied of the mushroom beta-glucans is lentinan. Lentinan is typically used parenterally and appears to have little antitumor activity when administered orally. Parenterally administered lentinan has been demonstrated to have immunomodulatory activity. Lentinan appears to stimulate such cells as macrophages, monocytes, neutrophils, NK (natural killer) cells and LAK (lymphokine-activated killer) cells. Stimulation of these cells by lentinan may release a number of different cytokines, including TNF (tumor necrosis factor)-alpha, IL (interleukin)-1, IL-2 and IL-6; lentinan may also stimulate the production of nitric oxide (NO) in macrophages. These effects may result in antimicrobial and

tumoricidal activities. Grifolan, schizophyllan and SSG have been shown to have similar effects when used parenterally.

The possible immunomodulatory effects of oral mushroom beta-glucans remain unclear. They may have immunological activity by virtue of their interaction with gut-associated lymphoid tissue (GALT). Immune cells associated with GALT, activated by contact with mushroom or other myco-beta-glucans in the gut, may migrate to other tissues where they might exert immunomodulatory effects. Further, there may be some digestion of myco-beta-glucans in the large intestine, via bacterial beta-glucosidases, to produce some oligosaccharides, which may be absorbed and may have immunomodulatory activity. However, this is unclear. There also may be substances in mushrooms other than beta-glucans that have immunomodulatory activity.

The possible antitumor and antimicrobial activities of the myco-beta-glucans are thought to be accounted for, in large part, by their possible immunomodulatory activities.

The mechanism of the possible cholesterol-lowering activity of the myco-beta-glucans is unclear. The myco-beta-glucans are somewhat similar in structure to oat beta-glucan. It is thought that the cholesterol-lowering effect of oat beta-glucan may be accounted for, in large part, by promoting the excretion of bile acids. Myco-beta-glucans may also promote the excretion of bile acids.

The mechanism of the possible glucose-regulatory activity of myco-beta-glucans is poorly understood.

PHARMACOKINETICS
Following ingestion, there is virtually no digestion of myco-beta-glucans in the small intestine. There are no beta-glucosidases among the digestive enzymes. Some digestion of myco-beta-glucans does take place in the large intestine via the action of bacterial beta-glucosidases. Some oligosaccharides (up to molecular weights of 20,000 daltons) that are produced via the bacterial beta-glucosidases may get absorbed. A large percentage of the ingested myco-beta-glucans is excreted in the feces.

INDICATIONS AND USAGE
The myco-polysaccharides may have anticarcinogenic, immune-modulating, antimicrobial, anti-inflammatory, cardioprotective, hepatoprotective, nephroprotective, hypoglycemic and anticaries effects.

RESEARCH SUMMARY
Many myco-polysaccharides, particularly those derived from *Lentinus edodes* (the shiitake mushroom), *Grifold frondosa* (the maitake mushroom), *Sclerotinia sclerotiorum* and *Schizophyllum commune*, have demonstrated anticarcinogenic effects in both animals and humans. The beta-glucan constituents of these polysaccharides are believed to be their

most active anticancer components. These beta-glucans are lentinan from *Lentinus edodes*, GRN from *Grifola frondosa*, SPG from *Schizophyllum commune* and SSG from *Sclerotinia sclerotiorum*.

In *in vitro* studies, lentinan demonstrated anticancer effects by significantly boosting the cytotoxic capabilities of macrophages, enhancing production of macrophage tumor necrosis factor-alpha. It also increased production of interleukin (IL)-1. GRN also produced macrophage-stimulating activity in mouse macrophages, as did (though to lesser extents) SPG and SSG.

In animal experiments, these beta-glucans have shown varying activity against sarcomas, mammary cancer, some chemically induced cancers, adenocarcinoma, colon cancer and some leukemias, among others.

In humans, lentinan and SPG are approved for clinical use in Japan. Injected lentinan has reportedly increased survival time in patients with gastric and colorectal cancers, while SPG has shown clinical activity against cervical cancer, prolonging survival time and time to recurrence in stage II, but not stage III, cervical cancer patients. Its efficacy against gastric cancer is low.

Lentinan, combined with some other anticancer agents, prolonged survival times in some patients with advanced cancers of different types, including gastric cancer. SPG similarly enhanced the efficacy of several cancer treatments, including surgery and radiotherapy. Combining these treatments with SPG resulted in significantly longer survival times. In one recently concluded multi-center prospective study of lentinan's use in advanced gastric cancer patients, the combination of lentinan, tegafur and cisplatin resulted in median survival of 297 days versus 199 days for those controls receiving the two cancer drugs without lentinan.

Some substances, other than the beta-glucans identified above, have been isolated from these mushrooms, which also show anticancer activity in *in vitro* and animal experiments. Research continues.

The non-specific (macrophage-activating) immune-enhancing effects of the myco-polysaccharides most likely account for much of their reported anti-inflammatory and antimicrobial activities. Preliminary trials of intravenous lentinan have not produced significant results in HIV-positive subjects. One recent study found that lentinan significantly stimulated expression of IL-2 receptors on peripheral blood mononuclear cells in patients with chronic hepatitis B.

Another recent study identified three antibacterial substances in shiitake mushrooms. They showed efficient activity against *Streptococcus spp.* and *Actinomyces spp.*, among others. They were far less effective against *Enterococcus spp.*, *Staphylococcus spp.* and some others.

Cordyceps sinensis has enhanced cellular immune function in subjects with chronic renal failure and has boosted natural killer activity in cells from both healthy individuals and some with leukemia. NK activities were also boosted by an extract of *Cordyceps sinensis* in mice with lung melanoma.

Ganoderma lucidum has immunologically active polysaccharides. Some of these have shown some activity against HIV-1 *in vitro* but not *in vivo*. Various extracts of the mushroom have exhibited some antibacterial activity *in vitro*, especially against *Micrococcus luteus*, and have been shown to have microbial additive effects with some antibiotics and antagonistic effects with others. Clearly, more research is needed before ganoderma preparations can be recommended for use with antibiotic drugs.

Recently, two patients with postherpetic neuralgia that had not yielded to other therapies and two patients with severe pain due to herpes zoster infection were said to receive dramatic pain relief upon administration of hot water soluble extracts of *Ganoderma lucidum* (36 to 72 grams dry weight per day). More recently still, various ganoderma polysaccharides have been isolated that show significant antiherpetic activity *in vitro* against both HSV-1 and HSV-2. Research is ongoing.

Various constituents of shiitake have shown effects that could be cardioprotective. Inhibition of platelet aggregation and some hypocholesterolemic effects have been noted *in vitro*. Dietary shiitake significantly lowered plasma-free cholesterol, triglycerides and phospholipids in spontaneously hypertensive rats, compared with controls. Shiitake, however, did not reduce blood pressure in these animals. Maitake, on the other hand, significantly lowered blood pressure but had no significant effect on lipids in this study. In some other animal studies, however, maitake did have favorable lipid effects.

A constituent of *Cordyceps sinensis* has been shown to have hypotensive and vasorelaxant effects in animal studies. Another extract has reportedly counteracted chemically induced arrhythmias in rats.

Ganoderma lucidum was said to significantly inhibit platelet aggregation in 15 healthy volunteers and 33 subjects with atherosclerotic disease.

Cordyceps sinensis protected animals from the nephrotoxic effects of cyclosporin A in one experiment. *Ganoderma lucidum* was hepatoprotective in another animal model.

Maitake and some of its constituents have shown some antidiabetic activity in animals. Blood glucose reductions were observed in genetically diabetic mice given these substances, compared with controls in which blood glucose levels rose with age. In an animal model of NIDDM, maitake again produced significant reductions in blood glucose levels, compared with controls. Researchers in this study concluded that maitake does not inhibit glucose absorption at the enteron but, rather, inhibits the metabolism of absorbed glucose.

Cordyceps sinensis extracts have also shown some ability to lower plasma glucose levels in animal models of diabetes. A *cordyceps sinensis* polysaccharide was said to have potent hypoglycemic effects, via intraperitoneal administration, in genetic diabetic mice.

Finally, a polysaccharide constituent of shiitake has been reported to have an anticaries effect. A significantly lower caries score was seen in shiitake-supplemented rats fed a cariogenic diet, compared with controls on the same diet but without shiitake extract.

CONTRAINDICATIONS, PRECAUTIONS, ADVERSE REACTIONS

CONTRAINDICATIONS

Myco-beta-glucans and myco-polysaccharides are contraindicated in those who are hypersensitive to mushrooms, to mushroom extracts and to any component in a mushroom-containing supplement, a mushroom extract-containing supplement, a mushroom polysaccharide-containing supplement or a mushroom beta-glucan-containing supplements.

PRECAUTIONS

Pregnant women and nursing mothers should avoid supplementation with mushroom extracts and should avoid mushroom polysaccharide-containing supplements and mushroom beta-glucan-containing supplements.

Those with cancer, immune deficiencies and other medical problems should only use mushroom supplementation, mushroom polysaccharide or mushroom beta-glucan supplements under medical supervision.

ADVERSE REACTIONS

The most commonly reported adverse reactions from the use of the various beta-glucan-containing fungal products are gastrointestinal, including nausea and epigastric distress. Eosinophilia has been reported in subjects taking 4 grams daily of shiitake mushroom powder. Contact dermatitis has also been reported in some cases, from the handling of shiitake mushrooms.

INTERACTIONS

DRUGS

Antibiotics and chemotherapeutic agents: In vitro studies, animal studies and parenteral use of the mushroom beta-glucans suggest that they may enhance the efficacy of various chemotherapeutic agents, as well as antibiotics.

However, it is unclear if oral use of these substances, either in concentrated forms or in the form of mushrooms, would produce similar interactions.

Antiplatelet drugs: Ganoderma may enhance the effect of antiplatelet drugs.

OVERDOSAGE

There are no reports of overdosage of any of the products mentioned in this monograph.

DOSAGE AND ADMINISTRATION

The beta-glucans lentinan, grifolan, schizophyllan and SSG are available in Japan. Lentinan and schizophyllan are approved in Japan as drugs for the treatment of cancer. Edible mushrooms rich in beta-glucans include the shiitake mushroom (*Lentinus edodes*), the maitake mushroom (*Grifola frondosa*), the himematsutake mushroom (*Agaricus blazei*), the button mushrooms (*Schizophyllum commune* and *Sclerotina sclerotiorium*), the wood ear mushroom (*Auricularia auricula*), the tremella mushroom (*Tremella fuciformis*), the poria mushroom (*Wolfporia cocos*) and the enoki mushroom (*Flammulina velutipes*). Huitlacoche (*Ustilago maydis*) is not a true mushroom, but it is an edible fungus and also rich in beta-glucans. Non-edible mushrooms that are rich in beta-glucans include the reishi mushroom (*Ganoderma lucidum*) and the coriolus mushroom (*Coriolus versicolor*). *Cordyceps sinensis* is a fungus, not a mushroom.

Nutritional supplements containing extracts of the above edible and non-edible mushrooms are available and are typically marketed with emphasis on their beta-glucan content.

One supplement contains a mixture of reishi, maitake, shiitake, hericium, cordyceps, coriolus, wood ear, tremella, poria and umbellatus/polyporus (*Grifola umbellatus*). There is no typical dose of this supplement.

A beta-glucan-enriched maitake supplement, called the maitake D fraction, is available. The maitake D fraction comprises a mixed beta-D-glucan fraction prepared from the maitake mushroom. The supplement is available in solid and liquid form. Maitake in the form of a crude dried mushroom is also available. Crude dried reishi mushrooms, reishi powders and reishi tinctures are available, as are crude dried shiitake mushrooms and shiitake powders. *Cordyceps sinensis* is available in powdered form. No specific doses of these products can be recommended at this time.

LITERATURE

Borchers AT, Stern JS, Hackman RM, Keen CL, Gershwin ME. Mushrooms, tumors, and immunity. *Proc Soc Exp Biol Med.* 1999; 221:281-293.

Chang R. Functional properties of edible mushrooms. *Nutr Rev.* 1996; 54:S91-S93.

Chang RY. Potential application of *Ganoderma* polysaccharides in the immune surveillance and chemoprevention of cancer. In: Royse DJ, ed. *Mushroom Biology and Mushroom Products*. 1996; Penn State Univ:153-159.

Chen AW, Miles PG. Biomedical research and the application of mushroom nutriceuticals from *Ganoderma lucidum*. In: Royse DJ, ed. *Mushroom Biology and Mushroom Products*. 1996; Penn State Univ:161-175.

Eo SK, Kim YS, Lee CK, Han SS. Antiherpetic activities of various protein bound polysaccharides isolated from Ganoderma lucidum. *J Ethnopharmacol*. 1999; 68:175-181.

Fujimiya Y, Suzuki Y, Oshiman K, et al. Selective tumoricidal effect of soluble proteoglucan extracted from the basidiomycete, *Agaricus blazei* Murill, mediated via natural killer cell activation and apoptosis. *Canc Immunol Immunotherapy*. 1998; 46:147-159.

Gordon M, Bihari B, Goosby E, et al. A placebo-controlled trial of the immune modulator, lentinan in HIV-positive patients: a phase I/II trial. *J Med*. 1998; 29:305-330.

He Y, Li R, Chen Q, et al. [Chemical studies on immunologically active polysaccharides of Ganoderma lucidum (Leyss ex Fr.) Karst.] [Article in Chinese.] *Chung Kuo Chung Yao Tsa Chih*. 1992; 17:226-228,256.

Kidd P. The use of mushroom glucans and proteoglycans in cancer treatment. *Altern Med Rev*. 2000; 5:4-27.

Kiho T, Yamane A, Hui J, et al. Polysaccharides in fungi. XXXVI. Hypoglycemic activity of a polysaccharide (CS-F30) from the cultural mycelium of Cordyceps sinensis and its effect on glucose metabolism in mouse liver. *Biol Pharm Bull*. 1996; 19:294-296.

Kubo K, Nanba H. Anti-diabetic mechanism of maitake (*Grifola frondosa*). In: Royse DJ, ed. *Mushroom Biology and Mushroom Products*. 1996; Penn State Univ:215-222.

Kuo YC, Tsai WJ, Shiao MS, et al. Cordyceps sinensis as an immunomodulatory agent. *Am J Chin Med*. 1996; 24:111-125.

Ladanyi A, Timar J, Lapis K. Effect of lentinan on macrophage cytotoxicity against metastatic tumor cells. *Cancer Immunol Immunother*. 1993; 36:123-126.

Levy AM, Kita H, Phillips SF, et al. Eosinophilia and gastrointestinal symptoms after ingestion of shiitake mushrooms. *J Allergy Clin Immunol*. 1998; 101:613-620.

Manzi P, Pizzoferrato L. Beta-glucans in edible mushrooms. *Food Chemistry*. 2000; 68:315-318.

Matsuoka H, Seo Y, Wakasugi H, et al. Lentinan potentiates immunity and prolongs the survival time of some patients. *Anticancer Res*. 1997; 17:2751-2755.

Mitamura T, Sakamoto S, Suzuki S, et al. Effects of lentinan on colorectal carcinogenesis in mice with ulcerative colitis. *Oncol Rep*. 2000; 7:559-601.

Mizuno M, Minato K, Ito H, et al. Anti-tumor polysaccharide from the mycelium of liquid-cultured Agaricus blazei mill. *Biochem Mol Biol Int*. 1999; 47:707-714.

Murata T, Hatayama I, Kakizaki I, et al. Lentinan enhances sensitivity of mouse colon 26 tumor to cis-diamminedichloroplatinum (II) and decreases glutathioline transferase expression. *Jpn J Cancer Res*. 1996; 87:1171-1178.

Nakano H, Namatame K, Nemoto H, et al. A multi-institutional prospective study of lentinan in advanced gastric cancer patients with unresectable and recurrent diseases: effect on prolongation of survival and improvement of quality of life. Kanagawa Lentinin Research Group. *Hepatogastroenterology*. 1999; 46:2662-2668.

Nakumara T. Shiitake (Lentinus edodes) dermatitis. *Contact Dermatitis*. 1992; 27:65-70.

Shouji N, Takada K, Fukushima K, Hirasawa M. Anticaries effect of a component from shiitake (an edible mushroom). *Caries Res*. 2000; 34:94-98.

Tari K, Satake I, Nakagomi K, et al. [Effect of lentinan for advanced prostate carcinoma.] [Article in Japanese.] *Hinyokika Kiyo*. 1994; 40:119-123.

Wan K. [Effects of lentinan of peripheral blood mononuclear cell expression of interleukin-2 receptor in patients with chronic hepatitis B *in vivo* and *in vitro*.] [Article in Chinese.] *Hunan I Ko Ta Hsueh Hsueh*. 1998; 23:90-92.

Wasser SP, Weis AL. Therapeutic effects of substances occurring in higher Basidiomycetes mushrooms: a modern prospective. *Crit Rev Immunol*. 1999; 19:65-96.

Yoon SY, Eo SK, Kim YS, et al. Antimicrobial activity of Ganoderma lucidum extract alone and in combination with some antibiotics. *Arch Pharm Res*. 1994; 17:438-442.

Myo-Inositol

DESCRIPTION

Myo-inositol, the major nutritionally active form of inositol, is vital to many biological processes of the body, participating in a diverse range of activities. *Myo*-inositol is one of nine distinct isomers of inositol. It is essential for the growth of rodents, but not for most animals, including humans. Humans can make *myo*-inositol endogenously, which they do from glucose, and, even though *myo*-inositol is sometimes referred to as a vitamin, it is not a vitamin for humans or most animals. However, the dietary intake of *myo*-inositol can influence the levels of circulating and bound *myo*-inositol in the body and may influence certain biological activities. Nutritional supplementation of this cyclitol may affect behavior and may have anti-depressant and anti-anxiety activities. For more information on Inositol supplementation, see Inositol Hexanicotinate.

Myo-inositol intake from the average diet is approximately one gram daily. The major dietary forms of *myo*-inositol are inositol hexaphosphate or phytic acid, which is widely found in cereals and legumes and associated with dietary fiber, and *myo*-inositol-containing phospholipids from animal and plant sources.

Myo-inositol is also known as inositol, hexahydroxycyclohexane, cyclohexanehexol, mouse antialopecia factor and, chemically, as cis-1,2,3,5-trans-4,6-cyclohexanehexol. *Myo*-inositol is abbreviated as Ins and sometimes as just I. It is represented by the following chemical structure:

myo-Inositol

Another naturally occurring isomer of inositol, D-*chiro*-inositol, has been found to have activity against insulin resistance. However, at present, D-*chiro*-inositol is neither available as a nutritional supplement nor as a drug. A hexanicotinate conjugate of *myo*-inositol, inositol niacinate or inositol nicotinate, is available in Europe as a drug for the treatment of circulatory problems.

ACTIONS AND PHARMACOLOGY

ACTIONS

Myo-inositol may have antidepressant and antianxiety activity.

MECHANISM OF ACTION

The mechanism of action of *myo*-inositol has yet to be fully elucidated. However, much is known about the biological roles of *myo*-inositol and some speculation can be made. *Myo*-inositol is metabolized to phosphatidylinositol, which makes up a small, but very significant, component of cell membranes. Phosphatidylinositol can be converted to phosphatidylinositol-4,5-bisphosphate, a key intermediate in biological signaling. Phosphatidylinositol-4,5-bisphosphate is the precursor of at least three second-messenger molecules. These are inositol-1,4,5-triphosphate, which modifies intracellular calcium levels, diacylglycerol, which regulates some members of the protein kinase C family, and phosphatidylinositol-3,4,5-triphosphate, which is involved in signal transduction.

Some of the second-messenger activity is related to activation of serotonin receptors. It is hypothesized that the mechanism of action of *myo*-inositol's possible benefit in the management of depression, panic attacks and obsessive-compulsive behavior may be explained by *myo*-inositol's role as a second-messenger precursor.

PHARMACOKINETICS

Myo-inositol is absorbed from the small intestine following ingestion and is transported by the portal circulation to the liver and then by the systemic circulation to various tissues in the body, including the brain. *Myo*-inositol crosses the blood-brain barrier.

Within the liver and the various tissues of the body, *myo*-inositol enters into a wide range of diverse biochemical pathways. *Myo*-inositol reacts with CDP-diacylglycerol to form the phospholipid phosphatidylinositol, which can be incorporated into membrane structure. Phosphatidylinositol, via kinase reactions, forms phosphatidyl-4,5-bisphosphate, which is the precursor to inositol-1,4,5-triphosphate, diacylglycerol, phosphatidylinositol-3,4,5-triphosphate, *myo*-inositol 1,3,4-triphosphate and *myo*-inositol 1,3,4,5-tetrakisphosphate, among others. The *myo*-inositol phosphates can be dephosphorylated via phosphatases.

It is believed that the mechanism of action of lithium is due, in part, to its inhibition of the phosphatase that converts *myo*-inositol-monophosphate back to *myo*-inositol.

INDICATIONS AND USAGE

Myo-inositol has exhibited positive effects in a number of studies related to depression, panic attacks and obsessive-compulsive disorder. On the other hand, it generally has not been effective in treating Alzheimer's disease, autism, schizophrenia and electroconvulsive therapy-induced memory impairment. The suggestion, from animal studies, that *myo*-inositol might be helpful in preventing neural tube defects has not been tested in humans.

RESEARCH SUMMARY

Inositol levels in cerebrospinal fluid are decreased, compared with general populations, in many suffering from depression. In one double-blind study, 28 depressed patients received placebo or high-dose (12 grams daily) *myo*-inositol for four weeks. Overall, significant improvement was achieved in the treatment group but not in the placebo group. There was improvement in both monopolar and bipolar depression in this pilot study. *Myo*-inositol, however, was not shown, in another study, to enhance or speed the response of depressed subjects to SSRIs (serotonin selective reuptake inhibitors). More research is needed in this area.

In another double-blind study, 21 patients with panic disorder, with or without agoraphobia, received 12 grams daily of *myo*-inositol or placebo for four weeks. Again, the treated group, overall, achieved improvement (frequency and severity of both panic attacks and agoraphobia declined significantly), compared with no significant improvement in the placebo group.

And in a third double-blind study, this one with a crossover component, 13 patients with obsessive-compulsive disorder (OCD) received 18 grams of inositol or placebo for six weeks each. Subjects improved significantly more, as reflected by significantly lower scores on the Yale-Brown Obsessive Compulsive Scale, when taking *myo*-inositol than when taking placebo. *Myo*-inositol, in a subsequent study, did not enhance the effects of SSRIs in subjects with treatment-refractory OCD. Again, more research is needed to confirm and further elucidate *myo*-inositol's role in treating OCD. Its effectiveness, to the extent demonstrated to date, combined with its general lack of serious side effects, make it an attractive potential therapy in these psychiatric disorders.

Myo-inositol has not demonstrated the same promise in Alzheimer's disease, autism, schizophrenia and electroconvulsive therapy-induced memory impairment. Studies related to these conditions have produced negative results. And in children with attention deficit disorder, *myo*-inositol aggravated rather than ameliorated symptoms in one small study.

In general, it appears that *myo*-inositol may be effective in many of the same disorders in which the SSRIs have shown some usefulness. This may not be surprising since *myo*-inositol has been shown to help reverse desensitization of serotonin receptors.

Myo-inositol is also being investigated for possible use in pediatric respiratory depression syndrome and for prevention of neural tube defects. Its usefulness with respect to the latter has been demonstrated in embryonic mice, but its use in humans may be curtailed or limited due to the fact that it has also been shown to induce uterine contractions.

CONTRAINDICATIONS, PRECAUTIONS, ADVERSE REACTIONS

CONTRAINDICATIONS
None known.

PRECAUTIONS
Because of lack of long-term safety data, *myo*-inositol should be avoided by pregnant women and nursing mothers. Also, high-dose *myo*-inositol may induce uterine contractions.

Because of the hypothetical possibility that *myo*-inositol may exacerbate hypomanic or manic symptoms in those with bipolar disorder, those with this condition should use supplemental *myo*-inositol with caution and under medical supervision.

ADVERSE REACTIONS
Myo-inositol supplementation is generally well tolerated. Gastrointestinal effects such as nausea and diarrhea are occasionally reported.

INTERACTIONS

DRUGS
Theoretically, high-dose *myo*-inositol may have additive effects with selective serotonin reuptake inhibitors (SSRIs) such as fluoxetine sertraline, paroxetine, fluvoxamine and citalopram, and with 5-hydroxytrytamine receptor agonists, such as sumatriptan.

NUTRITIONAL SUPPLEMENTS
No interactions known.

FOODS
Very small amounts of the inositol isomer, *scyllo*-inositol, are present in some foods. *Scyllo*-inositol has been reported to inhibit uptake of *myo*-inositol into the brain. Since the amount of *scyllo*-inositol intake is likely to be very little, this potential interaction is insignificant.

HERBS
Theoretically, high-dose *myo*-inositol may have additive effects with St. John's Wort.

OVERDOSAGE
Not reported.

DOSAGE AND ADMINISTRATION
For the management of depression and panic attacks, 12 grams of *myo*-inositol daily, in divided doses, were used in clinical studies. In the clinical studies performed with *myo*-inositol, effects, if any, were seen in about one month. Compliance with such doses may be a problem.

HOW SUPPLIED
Capsules — 500 mg
Powder
Tablets — 324 mg, 500 mg, 650 mg

LITERATURE
Barak Y, Levine J, Glassman A, et al. Inositol treatment of Alzheimer's disease: a double blind, cross-over placebo controlled trial. *Prog Neuropsychopharmacol Biol Psychiatry*. 1996; 20:729-735.

Benjamin J, Levine J, Fox M, et al. Double-blind, placebo-controlled, crossover trial of inositol treatment for panic disorder. *Am J Psyvhiatry*. 1995; 152:1084-1086.

Cohen RA, MacGregory LC, Spokes KC, et al. Effect of *myo*-inositol on renal Na-K-ATPase in experimental diabetes. *Metabol*. 1990; 39:1026-1032.

Colodny L, Hoffman RL. Inositol-clinical applications for exogenous use. *Altern Med Rev*. 1998; 3:432-447.

Downes CP. The cellular functions of *myo*-inositol. *Biochem Soc Trans*. 1989; 17:259-268.

Einat H, Belmaker RH, Kopilov M, et al. Rat brain monomines after acute and chronic *myo*-inositol treatment. *Eur Neuropsychopharmacol*. 1999; 10:27-30.

Einat H, Karbovski H, Korik J, et al. Inositol reduces depressive-like behaviors in two different models of depression. *Psychopharmacology*. 1999; 144:158-162.

Fox M, Levine J, Aviv A, Belmaker RH. Inositol treatment of obsessive-compulsive disorder. *Am J Psychiat*. 1996; 153:1219-1221.

Holub BJ. Metabolism and function of *myo*-inositol and inositol phospholipids. *Annu Rev Nutr*. 1986; 6:563-597.

Holub BJ. The cellular forms and functions of the inositol phospholipids and their metabolic derivates. *Nutr Rev*. 1987; 45:65-71.

Khandelwal M, Reece EA, Wu YK, Borenstein M. Dietary *myo*-inositol therapy in hyperglycemic-induced embryopathy. *Teratology*. 1998; 57:79-84.

Larner J, Allan G, Kessler C, et al. Phosphoinositol glycan derived mediators and insulin resistance. Prospects for diagnosis and therapy. *J Basic Clin Physiol Pharmacol*. 1998; 9:127-137.

Levine J. Controlled trials of inositol in psychiatry. *Eur Neuropsychopharmacol*. 1997; 7:147-155.

Levine J, Aviram A, Holan A, et al. Inositol treatment of action, *J Neural Transm*. 1997; 104:307-310.

Levine J, Barak Y, Gonzalues M, et al. Double-blind, controlled-trial of inositol treatment of depression. *Am J Psychiatry*. 1995; 152:792-794.

Levine J, Goldberger I, Rapaport A, et al. CSF inositol in schizophrenia and high-dose inositol treatment of schizophrenic. *Eur Neuropsychopharmacol*. 1994; 4:487-490.

Levine J, Kurtzman L, Rapoport A, et al. CSF inositol does not predict antidepressant response to inositol. *J Neural Transm*. 1996; 103:1457-1462.

Nestler JE, Jakabowicz DJ, Reamer P, et al. Ovulatory and metabolic effects of D-*chiro*-inositol in the polycystic overary syndrome. *N Engl J Med*. 1999; 340:1314-1320.

Seedat S, Stein DJ. Inositol augmentation of serotonin reuptake inhibitors in treatment-refractory obsessive-compulsive disorder: an open trial. *Int Clin Psychopharmacol*. 1999; 14:353-356.

NADH

DESCRIPTION

NADH is a natural substance found in most life forms and is necessary for energy production. NADH is located both in the mitochondria and cytosol of cells. It is a dinucleotide comprised of the nucleotide adenylic acid and a second nucleotide in which nicotinamide, a B vitamin, is the nitrogenous base. NADH is a key member of the electron transfer chain in mitochondria. The nicotinamide moiety is the portion of the dinucleotide that undergoes reversible reduction. NADH is the reduced form of the dinucleotide. The passage of electrons along the electron transport chain is coupled to the formation of ATP by the process known as oxidative phosphorylation.

NADH is synthesized by the body and thus is not an essential nutrient. It does require the essential nutrient nicotinamide for its synthesis, and its role in energy production is certainly an essential one. In addition to its role in the mitochondrial electron transport chain, NADH is produced in the cytosol. The mitochondrial membrane is impermeable to NADH, and this permeability barrier effectively separates the cytoplasmic from the mitochondrial NADH pools. However, cytoplasmic NADH can be used for biologic energy production. This occurs when the malate-aspartate shuttle introduces reducing equivalents from NADH in the cytosol to the electron transport chain of the mitochondria. This shuttle mainly occurs in the liver and heart.

NADH is the abbreviation for the reduced form of nicotinamide adenine dinucleotide. It is also known as coenzyme I. An older name was diphosphopyridine nucleotide reduced or DPNH. NADH has the following chemical structure:

NADH

ACTIONS AND PHARMACOLOGY

ACTIONS

The action of supplemental NADH is unclear.

MECHANISM OF ACTION

Any comments on the mechanism of action are speculative. NADH is a redox active substance and participates in biologic energy production. However, how the known roles of endogenous NADH relate to any possible action of supplemental NADH is not known. There is some evidence that a mitochondrial DNA mutation appears to cause a defective complex I in the mitochondria of Parkinson's disease patients. Complex I is comprised of NADH: ubiquinone oxidoreductase. Exogenous NADH may improve symptoms in some with ideopathic Parkinson's disease, and it is speculated that this is due to stimulation of levodopa biosynthesis.

PHARMACOKINETICS

There is scant pharmacokinetic data on supplemental NADH. It is unclear how much of an administered dose is absorbed and what the metabolic course is of any absorbed NADH. If NADH were to be transported into cells, it is highly unlikely that any would enter mitochondria.

INDICATIONS AND USAGE

There is very preliminary evidence suggesting that NADH might be useful in Parkinson's disease, chronic fatigue syndrome, Alzheimer's disease and cardiovascular disease.

RESEARCH SUMMARY

Reports that NADH may stimulate endogenous dopamine biosynthesis have led to its experimental use in Parkinson's disease. Some favorable results have been reported in case studies and open-label trials using both intravenous and oral NADH. In one open-label study of 885 subjects with Parkinson's disease, half received oral NADH and half received parenteral NADH with similar results. Some 80% of patients were said to have benefited clinically, with 19.3% showing good improvement, 58.8% moderate improvement and 21.8% non-responding. Younger patients and those with the shortest duration of disease showed the most improvement.

Only one very small double-blind study (with five Parkinson's patients) has been conducted to date. This was a short-term study. It found no benefit from NADH. More research is needed to determine the therapeutic role, if any, of NADH in Parkinson's disease.

Hope that NADH might be helpful in treating chronic fatigue syndrome was raised recently by a double-blind, placebo-controlled cross-over study of 26 patients. In the first phase of the study, subjects were randomly assigned to receive either 10 milligrams of NADH or a placebo for four weeks. After a four-week washout period, subjects were assigned to the alternate regimen for the final four-week trial period. Among the NADH-treated patients, 31% were judged to have notable improvement, while 8% of controls were similarly improved. Larger trials are indicated.

In another pilot study, 17 patients with dementia associated with Alzheimer's disease were treated with NADH for eight to 12 weeks. Researchers reported improvement in cognitive function in all 17 patients in this open-label trial, but they cautioned that "a double-blind, placebo-controlled study is necessary to demonstrate the clinical efficacy of NADH."

Yet another recent study sought to see whether oral NADH might lower blood pressure and affect lipids in a hypertensive animal model. This was a blinded, placebo-controlled, 10-week study. Systolic blood pressure was the same in the treated and placebo groups over the first month but thereafter was significantly reduced in the NADH group. Total cholesterol and LDL cholesterol were significantly reduced in the NADH group. No significant differences were noted in blood levels of glucose, insulin, triglyceride or HDL cholesterol. More research is warranted to see whether NADH might be useful in cardiovascular disease.

CONTRAINDICATIONS, PRECAUTIONS, ADVERSE REACTIONS

CONTRAINDICATIONS
None known.

PRECAUTIONS
Because of lack of long-term safety studies, NADH should be avoided by children, pregnant women and nursing mothers.

ADVERSE REACTIONS
There are a few reports of gastrointestinal side effects, including nausea and loss of appetite.

INTERACTIONS
There are no reported drug, nutritional supplement, food or herb interactions.

OVERDOSAGE
None reported.

DOSAGE AND ADMINISTRATION

Those who use NADH typically take either 5 milligrams once daily or 5 milligrams twice a day. Enteric-coated preparations are claimed to have better stability.

HOW SUPPLIED

Tablets — 2.5 mg, 5 mg

LITERATURE

Birkmayer JG. Coenzyme nicotinamide adenine dinucleotide: new therapeutic approach for improving dementia of the Alzheimer type. *Ann Clin Lab Sci.* 1996; 26:1-9.

Birkmayer JG, Vrecko C, Volc D, Birkmayer W. Nicotinamide adenine dinucleotide (NADH)—a new therapeutic approach to Parkinson's disease. Comparison of oral and parenteral application. *Acta Neurol Scand Suppl.* 1993; 146:32-35.

Bushehri N, Jarrell ST, Lieberman S, et al. Oral reduced B-nicotinamide adenine dinucleotide (NADH) affects blood pressure, lipid peroxidation, and lipid profile in hypertensive rats (SHR). *Geriatr Nephrol Urol.* 1998; 8:95-100.

Dizdar N, Kagedal B, Lindvall B. Treatment of Parkinson's disease with NADH. *Acta Neurol Scand.* 1994; 90:345-347.

Forsyth LM, Preuss HG, MacDowell AL, et al. Therapeutic effects of oral NADH on the symptoms of patients with chronic fatigue syndrome. *Ann Allergy Asthma Immunol.* 1999; 82:185-191.

Kuhn W, Muller T, Winkel R, et al. Parenteral application of NADH in Parkinson's disease: clinical improvement partially due to stimulation of endogenous levodopa biosynthesis. *J Neural Transm.* 1996; 103:1187-1193.

Swerdlow RH. Is NADH effective in the treatment of Parkinson's disease? *Drugs Aging.* 1998; 13:263-268.

Swerdlow RH, Parks JK, Miller SW, et al. Origin and functional consequences of the complex I defect in Parkinson's disease. *Ann Neurol.* 1996; 40:663-671.

Niacin (Nicotinic Acid)

TRADE NAMES

Niacinol (Tyler Encapsulations), Nicotinex (Fleming and Company), B-3-50 (Bio-Tech Pharmacal), Slo-Niacin (Upsher-Smith).

DESCRIPTION

The term niacin is used in two different ways. As a collective term, it refers to both nicotinic acid and nicotinamide. It is also used synonymously with nicotinic acid. In this monograph, the biochemistry and pharmacology of niacin—nicotinic acid and nicotinamide—will be discussed, as well as the actions of and indications for nicotinic acid. The actions of and indications for nicotinamide will be discussed in a separate monograph (see Nicotinamide). Nicotinic acid and nicotinamide have identical vitamin activities, but have very different pharmacological activities.

Niacin is a member of the B-vitamin family. It is sometimes referred to as vitamin B_3. Nicotinic acid was first discovered as an oxidation product of nicotine and thus, the origin of its name. In fact, much of the confusion caused by the use of the term niacin for both nicotinic acid and nicotinamide, as well as for nicotinic acid alone, was created by the attempt to dissociate nicotinic acid from its nicotine origins. Niacin, via its metabolites, is involved in a wide range of biological processes, including the production of energy, the synthesis of fatty acids, cholesterol and steroids, signal transduction, the regulation of gene expression and the maintenance of genomic integrity. Nicotinic acid, in pharmacological doses, is used as an antihyperlipidemic agent.

Niacin and substances that are convertible to niacin are found naturally in meat (especially red meat), poultry, fish, legumes and yeast. In addition to preformed niacin, some L-tryptophan found in the proteins of these foods is metabolized to niacin. Niacin is also present in cereal grains, such as corn and wheat. However, consumption of corn-rich diets has resulted in niacin deficiency in certain populations. The reason for this is that niacin exists in cereal grains in bound forms, such as the glycoside niacytin, which exhibit little or no nutritional availability. Interestingly, niacin deficiency is not common in Mexico and Central America even though the diets of those in these countries are based on corn. Alkaline treatment, such as soaking corn in a lime solution, the process used by the populations of Mexico and Central America in the production of corn tortillas, yields release of bound niacin and increased availability of the vitamin.

The well-known disorder of niacin deficiency is pellagra. The term pellagra is derived from the Italian words pelle agra meaning rough or smarting skin. Pellagra is characterized by the triad of dermatitis, diarrhea and dementia. A fourth d, death, is the final outcome of the disease, if not treated. The skin lesions are primarily located on sun-exposed areas of the face, hands, arms and feet. The dermatitis progresses from an erythematous, often pruritic rash, to vesicles and blisters with scales and fissures, and finally, to thickened, lichenified, hyperpigmented skin. Casal's necklace refers to characteristic advanced skin lesions of pellagra. Casal's necklace is named for Gaspar Casal, the physician to King Ferdinand of Spain, who first reported on the symptoms and signs of pellagra in modern times. He called the disease mal de la rosa (disease of the rose), because of the red and glossy color of the skin lesions. Casal attributed the disorder to the diets of the poor laborers; diets which were mainly comprised of corn. Although pellagra was commonly found in the United States through the 1930s, the disorder is rare today in industrialized countries. This is due, in large part, to the enrichment of refined flours with niacin.

Niacin deficiency, however, can and does occur under certain conditions. These conditions include alcoholism, malabsorption syndromes, cirrhosis and in those receiving total parenteral nutrition (TPN) with inadequate niacin. It may also occur in Hartnup's syndrome, an autosomal recessive disorder in which there is defective conversion of tryptophan to niacin; carcinoid syndrome, in which tryptophan metabolism is diverted to form 5-hydroxytryptamine, and in those receiving isoniazid for the treatment of tuberculosis.

The biochemical effects of niacin are principally mediated by its metabolite nicotinamide adenine dinucleotide or NAD^+. NAD^+ serves both coenzyme and substrate functions. NAD^+ was originally called cozymase and was also known as coenzyme I and DPN or diphosphopyridine nucleotide. The positive sign in NAD^+ refers to the fact that the nitrogen in the pyridine ring of niacin is positively charged in the NAD^+ structure. NAD^+ and its reduced form NADH (reduced nicotinamide dinucleotide) are the major hydrogen acceptor and donor, respectively, in many biological redox reactions. NAD^+ is used in metabolic reactions to transfer the potential free energy stored in carbohydrates, lipids and proteins to NADH, which is used to form ATP (adenosine triphosphate).

$NADP^+$ or nicotinamide adenine dinucleotide phosphate is formed from NAD^+ via a kinase-catalyzed phosphorylation. $NADP^+$ participates as a coenzyme in the oxidation of glucose 6-phosphate via the enzyme glucose 6-phosphate dehydrogenase. This is the oxidative reaction in the pentose phosphate pathway which produces, among other things, ribose 5-phosphate. During the oxidation of glucose 6-phosphate, $NADP^+$ is reduced to NADPH or reduced nicotinamide adenine dinucleotide phosphate. NADPH serves as the reducing agent in fatty acid and steroid biosyntheses and serves to maintain glutathione in its reduced form.

In addition to its coenzyme role in many metabolic reactions, NAD^+ also serves as a substrate in a number of biochemical reactions. The beta-N-glycosylic bond of NAD^+ can be cleaved by three types of enzymes. In the process, nicotinamide and ADP (adenosine diphosphate)-ribose are formed. One type of enzyme catalyzes mono(ADP-ribosyl)ation of proteins—a posttranslational modification—by transferring ADP-ribose from NAD^+ to target proteins. The enzymes are known as mono(ADP-ribosyl)transferases (mADPRTs). Mono(ADP-ribosyl)ation of endogenous proteins by bacterial toxins, such as diphtheria toxin and cholera toxin, accounts, in large part, for the pathogenic effects of these toxins. The physiological functions of endogenous mono(ADP-ribosyl)transferases are not clear. Another type of enzyme catalyzes poly(ADP-ribosyl)ation of target proteins. This enzyme is known as poly(ADP-ribose)polymerase or PARP. PARP is also known as poly(ADP-ribose) synthetase (PARS), poly(ADP-ribose)transferase (pADPRT) and PARP1. PARP is believed to be involved in DNA repair, among other things.

NAD^+ is also involved in the biosynthesis of signaling molecules. A third type of beta-N-glycosylic bond-cleaving enzymes catalyzes the formation of cyclic ADP-ribose (cADPR). Cyclic ADP-ribose is an intracellular calcium mobilizing agent. The enzyme that catalyzes the synthesis of cyclic ADP-ribose is called ADP-ribosyl cyclase. $NADP^+$ is also involved in the biosynthesis of signaling molecules. $NADP^+$ leads to the formation of $NAADP^+$ (nicotinic acid adenine dinucleotide phosphate) and cADPRP (2'-phospho cyclic ADP-ribose). $NAADP^+$ and cADPRP are also intracellular calcium mobilizing agents.

The enzyme poly(ADP-ribose) polymerase(PARP) is a highly abundant nuclear protein, the physiological role of which is not yet clear. PARP poly(ADP-ribosyl)ates various nuclear proteins as well as itself. PARP is thought to be involved in a number of biological processes, including

DNA repair and replication, cell differentiation and cellular apoptosis. DNA damage appears to enhance the activity of PARP. In damaged cells, PARP binds to DNA and becomes enzymatically activated. Once activated, PARP automodifies itself through poly(ADP-ribosyl)ation. This results in its inactivation and its dissociation from DNA breaks. This dissociation is necessary for DNA repair.

Recently, it has been found that NAD^+ plays a key role in life-span extension by calorie restriction in the yeast *Saccharomyces cerevisiae*. It does so by serving as the cofactor for an NAD^+-dependent histone deacetylase, an enzyme that removes acetyl groups from the lysine residues of histone proteins, thus promoting genomic silencing. Maintenance of genomic silencing may be critical to longevity either by repressing genomic instability or by preventing inappropriate gene expression. A similar mechanism may operate in metazoans, including humans.

As mentioned above, niacin is used either to refer to both nicotinic acid and nicotinamide or to nicotinic acid itself. Nicotinic acid, in addition to being known as niacin, is also known as pyridine-3-carboxylic acid, vitamin B_3, 3-pyridine-carboxylic acid, pyridine-beta-carboxylic acid, antipellagra vitamin and pellagra preventive factor. The molecular formula of nicotinic acid is $C_6H_5NO_2$. The molecular weight of nicotinic acid is 123.11 daltons and the structural formula is:

Nicotinic Acid

Nicotinamide is also known as pyridine-3-carboxamide, niacinamide and nicotinic acid amide. Its molecular formula is $C_6H_6N_2O$ and its molecular weight is 122.13 daltons.

ACTIONS AND PHARMACOLOGY

ACTIONS

Nicotinic acid has antihyperlipidemic activity and may have anti-atherogenic activity.

MECHANISM OF ACTION

Nicotinic acid in gram doses, but not nicotinamide, lowers serum levels of total cholesterol, low-density lipoprotein cholesterol (LDL-C), very low-density lipoprotein (VLDL) and triglycerides. High-dose nicotinic acid also increases serum levels of high-density lipoprotein cholesterol (HDL-C) and decreases serum levels of lipoprotein (a) [Lp(a)] and apolipoprotein B-100 (Apo B). The mechanism of the antihyperlipidemic action of nicotinic acid is not well understood. It is thought that this effect is mediated, in part, via decreases in the release of free fatty acids from adipose tissue, thereby decreasing the influx of free fatty acids into the liver, the hepatic reesterification of free fatty acids and the rate of production of hepatic very low-density lipoprotein (VLDL). A decrease in the hepatic production of VLDL reduces the level of circulating VLDL available for conversion to LDL. Another hypothesis holds that nicotinic acid directly inhibits hepatic synthesis or secretion of apolipoprotein B-containing lipoproteins. Still another hypothesis holds that nicotinic acid has the potential to cause a generalized inhibition of synthetic function in the liver. This mechanism may be considered a manifestation of nicotinic acid hepatotoxicity resulting in decreased LDL-cholesterol. However, this liver-damaging hypothesis would not explain the HDL-elevating effect of nicotinic acid. The mechanism by which nicotinic acid elevates HDL is unknown.

High dose nicotinic acid has been found to significantly decrease cardiovascular and cerebrovascular events in those with coronary heart disease. It is thought that this effect is due, in part, to nicotinic acid's antihyperlipidemic activity.

PHARMACOKINETICS

Both nicotinic acid and nicotinamide are efficiently absorbed from the stomach and small intestine. At low amounts, absorption is mediated by sodium-dependent facilitated diffusion. Passive diffusion is the principal mechanism of absorption at higher doses. Doses of up to three to four grams of nicotinic acid and niacinamide are almost completely absorbed. Nicotinic acid and nicotinamide are transported via the portal circulation to the liver and via the systemic circulation to the various tissues of the body. Nicotinic acid and nicotinamide enter most cells by passive diffusion and enter erythrocytes by facilitated transport.

Nicotinic and nicotinamide are metabolized through different pathways. Nicotinic acid is not directly metabolized to nicotinamide. It undergoes a number of metabolic steps to yield NAD^+ which in turn can be converted to nicotinamide. Nicotinamide can be directly converted to nicotinic acid. Nicotinic acid is metabolized to nicotinic acid mononucleotide (NicMN, nicotinic acid ribonucleotide). NicMN is also the first niacin metabolite to which dietary L-tryptophan is converted. NicMN is converted to nicotinic acid adenine dinucleotide (NicAD, desamido-NAD^+). NicAD is converted in turn to NAD+. NAD^+ has a number of metabolic opportunities. These include, the formation of nicotinamide, $NADP^+$, nicotinamide 5'-mononucleotide (NMN), cyclic ADP-ribose and nicotinic acid dinucleotide phosphate (NAADP). NAD^+ also serves as the substrate for mono-(ADP-ribosyl)ation and poly(ADP-ribosyl)ation reactions. Nicotinamide is converted to nicotinic acid via the enzyme nicotinamidase. Nicotinamide is also metabolized to NMN which in turn is converted to NAD^+.

In the liver, the principal catabolic product of high doses of nicotinic acid is the glycine conjugate of nicotinic acid called nicotinuric acid. The principal catabolic products of nicotinamide are N'-methylnicotinamide, N'-methyl-5-carboxamide-2-pyridone, N'-methyl-5-carboxamide-4-pyridone and nicotinamide-N-oxide.

High doses of nicotinic acid are excreted in the urine as unchanged nicotinic acid and the glycine conjugate of nicotinic acid nicotinuric acid. High doses of nicotinamide are excreted in the urine as unchanged nicotinamide, N'-methylnicotinamide, N'-methyl-5-carboxamide-2-pyridone, N'-methyl-5-carboxamide-4-pyridone and nicotinamide-N-oxide.

The pharmacokinetics of the various forms of nicotinic acid (immediate-release, intermediate-release, extended-release) differ in certain particulars. The time to reach peak serum concentrations of the immediate-release or crystalline form of nicotinic acid is approximately 45 minutes following ingestion. The time to reach peak serum concentrations of the extended-release form of nicotinic acid is from 4-5 hours following ingestion. Administration of nicotinic acid with food maximizes its availability. Nicotinic acid-induced flushing, which is due to vasodilation, occurs within 20 minutes following ingestion of immediate-release nicotinic acid and may last for up to one hour.

INDICATIONS AND USAGE

Nicotinic acid is effective in lowering cholesterol and triglycerides and appears to help protect against atherosclerosis. There is no little support for claims that nicotinic acid is effective in treating schizophrenia, diabetes, arthritis, hypertension, sexual dysfunction or migraine headaches. Claims that it is a ''detoxifier'' and aids in withdrawal from alcohol and narcotic drugs are similarly unsubstantiated.

RESEARCH SUMMARY

Nicotinic acid has been tested for its effects on cardiovascular-disease risk factors in a number of major trials. In the largest of these, the effect of nicotinic acid monotherapy on cardiovascular endpoints was investigated. The study included 8,341 men who had suffered myocardial infarction. In this randomized, six-year study, nicotinic acid, given in 1 gram doses three times a day, decreased cholesterol levels by 10% and triglyceride levels by 26%. There was a decrease of 27% in recurrent non-fatal heart attacks among the nicotinic-acid treated subjects. They also experienced 26% fewer cerebrovascular events.

In a five-year randomized, placebo-controlled study of 555 survivors of myocardial infarction, nicotinic acid, in combination with clofibrate, was found to significantly decrease total and cardiac mortality. Total mortality declined by 26%.

Nicotinic acid was given in 1 gram doses three times daily. Clofibrate was given in 1 gram doses twice daily.

In another well-controlled study of men aged 40 to 59 who had undergone coronary artery bypass, nicotinic acid used in combination with colestipol significantly decreased disease progression in some and significantly increased disease regression in some others, compared with placebo.

Various studies have shown that nicotinic acid can significantly lower total cholesterol, LDL-cholesterol, triglycerides and lipoprotein (a) levels. It can also increase HDL-cholesterol levels.

Nicotinic acid may be an effective and safe lipid-modifying agent even among those with diabetes. A recent report of the analysis of data from the Arterial Disease Multiple Intervention Trial (ADMIT), showed that those with and without diabetes who received crystalline nicotinic acid (3,000 milligrams/day) had significantly increased levels of HDL-cholesterol and decreased levels of LDL-cholesterol and triglycerides after 18 weeks of treatment. Glucose levels were only modestly increased among subjects with and without diabetes. Among those with diabetes, HbA_{1c} levels were unchanged in the nicotinic acid group, but decreased in the placebo group. No significant differences in nicotinic acid discontinuation or hypoglycemic therapy were noted in those with diabetes assigned to nicotinic acid vs placebo.

A newer extended-release nicotinic acid, used once daily, either as monotherapy or in combination with lipid-lowering drugs, has demonstrated the same favorable effects on lipids in clinical trials. This form may be less hepatotoxic than slow-release nicotinic acid.

CONTRAINDICATIONS, PRECAUTIONS, ADVERSE REACTIONS

CONTRAINDICATIONS

Niacin is contraindicated in those who are hypersensitive to any component of a niacin-containing product. High-dose nicotinic acid is contraindicated in those with hepatic dysfunction, unexplained elevations of serum aminotransferases (transaminases), active peptic ulcer disease and arterial bleeding.

PRECAUTIONS

Pregnant women and nursing mothers should avoid supplement doses of niacin greater than U.S. RDA amounts (20 milligrams daily) unless higher doses are prescribed by their physicians.

The use of nicotinic acid as an antihyperlipidemic agent should only be undertaken under medical supervision.

Those with a past history of hepatobiliary disease, jaundice, peptic ulcer disease or gastritis should exercise caution in the use of high-dose nicotinic acid. Those with a history of diabetes, renal dysfunction, cardiovascular disease (especially acute myocardial infarction and unstable angina) and gout should exercise caution in the use of high-dose nicotinic acid. Those who consume substantial amounts of alcohol should also exercise caution in the use of high-dose nicotinic acid.

Those who take high-dose nicotinic acid should have their serum aminotransferase levels monitored. Aspartate aminotransferase (AST, also known as SGOT or serum glutamate oxaloacetate transaminase) and alanine aminotransferase (ALT, also known as SGPT or serum glutamate pyruvate transaminase) levels should be determined prior to starting high-dose nicotinic acid therapy, then every 6-12 weeks for one year and after one year, periodically. High-dose nicotinic acid should be discontinued if the aminotransferase levels are equal to greater than three times the upper limit of normal.

Intermediate-release (extended-release) and slow-release forms of nicotinic acid should not be substituted for equivalent doses of immediate-release (crystalline) nicotinic acid. Cases of severe hepatic toxicity, including fulminant hepatic necrosis, have occurred in subjects who have substituted sustained-release nicotinic acid products for immediate-release nicotinic acid at equivalent doses. Those who switch from immediate-release nicotinic acid to sustained-release forms of nicotinic acid, should start off with low doses of sustained-release nicotinic acid and the dose should then be slowly increased in order to obtain the desired therapeutic response.

High-dose nicotinic acid may negatively effect glucose tolerance. Diabetics who take nicotinic acid for lipid-lowering, should have their serum glucose levels carefully monitored and the dose of their antidiabetic medications adjusted as necessary.

ADVERSE REACTIONS

Nicotinic acid can cause vasodilation of cutaneous blood vessels resulting in increased blood flow, principally in the face, neck and chest. This produces the niacin- or nicotinic acid-flush. The niacin-flush is thought to be mediated via the prostaglandin prostacyclin. Histamine may also play a role in the niacin-flush. Flushing is the adverse reaction first observed after intake of a large dose of nicotinic acid, and the most bothersome one. It is the principal reason for compliance issues with the use of high-dose nicotinic acid for the treatment of hyperlipidemia. Nicotinamide does not appear to be associated with flushing. However, high-dose nicotinamide does not possess antihyperlipidemic activity. The symptoms of flushing include a burning, tingling and itching sensation. A reddened flush occurs primarily on the face, arms and chest. Flushing is often accompanied by pruritis and headaches. In one study, 5% of subjects ingesting 50 milligrams of nicotinic acid experienced flushing, 50% experienced flushing after ingesting 100 milligrams of nicotinic acid and 100% of subjects ingesting 500 milligrams of nicotinic acid experienced flushing. In another study, 66% of subjects experienced a flushing sensation after ingestion of 50 milligrams of nicotinic acid. Based on these studies, the Food and Nutrition Board of the Institute of Medicine has established a LOAEL (lowest-observed-adverse-effect level) for niacin of 50 mg/day. Based on this LOAEL, the Tolerable Upper Intake Level (UL) for niacin, for adults, is set at 35 mg/day. To obtain this UL, the LOAEL of 50 mg/day was divided by an uncertainty factor (UF) of 1.5 and rounded off.

The flushing effect of nicotinic acid is transient and tolerance to this effect occurs with continued administration of the vitamin. The flushing effect, as mentioned above, is prostaglandin mediated, and tolerance results from reduction in prostaglandin levels with continued administration.

Other adverse reactions of nicotinic acid, include dizziness, palpitations, tachycardia, shortness of breath, sweating, chills, insomnia, nausea, vomiting, abdominal pain and myalgias. Nicotinic acid can cause hepatotoxicity. In the most severe cases, subjects develop liver dysfunction and fulminant hepatitis and may progress to stage 3 and 4 encephalopathy requiring liver transplantation. The most frequently observed manifestations of nicotinic acid-induced hepatitis are increased levels of serum aminotransferases (transaminases) and jaundice. Many, if not most of the subjects who developed hepatoxicity from nicotinic acid appeared to be taking the slow-release form. A recent double-blind comparison suggested that the slow-release form is more hepatotoxic than the immediate-release form. However, not all studies find this to be the case. Another recent study reported that both the slow release and immediate-release forms of nicotinic acid are hepatotoxic.

High-dose nicotinic acid (approximately 3 grams daily) has caused impaired glucose tolerance in otherwise healthy individuals. Further, glucose tolerance in diabetics may be worsened by nicotinic acid therapy. High doses of nicotinic acid (1.5 to 5 grams/day) have also caused ocular effects, including blurred vision, macular edema, toxic amblyopia and cystic maculopathy. Nicotinic acid-induced ocular effects do not appear to be common and appear to be reversible. Elevated uric acid levels have also occurred with nicotinic acid therapy.

INTERACTIONS
DRUGS
Alpha₁-blockers (doxazosin, prazosin, tamsulosin, terazosin): Concomitant use of high-dose nicotinic acid and an alpha₁-blocker may potentiate the hypotensive effect of the alpha₁-blocker and may cause postural hypotension.

Alpha-glucosidase inhibitors (acarbose, miglitol): High-dose nicotinic acid may antagonize the antidiabetic action of alpha-glucosidase inhibitors, requiring adjustment of their dosage.

Biguanides (metformin): High-dose nicotinic acid may antagonize the antidiabetic activity of metformin, requiring adjustment of its dosage,

Calcium channel blockers: Concomitant use of high-dose nicotinic acid and a calcium channel blocker may potentiate the hypotensive effect of the calcium channel blocker.

Cholestyramine: Concomitant use of high-dose nicotinic acid and cholestyramine may reduce the absorption of nicotinic acid. It is recommended that a 4 to 6 hour interval elapse between the ingestion of cholestyramine and the administration of nicotinic acid. Administration of high-dose nicotinic acid and cholestyramine may produce complementary antihyperlipidemic effects.

Colestipol: Concomitant use of high-dose nicotinic acid and colestipol may reduce the absorption of nicotinic acid. It is recommended that a 4 to 6 hour interval elapse between the ingestion of colestipol and the administration of nicotinic acid. Administraion of high-dose nicotinic acid and colestipol may produce complementary antihyperlipidemic effects.

Ganglionic blocking agents (mecamylamine HCL, trimethaphan): Nicotinic acid may potentiate the effects of ganglionic blocking agents resulting in postural hypotension.

Gemfibrozil: Adminisration of high-dose nicotinic acid and gemfibrozil may produce complementary antihyperlipidemic effects.

HMG-CoA reductase inhibitors or "statins" (atorvastatin, cerivastatin, fluvastatin, lovastatin, pravastatin, simvastatin): Concomitant administration of high-dose nicotinic acid and HMG-CoA reductase inhibitors have resulted in rare cases of rhabdomyolysis. Those receiving concomitant high-dose nicotinic acid and an HMG-CoA reductase inhibitor should be carefully monitored for any signs or symptoms of muscle pain, tenderness or weakness. Administration of high-dose nicotinic acid and a statin may produce complementary antihyperlipidemic effects.

Meglitinides (repaglinide): High-dose nicotinic acid may antagonize the antidiabetic action of repaglinide, a metglitinide analogue, requiring adjustment of its dosage.

Nicotine patch: Concomitant use of a transdermal nicotine patch and nicotinic acid may enhance the flushing reaction.

Nitrates: Concomitant use of high-dose nicotinic acid and a nitrate may potentiate the hypotensive effect of the nitrate.

NSAIDs (ibuprofen, etc.) and aspirin: The use of aspirin (80 to 325 milligrams), ibuprofen (200 to 400 milligrams), or other NSAIDs, taken 30 minutes to one hour before a dose of nicotinic acid, may blunt the flushing effect of high-dose nicotinic acid. Nicotinic acid induces the release of prostacyclin. Prostacyclin is thought to account for, in large part, nicotinic acid-induced flushing. Aspirin may also decrease the metabolic clearance of nicotinic acid.

Sulfonylureas (chlorpropamide, glimepiride, glipizide, glyburide): High-dose nicotinic acid may antagonize the antidiabetic action of sulfonylureas, requiring adjustment of their dosage.

Thiazolidinediones (pioglitazone, rosiglitazone): High-dose nicotinic acid may antagonize the antidiabetic action of thiazolidinediones, requiring adjustment of their dosage.

Warfarin: Extended-release (intermediate-release) forms of nicotinic acid have been associated with small but statistically significant increases in prothrombin time. Concomitant use of extended-release forms of nicotinic acid, as well as other forms of nicotinic acid, may enhance the anticoagulant activity of warfarin. INRs should be closely monitored in those taking high-dose nicotinic acid concomitantly with warfarin.

NUTRITIONAL SUPPLEMENTS
Red yeast rice: The nutritional supplement red yeast rice contains HMG-CoA reductase inhibitors including lovastatin. Concomitant administration of high-dose nicotinic acid and HMG-CoA reductase inhibitors, including lovastatin, have resulted in rare cases of rhabdomyolysis.

FOODS
Ethanol-containing beverages: Concomitant intake of nicotinic acid and ethanol-containing beverages may cause an increase in nicotinic acid-induced flushing.

Hot beverages and hot foods: Concomitant intake of hot beverages or hot foods and nicotinic acid may cause an increase in nicotinic acid-induced flushing.

OVERDOSAGE
There are no reports of niacin overdosage in the literature.

DOSAGE AND ADMINISTRATION
Niacin, as nicotinamide (niacinamide) is the principal form used for nutritional supplementation. It is available as a single ingredient product (see Nicotinamide) and in multivitamin and multivitamin/multimineral products. Typical supplemental dosage, ranges from 20 to 100 milligrams daily. Nicotinamide is also the form of niacin used in food fortification.

The Food and Nutrition Board of the Institute of Medicine of the National Academy of Sciences has recommended the following dietary reference intakes (DRIs) for niacin: (Preformed niacin refers to nicotinic acid and nicotinamide; niacin equivalents refer to nicotinic acid, to nicotinamide and the contribution to niacin obtained by conversion from dietary L-Tryptophan. The relative contribution of tryptophan is estimated as follows: 60 mg of L-tryptophan = one mg of niacin = 1 mg of niacin equivalents.)

Infants	Adequate Intakes (AI)
0—6 months	2 mg/day of preformed niacin ≈ 0.2 mg/Kg
7—12 months	4 mg/day of niacin equivalents ≈ 0.4 mg/Kg

Children	Recommended Dietary Allowances (RDA)
1—3 years	6 mg/day of niacin equivalents
4—8 years	8 mg/day of niacin equivalents

Boys	
9—13 years	12 mg/day of niacin equivalents
14—18 years	16 mg/day of niacin equivalents

Girls	
9—13 years	12 mg/day of niacin equivalents
14—18 years	14 mg/day of niacin equivalents

Men	
19 years and older	16 mg/day of niacin equivalents

Women	
19 years and older	14 mg/day of niacin equivalents

Pregnancy	
14—50 years	18 mg/day of niacin equivalents

Lactation	
14—50 years	17 mg/day of niacin equivalents

The U.S. RDA for niacin, which is used for determining percent daily values on nutritional supplement and food labels, is 20 milligrams.

Nicotinic acid is available as a single ingredient product. It is available both as an OTC product and as a prescription product. The use of nicotinic acid as an antihyperlipidemic agent should only be undertaken under medical supervision. Three different formulations are available for antihyperlipidemic use: immediate-release (crystalline) nicotinic acid, extended-release (intermediate-release) nicotinic acid and slow-release nicotinic acid. Recommended adult doses are up to 3 grams daily of the immediate-release form or 1 to 2 grams of the extended-release forms. It is recommended that nicotinic acid be started at low doses and slowly titrated to the desired therapeutic dose. Administration on an empty stomach is *not* recommended. The use of an NSAID taken ¹/₂ hour before nicotinic acid may blunt the flushing reaction. The flushing is less severe with extended-release and slow-release forms than it is with immediate-release forms. However, the slow-release form may lead to an increased incidence of gastrointestinal problems and hepatotoxicity. The intermediate-release form may be less hepatotoxic than the slow-release form.

HOW SUPPLIED

Capsules — 100 mg, 500 mg

Capsules, Extended Release — 125 mg, 250 mg, 400 mg, 500 mg

Elixir — 50 mg/5 mL

Tablets — 50 mg, 100 mg, 250 mg, 500 mg,

Tablets, Timed Release — 250 mg, 500 mg, 750 mg, 1000 mg

LITERATURE

Capuzzi DM, Guyton JR, Morgan JM, et al. Efficacy and safety of an extended-release niacin (Niaspan): a long-term study. *Am J Cardiol.* 1998; 82(12A):74U-81U.

Carlson LA, Rosenhamer G. Reduction of mortality in the Stockholm ischemic Heart Disease Secondary Prevention Study by combined treatment with clofibrate and nicotinic acid. *Acta Med Scand.* 1988; 223:405-418.

Canner PL, Berge KG, Wenger NK, et al. Fifteen year mortality in Coronary Drug Project patients: long-term benefit with niacin. *J Am Coll Cardiol.* 1986; 8:1245-1255.

Cervantes-Laurean D, McElvaney NG, Moss J. Niacin. In: Shils ME, Olson JA, Shike M, Ross AC, eds. *Modern Nutrition in Health and Disease.* 9ᵗʰ ed. Baltimore, MD: Williams and Wilkins; 1999:401-411.

Chojnowska-Jezierska J, Adamska-Dyniewska H. [Prolonged treatment with slow release nicotinic acid in patients with type II hyperlipidemia]. [Article in Polish]. *Pol Arch Med Wewn.* 1997; 98:391-399.

Colletti RB, Neufeld EJ, Roff NK, et al. Niacin treatment of hypercholesterolemia in children. *Pediatrics.* 1993; 92:78-82.

Dietary Reference Intakes for Thiamin, Riboflavin, Niacin, Vitamin B₆, Folate, Vitamin B₁₂, Pantothenic Acid, Biotin, and Choline. Washington, DC: National Academy Press; 1998.

Elam MB, Hunninghake DB, Davis KB, et al. Effect of niacin on lipid and lipoprotein levels and glycemic control in patients with diabetes and peripheral arterial disease: The ADMIT Study: A randomized trial. *JAMA.* 2000; 284:1263-1270.

Goldberg A, Alagona P Jr, Capuzzi DM, et al. Multiple-dose efficacy and safety of an extended-release form of niacin in the management of hyperlipidemia. *Am J Cardiol.* 2000; 85:1100-1105.

Gray DR, Morgan T, Chretian SD, Kashyap ML. Efficacy and safety of controlled-release niacin in dyslipoproteinemic veterans. *Ann Intern Med.* 1994; 121:252-258.

Guyton JR. Effect of niacin on atherosclerotic cardiovascular disease. *Am J Cardiol.* 1998; 82:18U-23U.

Guyton JR, Blazing MA, Hagar J, et al. Extended-release niacin vs gemfibrozil for the treatment of low levels of high-density lipoprotein cholesterol. Niaspan-Gemfibrozil Study Group. *Arch Int Med.* 2000; 160:1177-1184.

Henkin Y, Oberman A, Hurst DC. Niacin revisited: clinical observations on an important but underutilized drug. *Am J Med.* 1991; 91:239-246.

Illingworth DR, Stein EA, Mitchel YB, et al. Comparative effects of lovastatin and niacin in primary hypercholesterolemia. *Arch Intern Med.* 1994; 154:1586-1595.

Johansson JO, Egberg N, Asplund-Carlson A, Carlson LA. Nicotinic acid treatment shifts the fibrinolytic balance favorably and decreases plasma fibrinogen in hypertriglyceridaemic men. *J Cardiovasc Risk.* 1997; 4:165-171.

Lin S-J, Defossez P-A, Guarente L. Requirement of NAD and SIR2 for life-span extension by calorie restriction in *Saccharomyces cerevisiae. Science.* 2000; 289:2126-2128.

King JM, Crouse JR, Terry JG, et al. Evaluation of effects of unmodified niacin on fasting and postprandial plasma lipids in normolipidemic men with hypoalphalipoproteinemia. *Am J Med.* 1994; 97:323-331.

McKenney JM, Proctor JD, Harris S, Chinchili VM. A comparison of the efficacy and toxic effects of sustained-vs immediate-release niacin in hypercholesterolemic patients. *JAMA.* 1994; 271:672-677.

Rader JI, Calvert RJ, Hathcock JN. Hepatic toxicity of unmodified and time-release preparations of niacin. *Am J Med.* 1992; 92:77-81.

Saareks V, Mucha I, Sievi E, Riutta A. Nicotinic acid and pyridoxine modulate arachidonic acid metabolism in vitro and ex vivo in man. *Pharmacol Toxicol.* 1999; 84:274-280.

Tato F, Vega GL, Grundy SM. Effects of crystalline nicotinic acid-induced hepatic dysfunction on serum low-density lipoprotein cholesterol and lecithin cholesteryl acyl transferase. *Am J Cardiology.* 1998; 81:805-807.

Trueblood NA, Ramasamy R, Wang LF, Schaefer S. Niacin protects the isolated heart from ischemia-reperfusion injury. *Am J Physiol Heart Circ Physiol.* 2000; 279:H764-H771.

Tsalamandris C, Panagiotopoulos S, Sinha A, et al. Complementary effects of pravastatin and nicotinic acid in the treatment of combined hyperlipidaemia in diabetic and non-diabetic patients. *J Cardiovasc Risk.* 1994; 1:231-239.

Vispé S, Yung TMC, Ritchot J, et al. A cellular defense pathway regulating transcription through poly(ADP-ribosyl)ation in response to DNA damage. *Proc Natl Acad Sci USA.* 2000; 97:9886-9891.

Wang W, Basinger A, Neese RA, et al. Effects of nicotinic acid on fatty acid kinetics, fuel selection, and pathways of glucose production in women. *Am J Physiol Endocrinol Metab.* 2000; 279:E50-E59.

Ziegler M. New Functions of a long-known molecule. Emerging roles of NAD in cellular signaling. *Eur J Biochem.* 2000; 267:1550-1564.

Nickel

DESCRIPTION

Nickel is a hard, malleable and ductile metal with atomic number 28 and symbol Ni. It occurs in igneous rock and as a free metal and, together with iron, it is a component of the earth's core. Nickel also occurs in living organisms, mainly in plants.

Nickel is not currently considered an essential nutrient for humans. Nickel deficiency states have been reported in some animals. Rats and goats fed nickel-deficient diets have depressed growth, reproductive performance and plasma glucose, as well as abnormalities in mineral status. Nickel is conjectured to play a role in processes related to the vitamin B12-and folic acid-dependent pathway in methione metabolism.

The major dietary source of nickel is plant foods. Nickel-rich food items include nuts, beans, peas, grains and chocolate. Animal foods are low in nickel. Total daily dietary intakes of nickel vary depending on the amount of plant and animal foods consumed. Diets high in plant foods, such as the ones listed above, supply about 900 micrograms daily of nickel. Nickel intake in the United States ranges from 69 to 162 micrograms daily. A daily dietary requirement of 25 to 35 micrograms has been suggested.

Nickel allergies are not uncommon and usually manifested as hand eczema. The results of one open, prospective trial suggested that low-nickel diets may benefit some nickel-sensitive individuals.

ACTIONS AND PHARMACOLOGY

ACTIONS

The actions of dietary nickel are not known.

PHARMACOKINETICS

Little is known about the pharmacokinetics of dietary nickel in humans. Apparently nickel is poorly absorbed when ingested in typical diets. The mechanism of absorption is unclear. Following absorption, nickel is transported in blood bound to serum albumin. Nickel is not significantly accumulated by any tissue in the body, although the thyroid and adrenal glands have relatively high nickel concentrations compared with other tissues. Most of the absorbed nickel is excreted by the kidney as low-molecular weight complexes. Nickel is also lost in sweat and bile.

INDICATIONS AND USAGE

There is no indication for the use of supplemental nickel.

RESEARCH SUMMARY

Though decreased levels of nickel have been reported in some conditions, there is no evidence that supplemental nickel is of any benefit in any of these conditions.

CONTRAINDICATIONS, PRECAUTIONS, ADVERSE REACTIONS

CONTRAINDICATIONS

None known.

PRECAUTIONS

Those with nickel-sensitivity should avoid nickel supplementation.

ADVERSE REACTIONS

None known.

DOSAGE AND ADMINISTRATION

No recommendation.

Nickel is available in some multivitamin preparations, typically at a dose of about 5 micrograms. Nickel may also be present in colloidal or liquid mineral supplements.

LITERATURE

Nielsen FH. Ultratrace minerals. In: Shils ME, Olson JA, Shike M, Ross AC, eds. *Modern Nutrition in Health and Disease.* 9th ed. Baltimore MD: Williams and Wilkins; 1999; 283-303.

Uthus EO, Poellot RA. Dietary nickel and folic acid interact to affect folate and methionine metabolism in the rat. *Biol Trace Elem Res.* 1997; 58:25-33.

Veien NK, Hattel T, Laurberg G. Low nickel diet: an open prospective trial. *J Am Acad Dermatol.* 1993; 29:1001-1007.

Nicotinamide

DESCRIPTION

Nicotinamide (niacinamide) is one of the two principal forms of the B-complex vitamin niacin (see Niacin). The term niacin is used as a collective term to refer to both nicotinamide and nicotinic acid, the other principal form of niacin, or the term is used synonymously with nicotinic acid. Nicotinamide and nicotinic acid have identical vitamin activities, but they have very different pharmacological activities.

Nicotinamide, via its major metabolite NAD+ (nicotinamide adenine dinucleotide), is involved in a wide range of biological processes, including the production of energy, the synthesis of fatty acids, cholesterol and steroids, signal transduction and the maintenance of the integrity of the genome. Nicotinic acid, in pharmacological doses, is used as an antihyperlipidemic agent. It also causes vasodilation of cutaneous blood vessels resulting in the so-called niacin flush. Nicotinamide in pharmacological doses does not have antihyperlipidemic activity, nor does it cause a niacin-flush. There is evidence, however, that pharmacological doses of nicotinamide may prevent type 1 diabetes mellitus. And, interestingly, pyrazinamide, an important drug in the treatment of tuberculosis, is an analogue of and shares the same biochemical mechanism with nicotinamide.

Nicotinamide, in addition to being known as niacinamide, is also known as 3-pyridinecarboxamide, pyridine-3-carboxamide, nicotinic acid amide, vitamin B_3 and vitamin PP. Its molecular formula is $C_6H_6N_2O$ and its molecular weight is 122.13 daltons and the structural formula is:

Nicotinamide

Nicotinamide is the principal form of niacin used in nutritional supplements and in food fortification. See also Niacin (Nicotinic Acid).

ACTIONS AND PHARMACOLOGY

ACTIONS

Nicotinamide may have anti-diabetogenic activity in some. It may also have antioxidant, anti-inflammatory and anticarcinogenic activities. Nicotinamide has putatitive activity against osteoarthritis and granuloma annulare.

MECHANISM OF ACTION

Nicotinamide is being investigated as an agent for the possible prevention or delaying of the onset of type 1 diabetes mellitus (insulin-dependent diabetes mellitus or IDDM). The rationale for using nicotinamide to prevent type 1 diabetes mellitus is derived from human and animal studies as well as *in vitro* investigations. Nicotinamide has been found to prevent diabetes in alloxan- and streptozotocin-treated mice and rats and in non-obese diabetic (NOD) mice. *In vitro* studies have shown that nicotinamide can prevent macrophage- or interleukin-1beta-induced beta-cell damage. An intervention study in New Zealand using nicotinamide treatment showed a 50% reduction in the development of IDDM over a five-year period.

The mechanism of the possible anti-diabetogenic activity of nicotinamide is not well understood. The pathogenesis of IDDM involves the autoimmune destruction of beta-cells, which is accompanied by the appearance of beta-cell specific antibodies, such as islet cell antibodies (ICA) and antibodies to glutamic acid decarboxylase (GAD), many years before the onset of the disease. Macrophages and T lymphocytes are the first cells to appear in the islets of the pancreas during the development of autoimmune diabetes. It is thought that cytokines released by macrophages/monocytes, such as interleukin (IL)-12 and tumor necrosis factor (TNF)-alpha, might play a role in early beta-cell damage. IL-12 may play a role in the initiation of the autoimmune process by enhancing T helper 1 lymphocyte (Th1) responses. Nicotinamide has been shown to decrease the production of IL-12 and TNF-alpha in cultures of whole blood from prediabetic and diabetic subjects and also in healthy controls. Inhibition of IL-12 production by nicotinamide could play an important role in the modulation of the immune response leading to IDDM. Further, since the cytokine-inhibitory activity was observed in healthy controls, as well as in prediabetic and diabetic subjects, nicotinamide may have application in other autoimmune disorders.

Nicotinamide has been demonstrated, in one study, to affect glucose tolerance and insulitis in NOD mice, slowing down diabetes progression. In this study, nicotinamide decreased MHC class II expression (but not MHC class I), enhanced intercellular adhesion molecule-1 (ICAM-1) expression, counteracted the fall of superoxide dismutase (observed in untreated NOD mice) and increased the levels of interleukin (IL)-4, a T helper 2 lymphocyte (Th2) protective cytokine.

The anti-diabetogenic effect of nicotinamide may be due, in part, to an increase in the pool size of NAD^+ in beta-cells. NAD^+ is the principal metabolite of nicotinamide. It appears that the pool size of NAD^+ in beta-cells in pre-diabetics and diabetics is significantly reduced. Damage and destruction of beta-cells may occur via oxidative stress. Increased levels of reactive oxygen species in beta-cells may result in, among other things, oxidative damage to DNA resulting in DNA strand breaks. The enzyme poly(ADP-ribose)polymerase or PARP is believed to play a role in DNA repair. PARP uses NAD^+ as its substrate. In the context of a reduced level of NAD^+, PARP activity may essentially use most of the cellular NAD^+. This could result in cellular apoptosis. Nicotinamide is an inhibitor of PARP. It also has antioxidant activity and, of course, is metabolized to NAD^+. All of these effects may play some role in the possible anti-diabetogenic action of nicotinamide.

Nicotinamide has been shown to have antioxidant activity. *In vitro*, it has been found to inhibit protein oxidation and lipid peroxidation. It has also been found to inhibit reactive oxygen species-induced apoptosis, to inhibit phagocytic generation of reactive oxygen species, to scavenge reactive oxygen species and to inhibit the oxidative activity of nitric oxide.

Nicotinamide has demonstrated a number of anti-inflammatory activities. Nicotinamide has been shown to inhibit lipopolysaccharide-induced TNF-alpha in the mouse, in a dose-dependent manner. It is thought that this inhibition of TNF-alpha is mediated via inhibition, at the gene transcription level, of NF-Kappa B, which in turn inhibits TNF-alpha. Nicotinamide has also been shown to decrease the production of IL-12 and TNF-alpha in cultures of whole blood from prediabetic and diabetic subjects and also in healthy subjects.

Niacin deficiency has been found to inhibit DNA repair in cell culture models. NAD+ is the substrate for PARP, an enzyme thought to be involved in DNA repair. Extensive damage to DNA may result in depletion of NAD+ secondary to its use by PARP. Depletion of NAD+ may trigger cellular apoptosis. DNA repair by PARP, as well as its possible role in apoptosis, may contribute to protection against carcinogenesis. These mechanisms may account, in part, for the possible anticarcinogenic activity of nicotinamide. Nicotinamide, via NAD+, modulates the expression of the p53 tumor suppressor protein in human breast, lung, skin and lung cells. This is another mechanism for nicotinamide's possible anticarcinogenic activity.

A pilot study suggests that nicotinamide may be beneficial in some with osteoarthritis. The mechanism of this putative activity is unknown. The mechanism of the putative activity of nicotinamide in granuloma annulare is also unknown.

PHARMACOKINETICS

Nicotinamide is efficiently absorbed from the gastrointestinal tract. At low doses, absorption is mediated via sodium-dependent facilitated diffusion. Passive diffusion is the principal mechanism of absorption at higher doses. Doses of up to three to four grams of nicotinamide are almost completely absorbed. Nicotinamide is transported via the portal circulation to the liver and via the systemic circulation to the various tissues of the body. Nicotinamide enters most cells by passive diffusion and enters erythrocytes by facilitated transport.

Nicotinamide is metabolized to NAD+ which in turn has a number of metabolic opportunities, including the formation of nicotinamide, NADP+ (nicotinamide adenine dinucleotide phosphate), NMN (nicotinamide 5'-mononucleotide), cyclic ADP-ribose and NAADP (nicotinic acid dinucleotide phosphate). NAD+ also serves as the substrate for mono(ADP-ribosyl)ation and poly(ADP-ribosyl)ation. Poly(ADP-ribosyl)ation is catalyzed by PARP. Nicotinamide may be converted to nicotinic acid via the enzyme nicotinamidase.

In the liver, the principal catabolic products of high-dose nicotinamide are N'-methylnicotinamide, N'-methyl-5-carboxamide-2-pyridone, N'-methyl-5-carboxamide-4-pyridone and nicotinamide-N-oxide. High-dose nicotinamide is ex-creted in the urine as unchanged nicotinamide, N'-methylnicotinamide, N'-methyl-5-carboxamide-2-pyridone, N'-methyl-5-carboxamide-4-pyridone and nicotinamide-N-oxide.

INDICATIONS AND USAGE

Nicotinamide, unlike nicotinic acid, does not have significant effects on lipids, but it has been shown to be useful in some with type 1 (insulin-dependent) diabetes. There is preliminary evidence it might help some with generalized granuloma annulare and osteoarthritis. There is little evidence that it is helpful in rheumatoid arthritis or schizophrenia. There is a suggestion that it might aid in some cancer therapies. There is little evidence that it is useful in tinnitus.

RESEARCH SUMMARY

Nicotinamide was shown to protect the non-obese diabetic (NOD) mouse from type 1 (IDDM) diabetes if given early enough and at high enough doses. Nicotinamide might similarly intervene in human type 1 diabetes as evidenced, among other things, by its observed ability to protect isolated islets of Langerhans *in vitro* from various toxic agents. *In vitro* experiments also showed that nicotinamide could reduce beta cell impairment and death caused by macrophages and exposure to various cytokines involved in this autoimmune disease.

Since nicotinamide has not been shown to have significant, prolonged effects when introduced after the onset of type 1 diabetes, its efficacy has been researched as an interventive therapy. It shows some ability to extend the remission phase when administered to subjects newly diagnosed with the disease. During the remission phase, the need for exogenous insulin is decreased or obliterated, but insulin-dependence reasserts itself, usually within one year despite nicotinamide supplementation. On the other hand, nicotinamide appears to be far more effective as a preventive.

In one 5-year intervention study, nicotinamide was administered prior to the clinical onset of IDDM. Using antibody markers that predict the onset of IDDM within 5 years, 150 young subjects were selected to receive nicotinamide at a dose of 1.2 grams per square meter of body surface area daily. It was concluded that nicotinamide supplementation reduced the expected incidence of IDDM 50% over a 5-year period. A much larger multi-center intervention study is now underway.

There is one recent single-blind, placebo-controlled study indicating that nicotinamide improves insulin secretion and metabolic control in lean type 2 diabetic patients with secondary failure to sulfonylureas. Followup is needed.

There is a case study showing pronounced improvement in a patient with generalized granuloma annulare treated with high-dose (1,500 milligrams daily) niacinamide for six months. This patient's disease had previously resisted treatment with topical adrenal steroids, oral erythromycin and oral zinc.

A recent double-blind, placebo-controlled, pilot study examined the effect of nicotinamide in subjects with osteoarthritis. In the study, 72 subjects with osteoarthritis were randomly assigned to receive nicotinamide (500 milligrams six times per day) or placebo. The study lasted 12 weeks. Subjects who received nicotinamide reduced their non-steroidal anti-inflammatory (NSAID) medication by 13% compared with those in the placebo group. Pain levels were no different in the two groups. Nicotinamide reduced the sedimentation rate by 22% and increased joint mobility by 22% over controls. Followup is needed.

Some preliminary evidence suggests that nicotinamide may increase the irradiation response of experimental tumors. More research is needed in this area.

Nicotinamide produced effects no better than placebo when used in a double-blind trial involving 48 subjects with tinnitus.

CONTRAINDICATIONS, PRECAUTIONS, ADVERSE REACTIONS
CONTRAINDICATIONS
Nicotinamide is contraindicated in those hypersensitive to any component of a nicotinamide-containing preparation.

High-dose nicotinamide (doses greater than 500 milligrams/day) is contraindicated in those with liver disease and in those with active peptic ulcer disease.

PRECAUTIONS
Pregnant women and nursing mothers should avoid supplemental doses of nicotinamide greater than the U.S. RDA (20 milligrams/day), unless higher doses are prescribed by their physicians.

The use of nicotinamide for any medical indication requires medical supervision.

Those with a history of peptic ulcer disease, gastritis, liver disease, gallbladder disease, diabetes and gout, should exercise caution in the use of high-dose nicotinamide.

ADVERSE REACTIONS
In contrast to nicotinic acid, nicotinamide does not cause flushing and has only very rarely been associated with diabetogenic effects. There are rare reports of elevations in liver tests and liver damage, including jaundice and parenchymal liver cell injury. These reports were in those using very high doses of nicotinamide (10 grams or greater, daily).

Adverse reactions in those using high-dose nicotinamide, include nausea, vomiting, diarrhea, headache and dizziness.

INTERACTIONS
DRUGS
Carbamazepine: Concomitant use of nicotinamide and carbamazepine may decrease carbamazepine clearance.

OVERDOSAGE
Nicotinamide overdosage is not reported in the literature.

DOSAGE AND ADMINISTRATION
Nicotinamide is the form of niacin which is typically used for nutritional supplementation. It is also the form of niacin used in food fortification. It is available as a single ingredient product (immediate-release and sustained-release) and in multivitamin and multivitamin/multimineral products. Typical supplemental dosage ranges from 20 to 100 milligrams daily. Pre- and postnatal vitamin/mineral supplements typically deliver a dose of 20 milligrams daily.

HOW SUPPLIED
Capsules — 100 mg, 250 mg, 500 mg, 550 mg

Tablets — 100 mg, 250 mg, 500 mg

Tablets, Extended Release — 1000 mg, 1500 mg

LITERATURE
Akabane A, Kato I, Takasawa S, et al. Nicotinamide inhibits IRF-1mRNA induction and prevents IL-1 beta-induced nitric oxide synthase expression in pancreatic beta cells. *Biochem Biophys Res Commun.* 1995; 215:524-530.

Behme MT. Nicotinamide and diabetes prevention. *Nutr Rev.* 1995; 53:137-139.

Boyonoski AC, Gallacher LM, ApSimon MM, et al. Niacin deficiency increases the sensitivity of rats to the short and long term effects of ethylnitrosourea treatment. *Mol Cellular Biochem.* 1999; 193:83-87.

Chaplin DJ, Horsman MR, Trotter MJ. Effect of nicotinamide on the microregional hetereogeneity of oxygen delivery within a murine tumor. *J Natl Cancer Inst.* 1990; 82:672-676.

Crowley CL, Payne CM, Bernstein H, et al. The NAD+ precursors, nicotinic acid and nicotinamide protect cells against apoptosis induced by a multiple stress inducer, deoxycholate. *Cell Death Differ.* 2000; 7:314-326.

Elliott RB, Pilcher CC, Stewart A, et al. The use of nicotinamide in the prevention of type 1 diabetes. *Ann NY Acad Sci.* 1993; 696:333-341.

Gale EA. Molecular mechanisms of beta-cell destruction in IDDM: the role of nicotinamide. *Horm Res.* 1996; 45 Suppl1:39-43.

Greenbaum CJ, Kahn SE, Palmer JP. Nicotinamide's effect on glucose metabolism in subjects at risk for IDDM. *Diabetes.* 1996; 45:1631-1634.

Hiromatsu Y, Yang D, Miyake I, et al. Nicotinamide decreases cytokine-induced activation of orbital fibroblasts from patients with thyroid-associated ophthalmopathy. *J Clin Endocrinol Metab.* 1998; 83:121-124.

Hoorens A, Pipeleers D. Nicotinamide protects human beta cells against chemically-induced necrosis, but not against cytokine-induced apoptosis. *Diabetologia.* 1999; 42:55-59.

Jacobson EL, Shieh WM, Huang AC. Mapping the role of NAD metabolism in prevention and treatment of carcinogenesis. *Mol Cellular Biochem.* 1999; 193:69-74.

Jonas WB, Rapoza CP, Blair WF. The effect of niacinamide on osteoarthritis: a pilot study. *Inflamm Res.* 1996; 45:330-334.

Kamat JP, Devasagayam TP. Nicotinamide (vitamin B$_3$) as an effective antioxidant against oxidative damage in rat brain mitochondria. *Redox Rep.* 1999; 4:179-184.

Klaidman LK, Mukherjee SK, Hutchin TP, Adams JD. Nicotinamide as a precursor for NAD$^+$ prevents apoptosis in the mouse brain induced by tertiary-butylhydroperoxide. *Neurosci Lett.* 1996; 206:5-8.

Kolb H, Burkart V. Nicotinamide in type 1 diabetes. Mechanism of action revisited. *Diabetes Care.* 1999; 22 Supp 2:B16-B20.

Kretowski A, My liwiec J, Szelachowaska M, et al. Nicotinamide inhibits enhanced *in vitro* production of interleukin-12 and tumor necrosis factor-alpha in peripheral whole blood of people at high risk of developing Type 1 diabetes and people with newly diagnosed Type 1 diabetes. *Diabetes Res Clin Pract.* 2000; 47:81-86.

Kroger H, Hauschild A, Ohde M, et al. Nicotinamide and methionine reduce the liver toxic effect of methotrexate. *Gen Pharmacol.* 1999; 33:203-206.

Lewis CM, Canafax DM, Sprafka JM, Barbosa JJ. Double-blind randomized trial of nicotinamide on early-onset diabetes. *Diabetes Care.* 1992; 15:121-123.

Ma A, *Medenica* M. Response of generalized granuloma annulare to high-dose niacinamide. *Arch Dermatol.* 1983; 119:836-839.

McCarty MF, Russell AL. Niacinamide therapy for osteoarthritis—does it inhibit nitric oxide synthase induction by interleukin 1 in chondrocytes? *Med Hypotheses.* 1999; 53:350-360.

Melo SS, Arantes MR, Meirelles MS, et al. Lipid peroxidation in nicotinamide-deficient and nicotinamide-supplemented rats with streptozotocin-induced diabetes. *Acta Diabetol.* 2000; 37:33-39.

Miesel R, Kurpisz M, Kroger H. Modulation of inflammatory arthritis by inhibition of poly(ADPribose)polymerase. *Inflammation.* 1995; 19:379-387.

Olsson AR, Sheng Y, Pero RW, et al. DNA damage and repair in tumour and non-tumour tissues. *Br J Cancer.* 1996; 74:368-373.

Papaccio G, Ammendola E, Pisanti FA. Nicotinamide decreases MHC class II but not MHC class I expression and increases intercellular adhesion molecule-1 structures in non-obese diabetic mouse pancreas. *J Endocrinol.* 1999; 160:389-400.

Pero RW, Axelsson B, Siemann D, et al. Newly discovered anti-inflammatory properties of the benzamides and nicotinamides. *Mol Cellular Biochem.* 1999; 193:119-125.

Petley A, Macklin B, Renwick AG, Wilkin TJ. The pharmacokinetics of nicotinamide in humans and rodents. *Diabetes.* 1995; 44:152-155.

Polo V, Saibene A, Portiroli AE. Nicotinamide improves insulin secretion and metabolic control in lean type 2 diabetic patients with secondary failure to sulphonylureas. *Acta Diabetol.* 1998; 35:61-64.

Pozzilli P, Browne PD, Kolb H. Meta-analysis of nicotinamide treatment in patients with recent-onset IDDM. The Nicotinamide Trialists. *Diabetes Care.* 1996; 19:1357-1363.

Vidal J, Fernandez-Balsells M, Sesmilo G, et al. Effects of nicotinamide and intravenous insulin therapy in newly diagnosed type 1 diabetes. *Diabetes Care.* 2000; 23:360-364.

Wan FJ, Lin HC, Kang BH, et al. D-amphetamine-induced depletion of energy and dopamine in the rat striatum is attenuated by nicotinamide pretreatment. *Brain Res Bull.* 1999; 50:167-191.

Zimhony O, Cox JS, Welch JT, et al. Pyrazinamide inhibits the eukaryotic-like fatty acid synthetase I (FASI) of *Mycobacterium tuberculosis. Nature Med.* 2000; 6:1043-1047.

Nucleic Acids/Nucleotides

TRADE NAMES

R.N.A.-180 (The Key Company), RNA/DNA (Synergy Plus), DNA Boost Colloidal (Etherium Technology).

DESCRIPTION

DNA (deoxyribonucleic acid), the molecule that comprises the genome, and RNA (ribonucleic acid) are marketed as nutritional supplements. DNA, which makes up the genetic material, is comprised of units called nucleotides. A nucleotide consists of a base, a sugar and a phosphate group. The major bases in DNA are the purines adenine and guanine and the pyrimidines cytosine and thymine. The sugar moiety of the nucleotide is 2'-deoxyribose. RNA, which is more abundant in tissues than DNA by about an order of magnitude, is also comprised of nucleotide units. In the case of RNA, the major bases are again the purines adenine and guanine, and the pyrimidines are cytosine and uracil. One of the major differences between DNA and RNA is the presence of uracil in RNA and of thymine in DNA. The other major difference is in the sugar moiety. In RNA, the sugar moiety of the nucleotide is ribose, whereas in DNA it is deoxyribose.

For years, nucleic acids and nucleotides were not considered essential nutrients. It was thought that the body can synthesize sufficient nucleotides to meet its physiological demands via *de novo* nucleotide synthetic pathways. Some research during the last several years indicates that this may not be completely correct. There are certain conditions in which the body requires dietary nucleic acids/nucleotides to meet its physiological requirements. These conditions include rapid growth, limited food supply and metabolic stress. Under these conditions, metabolic demand exceeds the capacity of *de novo* synthesis. Under these conditions, dietary nucleosides, nucleotides and nucleic acids become conditionally essential nutrients. Dietary nucleotides may spare the energetic cost of *de novo* synthesis of nucleotides.

Dietary nucleic acids are found in plant and animal foods. The dietary intake of RNA is typically about an order of magnitude greater than DNA. The nucleotide salts disodium inosinate and disodium guanylate are present in many food products as seasoning substances, contributing to the dietary nucleotide intake. Interestingly, mother's milk is a rich source of nucleic acids, especially RNA, and nucleotides. There are a few medical foods and enteral supplements containing RNA and nucleotides, which are used for immune-enhancement under conditions of metabolic stress. RNA and nucleotides are sometimes referred to as immuno-nutrients. Nutritional supplements of RNA, DNA, nucleotides, nucleosides and bases are also being marketed.

ACTIONS AND PHARMACOLOGY

ACTIONS

Nucleic acids and nucleotides may have immune-enhancing and tissue-regenerating activities.

MECHANISM OF ACTION

Nucleotides have been demonstrated to affect a number of immune functions, including reversing malnutrition and starvation-induced immunosuppression, enhancing T-cell maturation and function, enhancing natural killer cell activity, improving delayed cutaneous hypersensitivity, aiding in resistance to such infectious agents as *Staphylococcus aureus* and *Candida albicans,* and modulating T-cell responses toward type 1 CD4 helper lymphocytes or Th1 cells. Mice fed a nucleotide-free diet have both impaired cellular and humoral immune responses. Addition of dietary nucleotides restores both types of responses. Both RNA, which can be considered a delivery form of nucleotides, and ribonucleotides were used in these studies. The mechanism of the immune-enhancing activity of nucleic acids/nucleotides is unclear.

RNA and nucleotides have been shown to have stimulatory effects on recovery from hepatectomy in animals. They have also been shown to stimulate intestinal repair, in animals. The mechanism of the tissue-regenerating effects of RNA and nucleotides is unclear. Possibly the regenerating activity may be explained, in part, by the nucleotides serving as precursors of nucleic acid synthesis via the salvage pathways of nucleotide synthesis. Utilization of the salvage pathways may spare the energetic cost of *de novo* nucleotide synthesis.

PHARMACOKINETICS

RNA is digested in the small intestine via the action of the pancreatic enzyme ribonuclease to the nucleotides adenosine-5' -monophosphate (AMP), guanosine-5'-monophosphate (GMP), cytidine-5' -monophosphate (CMP) and uridine-5'-monophosphate (UMP). These nucleotides are then hydrolyzed to the nucleosides adenosine, guanosine, cytidine and uridine, respectively, via the action of the enzymes alkaline phosphatase and nucleotidase. The nucleosides may be further hydrolyzed to the purine bases adenine and guanine and the pyrimidine bases cytosine and uracil.

The nucleosides are transported in the enterocytes by both facilitated diffusion and sodium-dependent carrier mediated processes. Under normal conditions, that is, under conditions where the body is not under metabolic stress, the nucleosides undergo extensive catabolism in the enterocytes. The end product of purine catabolism is uric acid. An end product of pyrimidine metabolism is beta-alanine. Nucleosides and bases that are not catabolized in the enterocytes are transported via the portal circulation to the liver, where they are also catabolized. A small percentage of ingested RNA and nucleotides reach the systemic circulation and is transported to various tissues of the body.

Even under normal conditions, a small percentage (from 2% to 5%) of dietary RNA and dietary nucleotides is incorporated into nucleic acids, especially in the small intestine, liver and skeletal muscle. This occurs via the salvage pathways of purine nucleotide and pyrimidine nucleotide synthesis. During conditions of metabolic stress, including trauma, rapid growth and limited food supply, there is apparently greater conversion of dietary RNA and nucleotides into tissue nucleotides and nucleic acids.

DNA is digested in the small intestine via the action of the pancreatic enzyme deoxyribonuclease to deoxynucleotides; these, in turn, are hydrolyzed to deoxynucleosides and finally to the pyrimidine bases cytosine and thymine and the purine bases adenine and guanine. The deoxynucleosides and bases are absorbed by the enterocytes and processed as described above for the nucleosides.

INDICATIONS AND USAGE

The nucleotides appear to be effective in boosting immune response in some circumstances. They may also promote tissue repair in some conditions. Claims that they are an effective treatment for Alzheimer's disease, depression, skin disorders, sexual dysfunction, fatigue and aging are unsubstantiated.

RESEARCH SUMMARY

Numerous studies have shown that nucleotides can help restore immune function in malnourished animals, can enhance the activity of T-cells and natural killer cells, and can increase resistance to some pathogenic agents. Infants fed formulas supplemented with nucleotides had a lower incidence of diarrhea, higher natural killer cell activity and higher antibody titers following *Haemophilus influenzae* type b vaccination, compared with unsupplemented controls. In another study, post-operative immune response, evidenced by several measures, was enhanced in patients with upper-gastrointestinal cancer who were given supplements of RNA, arginine and omega-3 fatty acids.

Nucleosides have promoted tissue repair in a number of animal studies. They have shortened recovery time in animals with liver injury and have enhanced healing of experimental intestinal ulcers. They have shortened recovery time following small and large bowel injuries.

CONTRAINDICATIONS, PRECUATIONS, ADVERSE REACTIONS

CONTRAINDICATIONS

Supplemental RNA, DNA, nucleotides and nucleosides are contraindicated in those hypersensitive to any component of products containing these substances.

PRECAUTIONS

Pregnant women and nursing mothers should avoid nucleic acid and nucleotide supplements unless recommended by their physicians.

Those with a history of hyperuricemia should be extremely cautious about use of nucleic acid and nucleotide supplements.

ADVERSE REACTIONS

No reports of adverse reactions.

DOSAGE AND ADMINISTRATION

Medical foods are available containing RNA as a delivery form of nucleotides/nucleosides, sometimes along with L-arginine and fish oils. These medical foods are used to support the immune system under conditions of metabolic stress.

RNA and DNA nutritional supplements are available, with RNA supplements being more popular. Typical doses range from 0.5 to 1.5 grams daily.

Brewer's yeast is a rich source of RNA (see Brewer's Yeast). Inosine is a nucleoside (see Inosine).

HOW SUPPLIED

RNA products are supplied as follows:

Tablets — 180 mg

DNA products are available as follows:

Liquid

Tablets

LITERATURE

Adjei AA, Yamamoto S. A dietary nucleoside-nucleotide mixture ihibits endotoxin-induced bacterial translocation in mice fed protein-free diet. *J Nutr.* 1995; 125:42-48.

Carver JD. Dietary nucleotides: effects on the immune and gastrointestinal systems. *Acta Paediatr Suppl.* 1999; 88:83-88.

Carver JD, Cox WI, Barness LA. Dietary nucleotide effects upon murine natural killer cell activity and macrophage activation. *J Parenter Enteral Nutr.* 1990; 14:18-22.

Carver JD, Walker A. The role of nucleotides in human nutrition. *Nutr Biochem.* 1995; 6:58-72.

De Jong JW, Vander Meer P, Owen P, Opie LH. Prevention and treatment of ischemic injury with nucleosides. *Bratisl Lek Listy.* 1991; 92(3-4):165-173.

Fanslow WC, Kulkarni AD, Van Buren CT, Rudolph FB. Effect of nucleotide restriction and supplementation of resistance to experimental murine candidiasis. *J Parenter Enteral Nutr.* 1988; 12:49-52.

Frank BS. *Nucleic Acid and Antioxidant Therapy of Aging and Degeneration.* New York, NT: Rainstone Publishing; 1977.

Grimble GK. Dietary nucleotides and gut mucosal defense. *Gut.* 1994; 35(Suppl 1):S46-S51.

Jackson CD, Weis C, Miller BJ, et al. Comparison of cell proliferation following partial hepatectomy in rats fed NIH-31 or semipurified AIN-76A diets: effects of nucleic acid supplementation. *Nutr Res.* 1995; 15:1487-1495.

Jyonouchi H, Sun S, Abiru T, et al. Dietary nucleotides modulate antigen-specific type 1 and type 2 T-cell responses in young C57BL/6 mice. *Nutrition.* 2000; 16:442-446.

Leach JL, Baxter JH, Molitor BE, et al. Total potentially available nucleosides of human milk by stage of lactation. *Am J Clin Nutr.* 1995; 61:1224-1230.

Pickering LK, Granoff DM, Erickson JR, et al. Modulation of the immune system by human milk and infant formula containing nucleotides. *Pediatrics.* 1998; 101:242-249.

Rudoph FB, Kulkarni AD, Fanslow WC, et al. Role of RNA as a dietary source of pyrimidines and purines in immune function. *Nutr.* 1990; 6:45-52.

Torres-Lopé z MI, Fernandez I, Fontana L, et al. Influence of dietary nucleotides on liver structural recovery and hepatocyte binuclearity in cirrhosis induced by thioacetamide. *Gut.* 1996; 38:260-264.

Tsujinaka T, Kishibuchi M, Iijima S, et al. Nucleotides and intestine. *J Parenter Enteral Nutr.* 1999; 23:S74-S77.

Yu VY. The role of dietary nucleotides in neonatal and infant nutrition. *Singapore Med J.* 1998; 39:145-150.

Oat Beta-D-Glucan

TRADE NAMES
PC Oat Beta Glucan (Schiff), NSC-24 Immune Enhancer (Nutritional Supply Corp.), Maitake Bio-Beta-Glucan (Nature's Answer).

DESCRIPTION
In 1998, the Food and Drug Administration (FDA) issued its final rule allowing health claims to be made on the labels of foods containing soluble fiber from whole oats (oat bran, oat flour and rolled oats), noting that these foods, in conjunction with a diet low in saturated fat and cholesterol, may reduce the risk of heart disease. In order to qualify for the health claim, the whole oat-containing food must provide at least 0.75 grams of soluble fiber per serving. The soluble fiber in whole oats comprises a class of polysaccharides known as beta-D-glucans.

Beta-D-glucans, usually referred to as beta-glucans, comprise a class of non-digestible polysaccharides widely found in nature in such sources as oats, barley, yeast, bacteria, algae and mushrooms.

Beta-glucans are located primarily in the cell walls. In oats, barley and other cereal grains, they are located primarily in the endosperm cell wall.

Oat beta-glucan is a soluble fiber. It is a viscous polysaccharide made up of units of the sugar D-glucose. Oat beta-glucan is comprised of mixed-linkage polysaccharides. This means that the bonds between the D-glucose or D-glucopyranosyl units are either beta-1, 3 linkages or beta-1, 4 linkages. This type of beta-glucan is also referred to as a mixed-linkage $(1\rightarrow3)$, $(1\rightarrow4)$-beta-D-glucan. Most of the oat bran beta-glucan molecules consist of cellotriose and cellotetraose blocks separated by $(1\rightarrow3)$-linkages. There is, however, a smaller amount of sequences of $(1\rightarrow4)$-linkages longer than the tetraose type. The $(1\rightarrow3)$-linkages break up the uniform structure of the beta-D-glucan molecule and make it soluble and flexible. In comparison, the nondigestible polysaccharide cellulose is also a beta-glucan but is non-soluble. The reason that it is non-soluble is that cellulose consists only of $(1\rightarrow4)$-beta-D-linkages. The percentages of beta-glucan in the various whole oat products are: oat bran, greater than 5.5%; rolled oats, about 4%; whole oat flour about 4%.

ACTIONS AND PHARMACOLOGY
ACTIONS
Oat beta-glucan may have hypocholesterolemic and glucose-regulating activity. It also has putative immunomodulatory activity.

MECHANISM OF ACTION
The exact mechanism of oat beta-glucan's possible hypocholesterolemic effect is not clear. Oat beta-glucan does not appear to have any effect on the biosynthesis of cholesterol. It appears to promote increased excretion of bile acids, which could explain, in large part, its possible cholesterol-lowering activity. Oat beta-glucan may also promote cholesterol clearance from the plasma via reverse cholesterol transport.

The mechanism of the possible glucose-regulatory activity of oat beta-glucan is also not well understood. Oat beta-glucan may delay gastric emptying time and consequently affect the rate of uptake of D-glucose from the small intestine. This may be one possible mechanism; the high viscosity of oat beta-glucan may delay absorption of glucose, which may be another possible mechanism. Oat beta-glucan has been found to have immunomodulatory activity in tissue culture and in mice. It appears to activate macrophages to release certain cytokines. Such activity, in mice, has been found to be protective against bacterial infection. It is unclear whether oat beta-glucan has immunomodulatory activity in humans.

PHARMACOKINETICS
Following ingestion, there is virtually no digestion of oat beta-glucan in the small intestine. Some digestion of oat beta-glucan does take place in the large intestine via bacterial beta-glucosidases. Some smaller oligosaccharides produced by the bacterial transformation of oat beta-glucan may get absorbed, but this is unclear. A large percentage of the ingested beta-glucan is excreted in the feces.

INDICATIONS AND USAGE
Oat beta-glucan has hypocholesterolemic effects and may also favorably affect some other lipids. It has demonstrated some immune-enhancing effects and may be helpful in some with diabetes.

RESEARCH SUMMARY
Evidence that oat beta-glucan can reduce cholesterol levels was sufficient to induce the FDA to allow health claims on whole oat products that provide at least 0.75 grams of soluble fiber per serving. The allowed health claim is that these products reduce the risk of heart disease by reducing levels of cholesterol.

In one study, mildly hypercholesterolemic subjects on a "typical" diet, in which 35% of calories was derived from fat, were given an oat beta-glucan extract containing 1% or 10% oat beta-glucan. There was a significant reduction in total cholesterol levels in those receiving the 10% oat beta-glucan preparation after three weeks. Cholesterol levels declined significantly in the 1% group, as well, but not as quickly. There was also a significant decline in LDL-cholesterol levels in both groups. Triglyceride and HDL-cholesterol levels were not significantly changed. Some other studies have reported similar results.

Improved glucose and insulin responses have been reported in a study of moderately hypercholesterolemic healthy subjects. Oat extracts containing 1% and 10% beta-glucan both demonstrated these beneficial effects on glucose tolerance factors.

NIDDM patients given varying concentrations of oat beta-glucan also had significantly improved glucose and insulin responses. Higher doses of the oat beta-glucan correlated with greater improvement.

There are *in vitro* and animal studies demonstrating that oat beta-glucan, like those extracted from yeast and other fungi, has favorable immunomodulatory activities. These include the ability to activate macrophages and stimulate their release of interleukin (IL)-1 and tumor necrosis factor (TNF)-alpha, among other activities

Intraperitoneal administration of oat beta-glucan has enhanced a non-specific resistance to bacterial challenge in mice. Survival times have been improved in mice pre-treated with oat beta-glucan and then challenged with *Staphylococcus aureus*. Similarly, resistance to *Eimeria vermiformis* has been significantly increased in immunosuppressed mice given oat beta-glucan intragastrically or parenterally.

CONTRAINDICATIONS, PRECAUTIONS, ADVERSE REACTIONS

CONTRAINDICATIONS
None known.

PRECAUTIONS
None known.

ADVERSE REACTIONS
Oat beta-glucans are generally well tolerated. Occasional flatulence is reported.

OVERDOSAGE
There are no reports of overdosage.

DOSAGE AND ADMINISTRATION
Dosage of oat beta-glucan required for a possible hypocholesterolemic effect ranges from 3 to 6 grams daily. This can be obtained from a whole oat product. There is some marketed oat beta-glucan nutritional supplements.

HOW SUPPLIED
Oat bran products are supplied as follows:

Chewable Tablet — 500 mg

Tablets — 500 mg, 850 mg, 1000 mg

Oat beta-glucan products are supplied as follows:

Capsules — 2.5 mg, 5 mg, 7.5 mg, 10 mg, 20 mg

LITERATURE

Anderson JW, Gustafson NJ. Hypocholesterolemic effects of oat and bean products. *Am J Clin Nutr.* 1988; 48:749-753.

Anderson JW, Story L, Sieling B, et al. Hypocholesterolemic effects of oat-bran or bean intake for hypercholesterolemic men. *Am J Clin Nutr.* 1984; 40:1146-1155.

Behall KM, Scholfield DJ, Hallfrisch J. Effect of beta-glucan level in oat fiber extracts on blood lipids in men and women. *J Am Coll Nutr.* 1997; 16:46-51.

Bell S, Goldman VM, Bistrian BR, et al. Effect of beta-glucan from oats and yeast on serum lipids. *Crit Rev Food Sci Nutr.* 1999; 39:189-202.

Braaten JT, Wood PJ, Scott FW, et al. Oat beta-glucan reduces blood cholesterol concentration in hypercholesterolemic subjects. *Eur J Clin Nutr.* 1994; 48:465-474.

Davidson MH, Dugan LD, Burns JH, et al. The hypocholesterolemic effects of beta-glucan in oatmeal and oat bran. A dose-controlled study. *JAMA.* 1991; 265:1833-1839.

Estrada A, Yun CH, Van Kessel A, et al. Immunomodulatory activities of oat beta-glucan in vitro and in vivo. *Microbiol Immunol.* 1997; 41:991-998.

Food and Drug Administration. Food labeling: health claims; soluble fiber from certain foods and coronary heart disease: final rule 21 CFR Part 101. *Federal Reg.* Feb 18,1998; 63(32): 8103.

Hallfrisch J, Scholfield DJ, Behall KM. Diets containing soluble oat extracts improve glucose and insulin responses of moderately hypercholesterolemic men and women. *Am J Clin Nutr.* 1995; 61:379-384.

Johansson L, Virkki L, Maunu S, et al. Structural characterization of water soluble beta-glucan of oat bran. *Carbohydrate Polymers.* 2000; 42:143-148.

Lia A, Andersson H, Mekki N, et al. Postprandial lipemia in relation to sterol and fat excretion in ileostomy subjects given oat-bran and wheat test meals. *Am J Clin Nutr.* 1997; 66:357-365.

Lia A, Hallmans G, Sandberg AS, et al. Oat beta-glucan increases bile acid excretion and a fiber-rich barley fraction increases cholesterol excretion in ileostomy subjects. *Am Clin Nutr J.* 1995; 62:1245-1251.

Wood PJ, Braaten JT, Scott FW, et al. Effect of dose and modifications of viscous properties of oat gum on plasma glucose and insulin following an oral glucose load. *Br J Nutr.* 1994; 72:731-743.

Octacosanol

TRADE NAMES
Octacosanol is available from numerous manufacturers generically. Branded products include Enduraplex (Nutrilabs), Prometabs (Viobin) and Prometol (Viobin).

DESCRIPTION

Octacosanol is a 28 carbon long-chain saturated primary alcohol. It is a constituent of vegetable waxes. Octacosanol is isolated from the wax found on green blades of wheat. It is the major long-chain alcohol isolated from the waxes of sugar cane and yams. It is also found in wheat germ oil.

Octacosanol is also known as l-octacosanol, n-octacosanol and octacosyl alcohol. It has the following chemical formula:

$$CH_3(CH_2)_{26}CH_2OH$$

Octacosanol (1-Octacosanol)

Octacosanol is a solid waxy substance that is insoluble in water. Octacosanol belongs to the family of fatty alcohols.

ACTIONS AND PHARMACOLOGY

ACTIONS

The action of octacosanol is unknown. It is the major long-chain alcohol in policosanol (see Policosanol), and policosanol appears to lower cholesterol and LDL-cholesterol levels. However, the role of octacosanol in the putative cholesterol-lowering activity of policosanol is unclear.

PHARMACOKINETICS

The absorption of octacosanol is variable and low. Octacosanol absorption, following ingestion, ranges from about 11% in rats and humans to about 28% in rabbits. Less octacosanol is absorbed on an empty stomach and more with food. The higher the lipid content of food, the greater the absorption. Octacosanol is absorbed from the small intestine into the lymph and from there enters the bloodstream. Distribution is mainly to the liver, digestive tract, skeletal muscle and adipose tissue. Octacosanol may be partly oxidized to the long-chain fatty acid, octacosanoic acid, which then undergoes beta-oxidation.

Following a single dose of octacosanol in experimental animals, peak plasma levels are observed between 30 minutes to two hours. Following a single dose of octacosanol in human volunteers, peak plasma levels are observed at one hour and four hours later. Bile is the main route of excretion. Renal excretion is negligible.

INDICATIONS AND USAGE

Octacosanol, like policosanol (see Policosanol), may have cholesterol-lowering effects but research will have to be done to confirm this. Similarly, there is preliminary evidence suggesting that octacosanol may increase physical endurance and that it may benefit some with Parkinson's disease. Octacosanol is not indicated for use in amyotrophic lateral sclerosis despite some claims of efficacy in this disorder.

RESEARCH SUMMARY

There is limited evidence that octacosanol itself may lower cholesterol levels. This needs to be researched. (See Policosanol.) There are claims that octacosanol is useful in building strength and endurance, and these claims have made the supplement popular with some body builders and athletes. There is preliminary evidence, limited to animal experiments, that octacosanol may increase voluntary exercise in the animals.

Evidence that octacosanol may help in the treatment of Parkinson's disease is very preliminary, and the use of this substance in a well-designed study of those suffering from amyotrophic lateral sclerosis showed no benefit. Neither neurologic nor pulmonary functions were improved.

CONTRAINDICATIONS, PRECAUTIONS, ADVERSE REACTIONS

CONTRAINDICATIONS

None known.

PRECAUTIONS

Octacosanol is not recommended for children, pregnant women and nursing mothers. Parkinson's disease patients taking carbidopa-levodopa may experience side effects (see Adverse Reactions).

ADVERSE REACTIONS

Side effects of octacosanol taken up to 20 milligrams daily are infrequent. Mild position-related nonrotational dizziness, increased nervous tension and worsening of carbidopa-levodopa-related dyskinesias have been reported in a few Parkinson's disease patients taking octacosanol.

INTERACTIONS

Carbidopa-levodopa: Octacosanol has been reported to worsen dyskinesias in a few Parkinson's disease patients taking carbidopa-levodopa.

No other nutritional supplement, herb or food interactions are known.

OVERDOSAGE

There are no reports of overdosage.

DOSAGE AND ADMINISTRATION

Typical doses used are 1 to 8 milligrams (1,000 to 8,000 micrograms) daily taken with food. A dose of 20 milligrams daily should not be exceeded. Octacosanol frequently comes in mixtures with other long-chain alcohols.

HOW SUPPLIED

Capsules — 2000 mcg, 8000 mcg, 20,000 mcg

Tablets — 1000 mcg, 2000 mcg, 5000 mcg

LITERATURE

Kabir Y, Kimura S. Distribution of radioactive octacosanol in response to exercise in rats. *Nahrung.* 1994; 38:373-377.

Kato S, Hasegawa S, Nagasawa J, et al. Octacosanol affects lipid metabolism in rats fed on a high-fat diet. *Br J Nutr.* 1995; 73:433-441.

Norris FH, Denys EH, Fallat RJ. Trial of octacosanol in amyotrophic lateral sclerosis. *Neurol.* 1986; 36:1263-1264.

Snider SR. Octacosanol in Parkinsonism. *Ann Neurol.* 1984; 16:723.

Ornithine Alpha-Ketoglutarate

DESCRIPTION

Ornithine alpha-ketoglutarate, abbreviated OKG, also known as ornithine 2-oxoglutarate or ornithine oxoglutarate (OGO), is a salt formed of two molecules of the non-protein amino acid, L-ornithine, and one molecule of the Krebs cycle dicarboxylic acid, alpha-ketoglutarate. OKG has been used both enterally and parenterally in burn, trauma, surgical and chronically malnourished patients. It appears to decrease protein catabolism and/or increase protein synthesis under these conditions. OKG is a popular nutritional supplement for athletes, among others.

ACTIONS AND PHARMACOLOGY

ACTIONS

OKG, under certain conditions, may have immunomodulatory and anticatabolic and/or anabolic actions. OKG is a delivery form of L-glutamine and L-arginine precursors.

MECHANISM OF ACTION

The actions of OKG can be attributed to the metabolites that the OKG components, L-ornithine and alpha-ketoglutarate, give rise to. These metabolites are L-arginine, L-glutamine, L-proline and polyamines. The metabolism of L-glutamine and L-arginine is altered in trauma, and this alteration is linked to immune dysfunction.

One of the major biochemical events that occurs following a burn injury is a fall in intramuscular L-glutamine. This amino acid is released from muscle tissue to meet the increased needs of other cells, in particular immune cells and intestinal cells. L-glutamine is now known to be essential for sustaining the proliferation and activation of immune cells. In the intestine it is essential for maintaining the integrity of the mucosal barrier and its metabolic and immune function. Immune and gastrointestinal dysfunctions occur when *de novo* L-glutamine synthesis is insufficient to maintain normal function of immune cells and enterocytes. Under these conditions, for example a burn injury, the normally non-essential (meaning the body can make it) L-glutamine becomes a conditionally essential amino acid (meaning the body can't make enough of it). OKG is a delivery form of L-glutamine.

L-arginine is also essential for immune cells. It is thought that the role of L-arginine in immunity is mediated by its metabolite nitric oxide. Burn injury and some other traumas affect the status of both L-glutamine and L-arginine in the various tissues of the body, especially muscle, the immune system and the gastrointestinal tract. As in the case of L-glutamine, *de novo* synthesis of L-arginine during these conditions is probably not sufficient for normal immune and gastrointestinal function, nor for normal protein synthesis. OKG, in addition to being a delivery form of L-glutamine, is also a delivery form of L-arginine or more precisely L-ornithine, which is converted to L-arginine.

It is unclear if OKG has immunomodulatory or anticatabolic/ anabolic actions under normal conditions.

See L-Glutamine and L-Arginine.

PHARMACOKINETICS

Following ingestion, OKG is absorbed from the small intestine from whence it is transported to the liver. In the liver, OKG enters various metabolic pathways. L-ornithine is a precursor in the synthesis of L-arginine and polyamines, among others. Alpha-ketoglutarate is metabolized to L-glutamine, among other molecules. OKG not metabolized by the liver is transported via the systemic circulation and distributed to various tissues of the body, including the brain, where it undergoes metabolic reactions similar to those above. Under conditions of trauma or burn injury, OKG may be metabolized in immune cells, enterocytes and muscle tissue to produce L-arginine and L-glutamine.

INDICATIONS AND USAGE

OKG has demonstrated significant usefulness in the nutritional support of burn and other trauma patients, as well as in chronically malnourished subjects and post-surgery in the elderly. It has been shown to speed wound healing. It has exhibited some immunomodulating effects. Claims that it enhances athletic performance have not been confirmed.

RESEARCH SUMMARY

OKG has shown significant effects related to nutritional support in burn, trauma, surgical, elderly and chronically malnourished subjects. These effects have been achieved with both enteral and parenteral administration. OKG has been shown, in varying conditions, to decrease muscle protein catabolism and/or increase muscle protein synthesis. It has also been shown to enhance wound healing. Its ability to increase synthesis of L-glutamine and L-arginine may account for these positive effects. In a recent double-blind, placebo-controlled study, 60 severely burned subjects were randomized to receive 20 grams of OKG daily or placebo for

21 days beginning mean four days post-injury. Significant improvement was achieved in the OKG-treated group, compared with controls, as measured by both biological and clinical end points. Previous studies of OKG-treated burn patients have reported shorter hospitalizations and fewer fatalities.

No conclusions can yet be drawn from scant, preliminary evidence that OKG may exert some positive effects on immunity. And there is no credible research to support claims that OKG can build muscle in healthy individuals or that it can enhance exercise/athletic performance.

CONTRAINDICATIONS, PRECAUTIONS, ADVERSE REACTIONS

CONTRAINDICATIONS

OKG is contraindicated in those with deficiency of ornithine-delta-aminotransferase (OAT). This is a genetic disease resulting in gyrate atrophy of the choroid and retina and progressive blinding chorioretinal degeneration. It is rare.

PRECAUTIONS

Pregnant women and nursing mothers should avoid supplemental OKG. OKG supplementation may potentially cause hypoglycemia in starved individuals. Those with eating disorders or those who are on very-low-calorie diets should exercise caution in using OKG.

ADVERSE REACTIONS

None reported for those using supplemental OKG.

DOSAGE AND ADMINISTRATION

There are no typical doses for OKG supplementation. Some athletes use about 2.5 grams before and after exercise, as well as before breakfast and at bedtime.

Doses of 20 to 30 grams daily, given enterally, have been used in burn and trauma patients.

HOW SUPPLIED

Powder — 3.5 mg/teaspoonful

LITERATURE

Czernichow B, Nsi-Emvo E, Galluser M, et al. Enteral supplementation with ornithine alpha ketoglutarate improves the early adaptive response to resection. *Gut.* 1997; 40:67-72.

De Bandt JP, Coudray-Lucas C, Lioret N, et al. A randomized controlled trial of the influence of the mode of enteral ornithine alpha-ketoglutarate administration in burn patients. *J Nutr.* 1998; 128:563-569.

Dumas F, De Bandt JP, Colomb V, et al. Enteral ornithine alpha-ketoglutarate enhances intestinal adaptation to massive resection in rats. *Metabolism.* 1998; 47:1366-1371.

Donati L, Ziegler F, Pongelli G, Signorini MS. Nutritional and clinical efficacy of ornithine alpha-ketoglutarate in severe burn patients. *Clin Nutr.* 1999; 18:307-311.

Duranton B, Schleiffer R, Gosse F, Raul F. Preventive administration of ornithine alpha-ketoglutarate improves intestinal mucosal repair after transient ischemia in rats. *Crit Care Med.* 1998; 26:120-125.

Jeevanandam M, Holaday NJ, Petersen SR. Ornithine-alpha-ketoglutarate(OKG) supplementation is more effective than its component salts in traumatized rats. *J Nutr.* 1996; 126:2141-2150.

Jeevanandam M, Petersen SR. Substrate fuel kinetics in enterally fed trauma patients supplemented with ornithine alpha-ketoglutarate. *Clin Nutr.* 1999; 18; 209-217.

Le Boucher J, Eurengbiol, Farges MC, et al. Modulation of immune response with ornithine A-ketoglutarate in burn injury: an arginine or glutamine dependency? *Nutrition.* 1999; 15; 773-777.

Le Bricon T, Cynober L, Baracos VE. Ornithine alpha-ketoglutarate limits muscle protein breakdown without stimulating tumor growth in rats bearing Yoshida ascites hepatoma. *Metabolism.* 1994; 43; 899-905.

Le Bricon T, Cynober L. Field CJ, Baracos VE. Supplemental nutrition with ornithine alpha-ketoglutarate in rats with cancer-associated cachexia: surgical treatment of the tumor improves efficacy of nutritional support. *Nutr.* J 1995; 125:2999-3010.

Robinson LE, Bussiere FI, Le Boucher J, et al. Amino acid nutrition and immune function in tumour-bearing rats: a comparison of glutamine-, arginine- and ornithine 2-oxoglutarate-supplemented diets. Clin Sci (Colch). 1999; 97:657-669.

Roch-Arveiller M, Fontagne J, Coudray-Lucas C, et al. Ornithine alpha-ketoglutarate counteracts the decrease of liver cytochrome p-450 content in burned rats. *Nutrition.*1999; 15:379-383.

Roch-Arveiller M, Tissat M, Coudray-Lucas C, et al. Immunomodulatory effects of ornithine alpha-ketoglutarate in rats with burn injuries. *Arch Surg.* 1996; 131:718-723.

Varanasi RV, Saltzman JR. Ornithine oxoglutarate therapy improves nutrition status. *Nutr Rev.* 1996; 53:96-97.

Pantethine

TRADE NAMES

Pantethine 500 (Westlake Laboratories)

DESCRIPTION

Pantethine is the disulfide dimer of pantetheine, the 4'-phosphate derivative of which is an intermediate in the conversion of the B vitamin pantothenic acid to coenzyme A (see Pantothenic Acid). Pantethine is found naturally in small quantities in most forms of life, and therefore, in food sources. Very large doses of pantethine have been found to have lipid-lowering effects, and pantethine is used in Europe and Japan as a lipid-lowering agent. Pantethine is marketed in the United States as a nutritional supplement.

Pantethine is also known as D-bis(N-pantothenyl-beta-aminoethyl)disulfide and (R)-N,N'-[dithiobis(ethyleneiminocarbonylethylene]bis(2,4-dihydroxy-3,3-dimethylbutyramide). Its molecular formula is $C_{22}H_{42}N_4O_8S_2$ and its molecular weight is 554.73 daltons. Pantetine is represented by the following chemical structure:

Pantethine

ACTIONS AND PHARMACOLOGY

ACTIONS

Pantethine may have lipid-modulating activity. It has putative antiatherogenic, ophthalmoprotective and detoxification activities.

MECHANISM OF ACTION

Pantethine has been found to decrease serum levels of total cholesterol, low-density lipoprotein cholesterol (LDL-C), apolipoprotein B and triglycerides. It has also been found to increase high-density lipoprotein cholesterol (HDL-C) and apolipoprotein A1 levels. The mechanism of the possible lipid-modulating activity of pantethine is not understood. In isolated hepatocytes, pantethine has been shown to inhibit both cholesterol and fatty acid synthesis. It is speculated that pantethine, by acting as a precursor of coenzyme A, may enhance the beta-oxidation of fatty acids. However, this has not been confirmed. Another hypothesis is that the lipid-modulating effect of pantethine may be mediated via its metabolite cysteamine. It is argued that there is little pantethine found in the serum following its ingestion and that most of a dose is metabolized to pantothenic acid and cysteamine. Since pantothenic acid does not possess lipid-modulatory activity, cysteamine might. This lipid-modulatory activity could occur via the inhibition of acetyl coenzyme A carboxylase activity and the stimulation of hepatic fatty acid oxidation, resulting in lowered triglyceride levels, and via the inhibition of HMG-CoA reductase activity, resulting in lowered cholesterol levels. Again, this has not been confirmed. Further, cysteamine, a treatment for cystinosis, has not been found to have lipid-lowering activity in those with this rare genetic disorder. Nor, does pantethine appear to be efficacious in the treatment of cystinosis.

The putative antiatherogenic activity may be accounted for, in large part, by pantethine's possible lipid-modulatory activity. In addition, pantethine may have antioxidant activity and also may decrease platelet aggregability. A few studies suggest that pantethine may have antioxidant activity. One *in vitro* study found inhibition of peroxidation of LDL, but only under certain concentrations.

The mechanism of pantethine's possible antioxidant activity is unclear. Other studies have reported that pantethine may decrease platelet aggregability. Possible mechanisms, include decreased thromboxane production and modulation of platelet membrane fluidity. Treatment with pantethine has been found to decrease the cholesterol content of platelet membranes. This could result in increased platelet membrane fluidity and decreased platelet aggregability.

Parenterally administered pantethine has been demonstrated to inhibit lens opacification, in some animal studies. The mechanism of this possible ophthalmoprotective effect is not understood. One possibility is that pantethine may inhibit the formation of protein aggregates in the lens of the eye by forming mixed disulfides with cysteine residues of certain lens proteins. There is no evidence that orally administered pantethine has any activity in inhibiting lens opacification.

Other animal experiments have demonstrated that pantethine protects the liver against certain hepatotoxins, such as carbon tetrachloride. Again, pantethine was administered parenterally in these studies. This hepatoprotective activity may be accounted for, in part, by the possible antioxidant activity of pantethine.

Pantethine has been shown to lower serum acetaldehyde in a small human study, following ethanol ingestion. Acetaldehyde is thought to mediate some of the hepatotoxic effects of ethanol. It is speculated that pantethine-induced lowering of blood acetaldehyde levels following alcohol ingestion is due, in part, to accelerated acetaldehyde oxidation by an interaction between hepatic aldehyde dehydrogenase and pantethine-related intermediates formed in the liver.

PHARMACOKINETICS

The pharmacokinetics of pantethine in humans are incomplete. Following ingestion, pantethine is absorbed from the small intestine into the enterocytes where some is reduced, via glutathione reductase, to pantetheine. Some pantetheine is metabolized in the enterocytes to coenzyme A and the rest, along with pantethine, is released by the enterocytes into the portal circulation. It appears that pantethine undergoes significant metabolism in the blood to pantothenic acid and cysteamine. These metabolites, along with pantethine and pantetheine, are transported to the liver where they are extracted by the hepatocytes and undergo various metabolic reactions. In the liver, some pantethine is reduced to pantetheine and the pantetheine pool in that organ is metabolized to coenzyme A. There appears to be significant first-pass extraction, as well as first-pass metabolism, of pantethine by the liver. There does not appear to be much pantethine circulating in the blood, following ingestion. Coenzyme A itself is catabolized by a number of hydrolytic steps resulting in the production of pantothenate and cysteamine. There is some evidence that pantethine is more efficiently converted to coenzyme A than is pantothenic acid.

INDICATIONS AND USAGE

Pantethine may favorably affect lipids and protect against cardiomuscular disease. There is evidence, in animal research, that it can inhibit cataract formation. It also exhibits some hepatoprotective effects in animal models. Additionally, it has been shown to protect against a number of toxins, including alcohol. Preliminary research suggests that pantethine may influence various central nervous system and adrenal junctions, but no useful conclusions can yet be drawn from these early investigations. There is no credible evidence that pantethine enhances exercise performance or that it inhibits hair loss and graying of hair.

RESEARCH SUMMARY

Several studies have shown that pantethine can significantly lower levels of both cholesterol and triglycerides. Doses used in these studies have ranged from 600 to 1,200 milligrams daily. In one of these studies, seven children and 65 adults suffering from hypercholesterolemia alone or combined with hypertriglyceridemia achieved significant reductions in total cholesterol, LDL-cholesterol, triglycerides and apo-B, as well as significant increases in HDL-cholesterol and apo-A1. They received 900-1,200 milligrams of pantethine daily for three to six months.

Pantethine has also proved helpful in treating diabetics with dyslipidemia, reducing triglyceride levels by 37% in one study (utilizing 600 milligram daily doses). In general, looking at all studies to date, pantethine typically reduces total cholesterol by 15-25% and triglycerides by 25-40%.

Additionally, there is *in vitro* and clinical evidence that pantethine can help maintain normal platelet functions, favorably affecting platelet lipid composition and cell membrane fluidity. These effects may provide further protection against atherosclerosis.

Animal research indicates that pantethine can inhibit cataract formation. This has been demonstrated in several animal models. Reversal of existing opacities has not been demonstrated. More research is needed to see whether these findings extend to humans.

There is also considerable animal data suggesting that pantethine may have significant hepatoprotective effects. It has demonstrated protection against carbon tetrachloride, halocarbon, autoxidized linoleate, acetaldehyde, ethanol and other hepatotoxins.

There is no evidence that pantethine can prevent hair loss or graying of hair. Similarly there is no evidence that pantethine can enhance athletic performance. A recent study showed that a combination of pantethine, pantothenic acid and allithiamin had no effect on exercise performance.

CONTRAINDICATIONS, PRECAUTIONS, ADVERSE REACTIONS

CONTRAINDICATIONS

Pantethine is contraindicated in those hypersensitive to any component of a pantethine-containing product.

PRECAUTIONS

Pregnant women and nursing mothers should avoid the use of pantethine.

The use of pantethine for its possible lipid-lowering effects should only be undertaken under medical supervision.

ADVERSE REACTIONS

Doses up to 1,200 milligrams daily have been well tolerated. There are a few reports of gastrointestinal effects, including nausea and heartburn.

INTERACTIONS

DRUGS

HMG-CoA reductase inhibitors (atorvastatin, cerivastatin, fluvastatin, lovastatin, pravastatin, simvastatin): Concomitant use of pantethine and a HMG-CoA reductase inhibitor may produce additive lipid-modulatory effects.

NUTRITIONAL SUPPLEMENTS

Nicotinic acid: Concomitant use of pantethine and high-dose nicotinic acid may produce additive lipid-modulatory effects.

OVERDOSAGE

There are no reports of pantethine overdosage in the literature.

DOSAGE AND ADMINISTRATION

Single component and combination products (e.g., with pantothenic acid) are available. Possible lipid-lowering dosage typically ranges from 600 to 1,200 milligrams daily, taken in divided doses. See Precautions.

HOW SUPPLIED

Capsules — 500 mg

Sublingual Tablets — 25 mg

LITERATURE

Arsenio L, Bodria P, Magnati G, et al. Effectiveness of long-term treatment with pantethine inpatients with dyslipidemia. *Clin Ther.* 1986; 8:537-545.

Bertolini S, Donati C, Elicio N, et al. Lipoprotein changes induced by pantethine in hyperlipoproteinemic patients: adults and children. *Int J Clin Pharmacol Ther Toxicol.* 1986; 24:630-637.

Bon GB, Cazzolato G, Zago S, Avogaro P. Effects of pantothine on in vitro peroxidation of low density lipoproteins. *Atherosclerosis.* 1985; 57:99-106.

Branca D, Scutari G, Siliprandi N. Pantethine and pantothenate effect on the CoA content of rat liver. *Internat J Vit Nutr Res.* 1984; 54:211-216.

Carrara P, Matturri L, Galbussera M, et al. Pantethine reduces plasma cholesterol and the severity of arterial lesions in experimental hypercholesterolemic rabbits. *Atherosclerosis.* 1984; 53:255-264.

Cighetti G, Del Puppo M, Paroni R, et al. Pantethine inhibits cholesterol and fatty acid syntheses and stimulates carbon dioxide formation in isolated rat hepatocytes. *J Lipid Res.* 1987; 28:152-161.

Clark JI, Livesey JC, Steele JE. Delay or inhibition of rat lens opacification using pantethine and WR-77913. *Exp Eye Res.* 1996; 62:75-84.

Congdon NT, West ST, Duncan DT, et al. The effect of pantethine and ultraviolet-B radiation on the development of lenticular opacity in the emory mouse. *Curr Eye Res.* 2000; 20:17-24.

Donati C, Barbi G, Cairo G, et al. Pantethine improves the lipid abnormalities of chronic hemodialysis patients: results of a multicenter clinical trial. *Clin Nephrol.* 1986; 25:70-74.

Donati C, Bertieri RS, Barbi G. [Pantethine, diabetes mellitus and atherosclerosis. Clinical study of 1045 patients]. [Article in Italian]. *Clin Ter.* 1989; 128:411-422.

Friberg G, Pande J, Ogun O, Benedek GB. Pantethine inhibits the formation of high-Tc protein aggregates in gamma B crystallin solutions. *Curr Eye Res.* 1996; 15:1182-1190.

Gaddi A, Descovich GC, Noseda G, et al. Controlled evaluation of pantethine, a natural hypolipidemic compound, in patients with different forms of hyperlipoproteinemia. *Atherosclerosis.* 1984; 50:73-83.

Galeone F, Scalabrino A, Giuntoli F, et al. The lipid-lowering effect of pantethine in hyperlipidemic patients: a clinical investigation. *Curr Ther Res.* 1983; 34:383-390.

Gensini GF, Prisco D, Rogasi PG, et al. Changes in fatty acid composition of the single platelet phospholipids induced by pantethine treatment. *Int J Clin Pharm Res.* 1985; 5:309-318.

Hayashi H, Kobayashi A, Terada H, et al. Effect of pantethine on action potential of canine papillary muscle during hypoxic perfusion. *Jap Heart J.* 1985; 26:289-296.

Hiramatsu N, Kishida T, Hamano T, Natake M. Effects of dietary pantethine levels on contents of fatty acids and thiobarbituric acid reactive substances in the liver of rats orally administered varying amounts of autoxidized linoleate. *J Nutr Sci Vitaminol (Tokyo).* 1991; 37:73-87.

Hoffman B, Lang A, Ostermann G, et al. Effect of pantethine on platelet functions *in vitro. Curr Ther Res.* 1987; 41:791-801.

Iida J, Nishimura K, Ukei S, Azuma I. Macrophage activation with pantethine and pantetheine-4'-phosphate. *Int J Vitam Nutr Res.* 1985; 55:405-411.

Kumerova AO, Silova AA, Utno Lia. [Effect of pantethine on post-heparin lipolytic activity and lipid peroxidation in the myocardium]. [Article in Russian]. *Biull Eksp Biol Med.* 1991; 111:33-35.

Maggi GC, Donati C, Criscuoli G. Pantethine: a physiological lipomodulating agent in the treatment of hyperlipidemias. *Curr Ther Res.* 1982; 32:380-386.

Nagiel-Ostaszewski I, Lau-Cam CA. Protection by pantethine, pantothenic acid and cystamine against carbon tetrachloride-induced hepatotoxicity in the rat. *Res Commun Chem Pathol Pharmacol.* 1990; 67:289-292.

Prisco D, Rogasi PG, Matucci M, et al. Effect of pantethine treatment on platelet aggregation and thromboxane A_2 production. *Curr Ther Res.* 1984; 35:700-706.

Vecsei L, Alling C, Widerlov E. Comparative studies of intracerebroventricularly administered cysteamine and pantethine in different behavioral tests and on brain catechols in rats. *Arch Int Pharmacodyn Ther.* 1990; 305:140-151.

Watanabe A, Hobara BS, Kobayashi M, et al. Lowering of blood acetaldehyde but not ethanol concentrations by pantethine following alcohol ingestion: different effects in flushing and nonflushing subjects. *Alcoholism: Clin Exper Res.* 1985; 9:272-276.

Webster MJ. Physiological and performance responses to supplementation with thiamin and pantothenic acid derivatives. *Eur J Appl Physiol.* 1998; 77:486-491.

Wittwer CT, Graves CP, Peterson MA, et al. Pantethine lipomodulation: evidence for cysteamine mediation *in vitro* and *in vivo. Atherosclerosis.* 1987; 68:41-49.

Yoon SB, Kajiyama K, Ogura R. [Effect of pantethine on adriamycin-induced cardiotoxicity]. [Article in Japanese]. *Kurume Igakkai Zasshi.* 1982; 45:598-606.

Pantothenic Acid

TRADE NAMES

Pantothenic acid is available generically from numerous manufacturers. Branded products include: Panto-250 (Bio-Tech Pharmacal).

DESCRIPTION

Pantothenic acid, a member of the B-vitamin family, is an essential nutrient in human nutrition. It is sometimes referred to as vitamin B_5. Pantothenic acid is involved in a number of biological reactions, including the production of energy, the catabolism of fatty acids and amino acids, the synthesis of fatty acids, phospholipids, sphingolipids, cholesterol and steroid hormones, and the synthesis of heme and the neurotransmitter acetylcholine. It also appears to be involved in the regulation of gene expression and in signal transduction. Roger J. Williams, the discoverer of pantothenic acid and a scientist who pioneered the use of nutrients for the prevention and treatment of disease, thought that pantothenic acid might be helpful in the management of certain medical disorders, such as rheumatoid arthritis.

The term pantothenic acid is derived from the Greek word pantos, meaning everywhere. Pantothenic acid is widely distributed in plant and animal food sources, where it occurs in both bound and free forms. Rich sources of the vitamin, include organ meats (liver, kidney), egg yolk, avocados, cashew nuts and peanuts, brown rice, soya, lentils, broccoli and milk. Royal jelly and brewer's yeast, both of which are used as nutritional supplements, are two of the richest sources of pantothenic acid. The richest sources of the vitamin are the ovaries of cod and tuna. Pantothenic acid is synthesized by intestinal microflora and this may also contribute to the body's pantothenic acid requirements.

Pantothenic acid deficiency in humans is rare. Symptoms of pantothenic acid deficiency, which has occurred under conditions of severe malnutrition, include numbness in the toes and painful burning in the feet (melalgia). Experimentally-induced pantothenic acid deficiency in humans, produced headache, fatigue, insomnia, intestinal disturbances, paresthesias of the hands and feet, impaired antibody production, an elevated sedimentation rate and an impaired eosinopenic response to ACTH. Most of these symptoms and signs resolved with administration of pantothenic acid.

The principal biologically active forms of pantothenic acid are coenzyme A (CoA) and acyl carrier protein (ACP). In both CoA and ACP, the business center of the molecule is the pantothenic acid metabolite 4'-phosphopantetheine. Coenzyme A is comprised of 4'-phosphopantetheine linked by an anhydride bond to the nucleotide adenosine 5'-monophosphate. 4'-Phosphopantetheine itself is comprised of pantothenic acid linked at one end, via an amide bond, to beta-mercaptoethylamine, derived from L-cysteine, and at the other end to a phosphate group. The sulfhydryl group of 4'-phosphopantetheine, which is the business end of the coenzyme, forms thioesters with acyl groups producing acyl-CoA derivatives, including acetyl-CoA.

Acetyl-CoA is produced via beta-oxidation of fatty acids, via the metabolism of carbohydrates—glucose 6-phosphate to pyruvate to acetyl-CoA—and via the catabolism of amino acids. Acetyl-CoA has a number of metabolic opportunities. It is metabolized in the tricarboxylic acid cycle to produce carbon dioxide, water and energy. It can also be metabolized to fatty acids, cholesterol and steroid hormones. Acetyl-CoA also participates in a number of acetylation reactions, including the formation of acetylcholine, melatonin, N-acetylglucosamine, N-acetylgalactosamine and N-acetylneuraminic acid. Finally, acetyl-CoA is involved in the acetylation of proteins and peptides. Histone acetylation is an epigenetic mechanism of gene regulation. In general, chro-

matin fractions enriched in actively transcribed genes are also enriched in highly acetylated core histones, whereas silent genes are associated with nucleosomes with a low level of acetylation. Nucleosomes are the fundamental units of chromosomes.

The other major form of pantothenic acid is acyl carrier protein or ACP. Acyl carrier protein (ACP) functions as a coenzyme in the fatty acid synthetase complex which is central to the *de novo* synthesis of fatty acids. The prosthetic group of acyl carrier protein is again, 4'-phosphopantetheine. 4'-Phosphopantetheine binds to acyl carrier protein via a phosphodiester linkage to a serine residue of acyl carrier protein. The function of ACP in fatty acid synthesis is analogous to that of coenzyme A in the beta-oxidation of fatty acids. ACP serves as an anchor to which the acyl intermediates are esterified. The acyl intermediates are esterified to the sulfhydryl group of 4'-phosphopantetheine. 4'-Phosphopantetheine is added to ACP in a posttranslational modification reaction which is catalyzed by a transferase enzyme acting on CoA. In the case of coenzyme A, the sulfhydryl groups are also esterified to acyl groups, such as the acetyl group. However, the 4'-phosphopantetheine part of the structure is not esterified to a serine residue in a protein (ACP), but is bound to the nucleotide adenosine 5'-monophosphate.

In addition to acetyl-CoA, other forms of CoA also play important biological roles. Malonyl-CoA supplies two-carbon units for the synthesis of fatty acids up until palmitic acid, and succinyl-CoA reacts with delta-aminolevulinic acid in the first reaction of heme biosynthesis. Myristoyl-CoA, derived from the 14-carbon saturated fatty acid myristic acid, is involved in the myristoylation of proteins; palmitoyl-CoA is involved in the palmitoylation of proteins, and farnesyl-CoA and geranylgeranyl-CoA are involved in protein isoprenylation. Protein isoprenylation, myristoylation and palmitoylation appear to play roles in signal transduction, among other biological activities.

The principal supplemental form of pantothenic acid is calcium D-pantothenate (D-calcium pantothenate). This marketed supplement is usually made synthetically. Dexpanthenol, the corresponding alcohol of pantothenic acid is also available. Dexpanthenol is a synthetic form which is not found naturally. Dexpanthenol is converted to pantothenic acid in the body, and therefore can be considered a provitamin form of pantothenic acid. Dexpanthenol is used topically to promote wound healing. It is also used in various cosmetic products.

In addition to being known as vitamin B_5, pantothenic acid is also known as D(+)-pantothenic acid, D-pantothenic acid, D(+)-N-(2,4-dihydroxy-3,3-dimethylbutyryl)-beta-alanine and (*R*)-*N*-(2,4-dihydroxy-3,3-dimethyl-1-oxobutyl)-beta-alanine. D-pantothenic acid is the biologically active enantiomer of the vitamin and is comprised of beta-alanine and a dihydroxy acid called pantoic acid. Its molecular formula is $C_9H_{17}NO_5$, its molecular weight is 219.24 daltons and its structural formula is as follows:

Pantothenic Acid

Dexpanthenol, the corresponding alcohol of pantothenic acid, is also known as pantothenol, provitamin B_5 and (*R*)-2,4-dihydroxy-*N*-(3-hydroxypropyl)-3,3-dimethylbutyramide. Its molecular formula is $C_9H_{19}NO_4$ and its molecular weight is 205.3 daltons.

ACTIONS AND PHARMACOLOGY

ACTIONS

Pantothenic acid may have antioxidant and radioprotective activities. It has putative anti-inflammatory, wound healing and antiviral activities. It also has putative activity in the management of rheumatoid arthritis.

MECHANISM OF ACTION

Pantothenic acid and its derivatives, 4'-phosphopantothenic acid, pantothenol and pantethine, have been shown, *in vitro*, to protect cells against lipid peroxidation. This protective effect does not appear to be due to the scavenging of the reactive oxygen species by pantothenic acid. It is thought that the antioxidant effect of pantothenic acid is due to its stimulation of increased cellular levels of coenzyme A. Coenzyme A may facilitate removal of lipid peroxides by increasing mobilization of fatty acids, and promote repair of plasma membranes by activating phospholipid synthesis. Pantothenic acid has also been shown to increase levels of cellular reduced glutathione. The mechanism by which pantothenic acid increases glutathione levels is unknown. However, increased levels of glutathione may play a large role in the protective effect of pantothenic acid against peroxidative damage of cell membranes.

Pantothenol has been demonstrated to protect rats against some of the deleterious effects of gamma radiation. The deleterious effects of gamma radiation occur via the generation of reactive oxygen species resulting in the peroxidation of lipid membranes. It is thought that the protective effects of pantothenol, which is a precursor of pantothenic acid, is due, in part, to its promotion of coenzyme A biosynthesis and to

its increasing cellular levels of reduced glutathione (see above).

There is some evidence that pantothenic acid may be helpful in the management of some with rheumatoid arthritis. The mechanism of this putative effect is unclear. Activated granulocytes play a role in the inflammatory response by production of reactive oxygen species. Pantothenic acid, in the form of calcium D-pantothenate, was found to significantly inhibit the release of myeloperoxidase from granulocytes *in vitro*, as well as to inhibit the production of reactive oxygen species by these cells. This effect of pantothenic acid as well as the antioxidant effect of the vitamin discussed above, may account, in part, for the putative action of pantothenic acid in rheumatoid arthritis.

Pantothenic acid has been shown to accelerate wound healing in experimental animals. The mechanism of the putative wound healing effect of pantothenic acid is unclear. In human dermal fibroblasts in culture, calcium D-pantothenate was demonstrated to accelerate the wound healing process by increasing the number of cells migrating into a wounded area, as well as their mean migration speed. Dexpanthenol (pantothenol), the corresponding alcohol of pantothenic acid, is used topically for the treatment of various minor skin disorders and to promote wound healing. Topical dexpanthenol has been found to improve stratum corneum hydration, reduce tranepidermal water loss and to stabilize the epidermal barrier function. The putative wound healing activity of pantothenic acid, may also be accounted for, in part, by its possible antiinflammatory activity.

PHARMACOKINETICS

Dietary sources of pantothenic acid include bound and unbound forms. The principal bound form of the vitamin is coenzyme A. The principal supplementary form of the vitamin is calcium D-pantothenate, Dietary coenzyme A is hydrolyzed in the intestine to dephospho-CoA, phosphopantetheine and pantetheine. Pantetheine, in turn, is hydrolyzed to pantothenic acid. Pantothenic acid is efficiently absorbed from the small intestine. Absorption at low intakes occurs via a sodium-dependent carrier-mediated active transport process, and at higher intakes, by passive diffusion. Pantothenic acid is transported via the portal circulation to the liver and via the systemic circulation to other tissues of the body. Uptake of pantothenic acid by most cells of the body is by a sodium-dependent process.

Pantothenic acid is metabolized to coenzyme A via a sequence of steps. Coenzyme A is a precursor of acyl carrier protein. Approximately 95% of CoA is found in the mitochondria. Coenzyme A is catabolized by a number of hydrolytic steps resulting in pantothenate and cysteamine. Unchanged pantothenate is the major urinary excretion product of pantothenic acid. In dogs, a glycosylated catabolite of the vitamin, pantothenyl-4'-beta-glucoside, has been identified in the urine. Glycosylated catabolites of pantothenic acid have not, to date, been reported in humans.

INDICATIONS AND USAGE

There is some dated evidence that pantothenic acid may be of some benefit in some with rheumatoid arthritis. Research results are mixed, but overall not encouraging, with respect to claims that pantothenic acid enhances exercise performance. There is some animal and *in vitro* evidence that pantothenic acid may aid in wound healing. However, one human clinical study did not show a wound healing effect for oral pantothenic acid. A topical form of the provitamin, dexpanthenol (pantothenol) is used for the treatment of minor skin disorders, including for the promotion of wound healing. There is preliminary evidence that pantothenic acid may be helpful in treating those with hepatitis A and a suggestion from animal studies that it may be helpful in some with Duchenne muscular dystrophy. There is no evidence that it prevents loss of hair and graying of hair.

RESEARCH SUMMARY

Decades ago there were reports that supplemental pantothenic acid could ameliorate some bone and cartilage disorders in acutely pantothenic acid-deficient young rats. Years later, it was noted that blood levels of pantothenic acid are significantly reduced in rheumatoid arthritis (RA) patients. A clinical trial tested 50 milligrams daily of injected calcium pantothenate. Blood levels rose to normal, and significant symptomatic relief was achieved in many of the test subjects. When the pantothenate was withdrawn, symptoms returned. The best results were achieved in a subgroup of vegetarians, and still better results were reported in vegetarians who were given a combination of pantothenic acid and royal jelly. (See Royal Jelly). This study was conducted in 1963.

In 1980, a double-blind, placebo-controlled study followed-up on the initial report. Subjects with various forms of arthritis were randomized to receive oral calcium pantothenate or placebo. Dosage was as follows: one tablet (500 milligrams) daily for two days, then one twice a day for three days, then one three times a day for four days and, finally, one four times a day thereafter.

Calcium pantothenate was no better than placebo in treating all forms of arthritis—except RA. In the subset of subjects with RA, pantothenic acid produced significant results. The researchers noted, in particular, that "highly significant effects were recorded for calcium pantothenate in reducing the duration of morning stiffness, degree of disability and severity of pain, whereas placebo produced no effects on these symptoms." As these researchers noted, further investigation is warranted.

There have been reports that pantothenic acid speeds wound healing in animal models. However, recent, double-blind, prospective, randomized trial found "no major improvement" of the human skin wound healing process. This 21-day study tested a combination of 1 gram of ascorbic acid and 0.2 grams of pantothenic acid daily on 49 subjects. Further investigation is needed to determine if oral pantothenic acid has any role in wound healing. A topical forms of the provitamin, pantothenol, appears to play some role in the management of minor skin disorders.

Claims that pantothenic acid enhances exercise performance rest, primarily, in the results of one study in which experienced distance runners received 2 grams of pantothenic acid daily for 14 days. Their performance was significantly better than that of equally well-trained distance runners who received placebo.

In another study, however, 1 gram of pantothenic acid daily for two weeks did not enhance the performance of distance runners compared with distance runners given placebo.

More recently, highly trained cyclists performed no better with a combination of 1 gram of allithiamin and 1.8 grams of a 55%/45% pantethine/pantothenic acid mixture than they did with placebo. The substances were administered for seven days prior to each exercise performance test. The researchers concluded: "we found the oral administration of these compounds to have no effect on any physiological or performance parameters during steady-state or high-intensity exercise."

There is preliminary evidence that pantothenic acid, in combination with pantetheine, may be helpful in the treatment of hepatitis A. Pantetheine is thought to be more active in this respect than pantothenic acid.

Administration of pantothenic acid increased skeletal muscle energy metabolism in the murine model of Duchenne muscular dystrophy, the mdx mouse. Reduced energy metabolism in slow-and fast-twitch skeletal muscle fibers has been reported in the mdx mouse. It is thought that this is due to a decreased oxidative utilization of glucose and free fatty acids. It is speculated that inefficiency of coenzyme A transport in the mitochondria might account for the reduced energy metabolism. Administration of pantothenic acid to mdx mice increased the cytoplasmic synthesis of CoA, and increased the thermogenic response to glucose, more in the muscles of mdx mice than in control muscles. Human studies are warranted.

CONTRAINDICATIONS, PRECAUTIONS, ADVERSE REACTIONS

CONTRAINDICATIONS

Pantothenic acid is contraindicated in those hypersensitive to any component of a pantothenic acid-containing product.

Dexpanthenol (pantothenol), the alcohol analog of pantothenic acid, is contraindicated in those hypersensitive to any component of a dexpanthenol-containing product. Oral and parenteral dexpanthenol are also contraindicated in those with ileus due to mechanical obstruction and those with hemophilia.

PRECAUTIONS
Pregnant women and nursing mothers should avoid doses of pantothenic acid greater than the U.S. RDA (10 milligrams/day) unless a higher dosage is prescribed by their physicians.

Those who have developed contact dermatitis from use of dexpanthenol may develop eczema from the use of oral pantothenic acid. Dexpanthenol, also known as pantothenol and provitamin B_5, in addition to being used for the treatment of various minor skin disorders, is an ingredient in many cosmetic products.

The use of pantothenic acid for any medical condition must be medically supervised.

ADVERSE REACTIONS
Contact dermatitis has been reported with topical use of dexpanthenol.

INTERACTIONS
NUTRITIONAL SUPPLEMENTS
Biotin: High doses of pantothenic acid may inhibit the absorption of biotin produced by the microflora in the large intestine. Pantothenic acid and biotin appear to use the same uptake carrier in colonocytes.

OVERDOSAGE
There are no reports of pantothenic acid overdosage in the literature.

DOSAGE AND ADMINISTRATION
The principal form of supplementary pantothenic acid is calcium D-pantothenate. Calcium D-pantothenate is available in multivitamin, multivitamin/multimineral and B-complex products, as well as single ingredient products. Typical doses of pantothenic acid range from 10-50 milligrams/day. Single ingredient tablets and capsules of pantothenic acid are available in doses ranging from 100 to 500 milligrams.

The Food and Nutrition Board of the Institute of Medicine of the U.S. National Academy of Sciences has recommended the following Dietary Reference Intakes (RDI) for pantothenic acid:

Infants	Adequate Intakes (AI)
0 through 6 months	1.7 milligrams/day ≈ 0.2 mg/Kg
7 through 12 months	1.8 milligrams/day ≈ 0.2 mg/Kg
Children	
1 through 3 years	2 milligrams/day
4 through 8 years	3 milligrams/day
Boys	
9 through 13 years	4 milligrams/day
14 through 18 years	5 milligrams/day
Girls	
9 through 13 years	4 milligrams/day
14 through 18 years	5 milligrams/day
Men	
19 years and older	5 milligrams/day
Women	
19 years and older	5 milligrams/day
Pregnancy	
14 through 50 years	6 milligrams/day
Lactation	
14 through 50 years	7 milligrams/day

There is no evidence of toxicity associated with the ingestion of pantothenic acid. Therefore, a lowest-observed-adverse-effect level (LOAEL) and an associated no-observed-adverse-effect level (NOAEL) cannot be determined.

The optimal intakes of pantothenic acid are not known.

The U.S. RDA for pantothenic acid, which is used for determining percent daily values on nutritional supplement and food labels, is 10 milligrams/day.

HOW SUPPLIED
Capsules — 100 mg, 250 mg, 500 mg

Capsules, Extended Release — 1000 mg

Liquid — 200 mg/5 mL

Tablets — 100 mg, 200 mg, 250 mg, 500 mg, 1000 mg

Tablets, Extended Release — 500 mg, 1000 mg

LITERATURE
Anon. Calcium pantothenate in arthritic conditions. A report from the General Practitioner Research Group. *Practitioner.* 1980; 224:208-211.

Aprahamian M, Dentinger A, Stock-Damge C, et al. Effects of supplemental pantothenic acid on wound healing: experimental study in rabbit. *Am J Clin Nutr.* 1985; 41:578-589.

Barton-Wright EC, Elliot WA. The pantothenic acid metabolism of rheumatoid arthritis. *Lancet.* 1963; 2:862-863.

Dietary Reference Intakes for Thiamin, Riboflavin, Niacin, Vitamin B6, Folate, Vitamin B12, Pantothenic Acid, Biotin, and Choline. Washington, DC: National Academy Press; 1998.

Even PC, Decrouy A, Chinet A. Defective regulation of energy metabolism in mdx-mouse skeletal muscles. *Biochem J.* 1994; 304:649-654.

Gehring W, Gloor M. Effect of topically applied dexpanthenol on epidermal barrier function and stratum corneum hydration. Results of a human *in vivo* study. *Arzneimittelforschung*. 2000; 50:659-663.

Hahn C, Roseler S, Fritzsche R, et al. Allergic contact reaction to dexpanthenol: lymphocyte transformation test and evidence for microsomal-dependent metabolism of the allergen. *Contact Dermatitis*. 1993; 28:81-83.

Kapp A, Zeak-Kapp G. Effect of Ca-pantothenate on human granulocyte oxidative metabolism. *Allerg Immunol (Leipz)*. 1991; 37:145-150.

Kehrl W, Sonnemann U. [Dexpanthenol nasal spray as an effective therapeutic principle for treatment of rhinitis sicca anterior]. [Article in German]. *Laryngorhinootologie*. 1998; 77:506-512.

Komar VI. [The use of pantothenic acid preparations in treating patients with viral hepatitis A]. [Article in Russian]. *Ter Arkh*. 1991; 63:58-60.

Kumerova AO, Utno LIa, Lipsberga ZE, Shkestere IIa. [Study of pantothenic acid derivatives as cardiac protectors in a model of experimental ischemia and reperfusion of the isolated heart]. [Article in Russian]. *Biull Eksp Biol Med*. 1992; 113:373-375.

Litoff D, Scherzer H, Harrison J. Effects of pantothenic acid supplementation on human exercise. *Med Sci Sports Exercise*. 1985; 17:287(Abstract 17).

Loftus EV Jr, Tremaine WJ, Nelson RA, et al. Dexpanthenol enemas in ulcerative colitis: a pilot study. *Mayo Clin Proc*. 1997; 72:616-620.

Moiseenok AG, Dorofeev BF, Omel'ianchik SN. [The protective effect of pantothenic acid derivatives and changes in the system of acetyl CoA metabolism in acute ethanol poisoning]. [Article in Russian]. *Farmakol Toksikol*. 1988; 51:82-86.

Nice C, Reeves AG, Brinck-Johnsen T, Noll W. The effects of pantothenic acid on human exercise capacity. *J Sports Med*. 1984; 24:26-29.

Plesofsky-Vig N. Pantothenic acid. In: Shils, ME, Olson JA, Shike M, Ross AC, eds. *Modern Nutrition in Health and Disease*. 9th ed. Baltimore MD: Williams and Wilkins; 1999:423-432.

Rychlik M. Quantification of free and bound pantothenic acid in foods and blood plasma by a stable isotope dilution assay. *J Agric Food Chem*. 2000; 48:1175-1181.

Sachs M, Asskali F, Lanaros C, et al. [The metabolism of panthenol in patients with postoperative intestinal atony]. [Article in German]. *Z Ernahrungswiss*. 1990; 29:270-283.

Slyshenkov VS, Moiseenok AG, Wojtczak L. Noxious effects of oxygen reactive species on energy-coupling processes in Ehrlich ascites tumor mitochondria and the protection by pantothenic acid. *Free Rad Biol Med*. 1996; 20:793-800.

Slyshenkov VS, Omelyanchik SN, Moiseenok AG, et al. Panthenol protects rats against some deleterious effects of gamma radiation. *Free Rad Biol Med*. 1998; 24:894-899.

Slyshenkov VS, Rakowska M, Moiseenok AG, Wojtczak L. Pantothenic acid and its derivatives protect Ehrlich ascites tumor cells against lipid peroxidation. *Free Rad Biol Med*. 1995; 19:767-772.

Slyshenkov VS, Rakowska M, Wojtczak L. Protective effect of pantothenic acid and related compounds against permeabilization of Ehrlich ascites tumor cells by digitonin. *Acta Biochim Pol*. 1996; 43:407-410.

Vaxman F, Olender S, Lambert A, et al. Effect of pantothenic acid and ascorbic acid supplementation on human skin wound healing process. A double-blind, prospective and randomized trial. *Eur Surg Res*. 1995; 27:158-166.

Webster MJ. Physiological and performance responses to supplementation with thiamin and pantothenic acid derivatives. *Eur J Appl Physiol*. 1998; 77:486-491.

Weimann BI, Hermann D. Studies on wound healing: effects of calcium-D-pantothenate on the migration, proliferation and protein synthesis of human dermal fibroblasts in culture. *Int J Vitam Nutr Res*. 1999; 69:113-119.

Williams RJ. *Biochemical Individuality*. New York, NY: John Wiley and Sons, Inc; 1963.

Para-Aminobenzoic Acid (PABA)

TRADE NAMES

PABA and para-aminobenzoate potassium are available from numerous manufacturers generically. Branded products for para-aminobenzoate potassium include M2 Potassium (Miller Pharmacal) and Potaba (Glenwood).

DESCRIPTION

Para-aminobenzoic acid or PABA is a non-protein amino acid that is widely distributed in nature. It is sometimes referred to as vitamin Bx, but it is neither a vitamin nor an essential nutrient for humans. PABA is an intermediate in the synthesis of folic acid in bacteria. The sulfonamide antibiotics are structurally similar to PABA and interfere with the synthesis of nucleic acids in sensitive micro-organisms by blocking the conversion of PABA to the co-enzyme dihydrofolic acid, a reduced form of folic acid. In humans, dihydrofolic acid is obtained from dietary folic acid; thus sulfonamides do not affect human cells. PABA is also known as 4-aminobenzoic acid. It is a solid substance with slight solubility in water. Its chemical structure is:

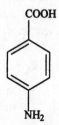

PABA (p-Aminobenzoic acid)

ACTIONS AND PHARMACOLOGY

ACTIONS

PABA may have antifibrosis activity.

MECHANISM OF ACTION

The mechanism of action of PABA's reputed antifibrosis effect in not known. It has been speculated that PABA mediates increased oxygen uptake at the tissue level, but this has never been established.

PHARMACOKINETICS

Following ingestion, PABA is passively absorbed mainly from the small intestine. From there, it enters the portal circulation. Some metabolism of PABA occurs in the liver. A major metabolite is N-acetyl PABA. PABA and its metabolites are mainly excreted in the urine. Small amounts are eliminated in the feces and in bile, milk and other secretions.

INDICATIONS AND USAGE

Pharmaceutical doses of PABA are indicated for Peyronie's disease, scleroderma, morphea and linear scleroderma. There is less evidence to indicate it for pemphigus and dermatomyositis. Claims that it can halt hair loss and restore color to graying hair are entirely anecdotal.

RESEARCH SUMMARY

A retrospective review reported on 32 Peyronie's disease patients treated for at least three months with 12 grams daily of a potassium PABA preparation (POTABA) and followed for 8 to 24 months. Improvement in penile discomfort was demonstrated in 8 of 18 patients, decreased plaque size was reported in 18 of 32 patients, improvement in penile angulation in 18 of 31 patients. No significant adverse effects were noted. Additional research is needed to confirm these findings.

Another retrospective review analyzed skin responses of scleroderma patients to potassium para-aminobenzoate therapy. Ninety percent of 224 patients treated with about 12 grams daily of potassium para-benzoate (POTABA) experienced mild, moderate or marked skin softening. Among a parallel group of 96 evaluable scleroderma patients who did not receive potassium para-benzoate, less than 20% had mild or moderate improvement at the end of follow-up. The difference in skin softening in the treated group, compared to the untreated group, was statistically significant, and no significant adverse events were reported. Again, these findings require confirmation. Clinical improvement was noted in two dermatomyositis patients treated with 15 to 20 grams of potassium para-benzoate daily. Adequate clinical trials are necessary before any conclusion can be drawn regarding the possible effectiveness of PABA for dermatomyositis.

There are anecdotal reports that PABA can halt hair loss and restore color to graying hair; there are at least as many reports that contradict these claims.

CONTRAINDICATIONS, PRECAUTIONS, ADVERSE REACTIONS

CONTRAINDICATIONS

PABA should not be administered to anyone taking sulfonamides or to anyone who is hypersensitive to it.

PRECAUTIONS

PABA should be avoided by children, pregnant women and nursing mothers. PABA should be used with caution in those with renal disease. If anorexia or nausea occurs, PABA should be stopped until the person is eating normally again. PABA should be stopped if hypersensitivity develops. Those taking pharmaceutical doses of PABA must be under medical supervision.

ADVERSE REACTIONS

Anorexia, nausea, vomiting, fever and rash have been reported in those taking PABA, particularly with larger doses. These symptoms resolve when PABA is stopped.

INTERACTIONS

Sulfonamides: PABA can decrease the effectiveness of sulfonamides and is contraindicated in anyone taking sulfonamides.

No other drug, nutritional supplement, herb or food interaction is known.

OVERDOSAGE

There are no known reports of overdosage.

DOSAGE AND ADMINISTRATION

In addition to PABA, the potassium salt of PABA called POTABA is available on prescription. POTABA is indicated for Peyronie's Disease and scleroderma. (See *Physicians' Desk Reference* for complete prescribing information.)

The dose for Peyronie's disease and scleroderma is high and must only be used under medical supervision. The dose used for these disorders is 12 grams daily taken in four to six divided doses with meals. The tablets must be dissolved in plenty of liquid to prevent gastrointestinal upset. Because of the high doses needed to achieve clinical efficacy, patient compliance is typically poor.

HOW SUPPLIED

PABA

Capsules — 100 mg, 250 mg
Extended Release Tablets — 500 mg
Tablets — 100 mg, 500 mg

AMINOBENZOATE POTASSIUM

Capsules — 60 mg, 500 mg
Powder — 2 gm/packet
Tablets — 500 mg

LITERATURE

Carson CC. Potassium para-aminobenzoate for treatment of Peyronie's disease: is it effective? *Tech Urol.* 1997; 3:135-139.

Hasche-Klunder R. Treatment of Peyronie's disease with para-aminobenzoacidic potassium. *Urologe[A].* 1978; 17:224-227.

Kierkegaard E, Nielsen B. Peyronie's diseases treated with K-para-aminobenzoate and vitamin E. *Ugeskr Laeger.* 1979; 141:2052-2053.

Physicians' Desk Reference. 54th edition. Montvale, NJ: Medical Economics Company; 2000.

Zarafonetis CJ, Dabich L, Skovronski JJ, et al. Retrospective studies in scleroderma: skin responses to potassium para-aminobenzoate therapy. *Clin Exp Rheumatol.* 1998; 6:261-268.

Zuckerman JE, Hollinger MA, Giri SN. Evaluation of antifibrotic drugs in bleomycin-induced pulmonary fibrosis in hamsters. *J Pharmacol Exp Ther.* 1980; 213:425-431.

Pectin

TRADE NAMES

Apple, grapefruit and citrus pectin products are available from many manufacturers; branded products include Modified Citrus Pectin Power (Nature's Herbs).

DESCRIPTION

Pectin is classified as a soluble fiber. It is found in most plants, but is most concentrated in citrus fruits (oranges, lemons, grapefruits) and apples. Pectin is obtained by the aqueous extraction of citrus peels and apple pulp under mildly acidic conditions. Pectin obtained from citrus peels is referred to as citrus pectin.

Pectin is widely used in the food industry as a gelling agent to impart a gelled texture to foods, mainly fruit-based foods such as jams and jellies. It also has pharmaceutical applications. Pectin is used in combination with the clay kaolin (hydrated aluminum silicate) for the management of diarrhea. It is used as a component in the adhesive part of ostomy rings. Pectin is also marketed as a nutritional supplement for the management of elevated cholesterol.

Chemically, pectin is a linear polysaccharide containing from about 300 to 1,000 monosaccharide units. D-Galacturonic acid is the principal monosaccharide unit of pectin. Some neutral sugars are also present in the substance. The D-galacturonic acid residues are linked together by alpha-1, 4 glycosidic linkages. The molecular weight of pectin ranges from 50,000 to 150,000 daltons. The galacturonic acid residues in pectin may be esterified with methyl groups. There are different types of pectin. Pectin in which more than 50% of the galacturonic acid residues are esterified is called high methoxyl or HM pectin. Pectin in which less than 50% of the galacturonic acid residues are esterified is called low methoxy or LM pectin. Pectin is a nondigestible polysaccharide. So-called modified citrus pectin is pectin that has been hydrolyzed and otherwise modified to make it more digestible and absorbable.

ACTIONS AND PHARMACOLOGY

ACTIONS

Pectin may have hypocholesterolemic and antithrombotic activities. It has a putative protective action against colorectal cancer.

MECHANISM OF ACTION

The mechanism of the possible hypocholesterolemic activity of pectin is not well understood. It appears that the viscosity of pectin is related to its possible hypocholesterolemic activity. Pectin preparations with high viscosity appear to be more effective in lowering cholesterol than are pectin preparations with lower viscosity. High-viscosity pectin is thought to lower cholesterol levels by raising the excretion of fecal bile acids and neutral sterols. High-viscosity pectin may interfere with the formation of micelles and/or lower the diffusion rate of bile acid and cholesterol-containing micelles through the bolus, consequently diminishing the uptake of cholesterol and bile acids.

Pectin has been found to alter the characteristics of the fibrin-network architecture, suggesting that it may have some antithrombotic activity. Fibrin networks, following pectin supplementation, were found to have lower tensile strength, and to be more lysable and permeable. Acetate supplementation was found to have similar activity on fibrin networks. It is thought that the acetate resulting from bacterial fermentation of pectin in the large intestine may account for pectin's possible effect on fibrin networks.

The putative protective activity of pectin against colorectal cancer may be accounted for by its fermentation in the large intestine to butyric acid. Butyric acid may upregulate apoptosis.

PHARMACOKINETICS

Following ingestion of pectin, very little of it gets digested in the small intestine. Some fermentation of pectin takes place in the large intestine via the action of bacteria. The final products of fermentation of pectin are the short-chain fatty acids, acetate, propionate and butyrate, as well as hydrogen and carbon dioxide. The short-chain fatty acids that escape colonic metabolism are transported via the portal circulation to the liver where they undergo metabolism. The short-chain fatty acids that are not metabolized in the liver enter the systemic circulation and are distributed to the various tissues of the body. Acetate appears to be the principal short-chain fatty acid to reach the systemic circulation from the liver.

INDICATIONS AND USAGE

Pectin appears to have hypocholesterolemic effects and may be antiatherogenic in some. It is used in some multi-ingredient preparations for the treatment of constipation and diarrhea. Claims that it is an effective antiobesity agent are unsubstantiated. There is a recent preliminary animal study suggesting that pectin could have some anticancer activity. (See also Modified Citrus Pectin.)

RESEARCH SUMMARY

Numerous studies have demonstrated that pectin has favorable effects on lipids. In a small early study, administration of 15 grams of pectin daily for three weeks resulted in a mean 13% reduction in plasma cholesterol levels. There was no effect on plasma triglyceride concentrations. Subsequently, giving 40 to 50 grams of pectin daily significantly lowered cholesterol levels in both normolipidemic and hyperlipidemic subjects. In another study, a pectin-supplemented diet (without other dietary or lifestyle changes), significantly reduced plasma cholesterol in volunteers evaluated to be at medium to high risk for coronary heart disease due to hypercholesterolemia. This was a double-blind, placebo-controlled trial. Treatment continued for 16 weeks. The pectin was credited with decreasing plasma cholesterol 7.6% and LDL-cholesterol 10.8%.

Pectin's adsorbent and bulk-forming properties have promoted its use in some multi-ingredient anticonstipation and antidiarrheal preparations.

Recently, pectin was found to be associated with higher apoptotic index in colonocytes of rats, suggesting that it might be useful in protecting against development of colorectal cancer. Followup is needed. Modified citrus pectin has also demonstrated some anti-carcinogenic activity. (See Modified Citrus Pectin.)

CONTRAINDICATIONS, PRECAUTIONS, ADVERSE REACTIONS

CONTRAINDICATIONS

Pectin is contraindicated in those hypersensitive to any component of a pectin-containing supplement.

PRECAUTIONS

Pregnant women and nursing mothers should avoid pectin supplementation.

ADVERSE REACTIONS

Pectin may cause such gastrointestinal symptoms as flatulence, cramps, gas and diarrhea.

INTERACTIONS

DRUGS

Lovastatin: Pectin when used concomitantly may decrease the absorption of lovastatin. There are no reports of interactions between pectin and other statins.

Clindamycin, Tetracycline, Digoxin: Concomitant use of a kaolin-pectin antidiarrheal suspension with clindamycin, tetracycline and digoxin has been reported to decrease the absorption of those drugs. However, it is unclear as to which component (kaolin or pectin or both) is responsible for this interaction. Kaolin (hydrated aluminum silicate) is known to adsorb a wide variety of drugs and other substances.

NUTRITIONAL SUPPLEMENTS

Caroteroids: Concomitant use of pectin and lycopene, lutein and beta-carotene has been reported to decrease the absorption of these carotenoids.

Minerals: Pectin may decrease the absorption of such minerals as zinc, copper, iron, calcium and magnesium if used concomitantly.

FOODS

Pectin may decrease the absorption of such minerals in foods as zinc, copper, iron and calcium.

Pectin, when used concomitantly with lovastatin, caused a paradoxical increase in LDL-cholesterol. It was thought that the pectin reduced the absorption of lovastatin.

DOSAGE AND ADMINISTRATION

There are no typical doses of pectin supplements. Doses of 10 to 15 grams daily have been used in studies showing cholesterol-lowering effects in hypercholesterolemic individuals. Pectin supplements should be used with plenty of fluid.

HOW SUPPLIED

Capsules — 500 mg

Powder

Tablets — 300 mg, 500 mg, 750 mg, 1000 mg

LITERATURE

Anderson JW, Jones AE, Riddell-Mason S. Ten different dietary fibers have significantly different effects on serum and liver lipids of cholesterol-fed rats. *J Nutr.* 1994; 124:78-83.

Avivi-Green C, Polak-Charcon S, Madar Z, Schwartz B. Dietary regulation and localization of apoptosis cascade proteins in the colonic crypt. *J Cell Biochem.* 2000; 77:18-29.

Cerda JJ, Normann SJ, Sullivan MP, et al. Inhibition of atherosclerosis by dietary pectin in microswine with sustained hypercholesterolemia. *Circulation.* 1994; 89:1247-1253.

Cerda JJ, Robbins FL, Burgin CW, et al. The effects of grapefruit pectin on patients at risk for coronary heart disease without altering diet or lifestyle. *Clin Cardiol.* 1988; 11:589-594.

Ebihara K, Kiriyama S, Manabe M. Cholesterol-lowering activity of various natural pectins and synthetic pectin-derivatives with different physico-chemical properties. *Nutr Rep Int.* 1979; 20:519-526.

Hillman LC, Peters SG, Fisher CA, Pomare EW. The effects of the fiber components pectin, cellulose and lignin on serum cholesterol levels. *Am J Clin Nutr*. 1985; 42:207-213.

Judd PA, Truswell AS. The hypocholesterolemic effects of pectins in rats. *Br J Nutr*. 1985; 53:409-425.

Kay RM, Truswell AS. Effects of citrus pectin on blood lipids and fecal steroid excretion in man. *Am J Clin Nutr*. 1977; 30:171-175.

Platt D, Raz A. Modulation of the lung colonization of B16-F1 melanoma cells by citrus pectin. *J Natl Cancer Inst*. 1992; 84:438-442.

Richter WO, Jacob BG, Schwandt P. Interaction between fibre and lovastatin. *Lancet*. 1991; 338:706.

Riedl J, Linseisen J, Hoffman J, Wolfran G. Some dietary fibers reduce the absorption of carotenoids in women. *J Nutr*. 1999; 129:2170-2176.

Rock CL, Swendseid ME. Plasma beta-carotene response in humans after meals supplemented with dietary pectin. *Am J Clin Nutr*. 1992; 55:96-99.

Terpstra AHM, Lapre JA, de Vries HT, Beynen AC. Dietary pectin with high viscosity lowers plasma and liver cholesterol concentration and plasma ester transfer protein activity in hamsters. *J Nutr*. 1998; 128:1944-1949.

Veldman FJ, Nair CH, Vorster HH, et al. Possible mechanism through which dietary pectin influences fibrin network architecture in hypercholesterolaemic subjects. *Thromb Res*. 1999; 93:253-264.

Perilla Oil

DESCRIPTION

Perilla oil is derived from the seed of the plant *Perilla frutescens*. Perilla oil is a very rich source of alpha-linolenic acid. About 50 to 60% of perilla oil is alpha-linolenic acid. Alpha-linolenic acid is an n-3 (omega-3) all-cis polyunsaturated fatty acid containing 18 carbon atoms and three double bonds. It is also known as ALA; ALA, 18:3n-3; 9,12, 15-octadecatrienoic acid and (Z,Z, Z)-9,12,15-octadecatrienoic acid. ALA has the following chemical formula:

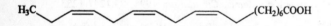

Alpha-linolenic acid

Alpha-linolenic acid is found in perilla oil as a triacylglycerol or triglyceride. The Mediterranean diet, high in ALA, appears to lower the risk of coronary artery disease and certain types of cancer.

ACTIONS AND PHARMACOLOGY

ACTIONS

Perilla oil may have anti-inflammatory, antithrombotic and anti-proliferative activities.

MECHANISM OF ACTION

The possible actions of perilla oil are probably dependent on the presence of ALA. ALA is metabolized to eicosapaentenoic acid (EPA) and docosahexaenoic acid (DHA). EPA is a precursor of the series-3 prostaglandins, the series-5 leukotrienes and the series-3 thromboxanes. These eicosanoids have anti-inflammatory and anti-atherogenic properties. The incorporation of metabolites of ALA in cell membranes may play a role in anti-inflammatory activity, inhibition of platelet aggregation and possibly in anti-proliferative actions of ALA.

PHARMACOKINETICS

ALA-laden triacylglycerols (TAGs), following ingestion, undergo hydrolysis via lipases to form monoglycerides and free fatty acids. Once formed, the monoglycerides and the free fatty acids are absorbed by the enterocytes. In the enterocytes, reacylation takes place reforming TAGs, which are then reassembled with phospholipids, cholesterol and apolipoproteins into chylomicrons. The chylomicrons are released into the lymphatics from whence they are transported to the systemic circulation. In the circulation, the chylomicrons are degraded by lipoprotein lipase, and the fatty acids, including ALA, are taken up in part by the endothelial cells where ALA is metabolized to phospholipids. ALA is transported via the circulation to various tissues in the body where it is metabolized to EPA, DHA and series-3 prostaglandins, series-5 leukotrienes and series-3 thromboxanes. Most of this metabolism occurs in cell membrane phospholipids.

An intake of from 3 to 4 grams daily of ALA is estimated to be equivalent to an intake of 0.3 grams daily of EPA, which one would get from a diet rich in fish.

INDICATIONS AND USAGE

Perilla oil may be indicated as a cardioprotective supplement, to help prevent blood clots and to ameliorate some of the symptoms of inflammatory bowel disease. Animal studies suggest that perilla oil might eventually prove useful in the prevention or management of some cancers.

RESEARCH SUMMARY

Perilla oil is a rich source of alpha-linolenic acid (ALA). Perilla oil has cardio-protective effects. It decreases platelet-activating factor, helping to prevent arterial blood clots.

One group of researchers suggests that perilla oil may be superior to either eicosapaentoic acid (EPA) or docahexaenoic acid (DHA) in ameliorating the colitis of experimental

Crohn's disease. Perilla oil may be a palatable alternative to those who find fish oils effective in colitis but cannot tolerate taking them for prolonged periods.

In animal experiments, perilla oil proved superior to either soybean or safflower oils in inhibiting mammary, colon and kidney cancers. In one animal study, a relatively small amount of perilla oil, constituting 25% of total dietary fat, significantly protected against colon cancer. In another recent animal study, perilla oil suppressed the development of liver cell carcinoma.

CONTRAINDICATIONS, PRECAUTIONS, ADVERSE REACTIONS

CONTRAINDICATIONS

None known.

PRECAUTIONS

Infants, young children, pregnant women and nursing mothers should only use perilla oil if recommended and monitored by a physician. Because of perilla oil's possible antithrombotic activity, hemophiliacs and those taking warfarin should exercise caution in its use. Perilla oil intake should be stopped in those having surgical procedures.

ADVERSE REACTIONS

Perilla oil may cause some mild gastrointestinal symptoms such as diarrhea.

INTERACTIONS

Interactions may occur between ALA in perilla oil and aspirin, other NSAIDs or herbs, such as *Allium sativum* (garlic) and *Ginkgo biloba* (ginkgo). Such interactions, if they were to occur, might be manifested by nosebleeds and increased susceptibility to bruising. If this does occur, consideration should be given to lowering or stopping intake.

OVERDOSAGE

There are no reports of overdosage.

DOSAGE AND ADMINISTRATION

One-gram capsules of perilla oil containing 55% ALA are available. A usual dose for any of the indications is about 6 grams daily in divided doses with meals. This provides an intake of 3.3 grams of ALA.

LITERATURE

Indu M. Ghafoorunissa n-3 Fatty acids in Indian diets: comparison of the effects of precursor (alpha-linolenic acid) vs product (long-chain n-3 polyunsaturated fatty acids). *Nutr Res.* 1992; 12:569-582.

Narisawa T, Fukaura Y, Yazawa K, et al. Colon cancer prevention with a small amount of dietary perilla oil high in alpha-linolenic acid in an animal model. *Cancer.* 1994; 73:2069-2075.

Oh-hashi K, Takehashi T, Watanabe S. Possible mechanisms for the differential effects high linoleate safflower oil and high alpha-linolenate perilla oil diets on platelet-activating factor

production by rat polymorphonuclear leukocytes. *J Lipid Mediat Cell Signal.* 1997; 17:207-220.

Shoda R, Matsuedo K, Yamato S, Umeda N. Therapeutic efficacy of n-3 fatty acid in experimental Crohn's disease. *J Gastroenterol.* 1995; 30 Suppl 8:98-101.

Phosphatidylcholine

DESCRIPTION

Phosphatidylcholine is a phospholipid that is a major constituent of cell membranes. Phosphatidylcholine is also known as 1, 2-diacyl-sn-glycero-3-phosphocholine, PtdCho and lecithin. It is represented by the following chemical structure:

R and R^1 = fatty acids residues

Phosphatidylcholine

The term lecithin itself has different meanings when used in chemistry and biochemistry than when used commercially. Chemically, lecithin is phosphatidylcholine. Commercially, it refers to a natural mixture of neutral and polar lipids. Phosphatidylcholine, which is a polar lipid, is present in commercial lecithin in concentrations of 20 to 90%. Most of the commercial lecithin products contain about 20% phosphatidylcholine.

Lecithins containing phosphatidylcholine are produced from vegetable, animal and microbial sources, but mainly from vegetable sources. Soybean, sunflower and rapeseed are the major plant sources of commercial lecithin. Soybean is the most common source. Plant lecithins are considered to be GRAS (generally regarded as safe). Egg yolk lecithin is not a major source of lecithin in nutritional supplements. Eggs themselves naturally contain from 68 to 72% phosphatidylcholine, while soya contains from 20 to 22% phosphatidylcholine.

The fatty acid makeups of phosphatidylcholine from plant and animal sources differ. Saturated fatty acids, such as palmitic and stearic, make up 19 to 24% of soya lecithin; the monounsaturated oleic acid contributes 9 to 11%; linoleic acid provides 56 to 60%; and alpha-linolenic acid makes up 6 to 9%. In egg yolk lecithin, the saturated fatty acids, palmitic and stearic, make up 41 to 46% of egg lecithin, oleic acid 35 to 38%, linoleic acid 15 to 18% and alpha-linolenic

0 to 1%. Soya lecithin is clearly richer in polyunsaturated fatty acids than egg lecithin. Unsaturated fatty acids are mainly bound to the second or middle carbon of glycerol.

Choline comprises about 15% of the weight of phosphatidyl-choline. (See monograph on Choline.)

ACTIONS AND PHARMACOLOGY
ACTIONS
Phosphatidylcholine may have hepatoprotective activity.

Phosphatidylcholine is important for normal cellular membrane composition and repair. Phosphatidylcholine is also the major delivery form of the essential nutrient choline. Choline itself is a precursor in the synthesis of the neurotransmitter acetylcholine, the methyl donor betaine and phospholipids, including phosphatidylcholine and sphingo-myelin among others. (See the Choline monograph for further discussion.) Phosphatidylcholine is involved in the hepatic export of very-low-density lipoproteins.

MECHANISM OF ACTION
Phosphatidylcholine's role in the maintenance of cell-membrane integrity is vital to all of the basic biological processes. These are: information flow that occurs within cells from DNA to RNA to proteins; the formation of cellular energy and intracellular communication or signal transduction. Phosphatidylcholine, particularly phosphatidylcholine rich in polyunsaturated fatty acids, has a marked fluidizing effect on cellular membranes. Decreased cell-membrane fluidization and breakdown of cell-membrane integrity, as well as impairment of cell-membrane repair mechanisms, are associated with a number of disorders, including liver disease, neurological diseases, various cancers and cell death.

PHARMACOKINETICS
Phosphatidylcholine is absorbed into the mucosal cells of the small intestine, mainly in the duodenum and upper jejunum, following some digestion by the pancreatic enzyme phospholipase, producing lysophosphatidylcholine (lysolecithin). Re-acylation of lysolecithin takes place in the intestinal mucosal cells, reforming phosphatidylcholine, which is then transported by the lymphatics in the form of chylomicrons to the blood. Phosphatidylcholine is transported in the blood in various lipoprotein particles, including very-low-density lipoproteins (VLDL), low-density lipoproteins (LDL) and high-density lipoproteins (HDL); it is then distributed to the various tissues of the body. Some phosphatidylcholine is incorporated into cell membranes.

Phosphatidylcholine is also metabolized to choline, fatty acids and glycerol. The fatty acids and glycerol either get oxidized to produce energy or become involved in lipogenesis. Choline is a precursor of acetylcholine. Serum choline levels peak between 2 to 6 hours after oral intake.

INDICATIONS AND USAGE
Phosphatidylcholine may be indicated to help restore liver function in a number of disorders, including alcoholic fibrosis, and possibly viral hepatitis. It may also be indicated for the treatment of some manic conditions. There is some evidence that Phosphatidylcholine may be useful in the management of Alzheimer's disease and some other cognitive disorders. A possible future role in cancer therapy is also suggested by recent research. It may also be indicated in some with tardive dyskinesia.

RESEARCH SUMMARY
Clinical studies have demonstrated that choline is essential for normal liver function. Phosphatidylcholine is a better delivery form and is also more tolerable than choline. But, in addition, research has shown that phosphatidylcholine, independent of its choline content, has striking hepatoprotective effects. In two animal studies using baboons fed diets high in alcohol, some supplemented with a soy-derived polyunsaturated lecithin (60% phosphatidylcholine) and some unsupplemented, both fibrosis and cirrhosis were largely prevented in the phosphatidylcholine group. Most of the unsupplemented animals in these studies, which continued for up to eight years, developed fibrosis or cirrhosis.

Because these researchers had previously found that choline, equal in amounts contained in the phosphatidylcholine-rich lecithin they subsequently used, had no comparable protective effects on the liver, they concluded that the polyunsaturated phospholipids themselves may have been responsible for the benefits observed.

In vitro studies have shown that these phospholipids increase hepatic collagenase activity and may thus help prevent fibrosis and cirrhosis by encouraging collagen breakdown. Several other mechanisms under investigation may also contribute.

Others have reported similarly encouraging results in animal models. Clearly, human trials are warranted.

In addition, phosphatidylcholine has demonstrated other protective effects in non-alcoholic liver disorders, including protection against various other toxic substances. Its benefits in viral hepatitis were reported some years ago by several different research groups in Europe and elsewhere. In one of these studies, individuals suffering from hepatitis type A and B were given 1.8 grams of phosphatidylcholine daily. Compared with unsupplemented controls, the phosphatidyl-choline group enjoyed quicker recoveries, fewer relapses and quicker normalization of liver function tests.

Researchers in Great Britain treated chronic active hepatitis C patients with 3 grams daily of phosphatidylcholine in double-blind fashion. The phosphatidylcholine patients had significantly reduced symptoms, compared with controls. All histologic evidence of the disease disappeared in some cases. These researchers, like others, have hypothesized that phosphatidylcholine's possible antiviral effects are related to the supplement's apparent ability to increase cellular membrane fluidity and repair the membranes of liver cells.

Phosphatidylcholine may help some with tardive dyskinesia, a neurological disorder characterized by defective cholinergic nerve activity. Both supplemental choline and phosphatidylcholine were found to reduce the muscular hyperactivity of this disorder by about 50% in some studies. However, one significant trial did not see a beneficial effect.

There is some very preliminary evidence that phosphatidylcholine may help control manic symptoms in some.

There has been hope, for some time, that phosphatidylcholine would demonstrate clear-cut benefits in cognitive disorders, such as age-related memory loss and Alzheimer's disease. There are a few reports that supplemental choline can improve short-term memory skills and enhance the memories of those who are initial poor learners.

Those with Alzheimer's disease have a diminished ability to synthesize and/or utilize the neurotransmitter acetylcholine, particularly in those areas of the brain related to memory, thus the hope that supplemental choline/phosphatidylcholine might be of benefit. A few studies have suggested some small benefit in memory restoration, but most have not. Research continues.

Recently it has been suggested that phosphatidylcholine might eventually have some therapeutic role in some cancers. There is no evidence of this to date, but animal studies indicate that deficiencies in choline and phosphatidylcholine may disrupt cell membrane signal transduction in ways that could lead to various cancers. There is ample evidence that liver cancer is promoted in various animals by choline-deficient diets, and it has been shown that excess choline can protect against liver cancer in a mouse model.

Phosphatidylcholine has been used to lower serum cholesterol levels, based on the premise that lecithin cholesterol acyltransferase (LCAT) activity has an important role in the removal of cholesterol from tissues. A few studies have shown reduction in serum cholesterol with phosphatidylcholine intake. The results were quite modest, and most studies have not shown any significant cholesterol-lowering activity.

CONTRAINDICATIONS, PRECAUTIONS, ADVERSE REACTIONS

CONTRAINDICATIONS

There are no reported or known contraindications of phosphatidylcholine supplementation.

PRECAUTIONS

Those with malabsorption problems may develop diarrhea or steatorrhea when using phosphatidylcholine supplements. Those with the antiphospholipid-antibody syndrome should exercise caution in the use of phosphatidylcholine supplements.

ADVERSE REACTIONS

No major side effects have been reported. Mild side effects have been noted occasionally such as nausea, diarrhea and increased salivation in some. This holds for all forms of phosphatidylcholine.

INTERACTIONS

There are no known interactions.

OVERDOSAGE

There are no reports of overdosage.

DOSAGE AND ADMINISTRATION

There are several forms of phosphatidylcholine supplements. Typical commercial lecithin supplements contain 20 to 30% phosphatidylcholine. Softgel capsules containing 55% and 90% phosphatidylcholine are available. Liquid concentrates containing 3 grams of phosphatidylcholine per 5 milliliters (one teaspoon) are also available.

Recommended doses range from 3 to 9 grams of phosphatidylcholine daily in divided doses.

LITERATURE

Atoba MA, Ayoola EA, Ogunseyinde O. Effects of essential phospholipid choline on the course of acute hepatitis-B infection. *Trop Gastroenterol.* 1985; 6:96-9.

Buko V, Lukivskaya O, Nikitin V, et al. Hepatic and pancreatic effects of polyenoylphosphatidylcholine in rats with alloxan-induced diabetes. *Cell Biochem Funct.* 1996; 14:131-137.

Canty DJ, Zeisel SH. Lecithin and choline in human health and disease. *Nutr Rev.* 1994; 52:327-339.

Cohen BM, Lipinski JF, Altesman RI. Lecithin in the treatment of mania: double-blind, placebo-controlled trials. *Am J Psychiatry.* 1982; 139:1162-1164.

Gelenberg AJ, Dorer DJ, Wojcik JD, et al. A crossover study of lecithin treatment of tardive dyskinesia. *J Clin Psychiatry.* 1990; 51:149-153.

Growdon JH, Gelenberg AJ, Doller J, et al. Lecithin can suppress tardive dyskinesia. *N Engl J Med.* 1978; 298:1029-1030.

Hanin I, Ansell GB, eds. *Lecithin. Technological, Biological and Therapeutic Aspects.* New York and London: Plenum Press; 1987.

Hirsch MJ, Growdon JH, Wurtman RJ. Relations between dietary choline or lecithin intake, serum choline levels, and various metabolic indices. *Metabolism.* 1978; 27:953-960.

Jackson IV, Nuttall EA, Ibe IO, Perez-Cruet J. Treatment of tardive dyskinesia with lecithin. *Am J Psychiatry.* 1979; 136:1458-1460.

Jenkins PJ, Portmann BP, Eddleston AL, Williams R. Use of polyunsaturated phosphatidylcholine in HBsAg negative chronic active hepatitis: results of prospective double-blind controlled trial. *Liver.* 1982; 2:7-81.

Kosina F, Budka K, Kolouch Z, et al. Essential cholinephospholipids in the treatment of virus hepatitis. *Cas Lek Cesk.* 1981; 120:957-960.

Lieber CS, Leo MA, Aleynik SI, et al. *Alcohol Clin Exp Res.* 1997; 21:375-379.

Lieber CS, De Carl LM, Mak KM, et al. Attenuation of alcohol-induced hepatic fibrosis by polyunsaturated lecithin. *Hepatol.* 1990; 12:1390-1398.

Little A, Levy R, Chuaqui-Kidd P, Hand D. A double-blind, placebo-controlled trial of high-dose lecithin in Alzheimer's disease. *J Neur Neurosurg Psych.* 1985; 48:736-742.

Visco G. Polyunsaturated phosphatidylcholine in association with vitamin B complex in the treatment of acute viral hepatitis B. results of a randomized double-blind clinical study. *Clin Ter.* 1985; 114:183-188.

Wurtman RJ, Hefti F, Melamed E. Precursor control of neurotransmitter synthesis. *Pharmac Rev.* 1981; 32:315-335.

Wurtman RJ, Hirsch MJ, Growdon JH. Lecithin consumption raises serum-free-choline levels. *Lancet.* 1977; 2(8028):68-69.

Phosphatidylserine

DESCRIPTION

Phosphatidylserine is a phospholipid that is a structural component of biological membranes of plants, animals and other life forms. Phosphatidylserine was first isolated from brain lipids called cephalins. The major cephalins are phosphatidylserine and phophatidylethanolamine. Another major phospholipid found in egg yolks and soya is phosphatidylcholine, also known, chemically, as lecithin. Phosphatidylserine is also isolated from soya and egg yolks.

Phosphatidylserine is made up of a glycerophosphate skeleton linked to two fatty acid molecules and the amino acid L-serine. It is an amphiphilic molecule because it is made up of the lipophilic fatty acid tails on one side and the hydrophilic head group containing phosphate and serine on the other side of the molecule. Phosphatidylserine is located in the internal layers of biologic membranes, facing the cytoplasm with its polar head group. In animal tissues, phosphatidylserine is formed from phosphatidylethanolamine by exchange of the ethanolamine head for L-serine. Phosphatidylethanolamine itself is synthesized from diacylglycerol and CDP-ethanolamine.

Phosphatidylserine is known chemically as 1,2-diacyl-sn-glycerol-(3)-L-phosphoserine. It is abbreviated as Ptd Ser, $Acyl_2$ Gro PSer and PS. Most commonly, it is called phosphatidylserine or PS. It has the following chemical structure:

Phosphatidylserine

The fatty acid composition of phosphatidylserine derived from bovine brain and soya lecithin differ. Phosphatidylserine from soya lecithin contains mainly polyunsatured fatty acids, while phosphatidylserine derived from bovine brain contains mainly saturated and monounsaturated fatty acids, as well as some docosahexaenoic acid.

Phosphatidylserine is involved in signal transduction activity as well as being a basic structural component of biologic membranes.

ACTIONS AND PHARMACOLOGY

ACTIONS

Supplemental phosphatidylserine may have cognition enhancing activity.

MECHANISMS OF ACTION

Since the action of phosphatidylserine has not been established, any discussion of the mechanism of action is speculative. However, some findings from animal studies are of interest. Cholinergic hypofunction is thought to account in part for the cognitive deficits found in Alzheimer's disease. The most commonly used drugs for the treatment of Alzheimer's disease are reversible acetylcholinesterase inhibitors. The rationale of these drugs is to increase acetylcholine levels in the brains of Alzheimer's patients, and they may be somewhat effective in some cases. Animal studies indicate that phosphatidylserine restores acetylcholine release in aging rats by maintaining an adequate supply of the molecule and is able to increase the availability of endogenous choline for *de novo* acetylcholine synthesis.

The hippocampus of the brain is believed to be important for cognitive processes and is affected in those with Alzheimer's disease. The dendritic spines of pyramidal cells, the post-synaptic target of the excitatory input to the hippocampus, have been proposed as a substrate for information storage. Age-dependent dendritic spine loss in pyramidal neurons has been reported in the human brain, and the extent of synaptic loss appears to correlate with the degree of cognitive impairment. Rat experiments indicate that phosphatidylserine treatment prevents the age-related reduction in dendritic spine density in rat hippocampus. Protein kinase C facilitation of acetylcholine release has been reported in rats. Phosphatidylserine was found to restore protein kinase C activity in aging rats. Stimulation of calcium uptake by brain synaptosomes and activation of protein kinase C are yet other speculative mechanisms of phosphatidylserine's putative cognition-enhancing action.

PHARMACOKINETICS

Pharmacokinetic studies of phosphatidylserine have been performed in rats. Little is known of the pharmacokinetics of oral phosphatidylserine in humans. In rats, it appears that there is extensive digestion of phosphatidylserine in the small intestine, producing, among other things, lysophosphatidylserine, a substance that contains only one fatty acid, and phosphatidylethanolamine.

Following absorption, lysophosphatidylserine is metabolized in intestinal mucosa cells, and its metabolites, which include some phosphatidylserine, enter the lymphatics draining the small intestine. It appears that only a small fraction of ingested phosphatidylserine reaches the systemic circulation as part of the phospholipid pool. The amount that reaches the brain, after either intraperitoneal injection or oral administration, is very small. Most of the behavioral and neurochemical effects noted in animal studies have been observed only after repeated intraperitoneal and oral phosphatidylserine dosing.

INDICATIONS AND USAGE

Phosphatidylserine has demonstrated some usefulness in treating cognitive impairment, including Alzheimer's disease, age-associated memory impairment and some non-Alzheimer's dementias. More research is needed before phosphatidylserine can be indicated for immune enhancement or for reduction of exercise stress.

RESEARCH SUMMARY

Several double-blind studies suggest that phosphatidylserine can help maintain cognitive function in older individuals and may be able to improve memory and learning skill in some. These results, while encouraging, are not, to date, dramatic.

Various animal experiments have also demonstrated some benefits including stimulation of brain catecholaminergic turnover and increased acetylcholine output from the cerebral cortex of adult and old rats, as well as enhanced neurotransmitter and central nervous system signal transduction. There is evidence that phosphatidylserine can help maintain the hippocampal dendritic spine population of aging rats. It has been suggested that these spines serve as a substrate for information storage. There are several studies demonstrating improved cognitive function in several animal models.

In the largest multicenter study to date of phosphatidylserine and Alzheimer's disease, 142 subjects aged 40 to 80 were given 200 milligrams of phosphatidylserine per day or placebo over a three-month period. Those treated with phosphatidylserine exhibited improvement on several items on the scales normally used to assess Alzheimer's status. The differences between placebo and experimental groups were small but statistically significant. Researchers directing a smaller study, also achieving statistical significance with respect to several measures, characterized the therapeutic effects of phosphatidylserine in their Alzheimer's subjects as "mild."

Phosphatidylserine has also shown some efficacy in some non-Alzheimer's dementias, in age-associated memory impairment and general mental deterioration. More clinical trials need to be conducted before anything conclusive can be said about phosphatidylserine in the treatment of cognition impairment. But, given the results to date and the fact that there are so few side effects associated with phosphatidylserine and so few treatment options for Alzheimer's disease, one research group concludes that "the therapeutic possibilities offered by phosphatidylserine should not be dismissed." There are some animal studies demonstrating positive immunomodulatory effects but, as yet, no human studies showing similar effects. There is preliminary research indicating that phosphatidylserine, at doses of 400 to 800 milligrams per day, can inhibit exercise-induced increases in cortisol.

CONTRAINDICATIONS, PRECAUTION, ADVERSE REACTIONS

CONTRAINDICATIONS

Phosphatidylserine supplementation is contraindicated in those hypersensitive to any component of the preparation.

PRECAUTIONS

Because of lack of long-term safety studies, phosphatidylserine should be avoided by children, pregnant women and nursing mothers. Those with the antiphospholipid-antibody syndrome should exercise caution in the use of phosphatidylserine and only take it under medical supervision and monitoring.

ADVERSE REACTIONS

Occasional gastrointestinal side effects, such as nausea and indigestion, are reported.

INTERACTIONS

There are no reported drug, nutritional supplement, food or herb interactions with phosphatidylserine.

OVERDOSAGE

There are no reports of overdosage.

LD$_{50}$ in rats is more than 5g/kg, and in rabbits is more than 2g/kg.

DOSAGE AND ADMINISTRATION

Phosphatidylserine supplements derived from both bovine brain and from soya lecithin are available. Phosphatidylserine derived from soya lecithin undergoes an enzymatic process that converts phosphatidylcholine to phosphatidylserine. Because of the hypothetical possibility of bovine spongiform encephalopathy, the soya-derived phosphatidylserine is preferred. Typical doses are 100 milligrams three time daily.

HOW SUPPLIED

Capsules — 50 mg, 100 mg, 500 mg

LITERATURE

Amaducc L, SMID Group. Phosphatidylserine in the treatment of Alzheimer's disease. Results of a multicenter study. *Psychopharmacol Bull.* 1988; 24:130-134.

Baer E, Maurukas J. Phosphatidyl serine. *J Biol Chem.* 1955; 212:25-38.

Blokland A, Honig W, Brouns F, Jolles J. Cognition-enhancing properties of subchronic phosphatidylserine (PS) treatment in middle-aged rats: comparison of bovine cortex PS with eggs PS and soybean PS. *Nutr.* 1999; 15: 778-783.

Casamenti F, Scali C, Pepeu G. Phosphatidylserine reverses the age-development decrease in cortical acetylcholine release: a microdialysis study. *Eur J Pharmac.* 1991; 194:11-16.

Crook T, Petrie W, Wells C, et al. Effects of phosphatidylserine in Alzheimer's disease. *Psychopharmacol Bull.* 1992; 28:61-66.

Crook TH, Tinklenberg J, Yesavage J, et al. Effects of phosphatidylserine in age-associated memory impairment. *Neurol.* 1991; 41:644-649.

Folch J. Brain cephalin, a mixture of phosphatides. Separation from it of phosphatidyl serine, phosphatidyl ethanolamine, and a fraction containing an inositol phosphatide. *J Biol Chem.* 1942; 146:35-41.

Monteleleone P, Maj M, Reinat L, et al. Blunting by chronic phosphatidylserine administration of the stress-induced activation of the hypothalamo-pituitary-adrenal axis in healthy men. *Eur J Pharmacol.* 1992; 41:385-388.

Nunzi MG, Milan F, Guidolin D, Toffano G. Dendritic spine loss in hippocampus of aged rats. Effect of brain phosphatidylserine. *Neurobiol Aging.* 1987; 8:501-510.

Pepeu G, Marconcini Pepeu I, Amaducc L. A review of phosphatidylserine pharmacological and clinical effects. Is phosphatidylserine a drug for the ageing brain? *Pharmacol Res.* 1996; 33:73-80.

Phosphatidylserine- a novel pharmacological approach to brain ageing. *Clin Trials J.* 1987; 24:1-130.

Villardita C, Grioli S, Salmeri G, et al. Multicentre clinical trial of brain phophatidylserine in elderly patients with intellectual deterioration. *Clinic Trials J.* 1987; 24:84-93.

Zanott A, Valzelli L, Toffano G. Chronic phosphatidylserine treatment improves spatial memory and passive avoidance in aged rats. *Psychopharmacol.* 1989; 99:316-321.

Phosphorus

DESCRIPTION

Phosphorus is an essential macromineral in human nutrition and plays pivotal roles in the structure and function of the body. Phosphorus, in its pentavalent phosphate form, is essential for the process of bone mineralization and makes up the structure of bone. Approximately 85% of phosphorus in the adult body is in bone. Phosphorus in the form of phospholipids makes up the structure of cellular membranes. Phosphorus also makes up the structure of nucleic acids and nucleotides, including adenosine triphosphate, among other things. Life has been said to be built around phosphorus.

The ability of cells to actively transport phosphate is recognized as a requirement for mineralization in bone. There is some recent evidence that phosphate may regulate the expression of a gene that might be involved in bone mineralization. Phosphate has been found to regulate the expression of the phosphorylated glycoprotein osteopontin. Osteopontin is thought to modulate hydroxyapatite crystal elongation, among other things.

Phosphorus is a non-metallic element with atomic number 15 and an average atomic weight of 30.97 daltons. Its symbol is P. Phosphorus occurs in nature as phosphates in the soil and, in particular, the mineral apatite. The total adult body content of phosphorus is about 700 grams. It accounts for about 2%-4% of the dry weight of most cells.

Phosphorus, mainly in the form of phosphates, is widely distributed in the food supply, and phosphorus intake from the normal diet is usually sufficient to meet the body's phosphorus needs. Milk and milk products are particularly rich sources of phosphorus. One liter of milk contains about 1,000 milligrams of phosphorus. Phosphorus deficiency states, however, do occur but usually they are caused by some disease process. For example, those with malabsorption syndromes and those with diseases causing renal tubular losses of phosphorus can become phosphorus depleted. In addition, those with malnutrition, alcoholics and critically ill patients, such as those being treated for diabetic ketoacidosis, are at risk for phosphorus deficiency, as well as phosphorus imbalance. The so-called refeeding syndrome can cause hypophosphotemia which may be life-threatening.

Phosphorus deficiency can result in anorexia, impaired growth, osteomalacia, skeletal demineralization, proximal muscle atrophy and weakness, cardiac arrhythmias, respiratory insufficiency, increased erythrocyte and lymphocyte dysfunction, susceptibility to infectious rickets, nervous system disorders and even death. Phosphate salts are used in the treatment of phosphorus deficiency. Besides their use for the treatment of phosphorus deficiency, phosphorus supplements are not widely used in the United States. The one exception is calcium phosphate, which is mainly used as a delivery form of calcium.

ACTIONS AND PHARMACOLOGY

ACTIONS

Supplemental phosphorus is used to treat phosphorus deficiency. Calcium phosphate is mainly used as a delivery form of calcium. Phosphorus has putative ergogenic (exercise performance-enhancement) activity.

MECHANISM OF ACTION

Phosphate salts are delivery forms of phosphorus and are used parenterally and orally under conditions of phosphate deficiency.

See Calcium for actions and mechanism of actions of that nutrient.

Short term phosphate-loading, using phosphate salts such as dibasic calcium phosphate ($CaHPO_4$), tribasic sodium phosphate (Na_3PO_4) or dibasic sodium and dibasic potassium phosphates, are used by some athletes who are not phosphorus deficient for performance enhancement.

The effectiveness of phosphate-loading is questionable. The mechanism proposed for this putative effect is attributed to the possible increase of 2, 3-diphosphoglycerate (2,3-DPG) with increased intake of phosphate. 2,3-DPG shifts the oxyhemoglobin dissociation curve to the right, thus allowing a greater unloading of oxygen at the tissue level. Although a few studies suggest that phosphate supplementation in phosphorus-sufficient subjects may increase 2,3-DPG levels in erythrocytes, most studies have reported that it does not have this effect.

PHARMACOKINETICS

Phosphorus supplements are inorganic phosphate salts of sodium, potassium or calcium. Calcium phosphate is a supplement used to supply both calcium and phosphorus. The efficiency of absorption of inorganic forms of phosphorus from the gastrointestinal tract ranges from 55% to 70% in adults. The efficiency of absorption of food phosphorus, which is a mixture of inorganic and organic forms of phosphorus, is similar. Organic forms of phosphorus are hydrolyzed by phosphatases, and therefore most phosphorus absorption occurs as absorption of inorganic phosphate.

Absorption of phosphate occurs by both a saturable, active transport process and by passive diffusion. The saturable, active transport process is stimulated by the active form of vitamin D, 1, 25 dihydroxycholecalciferol (1, 25 (OH_2) D_3). The absorption of phosphorus is mainly via the passive, concentration-dependent process.

Phosphorus is transported via the portal circulation to the liver where the hepatocytes extract a fraction of it for their metabolic requirements. Phosphorus is transported via the systemic circulation to the various tissues of the body, where it is used for the metabolic requirements of these tissues. Excretion of phosphorus is mainly via the kidneys. Phosphorus is freely filtered in the glomerulus. Greater than 80% of the filtered phosphorus is reabsorbed in the proximal tubule and a small amount in the distal tubule. Parathyroid hormone adjusts the renal clearance of phosphorus. In the healthy adult, urine phosphorus is essentially equal to absorbed phosphorus.

INDICATIONS AND USAGE

Apart from its use in conditions of phosphorus deficiency, supplemental phosphorus has produced mixed results in tests of its putative ability to enhance exercise performance.

RESEARCH SUMMARY

Oral, enteral and parenteral phosphorus are used as replacement therapy in hypophosphatemia, a condition seen in some with chronic alcoholism or diabetic ketoacidosis, among others.

Claims that supplemental phosphorus enhances athletic performance are supported by some studies and are refuted by others. The majority of studies provide some support. In an early study, phosphate loading in ten trained distance runners attenuated increases in blood lactate after exercise. In another study, 1,000 milligrams of tribasic sodium phosphate four times a day for six days significantly increased maximal oxygen uptake and ventilatory anaerobic threshold. Phosphate loading did not, however, significantly improve five-mile run times compared with placebo, in these subjects.

Tribasic sodium phosphate loading enhanced endurance performance in competitive cyclists and triathletes in a placebo-controlled study. Dosage was 1 gram of phosphate four times a day for three days prior to exercise testing. Another study has suggested that athletes on caloric-restricted diets may benefit from increased dietary phosphorus intake. Researchers have cited limited data indicating that low-phosphorus status may increase incidence of muscle cramps. Again, increased dietary intake of, rather than supplementation with, phosphorus has been suggested. Long-term phosphate supplementation may pose serious health risks.

Not all studies have found benefit from phosphate loading. In a double-blind trial, 1.24 grams of sodium acid phosphate and potassium phosphate, administered one hour before exercise, produced results no better than placebo in male subjects, in terms of leg power and performance on a high-intensity treadmill exercise. Calcium phosphate loading similarly failed to improve work tolerance or aerobic capacity among male runners, compared with placebo, and, in yet another trial, dibasic calcium phosphate loading was found to be ineffective as an ergogenic aid in subjects of different aerobic fitness levels.

More study will be needed to determine whether phosphate loading has significant benefits in exercise performance.

CONTRAINDICATIONS, PRECAUTIONS, ADVERSE REACTIONS

CONTRAINDICATIONS

Phosphorus supplements are contraindicated in those with hyperphosphatemia and in those with severely impaired renal function (less than 30% of normal). In addition, potassium phosphate is contraindicated in those with hyperkalemia, and calcium phosphate is contraindicated in those with hypercalcemia.

Inorganic phosphates are contraindicated in those with hypersensitivity to any component of an inorganic phosphate-containing supplement.

PRECAUTIONS

The use of supplementary phosphorus in those with phosphorus deficiency requires medical supervision.

Pregnant women and nursing mothers should avoid phosphorus intakes greater than RDA amounts.

Athletes who use supplementary phosphorus should avoid using such supplements for more than four to six days since they may cause hypocalcemia.

ADVERSE REACTIONS

The most common adverse reaction with use of sodium or potassium phosphate is diarrhea. The salts are less likely to cause diarrhea when they are used by phosphorus-deficient individuals than when used by those with normal phosphorus status. Other gastrointestinal symptoms that may occur include nausea, vomiting and stomach pain. Those with renal failure may develop hyperphosphatemia and hypocalcemia with potassium or sodium phosphate supplementation. Hyperphosphatemia can result in ectopic calcification. Prolonged use of high doses of inorganic phosphate salts may result in hypocalcemia even in healthy individuals with normal renal function.

INTERACTIONS

DRUGS

Aluminum-containing antacids: Aluminum-containing antacids are used in the treatment of hyperphosphatemia. Concomitant intake of aluminum-containing antacids and phosphorus will decrease absorption of phosphorus (in the phosphate form).

NUTRITIONAL SUPPLEMENTS

Zinc: Concomitant intake of zinc and phosphate salts (sodium phosphate, potassium phosphate, calcium phosphate) may decrease the absorption of zinc.

OVERDOSAGE

There are no reports of overdosage with oral phosphorus supplements in healthy individuals.

DOSAGE AND ADMINISTRATION

Sodium phosphate is available as monobasic sodium phosphate (NaH_2PO_4), dibasic sodium phosphate (Na_2HPO_4) and tribasic sodium phosphate (Na_3PO_4). Potassium phosphate is available as monobasic potassium phosphate (KH_2PO_4), dibasic potassium phosphate (K_2HPO_4) and tribasic potassium phosphate (K_3PO_4). There are also preparations which are mixtures of the different forms. Monobasic sodium and potassium phosphates are the least basic, and tribasic sodium and potassium phosphate are the most basic of these salts. Use of these salts for the treatment of phosphorus deficiency requires medical supervision.

Calcium phosphate salts used for nutritional supplementation are tribasic calcium phosphate ($Ca_3(PO_4)_2$) and dibasic calcium phosphate ($CaHPO_4$). These are used mainly as calcium supplements (see Calcium for dosage).

Some athletes use calcium phosphate for phosphate-loading.

Several homeopathic remedies are phosphate salts. They include kali phosphoricum (potassium phosphate), ferrum phosphoricum (iron phosphate), magnesia phosphorica (magnesium phosphate), natrum phosphoricum (sodium phosphate) and mixtures of phosphates called biochemic phosphates.

Milk is frequently recommended for phosphorus supplementation in phosphorus-deficient individuuals. One milliliter of milk contains approximately one milligram of phosphorus.

The Food and Nutrition Board of the Institute of Medicine of the National Academy of Sciences has recommended the following adequate intakes (AI) and Recommended Dietary Allowance (RDA) for phosphorus:

Infants	(AI)
0 through 6 months	100 mg/day
7 through 12 months	275 mg/day

Children	(RDA)
1 through 3 years	460 mg/day
4 through 8 years	500 mg/day
Boys	
9 through 18 years	1,250 mg/day
Girls	
9 through 18 years	1,250 mg/day
Men	
19 years and greater	700 mg/day
Women	
19 years and greater	700 mg/day
Pregnancy	
14 through 18 years	1,250 mg/day
19 through 50 years	700 mg/day
Lactation	
14 through 18 years	1,250 mg/day
19 through 50 years	700 mg/day

A NOAEL (No-Observed-Adverse-Effect Level) for phosphorus for adults is 10.2 grams/day.

Tolerable upper Intake Levels (UL) for phosphorus for adults is calculated by the Food and Nutrition Board by dividing the NOAEL for phosphorus by an uncertainty factor (UF) of 2.5.

Adults	(UL)
19 through 70 years	4.0 g/day
Infants	
0 through 12 months	Not possible to establish.
Children	
1 through 8 years	3.0 g/day
9 through 18 years	4.0 g/day
Older Adults	
Greater than 70 years	3.0 g/day
Pregnancy	
14 through 50 years	3.5 g/day
Lactation	
14 through 50 years	4.0 g/day

LITERATURE

Beck GR Jr, Zerler B, Moran E. Phosphate is a specific signal for induction of osteopontin gene expression. *Proc Natl Acad Sci USA.* 2000; 97:8352-8357.

Berner YN, Shike M. Consequences of phosphate imbalance. *Ann Rev Nutr.* 1988; 8:121-148.

Bredle DL, Stager JM, Brechue WF, Farber MO. Phosphate supplementation, cardiovascular function, and exercise performance in humans. *J Appl Physiol.* 1988; 65:1821-1826.

Cade R, Conte M, Zauner C, et al. Effects of phosphate loading on 2, 3-diphosphoglycerate and maximal oxygen uptake. *Med Sci Sports Exerc.* 1984; 16:263-268.

Dietary Reference Intake for Calcium, Phosphorous, Magnesium, Vitamin D and Fluoride. Washington, DC: National Academy Press; 1997.

Duffy DJ, Conlee RK. Effects of phosphate loading on leg power and high intensity treadmill exercise. *Med Sci Sports Exerc.* 1986; 18:674-677.

Galloway SD, Tremblay MS. Sexsmith JR, Roberts CJ. The effects of phosphate supplementation in subjects of different aerobic fitness levels. *Eur J Appl Physiol Occup Physiol.* 1996; 72:224-230.

Knochel JP. Phosphorus. In: Shils ME, Olson JA, Shike M, Ross AC, eds. *Modern Nutrition in Health and Disease.* 9th ed. Baltimore, MD: Williams and Wilkins; 1999:157-167.

Kreider RB, Miller GW, Schenk D, et al. Effects of phosphate loading on metabolic and myocardial responses to maximal and endurance exercise. *Int J Sport Nutr.* 1992; 2:20-47.

Kreider RB, Miller GW, Williams MH, et al. Effects of phosphate loading on oxygen uptake, ventilatory anaerobic threshold, and run performance. *Med Sci Sports Exerc.* 1990; 22:250-256.

Loghman-Adham M. Phosphate binders for control of phosphate retention in chronic renal failure. *Pediatr Nephrol.* 1999; 13:701-708.

Stewart I, McNaughton L, Davies P, Tristram S. Phosphate loading and the effects on VO2max in trained cyclists. *Res Q Exerc Sport.* 1990; 61:80-84.

Tremblay MS, Galloway SD, Sexsmith JR. Ergogenic effects of phosphate loading: physiological fact or methodological fiction? *Can J Appl Physiol.* 1994; 19:1-11.

Weisinger JR, Bellorí n-Font E. Magnesium and phosphorus. *Lancet.* 1998; 352:391-396.

Zorbas YG, Federenko YF, Naexu KA. Phosphate-loading test influences on endurance-trained volunteers during restriction of muscular activity and chronic hyperhydration. *Biol Trace Elem Res.* 1995; 48:51-65.

Phytostanols

DESCRIPTION

Phytostanols are saturated phytosterols. (See Phytosterols and Beta-Sitosterol.) That is, they have no double bonds in the sterol ring. Phytosterols, widely found in the plant kingdom, resemble cholesterol. Cholesterol, however, does not occur in plants. The cylcopentanoperhydrophenanthrene ring structure is common to all sterols; the differences among the various sterols are primarily in the structure of the side chains. Beta-sitostanol has the following chemical structure:

Beta-sitostanol

Phytosterols are present in the diet. Typical daily dietary intakes of phytosterols range from 100 to 300 milligrams. It is higher in vegetarians. Saturated phytosterols or phytostanols are also present in the diet in much smaller quantities, usually making up approximately 10 to 20% of the phytosterol intake. There are over 40 phytosterols, but beta-sitosterol is the most abundant one, comprising about 50% of dietary phytosterols. The next most abundant phytosterols are campesterol (about 33%) and stigmasterol (about 2 to 5%).

Phytostanols are potentially atherogenic like cholesterol, but except in the rare genetic disorders, cerebrotendinotic xanthomatosis and sitosterolemia, they are not. This is because so little of the phytosterols, and even less of the phytostanols, are absorbed. On the other hand, phytosterols can lower cholesterol levels. As early as 1951, it was shown that phytosterols lowered cholesterol in chickens, and subsequently they were found to lower cholesterol in other animals and in humans.

Recently, functional foods, containing phytostanols esterified with fatty acids, have entered the marketplace in the form of margarines, spreads and salad dressings. In the case of most of these products, the esterified phytostanols are derived from tall oil from the *Pinaceae* family. Tall oil is a byproduct of the pulp and paper industry. The phytosterols and phytostanols derived from tall oil undergo hydrogenation to produce mainly beta-sitostanol, campestanol and stigmastanol and then, in an esterification step with fatty acids derived from such vegetable oils as rapeseed oil, arrive at the finished product.

Phytostanols are also known as plant stanols and saturated plant sterols. Phytostanols themselves have extremely poor solubility in both aqueous and lipid media. Esterification of phytostanols with long-chain fatty acids increases their lipid solubility.

ACTIONS AND PHARMACOLOGY

ACTIONS
Phytostanols have cholesterol-lowering activity.

MECHANISM OF ACTION
The mechanism of the cholesterol-lowering activity of phytostanols is not fully understood. Phytostanols appear to inhibit the absorption of dietary cholesterol and the reabsorption (via the enterohepatic circulation) of endogenous cholesterol from the gastrointestinal tract. Consequently, the excretion of cholesterol in the feces leads to decreased serum levels of this sterol. Phytostanols do not appear to affect the absorption of bile acids.

It is believed that phytostanols displace cholesterol from bile salt micelles. Another proposed mechanism is the inhibition of the rate of cholesterol esterification in the intestinal mucosa. Much more research is needed on the mechanism of the cholesterol-lowering effect of phytostanols.

PHARMACOKINETICS
Supplemental esterified phytostanols, following ingestion, undergo hydrolysis in the small intestine catalyzed by such enzymes as cholesterol esterase to yield the phytostanols sitostanol, campestanol and stigmastanol. Less than 1% of ingested phytostanols are distributed rapidly and mainly to the liver where some proportion is glucuronidated. The phytostanols are excreted either in the free or glucuronidated form mainly via the biliary route. Virtually all of ingested phytostanols are excreted in the feces.

INDICATIONS AND USAGE
Phytostanols may be indicated for the management of hypercholesterolemia.

RESEARCH SUMMARY
In a double-blind study, 153 subjects with mild hypercholesterolemia were randomized to receive a control margarine or a margarine containing sitostanol ester (1.8 or 2.6 grams of sitostanol daily). The study continued for one year, at the conclusion of which there was a mean reduction in serum cholesterol of 10.2% in the sitostanol groups, compared with a 0.1% increase in the control group. LDL-cholesterol was reduced 14.1% in the sitostanol groups versus 1.1% in the control group. Sitostanol was significantly superior to the control margarine at both dose levels, but the higher dose was significantly more effective than the lower dose. Neither LDL-cholesterol nor triglycerides were affected by sitostanol.

In a more recent study, 318 mildly hypercholesterolemic subjects were randomized to receive margarine containing no phytostanols (placebo control) or margarines with 2 grams or

3 grams of stanol esters daily. Both stanol esters doses were effective, but the 3-gram dose was more effective, lowering total cholesterol by 6.4% and LDL-cholesterol by 10.1%. There was no effect on triglycerides or HDL-cholesterol.

Several other studies have confirmed these results. In a study of post-menopausal women with documented cardiovascular disease, stanol esters decreased total cholesterol by 13% and LDL-cholesterol by 20%, administered in a margarine that delivered 3 grams of sitostanol daily. These women were not taking lipid-lowering medication. In another study, stanol esters augmented the effects of simvastatin in further lowering LDL-cholesterol levels.

Recently, studies have been conducted to compare the relative efficacies of vegetable-oil stanol esters and wood stanol esters. They have found them to be equal in their LDL-cholesterol lowering effects.

Another study has compared a phytostanol ester-supplemented margarine with a soybean margarine that primarily contains sterol esters (see Phytosterols). Both of these, used in similar quantities, were equally significant in reducing LDL-cholesterol by 13%.

CONTRAINDICATIONS, PRECAUTIONS, ADVERSE REACTIONS
CONTRAINDICATIONS
Phytostanol supplementation is contraindicated in those with the rare genetic disorders sitosterolemia and cerebrotendinotic xanthomatosis.

PRECAUTIONS
Phytostanol supplementation should be avoided by pregnant women and nursing mothers.

ADVERSE REACTIONS
Adverse reactions reported with phytostanol or phytosterol ingestion are mainly mild gastrointestinal ones, including occasional indigestion, feeling of fullness, gas, diarrhea and constipation. Phytostanol supplementation is generally well tolerated.

INTERACTIONS
DRUGS
None known to date. Phytostanol supplementation may be additive to the cholesterol-lowering effects of such cholesterol-lowering drugs as the statins.

NUTRITIONAL SUPPLEMENTS AND FOOD
Some randomized trials have indicated that phytostanols, as well as phytosterols, may lower serum levels of alpha- and beta-carotene, lycopene and vitamin E, probably by interfering with their absorption. Neither vitamin A nor vitamin D levels appear to be affected by phytostanol ingestion. There are no data yet available on the effect of phytostanols on other carotenoids, flavonoids or polyphenols.

DOSAGE AND ADMINISTRATION
At present, phytostanols, in the form of fatty acid esters, are available in some functional foods, including margarines, spreads and salad dressing. Phytostanols and phytostanol esters are being developed as nutritional supplements in capsule form.

A few studies indicate a dose of 2 grams of phytostanols daily to be optimal. Doses used are 1.5 to 4.5 grams daily. Capsules, when available, should be taken with meals.

LITERATURE
Gylling H, Miettinen TA. Cholesterol reduction by different plant stand mixtures and with variable fat intake. *Metabolism.* 1999; 48:575-580.

Gylling H, Puska P, Vartiainen E, Miettinen TA. Retinol, vitamin D, carotenes and alpha-tocopherol in serum of a moderately hypercholesterolemic population consuming sitostanol ester margarine. *Atherosclerosis.* 1999; 145:279-285.

Gylling H, Puska P, Vartiainen E, Miettinen TA. Serum sterols during stanol ester feeding in a mildly hypercholesterolemic population. *J Lipid Res.* 1999; 4:593-600.

Gylling H, Radhakrishnan R, Miettinen TA. Reduction of serum cholesterol in post menopausal women with previous myocardial infarction and cholesterol malabsorption induced by dietary sitostanol ester margarine: women and dietary sitostanol. *Circulation.* 1997; 96:4226-4231.

Hallbrook T, Kristiannsson B, Hildebrand H, et al. [Phytosterolemia is an unknown but serious disease. Xanthomatosis in childhood is a warning signal.] *Lakartidningen.* 1996; 93:4275-4277.

Hallikainen MA, Sarkkinen ES, Uusitupa MIJ. Plant stanol esters affect serum cholesterol concentrations of hypercholesterolemic men and women in a dose-dependent manner. *J Nutr.* 2000; 130:767-776.

Hallikainen MA, Sarkkinen ES, Uusitupa MI. Effects of low-fat stanol ester enriched margarines on concentrations of serum carotenoids in subjects with elevated serum cholesterol concentrations. *Eur J Clin Nutr.* 1999; 53:966-969.

Hallikainen MA, Uusitupa MI. Effects of 2 low-fat stanol ester-containing margarines on serum cholesterol concentrations as part of a low-fat diet in hypercholesterolemic subjects. *Am J Clin Nutr.* 1999; 69:403-410.

Jones PJ, Ntanios FY, Rainini-Sarjaz M, Vanstone CA. Cholesterol-lowering efficacy of a sitostanol-containing phytosterol mixture with a prudent diet in hyperlipidemic men. *Am J Clin Nutr.* 1999; 69:1144-1150.

Law M. Plant sterol and stanol margarines and health. *BMJ.* 2000; 320:861-864.

Ling WH, Jones PJ. Enhanced efficacy of sitostanol-containing versus sitostanol-free phytosterol mixtures in altering lipoprotein cholesterol levels and synthesis in rats. *Atherosclerosis.* 1995; 118:319-331.

Miettinen TA Puska P, Gylling H, et al. Reduction of serum cholesterol with sitostanol-ester margarine in a mildly hypercholesterolemic population. *N Eng J Med.* 1995; 333:1308-1312.

Nakamura T, Matsuzawa Y. [Cerebrotendinous xanthomatosis and phytosterolemia.] [Article in Japanese.] *Tanpakushitsu Kakusan Koso.* 1998; 33:794-797.

Plat J, Mensink RP. Vegetable oil based versus wood based stanol ester mixtures: effects on serum lipids and hemostatic factors in non-hypercholesterolemic subjects. *Atherosclerosis.* 2000; 148:101-112.

Nguyen TT, Dale LC. Plant stanol esters and vitamin K. Mayo *Clin Proc.* 1999; 74:642-643.

Nguyen TT, Dale LC, von Bergmann K, et al. Cholesterol-lowering effect of stanol ester in a US population of mildly hypercholesterolemic men and women: a randomized controlled trial. *Mayo Clin Proc.* 1999; 74:1198-1206.

Normé n L, Dutta P, Lia A, Andersson H. Soy sterol esters and beta-sitostanol esters as inhibitors of cholesterol absorption in human small bowel. *Am J Clin Nutr.* 2000; 71:908-913.

Turnbull D, Frankos VH, Leeman WR, Jonker D. Short-term tests of estrogenic potential of plant stanols and plant stanol esters. *Regul Toxicol Pharmacol.* 1999; 29(2 Pt 1):211-215.

Vuorio AF, Gylling H, Turtola H, et al. Stanol ester margarine alone and with simvastatin lowers serum cholesterol in families with familial hypercholesterolemia caused by the FH—North Karelia mutation. *Arterioscler Thromb Vasc Biol.* 2000; 20:500-506.

Phytosterols

TRADE NAMES
Combination products include Phytosterol Complex w/Beta Sitosterol (Source Naturals).

DESCRIPTION
Phytosterols (also see Phytostanols and Beta-Sitosterol), widely found in the plant kingdom, are chemically similar to cholesterol. Cholesterol, however, only occurs in animals and is not found in plants. The cylclopentanoper-hydrophenanthrene ring structure of the sterol molecule is common to all sterols; the differences are primarily in the structure of the side chains.

Phytosterols are present in the diet. Typical daily dietary intakes of phytosterols range from 100 to 300 milligrams. It is higher in vegetarians. There are over 40 phytosterols, but beta-sitosterol is the most abundant one, comprising about 50% of dietary phytosterols. The next most abundant phytosterols are campesterol (about 33%) and stigmasterol (about 2 to 5%). Other phytosterols found in the diet include brassicasterol, delta-7-stigmasterol and delta-7-avenasterol.

Beta-sitosterol differs from cholesterol by the presence of an ethyl group at the 24th carbon position of the side chain. In the case of campesterol, this position is occupied by a methyl group. Chemically, the phytosterols are classified as 4-desmethylsterols of the cholestane series. Beta-sitosterol has the following chemical structure:

Beta-sitosterol

Phytosterols are potentially atherogenic like cholesterol, but except in the rare genetic disorders, sitosterolemia and cerebrotendinotic xanthomatosis, they are not. This is because so little of the phytosterols are absorbed. On the other hand, phytosterols can lower cholesterol levels. As early as 1951, it was shown that phytosterols lowered cholesterol in chickens, and subsequently they were found to lower cholesterol in humans. Recently, functional foods containing phytosterols have become available. These functional foods are in the form of margarines, spreads and salad dressings. In the case of most of these products, phytosterols are found esterified with long-chain fatty acids. These phytosterols are derived from soybean oil and are mainly beta-sitosterol, campesterol and stigmasterol.

Phytosterols are also known as plant sterols and, owing to their large sitosterol content, are sometimes called sitosterol. Phytosterols are virtually insoluble in aqueous media and are poorly soluble in lipid media. Esterification of phytosterols with long-chain fatty acids increases their lipid solubility.

ACTIONS AND PHARMACOLOGY
ACTIONS
Phytosterols have cholesterol-lowering activity.

MECHANISM OF ACTION
The mechanism of the cholesterol-lowering activity of phytosterols is not fully understood. Phytosterols appear to inhibit the absorption of dietary cholesterol and the reabsorption (via the enterohepatic circulation) of endogenous cholesterol from the gastrointestinal tract. Consequently, the excretion of cholesterol in the feces leads to decreased serum levels of this sterol. Phytosterols do not appear to affect the absorption of bile acids.

It is believed that phytosterols displace cholesterol from bile salt micelles. Another proposed mechanism is the possible inhibition of the rate of cholesterol esterification in the intestinal mucosa.

PHARMACOKINETICS

Supplemental esterified phytosterols, following ingestion, undergo hydrolysis in the small intestine, catalyzed by such enzymes as cholesterol esterase, to yield the phytosterols beta-sitosterol, campesterol and stigmasterol. Of course, unesterified phytosterols do not undergo hydrolysis. About 5% of the ingested beta-sitosterol and about 15% of the campesterol are absorbed and transported via the portal circulation to the liver where some fraction of these phytosterols is glucuronidated. The phytosterols are excreted either in the free or glucuronidated form mainly via the biliary route.

INDICATIONS AND USAGE

Phytosterols may be indicated for the management of hypercholesterolemia.

RESEARCH SUMMARY

Phytosterols have been compared with phytostanols to assess their relative efficacy in lowering total cholesterol and LDL-cholesterol. These studies confirm that both are effective in lowering these lipids. A recent review concluded that plant sterols and stanols, in the studies analyzed, reduce, on average, total cholesterol by 10% and LDL-cholesterol by 13%. They have no significant effect in either HDL-cholesterol or triglycerides. (See Phytostanols.)

CONTRAINDICATIONS, PRECAUTIONS, ADVERSE REACTIONS

CONTRAINDICATIONS

Phytosterol supplementation is contraindicated in those with the rare genetic disorders sitosterolemia and cerebrotendinotic xanthomatosis.

PRECAUTIONS

Phytosterol supplementation should be avoided by pregnant women and nursing mothers.

ADVERSE REACTIONS

Adverse reactions are mainly mild gastrointestinal ones, including occasional indigestion, feeling of fullness, gas, diarrhea and constipation. Phytosterol supplementation is generally well tolerated.

INTERACTIONS

DRUGS

None known to date. Phytosterol supplementation may be additive to the cholesterol-lowering effects of such cholesterol-lowering drugs as the statins.

NUTRITIONAL SUPPLEMENTS AND FOOD

Some randomized trials have indicated that phytosterols may lower serum levels of alpha- and beta-carotene, lycopene and vitamin E, probably by interfering with their absorption. Neither vitamin A nor vitamin D levels appear to be affected by phytosterol ingestion. There are no data yet available on the effect of phytosterols on other carotenoids (lutein, zeaxanthin), flavonoids or polyphenols.

OVERDOSAGE

No reports of overdosage.

DOSAGE AND ADMINISTRATION

Phytosterols are available in the form of fatty acid esters in some functional food products, including margarines, spreads and salad dressing. Unesterified phytosterols are available in capsules. Doses of the phytosterol esters range from 1.12 to 2.24 grams daily. Doses of the unesterified phytosterols are about 1 gram daily. Capsules, if used, should be taken with meals.

LITERATURE

Ayesh R, Westrate JA, Drewitt PN, Hepburn PA. Safety evaluation of phytosterol esters. Part 5. Faecal short-chain fatty acid and microflora content, faecal bacterial enzyme activity and serum female sex hormones in healthy hormolipidaemic volunteers consuming a controlled diet either with or without a phytosterol ester-enriched margarine. *Food Chem Toxicol.* 1999; 37:1127-1138.

Baker VA, Hepburn PA, Kennedy SJ, et al. Safety evaluation of phytosterol esters. Part 1. Assessment of oestrogenicity using a combination of in vivo and *in vitro* assays. Food *Chem Toxicol.* 1999; 37:13-22.

Hendriks HF, Westrate JA, van Vliet T, Meijer GW. Spreads enriched with three different levels of vegetable oil sterols and the degree of cholesterol lowering in normocholesterolaemic and mildly hypercholesterolaemic subjects. *Eur J Clin Nutr.* 1999; 53:319-327.

Hepburn PA, Horner SA, Smith M. Safety evaluation of phytosterol esters. Part 2. Subchronic 90-day oral toxicity study on phytosterol esters — a novel functional food. *Food Chem Toxicol.* 1999; 37:521-532.

Hallbrook T, Kristiannsson B, Hildebrand H, et al. [Phytosterolemia is an unknown but serious disease. Xanthomatosis in childhood is a warning signal.] *Lakartidningen.* 1996; 93:4275-4277.

Howell TJ, Mac Dougall DE, Jones PJ. Phytosterols partially explain differences in cholesterol metabolism caused by corn or olive oil feeding. *J Lipid Res.* 1998; 39:892-900.

Law M. Plant sterol and stanol margarines and health. *BMJ.* 2000; 320:861-864.

Ling WH, Jones PJ. Dietary phytosterols: a review of metabolism, benefits and side effects. *Life Sci.* 1995; 57:195-206.

Moghadasian MH, Frohlich JJ. Effects of dietary phytosterols on cholesterol metabolism and atherosclerosis: clinical and experimental evidence. *Am J Med.* 1999; 107:588-594.

Moghadasian MH, Mc Manus BM, Pritchard PH, Frohlich JJ. "Tall oil"-derived phytosterols reduce atherosclerosis in ApoE-deficient mice. *Arterioscler Thomb Vasc Biol.* 1997; 17:119-126.

Jones PJ, Howell T, MacDougall DE, et al. Short-term administration of tall oil phytosterols improves plasma lipid profiles in subjects with different cholesterol levels. *Metabolism.* 1998; 47:751-756.

Jones PJ, Mac Dougall DE, Ntanios F, Vanstone CA. Dietary phytosterols as cholesterol-lowering agents in human diet. *Can J Physiol Pharmacol.* 1997; 75:217-227.

Nakamura T, Matsuzawa Y. [Cerebrotendinous xanthomatosis and phytosterolemia.] [Article in Japanese.] *Tanpakushitsu Kakusan Koso.* 1998; 33:794-797.

Normé n L, Dutta P, Lia A, Andersson H. Soy sterol esters and beta-sitostanol esters as inhibitors of cholesterol absorption in human small bowel. *Am J Clin Nutr.* 2000; 71:908-913.

Ntanios FY, Mac Dougall DE, Jones PJ. Gender effects of tall oil versus soybean phytosterols as cholesterol-lowering agents in hamsters. *Can J Physiol Pharmacol.* 1988; 76:780-787.

Sierksma A, Westrate JA, Meijer GW. Spreads enriched with plant sterols, either esterified 4,4-dimethylsterols or free 4-desmethylsterols, and plasma total-and LDL-cholesterol concentrations. *Br J Nutr* 1999. 82:273-282.

Waalkens-Beredsen DH, Wolterbeek AP, Wijnands MV. et al. Safety evaluation of phytosterol esters. Part 3. Two generation study in rats with phytosterol ester — a novel functional food. *Food Chem Toxicol.* 1999; 37:683-696.

Westrate JA, Ayesh R, Bauer-Plank C, Drewitt PN. Safety evaluation of phytosterol esters. Part 4. Faecal concentrations of bile acids and neutral sterols in healthy normolipidaemic volunteers consuming a controlled diet either with or without a phytosterol ester-enriched margarine. *Food Chem Toxicol.* 1999; 37:1063-1071.

Westrate JA. Ayesh R, Meijer GW. Plant sterl-enriched margarines and reduction of plasma total-and LDL-cholesterol concentrations in normocholesterolaemic subjects. *Eur J Clin Nutr.* 1998; 52:334-343.

Piperine

DESCRIPTION

Piperine is an alkaloid found naturally in plants belonging to the *Piperaceae* family, such as *Piper nigrum* L, commonly known as black pepper, and *Piper longum* L, commonly known as long pepper. Piperine is the major pungent substance in these plants and is isolated from the fruit of the black pepper and long pepper plants. Piperine comprises 1 to 99% of these plants. The term black pepper is used both for the plant *Piper nigrum* and the spice that is mainly in the fruit of the plant.

Piperine is a solid substance essentially insoluble in water. It is a weak base that is tasteless at first, but leaves a burning aftertaste. Piperine belongs to the vanilloid family of compounds, a family that also includes capsaicin, the pungent substance in hot chili peppers. Its molecular formula is $C_{17}H_{19}NO_3$, and its molecular weight is 285.34 daltons. Piperine is the trans-trans stereoisomer of 1-piperoylpiperidine. It is also known as (E, E)-1-piperoylpiperidine and (E, E)-1-[5-(1, 3-benzodioxol-5-y1)-1-oxo-2, 4-pentdienyl] piperidine. It is represented by the following chemical structure:

Piperine

Black pepper and long pepper have been used in Ayurvedic medicine for the treatment of various diseases. One such preparation is known by the Sanskrit name trikatu and consists of black pepper, long pepper and ginger. Another preparation, known by the Sanskrit name pippali, consists of long pepper. It is thought that piperine is one of the major bioactive substances of these Ayurvedic remedies. Black pepper has also been used in traditional Chinese medicine to treat seizure disorders. A derivative of piperine, antiepilepsirine, has also been used in China to treat seizure disorders. Some recent research suggests that piperine may enhance the bioavailability of some drugs and nutritional substances.

ACTIONS AND PHARMACOLOGY

ACTIONS

Piperine may have bioavailability-enhancing activity for some nutritional substances and for some drugs. It has putative anti-inflammatory activity and may have activity in promoting digestive processes.

MECHANISM OF ACTION

Piperine has been demonstrated to increase the serum levels and lengthen the serum half lives of some nutritional substances, such as coenzyme Q_{10} and beta-carotene. The mechanism of this action is unknown. It is speculated that piperine may act as a so-called thermonutrient and increase the absorption of certain nutritional substances from the gastrointestinal tract by producing a local thermogenic action. There is no evidence for this.

Piperine has also been found to increase the serum levels and lengthen the serum half lives of some drugs, such as propanolol and theophylline. The mechanism is thought to be by inhibition of certain enzymes involved in the biotransformation of the affected drugs. Piperine has been found to be a nonspecific inhibitor of drug and xenobiotic metabolism. It appears to inhibit many different cytochrome P450 isoforms, as well as UDP-glucuronyltransferase and hepatic arylhydrocarbon hydroxylase and other enzymes involved in drug and xenobiotic metabolism.

The mechanism of piperine's putative anti-inflammatory activity may be accounted for, in part, by piperine's possible antioxidant activity. There are a few studies suggesting that piperine may inhibit lipid peroxidation. Piperine has been shown to stimulate the secretion of the digestive enzymes pancreatic amylase, trypsin, chymotrypsin and lipase in rats. However, piperine appears to have this activity when administered with other spice bioactives, such as capsaicin and curcumin, and not when administered by itself.

PHARMACOKINETICS
The pharmacokinetics of piperine in humans remains incompletely understood. In rats, piperine is absorbed following ingestion, and some metabolites have been identified: piperonylic acid, piperonyl alcohol, piperonal and vanillic acid are found in the urine. One metabolite, piperic acid, is found in the bile. Human pharmacokinetic studies are needed.

INDICATIONS AND USAGE
Piperine, in appropriate doses, may be useful in increasing the bioavailability of some drugs and nutrients. There is very preliminary evidence suggesting that piperine may aid in the digestion of food. There is also preliminary evidence that it may have some anticonvulsant, anticarcinogenic and anti-inflammatory properties. On the other hand, there is also preliminary evidence that it might be carcinogenic and cytotoxic in some circumstances and that it might interfere with reproductive processes and have negative effects on sperm.

RESEARCH SUMMARY
There are in vitro, animal and human studies demonstrating that piperine can significantly increase the bioavailability of numerous drugs and some nutritional supplements. Reportedly, it has demonstrated this effect with some antimicrobial, antiprotozoal, antihelmintic, antihistaminic, non-steroidal anti-inflammatory, muscle-relaxant and anticancer drugs, among others. It has also increased the bioavailability of coenzyme Q10, curcumin and beta-carotene.

In humans given 2-gram doses of curcumin alone, levels of curcumin in serum were undetectable to very low one hour post-administration. Concomitant administration of 20 mg of piperine was said to significantly increase absorption and bioavailability (by 2000%). Similar results were reported in rats.

In a double-blind crossover study, 5 mg of piperine daily for 14-day periods resulted in significant increases in serum beta-carotene levels. The same dose of piperine produced similar results in another study, this one involving coenzyme Q10.

The claim that piperine may aid in the digestion of food is based on some experimental animal data showing that dietary piperine seems to enhance pancreatic amylase lipase, trypsin and chymotrypsin activity.

The claim that piperine may have some anticonvulsant activity comes, in part, from China, where the substance is used in an effort to treat some forms of epilepsy. In mice, piperine injected intraperitoneally inhibited clonic convulsions induced by kainate. It did not significantly block seizure activity induced by L-glutamate, N-methyl-D-aspartate or guanidinosuccinate.

In a rat intestinal model, piperine was said to provide protection against oxidative changes induced by a number of chemical carcinogens. In another study, this one in vitro, piperine reportedly reduced the cytotoxicity of aflatoxin B1 in rat hepatoma cells.

Piperine exhibited significant anti-inflammatory activity in carageenan-induced rat paw edema and in some other experimental models of inflammation. In one animal study, piperine reduced liver lipid peroxidation, acid phosphatase and edema induced by carageenan.

On the negative side, piperine has shown some evidence of being mutagenic and potentially carcinogenic under some circumstances. It has reportedly given rise to mutagenic products on reaction with nitrites. This causes concern since nitrites and piperine may be consumed simultaneously. Risk might increase with high-dose piperine supplementation. In another study, piperine appeared to enhance the bioavailability of aflatoxin B1 in rat tissues. And in yet another study, piperine was found to be cytotoxic to cultured brain neurons. Piperine was said to be non-mutagenic, however, in a study examining effects of the substance on the germ cells of Swiss albino mice.

In a recent study utilizing albino rats, piperine, given at doses of 5 and 10 mg/kg body weight for 30 days, resulted (at the 10-mg/kg dose level) in significant reduction in the weights of testes and accessory sex organs as well as severe damage to seminiferous tubules. The 5-mg/kg dose resulted in partial degeneration of germ cells.

Decreased mating performance, decreased fertility and anti-implantation activity, along with some other adverse reproductive events, were observed in mice given very high doses of piperine.

CONTRAINDICATIONS, PRECAUTIONS, ADVERSE REACTIONS

CONTRAINDICATIONS

Piperine is contraindicated for those who are hypersensitive to any component of a piperine-containing preparation.

PRECAUTIONS

Pregnant women and nursing mothers should avoid piperine supplementation.

Piperine at doses generally higher than 15 mg daily may affect the metabolism of a wide range of drugs and xenobiotics (see Interactions). In some cases, doses lower than 15 mg daily may affect the metabolism of these substances. Those using the drugs listed in Interactions should exercise caution in the use of piperine supplements.

Piperine may form mutagenic and possibly carcinogenic substances with nitrites. Those who eat processed food containing nitrites and nitrates as food preservatives should exercise caution in the use of piperine supplements.

ADVERSE REACTIONS

The typical dose of piperine in nutritional formulas is 5 milligrams, and doses of 15 milligrams daily are rarely exceeded. No adverse reactions have been reported with these doses. Piperine, if exposed to the tongue, is tasteless at first but leaves a burning aftertaste.

INTERACTIONS

DRUGS

Piperine, usually at a dose of 20 mg or greater, has been shown to inhibit the metabolism of the following drugs: propanolol, theophylline, phenytoin, sulfadiazene, rifampicin, isoniazid, ethambutol, pyrazinamide and dapsone. This list is not inclusive. Piperine is a nonspecific inhibitor of drugs and xenobiotics. Most drugs metabolized via cytochrome P450 enzymes would likely be affected by piperine.

NUTRITIONAL SUPPLEMENTS

Piperine at a dose of 5 mg daily has been found to enhance the absorption of beta-carotene and coenzyme Q_{10}. At a dose of 20 mg daily, it has been found to enhance the absorption of curcumin. Piperine may also enhance the absorption of vitamin B_6, vitamin C and the mineral selenium in the form of L-selenomethionine.

FOOD

Piperine may enhance the absorption of beta-carotene, vitamin B_6, Vitamin C and L-selenomethionine found in certain foods.

DOSAGE AND ADMINISTRATION

Piperine is available in stand-alone supplements and in combination products. A typical dose is 5 mg daily. Doses higher than 15 mg daily should be avoided.

LITERATURE

Atal CK, Dubey RK, Singh J. Biochemical basis of enhanced drug bioavailability by piperine: evidence that piperine is a potent inhibitor of drug metabolism. *J Pharmacol Exp Ther.* 1985; 232:258-262.

Badmaev V, Majeed M, Norkus EP. Piperine, an alkaloid derived from black pepper increases serum response of beta-carotene during 14-days of oral beta-carotene supplementation. *Nutr Res.* 1999; 19:381-388.

Badmaev V. Majeed M, Prakash L. Piperine derived from black pepper increases the plasma levels of coenzyme Q_{10} following oral supplementation. *J Nutr Biochem.* 2000; 11:109-113.

Bano G, Raina RK, Zutshi U, et al. Effect of piperine on bioavailability and pharmacokinetics of propanolol and theophylline in healthy volunteers. *Eur J Clin Pharmacol.* 1991; 41:615-617.

D'Hooge R, Pei YQ, Raes A, et al. Anticonvulsant activity of piperine on seizures induced by excitatory amino acid receptor agonists. *Arzneimittelforschung.* 1996; 46:557-560.

Dhuley JN, Raman PH, Mujumdar AM, Naik SR. Inhibition of lipid peroxidation by piperine during experimental inflammation in rats. *Indian J Exp Biol.* 1993; 31:443-445.

Karekar VR, Mujumdar AM, Joshi SS, et al. Assessment of genotoxic effect of piperine using Salmonella typhimurium and somatic and somatic and germ cells of Swiss albino mice. *Arzneimittelforschung.* 1996; 46:972-975.

Khajuria A, Thusu N, Zutshi U, Bedi KL. Piperine modulation of carcinogen induced oxidative stress in intestinal mucosa. *Mol Cell Biochem.* 1998; 189:113-118.

Khajuria A, Zutshi U, Bedi KL. Permeability characteristics of piperine on oral absorption — an active alkaloid from peppers and a bioavailability enhancer. *Ind J Exp Biol.* 1998; 36:46-50.

Majeed M, Badmaev V, Rajendran R. Use of piperine as a bioavailability enhancer. United States Patent No. 5,972,382. Oct. 26, 1999.

Malini T, Manimaran RR, Arunakaran J, et al. Effects of piperine on testis of albino rats. *J Ethnopharmacol.* 1999; 64:219-225.

Mujumdar AM, Dhuley JN, Deshmukh VK, et al. Anti-inflammatory activity of piperine. *Jpn J Med Sci Biol.* 1990; 433:95-100.

Pei YQ. A review of pharmacology and clinical use of piperine and its derivatives. *Epilepsia.* 1983; 24:177-182.

Platel K, Srinivasan K. Influence of digestive spices and their active principles on pancreatic digestive enzymes in albino rats. *Nahrung.* 2000; 44:42-46.

Shenoy NR, Choughuley AS. Characterization of potentially mutagenic products from the nitrosation of piperine. *Cancer Lett.* 1992; 64:235-239.

Shoba G, Joy D, Joseph TM, et al. Influence of piperine on the pharmacokinetics of curcumin in animals and human volunteers. *Planta Med.* 1998; 64:353-356.

Unchern S, Nagata K, Saito H, Fukuda J. Piperine, a pungent alkaloid, is cytotoxic to cultured neutrons from the embryonic rat brain. *Biol Pharm Bull.* 1994; 17:403-406.

Policosanol

DESCRIPTION

Policosanol is the generic term used for a mixture of long-chain primary aliphatic saturated alcohols. These alcohols are derived from the waxes of such plants as sugar cane (*Saccharum officinarium*) and yams (*e.g. Dioscorea opposita*). They are also found in beeswax. The main long-chain alcohol in policosanol is the 28 carbon 1-octanosol, and next most abundant is the 30 carbon 1-triacontanol. Other long-chain alcohols present in much lower concentrations are: 1-docosanol (C_{22}), 1-tetracosanol (C_{24}), 1-hexacosanol (C_{26}), 1-heptacosanol (C_{27}), 1-nonacosanol (C_{29}), 1-dotriacontanol (C_{32}) and 1-tetracontanol (C_{34}). These long-chain alcohols are solid waxy substances and are soluble in water. They are known collectively as fatty alcohols.

ACTIONS AND PHARMACOLOGY

ACTIONS

Policosanol may reduce total serum cholesterol and low-density lipoprotein-cholesterol (LDL-C) levels in some.

MECHANISM OF ACTION

The mechanism of action of reported cholesterol-lowering activity is unknown. Some animal studies suggest that policosanol may inhibit cholesterol syntheses in the liver. It is also unclear if the putative cholesterol-lowering activity is due to octacosanol. The long-chain alcohols appear to have different biological activities, and octacosanol by itself may not have the same activities as policosanol. They may work synergistically.

PHARMACOKINETICS

Pharmacokinetic studies have been performed on octacosanol, the major alcohol in policosanol, in experimental animals and human volunteers. The absorption of octacosanol is variable and low. Octacosanol absorption ranges from about 11% in rats and humans to about 28% in rabbits. Octacosanol is absorbed from the small intestine into the lymph and from there enters the blood stream.

Distribution is primarily to the liver digestive tract, skeletal muscle and adipose tissues. Octacosanol may be partly oxidized to the long-chain saturated fatty acid, octacosanoic acid which undergoes beta-oxidation.

Following a single dose of octacosanol in experimental animals, peak plasma levels are seen between 30 minutes to 2 hours. Following a single dose of octacosanol in human volunteers, peak plasma levels are seen at one hour and four hours later. Bile is the main route of excretion. Renal excretion is negligible.

INDICATIONS AND USAGE

Policosanol may be indicated for reducing cholesterol levels. There is preliminary evidence that it can reduce platelet aggregation in both healthy and hypercholesterolemic individuals and that it may be of benefit in individuals with intermittent claudication. Reports that it can boost energy and enhance sexual performance are anecdotal.

RESEARCH SUMMARY

A mixture of higher aliphatic primary alcohols derived from sugar cane wax has become popular in such places as Cuba for its reputed cholesterol-lowering benefits, energizing effects and enhancement of sexual function. It is also the source of another increasingly popular supplement—octacosanol (the primary long-chain alcohol in policosanol).

There are a number of animal studies suggesting that policosanol can lower cholesterol, that it can inhibit experimentally induced atherosclerotic lesions of cerebral ischemia, that it can help prevent the peroxidation of lipoprotein and inhibit platelet aggregation.

Human studies have been increasing. In one recent study, patients with LDL-cholesterol greater than 160 mg/dl were randomized in double-blind fashion to receive policosanol (10 milligrams daily), lovastatin (20 milligrams daily) or simvastatin (10 milligrams daily). After eight weeks of therapy, LDL-cholesterol was reduced 24% in the policosanol groups, 22% in the lovastatin group and 15% with simvastatin. HDL-cholesterol increased significantly in the policosanol group but not in the other two groups. Policosanol was judged to be "a safe and effective cholesterol reducing agent."

In another recent double-blind study of policosanol's possible effects in hypercholesterolemia, patients received 5 milligrams of policosanol or placebo daily for 12 weeks followed by 10 milligrams of policosanol or placebo for a subsequent 12 weeks. Policosanol (5 and 10 milligrams daily) appeared to significantly reduce LDL-cholesterol (18.2% and 25.6% respectively) and reduce cholesterol (13% and 17.4%). It appeared to raise HDL-cholesterol (15.5% and 28.4%). Triglycerides were unchanged in the first 12-week period but were significantly reduced (5.2%) by the end of the second 12-week period. Side effects were few and minor. There were 11 serious (7 of these were vascular) adverse events among those taking policosanol.

Policosanol appears to significantly reduce platelet aggregation in both healthy and hypercholesterolemic individuals, apparently proving as effective (at 20 milligrams daily doses) as aspirin (100 milligrams per day). The substance also appears to demonstrate beneficial effect in patients with intermittent claudication. Long-term therapy (20 months) using 5 milligrams of policosanol twice a day resulted in significant improvement in treadmill exercise performance and exercise — ECG responses in a group of coronary heart disease patients. The addition of 125 milligrams of aspirin daily further enhanced these results. It is hoped that others will confirm these very promising, largely Cuban studies.

Policosanol's reputed efficacy in boosting energy and enhancing sexual function, particularly male sexual function, is entirely anecdotal.

CONTRAINDICATIONS, PRECAUTIONS, ADVERSE REACTION

CONTRAINDICATIONS

Hypersensitivity to any component of policosanol.

PRECAUTIONS

Policosanol is not recommended for children, pregnant women and nursing mothers. Because of possible antithrombotic activity, those taking warfarin and hemophliacs should exercise caution in the use of policosanol. Policosanol supplementation should be stopped before any surgery.

ADVERSE REACTIONS

Mild gastrointestinal side effects, skin rash, headache, insomnia and weight loss have been reported. The incidence of these adverse reactions is low. Policosanol is generally well tolerated.

Except for possible lowering of serum total cholesterol and LDL-cholesterol, policosanol does not appear to affect any other laboratory test results.

INTERACTIONS

Aspirin: Policosanol showed a synergism with the antithrombotic properties of aspirin in different experimental models.

No adverse interactions have been found with policosanol use in combination with beta-blockers, diuretics, calcium-channel blockers, NSAIDs, anxiolytics, oral hypoglycemic agents, digoxin, nitroglycerin, neuroleptics or anti-depressants.

No known adverse interactions with nutritional supplements, herbs or foods.

OVERDOSAGE

There are no reports of overdosage. A single dose of 1 gram (50 times the maximum recommended dose) was well tolerated by healthy volunteers. Oral LD_{50} in mice, rats and rabbits is higher than 5 grams per kilogram. Policosanol did not induce genotoxic changes in somatic or germ cells, and it does not act as a mutagenic agent. Teratogenic and carcinogenic testing to date have been negative.

DOSAGE AND ADMINISTRATION

The recommended starting dose of policosanol is 5 milligrams daily taken once a day at dinner time. An effect may take up to 12 weeks to be observed. The dose can be doubled to 5 milligrams twice a day, taken at lunch and dinner time. A dose of 20 milligrams daily should not be exceeded.

LITERATURE

Arruzazabala, ML, Carbajal D, Mas R, et al. Cholesterol-lowering effects of policosanol in rabbits. *Biol Res.* 1994; 27:205-208.

Arruzazabala ML, Mas R, Molina V, et al. Effect of policosanol on platelet aggregation in type II hypercholesterolemic patients. *Int J Tissue React.* 1998; 20:119-124.

Arruzazabala ML, Valdes S, Mas R, et al. Comparative study of policosanol, aspirin and the combination therapy policosanol-aspirin on platelet aggregation in healthy volunteers. *Pharmacol Res.* 1997; 36:293-297.

Castano G, Mas R, Roca J, et al. A double-blind, placebo-controlled study of the effects of policosanol in patients with intermittent claudication. *Angiology.* 1999; 50:123-130.

Hernandez F, Illnait J, Mas R, et al. Effect of policosanol on serum lipids and lipoproteins in healthy volunteers. *Current Therap Res.* 1992; 52:568-575.

Mas R, Castano G, Illnait J, et al. Effects of policosanol in patients with type II hypercholesterolemia and additional coronary risk factors. *Clin Pharmaco Ther.* 1999; 64:439-447.

Menendez R, Frago V, Amor GM, et al. Oral administration of policosanol inhibits in vitro copper ion-induced rat lipoprotein peroxidation. *Physiol Behav.* 1999; 67: 1-7.

Prat H, Roman O, Piro E. Comparative effects of policosanol and two HMG-CoA reductase inhibitors on type II hypercholesterolemia. *Rev Med Chil.* 1999; 127:286-294.

Stusser R, Batista J, Padron R, et al. Long-term therapy with policosanol improves treadmill exercise- ECG testing performance of coronary heart disease patients. *Int J Clin Pharmacol Ther.* 1998; 36:469-473.

Torres O, Agramante AJ, Illnait J, et al. Treatment of hypercholesterolemia in NIDDM with policosanol. *Diabet Care.* 1995; 18:393-396.

Potassium

TRADE NAMES

Potassium is available generically from numerous manufacturers as an OTC product. Branded products include: Potassium Fortified (Rexall Consumer), Potassium '99' (McGuff), Glu-K (Western Research Labs), K-99 (Bio-Tech Pharmacal), K-Glucon (Wesley Pharmacal).

DESCRIPTION

Potassium is an essential macromineral in human nutrition with a wide range of biochemical and physiological roles. Among other things, it is important in the transmission of nerve impulses, the contraction of cardiac, skeletal and smooth muscle, the production of energy, the synthesis of nucleic acids, the maintenance of intracellular tonicity and the maintenance of normal blood pressure. In 1928, it was first suggested that high potassium intake could exert an anti-hypertensive effect. Accumulating evidence suggests that diets high in potassium may be protective not only against hypertension, but also strokes and cardiovascular disease and possibly other degenerative diseases, as well.

Potassium is a metallic element with atomic number 19 and an average atomic weight of 39.09 daltons. Its symbol is K. It is an alkali metal and belongs to the same group as lithium, sodium, rubidium, cesium and francium. The only non-alkali element that it shares some similarities with is thallium. The thallous cation is similar in size to the potassium cation, which is the basis of the use of thallium for myocardial perfusion imaging. The thallous cation is considered a potassium cation analogue. Potassium exists physiologically in its univalent cationic state. It is the principal intracellular cation with an intracellular concentration of about 145 milliequivalents or millimoles per liter. This is 30 to 40 times greater than its extracellular concentration, which is normally 3.5 to 5.0 milliequivalents or millimoles per liter. About 98% of the body's potassium is in intracellular fluid.

The major cause of potassium deficiency is excessive losses of potassium through the alimentary tract or through the kidneys. Potassium depletion typically occurs as a consequence of prolonged use of oral diuretics, from severe diarrhea and from primary or secondary hyperaldosteronism, diabetic ketoacidosis or in those on long-term total parenteral nutrition who have received inadequate potassium. Signs and symptoms of potassium deficiency include hypokalemia, metabolic alkalosis, anorexia, weakness, fatigue, listlessness and cardiac dysrhythmias. Prominent U-waves are seen in the electrocardiograms of those with hypokalemia.

The intake of potassium in the American diet ranges from about 1,560 to 4,680 milligrams (40 to 120 milliequivalents or millimoles) daily. The potassium intake of vegetarians is at the high end. Foods that are rich in potassium are fresh vegetables and fruits. A medium-size banana supplies 630 milligrams of potassium or about 75 milligrams per inch; a medium orange, 365 milligrams; half a cantaloupe, 885 milligrams; half an avocado, 385 milligrams; raw spinach, 780 milligrams per three to four ounces; raw cabbage, 230 milligrams a cup; raw celery, 300 milligrams a cup. Some vegetable juices supply up to 800 milligrams per serving. A dietary intake of about 3.5 grams of potassium is considered to be a desirable intake of potassium for adults.

ACTIONS AND PHARMACOLOGY

ACTIONS

Supplementary potassium is used to treat potassium depletion states, e.g., from prolonged use of diuretics. It is also used to prevent potassium depletion in those on diuretics. Potassium may also have antihypertensive and cerebrovascular- and cardiovascular-protective activities.

MECHANISM OF ACTION

Potassium chloride, in the form of potassium-rich foods or potassium chloride supplements, is used in the management of potassium-deficiency associated with metabolic alkalosis. The fundamental cause of the deficiency is also treated whenever possible. Potassium deficiency may also be associated with metabolic acidosis, e.g., in those with renal tubular acidosis. In those cases, potassium salts other than potassium chloride are used, including potassium citrate, potassium acetate or potassium carbonate.

Potassium supplementation has been demonstrated to bring about small but significant reductions in blood pressure in those with mild to moderate hypertension. The mechanism of this effect is unclear. Possible mechanisms for this antihypertensive effect include a decrease in plasma renin activity, effects on resistance vessels related either to a high potassium concentration or to a decrease in the number of angiotensin II receptors and natriuresis (potassium inhibits sodium reabsorption in the proximal tubules).

The mechanism by which increased potassium intake may prevent stroke is not known. Possible mechanisms include potassium's hypotensive effect, inhibition of free radical formation, prevention of vascular smooth muscle proliferation and prevention of arterial thrombosis. In *in vitro* and in animal studies, elevation of extracellular potassium concentration within the physiological range has been shown to inhibit free radical formation from macrophages and endothelial cells, as well as to inhibit proliferation and thymidine incorporation of vascular smooth muscle cells and to reduce platelet sensitivity to thrombin and other agonists. High potassium diets have also been shown to reduce oxidative stress on the endothelium of high sodium chloride-fed stroke-prone spontaneously hypertensive rats independent of blood pressure changes.

PHARMACOKINETICS

The efficiency of absorption of supplementary potassium from the gastrointestinal tract is high. Greater than 90% of an ingested dose of potassium is absorbed. The efficiency of absorption of dietary potassium is similar. Potassium is delivered to the liver via the portal circulation and the rest of the body via the systemic circulation. Insulin and catecholamines promote potassium transport into cells. Potassium is lost from the body in the urine and, to a lesser degree, in gastrointestinal secretions.

INDICATIONS AND USAGE

Potassium may be useful in the prevention and treatment of hypertension in some, notably African Americans. Epidemiological studies have suggested that high dietary intake of potassium may protect many populations against stroke. More recent analyses suggest that this protection may be restricted to black men and hypertensive men. There is experimental data indicating that high potassium intake may have a number of cardioprotective effects. There is no credible evidence that supplemental potassium has anticarcinogenic effects or that it can enhance athletic performance other than, possibly, in those who are potassium deficient.

RESEARCH SUMMARY

Epidemiological studies have shown an inverse relationship between potassium intake and blood pressure. A major meta-analysis designed to assess the effects of potassium supplements on blood pressure examined data from 33 randomized, controlled trials involving 2,609 subjects. The researchers concluded that low potassium intake may be an important contributor to hypertension and that increased potassium intake can both prevent and treat hypertension, particularly in those who cannot or will not reduce their sodium intake.

The study found that potassium supplementation resulted in a significant reduction in mean systolic blood pressure of 3.11 mmHg and a significant reduction in mean diastolic blood pressure of 3.42 mmHg. Greater reductions were also seen in black Americans, compared with Caucasians. Better results were reported in hypertensives than in normotensives, but effects in the latter were sufficient to suggest that supplemental potassium may help significantly prevent hypertension.

Studies have shown that diets high in potassium, magnesium and fiber reduce the risk of strokes. Other studies have reported an inverse relationship between potassium intake and stroke. One of these studies found that, among men with the highest potassium intakes, risk of any type of stroke was 38% lower than among those with the lowest potassium intakes. Potassium supplementation has specifically been inversely associated with the risk of stroke, especially among hypertensive men.

In perhaps the best analysis to date, increased potassium intake was significantly associated with decreased risk of stroke mortality — but only among black men and hypertensive men. Research is ongoing.

There are an abundance of *in vitro* and animal data suggesting that high potassium intake may protect against cardiovascular disease. Various studies have reported that potassium reduces vascular and plasma lipids, macrophage adherence to the vascular wall and endothelial permeability in hypertensive animals. Other animal studies have demonstrated that potassium can reduce atherosclerotic cholesterol ester deposition in the aorta. Research continues.

CONTRAINDICATIONS, PRECAUTIONS, ADVERSE REACTIONS

CONTRAINDICATIONS

Potassium supplements are contraindicated in those with hyperkalemia.

Potassium supplements are also contraindicated in those with hypersensitivity to any component of a potassium-containing supplement.

PRECAUTIONS

The use of potassium supplements in those with potassium deficiency requires medical supervision.

Pregnant women and nursing mothers should avoid potassium supplements unless they are prescribed by their physicians.

ADVERSE REACTIONS

The most common adverse reactions of potassium supplements are gastrointestinal ones and include nausea, vomiting, abdominal discomfort, flatulence and diarrhea. Taking potassium supplements with meals may reduce these adverse reactions. Rashes are occasionally reported. The most serious adverse reaction is hyperkalemia. Hyperkalemia is rare in those with normal renal function.

INTERACTIONS

DRUGS

Angiotensin Converting Enzyme (ACE) inhibitors (benazepril, captopril, enalapril, fosinopril, lisinopril, moexipril, perindopril, quinapril, ramipril, trandolapril): ACE inhibitors will produce some potassium retention by inhibiting aldosterone production. Potassium supplements should be given to those receiving ACE inhibitors only with close monitoring.

Potassium sparing diuretics (amiloride, triamterene, spironolactone): The concomitant administration of a potassium-sparing diuretic and a potassium supplement can produce severe hyperkalemia.

OVERDOSAGE

The use of oral potassium supplements in those with normal renal function very rarely causes serious hyperkalemia. However, overdoses with oral potassium supplements in those with normal renal function have been reported. For example, a 46 year-old woman ingested 31 grams of potassium chloride in a suicide attempt and developed severe hyperkalemia associated with life-threatening arrhythmias. The woman died two weeks later as a result of cerebral anoxia during cardiopulmonary arrest. Oral doses greater than 18 grams of potassium taken at one time may lead to severe hyperkalemia in those with normal renal function.

DOSAGE AND ADMINISTRATION

The use of potassium supplements in those with potassium deficiency requires medical supervision.

There are several potassium supplemental forms available, including potassium chloride, potassium citrate, potassium gluconate, potassium bicarbonate, potassium aspartate and potassium orotate.

Multivitamin, multimineral supplements do not contain more than 99 milligrams of potassium per serving. One milliequivalent or millimole is equal to 39.09 milligrams.

High-potassium (up to 800 milligrams per serving), low-sodium vegetable juices are available. Some soft drinks are rich in potassium. Some soft drinks contain potassium gluconate which has a less bitter taste than some other potassium supplements. Salt substitutes are high in potassium.

Potassium-rich foods and drinks are the best ways to increase potassium intake.

HOW SUPPLIED

Potassium acetate is available in the following forms and strengths for Rx use:

Injection — 2 meq/mL, 4 meq/mL

Potassium chloride is available in the following forms and strengths for OTC use:

Tablets — 75 mg, 95 mg, 99 mg, 180 mg

Potassium chloride is available in the following forms and strengths for Rx use:

Injection — 2 meq/mL, 10 meq/50 mL, 20 meq/50 mL, 10 meq/100 mL, 20 meq/100 mL, 30 meq/100 mL, 40 meq/100 mL
Liquid — 20 meq/15 mL, 40 meq/15 mL
Powder for Reconstitution — 20 meq, 25 meq
Tablet, Extended Release — 8 meq, 10 meq, 20 meq

Potassium gluconate is available in the following forms and strengths:

Tablets — 486 mg, 500 mg, 550 mg, 595 mg, 610 mg, 620 mg

LITERATURE

Addison WLT, The use of sodium chloride, potassium chloride, sodium bromide and potassium bromide in cases of arterial hypertension which are amenable to potassium chloride. *Can Med Assoc J.* 1928; 18:281-285.

Cappuccio FP, MacGregor GA. Does potassium supplementation lower blood pressure? A meta-analysis of published trials. *J Hypertens.* 1991; 9:465-473.

Fang J, Madhavan S, Alderman MH. Dietary potassium intake and stroke mortality. *Stroke.* 2000; 31:1532-1537.

Hermans JJ, Fischer MA, Schiffers PM, Struijker-Boudier HA. High dietary potassium chloride intake augments rat renal mineralocorticoid receptor selectivity via 11beta-hydroxysteroid dehydrogenase. *Biochim Biophys Acta.* 1999; 1472:537-549.

Hermansen K. Diet, blood pressure and hypertension. *Br J Nutr.* 2000; 83 Suppl:S113-S119.

Ishimitsu T, Tobian L. High potassium diets reduce endothelial permeability in stroke-prone spontaneously hypertensive rats. *Clin Exp Pharmacol Physiol.* 1997; 23:241-245.

Ishimitsu T, Tobian L, Sugimoto K, Everson T. High potassium diets reduce vascular and plasma lipid peroxides in stroke-prone spontaneously hypertensive rats. *Clin Exp Hypertens.* 1996; 18:659-673.

Ishimitsu T, Tobian L, Sugimoto K, Lange JM. High potassium diets reduce macrophage adherence to vascular wall in stroke-prone spontaneously hypertensive rats. *J Vasc Res.* 1995; 32:406-412.

Ishimitsu T, Tobian L, Uehara Y, et al. Effect of high potassium diets on the vascular and renal prostaglandin system in stroke-prone spontaneously hypertensive rats. *Prostaglandins Leukot Essent Fatty Acids.* 1995; 53:255-260.

Jin L, ChaoL, Chao J. Potassium supplement upregulates the expression of renal kalikrein and bradykinin B_2 receptor in SHR. *Am J Physiol.* 1999; 276:F476-F484.

Khaw K-T, Barrett-Conner E. Dietary potassium and stroke-associated mortality. *N Engl J Med.* 1987; 316:235-240.

Krishna GG, Miller E, Kapoor S. Increased blood pressure during potassium depletion in normotensive men. *N Eng J Med.* 1989; 320:1177-1182.

Lin H, Young DB. Interactions between plasma potassium and epinephrine in coronary thrombosis in dogs. *Circulation.* 1994; 89:331-338.

Ma G, Young DB, Clower BR. Inverse relationship between potassium intake and coronary artery disease in the cholesterol-fed rabbit. *Am J Hypertens.* 1999; 12:821-825.

McCabe RD, Backarich MA, Srivastava K, Young DB. Potassium inhibits free radical formation. *Hypertension.* 1994; 24:77-82.

McCabe RD, Young DB. Potassium inhibits cultural vascular smooth muscle proliferation. *Am J Hypertens.* 1994; 7:346-350.

Sugimoto T, Tobian L, Ganguli MC. High potassium diets protect against dysfunction of endothelial cells in stroke-prone spontaneously hypertensive rats. *Hypertension.* 1988:11:579-585.

Sugimoto K, Tobian L, Ishimutsu T, Lange JM. High potassium diets greatly increase growth-inhibiting agents in aortas of hypertensive rats. *Hypertension.* 1992; 19:749-752.

Tannen RL. Effects of potassium on blood pressure control. *Ann Intern Med.* 1983; 98(part 2):773-780.

Tobian L. Salt and hypertension. Lessons from animal models that relate to human hypertension. *Hypertension.* 1991; 17:152-158.

West SG, Light KC, Hinderliter AL, et al. Potassium supplementation induces beneficial cardiovascular changes during rest and stress in salt sensitive individuals. *Health Psychol.* 1999; 18:229-240.

Whelton PK, He J, Cutler JA, et al. Effects of oral potassium on blood pressure. Meta-analysis of randomized controlled clinical triglyceride trials. *JAMA.* 1997; 277:1624-1632.

Young DB, Lin H, McCabe RD. Potassium's cardiovascular protective mechanisms. *Am J Physiol.* 1995; 268:R825-R837.

Young DB, Ma G. Vascular protective effects of potassium. *Semin Nephrol.* 1999; 19:477-486.

Zhou MS, Nishida Y, Yoneyama H, et al. Potassium supplementation increases sodium excretion in hypertensive Dahl rats. *Clin Exp Hypertens.* 1999; 21:1397-1411.

Prebiotics

DESCRIPTION

Prebiotics are defined as nondigestible food ingredients that may beneficially affect the host by selectively stimulating the growth and/or the activity of a limited number of bacteria in the colon. Thus, to be effective, prebiotics must escape digestion in the upper gastrointestinal tract and be used by a limited number of the microorganisms comprising the colonic microflora. Prebiotics are principally oligosaccharides. They mainly stimulate the growth of bifidobacteria, for which reason they are referred to as bifidogenic factors.

The following describes the various oligosaccharides which are classified as prebiotics.

FRUCTO-OLIGOSACCHARIDES

Fructo-oligosaccharides or FOS (see Fructo-Oligosaccharides) typically refer to short-chain oligosaccharides comprised of D-fructose and D-glucose, containing from three to five monosaccharide units. FOS, also called neosugar and short-chain FOS (sc FOS), are produced on a commercial scale from sucrose using a fungal fructosyltransferase enzyme. FOS are resistant to digestion in the upper gastrointestinal tract. They act to stimulate the growth of *Bifidobacterium* species in the large intestine. FOS are marketed in the United States in combination with probiotic bacteria and in some functional food products.

INULINS

Inulins (see Inulins) refer to a group of naturally-occurring fructose-containing oligosaccharides. Inulins belong to a class of carbohydrates known as fructans. They are derived from the roots of chicory *(Cichorium intybus)* and Jerusalem artichokes. Inulins are mainly comprised of fructose units and typically have a terminal glucose. The bond between fructose units in inulins is a beta-(2-1) glycosidic linkage. The average degreee of polymerization of inulins marketed as nutritional supplements is 10 to 12. Inulins stimulate the growth of *Bifidobacterium* species in the large intestine.

ISOMALTO-OLIGOSACCHARIDES

Isomalto-oligosaccharides comprise a mixture of alpha-D-(1→6)-linked glucose oligomers, including isomaltose, panose, isomaltotetraose, isomaltopentaose, nigerose, kojibiose, isopanose and higher branched oligo-saccharides. Isomalto-oligosaccharides are produced by various enzymatic processes. They act to stimulate the growth of *Bifidobacterium* species and *Lactobacillus* species in the large intestine. Isomalto-oligosaccharides are marketed in Japan as dietary supplements and in functional foods. They are being developed in the United States for similar uses.

LACTILOL

Lactilol is a disaccharide analogue of lactulose. Its pharmaceutical use is in the treatment of constipation and hepatic encephalopathy. Lactilol is also used in Japan as a prebiotic. It is resistant to digestion in the upper gastrointestinal tract and it is fermented by a limited number of colonic bacteria, resulting in an increase in the biomass of bifidobacteria and lactobacilli in the colon. Lactilol is known chemically as 4-0-(beta-D-galactopyranosyl)-D-glucitol. Lactilol is not approved for the treatment of hepatic encephalopathy or constipation in the U.S., and its use as a prebiotic is considered experimental. Lactilol is used in Europe as a food sweetener.

LACTOSUCROSE

Lactosucrose is a trisaccharide comprised of D-galactose, D-glucose and D-fructose. Lactosucrose is produced enzymatically by the enzymatic transfer of the galactosyl residue in lactose to sucrose. Lactosucrose is resistant to digestion in the stomach and small intestine. It is selectively utilized by intestinal *Bifidobacterium* species resulting in significant induction of growth of these bacteria in the colon. Therefore, under physiological conditions, lactosucrose acts on the intestinal microflora as a growth factor for *Bifidobacterium* species. Lactosucrose is also known as 4G-beta-D-galactosylsucrose. It is widely used in Japan as a dietary supplement and in functional foods, including yogurt. Lactosucrose is being developed in the United States for similar uses.

LACTULOSE

Lactulose (see Lactulose) is a semisynthetic disaccharide comprised of the sugars D-lactose and D-fructose. The sugars are joined by a beta-glycosidic linkage, making it resistant to hydrolysis by human digestive enzymes. Lactulose is, however, fermented by a limited number of colonic bacteria. This can lead to changes in the colonic ecosystem in favor of bacteria, such as lactobacilli and bifidobacteria, which may confer some health benefits. Lactulose is a prescription drug in the United States for the treatment of constipation and hepatic encephalopathy. It is marketed in Japan for use as a dietary supplement and in functional foods. Its use in the United States as a prebiotic substance is still experimental.

PYRODEXTRINS

Pyrodextrins comprise a mixture of glucose-containing oligosaccharides that is derived from the hydrolysis of starch. Pyrodextrins have been found to promote the proliferation of *Bifidobacterium* species in the large intestine. They are resistant to digestion in the upper gastrointestinal tract. Pyrodextrins are being developed for the nutritional supplement market place.

SOY OLIGOSACCHARIDES

Soy oligosaccharides refer to oligosaccharides found in soybeans and also in other beans and peas. The two principal soy oligosaccharides are the trisaccharide raffinose and the tetrasaccharide stachyose. Raffinose is comprised of one molecule each of D-galactose, D-glucose and D-fructose. Stachyose is comprised of two molecules of D-galactose, one molecule of D-glucose and one molecule of D-fructose. Soy oligosaccharides act to stimulate the growth of *Bifidobacterium* species in the large intestine. They are marketed in Japan as dietary supplements and in functional foods. They are being developed in the United States for similar uses.

TRANSGALACTO-OLIGOSACCHARIDES

Transgalacto-oligosaccharides (TOS) are a mixture of oligosaccharides consisting of D-glucose and D-galactose. TOS are produced from D-lactose via the action of the enzyme beta-galactosidase obtained from *Aspergillus oryzae*. TOS are resistant to digestion in the upper gastrointestinal tract and stimulate the growth of bifidobacteria in the large intestine. TOS are marketed in Japan and Europe as dietary supplements and are used in functional foods. They are being developed for similar use in the United States. (See Transgalacto-Oligosaccharides).

XYLO-OLIGOSACCHARIDES

Xylo-oligosaccharides are comprised of oligosaccharides containing beta $(1 \rightarrow 4)$ linked xylose residues. The degree of polymerization of xylo-oligosaccharides is from two to four. Xylo-oligosaccharides are obtained by enzymatic hydrolysis of the polysaccharide xylan. They are marketed in Japan as prebiotics and are being developed for similar use in the United States.

ACTIONS AND PHARMACOLOGY

ACTIONS

Prebiotics may have anticarcinogenic, antimicrobial, hypolipidemic and glucose-modulatory activities. They may also have activity in improving mineral absorption and balance and may have anti-osteoporotic activity.

MECHANISM OF ACTION

The possible anticarcinogenic activity of prebiotics is not well understood. It may be accounted for, in part, by the possible anticarcinogenic activity of butyrate. Butyrate, along with other short-chain fatty acids, is produced by bacterial fermentation of the various prebiotic oligosaccharides in the colon. Some studies suggest that butyrate may induce growth arrest and cell differentiation and may also upregulate apoptosis, three activities which could be significant for its possible anticarcinogenic activity. The prebiotic oligosaccharides may also aid in increasing the concentrations of calcium and magnesium in the colon. Elevated concentrations of these cations in the colon may help to control the rate of cell turnover. Elevated concentrations of calcium in the colon may help to control the formation of insoluble bile or salts of fatty acids. This might reduce the potential damaging effects of bile or fatty acids on colonocytes. The prebiotics may stimulate the growth of bifidobacteria and lactobacilli in the large intestine. There are *in vitro* and animal data suggesting that these bacteria can bind to and inactivate some carcinogens, can directly inhibit the growth of some tumors and can inhibit bacteria that may convert precarcinogens into carcinogens.

The possible antimicrobial activity of the prebiotics may be accounted for by their growth-promoting effects on bifidobacteria and lactobacilli. These bacteria can reinforce the barrier function of the intestinal mucosa, helping in the prevention of the attachment of pathogenic bacteria, essentially by crowding them out. These bacteria may also produce antimicrobial substances and stimulate antigen specific and nonspecific immune responses.

The prebiotics may lower triglyceride levels in some. The mechanism of this possible effect is unclear. Decreased hepatocyte *de novo* synthesis of triglycerides is one hypothetical possibility. The prebiotics may also lower total cholesterol and LDL-cholesterol levels in some. Again, the mechanism of this possible effect is unclear. Propionate, a product of oligosaccharide fermentation in the colon, may inhibit HMG-CoA reductase, the rate limiting step in cholesterol synthesis.

The possible effects of the prebiotics on blood glucose may be accounted for in a few ways. The oligosaccharides may delay gastric emptying and/or shorten small intestinal tract transit time. This may be via the short-chain fatty acids produced from the oligosaccharides in the colon. Short-chain fatty acids may be involved in the so-called "ileocolonic brake," which refers to the inhibition of gastric emptying by nutrients reaching the ileo-colonic junction. Short-chain fatty acids may also stimulate contractions of the ileum and shorten ileal emptying. In addition, propionate may inhibit gluconeogenesis by its metabolic conversion to methylmalonyl-CoA and succinyl-CoA. These metabolites could inhibit pyruvate carboxylase. Propionate may also reduce plasma levels of free fatty acids. High levels of free fatty acids lower glucose utilization and induce insulin resistance. Finally, propionate may enhance glycolysis via depletion of citrate in hepatocytes. Citrate is an allosteric inhibitor of phosphofructokinase. In short, the mechanism of the possible effects of prebiotics on glucose tolerance are not well understood.

The oligosaccharides may bind/sequester such minerals as calcium and magnesium in the small intestine. The short-chain fatty acids formed from the bacterial fermentation of the oligosaccharides may facilitate the colonic absorption of calcium and, possibly, also magnesium ions. This could be beneficial in the prevention of osteoporosis and osteopenia.

PHARMACOKINETICS
Following ingestion, the prebiotic oligosaccharides reach the colon with very little of them being digested in the upper gastrointestinal tract. The oligosaccharides are fermented by bifidobacteria, lactobacilli and some other bacteria in the colon to produce the short-chain fatty acids acetate, propionate and butyrate; the gases hydrogen, hydrogen sulfide, carbon dioxide and methane; and lactate, pyruvate, succinate and formate. Acetate, propionate and butyrate that are not metabolized in colonocytes are absorbed from the colon and transported via the portal circulation to the liver. These short-chain fatty acids are extensively metabolized in hepatocytes. Acetate, propionate and butyrate that are not metabolized in hepatocytes are transported by the circulation to various tissues where they undergo further metabolism. Butyrate is an important respiratory fuel for colonocytes.

INDICATIONS AND USAGE
Some prebiotics are used, pharmaceutically, for the treatment of constipation and hepatic encephalopathy. Prebiotics may protect against some intestinal pathogens and may be helpful in some inflammatory bowel disease. They may have some anticarcinogenic effects and may exert favorable lipid effects in some. They may, in some instances, enhance mineral absorption and might help protect against osteoporosis. There is some preliminary research that certain prebiotics might be of some benefit in diabetes mellitus.

RESEARCH SUMMARY
Lactulose is a prescription drug in the United States. It is used to treat constipation and hepatic encephalopathy. Lactilol, similarly, is used pharmaceutically in Europe and elsewhere to treat the same conditions. These prebiotics, as well as several others, including transgalacto-oligosaccharides (TOS), fructo-oligosaccharides (FOS) and various of the experimental prebiotics, have shown benefits in favorably modulating the microbial ecology of the gut, protecting against various intestinal pathogens and, in some instances, boosting gastrointestinal immunity. Lactulose has exhibited some ability to ameliorate symptoms of idiopathic, as well as infectious, inflammatory bowel disease.

Both lactulose and inulins have suppressed experimentally induced colonic aberrant crypt foci in rats, and lactulose helped protect colonic mucosa against a known colon carcinogen in another study. FOS has also shown experimental anticarcinogenic effects, significantly reducing incidence of colon tumors, for example, in one animal study.

In one clinical study, patients who had undergone endoscopic removal of colorectal polyps were administered antioxidant vitamins or lactulose to see if these substances could reduce the recurrence rate of adenomatous polyps. The study continued for five years. During this period polyps recurred in 5.7% of those taking the vitamins (A, C and E) and in 14.7% of those taking lactulose. The recurrence rate in untreated controls was 35.9%.

TOS have exerted hypocholesterolemic effects in animals. They have also shown some preliminary, experimental ability to lower triglycerides. A fermented milk product containing FOS lowered LDL-cholesterol levels in male subjects with borderline elevated serum cholesterol levels in a double-blind, placebo-controlled study. There is a small study in which inulins reportedly lowered plasma total cholesterol and triglyceride levels significantly in healthy male volunteers. Results have been mixed, however, with respect to prebiotic effects on lipids, and more research is needed.

TOS have demonstrated positive effects on calcium absorption and have prevented bone loss in some animal research. Lactulose has significantly stimulated calcium absorption in postmenopausal women in preliminary clinical work.

Lactulose and some of the other prebiotics have also shown some ability to improve glucose tolerance and have other effects on carbohydrate metabolism that could prove helpful in some with diabetes mellitus. This research, too, is very preliminary and ongoing.

CONTRAINDICATIONS, PRECAUTIONS, ADVERSE REACTIONS

CONTRAINDICATIONS

Prebiotics are contraindicated in those who are hypersensitive to any component of a prebiotic-containing supplement.

Some lactulose preparations contain galactose. Therefore, lactulose is contraindicated in those who require a low galactose diet.

PRECAUTIONS

In the United States, lactulose is a prescription drug. Its use requires medical supervision. Its use as a dietary supplement is considered experimental.

Those with lactose intolerance should exercise caution in the use of lactulose, lactilol and transgalacto-oligosaccharides.

Those who develop gastrointestinal symptoms (flatus, bloating, diarrhea) with the use of dietary fiber should exercise some degree of caution in the use of prebiotics. Those receiving whole body radiation or radiation to the gastrointestinal tract should avoid prebiotic supplements.

Pregnant women and nursing mothers should only use prebiotic supplements if prescribed by their physicians.

ADVERSE REACTIONS

Doses of prebiotic oligosaccharides up to 10 grams daily are well tolerated. Higher doses may cause gastrointestinal symptoms, such as flatulence, bloating and diarrhea.

INTERACTIONS

NUTRITIONAL SUPPLEMENTS

Alpha-galactosidase: Concomitant use of alpha-galactosidase (see Supplemental Enzymes) and soy oligosaccharides may decrease the effectiveness of the soy oligosaccharides.

Minerals (calcium, magnesium): Concomitant intake of calcium or magnesium and prebiotics may enhance the colonic absorption of these minerals.

Probiotics: Concomitant intake of probiotics and prebiotics may enhance the possible effectiveness of both the probiotics and the prebiotics.

FOODS

Prebiotic oligosaccharides may enhance the colonic absorption of calcium and magnesium in foods.

DOSAGE AND ADMINISTRATION

Fructo-oligosaccharides, (FOS) and inulins are available in nutritional supplements and in functional foods. Dosage is variable for both FOS and inulins and ranges from 4 to 10 grams. Those who use more than 10 grams daily of FOS or inulins should split the dosage throughout the day. Doses higher than 30 grams daily of FOS or inulins may cause significant gastrointestinal discomfort (flatulence, bloating, cramping, diarrhea).

LITERATURE

Amarowicz R. [Nutritional importance of oligosaccharides]. [Article in Polish]. *Rocz Panstw Zakl Hig.* 1999; 50:89-95.

Flickinger EA, Wolf BW, Garleb KA, et al. Glucose-based oligosaccharides exhibit different in vitro fermentation patterns and affect in vivo apparent nutrient digestibility and microbial populations in dogs. *J Nutr.* 2000; 130:1267-1273.

Gibson GR. Dietary modulation of the human gut microflora using prebiotics. *Br J Nutr.* 1998; 80:S209-S212.

Grizard D, Barthomeuf C. Non-digestible oligosaccharides used as prebiotic agents: mode of production and beneficial effects on animal and human health. *Reprod Nutr Dev.* 1999; 39:563-588.

Macfarlane GT, Cummings JH. Probiotics and prebiotics: can regulating the activities of intestinal bacteria benefit health. *West J Med.* 1999; 171:187-191.

Murosaki S, Muroyama K, Yamamoto Y, et al. Immunopotentiating activity of nigerooligosaccharides for the T helper 1-like immune response in mice. *Biosci Biotechnol Biochem.* 1999; 63:373-378.

Ohkusa T, Ozaki Y, Sato C, et al. Long-term ingestion of lactosucrose increases *Bifidobacterium sp.* in human fecal flora. *Digestion.* 1995; 56:415-420.

Roberfroid MB. Chicory fructooligosaccharides and the gastrointestinal tract. *Nutrition.* 2000; 16:677-679.

Roberfroid MB. Health benefits of non-digestible oligosaccharides. *Adv Exp Med Bull.* 1997; 427:211-219.

Roberfroid MB. Prebiotics and synbiotics: concepts and nutritional properties. *Br J Nutr.* 1998; 80:S197-S202.

Roberfroid MB. Prebiotics and probiotics: are they functional foods. *Am Clin Nutr.* 2000; 71 (6 Suppl):1682S-1687S, discussion 1688S-1690S.

Soontornchai S, Sirichakwal P, Puwastien P, et al. Lactilol tolerance in healthy Thai adults. *Eur J Nutr.* 2000; 38:218-226.

Teramoto F, Rokutan K, Kawakami Y, et al. Effect of 4G-beta-D-galactosylsucrose (lactosucrose) on fecal microflora in patients with chronic inflammatory bowel disease. *J Gastrenterol.* 1996; 31:33-39.

Wang X-D, Rakshit SK. Biosynthesis of nutraceutical iso-oligosaccharides by multiple forms of transferase produced by *Aspergillus foetidus. Nahrung.* 2000; 44:207-210.

For additional Literature, see Fructo-Oligosaccharides, Inulins, Lactulose, Transgalacto-Oligosaccharides.

Pregnenolone

TRADE NAMES

Pregnenolone is available from numerous manufacturers generically. Branded products include MaxiLife Pregnenolone (Twinlab).

DESCRIPTION

Pregnenolone is a steroid naturally found in animal tissues, especially in the gonads, adrenal gland and brain. Pregnenolone is synthesized from cholesterol and is a precursor for the biosynthesis of steroid hormones. In the adrenal gland, pregnenolone is a precursor to the mineralocorticoid aldosterone, the glucocorticoid cortisol, as well as dehydroepiandrosterone (DHEA) and progesterone. In the ovary, pregnenolone is a precursor to estrogens and progesterone, and, in the testis, pregnenolone is a precursor to testosterone.

Pregnenolone and its metabolite pregnenolone sulfate are now known to be synthesized in the brain either *de novo* from cholesterol or from other metabolites. Pregnenolone and pregnenolone sulfate found in the brain and central nervous system are referred to as neurosteroids.

Pregnenolone is known chemically as 3-Hydroxypregn-5-en-20-one; delta 5-pregnen-3 beta-ol-20-one, and 17 beta-(1-ketoethyl)-delta 5-androstene-3 beta-ol. Its abbreviation is PREG and the abbreviation of its metabolite, progesterone sulfate, is PREG S. Pregnenolone is a lipophilic solid substance that is sparingly soluble in water. Pregnenolone has the following chemical structure:

Pregnenolone

ACTIONS AND PHARMACOLOGY

ACTIONS

Supplemental pregnenolone has putative memory-enhancing activity.

MECHANISM OF ACTION

Memory enhancement has been observed in aged animals when given pregnenolone or pregnenolone sulfate. Pregnenolone sulfate is both a gamma-aminobutyrate (GABA) antagonist and a positive allosteric modulator at the N-methyl-D-asparatate (NMDA) receptor and may reinforce neurotransmitter systems that may decline with age.

Pregnenolone sulfate was found to stimulate acetylcholine release in the adult rat hippocampus. Acetylcholine release may be due to pregnenolone sulfate's negative modulation of the GABA (A) receptor complex and positive modulation of the NMDA receptor. While a modest increase in acetylcho-line release facilities memory processes, elevation of acetyl-choline beyond an optimal level is ineffective in doing so.

PHARMACOKINETICS

Little is known about the pharmacokinetics (PK) of pregnenolone in humans. Some PK studies have been done in animals. The absorption of pregnenolone, similar to the absorption of most steroids, is variable. It appears that some pregnenolone is absorbed from the small intestine and distributed throughout the body. How much is taken up by the liver and metabolized is unclear. Likewise, it is unclear how much of an ingested pregnenolone dose is taken up by the brain. Metabolites of injected pregnenolone in the rat brain include pregnenolone sulfate, progesterone, 5 alpha-pregnane-3, 20-dione, 3 alpha-hydroxy-5 alpha-pregnan-20-one or allopregnanolone and DHEA. In other tissues, pregnenolone may be metabolized to DHEA, testosterone, estrogens, cortisol and aldosterone.

INDICATIONS AND USAGE

Pregnenolone may have some efficacy as a memory enhancer; this has so far been demonstrated in various animal models but not yet in humans. There are unsubstantiated claims that pregnenolone is useful in Alzheimer's disease, some forms of cancer and arthritis, in degenerative diseases associated with aging in general and in obesity.

RESEARCH SUMMARY

There are several studies showing a correlation between deficiencies in cognitive performance in aged animals and low pregnenolone levels in the brains of these animals, especially in the hippocampus. Performance or memory tests have been shown to improve in these animals when hippocampal pregnenolone levels were increased via intraperitoneal or bilateral intrahippocampal injection of pregnenolone sulfate.

There is direct evidence from many of these studies that pregnenolone sulfate stimulates release of acetylcholine in the hippocampus. There is additional evidence that suggests that exogenous pregnenolone can reinforce neurotransmitter systems that normally decline with age. A "global stimulatory effect on central cholinergic neurotransmission" has been suggested by one research group.

Though significant favorable results have been obtained with respect to memory enhancement in aged animals, human studies have yet to commence. These are warranted. Meanwhile, claims that supplemental pregnenolone is helpful in Alzheimer's disease are unsubstantiated. And there is no credible evidence that pregnenolone is useful in the treatment of arthritis, cancer, degenerative diseases or obesity.

CONTRAINDICATIONS, PRECAUTIONS, ADVERSE REACTIONS

CONTRAINDICATIONS

Pregnenolone is contraindicated in those with prostate, breast and uterine cancer.

PRECAUTIONS

Pregnenolone should be avoided by children, pregnant women and nursing mothers.

Because of the theoretical possibility that pregnenolone may lower seizure threshold—pregnenolone sulfate negatively modulates GABA (A) receptors in animals—those with seizure disorders should avoid pregnenolone.

ADVERSE REACTIONS

To date there are no reported significant adverse effects. Mild gastrointestinal effects, such as nausea, have been noted. However, pregnenolone may be converted to steroids such as DHEA, and DHEA does cause various adverse effects such as acne and hair loss, especially in women.

INTERACTIONS

There are no reported drug, nutritional supplement, food or herb interactions to date.

OVERDOSAGE

No reported overdosage.

DOSAGE AND ADMINISTRATION

Typical pregnenolone doses are 5 to 50 milligrams daily. The safety of taking pregnenolone at any dose, especially long term, is unknown.

HOW SUPPLIED

Capsules — 10 mg, 25 mg, 30 mg, 50 mg.

LITERATURE

Akawa Y, Baulieu EE. Neurosteroids: behavioral aspects and physiological implications. *J Soc Biol.* 1999; 193:293-298.

Barrot M, Vallee M, Gingras MA, et al. The neurosteroid pregnenolone sulfate increases dopamine release and the dopaminergic response to morphine in the rat nucleus accumbens. *Eur J Neurosci.* 1999; 10:3757-3760.

Darnaudery M, Koehl M, Pallares M, et al. The neurosteroid pregnenolone sulfate increases cortical acetylcholine release: a microdialysis study in freely moving rats. *J Neurochem.* 1998; 71:2018-2022.

Darnaudery M, Koehl M, Piazza PV, et al. Pregnenolone sulfate increases hippocompal acetylcholine release and spatial recognition. *Brain Res.* 2000; 852:173-179.

Kokate TG, Juhng KN, Kirkby RD, et al. Convulsant actions of the neurosteroid pregnenolone sulfate in mice. *Brain Res.* 1999; 831:119-124.

Legrand A, Alfonso G. Pregnenolone reverses the age-dependent accumulation of glial fibrillary acidic protein within astrocytes of specific regions of the rat brain. *Brain Res.* 1998; 802:125-133.

Pallares M, Darnaudery M, Day J, et al. The neurosteroid pregnenolone sulfate infused into the nucleus basalis increases both acetylcholine release in the frontal cortex or amygdala and spatial memory. *Neuroscience.* 1998; 87:551-558.

Vallee M, Mayo W, Darnaudery M, et al. Neurosteroids: deficient cognitive performance in aged rats depends on low pregnenolone sulfate levels in the hippocampus. *Proc Natl Accd Sci.* 1997; 94:14865-14870.

Probiotics

TRADE NAMES

Mega Dophilus (Natren), Healthy Trinity (Natren), Bifido Factor (Natren), Digesta Lac (Natren), Life Start (Natren), Probiata (Wakunaga Consumer).

DESCRIPTION

Probiotics are defined as live microorganisms, including *Lactobacillus* species, *Bifidobacterium* species and yeasts, that may beneficially affect the host upon ingestion by improving the balance of the intestinal microflora. The dietary use of live microorganisms has a long history. Mention of cultured dairy products is found in the Bible and the sacred books of Hinduism. Soured milks and cultured dairy products, such as kefir, koumiss, leben and dahi, were often used therapeutically before the existence of microorganisms was recognized. The use of microorganisms in food fermentation is one of the oldest methods for producing and preserving food. Much of the world depends upon various fermented foods that are staples in the diet.

Élie Metchnikoff, the father of modern immunology, spoke highly about the possible health benefits of the lactic acid-bacteria (LAB) *Lactobacillus bulgaricus* and *Streptococcus thermophilus* in his writings at the turn of the last century. He wrote in his book, *The Prolongation of Life,* that consumption of live bacteria, such as *Lactobacillus bulgaricus* and *Streptococcus thermophilus,* in the form of yogurt was beneficial for gastrointestinal health, as well as for health in general, and for longevity. Some recent research suggests that certain live microorganisms may have immuno-modulatory and anticarcinogenic effects, as well as other health benefits. There is presently much active research focusing on the development of target-specific probiotics containing well-characterized bacteria that are selected for their health-enhancing characteristics. These new probiotics are entering the marketplace in the form of nutritional supplements and functional foods, such as yogurt functional food products.

The gastrointestinal tract represents a complex ecosystem in which a delicate balance exists between the intestinal microflora and the host. The microflora are principally comprised of facultative anaerobes and obligate anaerobes. Approximately 95% of the intestinal bacterial population in humans is comprised of obligate anaerobes, including *Bifidobacterium, Clostridium, Eubacterium, Fusobacterium, Peptococcus, Peptostreptococcus* and *Bacteroides*. Approximately 1% to 10% of the intestinal population is comprised of facultative anaerobes, including *Lactobacillus, Escherichia coli, Klebsiella, Streptococcus, Staphylococcus* and *Bacillus*. Aerobic organisms are not present in the intestinal tract of healthy individuals with the exception of *Pseudomonas*, which is present in very small amounts. Most of the bacteria are present in the colon where the bacterial concentration ranges between 10^{11} to 10^{12} colony-forming units (CPU) per milliliter.

The intestinal microflora are important for maturation of the immune system, the development of normal intestinal morphology and in order to maintain a chronic and immunologically balanced inflammatory response. The microflora reinforce the barrier function of the intestinal mucosa, helping in the prevention of the attachment of pathogenic microorganisms and the entry of allergens. Some members of the microflora may contribute to the body's requirements for certain vitamins, including biotin, pantothenic acid and vitamin B_{12}. Alteration of the microbial flora of the intestine, such as may occur with antibiotic use, disease and aging, can negatively affect its beneficial role.

The probiotics that are marketed as nutritional supplements and in functional foods, such as yogurts, are principally the *Bifidobacterium* species and the *Lactobacillus* species. Probiotics are sometimes called colonic foods. Most of the presently available probiotics are bacteria. *Saccharomyces boulardii* is an example of a probiotic yeast.

The following describe the various bacteria and yeasts used as probiotics:

BIFIDOBACTERIUM

Bifidobacteria are normal inhabitants of the human and animal colon. Newborns, especially those that are breast-fed, are colonized with bifidobacteria within days after birth. Bifidobacteria were first isolated from the feces of breast-fed infants. The population of these bacteria in the colon appears to be relatively stable until advanced age when it appears to decline. The bifidobacteria population is influenced by a number of factors, including diet, antibiotics and stress. Bifidobacteria are gram-positive anaerobes. They are non-motile, non-spore forming and catalase-negative. They have various shapes, including short, curved rods, club-shaped rods and bifurcated Y-shaped rods. Their name is derived from the observation that they often exist in a Y-shaped or bifid form. The guanine and cytosine content of their DNA is between 54 mol% and 67mol%. They are saccharolytic

organisms that produce acetic and lactic acids without generation of CO_2, except during degradation of gluconate. They are also classified as lactic acid bacteria (LAB). To date, 30 species of bifidobacteria have been isolated. Bifidobacteria used as probiotics include *Bifidobacterium adolescentis, Bifidobacterium bifidum, Bifidobacterium animalis, Bifidobacterium thermophilum, Bifidobacterium breve, Bifidobacterium longum, Bifidobacterium infantis* and *Bifidobacterium lactis*. Specific strains of bifidobacteria used as probiotics include *Bifidobacterium breve* strain Yakult, *Bifidobacterium breve* RO7O, *Bifidobacterium lactis* Bb12, *Bifidobacterium longum* RO23, *Bifidobacterium bifidum* RO71, *Bifidobacterium infantis* RO33, *Bifidobacterium longum* BB536 and *Bifidobacterium longum* SBT-2928.

LACTOBACILLUS

Lactobacilli are normal inhabitants of the human intestine and vagina. Lactobacilli are gram-positive facultative anaerobes. They are non-spore forming and non-flagellated rod or coccobacilli. The guanine and cytosine content of their DNA is between 32 mol% and 51 mol%. They are either aerotolerant or anaerobic and strictly fermentative. In the homofermentative case, glucose is fermented predominantly to lactic acid. Lactobacilli are also classified as lactic acid bacteria (LAB). To date, 56 species of the genus *Lactobacillus* have been identified. Lactobacilli used as probiotics include *Lactobacillus acidophilus, Lactobacillus brevis, Lactobacillus bulgaricus, Lactobacillus casei, Lactobacillus cellobiosus, Lactobacillus crispatus, Lactobacillus curvatus, Lactobacillus fermentum, Lactobacillus GG (Lactobacillus rhamnosus* or *Lactobacillus casei* subspecies *rhamnosus), Lactobacillus gasseri, Lactobacillus johnsonii, Lactobacillus plantarum* and *Lactobacillus salivarus. Lactobacillus plantarum* 299v strain originates from sour dough. *Lactobacillus plantarum* itself is of human origin. Other probiotic strains of *Lactobacillus* are *Lactobacillus acidophilus* BG2FO4, *Lactobacillus acidophilus* INT-9, *Lactobacillus plantarum* ST31, *Lactobacillus reuteri, Lactobacillus johnsonii* LA1, *Lactobacillus acidophilus* NCFB 1748, *Lactobacillus casei* Shirota, *Lactobacillus acidophilus* NCFM, *Lactobacillus acidophilus* DDS-1, *Lactobacillus delbrueckii* subspecies *delbrueckii, Lactobacillus delbrueckii* subspecies *bulgaricus* type 2038, *Lactobacillus acidophilus* SBT-2062, *Lactobacillus brevis, Lactobacillus salivarius* UCC 118 and *Lactobacillus paracasei* subsp *paracasei* F19.

LACTOCOCCUS

Lactococci are gram-positive facultative anaerobes. They are also classified as lactic acid bacteria (LAB). *Lactococcus lactis* (formerly known as *Streptococcus lactis*) is found in dairy products and is commonly responsible for the souring of milk. Lactococci that are used or are being developed as probiotics include *Lactococcus lactis, Lactococcus lactis* subspecies *cremoris* (*Streptococcus cremoris*), *Lactococcus lactis* subspecies *lactis* NCDO 712, *Lactococcus lactis* subspecies *lactis* NIAI 527, *Lactococcus lactis* subspecies *lactis* NIAI 1061, *Lactococcus lactis* subspecies *lactis* biovar diacetylactis NIAI 8 W and *Lactococcus lactis* subspecies *lactis* biovar diacetylactis ATCC 13675.

SACCHAROMYCES

Saccharomyces belongs to the yeast family. The principal probiotic yeast is *Saccharomyces boulardii*. *Saccharomyces boulardii* is also known as *Saccharomyces cerevisiae* Hansen CBS 5296 and *S. boulardii*. *S. boulardii* is normally a nonpathogenic yeast. *S. boulardii* has been used to treat diarrhea associated with antibiotic use.

STREPTOCOCCUS THERMOPHILUS

Streptococcus thermophilus is a gram-positive facultative anaerobe. It is a cytochrome-, oxidase- and catalase-negative organism that is nonmotile, non-spore forming and homofermentative. *Streptococcus thermophilus* is an alpha-hemolytic species of the *viridans* group. It is also classified as a lactic acid bacteria (LAB). *Steptococcus thermophilus* is found in milk and milk products. It is a probiotic and used in the production of yogurt. *Streptococcus salivarus* subspecies *thermophilus* type 1131 is another probiotic strain.

ENTEROCOCCUS

Enterococci are gram-positive, facultative anaerobic cocci of the Streptococcaceae family. They are spherical to ovoid and occur in pairs or short chains. Enterococci are catalase-negative, non-spore forming and usually nonmotile. Enterococci are part of the intestinal microflora of humans and animals. *Enterococcus faecium* SF68 is a probiotic strain that has been used in the management of diarrheal illnesses.

ACTIONS AND PHARMACOLOGY

ACTIONS

Probiotics may have antimicrobial, immunomodulatory, anticarcinogenic, antidiarrheal, antiallergenic and antioxidant activities.

MECHANISM OF ACTION

Lactobacillus plantarum 299v, which is derived from sour dough and which is used to ferment sauerkraut and salami, has been demonstrated to improve the recovery of patients with enteric bacterial infections. This bacterium adheres to reinforce the barrier function of the intestinal mucosa, thus preventing the attachment of the pathogenic bacteria to the intestinal wall. *Bifidobacterium breve* was found to eradicate *Campylobacter jejuni* from the stools of children with enteritis, although less rapidly than in those treated with erythromycin. *Lactobacillus* GG was found to eradicate *Clostridium difficile* in patients with relapsing colitis, and supplementation of infant formula milk with *Bifidobacterium*

bifidum and *Streptococcus thermophilus* reduced rotavirus shedding and episodes of diarrhea in hospitalized children.

The antimicrobial activity of probiotics is thought to be accounted for, in large part, by their ability to colonize the colon and reinforce the barrier function of the intestinal mucosa. Probiotics, such as *Lactobacillus bulgaricus,* which do not adhere as well to the intestinal mucosa, are much less effective against enteric pathogens. In addition, some probiotics have been found to secrete antimicrobial substances. These substances are known as bacteriocins. Such a bacteriocin has been isolated from *Lactobacillus plantarum* ST31, a probiotic derived from sour dough. The substance was found to be a 20 amino acid peptide. A different bacteriocin was isolated from another strain of *Lactobacillus plantarum*. The bacteriocin has 27 amino acids and contains lanthionine residues. This type of bacteriocin is classified as a lantibiotic.

Lactobacillus casei has been demonstrated to increase levels of circulating immunoglobulin A (IgA) in infants infected with rotavirus. This has been found to be correlated with shortened duration of rotavirus-induced diarrhea. *Lactobacillus* GG has also been shown to potentiate intestinal immune response to rotavirus infection in children. *Lactobacillus acidophilus* and *Bifidobacterium bifidum* appear to enhance the nonspecific immune phagocytic activity of circulating blood granulocytes. This effect may account, in part, for the stimulation of IgA responses in infants infected with rotavirus. In healthy individuals, *Lactobacillus salivarius* UCC118 and *Lactobacillus johnsonii* LA1 were demonstrated to produce an increase in the phagocytic activity of peripheral blood monocytes and granulocytes. Also, *Lactobacillus johnsonii* LA1, but not *Lactobacillus salivarius* UCC118, was found to increase the frequency of interferon-gamma-producing peripheral blood monocytes.

Lactobacillus GG has been shown to inhibit chemically induced intestinal tumors in rats. The probiotic appears to alter the initiation and/or promotional events of the chemically-induced tumors. *Lactobacillus* GG also binds to some chemical carcinogens.

Saccharomyces boulardii has been shown to prevent antibiotic-associated diarrhea and also to prevent diarrhea in critically ill tube-fed patients. The mechanism of this antidiarrheal effect is not well understood. *S. boulardii* has been found to secrete a protease which digests two protein exotoxins, toxin A and toxin B, which appear to mediate diarrhea and colitis caused by *Clostridium difficile*. The protective effects of *S. boulardii* on *C. difficile*-induced inflammatory diarrhea may, in part, be due to proteolytic digestion of toxin A and toxin B by a secreted protease.

Dietary antigens may induce an immunoinflammatory response that impairs the barrier function of the intestine, resulting in aberrant absorption of intralumenal antigens. This may account, in part, for food allergies. Probiotics that colonize the colon may be helpful in the management of some with food allergies by reinforcing the barrier function of the intestinal mucosa. *Lactobacillus rhamnosus* GG and *Bifidobacterium lactis* Bb12 were found to produce significant improvement of atopic eczema in children with food allergies. The decrease in the signs and symptoms of atopic eczema occurred in parallel with a reduction in the concentration of circulating CD4+ T lymphocytes and an increase in transforming growth factor beta1 (TGF-beta1), indicating suppressive effects on T cell functions in this disorder. These probiotics may help restore the Th1/Th2 balance in atopic eczema.

Lactobacillus GG was found to scavenge superoxide anion radicals, inhibit lipid peroxidation and chelate iron *in vitro*. The iron chelating active of *Lactobacillus* GG may account, in part, for its antioxidant activity. Other lactic acid bacteria, including strains of *Lactobacillus acidophilus*, *Lactobacillus bulgaricus*, *Bifidobaterium longum* and *Streptococcus thermophilus*, have also demonstrated antioxidative ability. Mechanisms include chelation of metal ions (iron, copper), scavenging of reactive oxygen species and reducing activity.

PHARMACOKINETICS

The effectiveness of probiotics is related to their ability to survive in the acidic stomach environment and the alkaline conditions in the duodenum, as well as their ability to adhere to the intestinal mucosa of the colon and to colonize the colon. Some probiotics, such as *Lactobacillus* GG and *Lactobacillus plantarum* 299v, are better able to colonize the colon than others. After passage through the stomach and the small intestine, those probiotics that do survive become established transiently in the colon.

INDICATIONS AND USAGE

Probiotics have been used with some benefit in the prevention and treatment of some gastrointestinal disorders, including antibiotic-associated diarrhea and some infectious and viral diarrheas, most notably rotavirus-induced diarrhea in infants and children, lactose intolerance, sucrase and maltase deficiencies and inflammatory bowel disease. Probiotics may be of benefit in some with food allergies, but supporting evidence is preliminary. They may favorably modulate immunity in some circumstances and may have anticarcinogenic effects. There is the suggestion in some preliminary research that they may have some hypocholesterolemic activity. There is some evidence to support the use of probiotics to re-colonize the vaginas of women with recurrent vaginosis.

RESEARCH SUMMARY

Among the probiotics, only *S. boulardii, E. faecium* and *Lactobacillus sp.* have been useful in preventing antibiotic-

related diarrhea. In one double-blind study, 180 hospitalized patients on antibiotic therapy were randomized to receive placebo or *S. boulardii* supplementation. Incidence of diarrhea was significantly lower among those receiving the probiotic, compared with controls (9% and 22%, respectively). These results have been confirmed in other controlled studies.

Lactobacillus GG significantly reduced the severity and duration of rotavirus diarrhea in infants in a double-blind, placebo-controlled study. Other researchers have demonstrated that the incidence of acute diarrhea and rotavirus shedding can be significantly reduced among infants admitted to the hospital by adding *Bifidobacterium bifidum* and *Streptococcus thermophilus* to infant formula. *Lactobacillus* GG has been shown helpful in the treatment of diarrhea associated with relapsing colitis due to *Clostridium difficile*. These studies, however, were small and uncontrolled. In a double-blind, placebo-controlled trial, *Saccharomyces boulardii* was significantly superior to placebo in treating diarrhea despite having no apparent effect on *Clostridium difficile* toxin. The use of probiotics in the attempted prevention and treatment of traveler's diarrhea, most commonly caused by enterotoxigenic *E. coli*, has produced inconclusive results. More study is needed.

Reduced fecal concentrations of various probiotics have been noted, although without conclusive power, in some with active ulcerative colitis, Crohn's disease, active pouchitis and some other inflammatory gastrointestinal conditions. *Lactobacillus* species prevented development of spontaneous colitis in interleukin 10-deficient mice. *Lactobacillus plantarum* ameliorated colitis that was already established in the same animal model.

In a clinical trial, subjects with chronic relapsing pouchitis given a probiotic preparation for nine months, consisting of *L. casei, L. plantarum, L. acidophilus* and *L. delbruekii* subspecies *bulgaricus*, had significantly fewer relapses than did unsupplemented subjects receiving placebo. No side effects were seen. Some researchers believe that *Lactobacillus* GG may also be useful in treating pouchitis.

Some lactic acid bacteria, including *L. plantarum, L. rhamnosus, L. casei* and *Lactobacillus bulgaricus*, have demonstrated immuno-regulatory effects that might help protect against some allergic disorders. There is some evidence that some of these probiotic strains can reduce the intestinal inflammation associated with some food allergies, including cow's milk allergy among neonates. Breast-fed infants of nursing mothers given *Lactobacillus* GG had significantly improved atopic dermatitis, compared with infants not exposed to this probiotic.

There are *in vitro*, animal and some preliminary human data suggesting that some probiotics can bind and inactivate some carcinogens, can directly inhibit the growth of some tumors and can inhibit bacteria that may convert precarcinogens into carcinogens. *L. acidophilus* and *L. casei* have exhibited the latter activity in human volunteers. There is some preliminary evidence that *L. casei* may have reduced the recurrence of bladder tumors in humans. Confirmatory trials are needed. Animal work has suggested that some lactic-acid bacteria might help protect against colon cancer. Again, more research is needed.

Dairy products containing *L. acidophilus* have been credited with lowering cholesterol levels in some animal experiments. It has been hypothesized that bacterial assimilation of cholesterol in the intestine might reduce cholesterol stores available for absorption into the blood. To date, there is no credible evidence showing that any of the probiotics can lower cholesterol levels in humans. More study may be warranted. Yogurt has been used for some time as an "alternative" treatment for vaginitis. In an early test of this hypothesis, women with recurrent candidal vaginitis were treated with yogurt for six months. This was a crossover trial with subjects serving as their own controls. Daily ingestion of 8 ounces of yogurt significantly decreased both candidal colonization and infection.

Recently *L. acidophilus, L. crispatus* and *L. delbrueckii* subspecies *delbrueckii* all inhibited bacterial vaginosis-associated bacterial species *in vitro*. The researchers concluded that these probiotics might be useful for vaginal recolonization in women with recurrent vaginosis.

Owing to the fact that yogurt and some other probiotic-containing products are foods, rather than regulated pharmaceuticals, and owing to the fact that the probiotic content and potential of these food products may be highly variable, some researchers and clinicians have questioned the use of these products to treat vaginitis. In any event, larger better controlled studies are needed to further evaluate their reliability and efficacy in this context.

CONTRAINDICATIONS, PRECAUTIONS, ADVERSE REACTIONS

CONTRAINDICATIONS
Probiotics are contraindicated in those hypersensitive to any component of a probiotic-containing product.

PRECAUTIONS
Pregnant women and nursing mothers should only use probiotic nutritional supplements if recommended by their physicians.

The use of probiotics for the treatment of any disorder must be medically supervised.

ADVERSE REACTIONS
The most common adverse reactions with use of probiotics are gastrointestinal and include flatulence and constipation. Probiotics are generally well tolerated.

Four cases of *Saccharomyces boulardii* fungemia have been reported. All of the patients had indwelling catheters, and the fungemia was thought to be due to catheter contamination.

There are a few reports of *Lactobacillus* bacteremia and endocarditis. In all cases, there were underlying conditions, including cancer, diabetes mellitus and recent surgery. There is one death reported secondary to *Lactobacillus* bacteremia.

There is one report of meningitis caused by *Bifidobacterium* in an infant.

INTERACTIONS

NUTRITIONAL SUPPLEMENTS
Prebiotics: Concomitant use of prebiotics and probiotics may enhance the effectiveness of the probiotics. See Prebiotics. See Symbiotics.

DOSAGE AND ADMINISTRATION
There are many probiotic products available. These products contain various *Lactobacillus* strains, various *Bifidobacterium* strains, combinations of lactobacilli and bifidobacteria and combinations of probiotics and prebiotics. Typical doses of probiotics range from one to ten billion colony-forming units (CFU) a few times a week. Probiotics need to be consumed at least a few times a week to maintain their effect on the intestinal microecology.

The development of probiotic-containing yogurt products is actively being pursued by major food companies. These yogurt products are functional yogurt food products.

LITERATURE
Arunachalam K, Gill HS, Chandra RK. Enhancement of natural immune function by dietary consumption of bifidobacterium lactis. *Eur J Clin Nutr.* 2000; 54:263-267.

Arunachalam KD. Role of bifidobacteria in nutrition, medicine and technology. *Nutr Res.* 1999; 19:1559-1597.

Bielecka M, Biedrzycka E, Biedrzycka E, et al. Interaction of Bifidobacterium and Salmonella during associated growth. *Int J Food Microbiol.* 1998; 45:151-155.

Bleichner G, Blehaut H, Mentec H, Moyse D. *Saccharomyces boulardii* prevents diarrhea in critically ill tube-fed patients. A multicenter, randomized, double-blind, placebo-controlled trial. *Intensive Care Med.* 1997; 23:517-523.

Blum S, Reniero R, Schiffrin EJ, et al. Adhesion studies for probiotics: need for validation and refinement. *Trends Food Sci Technol.* 1999; 10:405-410.

Castagliuolo I, Riegler MF, Valenick L, et al. *Saccharomyces boulardii* protease inhibits the effects of *Clostridium difficile* toxins A and B in human colonic mucosa. *Infect Immun.* 1999; 67:302-307.

Czerucka D, Rampal P. Effect of *Saccharomyces boulardii* on cAMP- and Ca^{2+}-dependent Cl^- secretion in T84 cells. *Dig Dis Sci.* 1999; 44:2359-2368.

Dugas B, Mercenier A, Lenoir-Wijnkoop I, et al. Immunity and probiotics. *Immunol Today.* 1999; 20:387-390.

Elmer GW, McFarland LV, Surawicz CM, et al. Behavior of *Saccharomyces boulardii* in recurrent *Clostridium difficile* disease patients. *Aliment Pharmacol Ther.* 1999; 13:1663-1668.

Fredenucci I, Chomarat M, Boucaud C, Flandrois JP. *Saccharomyces boulardii fungemia* in a patient receiving Ultra-levure therapy. *Clin Infect Dis.* 1998; 27:222-223.

Gionchetti P, Rizzello F, Venturi A, Campieri M. Probiotics in infective diarrhoea and inflammatory bowel diseases. *J Gastroenterol Hepatol.* 2000; 15:489-493.

Gomes AMP, Malcata FX. *Bifidobacterium* spp. and *Lactobacillus acidophilus*: biological, biochemical, technological and therapeutical properties relevant for use as probiotics. *Trends Food Sci Technol.* 1999; 10:139-157.

Herias MV, Hessle C, Telemo E, et al. Immunomodulatory effects of *Lactobacillus plantarum* colonizing the intestine of gnotobiotic rats. *Clin Exp Immunol.* 1999; 116:283-290.

Hilton E, Isenberg HD, Alperstein P, et al. Ingestion of yogurt containing *Lactobacillus acidophilus*. *Ann Int Med.* 1992; 116:353-357.

Jahn HU, Ullrich R, Schneider T, et al. Immunological and trophical effects of *Saccharomyces boulardii* on the small intestine in healthy human volunteers. *Digestion.* 1996; 57:95-104.

Kimoto H, Kurisaki MN, Tsuji, et al. Lactococci as probiotic strains: adhesion to human enterocyte-like Caco-2 cells and tolerance to low pH and bile. *Lett Applied Microbiol.* 1999; 29:313-316.

Kirjavainen PV, Ouwehand AC, Isolauri E, Salminen SJ. The ability of probiotic bacteria to bind to human intestinal mucus. *FEMS Microbiol Lett.* 1998; 167:185-189.

Lactobacillus GG. *Nutrition Today.* 1996; 31:1S-52S.

Lin M-Y, Yen C-L. Antioxidative ability of lactic acid bacteria. *J Agric Food Chem.* 1999; 47:1460-1466.

Mack DR, Michail S, Wei S, et al. Probiotics inhibit enteropathogenic *E. coli* adherence in vitro by inducing intestinal mucin gene expression. *Am J. Physiol.* 1999; 276(4 Pt 1):G941-G950.

Majamaa H, Isolauri E. Probiotics: a novel approach in the management of food allergy. *J Allergy Clin Immunol.* 1997; 99:179-185.

Matilla-Sandholm T, Blum S, Collins JK, et al. Probiotics: towards demonstrating efficacy. *Trends Food Sci Technol.* 1999; 10:393-399.

Mattila-Sandholm T. The PROBDEMO project: demonstration of the nutritional functionality of probiotic foods. *Trends Food Sci Technol.* 1999; 10:385-386.

McFarland LV, Surawicz CM, Greenberg RN, et al. A randomized placebo-controlled trial of *Saccharomyces boulardii* in combination with standard antibiotics for *Clostridium difficile* disease. *JAMA.* 1994; 271:1913-1918.

Metchnikoff E. *The Prolongation of Life: Optimistic Studies.* The English translation. Mitchell PC, ed. 1908; New York:GP Putnam's Sons; 1908

O'Brien J, Crittenden R, Ouwehand AC, Salminen S. Safety evaluation of probiotics. *Trends Food Sci Technol.* 1999; 10:418-424.

Ouwehand AC, Tölkkö S, Kulmala J, et al. Adhesion of inactivated probiotic strains to intestinal mucus. *Lett Applied Microbiol.* 2000; 31:82-86.

Pletinex M, Legein J, Vandenplas Y. Fungemia with *Saccharomyces boulardii* in a 1-year old girl with protracted diarrhea. *J Pediatr Gastroenterol Nutr.* 1995; 21:113-115.

Saavedra J. Probiotics and infectious diarrhea. *Am J Gastroenterol.* 2000; 95 (1 Suppl):S16-S18.

Saxelin M, Grenov B, Svensson U, et al. The technology of probiotics. *Trends Food Sci Technol.* 1999; 10:387-392.

Shortt C. The probiotic century: historical and current perspectives. *Trends Food Sci Technol.* 1999; 10:411-417.

Symposium: Probiotic Bacteria: Implications for Human Health. *J Nutr.* 2000; 130:382S-409S.

Todorov S, Onno B, Sorokine O, et al. Detection and characterization of a novel antibacterial substance produced by *Lactobacillus plantarum* ST31 isolated from sourdough. *Int J Food Microbiol.* 1999; 48:167-177.

Turner DL, Brennan L, Meyer HE, et al. Solution structure of *plantaricin C*, a novel lantibiotic. *Eur J Biochem.* 1999; 264: 833-839.

Vaughan EE, Heilig HGHJ, Zoetendal EG, et al. Molecular approaches to study probiotic bacteria. *Trends Food Sci Technology.* 1999; 10:400-404.

Wollowski I, Ji S-T. Bakalinsky AT, et al. Bacteria used for the production of yogurt inactivate carcinogens and prevent DNA damage in the colon of rats. *J Nutr.* 1999; 129:77-82.

Propolis

TRADE NAMES

Bee Propolis (Twinlab, Rainbow Light, Nature's Answer), Propolis Power (Nature's Herbs).

DESCRIPTION

Propolis, also known as bee glue and bee propolis, is a brownish resinous substance collected by bees, mainly from poplar and conifer buds, and used to seal their hives.

Because of antimicrobial properties of propolis, it helps keep hives free of germs. Propolis has a long history of use in folk medicine and was even used as an official drug in London in the 1600s. Over time, propolis has been used for many purposes and marketed as lozenges, cough syrups, toothpastes, mouth rinses, lipsticks, cosmetics and even for the varnishing of Stradivarius violins. It appears to have antimicrobial and anti-inflammatory activities.

The composition of propolis is variable, depending on the locale and variety of trees and other plant species used for the collection. For example, unique constituents have been identified in propolis collected in Cuba and Brazil. The main chemical classes found in propolis are flavonoids, phenolics and terpenes. The flavonoids include quercetin, apegenin, galangin, kaempferol, luteolin, pinocembrin, pinostrobin and pinobanksin. The phenolic ester (caffeic acid phenethyl ester or CAPE) present in propolis is receiving much attention in the medical research community because of its potential for the treatment of a number of disorders, including spinal cord injury. Most of the substances in propolis are poorly soluble in water.

ACTIONS AND PHARMACOLOGY

ACTIONS

A list of possible actions of propolis includes: antibacterial, antifungal, antiviral (including anti HIV-1 activity), antioxidant, anticarcinogenic, antithrombotic and immunomodulatory.

MECHANISM OF ACTION

The mechanism of the possible actions of propolis may be understood by reviewing research findings on some of the individual compounds found in it. It is difficult to study the mechanism of actions of more than one compound at a time. Therefore, the following descriptions apply only to single compounds. The contribution of any single compound to the possible action of such a complex substance as propolis is difficult to know.

Caffeic acid phenethyl ester (CAPE) inhibits the lipoxygenase pathway of arachidonic acid, resulting in anti-inflammatory activity. CAPE is also known to have anticarcinogenic, antimitogenic and immunomodulatory properties. CAPE has been found to completely inhibit the activation of the nuclear transcription factor NF-Kappa B by tumor necrosis factor (TNF), as well as by other pro-inflammatory agents. The inhibition of NF-Kappa B activation may provide the molecular basis for its immunomodulatory, anticarcinogenic, anti-inflammatory and antiviral activities. It is possible that CAPE exerts its effects by inhibiting reactive oxygen species (ROS) production. ROS are known to play a major role in the activation of NF-Kappa B.

Compounds in propolis found to have antibacterial activity include a polyisoprenylated benzophenone, galangin, pinobanksin and pinocembrin. The exact mechanism of antimicrobial action of these compounds is not known.

INDICATIONS AND USAGE

There is evidence that propolis has some broad antimicrobial activity and that it may have anti-inflammatory effects that could make it useful in the treatment of some forms of arthritis, among other disorders. There is also some evidence of anti-cancer activity.

RESEARCH SUMMARY

In vitro and animal studies of propolis and derivative constituents have shown anti-bacterial, anti-viral and anti-fungal effects. It shows activity in culture against a broad spectrum of pathogens, including influenza and herpes viruses, as well as HIV and various fungal and bacterial organisms.

In a study of school children, an aqueous propolis extract was judged effective in reducing the incidence and intensity of acute and chronic rhinopharyngitis. In another study involving 10 volunteers, it exerted activity against oral bacteria. A Cuban study concluded that propolis is more effective than tinidazole against giardia.

Propolis has a high concentration of caffeic acid esters that some believe may give it some antitumor properties. In two studies, extracts of propolis fed to rats have inhibited azoxymethane-induced colonic tumors.

In vitro studies have shown propolis-related anti-inflammatory effects. Various extracts of propolis have also shown anti-inflammatory activity in animal models, particularly against adjuvant-induced arthritis.

More research is needed to further explore these preliminary findings.

CONTRAINDICATIONS, PRECAUTIONS, ADVERSE REACTIONS

CONTRAINDICATIONS

Propolis is contraindicated in those who are allergic or hypersensitive to any of its components.

PRECAUTIONS

Pregnant women and nursing mothers should avoid using propolis supplements.

ADVERSE REACTIONS

There are reported adverse reactions in those using topical preparations of propolis. These reactions are manifested as a dermatitis. There are reports of hypersensitivity reactions to ingested propolis, including rhinitis, conjunctivitis, skin rashes and bronchospasm.

OVERDOSAGE

No reported overdosage of propolis.

DOSAGE AND ADMINISTRATION

No typical dose. Propolis is available in several different preparations, including lozenges, tablets, creams, gels, mouth rinses, toothpastes and cough syrups.

HOW SUPPLIED

Capsules — 120 mg, 500 mg, 650 mg

Liquid

Lozenge — 50 grains

Tablets — 500 mg

LITERATURE

Burdock GA. Review of the biological properties and toxicity of bee propolis (propolis). *Food Chem Toxicol.* 1998; 36:347-363.

Chopra S, Pillai KK, Husain SZ, Giri DK. Propolis protects against doxorubicin-induced myocardiopathy in rats. *Exp Mol Pathol.* 1995; 62:190-198.

El-Ghazaly MA, Khayyal MT. The use of aqueous propolis extract against radiation-induced damage. *Drugs Exp Clin Res.* 1995; 21:229-236.

Grange JM, Davey RW. Antibacterial properties of propolis (bee glue). *J.R Soc Med.* 1990; 83:159-160.

Harish Z, Rubinstein A, Golodner M, et al. Suppression of HIV-1 replication by propolis and its immunoregulatory effect. *Drugs Exp Clin Res.* 1997; 23:89-96.

Khayyal MT, el-Ghazaly MA, el-Khatib AS. Mechanism involved in the anti-inflammatory effect of propolis extract. *Drugs Exp Clin Res.* 1993; 19:197-203.

Kujumgiev A, Tsverkova I, Serkedjieva Y, et al. Antibacterial, antifungal and antiviral activity of propolis of different geographic origins. *J Ethnopharmacol.* 1999; 64:235-240.

Ledon N, Casaco A, Gonzales R, et al. Antipsoriatic, anti-inflammatory and analgesic effects of an extract of red propolis. *Chung Kuo Yao Li Hsueh Pao.* 1997; 18:274-276.

Lin SC, Lin YH, Chen CF, et al. The hepatoprotective and therapeutic effects of propolis ethanol extract on chronic alcohol-induced liver injuries. *Am J Chin Med* 1997; 25:325-332.

Matsuno T, Jung SK, Matsumoto Y, et al. Preferential cytotoxicity to tumor cells of 3, 5-diprenyl-4-hydroxycinnamic acid (artipillin C) isolated from propolis. *Anticancer Res.* 1997; 17(5A):3565-3568.

Mirzoeva OK, Calder PC. The effect of propolis and its components on eicosanoid production during the inflammatory response. *Prostaglandins Leukot Essent Fatty Acids.* 1996; 55:441-449.

Mirzoeva OK, Grishanin RN, Calder PC. Antimicrobial actin of propolis and some of its components: the effects on growth, membrane potential and motility of bacteria. *Microbiol Res.* 1997; 152:239-246.

Natarajan K, Singh S, Burke TR Jr, et al. Caffeic acid phenethyl ester is a potent and specific inhibitor of activation of nuclear transcription factor NF-Kappa B. *Proc Natl Acad Sci.* 1996; 93:9090-9095.

Ozturk F, Kurt E, Cerci M, et al. The effect of propolis extract in experimental chemical corneal injury. *Ophthalmic Res.* 2000; 32:13-18.

Park EH, Kahng JH. Suppressive effects of propolis in rat adjuvant arthritis. *Arch Pharm Res.* 1999; 22:554-558.

Rao CV, Desai D, Simi B, et al. Inhibitory effect of caffeic acid esters on azoxymethane-induced biochemical change and aberrant crypt foci formation in rat colon. *Cancer Res.* 1993; 53:4182-4188.

Psyllium

TRADE NAMES

Konsyl and Konsyl-D (Konsyl Pharmaceuticals), Serutan (Lee Pharmaceuticals), Perdiem and Fiberall (Novartis Consumer), Syllact (Wallace Labs), Genfiber (Zenith Goldline), Modane (Savage), Metamucil (Procter & Gamble).

DESCRIPTION

In 1998, the Food and Drug Administration (FDA) issued its final rule allowing health claims to be made on the labels of foods containing soluble fiber from whole oats (see Oat Beta-D-Glucan), noting that these foods, in conjunction with a diet low in saturated fat and cholesterol, may reduce the risk of heart disease. Shortly afterward, the FDA amended this to include the soluble fiber psyllium in the health claim. The FDA requires that there be at least 1.7 grams of soluble fiber from psyllium seed husk per serving in any food for which this health claim is made. To achieve heart-health benefits, the consumption of 7 grams of soluble fiber from psyllium are required.

Psyllium or *Plantago ovata* Forsk is an annual plant grown primarily in India, southern Europe and the United States. Psyllium is cultivated primarily for its use as a laxative or as a dietary fiber ingredient in foods, such as ready-to-eat cereals. It is also known as blond psyllium, Indian psyllium and plantain. Although the seed alone contains the bioactive mucilage polysaccharide, the refined psyllium seed husk, known as the Ispaghula husk, is the psyllium component principally used as the soluble fiber source for laxatives, ready-to-eat cereals and nutritional supplements.

The term psyllium is used interchangeably for the seed husk, the seed and the plant. Psyllium seed husk is comprised primarily of xylans. Xylans are polysaccharides built from the five-carbon sugar D-xylose. Xylans in psyllium seed husk occur in association with cellulose. The soluble fiber derived from psyllium seed husk is also known as psyllium hydrophilic mucilloid, psyllium hydrocolloid and psyllium seed gum. It is a white to cream-colored, slightly granular powder with a slight acid taste.

ACTIONS AND PHARMACOLOGY
ACTIONS
Psyllium may have hypocholesterolemic, glucose-regulatory and bowel-regulatory actions.

MECHANISM OF ACTION
The mechanism of psyllium's possible hypocholesterolemic activity is not fully understood. The bioactive agent of psyllium is a soluble, viscous xylan fiber. It is thought that this polysaccharide stimulates the conversion of cholesterol to bile acids and that it stimulates fecal excretion of bile acids. Psyllium may also decrease the intestinal absorption of cholesterol.

Some studies indicate that psyllium may improve glycemic control in type 2 diabetics. The mechanism of the effect is unclear. Psyllium may delay the absorption of carbohydrates by increasing gastric-emptying time and/or decreasing small intestinal transit time.

The laxative effect of psyllium is thought to be due to the swelling of psyllium from absorption of water with consequent increase in stool bulk and stimulation of peristalsis.

PHARMACOKINETICS
Following ingestion of psyllium, very little is digested in the small intestine. The psyllium polysaccharides are resistant to hydrolysis by the digestive enzymes. Some fermentation of the psyllium polysaccharides takes place in the large intestine via the action of colonic bacteria. The products of fermentation include the short-chain fatty acids acetate, propionate and butyrate, as well as hydrogen and carbon dioxide. The short-chain fatty acids that escape colonic metabolism are transported via the portal circulation to the liver, where they undergo metabolism.

INDICATIONS AND USAGE
The FDA allows a health claim for psyllium to the effect that, in conjunction with a low-fat diet, it may reduce risk of heart disease if used in adequate amounts. Numerous studies have shown that psyllium is effective in lowering total cholesterol and LDL-cholesterol levels in some with hypercholesterolemia. It is also helpful in some with constipation and may have benefit in some with diabetes. Claims that it is useful in preventing and treating anal fissures and hemorrhoids appear related to psyllium's efficacy in preventing and treating constipation. There is no credible evidence to support claims that psyllium is helpful in those with psoriasis or that it is effective in treating obesity.

RESEARCH SUMMARY
A recent meta-analysis of eight controlled trials investigating the effects of psyllium on lipids concluded that this supplement significantly lowered serum total and LDL-cholesterol concentrations in both male and female subjects who consumed a low-fat diet. Consumption of 10.2 grams of psyllium per day lowered serum total cholesterol 4% and LDL-cholesterol by 7%, compared with controls also consuming a low-fat diet but not supplementing with psyllium. No significant effects were seen in this meta-analysis on either serum HDL-cholesterol or triacylglycerol concentrations.

In one recent animal model of hypertension induced by salt ingestion, psyllium supplementation significantly attenuated salt-accelerated hypertension. The proposed possible mechanism of action was increased fecal excretion of sodium taken up by the psyllium.

In a recent study, psyllium was used adjunctively with a traditional diabetes diet to treat men with mild-to-moderate hypercholesterolemia and type 2 diabetes. Subjects were randomized to receive 5.1 grams of psyllium or cellulose placebo twice daily for eight weeks. Those receiving psyllium had significant improvement in glucose and lipid values compared with controls. Concentrations of serum total and LDL-cholesterol were 8.9% and 13% lower, respectively, in the psyllium group than in the control group.

Psyllium has been used for some time as a major ingredient in bulk laxatives. The FDA has approved this use, and the German Commission E has indicated that psyllium may be helpful in those with chronic constipation and some of the possible complications of constipation, including anal fissures and hemorrhoids. It may also be useful in some forms of diarrhea and in those who have had anal/rectal surgery. Some pregnant women are said to benefit from it as well.

CONTRAINDICATIONS, PRECAUTIONS, ADVERSE REACTIONS
CONTRAINDICATIONS
Psyllium is contraindicated in those hypersensitive to psyllium or to any component of a psyllium-containing product. It is also contraindicated in those with intestinal obstruction, fecal impaction, difficulty in swallowing and esophageal narrowing.

PRECAUTIONS
Pregnant women and nursing mothers should only use psyllium supplements if recommended by their physicians.

Supplemental psyllium must be taken with adequate amounts of fluids. Inadequate fluid intake may cause psyllium to swell and block the throat, esophagus or intestines.

Supplemental psyllium should not be taken right before going to bed.

ADVERSE REACTIONS

The most common adverse reactions are flatulence and abdominal distention. Potentially severe allergic reactions, including anaphylaxis, have been reported. These are not common.

INTERACTIONS

DRUGS

Concomitant use of psyllium and lithium may reduce the absorption of lithium. Concomitant use of psyllium and carbamazepine, digoxin and warfarin may reduce the absorption of those drugs.

Psyllium may enhance the cholesterol-lowering action of cholestyramine.

NUTRITIONAL SUPPLEMENTS

Psyllium may decrease the absorption of such minerals as zinc, copper, iron, calcium and magnesium if used concomitantly.

OVERDOSAGE

No reports.

DOSAGE AND ADMINISTRATION

Psyllium supplements are typically used in powder form, along with adequate amounts of fluids.

A dose of at least 7 grams daily taken with adequate amounts of fluid (water, juice) is used by some for management of elevated cholesterol.

There are a number of psyllium products used for constipation. The usual dose is about 3.5 grams twice a day. Again, the psyllium should be taken with adequate amounts of fluid.

Psyllium is a component of several ready-to-eat cereals.

HOW SUPPLIED

Capsules — 560 mg, 566 mg, 600 mg, 610 mg, 630 mg, 660 mg

Granules for Reconstitution

Powder for Reconstitution

Wafers

LITERATURE

Anderson JW, Allgood LD, Lawrence A, et al. Cholesterol-lowering effects of psyllium intake adjunctive to diet therapy in men and women with hypercholesterolemia: meta-analysis of 8 controlled studies. *Am J Clin Nutr.* 2000; 71:472-479.

Anderson JW, Allgood LD, Turner J, et al. Effects of psyllium on glucose and serum lipid responses in men with type 2 diabetes and hypercholesterolemia. *Am J Clin Nutr.* 1999; 70:466-473.

Anderson JW, Davidson MH, Blonde L, et al. Long-term cholesterol-lowering effects of psyllium as an adjunct in the treatment of hypercholesterolemia. *Am J Clin Nutr.* 2000; 71:1433-1438.

Lantner RR, Espiritu BR, Zumerchik P, Tobin MC. Anaphylaxis following ingestion of a psyllium-containing cereal. *JAMA.* 1990; 264:2534-2536.

Levin EG, Miller VT, Muesing RA, et al. Comparison of psyllium hydrophilic mucilloid and cellulose in the treatment of mild to moderate hypercholesterolemia. *Arch Intern Med.* 1990; 150:1822-1827.

Turley SD, Daggy BP, Dietschy JM. Effect of feeding psyllium and cholestyramine in combination on low density lipoprotein metabolism and fecal bile acid excretion in hamsters with dietary-induced hypercholesterolemia. *J Cardiovasc Pharmacol.* 1996; 27:71-79.

Pycnogenol

TRADE NAMES

Pycnogenol Plus (Quantum), Pycnogenol Power (Nature's Herbs).

DESCRIPTION

The term pycnogenol refers to a specific mixture of procyanidins extracted from the bark of the French maritime pine, *Pinus maritima*. The French maritime pine grows in Bay of Biscay in the Landes de Gascogne in France. Although the term pycnogenol is now confined to procyanidins from the French maritime pine, the term was originally intended to serve as scientific name for this class of flavonoids.

Procyanidins are derivatives of the flavan-3-ol class of flavonoids. This class includes epicatechin and catechin. Procyanidins consisting of dimers of catechin and oligomers of epicatechin and catechin are found in pycnogenol. Pycnogenol has a high amount of oligomers containing 5 to 7 units. Procyanidin oligomers are also known as oligomeric procyanidins (OPC) oligomeric proanthocyanidins (also OPCs) and procyanidolic oligomers (PCOs). In addition to OPCs, pycnogenol contains catechin, epicatechin and taxifolin, and such phenolic acids as caffeic, ferulic and para-hydroxybenzoic acids as minor constituents. It also contains glycosylation products of flavonols and phenolic acids as minute constituents. Pycnogenol is abbreviated PYC.

Procyanidins, including oligomeric procyanidins, are also found in such foods as cocoa and chocolate, grape seeds, apples, peanuts, almonds, cranberries and blueberries. They are also found in such medicinal herbs as "Sangre de drago" (*Croton lechleri*).

Procyanidins are also known as leucocyanidins. Procyanidins and prodelphinidins comprise a class of polyphenolic compounds called proanthocyanidins. Whereas procyanidins are oligomers of catechin and epicatechin and their gallic acid esters, prodelphinidins are oligomers of gallocatechin and epigallocatechin and their galloylated derivatives. Proanthocyanidins are also known as condensed tannins.

ACTIONS AND PHARMACOLOGY

ACTIONS

Pycnogenol has antioxidant activity. It may also have anti-inflammatory activity and has putative cardiovascular-protective activity.

MECHANISM OF ACTION

Pycnogenol has demonstrated a number of antioxidant activities in the laboratory. These include scavenging of the superoxide radical anion, the hydroxyl radical, the lipid peroxyl radical, the peroxynitrite radical and singlet oxygen. It has also been shown to protect low-density lipoprotein (LDL) from oxidation. The oligomeric procyanidins appear to have especially potent antioxidant activity when compared with smaller molecules, such as catechin and epicatechin. The extent of the antioxidant potential of pycnogenol in *vivo* is unclear. Some studies suggest that the antioxidant potential is at least partially available *in vivo*. Pycnogenol has been shown to have anti-inflammatory activity, again in the laboratory. This activity is thought to be due, in large part, to pycnogenol's capacity as a scavenger of reactive oxygen and reactive nitrogen species.

Pycnogenol appears to inhibit the activation of the transcription factors NF-kappa B and AP-1. NF-kappa B and AP-1 upregulate the expression of several inflammatory mediators such as intercellular adhesion molecule-1 (ICAM-1). NF-kappa B is itself activated by reactive oxygen species. Pycnogenol has been found to inhibit the inducible expression of ICAM-1. Inhibition of ICAM-1 may be accounted for by inhibition, by pycnogenol, of the activation of NF-Kappa B and AP-1. Further, the inflammatory cytokine interferon-gamma (IFN-gamma) may upregulate ICAM-1 expression in keratinocytes. This has been noted in some inflammatory skin conditions, such as lupus erythematous, atopic dermatitis and psoriasis. Pycnogenol appears to inhibit IFN-gamma activation of STAT (signal transducer and activator of transcription) 1. Inhibition of ICAM-1 expression by pycnogenol could account for possible anti-inflammatory and anti-atherogenic activities of pycnogenol.

PHARMACOKINETICS

Little is known about the pharmacokinetics of pycnogenol in humans. It appears that at least some of it is absorbed. However, the extent of absorption appears to vary widely, not only among the various components of pycnogenol, but also among subjects.

Some of the components of pycnogenol (e.g., catechin) appear to undergo extensive glucuronidation and sulfation following and/or during absorption. The glucuronides and sulfates are excreted in the urine.

INDICATIONS AND USAGE

Claims made for pycnogenol are sweeping. It has been demonstrated to have free-radical-scavenging properties, but far from established are claims that it is useful in immune and neuro-degenerative disorders, that it is an effective anti-allergen, anticancer agent, antidiabetic agent and that it speeds healing of injuries, fights arthritis and is useful in cirrhosis of the liver and aging. Clinical trials are in short supply. Current research suggests that pycnogenol might have some cardioprotective effects and might be helpful in some vascular disorders. It is possible that some immune-modulating, anti-inflammatory and anticancer effects will emerge.

RESEARCH SUMMARY

In vitro studies have demonstrated that pycnogenol can protect some cells from lipid peroxidation and damage induced by various oxidative toxins.

In vivo, pycnogenol has shown some ability to minimize ischemic reperfusion injury in an animal model. There is some preliminary suggestion that pycnogenol may exhibit vasorelaxation activity, inhibit angiotensin-converting enzyme and enhance microcirculation by promoting increased capillary resistance. It may inhibit platelet aggregation and LDL-cholesterol oxidation. It may help maintain levels of some other antioxidants, principally vitamins C and E. Many of these effects have only been demonstrated *in vitro*.

In one of the few clinical trials of pycnogenol, the substance significantly inhibited smoking-induced platelet aggregation, more significantly with doses of 200 mg than with doses of 100 or 150 mg of pycnogenol. A single 200 mg dose of pycnogenol was reported to significantly inhibit platelet aggregation for longer than three days in smokers.

Pycnogenol has reportedly met with some success in treating certain vascular disorders, including varicose veins and chronic venous insufficiency. Pycnogenol has also inhibited some localized inflammation experimentally induced in animals.

Using doses of pycnogenol higher than could likely be administered to humans, researchers have restored some immune functions in an animal model of HIV-infection. In other animals, oral feeding of pycnogenol has resulted in significant improvement in T- and B-cell function. Natural killer cell cytotoxicity has been enhanced in animals given pycnogenol. Clinical trials are needed.

Pycnogenol has shown preliminary chemoprotective effects against NKK, a tobacco-specific nitrosamine, in rats exposed to this substance.

CONTRAINDICATIONS, PRECAUTIONS, ADVERSE REACTIONS.

CONTRAINDICATIONS

Pycnogenol is contraindicated in those with known hypersensitivity to any of the ingredients of a pycnogenol-containing product.

PRECAUTIONS

Pycnogenol supplementation should be avoided by pregnant women and nursing mothers.

ADVERSE REACTIONS

None reported.

INTERACTIONS

DRUGS

The use of pycnogenol and dextroamphetamine appeared superior to dextroamphetamine alone in the management of attention deficit-hyperactivity disorder, in one case report.

OVERDOSAGE

There are no reports of overdosage.

DOSAGE AND ADMINISTRATION

Dosage ranges from 25 to 200 mg daily.

HOW SUPPLIED

Capsules — 30 mg, 50 mg, 75 mg, 100 mg

Cream

Lotion

Tablets — 25 mg, 30 mg, 50 mg, 75 mg, 100 mg

LITERATURE

Bito T, Roy S, Sen CK, Packer L. Pine bark extract pycnogenol downregulates IFN-gamma-induced adhesion of T cells to human keratinocytes by inhibiting inducible ICAM-1 expression. *Free Rad Biol Med.*2000; 28:219-227.

Heimann SW. Pycnogenol for ADHD. *J Am Acad Child Adolesc Psychiatry.* 1999; 38:357-358.

Huynh HT, Teel RW. Effects of pycnogenol on the microsomal metabolism of the tobacco-specific nitrosamine NNK as a function of age. *Cancer Lett.*1998; 132:135-139.

Liu FJ, Zhang YX, Lau BH. Pycnogenol enhances immune and haemopoietic functions in senescence-accelerated mice. *Cell Mol Life Sci.* 1998; 54:1168-1172.

Packer LK, Rimbach G, Virgili F. Antioxidant activity and biological propertes of a procyanidin-rich extract from pine (*Pinus maritima*) bark, pycnogenol. *Free Rad Biol Med.* 1999; 27:704-724.

Putter M, Grotemeyer KH, Wurthwein G, et al. Inhibition of smoking-induced platelet aggregation by aspirin and pycnogenol. *Thromb Res.*1999; 95:155-161.

Pyruvate

TRADE NAMES

Pyruvate is available in generic formulations from numerous manufacturers. Branded products include Pyruvate Burn (Gen), Pyruvate Fuel (Twinlab), Pyruvate 1000 (Pinnacle), Diet Pyruvate (Source Naturals).

DESCRIPTION

Pyruvate is the anionic form of the three-carbon organic acid, pyruvic acid. Pyruvate is a key intermediate in the glycolytic and pyruvate dehydrogenase pathways, which are involved in biological energy production. Pyruvate is widely found in living organisms. It is not an essential nutrient since it can be synthesized in the cells of the body. Pyruvate, however, is consumed in the diet. The average daily intake of this substance ranges between about 100 milligrams and 1 to 2 grams. Certain fruits and vegetables are rich in pyruvate. For example, an average-size red apple contains approximately 450 milligrams. Dark beer and red wine are also rich sources of pyruvate.

Recent research suggests that pyruvate in supraphysiological concentrations may have a role in cardiovascular therapy, as an inotropic agent. Supraphysiological amounts of this dietary substance may also have bariatric and ergogenic applications.

Pyruvate is also known as 2-oxopropanoate, alpha-ketopropionate, acetylformate and pyroracemate. Pyruvate and pyruvic acid are frequently use interchangeably, even though pyruvate is the anion of pyruvic acid and the form that occurs in living organisms. Pyruvic acid is represented by the following chemical structure:

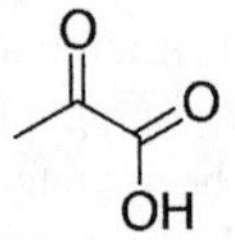

Pyruvic Acid

ACTIONS AND PHARMACOLOGY

ACTIONS

Pyruvate is a biological fuel source. It may also have cardiac and skeletal muscle inotropic activity as well as bariatric activity. Pyruvate also has antioxidant activity.

MECHANISM OF ACTION

Pyruvate serves as a biological fuel by being converted to acetyl coenzyme A, which enters the tricarboxylic acid or Krebs cycle where it is metabolized to produce ATP aerobically. Energy can also be obtained anaerobically from pyruvate via its conversion to lactate.

At supraphysiological levels, pyruvate increases contractile function of hearts when metabolizing glucose or fatty acids. This inotropic effect is striking in hearts stunned by ischemia/reperfusion. The inotropic effect of pyruvate requires intracoronary infusion.

Among possible mechanisms for this effect are increased generation of ATP and an increase in ATP phosphorylation potential. Another is activation of pyruvate dehydrogenase, promoting its own oxidation by inhibiting pyruvate dehydrogenase kinase. Pyruvate dehydrogenase is inactivated in ischemia myocardium. Yet another is reduction of cytosolic inorganic phosphate concentration. There are other possible mechanisms, such as enhanced sarcoplasmic reticular ion uptake, and release and reactive oxygen species scavenging.

Supraphysiological levels of pyruvate are reported to enhance aerobic endurance capacity. Again, the mechanism of this action is far from being well understood. Some studies indicate that pyruvate at supraphysiological levels increases the transport of glucose into muscle cells in a process known as blood glucose extraction. This could spare skeletal muscle glycogen stores.

The mechanism by which supraphysiological levels of pyruvate may lead to fat loss is unclear. Rats that consumed a diet supplemented with pyruvate and dihydroxyacetone reportedly had a lower respiratory quotient (RQ), indicating an increased utilization of fat as an energy source, as well as elevated resting metabolic rate. In addition, the rats that received pyruvate and dihydroxyacetone had elevated levels of thyroxine, lower levels of plasma insulin and lower rates of lipid synthesis in adipose tissue. Fat oxidation may be enhanced in some obese individuals administered pyruvate.

Regarding pyruvate's antioxidant action, pyruvate is known to scavenge such reactive oxygen species as hydrogen peroxide and lipid peroxides. This is a direct antioxidant effect. Indirectly, supraphysiological levels of pyruvate may increase cellular reduced glutathione.

PHARMACOKINETICS

Pyruvate is absorbed from the gastrointestinal tract from whence it is transported to the liver via the portal circulation. In the liver, pyruvate is metabolized via several pathways. Pyruvate may be converted to acetyl coenzyme A, which can enter the tricarboxylic acid or Krebs cycle for aerobic production of ATP. Energy can also be obtained from pyruvate anaerobically via its reduction to lactate. Via an aminotransferase reaction, pyruvate may be converted to L-alanine. And via its conversion to oxaloacetate by pyruvate carboxylase, it can become a precursor in the synthesis of glucose and glycogen by the process known as gluconeogenesis. Pyruvate not metabolized in the liver can be transported

via the systemic circulation to other tissues in the body and undergo similar metabolic processes as described above.

INDICATIONS AND USAGE

Pyruvate may help some obese individuals lose weight. There is also the suggestion in current research that it might help some overweight individuals lower their blood pressure, and it may favorably modify lipid profiles. It also appears to enhance exercise endurance in some and may be protective in others with cardiac ischemia. There is a suggestion in animal work that it might have an ability to reduce insulin resistance.

RESEARCH SUMMARY

Obese women were given a 1000-calorie liquid diet that included 30 grams of pyruvate daily or placebo in the form of matching liquid diet without pyruvate for 21 days. The pyruvate-supplemented women lost significantly more weight, including weight in the form of fat, than did the controls.

In a subsequent trial, hyperlipidemic subjects were randomized to receive 36 to 53 grams of pyruvate daily or 21 to 37 grams of polyglucose as placebo. There was a significant reduction in plasma cholesterol and LDL concentrations in the pyruvate-treated subjects but not in the controls. Plasma HDL cholesterol and triglyceride concentrations did not show significant change. Resting heart rate, diastolic blood pressure and rate-pressure product decreased 9%, 6% and 12% respectively in the treated group, but were unchanged in the untreated group.

In a recent double-blind study, a much lower dose of pyruvate was tested in overweight men and women. Twenty-six subjects were randomized to receive 6 grams of pyruvate daily or placebo. All subjects participated in 45 to 60 minutes of aerobics three times a week. At the conclusion of the six-week trial, there were significant decreases in body weight, body fat and percent body fat in the pyruvate group, compared with controls.

Pyruvate has also shown some ability to enhance exercise endurance capacity. Used in combination with dihydroxyacetone (DHA), pyruvate (100 grams for seven days) significantly enhanced submaximal arm endurance capacity in untrained males (20 to 26 years old). This placebo-controlled study demonstrated a pyruvate ability to significantly increase arm muscle glucose extraction before and during exercise.

A follow-up study demonstrated similar positive effects in enhancing leg exercise endurance. On the other hand, a recent study showed no pyruvate effect on anaerobic performance and body composition in football players except when it was combined with creatine. More research in needed.

There is evidence from *in vitro*, animal and preliminary human research that pyruvate, in doses and modes of administration not relevant to supplementation, may be effective in some with cardiac ischemia through its inhibition of free-radical generation, among other things.

A study in female Zucker obese rats showed that pyruvate can favorably alter metabolism in these animals; it appeared to reduce the insulin resistance that spontaneously develops in this animal model.

CONTRAINDICATIONS, PRECAUTIONS, ADVERSE REACTIONS

CONTRAINDICATIONS
None known.

PRECAUTIONS
Pregnant women and nursing mothers should avoid pyruvate supplementation.

ADVERSE REACTIONS
Those taking large doses of supplemental pyruvate—usually greater than 5 grams daily—have reported gastrointestinal symptoms, including abdominal discomfort and bloating, gas and diarrhea. One child receiving pyruvate intravenously for restrictive cardiomyopathy died.

INTERACTIONS
Acetyl-L-carnitine has been reported to reverse the age-related decrease in mitochondrial pyruvate metabolism in rats.

OVERDOSAGE
There are no reports of overdosage with supplemental pyruvate.

DOSAGE AND ADMINISTRATION
Dosage has been variable. The most current research suggests a dose of 5 to 6 grams daily for a possible bariatric action or for athletic use.

HOW SUPPLIED
Capsules — 325 mg, 500 mg, 650 mg, 750 mg

Powder — 3 g/teaspoonful

Tablets — 500 mg, 1000 mg

LITERATURE
Hermann H-P, Pieske B, Schwarzmü ller E, et al. Haemodynamic effects of intracoronary pyruvate in patients with congestive heart failure: an open study. *Lancet.* 1999; 353:1321-1323.

Ivy JL. Effect of pyruvate and dihydroxyacetone on metabolism and aerobic endurance capacity. *Med Sci Sports Exer.* 1998; 30:837-843.

Ivy JL, Cortez MY, Chandler RM, et al. Effects of pyruvate on the metabolism and insulin resistance of obese Zucker rats. *Am J Clin Nutr.* 1994; 59:331-337.

Kalman D, Colker CM, Wilets I, et al. The effects of pyruvate supplementation on body composition in overweight individuals. *Nutrition.* 1999; 15:337-340.

Mallet RT. Pyruvate: metabolic protector of cardiac performance. *Proc Soc Exp Biol Med.* 2000; 223:136-148

Mallet RT, Sun J. Mitochondrial metabolism of pyruvate is required for its enhancement of cardiac function and energetics. *Cardiovasc Res.* 1999; 42:149-161.

Matthys D, Van Coster R, Verhaaren H. Fatal outcome of pyruvate loading test in child with restrictive cardiomyopathy. *Lancet.* 1991; 338:1020-1021.

Robertson RJ, Stanko RT, Goss FL. Blood glucose extraction as a mediator of perceived exertion during prolonged exercise. *Eur J Appl Physiol.* 1990; 61:100-105.

Stanko RT, Arch JE. Inhibition of regain in body weight and fat with addition of 3-carbon compounds to the diet with hyperenergetic refeeding after weight reduction. *Int J Obes Relat Metab Disord.* 1996; 20:925-930.

Stanko RT, Mullick P, Clarke MR, et al. Pyruvate inhibits growth of mammary adenocarcinoma 13762 in rats. *Cancer Res.* 1994; 54:1004-1007.

Stanko RT Reynolds HR, Hoyson R, et al. Pyruvate supplementation of a low-cholesterol, low-fat diet: effects on plasma lipid concentrations and body composition in hyperlipidemic patients. *Am J Clin Nutr.* 1994; 59:423-427.

Stanko RT, Reynolds HR, Lonchar KD, Arch JE. Plasma lipid concentrations in hyperlipidemic patients consuming a high-fat diet supplemented with pyruvate for 6 weeks. *Am J Clin Nutr.* 1992; 56:950-954.

Stanko RT, Tietze DL, Arch JE. Body composition, energy utilization, and nitrogen metabolism with a 4.25 MJ/d low-energy diet supplemented with pyruvate. *Am J Clin Nutr.* 1992; 56:630-635.

Quercetin

DESCRIPTION
Quercetin belongs to a group of polyphenolic substances known as flavonoids. Quercetin is a member of the class of flavonoids called flavonols. It is widely distributed in the plant kingdom in rinds and barks. Especially rich sources of quercetin include onions, red wine, green tea and St. John's wort.

Quercetin is typically found in plants as glycone or carbohydrate conjugates. Quercetin itself is an aglycone or aglucon. That is, quercetin does not possess a carbohydrate moiety in its structure. Quercetin glycone conjugates include rutin and thujin. Rutin is also known as quercetin-3-rutinoside. Thujin is also known as quercitrin, quercetin-3-L-rhamnoside, and 3-rhamnosylquercetin. Onions contain conjugates of quercetin and the carbohydrate isorhamnetin, including quercetin-3,4'-di-O-beta glucoside, isorhamnetin-4'-0-beta-glucoside and quercetin-4'-0-beta-glucoside. Quercetin itself is practically insoluble in water. The quercetin carbohydrate conjugates have much greater water solubility then quercetin.

Quercetin is known chemically as 2-(3, 4-dihydroxyphenyl)-3,5,7-trihydroxy-4H-1-benzopyran-4-one and 3,3',4'5,7-pentahydroxy flavone. It is also known as meletin and sophretin and is represented by the following structural formula:

Quercetin

ACTIONS AND PHARMACOLOGY

ACTIONS

Quercetin may have antioxidant, anti-inflammatory, antivral, immunomodulatory, anticancer and gastroprotective activities. It may also have anti-allergy activity and activity in preventing secondary complications of diabetes.

MECHANISMS OF ACTION

Quercetin is a phenolic antioxidant and has been shown to inhibit lipid peroxidation. The putative anti-ulcer and gastroprotective effects of quercetin may, in part, be accounted for by this activity. *In vitro* and animal studies have shown that quercetin inhibits degranulation of mast cells, basophils and neutrophils. Such activity could account, in part, for quercetin's putative anti-inflammatory, anti-allergy and immunomodulating activities. Other *in vitro* and animal studies suggest that quercetin inhibits tyrosine kinase and nitric oxide synthase and that it modulates the activity of the inflammatory mediator, NF-kappaB. The mechanisms of anti-viral (in some cases enhanced with vitamin C) and anti-cancer activity that have been observed, again in *in vitro* and in animal studies, are unknown.

Aldose reductase, also known as alditol: NADP+ oxidoreductase, is the first enzyme of the polyol pathway. Hyperglycemia enhances the flow rate of the polyol pathway and this has been linked to such diabetic complications as cataracts,

retinopathy, neuropathy and nephropathy. Quercetin is known to inhibit aldose reductase.

PHARMACOKINETICS

About 25% of an ingested dose of quercetin is absorbed from the small intestine and is transported to the liver via the portal circulation, where it undergoes significant first pass metabolism. Quercetin and its metabolites are distributed from the liver to various tissues in the body. Quercetin is strongly bound to albumin in the plasma. Peak levels of plasma quercetin occur from 0.7 to 7 hours following ingestion, and the elimination half-life of quercetin is approximately 25 hours.

Regarding pharmacokinetics of the quercetin glycoside conjugates, it appears that the main determinant of absorption of these conjugates is the nature of the sugar moiety. For example, quercetin glucoside is absorbed from the small intestine, whereas quercetin rutinoside is absorbed from the colon after removal of the carbohydrate moiety by bacterial enzymes.

INDICATIONS AND USAGE

It has been claimed that quercetin protects against heart attacks and stroke, but recent research found no support for this claim. Quercetin may, however, have benefit in some allergies, in conditions characterized by capillary fragility, in chronic prostatis and in some cancers. It may have beneficial effects on immunity and may have gastro-protective effects. It may also protect against the development of such diabetic complications as cataracts, retinopathy, neuropathy and nephropathy.

RESEARCH SUMMARY

Epidemiological evidence has suggested for some time that dietary intake of flavonols and flavones is inversely associated with coronary heart disease. It has been hypothesized that the ability of flavonoids to inhibit lipid peroxidation, demonstrated both *in vitro* and in various animal models, might, at least partially, account for this association.

More recently, however, a double-blind, placebo-controlled study compared one-gram daily of oral quercetin with placebo in 27 healthy subjects. This dose was said to be about 50-fold greater than dietary intakes associated, epidemiologically, with reduced risk of coronary heart disease mortality. The study continued for 28 days, during which period subjects receiving quercetin achieved plasma quercetin levels 23-fold higher than levels in those on placebo.

The results showed no quercetin effect on serum total cholesterol, LDL-cholesterol, HDL-cholesterol or triglyceride levels. Nor was there any effect on other factors considered to be indicators of risk for cardiovascular/thrombogenic disease, including platelet aggregation, platelet thromboxane B$_2$ production, blood pressure and resting heart rate. There was no effect on levels of (n-6) or (n-3) polyunsaturated fatty acids in serum or platelet phospholipids.

The researchers noted that the previous studies indicating that flavonoids, including quercetin, might be beneficial in heart disease were all performed *in vitro* or in animal models. They further observed that prior studies showing a quercetin platelet aggregation-inhibiting effect, for example, used doses far higher than those used in this study and thus amounts greatly in excess of those present in normal diet.

The researchers concluded: "Our results suggest that any protective effect of foods containing quercetin may be mediated via effects on risk factors other than those we have measured.... Alternatively, the protective effect of quercetin-containing foods may be due to factors other than quercetin in those foods."

Another recent study increased plasma quercetin concentrations in 18 healthy subjects, via increased intake of quercetin-rich foods, such as onions. But, again, there was no effect on platelet aggregation, thromboxane B$_2$ production, factor VII or other hemostatic variables.

Quercetin is one of several flavonoids that have effects on mast cells and basophils; thus, some research suggests, it might be useful in some allergies, such as hay fever. Quercetin can help prevent the release of histamine and other mediators of allergic reactions, possibly by stabilizing cell membranes so that they are less reactive to allergens. Quercetin also exhibits anti-inflammatory properties, inhibiting formation of inflammatory prostaglandins and leukotrienes.

It was suggested in an open-label study that quercetin might be helpful in category III chronic prostatitis syndromes (nonbacterial chronic prostatitis and prostatodynia). Recently, this was confirmed in a prospective, randomized, double-blind, placebo-controlled trial.

Thirty men with these disorders received either placebo or 500 milligrams of quercetin twice daily for one month. Significant improvement was achieved in the treated group, as measured by the National Institutes of Health chronic prostatitis score. Some 67% of the treated subjects had at least 25% improvement in symptoms, compared with 20% of the placebo group achieving this same level of improvement.

In a follow up, unblind, open-label study, 17 additional men received the same amount of quercetin for one month, but this time the quercetin was combined with bromelain and papain, which may enhance its absorption. In this study, 82% achieved a minimum 25% improvement score.

Several of quercetin's activities, including anti-inflammatory, anti-oxidant and immune-modulating actions, are believed to play roles in achieving these effects. There was evidence that quercetin prevented oxidative-mediated cellular injury, which the researchers suggested would apply whether the injury was due to infective, inflammatory or auto-immune mechanisms.

The researchers concluded: "Few therapies have shown durable efficacy with these disorders. Quercetin is efficacious, inexpensive, well tolerated and safe."

Fears that quercetin might be carcinogenic have not been supported by recent research. On the contrary, quercetin appears to have some anti-cancer effects, as demonstrated *in vitro* and in some animal models. Several processes that contribute to some cancers have been inhibited by quercetin. Some experiments have suggested a chemopreventive role for quercetin in colorectal carcinogenesis. Quercetin is reported to be one of very few substances that inhibit an animal model of basophil leukemia.

These preliminary results, as well as tentative findings that quercetin can have favorable immune-modulating and (in combination with vitamin C) some anti-viral activity (against picomaviruses) need more vigorous follow up studies.

There are reports that quercetin may have some gastroprotective effects in animal models. High-dose quercetin promoted mucus production and helped diminish the severity of gastric lesions in animals injured with absolute thanol. Thiobarbituric acid reactive substances in gastric mucosa, a measure of lipid peroxidation, was significantly decreased by quercetin in ethanol-injured animals. Whether these findings will have relevance in humans remains to be seen.

Finally, quercetin has been shown to inhibit aldose reductase, the first enzyme in the polyol pathway. Experimental data link glucose metabolism via this pathway to long-term diabetic complications, such as cataract, nephropathy, retinopathy and neuropathy. Again, whether inhibition of aldose reductase will have any relevance in humans remains to be proven by well-controlled clinical trials.

CONTRAINDICATIONS, PRECAUTIONS, ADVERSE REACTIONS

CONTRAINDICATIONS

None known.

WARNINGS AND PRECAUTIONS

Because of lack of long-term safety data, quercetin should be avoided by pregnant women and nursing mothers.

ADVERSE REACTIONS

Adverse effects reported with oral quercetin include gastrointestinal effects such as nausea, and rare reports of headache and mild tingling of the extremities. Oral quercetin is generally well tolerated. Intravenous administration of quercetin has been associated with nausea, vomiting, diaphoresis, flushing and dyspnea.

INTERACTIONS

DRUGS

Quinolone Antibiotics: Quercetin binds, *in vitro*, to the DNA gyrase site in bacteria. Therefore, theoretically, it can serve as a competitive inhibitor to the quinolone antibiotics which also bind to this site.

Cisplatin: Because of the theoretical risk of genotoxicity in normal tissues in those using cisplatin along with quercetin, those taking cisplatin should avoid quercetin supplements.

NUTRITIONAL SUPPLEMENTS

Bromelain and papain are reported to increase absorption of quercetin.

OVERDOSAGE

There are no reports of overdosage with oral quercetin. Intravenous administration of doses greater than 945 milligram per square meter has been associated with nephrotoxicity.

DOSAGE AND ADMINISTRATION

Doses of quercetin used range from 200 to 1,200 milligrams daily.

In the study showing possible benefit of quercetin for chronic prostatitis (see Research Summary), a quercetin dose of 500 milligrams was used, administered twice a day for one month.

HOW SUPPLIED

Capsules — 250 mg, 300 mg, 500 mg

Tablets — 50 mg, 250 mg, 500 mg

LITERATURE

Alarcon de la Lastra C. Martin MJ, Motilve V. Antiulcer and gastroprotective effects of quercetin: a gross and histologic study. *Pharmacol.* 1994; 48:56-62.

Boulton DW, Walle UK, Walle T. Extensive binding of the bioflavonoid quercetin to human plasma proteins. *J Pharm Pharmacol.* 1998; 50:243-249.

Conquer JA, Maiani G, Azzini E, et al. Supplementation with quercetin markedly increases plasma quercetin concentration without effect on selected risk factors for heart disease in healthy subjects. *J Nutr.* 1998; 128:593-597.

Costantino L, Rastelli G, Gamberini MC, et al. 1-Benzopyran-4-one antioxidants as aldose reductase inhibitors. *J Med Chem.* 1999; 42:1881-1893.

de Vries JH, Jenssen PL, Hollman PC, et al. Consumption of quercetin and kaempferol in free-living subjects eating a variety of diets. *Cancer Lett.* 1997. 114:141-144.

Ferry DR, Smith A, Malkhandi J, et al. Phase I clinical trial of the flavonoid quercetine: phonmacokinetics and evidence for tyrosine kinase inhibition. *Clin Cancer Res.* 1996; 2:659-668.

Hilliard JJ, Krause HM, Bernstein JI, et al. A comparison of active site binding of 4-quinolones and novel flavone gyrase inhibitors to DNA gyrase. *Adv Exp Med Biol.* 1995; 390:59-69.

Hollman PC, Bijsman MN, van Gameren Y, et al. The sugar moiety is a major determinant of the absorption of dietary flavonoid glycosides in man. *Free Rad Res.* 1999; 31:569-573.

Hollman PC, de Vries JH, van Leeuwen SD, et al. Absorption of dietary quercetin glycosides and quercetin in healthy ileostomy volunteers. *Am J Clin Nutr.* 1995; 62:1276-1282.

Hollman PCH, van Trijp JMP, Mengelers MJB, et al. Bioavailability of the dietary antioxidant flavonol quercetin in man. *Cancer Lett.* 1997; 114:139-140.

Hollman PCH, Gaag MVD, Mengelers MJB, et al. Absorpotion and disposition kinetics of the dietary antioxidant quercetin in man. *Free Red Biol Med.* 1996; 21:703-707.

Ito N, Hagiwara A, Tamano S, et al. Lack of carcinogencity of quercetin in F344/DuCrj rats. *Jpn J Cancer Res.* 1989; 80:317-325.

Martin MJ, La-Casa C, Alarcon-de-la-Lastra C, et al. Antioxidant mechanisms involved in gastroprotective effects of quercetin. *Z Naturforsch[C].* 1998; 53:82-88.

Middleton Jr E, Anne S. Quercetin inhibits lipopolysaccharide-induced expression of endothelial cell intracellular adhesion molecule-1. *Int Arch Allergy Immunol.* 1995; 107:435-436.

Sato M, Miyazaki T, Kambe F, et al. Quercetin, a bioflavonoid, inhibits the induction of interlenkin 8 and monocyte chemoattractant protein-1 expression by tumor necrosis factor-alpha in cultured human synovial cells. *J Rheumatol.* 1997; 24:1680-1684.

Shoskes DA. Effect of the bioflavonoids quercetin and curcumin on ischemic renal injury: a new class of renoprotective agents. *Transplantation.* 1998; 66:147-152.

Shoskes DA, Zeitlin SI, Shahed A, Rajfer J. Quercetin in men with category III chronic prostatitis: a preliminary prospective double-blind, placebo-controlled trial. *Urology.* 1999; 54:960-963.

Stavric B. Quercetin in our diet: from potent mutagen to probable anticarcinogen. *Clin Biochem.* 1994; 27:245-248.

Varma SD, Kinoshita JH. Inhibition of lens aldose reductase by flavonoids. Their possible role in the prevention of diabetic cataracts. *Biochem Pharmacol.* 1976; 25:2505-2513.

Red Yeast Rice

TRADE NAMES

Cholesterol Management (Reese Pharmaceutical), Cholestin (Pharmanex), Cholestol (Nutura), CholesteSure (Natrol)

DESCRIPTION

Red yeast rice refers to the product of fermentation of rice with various strains of the yeast *Monascus purpureus* (Went). Red yeast rice has been used for centuries in China in foods and in medicines. It was introduced in the U.S. during the latter half of the 1990s as a dietary supplement for the promotion of healthy serum lipid levels. However, because it contains the HMG-CoA reductase inhibitor lovastatin, among other things, the U.S. FDA has contended that it is not a dietary supplement, but an unapproved drug. Presently, it is unclear what the final determination of this product will be; dietary supplement or unapproved drug.

The use of red yeast rice was apparently first noted in the Tang dynasty and was introduced to Taiwan by wine makers of Fukien about a century ago. It is used by the Chinese as a coloring agent in the preparation of foods, including fish, fish sauce, fish paste, rice wine (fu chiu), red soybean curd (hung-lu chiu, a cheese-like product used as a spice), pickled vegetables and salted meats. In addition to adding color, it adds flavor to foods. It has also been used in Chinese folk medicine for treating indigestion, diarrhea, and for improving blood circulation, among other things.

In addition to natural pigments such as monascorubin and monascin (azaphilone derivatives), red yeast rice contains starch, fatty acids (oleic, linoleic, linolenic, palmitic, stearic), phytosterols (beta-sitosterol, stigmasterol), isoflavones and monacolins. Monacolins possess hydroxymethyglutaryl coenzyme A (HMG-CoA) reductase-inhibitory activity. HMG-CoA reductase inhibitors are commonly known as statins. The first statin introduced in the U.S., for use as a cholesterol lowering agent, was lovastatin. Lovastatin was originally derived from *Monascus ruber*, and was first called monacolin K. Monacolin K is a lactone which is converted in the body to the active form of the statin, the corresponding beta-hydroxy acid of monacolin K (lovastastin, mevinolin).

The proprietary red yeast rice product that was first introduced in the U.S. was processed to yield 0.4% HMG-CoA reductase inhibitors in the final product. In addition to monacolin K or lovastatin, which comprises 0.2% of this product, it contains the corresponding beta-hydroxy acid of monacolin K at a concentration of 0.1%, and much smaller amounts of dihydromonacolin, monacolin I, monacolin II (hydroxy acid form), monacolin III, monacolin IV, monacolin V and monacolin VI, to give a total of 9 HMG-CoA reductase inhibitors. Traditional red yeast rice does not contain as high an amount of these substances. The yeast in red yeast rice is inactive.

The legal status surrounding red yeast rice as a dietary supplement has become an ongoing battle. In May, 1998, the FDA determined that the proprietary red yeast rice was an unapproved drug and not a dietary supplement. The FDA argued that although red yeast rice had been used as a food product for many years, neither it nor lovastatin were marketed as dietary supplements prior to the drug approval of the lovastatin drug product in 1987. They further argued that because of that situation, the product would not be covered under the Dietary Supplement Health and Education Act (DSHEA) which was passed in 1994. This meant that the product would be regulated by the FDA.

The manufacturer of the proprietary product argued that the FDA approved the lovastatin drug product and not the drug active (lovastatin) and also, that the product is a food product that had been used for centuries in China and thus, would fall under DSHEA. In February, 1999, the Federal District Court in Utah ruled against the FDA, stating that the proprietary red yeast rice product was not a drug but a dietary supplement. This decision came about as a result of a law suit brought by the manufacturer against the FDA. In the most recent legal turn of events, the 10th U.S. Circuit Court of Appeals ruled on July 24, 2000 that the proprietary red yeast product *is* subject to regulation by the U.S. FDA. The future of red yeast rice as a dietary supplement is unclear. Lovastatin has the following structural formula:

Lovastatin

Red yeast rice is known by various names, including Chinese red yeast rice, red rice, *Monascus purpureus*-fermented rice, red yeast, anka, ang-kak, ankak, angquac, beni-koji, beni-Jiuqu, aga-Jiuqu, aka-koji, xuezhikang, hung-chu and hongqu.

ACTIONS AND PHARMACOLOGY

ACTIONS

Red yeast rice may have hypocholesterolemic and hypotriglyceridemic activities in some.

MECHANISM OF ACTION

The mechanism of the hypolipidemic activity of red yeast rice is not entirely clear. The possible hypocholesterolemic activity of red yeast rice can be accounted for, in part, by the presence of HMG-CoA reductase inhibitors, especially monacolin I (lovastatin, mevinolin) and its corresponding beta-hydroxy acid, monacolin II. Lovastatin is converted in the body to its corresponding beta-hydroxy acid, which is the form that inhibits HMG-CoA reductase. HMG-CoA reductase catalyzes the conversion of HMG-CoA to mevalonate, which is an early and rate limiting step in cholesterol biosynthesis. Lovastatin is known to lower plasma total cholesterol, low-density lipoprotein cholesterol (LDL-C), the total cholesterol/HDL-C ratio and the LDL-C/HDL-C ratio. Lovastatin may also produce a modest increase in HDL-cholesterol and modest decreases in VLDL-C and triglyceride levels in some.

LDL is formed from VLDL and is principally catabolized via the high affinity LDL receptor. Lovastatin's mechanism in lowering LDL appears to also involve reduction of VLDL-C levels and upregulation of the LDL receptor, resulting in reduced production of LDL-C, as well as increased catabolism of LDL-C.

The hypolipidemic effects of red yeast rice have been found to be greater than those obtained from equivalent doses of the pharmaceutical form of lovastatin. To be clear about this, the amount of lovastatin delivered by red yeast rice is typically 7.2 milligrams. The amount of lovastatin in the pharmaceutical form of lovastatin ranges from 10 to 40 milligrams. It is unclear why a lovastatin dose of 7.2 milligrams in red yeast rice appears to have more potent lipid-lowering activity than higher doses of pharmaceutical lovastatin. It is speculated that other substances in red yeast rice besides the HMG-CoA reductase inhibitors, may have lipid-lowering activity themselves or may work synergistically with the HMG-CoA reductase inhibitors. What these substances are and how they may work synergistically with the HMG-CoA reductase inhibitors, is entirely unclear. Beta-sitosterol (see Beta-Sitosterol) is found in red yeast and it is known to have hypocholesterolemic activity. However, the amount of this substance found in red yeast rice is too small to make much of a cholesterol-lowering contribution.

PHARMACOKINETICS

There is little on the pharmacokinetics of red yeast rice in humans. However, the pharmacokinetics of lovastatin, which appears to be the principal bioactive substance in red yeast rice, are known. The efficiency of absorption of lovastatin is approximately 30%. The efficiency of absorption is greater when it is given with food. Following absorption, lovastatin is transported to the liver via the portal circulation where it undergoes extensive first-pass extraction. The liver is the principal site of action of lovastatin. Less than 5% of an oral dose of lovastatin reaches the systemic circulation. Lovastatin is metabolized in the liver to its corresponding beta-

hydroxy acid, which is the active HMG-CoA reductase inhibitor. In addition to the beta-hydroxy acid of lovastatin, lovastatin is metabolized to a few other metabolites, including its 6'-hydroxy derivative. Lovastatin is metabolized by the cytochrome P450 3A4 system. Excretion is mainly via the biliary route. Approximately 83% of an oral dose of lovastatin is excreted in the feces (biliary excretion and unabsorbed lovastatin), and approximately 10% is excreted in the urine.

INDICATIONS AND USAGE

Red yeast rice may have favorable effects on lipids, lowering cholesterol and triglycerides in some. However, there is an ongoing legal issue regarding the status of red yeast rice, particularly those preparations that contain statins, as a dietary supplement.

RESEARCH SUMMARY

Recent clinical studies have demonstrated that red yeast rice can significantly lower triglyceride and cholesterol levels in some individuals. In one multi-center, randomized, single-blind trial of the substance in 502 patients with hyperlipidemia, there was a 17% reduction of total cholesterol in the treated group. LDL-cholesterol was reduced an average of 24.6%, and serum triglyceride levels fell an average of 19.8%. HDL-cholesterol rose by 12.8% in the treatment group.

These results were measured after four weeks of treatment. Dosage was 600 milligrams of red yeast rice twice daily for a total of 1,200 milligrams daily. At the end of eight weeks of red yeast rice supplementation, still better results were reported for the treatment group: total cholesterol reduced by 22.7%, LDL-cholesterol reduced by 30.9%, triglycerides reduced by 34.1%, HDL-cholesterol increased by 19.9%.

In another recent study, this one conducted in a double-blind, placebo-controlled fashion, 83 hyperlipidemic subjects who were not being treated with lipid-lowering drugs were randomized to receive red yeast rice, 2.4 grams daily, or placebo. Subjects were instructed to consume a diet deriving 30% of energy from fat (with no more than 10% of this from saturated fat and no more than 300 milligrams of cholesterol daily).

The study continued for 12 weeks. Red yeast rice was found to significantly reduce total cholesterol, LDL-cholesterol and total triacylglycerol concentrations, compared with placebo. HDL-Cholesterol was not affected in this study. Research is ongoing. Also ongoing, is the legal issue regarding the status of lipid-lowering red yeast rice as a dietary supplement.

CONTRAINDICATIONS, PRECAUTIONS, ADVERSE REACTIONS

CONTRAINDICATIONS

Red yeast rice is contraindicated in those who are hypersensitive to any component of a red yeast rice-containing product. Red yeast rice is also contraindicated in pregnant women, nursing mothers, women of childbearing age who are likely to conceive, those with active liver disease and those with unexplained aminotransferase (transaminase) elevations.

PRECAUTIONS

Since the principal bioactive substance in red yeast rice is lovastatin, all of the warnings, precautions and interactions of pharmaceutical lovastatin apply to red yeast rice, as well.

The use of red yeast rice for the management of hyperlipidemia must be medically supervised.

Those with a past history of liver disease and those who routinely use alcoholic beverages should exercise caution in the use of red yeast rice.

Lovastatin and other HMG-CoA reductase inhibitors occasionally cause myopathy. This is manifested as muscle pain or weakness associated with elevated levels of creatine kinase. Rhabdomyolysis with or without acute renal failure secondary to myoglobinuria, has been reported rarely and can occur at any time. Those using red yeast rice should report promptly to their physicians unexplained muscle pain, tenderness or weakness.

Bleeding and/or increased INR values have been reported in a few patients taking warfarin concomitantly with lovastatin.

Persistant increases (to more than 3 times the upper limit of normal) in serum aminotransferases (transaminases) occurred in 1.9% of adults who received lovastatin for at least one year in some early clinical trials. It is recommended that liver tests be performed before starting red yeast rice, at 6 and 12 weeks after starting its use, and periodically thereafter.

Lovastatin has been reported to lower coenzyme Q (CoQ_{10}) levels.

ADVERSE REACTIONS

In clinical studies of red yeast rice, few adverse reactions were reported. Adverse reactions reported, included flatulence and heartburn. There is one report of anaphylaxis resulting from inhalation of red yeast rice. Adverse reactions from the pharmaceutical form of lovastatin, include elevated liver tests, elevated creatine kinase levels (noncardiac), myopathy and liver dysfunction. Overall, lovastatin is generally well tolerated; adverse reactions usually have been mild and transient.

INTERACTIONS

DRUGS

Azole antifungals (fluconazole, ketoconazole, itraconazole): Concomitant use of red yeast rice and an azole antifungal may increase the risk of myopathy.

Cyclosporine: Concomitant use of red yeast rice and cyclosporine may increase the risk of myopathy.

Fibrates (clofibrate, fenofibrate): Concomitant use of red yeast rice and a fibrate may increase the risk of myopathy.

Gemfibrozil: Concomitant use of red yeast rice and gemfibrozil may increase the risk of myopathy.

Macrolide antibiotics (clarithromycin, erythromycin): Concomitant use of red yeast rice and certain macrolide antibiotics may increase the risk of myopathy.

Nefazodone: Concomitant use of red yeast rice and nefazodone may increase the risk of myopathy.

Protease inhibitors (amprenavir, indinavir, nelfinavir, ritonavir, saquinavir): Concomitant use of red yeast rice and a protease inhibitor may increase the risk of myopathy.

Statins (atorvastatin, cerivastatin, fluvastatin, lovastatin, pravastatin, simvastatin): Concomitant use of red yeast rice with a pharmaceutical statin may increase the risk of adverse reactions.

Warfarin: Concomitant use of red yeast rice and warfarin may result in an increase in the INR as well as bleeding.

NUTRITIONAL SUPPLEMENTS

Nicotinic acid: Concomitant use of red yeast rice and high doses of nicotinic acid may increase the risk of myopathy.

FOODS

Grapefruit juice: Grapefruit juice contains some substances, such as the furanocoumarin bergamottin, which inhibit cytochrome P450 3A4, the enzyme that metabolizes lovastatin, among other substances. Therefore, concomitant use of red yeast rice and grapefruit juice may increase the risk of myopathy.

Meals: When lovastatin was given under fasting conditions, plasma concentrations of lovastatin and its active metabolite were on the average two-thirds those found when lovastatin was administered immediately following a meal.

OVERDOSAGE

There are no reports of overdosage with red yeast rice. A few cases of accidental overdosage have been reported with the pharmaceutical form of lovastatin. The maximum dose taken was 5-6 grams. No patients had any specific symptoms and they completely recovered.

DOSAGE AND ADMINISTRATION

Red yeast rice is currently available in single ingredient and combination products. The red yeast rice dietary supplements are standardized to 0.4% HMG-CoA reductase inhibitors, with 0.3% coming from lovastatin equivalents. A dose of 2,400 milligrams daily delivers 9.6 milligrams of HMG-CoA reductase inhibitors, including 7.2 milligrams of lovastatin equivalents. Red yeast rice typically comes in 600 milligram capsules. The usual dose has been 2,400 milligrams daily. See Precautions.

HOW SUPPLIED

Capsules — 400 mg, 600 mg

Tablets, Extended Release — 600 mg

LITERATURE

Baens-Arcega L, Ardisher AG, Beddows CG, et al. Indigenous amino acid/peptide sauces and pastes with meat-like flavors. Chinese soy sauce, Japanese shoyu, Japanese miso, Southeast Asian fish sauces and pastes, and related fermented foods. In: Steinkraus KH, ed. *Handbook of Indigenous Fermented Foods.* 2nd ed. New York, NY: Marcel Dekker, Inc; 1996:625-633.

Endo A. Monacolin K. A new hypocholesterolemic agent produced by a *Monascus* species. *J Antibiot (Tokyo).* 1979; 32:852-854.

Havel RJ. Dietary supplement or drug? The case of Cholestin (editorial). *Am J Clin Nutr.* 1999; 69:175-176.

Heber D, Yip I, Ashley JM, et al. Cholesterol-lowering effects of a proprietary Chinese red-yeast-rice dietary supplement. *Am J Clin Nutr.* 1999; 69:231-236.

Kou W, Lu Z, Guo J. [Effect of xuezhikang on the treatment of primary hyperlipidemia]. [Article in Chinese]. *Chung Hua Nei Ko Tsa Chih.* 1997; 36:529-531.

Li C, Wang Y, et al. *Monascus purpureus*-fermented rice (red yeast rice): a natural food product that lowers blood cholesterol in animal models of hypercholesterolemia. *Nutr Res.* 1998; 18:71-81.

SoRelle R. Appeals Court says Food and Drug Administration can regulate Cholestin. *Circulation.* 2000; 102:E9012-E9013.

Wigger-Alberti W, Bauer A, Hipler UC, Elsner P. Anaphylaxis due to *Monascus purpureus*-fermented rice (red yeast rice). *Allergy* 1999; 54:1330-1331.

Zhang ML, Pong CX, Chang MN. *Methods and Compositions Employing Red Yeast Fermentation Products.* International patent publication number: WO 98/14177. International publication date: 9 April 1998.

Resveratrol

TRADE NAMES

Protykin Resveratrol (Natrol), Resveratrol Antioxidant Protection (Source Naturals).

DESCRIPTION

Resveratrol is a naturally occurring phytoalexin produced by some higher plants in response to injury or fungal infection. Phytoalexins are chemical substances produced by plants as a defense against infection by pathogenic microorganisms, such as fungi. Alexin is from the Greek, meaning to ward off or to protect. Resveratrol may also have alexin-like activity

for humans. Epidemiological, *in vitro* and animal studies suggest that a high resveretrol intake is associated with a reduced incidence of cardiovascular disease, and a reduced risk for cancer.

Resveratrol is found in grapevines (*Vitis vinifera* L). It occurs in the vines, roots, seeds and stalks, but its highest concentration is in grape skins. Wine also contains resveratrol. The concentration of resveratrol in red wine is much higher than that of white wine. The main difference between red and white wine production, besides the grapes used, is that for red wine the skins and seeds are involved in the process, while white wine is mainly prepared from the juice, essentially avoiding the use of grape skins and seeds. During the wine making process, resveratrol, as well as other polyphenols, including quercetin, catechins, gallocatechins, procyanidins and prodelphidins (condensed tannins), are extracted from the grape skins via a process called maceration.

Resveratrol, as well as the other polyphenols in wine, is thought to account in large part for the so-called French Paradox. The French Paradox—the finding that the rate of coronary heart disease mortality in France is lower than observed in other industrialized countries with a similar risk factor profile—has been attributed to frequent consumption of red wine.

In addition to grapes and wine, dietary sources of resveratrol include peanuts and mulberries. Resveratrol is also found in significant amounts in the dried roots and stems of the plant *Polygonium cuspidatum* Sieb. Et Zucc., also known as the Japanese knotweed. The dried root and stem of this plant is used in traditional Chinese and Japanese medicine as a circulatory tonic, among other things. This traditional Chinese and Japanese remedy is also known as Hu Zhang, Hu Chang, tiger cane, kojo-kon and hadori-kon. Most of the resveratrol-containing supplements which are marketed in the U.S. contain extracts of the root of *Polygonium cuspidatum*. Darakchasava, an ayurvedic herbal remedy, has as its principal ingredient *Vitis vinifera* L, and therefore, contains resveratrol. It is mainly used in ayurvedic medicine as a cardiotonic.

Resveratrol, which is also known as 3,4',5 trihydroxystilbene and 3,4',5-stilbenetriol, exists in *cis*- and *trans*-stereoisomeric forms. Resveratrol is the parent molecule of a family of polymers called viniferins. *Cis*- and *trans*-resveratrol occur naturally as do their glucosides. Resveratrol-3-O-beta-D-glucoside is also known as piceid, and the respective *cis*- and *trans*-glucosides are called *cis*-piceid and *trans*-piceid. The molecular formula of resveratrol is $C_{14}H_{12}O_3$ and its molecular weight is 228.25 daltons. It is represented by the following structural formula:

Resveratrol

The stereoisomer of resveratrol found in grapes and peanuts is the *trans*-form. Both *cis*- and *trans*-resveratrol are found in *Polygonium cuspidatum*. Therefore, dietary supplements containing resveratrol, which are principally derived from this plant, contain both stereoisomers. The amount of resveratrol (*trans*-resveratrol) in peanuts ranges from 0.02 to 1.79 micrograms per gram. Red wine contains from 0.6 to 0.8 micrograms per milliliter, and fresh grape skin, approximately 50 to 100 micrograms per gram. A glass of red wine delivers on the average, between 600 to 700 micrograms of resveratrol.

ACTIONS AND PHARMACOLOGY

ACTIONS
Resveratrol may have cardioprotective and antiproliferative actions.

MECHANISM OF ACTION
Resveratrol has several activities that may account for its possible cardioprotective action. These include inhibition of the oxidation of low-density lipoprotein (LDL), inhibition of smooth muscle cell proliferation and inhibition of platelet aggregation. Resveratrol has also been found to reduce the synthesis of lipids in rat liver and to inhibit the production of proatherogenic eicosanoids by human platelets and neutrophils.

Resveratrol's antioxidant activity may play an important role in its possible cardioprotective action. Above, was mentioned its ability to inhibit the oxidation of LDL. Resveratrol also has been found to exert a strong inhibitory effect on superoxide anion and hydrogen peroxide production by macrophages stimulated by lipopolysaccharides or phorbol esters. It also has been demonstrated to decrease arachidonic acid release induced by lipopolysaccharides or phorbol esters, or by exposure to superoxide or hydrogen peroxide. It has hydroxyl-radical scavenging activity and has recently been found to possess glutathione-sparing activity.

In a rat study of the effect of resveratrol on ischemia-reperfusion, it was found that the substance had a dramatic effect against ischemia-reperfusion-induced arrhythmias and mortality. Resveratrol pretreatment both reduced the inci-dence and duration of ventricular dysrhythmias, including ventricular tachycardia and ventricular fibrillation. Resveratrol pretreatment also increased nitric oxide and decreased lactate dehydrogenase levels in the carotid blood. In this example, the cardioprotective effect of resveratrol may be correlated with its antioxidant activity, upregulation of nitric oxide synthesis and protection against endothelial dysfunction.

Resveratrol's possible phytoestrogenic activity may also contribute to its possible cardioprotective action. Resveratrol appears to act as a mixed agonist/antagonist for estrogen receptors alpha and beta. It has been found to bind estrogen receptor beta and estrogen receptor alpha with comparable affinity but with 7,000-fold lower affinity than estradiol. Resveratrol differs from other phytoestrogens, which bind estrogen receptor beta with higher affinity than they bind estrogen receptor alpha. Resveratrol also shows estradiol antagonistic behavior for estrogen receptor alpha with some estrogen receptors. It does not show estradiol antagonistic activity with estrogen receptor beta.

Resveratrol's possible antiproliferative activity also may be accounted for in several different ways. Resveratrol's antioxidant activity was discussed above. It also has antimutagenic activity, as illustrated by its dose-dependent inhibition of the mutagenic response induced by treatment of *Salmonella typhimurium* strain TM677 with 7,12-dimethylbenz(*a*)anthracene (DMBA). Resveratrol has been found to inhibit cellular events associated with tumor initiation, promotion and progression. It has been found to inhibit cyclooxygenase (COX) activities in different cancer models, suggesting an effect at the level of tumor promotion. It has also been found to reverse tumor-promoter-induced inhibition of gap-junctional intracellular communication in rat epithelial cells. Inhibition of gap-junctional intracellular communication is an important mechanism of tumor promotion.

Resveratrol has demonstrated inhibition of growth of several cancer cell lines and tumors, suggesting that it has an inhibitory effect on cancer promotion/progression. It has been found to inhibit ribonucleotide reductase, DNA polymerase, the transcription of COX-2 in human mammary epithelial cells and the activity of ornithine decarboxylase. Ornithine decarboxylase is a key enzyme of polyamine biosynthesis, which is enhanced in tumor growth.

Resveratrol has also been found to induce phase II metabolizing enzymes which are involved in the detoxification of carcinogens, to upregulate apoptosis, to inhibit the progression of cancer by inducing cell differentiation and to inhibit protein kinase D and possibly protein kinase C. Recently, resveratrol has been shown to inhibit both NF-kappaB activation and NF-kappaB-dependent gene expression via its ability to inhibit IkappaB kinase activity, the key regulator of NF-kappaB activation. This appears to upregulate apoptosis.

It is clear that resveratrol has a wide range of activities that may account for its possible antiproliferative action. It is also clear that the mechanism of this possible action is far from being understood.

PHARMACOKINETICS

From animal studies and from limited human studies, it appears that resveratrol is absorbed from the gastrointestinal tract following its ingestion. However, the efficiency of its absorption, as well as its distribution, metabolism and excretion, are not well understood. Much research needs to be done in order to elucidate the pharmacokinetics of resveratrol in its various forms.

INDICATIONS AND USAGE

Epidemiological, *in vitro* and animal studies suggest that resveratrol has anti-atherosclerotic activity and that it might have some immune-stimulating and anti-cancer effects. Human studies are few in number and inconclusive due to short duration and poor design.

RESEARCH SUMMARY

There has been a suggestion from epidemiological data for some time that moderate consumption of red wine is associated with a reduced incidence of mortality and morbidity from coronary heart disease. *In vitro* and animal work has strongly suggested that resveratrol and other polyphenols found in grapes and wines are at least partially responsible for often-observed anti-platelet aggregating anti-inflammatory and anti-oxidant effects.

Red wine has been shown, in some experiments, to be more effective than other alcoholic beverages in decreasing some of the risk factors of coronary heart disease. Compared, in one study, with ethanol, resveratrol had superior anti-platelet-aggregation effects; it was superior in this respect, as well, to catechin, epicatechin, alpha-tocopherol, hydroquinone and butylated hydroxytoluene. Resveratrol also inhibited the synthesis of thromboxane B2 and hydroxyheptadecatrienoate from arachidonate in a dose-dependent manner.

Other studies, in animals and *in vitro*, have shown that resveratrol can inhibit the oxidation of LDL-cholesterol and, more recently, that it can reduce smooth-muscle-cell proliferation, believed to be one of the requisites of atherogenesis, by 70-90%, in a dose-dependent pattern. Red wine extract and resveratrol have shown equally significant cardioprotective effects in animal models of myocardial ischemic reperfusion injury.

Additional evidence suggests that resveratrol also has estrogenic effects that may also provide cardiovascular protection. Bearing a structural resemblance to diethylstilbestrol, *trans*-resveratrol is a phytoestrogen found to have variable degrees of estrogen-receptor agonisms in different test systems.

The clinical data that would confirm or refute the relevance of these findings are largely lacking. In one small, short-term study, 24 healthy human subjects aged 26-45 consumed red wine, white wine, commercial grape juice and the same grape juice fortified with resveratrol over periods of 4 weeks. Results were mixed and conflicting, suggesting some positive benefit from resveratrol while also suggesting lack of activity in other measures related to coronary heart disease. The researchers themselves acknowledged multiple weaknesses in their study design. Further, better-controlled, longer-term studies are needed to determine whether red wine, high-resveratrol grape juice, or resveratrol supplements are efficacious in preventing atherosclerosis or in ameliorating it once it is present.

More preliminary yet are findings of some resveratrol-related anti-cancer and immune-stimulating effects. In a number of mostly *in vitro* studies, resveratrol has demonstrated an ability to inhibit tumor initiation, promotion and progression. Some of its antiproliferative activity is attributed to its observed ability to inhibit ribonucleotide reductase and DNA synthesis in mammalian cells. It has been shown to induce apoptotic cell death in human leukemia cell lines, as well as in some breast carcinoma cells.

Its antiestrogenic activity is also believed to play a role in its inhibition of human breast cancer cells *in vitro*. A partial estrogen-receptor agonist itself, resveratrol is believed by some researchers to be an estrogen-receptor antagonist in the presence of estrogen, resulting in breast cancer inhibition.

Finally, resveratrol has recently shown activity against herpes simplex virus types 1 and 2 in a dose-dependent manner. It appears to disrupt a critical early event in the viral reproduction cycle. More research is needed.

CONTRAINDICATIONS, PRECAUTIONS, ADVERSE REACTIONS

CONTRAINDICATIONS

Resveratrol is contraindicated in those hypersensitive to any component of a resveratrol-containing product.

PRECAUTIONS

Pregnant women and nursing mothers should avoid the use of resveratrol-containing supplements. They should also avoid the use of wine as a resveratrol source. Purple grape juice is a good and safe source of resveratrol, as well as other polyphenolic antioxidants.

DOSAGE AND ADMINISTRATION

Resveratrol, marketed as a nutritional supplement, is typically an extract of *Polygonum cuspidatum* (see Description). Such an extract contains both *cis-* and *trans*-resveratrol. The extracts are usually standardized to deliver about 8% resveratrol in its various forms. Many of the products currently marketed have resveratrol in combination with other phytonutrients and vitamins. Some supplements deliver 16 milligrams per serving or higher. There is no typical dosage. Functional food products containing resveratrol are being developed.

HOW SUPPLIED

Capsules — 15 mg, 50 mg, 200 mg

Tablets — 10 mg

LITERATURE

Bowers JL, Tyulmenkov VV, Jernigan SC, Klinge CM. Resveratrol acts as a mixed agonist/antagonist for estrogen receptors alpha and beta. *Endocrinology*. 2000; 141:3657-3667.

Burkitt MJ, Duncan J. Effects of *trans*-resveratrol on copper-dependent hydroxyl-radical formation and DNA damage: Evidence for hydroxyl-radical scavenging and a novel. Glutathione-sparing mechanism of action. *Arch Biochem Biophys*. 2000; 381:253-263.

Cao G, Prior RL. Red wine in moderation: Potential health benefits independent of alcohol. *Nutr Clin Care*. 2000; 3:76-82.

Chun YJ, Kim MY, Guengerich FP. Resveratrol is a selective human cytochrome P450 1A1 inhibitor. *Biochem Biophys Res Commun*. 1999; 262:20-24.

Cichewicz RH, Kouzi SA, Hamann MT. Dimerization of resveratrol by the grapevine pathogen. *Botrytis cinerea*. *J Natl Prod*. 2000; 63:29-33.

Ciolino HP, Yeh GC. Inhibition of aryl hydrocarbon-induced cytochrome P450 1A1 enzyme activity and CYP1A1 expression by resveratrol. *Mol Pharmacol*. 1999; 56:760-767.

Doherty JJ, Fu MM, Stiffer BS, et al. Resveratrol inhibition of herpes simplex virus replication. *Antiviral Res*. 1999; 43:145-155.

Dubash BD, Zheng BL, Kim CH, et al. Inhibitory effect of resveratrol and related compounds on the macromolecular synthesis in HL-60 cells and the metabolism of 7,12-dimethylbenz[a]anthracene by mouse liver microsomes. In: Shahidi F, Ho C-T, eds. *Phytochemicals and Phytopharmaceuticals*. Champaign, IL: AOCS Press; 2000:314-320.

Fontecave M, Lepoivre M, Elleingand E, et al. Resveratrol, a remarkable inhibitor of ribonucleotide reductase. *FEBS Lett*. 1998; 421:277-279.

Frémont L. Biological effects of resveratrol. *Life Sci*. 2000; 66:663-673.

Frémont L, Belguendouz L, Delpal S. Antioxidant activity of resveratrol and alcohol-free wine polyphenols related to LDL oxidation and polyunsaturated fatty acids. *Life Sci*. 1999; 64:2511-2521.

Gehm BD, McAndrews JM, Chien P-Y, Jameson JL. Resveratrol, a polyphenolic compound found in grapes and wine, is an agonist for the estrogen receptor. *Proc Natl Acad Sci USA*. 1997; 94:14138-14143.

Holmes-McNary M, Baldwin AS Jr. Chemopreventive properties of trans-resveratrol are associated with inhibition of activation of the IkappaB kinase. *Cancer Res*. 2000; 60:3477-3483.

Hsieh TC, Juan G, Darzynkiewicz Z, Wu JM. Resveratrol increases nitric oxide synthase, induces accumulation of p53 and p21 (WAF1/CIP1), and suppresses cultured bovine pulmonary artery endothelial cell proliferation by perturbing progression through S and G2. *Cancer Res*. 1999; 59:2596-2601.

Hung L-M, Chen J-K, Huang S-S, et al. Cardioprotective effect of resveratrol, a natural antioxidant derived from grapes. *Cardiovascular Res*. 2000; 47:549-555.

Jang M, Cai L, Udeani GO, et al. Cancer chemopreventive activity of resveratrol, a natural product derived from grapes. *Science*. 1997; 275:218-220.

Jang M, Pezzuto JM. Cancer chemopreventive activity of resveratrol. *Drugs Exp Clin Res*. 1999; 25:65-77.

Kirk RI, Deitch JA, Wu JM, Lerea KM. Resveratrol decreases early signaling events in washed platelets but has little effect on platelet aggregation in whole blood. *Blood Cells Mol Dis*. 2000; 26:144-150.

Martinez J, Moreno JJ. Effect of resveratrol, a natural polyphenolic compound, on reactive oxygen species and prostaglandin production. *Biochem Pharmacol*. 2000; 59:865-870.

Nielsen M, Ruch RJ, Vang O. Resveratrol reverses tumor-promoter-induced inhibition of gap-junctional intercellular communication. *Biochem Biophys Res Commun*. 2000; 275:804-809.

Pace-Asciak CR, Hahn S, Diamandis EP, et al. The red wine phenolics trans-resveratrol and quercetin block human platelet aggregation and eicosanoid synthesis: implications for protection against coronary heart disease. *Clin Chim Acta*. 1995; 235:207-219.

Paul B, Masih I, Deopujari J, Charpentier C. Occurrence of resveratrol and pterostilbene in age-old darakchasava, an ayurvedic medicine from India. *J Ethnopharmacol*. 1999; 68:71-76.

Pinto MC, García-Barrado JA, Macías P. Resveratrol is a potent inhibitor of the dioxygenase activity of lipoxygenase. *J Agric Food Chem*. 1999; 47:4842-4846.

Ray PS, Maulik G, Cordis GA, et al. The red wine antioxidant resveratrol protects isolated rat hearts from ischemia reperfusion injury. *Free Rad Biol Med*. 1999; 27:160-169.

Sanders TH, McMichael RW Jr, Hendrix KW. Occurrence of resveratrol in edible peanuts. *J Agric Food Chem*. 2000; 48:1243-1246.

Schneider Y, Vincent F, Duranton B, et al. Anti-proliferative effect of resveratrol, a natural component of grapes and wine, on human colonic cancer cells. *Cancer Lett.* 2000; 158:85-91.

Soleas GJ, Diamandis EP, Goldberg DM. Resveratrol: A molecule whose time has come? And gone? *Clin Biochem.* 1997; 30:91-113.

Stewart JR, Christman KL, O'Brian CA. Effects of resveratrol on the autophosphorylation of phorbol ester-responsive protein kinases. *Biochem Pharmacol.* 2000; 60:1355-1359.

Subbaramaiah K, Chung WJ, Michaluart P, et al. Resveratrol inhibits cyclooxygenase-2 transcription and activity in phorbol ester-treated human mammary epithelial cells. *J Biol Chem.* 1998; 273:21875-21882.

Subbaramaiah K, Michaluart P, Chung WJ, et al. Resveratrol inhibits cyclooxygenase-2 transcription in human mammary epithelial cells. *Ann NY Acad Sci.* 2000; 889:214-223.

Tang W, Eisenbrand G. *Chinese Drugs of Plant Origin.* Berlin: Springer-Verlag; 1992; 787-791.

Tessitore L, Davit A, Sarotto I, Caderni G. Resveratrol depresses the growth of colorectal aberrant crypt foci by affecting *bax* and *p21*CIP expression. *Carcinogenesis.* 2000; 21:1619-1622.

Tomera JF. Current knowledge of the health benefits and disadvantages of wine consumption. *Trends Food Sci Technol.* 1999; 10:129-138.

Tsai SH, Lin-Shiau SY, Lin JK. Suppression of nitric oxide synthase and the down-regulation of the activation of NFkappaB in macrophages by resveratrol. *Br J Pharmacol.* 1999; 126:673-680.

Zou J, Huang Y, Chen Q, et al. Suppression of mitogenesis and regulation of cell cycle traverse by resveratrol in cultured smooth muscle cells. *Int J Oncol.* 1999; 15:647-651.

Riboflavin (Vitamin B2)

TRADE NAMES

Ribo-100-T.D. (The Key Company), Ribo-2 (Tyson Neutraceuticals).

DESCRIPTION

Riboflavin or vitamin B2 is an essential nutrient in human nutrition and plays a key role in the production of energy. It is the precursor of flavin mononucleotide (FMN, riboflavin monophosphate) and flavin adenine dinucleotide (FAD). FMN and FAD serve as cofactors for a family of proteins called flavoenzymes. Flavoenzymes catalyze a wide range of biochemical reactions, typically of the redox type. They are key elements in cellular respiration, among other things. In cellular respiration, FAD and FMN act as intermediate hydrogen acceptors in the mitochondrial electron transport chain, accepting hydrogens derived from foodstuffs, and passing on electrons to the cytochrome system. During this process, cellular energy is produced. Recent research suggests that riboflavin may be effective in the prophylaxis of

migraine headaches in some with altered cerebral bioenergetics.

Riboflavin deficiency or ariboflavinosis was originally known as *pellagra sin pellagra.* The most common cause of riboflavin deficiency is dietary inadequacy, which occurs in those who do not consume rich dietary sources of the vitamin, such as organ meats, eggs, milk, cheese, yogurt, leafy green vegetables and whole grains. Deficiency of the vitamin can occur in the elderly subsisting on tea or coffee, toast and cookies. Riboflavin deficiency also occurs in those with chronic liver disease, chronic alcoholics and those who receive total parenteral nutrition (TPN) with inadequate riboflavin. Marginal riboflavin deficiency, in the context of nucleoside analog antiretroviral therapy, has been known to cause severe lactic acidosis.

The signs and symptoms of riboflavin deficiency include, cheilosis (fissuring of the vermilion surfaces of the lips), angular stomatitis, glossitis (magenta tongue), seborrheic dermatitis (particularly affecting the scrotum or labia majora and the nasolabial folds), sore throat, hyperemia and edema of the pharyngeal and oral mucous membranes and a normochromic, normocytic anemia associated with pure erythrocyte cytoplasia of the bone marrow. Isolated riboflavin deficiency is rare. Typically, riboflavin deficiency is accompanied by deficiency of other vitamins and other nutrients. Futher, the skin and mucosal signs of riboflavin deficiency may be difficult to interpret in the elderly. Esophageal lesions in the Turkoman people of Iran have been related to chronic riboflavin deficiency, and the greater incidence of esophageal cancer in this group has created interest in the relationship between esophageal cancer and riboflavin deficiency.

Riboflavin, in addition to being known as vitamin B2, is also known as riboflavine, 7, 8-dimethyl-10- (1¹-D-ribityl)isoalloxazine, 7, 8-dimethyl-10- (D-ribo-2, 3, 4, 5-tetrahydroxypentyl)isoalloxazine and 7, 8-dimethyl-10-ribitylisoalloxazine. Its molecular formula is $C_{17}H_{20}N_4O_6$ and its molecular weight is 376.4 daltons. It has the following structure:

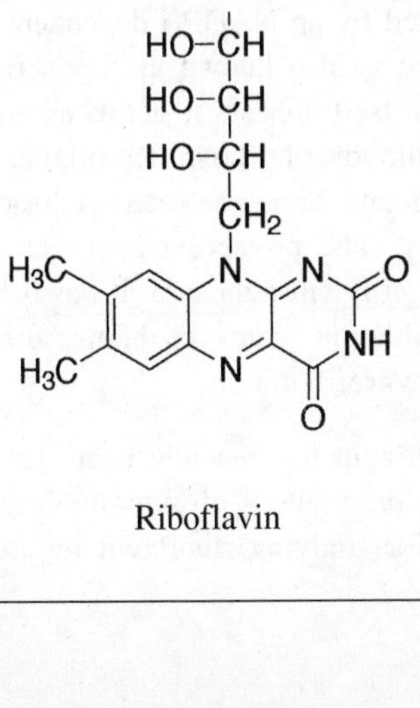

Riboflavin

Riboflavin is an orange powder, and water solutions have intense greenish yellow fluorescence. The 5^1-hydroxymethyl group of the ribityl side chain of riboflavin is metabolized in the body to form the coenzyme flavin mononucleotide or FMN. FMN is also known as riboflavin monophosphate, riboflavin-5^1-phosphate and riboflavin-5^1-(dihydrogen phosphate). FMN is metabolized in the body to form flavin adenine dinucleotide (FAD).

ACTIONS AND PHARMACOLOGY

ACTIONS

Riboflavin has antioxidant activity. It may have activity in the prophylaxis of migraine headaches and may have activity against esophageal cancer. It has putative anti-atherosclerotic activity and putative antimalarial activity.

MECHANISM OF ACTION

The antioxidant activity of riboflavin is principally derived from its role as a precursor of FAD and the role of this cofactor in the production of the antioxidant reduced glutathione. Reduced glutathione is the cofactor of the selenium-containing glutathione peroxidases (see Selenium), among other things. The glutathione peroxidases are major antioxidant enzymes. Reduced glutathione is generated by the FAD-containing enzyme glutathione reductase. Riboflavin deficiency is reported to be associated with compromised oxidant defense resulting in increased lipid peroxidation. Increased lipid peroxidation under conditions of riboflavin deficiency, may be accounted for, in large part, by decreased regeneration of reduced glutathione which is necessary for the function of the antioxidant glutathione peroxidases. Riboflavin deficiency may also affect the mitochondrial pool of reduced glutathione which in turn may affect the activities of the flavoenzymes NADPH-cytochrome P450 reductase and NADPH-cytochrome b reductase. Elevated riboflavin levels have been reported to provide protection against oxidative forms of hemeproteins. Oxidative forms of hemeproteins have been implicated in reperfusion injury. Riboflavin has also been shown to protect against reperfusion injury in isolated rabbit hearts. The protection by riboflavin against oxidative damage caused by oxidized forms of hemeproteins may be mediated by an NADPH-dependent methemoglobin reductase which is also known as flavin reductase. In this case, riboflavin itself appears to act as an antioxidant via its conversion to dihydroriboflavin. Riboflavin has been found to protect lung and brain, as well as heart, from cellular oxidative injury, The protection has been proposed to be mediated through flavin reductase. It has been demonstrated that higher oxidation states of hemeproteins are rapidly reduced by dihydroriboflavin.

High-dose riboflavin has recently been demonstrated to be effective in the prophylaxis of migraine headaches in some. The rationale for studying riboflavin for migraine prophy-

laxis came from the findings, in migraine sufferers, of a decreased mitochondrial phosphorylation potential between migraine attacks. This indicates that those with a history of migraines have decreased brain mitochondrial energy reserve between attacks. The studies were conducted using ^{31}P-NMR spectroscopy. Riboflavin is the precursor of flavin adenine mononucleotide (FMN) and flavin adenine dinucleotide (FAD), which are required for the activity of flavoenzymes involved in the electron transport chain and in the production of cellular energy. Riboflavin's effect on cerebral bioenergetics is a possible mechanism of riboflavin's antimigraine activity. There are most likely other mechanisms at work, as well.

Riboflavin deficiency has been associated with an increased incidence of esophageal cancer in certain parts of the world. Riboflavin supplementation has been found to reduce the prevalence of micronuclei in esophageal cells in a study performed in Huixan, People's Republic of China. Micronuclei are considered precancerous lesions. People living in this region have a high risk of esophageal cancer and poor riboflavin status. It remains unclear, however, whether riboflavin supplementation can decrease the incidence of esophageal cancer. The mechanism of the possible anticarcinogenic activity of riboflavin is also unclear. Riboflavin deficiency has been found to enhance the carcinogenicity of certain xenobiotics, such as azo dyes. The azo dyes are inactivated by a microsomal hydroxylase enzyme system that uses FAD. Riboflavin, as FAD, plays a key role in glutathione metabolism (see above). Glutathione is involved in the detoxification of xenobiotic substances. Riboflavin is also important for the maintenance of epithelial integrity.

The putative anti-atherosclerotic activity of riboflavin may be accounted for, in part, by its role in the metabolism of homocysteine. Elevated serum homocysteine is considered to be an independent risk factor for coronary heart disease. Vitamin B_6, folate and vitamin B_{12} are involved in the metabolism of homocysteine. The riboflavin metabolites FMN and FAD serve as cofactors for enzymes involved in the metabolism of vitamin B_6, folate and vitamin B_{12}. FMN serves as a cofactor for pyridoxine-5^1-phosphate oxidase, which is important for the formation of the active form of vitamin B_6, pyridoxal-5^1 - phosphate. FAD is a cofactor for methylenetetrahydrofolate reductase, which is important for the formation of 5-methyltetrahydrofolate. FMN and FAD are involved in vitamin B_{12} metabolism and serve as cofactors for methionine synthase reductase. Studies on riboflavin deficient subjects are needed to evaluate the usefulness of riboflavin supplementation in hyperhomocysteinemia. Riboflavin may also have anti-atherosclerotic activity secondary to its antioxidant action. Riboflavin, in the form of FAD, is necessary for the formation of reduced glutathione via the FAD-containing enzyme glutathione reductase. Glutathione is the cofactor of the glutathione peroxidases, antioxidant enzymes which protect against lipid peroxidation and oxidation of low-density lipoprotein (LDL). Oxidized-LDL is thought to be a key etiological factor in the pathophysiology of atherosclerosis.

Recently, riboflavin has been demonstrated to have antimalarial activity. The malarial parasite ingests a significant proportion of host cell hemoglobin in an acidic organelle called the food vacuole. The acidic pH of the food vacuole is favorable to the oxidation of hemoglobin to methemoglobin. The malarial parasite also digests hemoglobin and polymerizes the released free heme into hemozoin, also in the food vacuole. It has recently been shown that treatment of erythrocytes infected with *Plasmodium falciparum* with riboflavin decreased the production of methemoglobin and hemozoin, decreased the size of the food vacuole and inhibited asexual parasite growth in cultures. It is thought that the mechanism of the possible antimalarial action of riboflavin is via its acting as a substrate for the enzyme NADPH-methemoglobin reductase. During this reaction, methemoglobin is reduced while riboflavin is oxided to dihydroriboflavin. Thus, riboflavin acts as a reducing agent. Reduction of methemoglobin is correlated with inhibition of hemazoin formation and food vacuole development and arrest of asexual development to schizogony. It is thought that the reduction of methemoglobin plays a role in limiting the amount of hemoglobin which is available to the malarial parasite for further processing. The effects of riboflavin in this recent research differ from earlier studies showing that riboflavin deficiency has an antimalarial effect. The mechanism of antimalarial activity of riboflavin deficiency may be accounted for by a decrease in the activity of reductive enzymes, such as riboflavin reductase, which require riboflavin as a cofactor. This decreased activity lowers glutathione levels. This results in increased oxidative stress and lipid peroxidation, conditions detrimental to the malarial parasite. The use of high-dose riboflavin as an antimalarial strategy appears more attractive than that of causing riboflavin deficiency to treat malaria. Riboflavin deficiency may not only be detrimental to the malarial parasite, but can be detrimental to the host, as well. Continued research in this most important area is warranted and needed to determine, among other things, which approach—riboflavin treatment or riboflavin deficiency—should be the one to pursue regarding a possible new treatment of malaria.

PHARMACOKINETICS

In food, riboflavin is found mainly in the form of flavin mononucleotide (FMN, riboflavin-5¹-phosphate) and flavin adenine dinucleotide (FAD). Riboflavin is used for food fortification. Riboflavin and riboflavin-5¹-phosphate are the principal nutritional supplement forms of riboflavin, with riboflavin being the major form. Coenzyme forms of riboflavin (FAD, FMN) that are not covalently bound to proteins are released from proteins in the acid environment of the stomach. Covalently bound forms or riboflavin (e.g., in mitochondrial succinate dehydrogenase) are released from the proteins they are bound to following proteolysis. FAD and FMN are converted to riboflavin in the small intestine via the action of pyrophosphatase and phosphatase, respectively. Riboflavin is mainly absorbed in the proximal small intestine by a saturable transport system. The rate of absorption increases when riboflavin is ingested with food. The presence of bile salts appears to facilitate absorption of riboflavin. The maximal amount of riboflavin that is absorbed from a single oral dose appears to be about 27 milligrams. The amount of absorption of riboflavin-5¹-phosphate and FAD appears to be very low. During the process of absorption, riboflavin, in part, appears to be converted to FMN which is either used by the enterocytes for their metabolic requirements, or converted back to riboflavin for further processing. Riboflavin is transported via the portal circulation to the liver and by the systemic circulation to the various tissues of the body.

A large percentage of serum riboflavin is carried by immunoglobulins. Some serum riboflavin is carried by albumin. Riboflavin is transported into cells via facilitated diffusion at physiological concentrations, and by passive diffusion at higher concentrations. Within cells, riboflavin is converted to FMN via flavokinase. FMN is converted to FAD via FAD synthetase. FAD is the predominant form of riboflavin in tissues.

Very little riboflavin is stored in tissues. Riboflavin in excess of body requirements is excreted mainly by the kidneys. A number of riboflavin metabolites are also found in the urine, including 7-hydromethylriboflavin, 8-hydroxymethylriboflavin, 8 alpha-sulfonylriboflavin, 5¹-riboflavinyl peptide, 10-hydroxyethylflavin, lumiflavin, 10-formylmethylflavin and carboxymethylflavins. A significant percentage of large intakes of riboflavin—greater than 30 milligrams in a single dose—is excreted in the feces.

INDICATIONS AND USAGE

Riboflavin has been found to be an effective migraine prophylaxis in some. Riboflavin supplementation has resulted in full recovery of several patients who developed a sometimes fatal syndrome characterized by lactic acidosis and hepatic steatosis caused by treatment with nucleoside reverse-transcriptase inhibitors. Riboflavin has significant antioxidant-promoting activity which, experimentally, has protected against cardiac injury produced by reperfusion following ischemia. It has also exhibited notable ability to inhibit lipid oxidation and has protected against a number of oxidative injuries in the laboratory. It has demonstrated some activity against esophageal cancer. Intriguingly, riboflavin deficiency has been shown to be protective against malaria in both animals and humans. On the other hand, high doses of riboflavin may have antimalarial activity.

RESEARCH SUMMARY

Riboflavin has been called "a significant breakthrough" in migraine prophylaxis with "an outstanding efficacy-side effect profile" by one recent reviewer of migraine research developments.

In an open study, high-dose riboflavin showed significant effectiveness as a migraine prophylaxis. In a subsequent randomized trial, 400 milligrams of riboflavin and placebo were tested for three months in 55 migraine patients. In the riboflavin group, 59% improved by at least 50%, compared with 15% of the placebo group showing at least 50% improvement.

Recently, both riboflavin and beta-blockers were tested for their effects on the intensity dependence of auditory evoked cortical potentials. Intensity dependence is usually increased during migraines. In this study, the beta-blockers significantly decreased the intensity dependence, and this decrease correlated with significant clinical improvement. Riboflavin treatment did not affect intensity dependence but was, nonetheless, also associated with significant improvement. Thus, given that the two agents apparently act via two distinct pathophysiological mechanisms, the researchers concluded that a combination of the two treatments might enhance their efficacy without increasing central nervous system side effects. This hypothesis warrants investigation.

A 46-year-old woman who had been treated for AIDS with triple anti-retroviral therapy for four months developed lactic acidosis and marked hepatic steatosis. Suspecting that a riboflavin deficiency induced by amitriptyline, which she was also taking (see Interactions), might be contributing to these potentially life-threatening metabolic abnormalities, the physicians treated her with 50 milligrams of riboflavin daily. This was followed by rapid recovery.

Subsequently, these researchers similarly identified two other HIV-infected patients with less severe lactic acidosis. These patients had also been on triple drug therapy. Riboflavin again rapidly resolved the acidosis. This condition, they believed, results, in part, from impaired mitochondrial DNA replication caused by the HIV drug therapies.

Another researcher has also reported that 50 milligrams of riboflavin daily resolved the severe lactic acidosis of a 35-year-old pregnant HIV-infected patient. Blood lactate levels returned to normal within four days of beginning treatment. This syndrome is a rare complication of treatment with nucleoside reverse-transcriptase inhibitors, but, since it can be fatal, it is a significant one, as is riboflavin's apparent role in resolving it.

Riboflavin's antioxidant-promoting activity has been shown to provide protection against oxidative damage caused by oxidized forms of hemeproteins. In an animal model of ischemic reperfusion injury, riboflavin was significantly cardioprotective. In an *in vivo* animal experiment, it protected rat lungs from the oxidative injury initiated by injection of cobra venom factor. It also significantly protected rat brains from swelling after four hours of ischemia. Riboflavin is the precursor of co-enzymes that are required in potent antioxidant processes. Some researchers have concluded that riboflavin nutriture plays a crucial role in inactivation of lipid peroxides. Riboflavin supplementation has been shown to prevent hepatic lipid peroxidation both in *in vitro* and in animal studies.

Some studies have shown a synergy between Vitamin E and riboflavin as antioxidants. Riboflavin, for example, diminished lipid peroxidation and prevented the oxidation of Vitamin E in the livers of experimental animals. It has been suggested that riboflavin has a sparing effect on vitamin E or may help regenerate Vitamin E via production of reduced glutathione.

There is an epidemiological association between riboflavin and esophageal cancer. The incidence of this cancer is particularly high in parts of the world (some areas of China, Iran and Africa) where riboflavin deficiency is high. One study suggested that riboflavin supplementation might reduce the number of precancerous cells in the esophagus. This needs followup.

There is a finding, in both animals and humans, that a deficiency in riboflavin has significant antimalarial effects. Dietary riboflavin deficiency dramatically decreases malarial parasitemia with concomitant diminution of symptoms. Further, specific riboflavin antagonists have demonstrated antimalarial activity. Whether these findings can become the basis for a new pharmacological approach to the treatment of this challenging disease remains to be seen. On the other hand, a recent study reported that high doses of riboflavin may have antimalarial activity. Further research is necessary and warranted in order to resolve these seemingly contradictory findings.

CONTRAINDICATIONS, PRECAUTIONS, ADVERSE REACTIONS
CONTRAINDICATIONS
Riboflavin is contraindicated in those hypersensitive to any component of a riboflavin-containing product.

PRECAUTIONS

The use of riboflavin for the treatment of riboflavin deficiency or for any medical indication must be medically supervised.

Most pre- and postnatal vitamin/mineral supplements deliver 3.4 milligrams daily of riboflavin. Pregnant women and nursing mothers should avoid intakes of riboflavin greater than this amount unless higher amounts are prescribed by their physicians.

High dose intake of riboflavin may interfere with the Abbott TDX drugs-of-abuse assay.

Riboflavin absorption is increased in hypothyroidism and decreased in hyperthyroidism.

Those who use nucleoside reverse-transcriptase inhibitors (see Interactions) should be aware that even mild riboflavin deficiency may increase the risk of lactic acidosis.

ADVERSE REACTIONS

Riboflavin is well tolerated. Doses of 400 milligrams daily for four months were found to cause diarrhea and polyuria in two out of 28 subjects who participated in a migraine prophylaxis study. Riboflavin supplements impart a yellow-orange discoloration to urine. This color has no pathological implication.

INTERACTIONS

DRUGS

Cholestyramine: Concomitant intake of cholestyramine and riboflavin may decrease the absorption of riboflavin.

Chlorpromazine: Chlorpromazine may inhibit the conversion of riboflavin to FMN and FAD.

Colestipol: Concomitant intake of colestipol and riboflavin may decrease the absorption of riboflavin.

Doxorubicin: Doxorubicin may inhibit the conversion of riboflavin to FMN and FAD.

Metoclopramide: Metoclopramide may decrease the absorption of riboflavin.

Nucleoside reverse-transcriptase inhibitors (didanosine, lamivudine, stavudine, zidovudine): Riboflavin has been found to reverse nucleoside analogue-induced lactic acidosis in patients with mild riboflavin deficiencies. These mild riboflavin deficiencies may result from the use of drugs, such as amitriptyline, which may adversely affect riboflavin status.

Oral Contraceptive Agents: Use of oral contraceptive agents may result in decreased serum levels of riboflavin.

Probenecid: Probenecid may inhibit the absorption of riboflavin. It may also inhibit renal tubular secretion of riboflavin.

Propantheline bromide: Propantheline bromide may enhance the absorption of riboflavin by allowing the vitamin to remain at intestinal absorption sites for longer periods of time.

Quinacrine: Quinacrine may inhibit the conversion of riboflavin to FMN and FAD.

Tricyclic Antidepressants (amitriptyline, imipramine): Tricyclic antidepressant drugs may inhibit the conversion of riboflavin to FMN and FAD.

NUTRITIONAL SUPPLEMENTS

Boron: Boric acid may induce riboflavin deficiency, since it displaces riboflavin from plasma-binding sites and results in increased urinary excretion of the vitamin. Most forms of boron (see Boron) used for nutritional supplementation are readily converted to boric acid. High intakes of these boron supplements may result in riboflavin deficiency.

Psyllium: Concomitant intake of psyllium and riboflavin may decrease the absorption of riboflavin.

Vitamin E: Riboflavin may potentiate the antioxidant effect of Vitamin E.

FOODS

Concomitant intake of riboflavin with food enhances the absorption of riboflavin.

OVERDOSAGE

There are no reports of riboflavin overdosage in the literature.

DOSAGE AND ADMINISTRATION

Riboflavin and riboflavin 5¹-monophosphate are the principal forms of riboflavin supplements, with riboflavin being the major available form. Riboflavin is typically present in multivitamin, multivitamin/multimineral and B-complex preparations. Riboflavin is also available as a single ingredient supplement. Typical doses range from 1.7 to 10 milligrams daily. Pre- and postnatal supplements usually deliver riboflavin at a dose of 3.4 daily. In the migraine prophylaxis studies, 400 milligrams daily of riboflavin were used. Use of riboflavin for any medical indication must be medically supervised. Doses of riboflavin greater than 30 milligrams should be taken in divided doses.

The Food and Nutrition Board of the Institute of Medicine of the National Academy of Sciences recommends the following dietary reference intakes (DRI) for riboflavin:

Infants	Adequate Intakes (AI)	
0-6 months	0.3 mg/day	0.04 mg/kg

7-12 months	0.4 mg/day	0.04 mg/kg
		Recommended Dietary Allowances (RDA)
Children		
1-3 years		0.5 mg/day
4-8 years		0.6 mg/day
Boys		
9-13 years		0.9 mg/day
14-18 years		1.3 mg/day
Girls		
9-13 years		0.9 mg/day
14-18 years		1.0 mg/day
Men		
19 years and older		1.3 mg/day
Women		
19 years and older		1.1 mg/day
Pregnancy		
14-50 years		1.4 mg/day
Lactation		
14-50 years		1.6 mg/day

The U.S. RDA for riboflavin, which is used for determining percent daily values on nutritional supplement and food labels, is 1.7 milligrams.

HOW SUPPLIED

Capsules — 50 mg, 100 mg

Enteric Coated Tablets — 5 mg

Tablets — 10 mg, 25 mg, 50 mg, 100 mg, 250 mg, 400 mg

Tablets, Extended Release — 250 mg

LITERATURE

Akomporg T, Ghori N, Halder K. In vitro activity of riboflavin against the human malaria parasite Plasmodium faciparum. *Antimicrob Agents Chemother.* 2000; 44:88-96.

Christensen HN. Riboflavin can protect tissues from oxidative injury. *Nutr Rev.* 1998; 51:149-150.

Dietary Reference Intakes for Thiamin, Riboflavin, Niacin, Vitamin B6, Folate, Vitamin B12, Pantothenic Acid, Biotin, and Choline. Washington, DC: National Academy Press; 1998.

Dutta P, Pinto JT, Rivlin RS. Antimalarial effects of riboflavin deficiency. *Lancet.* 1985; 2:1040-1043.

Fraaije MW, van den Heuvel RH, van Berkel WJ, Mattevi A. Covalent flavinylation is essential for efficient redox catalysis in vanillyl-alcohol oxidase. *J Biol Chem.* 1999; 274:35514-35520.

Fraaije MW, Mattevi A. Flavoenzymes: diverse catalysts with recurrent features. *Trends Biochem Sci.* 2000; 25:126-132.

Fouty B, Frerman F, Reves R. Riboflavin to treat nucleoside analogue-induced lactic acidosis. *Lancet.* 1998; 352:291-292.

Huang S-N, Swaan PW. Involvement of a receptor-mediated component in cellular translocation of riboflavin. *J Pharmacol Exp Therap.* 2000; 294:117-125.

Hustad S, Ueland PM, Vollset SE, et al. Riboflavin as a determinant of plasma total homocysteine: effect modification by the methylenetetrahydrofolate reductase C677T polymorphism. *Clin Chem.*2000; 468:1065-1071.

Kunsman GW, Levine B, Smith ML. Vitamin B2 interference with TDx drugs-of abuse assays. *J Forensic Sci.* 1998; 43:1225-1227.

Lakshmi AV, Ramalakshmi BA. Effect of pyridoxine or riboflavin supplementation on plasma homocysteine levels in women with oral lesions. *Natl Med J India.* 1998; 11:171-172.

Luzzati R, Del Bravo P, Di Perri G, et al. Riboflavine and severe lactic acidosis. *Lancet.* 1999; 353:901-902.

McCormick DB. Riboflavin. In: Shils ME, Olson JA, Shike M, Ross AC, eds. *Modern Nutrition in Health and Disease.* 9th ed. Baltimore, MD: Williams and Wilkins; 1999:391-399.

Munoz N, Hayashi M, Bang LJ, et al. Effect of riboflavin, retinol, and zinc on micronuclei of buccal mucosa and of esophagus: a randomized double-blind intervention study in China. *J Natl Cancer Inst.*1987; 79:687-691.

Rivlin RS. Riboflavin. *Adv Exp Med Biol.* 1986; 206:349-355.

Rivlin RS, Dutta P. Vitamin B2 (riboflavin). Relevance to malaria and antioxidant activity. *Nutrition Today.* 1995; 30:62-67.

Sándor PS, Áfra J, Ambrosini A, Schoenen J. Prophylactic treatment of migraine with beta-blockers and riboflavin: differential effects on the intensity dependence of auditory evoked cortical potentials. *Headache.* 2000; 40:30-35.

Schoenen J. [Anti-migraine treatment: present and future]. [Article in French]. *Rev Med Liege.* 1999; 54:79-86.

Schoenen J, Jacquy J, Lenaerts M. Effectiveness of high-dose riboflavin in migraine prophylaxis. A randomized controlled trial. *Neurology.* 1998; 50:466-470.

Thurnham DI, Zheng SF, Munoz N, et al. Comparison of riboflavin, Vitamin A, and zinc status of Chinese populations at high and low risk for esophageal cancer. *Nutr Canc.* 1985; 7:131-143.

Wahrendorf J, Munoz N, Lu JB, et al. Blood, retinol and zinc riboflavin status in relation to precancerous lesions of the esophagus: findings from a vitamin intervention trial in the People's Republic of China. *Cancer Res.* 1988; 48:2280-2283.

Royal Jelly

TRADE NAMES

Royal Jelly is available from numerous manufacturers generically. It is also available in combination products. Branded products include Premium Royal Jelly (American Health).

DESCRIPTION

Royal jelly, also known as gelee royale and RJ, is the milky-white gelatinous substance secreted from the cephalic glands of nurse worker bees *(Apis mellifera)* for apparently the sole purpose of stimulating the growth and development of the queen bee. Without royal jelly, the queen bee would be no different from the worker bees and would live about as long (seven to eight weeks). With royal jelly, the queen bee can live five to seven years. This fact explains the popular belief that royal jelly has rejuvenating qualities.

Royal jelly, however, has not lived up to expectations that it is an important anti-aging substance. But it is not without medical interest. Royal jelly consists of an emulsion of proteins, sugars, lipids and some other substances in a water base. Proteins make up about 13% of royal jelly. Most of the proteins comprise a family called major royal jelly proteins. One protein in royal jelly called royalsin possesses antibiotic properties against gram-positive, but not gram-negative, bacteria. About 11% of royal jelly is made up of sugars, such as fructose and glucose, similar to those found in honey. Lipids comprise about 5% of the substance and consist mainly of medium-chain hydroxy fatty acids, such as trans-10-hydroxy-2-decenoic acid, which is also thought to possess antimicrobial properties.

Royal jelly also contains vitamins, such as pantothenic acid, minerals and phytosterols. Neopterin, or 2-amino-6- (1,2,3-trihydroxypropyl)-4 (3H)-pteridinone, was initially isolated from royal jelly. Neopterin is also found in humans, and, although its precise role is not known, it appears to play an important role in the human immune system.

Melbrosia, a mixture of royal jelly and bee pollen, is sometimes used by menopausal women to manage climacteric symptoms.

ACTIONS AND PHARMACOLOGY

ACTIONS

Royal jelly may have hypolipidemic, antibacterial, anti-inflammatory and antiproliferative activities.

MECHANISM OF ACTION

The mechanism of actions of royal jelly is not known. The possible antibacterial activity of some royal jelly proteins, while of interest for topical use, is unlikely to be expressed when ingested.

PHARMACOKINETICS

There are no reported pharmacokinetic studies of royal jelly. Proteins, carbohydrates and lipids in royal jelly should be digested, absorbed and metabolized in the same way that other such substances found in food are digested, absorbed and metabolized.

INDICATIONS AND USAGE

Royal jelly may have favorable lipid effects, including cholesterol-lowering effects. There is very preliminary evidence that it may have some antibiotic, immunomodulatory, anti-inflammatory, wound-healing and anti-cancer effects.

RESEARCH SUMMARY

A meta-analysis of royal jelly's reported effects on serum lipids in experimental animals and in humans found significant, positive results. The substance significantly decreased serum and liver total lipids and cholesterol in rats and mice, and retarded the formation of atheromas in the aortas of rabbits fed hyperlipidemic diets. Meta-analysis of controlled human studies also showed significant reduction in total serum lipids and cholesterol, and, in those with hyperlipidemia, it normalized HDL- and LDL-cholesterol determined from decreases in beta/alpha lipoproteins. The author of this meta-analysis concluded: "The best available evidence suggests that royal jelly, at approximately 50 to 100 milligrams per day, decreased total serum cholesterol levels by about 14% and total serum lipids by about 10% in the group of patients studied."

One group of researchers has reported that a royal jelly extract has potent antibiotic effects against gram-positive bacteria, but not against gram-negative bacteria. Royal jelly has exhibited immunomodulating effects in an animal model, stimulating antibody production and immunocompetent cell proliferation.

It has been claimed, anecdotally, for some time that royal jelly has anti-inflammatory effects and wound-healing properties. These claims were given preliminary support in a study of streptozotocin-diabetic rats. The researchers were looking for a hypoglycemic effect from royal jelly; none was found, but the researchers noted that royal jelly showed some anti-inflammatory activity and that it shortened healing time in desquamated skin lesions.

There have been scattered repots that royal jelly and its constituent 10-hydroxy-2-decenoic acid might have anti-cancer effects. There was one report that both provided complete protection against transplantable mouse leukemia. Tumor growth inhibition of other cancers has been associated with royal jelly supplementation in other animal models. More research is needed.

CONTRAINDICATIONS, PRECAUTIONS, ADVERSE REACTIONS

CONTRAINDICATIONS

Royal jelly is contraindicated in those allergic or hypersensitive to any of its components.

PRECAUTIONS

Pregnant women and nursing mothers should avoid using royal jelly supplements.

ADVERSE REACTIONS

Adverse reactions have included eczema, rhinitis, urticaria and bronchospasm. There is one report of a woman developing hemorrhagic colitis following use of royal jelly for approximately one month. Acute asthma, anaphylaxis and, in one case, death secondary to royal jelly-induced asthma have also been reported.

OVERDOSAGE

No reported overdosage of royal jelly.

DOSAGE AND ADMINISTRATION

Those who use royal jelly take 50 to 100 milligrams daily. Royal jelly is also available in cosmetic formulations. Those who are allergic or hypersensitive to royal jelly may develop dermatitis conditions from topical use.

HOW SUPPLIED

Capsules — 100 mg, 200 mg, 300 mg, 500 mg, 1000 mg, 1500 mg, 2000 mg

Chewable Tablets — 100 mg

Elixir — 167 mg/5 ml, 667 mg/5 ml

Liquid — 659 mg/teaspoonful (in a honey base)

LITERATURE

Bullock RJ, Rohan A, Straatmans JA. Fatal royal jelly-induced asthma. *Med J Aust.* 1999; 160:44.

Fujii A, Kobayashi S, Kuboyama N. Augmentation of wound healing by royal jelly (RJ) in streptozoticin-diabetic rats. *Jpn J Pharmacol.* 1990; 53:331-337.

Fujiwara S, Imai J, Fujiwara M, et al. A potent antibacterial protein in royal jelly. Purification and determination of the primary structure of royalisin. *J Biol Chem.* 1990; 265:11333-11337.

Gene M, Aslan A. Determination of trans-10-hydroxy-2-decenoic acid content in pure royal jelly products by column liquid chromatography. *J Chromatogr.* 1999; 839:265-268.

Hamerlinck FF. Neopterin: a review. *Exp Dermatol.* 1999; 8:167-176.

Harwood M, Harding S, Beasley R, Frankish PD. Asthma following royal jelly. *N Z Med J.* 1996; 109:325..

Ishiwata H, Takeda Y, Yamada T, et al. Determination and confirmation of methyl p-hydroxybenzoate in royal jelly and other foods produced by the honey bee. *Food Addit Contam,* 1999; 12:281-285.

Leung R, Ho A, Chan J, et al. Royal jelly consumption and hypersensitivity in the community. *Clin Exp Allergy.* 1997; 27:333-336.

Orsolic SL, Tadic Z, Njari B, et al. A royal jelly as a new potential immunomodulator in rats and mice. *Comp Immunol Microbiol Infect Dis.* 1996; 19:31-38.

Shen X, Lu R, He G. [Effects of lyophilized royal jelly on experimental hyperlipidemia and thrombosis.] [Article in Chinese.] *Chung Hua Yu Fang I Hsueh Tsa Chih.* 1995; 29:27-29.

Szanto E, Gruber D, Sator M, et al. [Placebo-controlled study of melbrosia in treatment of climacteric symptoms.] [Article in German.] *Wien Med Wochenschr.* 1994; 144:130-134.

Tamura T, Fujii A, Kuboyama N. [Antitumor effects of royal jelly.] [Article in Japanese.] *Nippon Yakurigaku Zasshi.* 1987; 89:73-80.

Thien FC, Leung R, Baldo BA, et al. Asthma and anaphylaxis induced by royal jelly. *Clin Exp Allergy.* 1996; 26:216-222.

Vittek J. Effects of royal jelly on serum lipids in experimental animals and humans with atherosclerosis. *Experientia.* 1995; 51:927-935.

Yonei Y, Shibagaki K, Tsukada N, et al. Case report: hemorrhagic colitis associated with royal jelly intake. *J Gastroenterol Hepatol.* 1997; 12:495-499.

Rutin

DESCRIPTION

The flavonoid rutin is a flavonol glycoside comprised of the flavonol quercetin (see Quercetin) and the disaccharide rutinose. Rutin is found in many plants, especially the buckwheat plant *Fagopyrum esculentum* Moench, the flour of which is used to make pancakes. Other rich dietary sources of rutin include black tea and apple peels.

Rutin is a solid substance, pale yellow in appearance and only slightly soluble in water. It is, however, much more soluble in water than its aglycone quercetin. Rutin's molecular formula is $C_{27}H_{30}O_{16}$, its molecular weight is 610.53 daltons, and its structural formula is:

Rutin

The disaccharide moiety of rutin, rutinose, is comprised of the sugars rhamnose (6-deoxy-L-mannose) and glucose. Many names are used for rutin in the literature. They include rutoside, quercetin-3-rutinoside and sophorin. Also, 3, 3', 4', 5, 7-pentahydroxyflavone-3-rutinoside, 3-rhamnosyl-glucosyl quercetin and 3-[[6-O-(6-deoxy-alpha-L-mannopyranosyl)-beta-D-glucopyranosyl] oxy]-2-(3, 4-dihydroxyphenyl)-5,7-dihydroxy-4*H*-1-benzopyran-4-one.

ACTIONS AND PHARMACOLOGY
ACTIONS
Rutin may have antioxidant, anti-inflammatory, anticarcinogenic, antithrombotic, cytoprotective and vasoprotective activities.

MECHANISM OF ACTION
Many, if not most, of rutin's possible activities can be accounted for, in part, by rutin's antioxidant activity. Rutin is a phenolic antioxidant and has been demonstrated to scavenge superoxide radicals. Rutin can chelate metal ions, such as ferrous cations. Ferrous cations are involved in the so-called Fenton reaction, which generates reactive oxygen species. Rutin may also modulate the respiratory burst of neutrophils. The *in vivo* antioxidant activity of rutin is most likely due to its aglycone quercetin, to which it is metabolized following ingestion. Although most studies show rutin to inhibit lipid peroxidation, a few studies do not. Rutin may also help maintain levels of the biological antioxidant reduced glutathione. Importantly, under certain conditions, rutin or its metabolite quercetin may become a pro-oxidant. For example, nitrosation of rutin/ quercetin may produce a pro-oxidant molecule that may have mutagenic potential.

PHARMACOKINETICS
The pharmacokinetics of rutin in humans is still under investigation. It appears that only about 17% of an ingested dose is absorbed. Absorption appears to occur mainly from the colon following the removal of the carbohydrate moiety by bacterial enzymes to form quercetin. Quercetin may undergo glucuronidation in the colonocytes. It is unclear to what extent there is absorption of quercetin glycosides. Quercetin and glucuronide conjugates of quercetin are transported to the liver via the portal circulation, where they undergo significant first pass metabolism. Metabolites may include isorhamnetin, kaempferol and tamarixetin. Quercetin itself may undergo glucuronidation and sulfation. Quercetin and its metabolites are distributed from the liver to various tissues in the body. Quercetin is strongly bound to albumin in the plasma.

INDICATIONS AND USAGE
Rutin may be useful in the management of venous edema. It may help strengthen capillaries, protect against some toxins and have anti-inflammatory effects, as well as some anti-cancer effects. It may also help prevent the oxidation of vitamin C and have some positive lipid effects.

RESEARCH SUMMARY
Some of the earliest research related to rutin found that, in daily doses of 200 to 600 mg, it is useful in treating some with conditions characterized by capillary fragility and attendant easy bruising. There was the suggestion in some of this early work that it might help decrease the incidence of cerebral hemorrhage, though no research was conducted to specifically confirm this. An early placebo-controlled study reported a significant reduction in mid-cycle menstrual bleeding in rutin-supplemented women.

Several placebo-controlled trials have demonstrated that rutin has significant efficacy in diminishing the venous edema that is an early sign of chronic venous disease of the leg.

Rutin's anti-inflammatory potential has been demonstrated in a number of animal studies. In experimentally induced colitis, both pre- and post-induction treatment with rutin conferred significant preventive and healing effects. Rutin was shown to increase colonic glutathione levels, thus reducing oxidative tissue damage in this inflammatory condition. It has also shown cytoprotective effects against ethanol injury in an animal model of ethanol-induced gastric lesions.

Rutin's radical-scavenging and, possibly, its iron-chelating abilities were said, in other animal studies, to significantly protect against asbestos-induced oxidative cellular injury.

Very preliminary animal research has found some evidence that rutin can inhibit some cancerous and pre-cancerous conditions, including chemically induced colonic neoplasia. Results, however, have been mixed. Far more research is required.

Although in most studies rutin has been found to inhibit lipid peroxidation, in one study rutin was not found to block cellular lipid peroxidation. However, according to the researchers, rutin may still potentially play a positive role in helping to prevent atherogenesis by inhibiting the depletion of cellular glutathione and ATP, thus perhaps reducing the cytotoxicity of oxidized LDL-cholesterol.

Finally, there is some evidence suggesting that rutin, taken with vitamin C, may help inhibit the oxidation of vitamin C and thus make it safer and more useful in some conditions. More research is needed to elucidate the relationship between the flavonoids and vitamin C.

CONTRAINDICATIONS, PRECAUTIONS, ADVERSE REACTIONS
CONTRAINDICATIONS
Rutin is contraindicated in those who are hypersensitive to any component of a rutin-containing product.

PRECAUTIONS.
Pregnant women and nursing mothers should avoid using rutin supplements.

There is some suggestion that rutin may undergo nitrosation with, for example, nitrates and nitrites found in some processed meat products to form potentially mutagenic substances. Those who supplement with rutin should avoid using it concomitantly with such products.

ADVERSE REACTIONS.

Rutin is generally well tolerated. Adverse reactions include gastrointestinal ones, such as nausea. There are rare reports of headache and mild tingling of the extremities.

INTERACTIONS

DRUGS

Quinolone antibiotics: Quercetin binds *in vitro* to the DNA gyrase site in bacteria. Therefore, theoretically, it can serve as a competitive inhibitor to the quinolone antibiotics, which also bind to this site.

NUTRITIONAL SUPPLEMENTS

Vitamin C: The interaction between flavonoids, such as rutin and quercetin, and vitamin C is unclear. It has been believed for some time that flavonoids work synergistically with vitamin C, enhancing the absorption of the vitamin and preventing it from oxidation. However, recent research indicates that flavonoids may actually inhibit the uptake of vitamin C into cells. More research is necessary in order to clarify this issue.

FOODS

Rutin may undergo nitrosation with nitrites and nitrates found in some processed meat products to form potentially mutagenic substances.

DOSAGE AND ADMINISTRATION

Typical doses used are 500 mg once or twice daily. Those with venous insufficiency/varicose veins often use 500 mg taken twice daily.

HOW SUPPLIED

Tablets — 50 mg, 250 mg, 500 mg,

LITERATURE

Clement DL. Management of venous edema: insights from an international task force. *Angiology*. 2000; 51:13-17.

Cruz T, Galvez J, Ocete MA, et al. Oral administration of rutoside can ameliorate inflammatory bowel disease in rats. *Life Sci*. 1998; 62:687-695.

Deschner EE, Ruperto JF. Wong GY, Newmark HL. The effect of dietary quercetin and rutin on AOM-induced acute colonic epithelial abnormalities in mice fed a high-fat diet. *Nutr Cancer*. 1993; 20:199-204.

Drewa G, Schachtschabel DO, Palgan K, et al. The influence of rutin on the weight, metastasis and melanin content of B16 melanotic melanoma in C57BL/6 mice. *Neoplasma*. 1998; 45:266-271.

Galvez J, Cruz T, Crespo E, et al. Rutoside as mucosal protective in acetic acid-induced rat colitis. *Planta Med*. 1997; 63:409-414.

Kostyuk VA, Potapovich AI. Antiradical and chelating effects in flavonoid protection against silica-induced cell injury. *Arch Biochem Biophys*. 1998; 355:43-48.

Kostyuk VA, Potapovich AI, Speransky SD, Maslova GT. Protective effect of natural flavonoids on rat peritoneal macrophages injury caused by asbestos fiber. *Free Rad Biol Med*. 1996; 21:487-493.

Olthof MR, Hollman PC, Vree TB, Katan MB. Bioavailabilities of quercetin-3-glucoside and quercetin-4'-glucoside do not differ in humans. *J Nutr*. 2000; 130:1200-1203.

Park JB, Levine M. Intracellular accumulation of ascorbic acid is inhibited by flavonoids via blocking of dehydroascorbic acid and ascorbic acid uptakes in HL-60, U937 and Jurkat cells. *J Nutr*. 2000; 130:1297-1302.

Perez Guerrero C, Martin MG, Marhuenda E. Prevention by rutin of gastric lesions induced by ethanol in rats: role of endogenous prostaglandins. *Gen Pharmacol*. 1994; 25:575-580.

Rueff J, Gaspar J, Laires A. Structural requirements for mutagenicity of flavonoids upon nitrosation. A structure-activity study. *Mutagenesis*. 1995; 10:325-328.

Schmitt A, Savayre R, Delchambre J, Negre-Salvayre A. Prevention by alpha-tocopherol and rutin of glutathione and ATP depletion induced by oxidized LDL in cultured endothelial cells. *Br J Pharmacol*. 1995; 116:1985-1990.

Webster RP, Gawde MD, Bhattacharya RK, Protective effect of rutin, a flavonol glycoside, on the carcinogen-induced DNA damage and repair enzymes in rats. *Cancer Lett*. 1996; 109:185-191.

S-Adenosyl-L-Methionine (SAMe)

TRADE NAMES

SAMe is available from numerous manufacturers generically. Branded products include SAMe Rx-Mood (Nature's Plus), Sam-Sulfate (Natrol).

DESCRIPTION

S-adenosyl-L-methionine (SAMe) is a natural substance present in the cells of the body. It is a direct metabolite of the essential amino acid L-methionine. It is variously known as ademetionine, S-adenosylmethione, SAM, SAMe and SAM-e. It is represented structurally as:

NH$_2$

S-Adenosylmethionine

SAMe is used as a drug in Europe for the treatment of depression, liver disorders, osteoarthritis and fibromyalgia. Recently, SAMe has been introduced into the United States as a dietary supplement for the support of bone and joint health, as well as mood and emotional well being.

ACTIONS AND PHARMACOLOGY

ACTIONS
SAMe plays a crucial biochemical role in the body by donating a one-carbon methyl group in a process called transmethylation. SAMe, formed from the reaction of L-methionine and adenosine triphosphate catalyzed by the enzyme S-adenosylmethionine synthetase, is the methyl-group donor in the biosynthesis of both DNA and RNA nucleic acids, phospholipids, proteins, epinephrine, melato-nin, creatine and other molecules.

Supplemental SAMe may have anti-depressant and hepato-protective activities.

MECHANISM OF ACTION
The mechanism of action of supplemental SAMe is unclear. Much is known, however, of the mechanism of action of endogenous SAMe.

Methylation of DNA is critical in the biological phenomenon known as gene silencing. Gene silencing helps suppress genes that may give rise to cancer or those that may carry information for endogenous retroviruses. Methylation of RNA, particularly transfer RNA, is similarly important in safeguarding the form and function of these molecules in protein synthesis.

SAMe is the methyl donor to phosphatidylethanolamine in the formation of phosphatidylcholine (PC). PC is a major component of cell membranes and is vital for maintenance of cellular membrane fluidity, important in sustaining the bioenergetics and information-processing functions of cells.

SAMe is also involved in the methylation of histones, major elements in chromosomal structure. This methylation is believed to play a key role in the regulation of DNA transcription, the process by which RNA is formed. The carbon and nitrogen atoms of L-carnitine are derived from methylated lysine residues, which are formed by methylating certain proteins with SAMe's methyl group.

SAMe's importance in the body is further emphasized by the fact that it is also the methyl donor for the synthesis of epinephrine (adrenaline), creatine, melatonin, glutathione, the polyamines spermine and spermidine, and the amino acids L-cysteine and taurine, all of which play vital roles in human health.

PHARMACOKINETICS
SAMe is absorbed from the small intestine following oral intake. Absorption is better on an empty stomach, and enteric-coated tablets are better absorbed than non-enteric-coated varieties. Peak plasma concentrations obtained with enteric-coated tablet formulations are dose related, with a peak concentration of 0.5 to 1 mg/L achieved three to five hours after single doses in the range of 400 to 1,000 milligrams.

Limited trials in healthy volunteers show low bioavailability following oral intake of SAMe. This indicates significant first-pass metabolism in the liver. SAMe is mainly metabo-lized in the liver (about 50%).

SAMe is metabolized to S-adenosylhomocysteine, which in turn is metabolized to homocysteine. Homocysteine can either be metabolized to cystathionine and then cysteine or to methionine. The cofactor in the metabolism of homocysteine to cysteine is vitamin B$_6$. Cofactors for the metabolism of homocysteine to methionine are folic acid, vitamin B12 and trimethylglycine (betaine).

Orally administered SAMe follows the same metabolic pathways as the natural compound found in cells. SAMe crosses the blood-brain barrier with slow accumulation in the cerebrovascular fluid. It can also get into joint synovial fluid.

One study showed that 15% of a 200 milligram-dose of SAMe was excreted in urine within 48 hours and that an additional 23% was eliminated in feces within 72 hours. The remainder was believed to be incorporated in stable metabol-ic pools (phosphatidylcholine, DNA, RNA, proteins and creatine, among others).

The pharmacokinetics of SAMe are similar whether in healthy individuals or in those with chronic liver disease.

INDICATIONS AND USAGE

SAMe may be indicated for the promotion and support of mood and emotional well-being. It is being used by some for the treatment of depression. It may also be indicated for the support of joint health, mobility and joint comfort. It is used for the treatment of osteoarthritis; there is, as yet, little convincing evidence that it is useful in any other form of arthritis. It is also used in some liver conditions, including various forms of cirrhosis and cholestasis, and there is a very preliminary indication that it might be useful in lowering lipids.

RESEARCH SUMMARY

A number of studies have now demonstrated an association between various neuropsychiatric disorders and deficient SAMe metabolism. SAMe's possible influence on mono-amine neurotransmitter metabolism, in particular, has focused attention on its possible role in depression. This has resulted in a series of small studies using oral and parenteral SAMe to treat depression. The results are preliminary but promising.

In a meta-analysis of the most significant clinical studies, SAMe's efficacy was shown to exceed that of placebo and to equal or slightly better that of tricyclic antidepressants. (There is no reliable data comparing SAMe with the selective serotonin reuptake inhibitors.) Parenteral administration was only slightly more effective than oral.

SAMe, unlike traditional antidepressants, has few side effects and a rapid onset of action (usually within one or two weeks compared with three to four weeks or longer for standard antidepressants). SAMe rarely produces the side effects common to many other anti-depressants, such as insomnia, nervousness, nausea and sexual dysfunction. SAMe should only be used in bipolar disorder under strict medical supervision, if at all.

SAMe's possible role in ameliorating a number of other neurological disorders is suggested by some early research but is far from proved. These disorders include Alzheimer's dementia and other clinical dementia syndromes. SAMe has been shown to have some positive effect on mood and depression associated with Parkinson's disease and chronic epileptic seizures.

SAMe is depleted in liver disease, and its replenishment through supplementation has been demonstrated in several studies. Its methylating properties promote the fluidity of liver lipid membranes. SAMe has been shown to improve functions measured by standard liver and liver-function tests, to increase hepatic glutathione levels in patients with both alcohol and non-alcoholic cirrhosis, to restore normal hepatic function in various forms of cholestasis and prevent or reverse hepatoxicity induced by drugs, alcohol and various chemicals.

There is some hope that SAMe might make a significant contribution to the treatment of osteoarthritis, as well, and without the side effects that characterize most of the non-steroidal anti-inflammatory drugs. Again, early results are encouraging but not yet conclusive. The same is true of SAMe's possible role in alleviating fibromyalgia. There is still no credible evidence, however, to support claims that SAMe can reverse cartilage degeneration. Nor is there other than the scantiest evidence that SAMe will be effective in any form of arthritis other than osteoarthritis.

SAMe is used as a cytoprotective agent against liver toxicity and there hope that it might one day be used as a chemopreventive agent against liver tumors. Some animal experiments suggest the possibility that it could be useful for that purpose through its apparent ability to inhibit the expression of some oncogene functions.

There is a single study, apparently without followup, showing that SAMe might be an effective agent for lowering lipids in humans.

CONTRAINDICATIONS, PRECAUTIONS, ADVERSE REACTIONS

CONTRAINDICATIONS

None known.

PRECAUTIONS

Sufferers of bipolar disorder (manic-depressive illness) should not use SAMe unless under medical supervision. Those who are taking anti-depressant medications should confer with their physicians before taking SAMe in place of or in addition to those medications. They should continue to be monitored by their physician. SAMe is not recommended for use in children. It should only be used by pregnant women with a physician's approval and under a physician's supervision. Nursing mothers should avoid SAMe supplementation.

There is no evidence that SAMe is either mutagenic or carcinogenic. But since nucleic acid methylation patterns may change in those with cancer, the use of SAMe by cancer patients should be discussed with their physicians. SAMe may one day be shown to be effective in preventing and possibly even treating some forms of cancer but, in the meantime, because it is an active methylating agent, some caution is advised in those who have cancer.

Those undergoing gene therapy should avoid supplemental SAMe.

ADVERSE REACTIONS

Although classified and sold as a drug in Europe, SAMe is marketed in the United States as a dietary supplement. There are so far no reports of serious adverse events in those taking this supplement in doses up to 1,600 mg per day over long periods of time. Side effects that have been reported include mild gastrointestinal upsets (such as stomach pain, nausea, diarrhea and flatulence), anxiety, hyperactive muscle movement, insomnia and hypomania. When these side effects occur they often diminish with time or resolve with lower doses or cessation of use. There are no documented cases of allergies to SAMe.

INTERACTIONS

There are so far no reported adverse interactions with SAMe and other drugs, dietary supplements or foods.

OVERDOSAGE

No overdosage reported.

DOSAGE AND ADMINISTRATION

SAMe is highly unstable at temperatures above 0 degree C. Since the 1970s, certain salts of SAMe have become available that are stable at higher temperatures. These forms, which are clearly more desirable, include SAMe paratoluene sulfonates (SAMe tosyls). These more stable forms have been used in many of the SAMe studies, but they are not always the forms that are found in the supplement marketplace. Another temperature-stable form is SAMe 1,4 butanedisulfonate. Even these temperature-stable forms must be kept very dry since moisture can cause hydrolysis. Stable, enteric-coated tablets are recommended.

SAMe is most frequently available in 200 mg tablets. The usual oral dose for use in depression has been in the range of 400 to 1,600 milligrams daily in divided doses. For liver problems, usual doses reported are up to 1,600 mg daily in divided doses. For bone and joint health, the daily dose is typically 200 to 1,200 milligrams in divided doses. SAMe should always be taken on an empty stomach, i.e. one hour before meals or two hours after meals. It is often reported in the literature that these doses can usually be cut in half when a positive effect is achieved. Effects, if any, are usually evident within two weeks of starting supplementation.

It is advisable to take SAMe with supplemental B_6, B_{12}, folic acid and possibly trimethylglycine (particularly in those with elevated homocysteine levels). Some SAMe supplements come with B_6, B_{12} and folic acid. These other nutrients help metabolize homocysteine which, at elevated levels, increases the risk of cardiovascular disease and some other disorders.

HOW SUPPLIED

Capsules — 50 mg, 100 mg, 200 mg

Enteric Coated Tablets — 200 mg

Tablets — 100 mg, 200 mg

LITERATURE

Almasio P, Bortolini M, et al. Role of S-adenosyl-l-methionine in the treatment of intrahepatic cholestasis. *Drugs.* 1990; 40 (Suppl 3):111-123.

Baldessarini RJ. Neuropharmacology of S-adenosyl-l-methionine. *Am J Med.* 1987; 83 (Suppl 5A):95-105.

Bell KM, Plon L, Bunney Jr. WE, Potkin SG. S-adenosylmethionine treatment of depression: a controlled clinical trial. *Am J Psychiatry.* 1988; 145:1110-1114.

Berger R, Nowak H. A new medical approach to the treatment of osteoarthritis. Report of an open phase IV study with ademetionine. *Am J Med.* 1987; 83 (Suppl 5A):84-88.

Bombardieri G, Pappalardo G, et al. Intestinal absorption of S-adenosyl-l-methionine in humans. *Int J Clin Pharm Ther Tox.* 1983; 21:186-188.

Bottiglieri T, Godfrey P, et al. Cerebrospinal fluid S-adenosylmethionine in depression and dementia: effects of treatment with parenteral and oral S-adenosylmethionine. *J Neuro Neurosurg Psych.* 1990; 53:1096-1098.

Bottiglieri T, Hyland K, Reynolds EH. The clinical potential of ademetionine (S-adenosylmethionine) in neurological disorders. *Drugs.* 1994; 48(2):137-152.

Bottiglieri T, Hyland K. S-adenosylmethionine levels in psychiatric and neurological disorders: a review. *Acta Neurol Scand.* 1994; (Suppl) 154:19-26.

Bradley JD, Flusser D, et al. A randomized double blind, placebo controlled trial of intravenous loading with S-adenosylmethionine (SAM) followed by oral SAMe therapy in patients with knee osteoarthritis. *J Rheumatol.* 1994; 21:905-911.

Bressa GM. S-adenosyl-l-methionine (SAMe) as antidepressant: meta-analysis of clinical studies. *Acta Neurol Scand.* 1994; (Suppl) 154:7-14.

Carney MWP, Toone BK, Reynolds EH. S-adenosylmethionine and affective disorders. *Am J Med.* 1987; 83 (Suppl 5A):104-106.

Caruso I, Pietrogrande V. Italian double-blind multicenter study comparing S-adenosylmethionine, naproxen and placebo in the treatment of degenerative joint disease. *Am J Med.* 1987; 83 (Suppl 5A):66-71.

Chawla RK, Bonkovsky HL, Galambos JT. Biochemistry and pharmacology of S-adenosyl-l-methionine and rationale for its use in liver disease. *Drugs.* 1990; 40 (Suppl 3): 98-110.

Di Padova C. S-adenosylmethionine in the treatment of osteoarthritis. Review of the clinical studies. *Am J Med.* 1987; 83 (Suppl 5A):60-65.

Fava M, Giannelli A, et al. Rapidity of onset of the antidepressant effect of parenteral S-adenosyl-l-methionine. *Psych Res.* 1995; 56:295-297.

Frezza M. A meta-analysis of therapeutic trials with ademetionine in the treatment of intrahepatic cholestasis. *Ann Ital Med Int.* 1993; 8:48S-51S.

Friedel HA, Goa KL, Benfield P. S-adenosyl-L-methionine. A review of its pharmacological properties and therapeutic potential in liver dysfunction and affective disorders in relation to its physiological role in cell membranes. *Drugs.* 1989; 38(3):389-416.

Galeone F, Salvadorini F, et al. Effect of intravenous injection of CDP-choline, S-adenosylmethionine and citiolone in subjects with hyperlipidemia. *Artery.* 1979; 5:157-169.

Jacobsen S, Danneskiold-Samsoe B, Bach Andersen R. Oral S-adenosylmethionine in primary fibromyalgia. Double-blind clinical evaluation. *Scan J Rheumatol.* 1991; 20:294-302.

Kagan BL, Sultzer MD, Rosenlicht N, Gerner RH, Gerner RH. Oral S-adenosylmethionine in depression: a randomized double-blind, placebo-controlled trial. *Am J Psychiatry.* 1990; 147:591-595.

Kaye GL, Blake JC, Burroughs AK. Metabolism of exogenous S-adenosyl-L-methionine in patients with liver disease. *Drugs.* 1990; 40 (Suppl 3):124-128.

Konig B. Long-term (two year) clinical trial with S-adenosylmethionine for the treatment of osteoarthritis. *Am J Med.* 1987; 83 (Suppl 5A):89-94.

Muller-Fassbender H. Double-blind clinical trial of S-adenosylmethionine versus ibuprofen in the treatment of osteoarthritis. *Am J Med.* 1987; (Suppl 5A):81-83.

Pascale RM, Marras V, et al. Chemoprevention of rat liver carcinogenesis by S-adenosyl-l-methionine: a long-term study. *Can Res.* 1992; 52:4979-4986.

Salmaggi P, Bressa GM, et al. Double-blind, placebo-controlled study of S-adenosyl-l-methionine in depressed postmenopausal women. *Psychother Psychosom.* 1993; 59:34-40.

Stramentinoli G. Pharmacologic aspects of S-adenosylmethionine. *Am J Med.* 1987; 83 (Suppl 5A):35-42.

Secoisolariciresinol Diglycoside (SDG)

DESCRIPTION

Secoisolariciresinol diglycoside, or SDG, is a plant lignan most notably found in flaxseed (linseed). SDG is classified as a phytoestrogen since it is a plant-derived, nonsteroid compound that possesses estrogen-like activity. SDG has weak estrogenic activity. The level of SDG in flaxseed typically varies between 0.6% and 1.8%.

Lignans are one of the two major classes of phytoestrogens; the other class is the isoflavones. Plant lignans are polyphenolic substances derived from phenylalanine via dimerization of substituted cinnamic alcohols. Mammalian lignans are lignans derived from plant lignans. For example, following ingestion, SDG is converted to the aglycone secoisolariciresinol, which is then metabolized to the mammalian lignans enterolactone and enterodiol. Most of the effects of oral SDG are mediated by enterolactone and enterodiol.

The molecular formula of SDG is $C_{32}H_{46}O_{16}$, and its molecular weight is 686.71 daltons. The aglycone of SDG is also known as 2, 3-bis (3-methoxy-4-hydroxybenzyl) butane-1, 4-diol. Enterolactone is also known as trans-2, 3-bis [(3-hydroxylphenyl) methyl]-butyrolactone. It is represented by the following structural formula:

Secoisolariciresinol diglycoside

ACTIONS AND PHARMACOLOGY

ACTIONS

SDG has estrogenic and antioxidant activities. It may also have antiestrogenic, anticarcinogenic, antiatherogenic and antidiabetic activities.

MECHANISM OF ACTION

SDG, as well as its mammalian lignan metabolites, enterolactone (EL) and enterodiol (ED), have weak estrogenic activity as measured in *in vivo* and *in vitro* assays.

SDG, EL and ED have a number of antioxidant activities, including inhibition of lipid peroxidation and scavenging of hydroxy radicals. SDG also has anti-platelet-activation factor (PAF) activity. PAF can induce the release of reactive oxygen species from neutrophils. SDG, via its metabolite EL, has been found to inhibit estrogen synthase (aromatase) and to stimulate the synthesis of sex hormone binding globulin (SHBG). Both of these actions could account for the possible anti-estrogen activity of SDG.

The possible anticarcinogenic, antiatherogenic and antidiabetic activities of SDG are thought to be due, in large part, to the antioxidant activities of its metabolites EL and ED.

PHARMACOKINETICS

SDG, following ingestion, is transported to the large intestine, where it is hydrolyzed by bacteria to the aglycone secoisolariciresinol. Secoisolariciresinol, in turn, is metabolized by bacteria in the large intestine to the mammalian lignans EL and ED. EL and ED are absorbed from the large intestine. Little is known about the distribution of EL and ED to the various tissues of the body. It is known that ED and EL undergo conjugation in the liver with glucuronate and sulfate. The glucuronate and sulfate conjugates of ED and EL are excreted in the urine and in the bile.

There appears to be considerable individual variation in the absorption and metabolism of the SDG metabolites ED and EL.

INDICATIONS AND USAGE

There is evidence in *in vitro* and animal research that SDG may have some ability to reduce cholesterol levels and protect against atherosclerosis; it may also have some anticancer and antidiabetic effects.

RESEARCH SUMMARY

Rabbits fed a high-cholesterol diet supplemented with flaxseed had 46% less atherosclerotic development than rabbits fed the same diet without flaxseed. Still better results were obtained (73% reduction in atherosclerosis) when the diet was supplemented with SDG instead of flaxseed. These effects were associated with reduced serum levels of cholesterol and LDL-cholesterol and increased levels of HDL-cholesterol.

SDG has exhibited a number of anticancer effects in *in vitro* and animal studies. SDG-treated rats were significantly protected against experimentally induced mammary cancer in one experiment. Subsequently, it was demonstrated that SDG significantly inhibited experimentally induced mammary tumor multiplicity in a dose-dependent fashion in rats, with more inhibition at higher doses. Flaxseed alone did not significantly affect tumor size, multiplicity or incidence in this study, but both flaxseed and SDG delayed progression of tumorigenesis. In another recent animal study, supplemental SDG decreased metastatic pulmonary melanoma tumor size in a dose-dependent fashion, compared with controls. Research continues.

In an animal model of human type 1 diabetes, SDG was said to significantly prevent this form of diabetes. Prevention was associated with a decrease in the serum and pancreatic lipid peroxidation product malondialdehyde. The researcher concluded that IDDM is mediated through oxidative stress and that SDG reduces this stress and thus helps prevent development of diabetes. In another experiment, SDG significantly prevented the development of streptozotocin-induced diabetes in rats. Clinical trials are needed.

CONTRAINDICATIONS, PRECAUTIONS, ADVERSE REACTIONS

CONTRAINDICATIONS
SDG is contraindicated in those who are hypersensitive to any component of an SDG-containing product.

PRECAUTIONS
Pregnant women and nursing mothers should avoid the use of SDG supplementation.

Women with estrogen receptor-positive tumors should discuss the advisability of the use of SDG-containing products with their physicians before deciding to use them.

OVERDOSAGE
There are no reports of overdosage.

DOSAGE AND ADMINISTRATION
SDG nutritional supplements are currently being developed, and there are no dosage recommendations at present.

SDG is present in flaxseed at levels of 0.6% to 1.8% and in much smaller amounts in flaxseed oil.

LITERATURE
Kitts DD, Yuan YV, Wijewickreme AN, Thompson LU. Antioxidant activity of the flaxseed lignan secoisolariciresinol diglycoside and its mammalian lignan metabolites enterodiol and enterolactone. *Mol Cell Biochem.* 1999; 202:91-100.

Li D, Yee JA, Thompson LU, Yan L. Dietary supplementation with secoisolariciresinol diglycoside (SDG) reduces experimental metastasis of melanoma cells in mice. *CancerLetters.* 1999; 142:91-96.

Pool-Zobel BL, Adlercreutz H, Glei M, et al. Isoflavonoids and lignans have different potentials to modulate oxidative genetic damage in human colon cells. *Carcinogenesis.* 2000; 21:1247-1252.

Prasad K. Hydroxyl radical-scavenging property of secoisolariciresinol diglucoside isolated from flax-seed. *Mol Cell Biochem.* 1997; 168:117-123.

Prasad K. Oxidative stress as a mechanism of diabetes in diabetic BB prone rats: effect of secoisolariciresinol diglucoside (SDG). *Mol Cell Biochem.* 2000; 209:89-96.

Prasad K. Reduction of serum cholesterol and hypercholesterolemic atherosclerosis in rabbits by secoisolariciresinol diglucoside isolated from flaxseed. *Circulation.* 1999; 99:1355-1362.

Prasad K, Mantha SV, Muir AD, Westcott ND. Protective effect of secoisolariciresinol diglucoside against streptozotocin-induced diabetes and its mechanism. *Mol CellBiochem.* 2000; 206:141-150.

Schottner M, Spiteller G. Lignans interfering with 5alpha-dihydrotestosterone binding to human sex hormone-binding globulin. *J Nat Prod.* 1998; 61:119-121.

Thompson LU, Seidl MM, Rickard SE, et al. Antitumorigenic effect of a mammalian lignan precursor from flaxseed. *Nutr Cancer.* 1996; 26:159-165.

Selenium

TRADE NAMES

Sele-Pak (Solopak Laboratories), Selepen (American Pharmaceutical Parners), Selenium Oceanic (Freeda Vitamins), Selenomax (Mason Vitamins).

DESCRIPTION

Selenium is an essential trace element in human and animal nutrition. It is involved in the defense against the toxicity of reactive oxygen species, in the regulation of thyroid hormone metabolism and the regulation of the redox state of cells. Recognition of the vital importance of selenium in human and animal nutrition was long impeded by its very real toxic potential and by fears that selenium might be carcinogenic, fears that have now been largely displaced by some evidence suggesting just the opposite—that selenium may provide protection against some cancers.

The amount of selenium in food is a function of the selenium content of the soil. Selenium enters the food chain through incorporation into plant proteins as the amino acids L-selenocysteine and L-selenomethionine. Selenium, like most trace elements and minerals, is not evenly distributed in the world's soil. Because of the uneven global distribution of selenium, disorders of both selenium deficiency and selenium excess are known. China has regions with both the lowest and highest selenium-containing soils in the world.

Marco Polo gave the first account of selenium toxicity, which he observed during his travels in western China in the 13th century. He linked the sloughing off of the hooves of horses to their consumption of certain plants in the regions. The soils of those areas are now known to contain the highest concentrations of selenium in the world. Soils rich in selenium are referred to as being seleniferous, and the condition of chronic selenium toxicity is known as selenosis. In the 1970s, a human cardiomyopathy endemic to certain areas of China was shown to be linked to dietary selenium deficiency. This disorder, known as Keshan disease, is endemic to those areas of China with some of the most selenium-poor soils in the world. Keshan disease is now treated and prevented by selenium supplementation.

Kashin-Beck disease, also known as ''big joint disease,'' is an osteoarthropathy that is found in areas in China where the soil is selenium-poor. It is also linked to dietary selenium deficiency. Kashin-Beck disease is found in Tibet, Siberia and North Korea, also in areas where the soil is selenium-poor and in which dietary selenium-deficiency is endemic.

Selenium is a metalloid element with atomic number 34 and an atomic weight of 78.96 daltons. It belongs to the sulfur group of elements, which also includes oxygen, tellurium and polonium. Its atomic symbol is Se. Selenium was discovered in 1817 by Berzelius who named it after Selene, the Greek goddess of the moon.

The essentiality of selenium for animals was first reported in 1957. It was found that selenium administered to vitamin E-deficient rats prevented liver necrosis. Subsequently, it was found that selenium could prevent a number of disorders of farm animals. Isolated selenium deficiency in humans has not been described. Selenium deficiency appears to cause an illness or disorder in combination with a co-factor. In the case of Keshan disease, the co-factor appears to be the Coxsackievirus. It has been shown that infection of mice on a selenium-deficient diet with a nonvirulent Coxsackievirus selects a stable cardiovirulent strain. In the case of Kashin-Beck osteoarthropathy, the co-factor appears to be iodine deficiency.

Selenium is found in human and animal tissues as L-selenomethionine or L-selenocysteine. L-selenomethionine is incorporated randomly in proteins in place of L-methionine. These proteins are called selenium-containing proteins. Only a small fraction of L-methionine in proteins is present as L-selenomethionine. On the other hand, the incorporation of L-cysteine into proteins known as selenoproteins is not random. That is, in contrast to L-selenomethionine, which randomly substitutes for L-methionine, L-selenocysteine does not randomly substitute for L-cysteine. In fact, L-selenocysteine has its own triplet code and is considered to be the 21st genetically coded amino acid.

The selenoproteins are comprised of four selenium-dependent glutathione peroxidases (GSHPx-1, GSHPx-2, GSHPx-3 and GSHPx-4), three selenium-dependent iodothyronine deiodinases, three thioredoxin reductases, selenoprotein P, selenoprotein W and selenophosphate synthetase. The glutathione peroxidases, and possibly selenoprotein P and selenoprotein W, are antioxidant proteins. The selenium-dependent iodothyronine deiodinases convert thyroxine to triiodothyronine, thus regulating thyroid hormone metabolism. The thioredoxin reductases reduce intramolecular disulfide bonds and regenerate vitamin C from its oxidized state, among other things.

ACTIONS AND PHARMACOLOGY

ACTIONS

Selenium has antioxidant activity. Selenium may also have immunomodulatory, anticarcinogenic and anti-atherogenic activities. It may have activity in detoxification of some metals and other xenobiotics and activity in fertility enhancement in males.

MECHANISM OF ACTION

The antioxidant activity of selenium is mainly accounted for by virtue of its role in the formation and function of the selenium-dependent glutathione peroxidases (GSHPx). Glutathione peroxidases use reducing equivalents from gluta-thione to detoxify hydroperoxides. There are four different glutathione peroxidases. GSHPx-1 is present in most cells of the body. GSHPx-2 (originally known as GSHPx-GI) is mainly found in the cells of the gastrointestinal tract. GSHPx-3 is an extracellular glutathione peroxidase. GSHPx-4 is a membrane-bound hydroperoxide glutathione peroxidase. GSHPx-4 is also known as phospholipid hydroperoxide or PHGPx. GSHPx-4 can detoxify phospholipid hydroperoxides and, along with d-alpha-tocopherol, helps prevent oxidative damage to membranes. GSHPx-3, the extracellular glutathione peroxidase, eliminates peroxides in the extracellular fluid.

Glutathione peroxidases detoxify hydrogen peroxide and fatty acid-derived hydroperoxides. This is the antioxidant role of these enzymes. However, recent research indicates that reactive oxygen species play important roles in signal transduction processes. Therefore, by affecting the concentrations of reactive oxygen species in cells, the glutathione peroxidases may also be considered to play regulatory roles in signal transduction.

Antioxidant activity of selenium can also be accounted for by its role in the selenium-dependent thioredoxin reductases. These enzymes reduce intramolecular disulfide bonds and regenerate ascorbic acid from dehydroascorbic acid. Thioredoxin reductases can also affect the redox regulation of a variety of factors, including ribonucleotide reductase (the enzyme that converts ribonucleoside diphosphates to deoxyribonucleoside diphosphates), the glucocorticoid receptor and the transcription factors AP-1 and NF-KappaB.

Selenium deficiency appears to depress the effectiveness of various components of the immune system. In humans, selenium deficiency has been associated with depressed IgG and IgM antibody titers. In animal models, selenium deficiency has resulted in depressed neutrophil activity, decreased Candidacidal activity by neutrophils and depressed cellular immunity. Selenium supplementation in humans has resulted in increased natural killer cell activity. The possible immunomodulatory effects of selenium are not well understood. Selenium's antioxidant activity may play some role, perhaps a major one, in these possible effects. It is postulated that selenium's possible effect on boosting cellular immunity may be due to upregulation of the expression of the T-cell high-affinity interleukin (IL)-2 receptor, providing a vehicle for enhanced T-cell responses, as well as prevention of oxidative-stress-induced damage to immune cells. Enhanced cellular immunity may explain the possible stimulatory effects of selenium on antibody production.

The possible anticarcinogenic activity of selenium may be accounted, for, in part, by its antioxidant activity as well as its possible immune-enhancing activity. Selenium has been shown to upregulate apoptosis in tumor cells *in vitro* and increase macrophage killing and protect against oxidative DNA damage, again, *in vitro*. Animal studies suggest that selenium may have anti-angiogenic activity. A possible mechanism for selenium's possible anti-angiogenic activity is its inhibitory effect on the expression of vascular endothelial growth factors (VEGFs). This has been observed in some animal studies. Selenium, in cell culture, has also been found to inhibit the gelatinolytic activity of matrix metalloproteinase-2 (MMP-2).

Some epidemiological studies have shown an inverse relationship between coronary heart disease and selenium intake. The possible anti-atherogenic activity of selenium may be accounted for, in part, by its antioxidant activity. Glutathione peroxidase may protect low density lipoprotein (LDL) from oxidation. Oxidized-LDL is thought to be a crucial etiological factor in atherogenesis. Selenium may decrease platelet aggregation. Selenium deficiency results in lipoperoxide accumulation. Lipoperoxides impair prostacyclin synthesis and promote thromboxane synthesis, which can increase platelet aggregation.

Selenium has been demonstrated to antagonize the effects of a number of toxic metals, including cadmium and arsenic. Selenium inhibits the growth stimulatory effect of cadmium on human prostatic epithelium *in vitro*. The mechanism of the possible antagonistic action of selenium against various toxic metals and other xenobiotics is unclear. One possibility is that it forms inactive complexes with these substances.

Selenium may have fertility enhancing effects for males. Phospholipid hydroperoxide glutathione peroxidase (GSHPx-4), in addition to its antioxidant role in sperm, also appears to be responsible for maintaining the structure of sperm, at least in mouse sperm.

PHARMACOKINETICS

There are various forms of supplemental selenium, including high-selenium yeast, L-selenomethionine, sodium selenate and sodium selenite. High-selenium yeast contains L-selenomethionine in proteins. Proteins in high-selenium yeast are enzymatically digested in the small intestine to yield amino acids, oligopeptides and L-selenomethionine. L-selenomethionine is efficiently absorbed from the small intestine via a similar mechanism to that of L-methionine. L-selenomethionine is transported via the portal circulation to the liver where a fraction is extracted by the hepatocytes and the remaining amount is transported by the circulation to the various tissues of the body. L-selenomethionine enters the L-methionine pool in the hepatocytes and other cells of the body and shares the same metabolic fate of L-methionine until it is metabolized by the transsulfuration pathway. That is, L-selenomethionine participates in the synthesis of proteins and in the formation of seleno-adenosylmethionine (the selenium form of S-adenosylmethionine or SAMe), homoselenocysteine and L-selenocysteine, among other metabolites.

The metabolism of L-selenocysteine is different in several particulars from that of L-cysteine. L-selenocysteine is converted to hydrogen selenide via the enzyme selenocysteine beta-lyase. Hydrogen selenide can be metabolized to selenophosphate via selenophosphate synthetase or it can be methylated. The methylated metabolites are excreted in the urine. Selenophosphate is the precursor of L-selenocysteine in proteins or of selenium nucleosides in transfer RNA. The incorporation of L-selenocysteine in proteins is via seryl-transfer RNA. Selenocysteine synthase converts seryl-transfer RNA to selenocysteyl-transfer RNA. The L-selenocysteine residues found in all of the selenoproteins is derived from selenocysteyl-transfer RNA.

Free L-selenomethione is absorbed, distributed, and metabolized as described above. The inorganic forms of selenium, selenate and selenite, are also efficiently absorbed from the gastrointestinal tract. The fractional absorption of these inorganic forms is greater than 50%. Selenate or selenite is delivered to the liver via the portal circulation. A fraction is extracted by the hepatocytes and the rest is delivered via the systemic circulation to the various cells of the body. Within cells, these inorganic salts are converted to hydrogen selenide, and the further metabolism of hydrogen selenide is as described above.

Selenium homeostasis is achieved via regulation of its excretion by the kidneys. As selenium intake increases, urinary excretion of selenide metabolite increases. At very high intakes of selenium, volatile forms are exhaled. The odor of the exhaled forms of selenium is garlic-like. The excretory metabolites of selenium are mainly methylated metabolites of selenide. The principal urinary metabolites are methyselenol and trimethylselonium. Selenium excreted in the breath is mainly in the form of dimethylselenide.

INDICATIONS AND USAGE

Low dietary intake of selenium is associated with increased risk of some cardiomyopathies, ischemic heart disease and cardiovascular disease generally. Low intakes are also associated with increased incidence of some cancers, including prostate, lung, colorectal, gastric and skin cancers. Selenium supplementation has diminished these risks in some populations. Selenium has demonstrated useful immune-enhancing effects in *in vitro*, animal and human studies. It is essential for healthy immune function. It may

also have some anti-inflammatory benefits and could be useful in some with rheumatoid arthritis. It has the ability to detoxify some metals and xenobiotics. Selenium appears to play an important role in maintaining the viability of sperm cells, and supplemental selenium may thus be helpful in some infertile men. There is very preliminary evidence that high doses of selenium might promote modest weight gain. Reports that selenium can inhibit graying of hair are anecdotal.

RESEARCH SUMMARY

Epidemiological data indicate that low dietary intake of selenium is associated with increased incidence of several cancers, including lung, colorectal, skin and prostate cancers. There are *in vitro*, animal and human data showing that supplemental selenium can protect against some cancers. Much interest is now focusing on these findings, given gathering evidence that selenium intakes may actually be declining in some parts of the world, including some areas of the United States and the United Kingdom and other European countries.

There was one large cohort study, however, in which no significant selenium/cancer association was observed. Selenium in this study, however, was measured via selenium content in toenails. Some believe that this is not a reliable indicator of selenium status.

Studies to date indicate that diminished selenium status is not, in itself, carcinogenic but, rather, increases susceptibility to malignancy in the presence of carcinogens. Some studies have also shown that low selenium status predicts a poorer outcome in those who have some cancers. Findings however, are not entirely consistent.

In a recent well-controlled, large study conducted between 1983 and 1993, selenium supplementation (200 micrograms daily delivered via high-selenium brewer's yeast tablets) significantly diminished total cancer mortality (by 52% compared with controls). It did not significantly affect the incidence of basal and squamous cell carcinomas of the skin but did significantly reduce the incidence of lung, colorectal and prostate cancers. A total of 1,312 subjects (mostly men), aged 18-80 years, were enrolled in the study. Subjects had a history of basal cell or squamous cell carcinomas. Subjects, enrolled at seven dermatology clinics in the eastern United States, were treated for a mean of 4.5 years and were followed up for 6.4 years.

Another long-term study, this one conducted in China, employed 200 micrograms of selenium daily over a four-year period. Those thus supplemented had a significantly lower incidence of primary liver cancer than did unsupplemented controls.

Some investigators have suggested that pharmacological doses of selenium, much higher than those used in typical supplements, might be effective in some established cancers. "Selenium compounds," one group has speculated, "that are able to generate a steady stream of methylated metabolites, in particular of the monomethylated species, are likely to have good chemopreventive potential."

More research is needed. A large study sponsored by the National Cancer Institute is now underway.

Keshan disease is a cardiomyopathy endemic in regions of China where selenium deficiency is prevalent. The Coxsackieviruses are co-factors with selenium deficiencies in this disease. A selenium-deficient environment in heart tissue appears to select for a cardiovirulent mutant of these viruses. *In vitro* animal and human data show that supplemental selenium can protect against this cardiomyopathy. Cardiomyopathies caused by long-term total parenteral nutrition (TPN) can also be prevented with adequate selenium supplementation.

Epidemiological data have demonstrated an inverse relationship between blood selenium levels and incidence of cardiovascular disease. Diminished selenium status has been associated with increased risk of myocardial infarction. Selenium has shown some ability to protect against oxidative damage to blood vessels. This damage is believed to play a role in the formation of atheromatous plaques. Selenium confers further protection by inhibiting peroxidation of some lipids. Still other heart benefits may accrue from selenium's demonstrated ability to inhibit platelet aggregation, modulate prostaglandin synthesis and protect against heavy metals.

Despite the foregoing positive evidence, large controlled prevention trials are still needed before selenium's preventive and therapeutic roles in cardiovascular disease can be properly assessed.

Selenium has been found to be essential for healthy immune function. Some viruses that are normally benign become pathogenic in those who are selenium deficient. This mechanism has been hypothesized by some to account for new mutant strains of influenza virus in China each year. Selenium has been shown to play important roles in T-cells and natural killer cells among other immune components. Deficiencies in selenium are associated with numerous adverse effects on immune function, including decreased CD4/ CD8 T-lymphocyte ratios and impaired phagocyte function.

Selenium supplementation has been shown to enhance T-cell responses, to stimulate antibody production and to partially reverse age-related cellular immunosuppression. Selenium supplementation has increased responsiveness to interleukin-2 (IL-2) in some studies. Supplementation also protects immune cells from oxidative damage in some instances. In one study, selenium supplementation reduced the incidence of hepatitis-B-induced hepatoma among those with low selenium status. Selenium status is predictive of survival time in some with AIDS, according to another study. Some have suggested that human immunodeficiency virus (HIV) may have been abetted in crossing the species barrier into humans in areas of Africa where selenium deficiency was prevalent. More research is needed and is ongoing with respect to supplemental selenium's role in immune function.

Selenium's anti-inflammatory effects are also related, at least in part, to its effects on immunity. Supplemental selenium can help protect some against Kashin-Beck Disease, a form of arthritis that afflicts many in selenium-deficient areas of China and other parts of Asia. There is some preliminary evidence that selenium, in combination with vitamin E, might alleviate articular pain and morning stiffness in some with arthritis.

In animal experiments, supplemental selenium has protected against some of the adverse effects of UV-radiation. In a mouse study, selenium significantly reduced the incidence of and mortality from non-melanoma skin cancers secondary to UV-exposure.

Selenium plasma levels have been found to be low in some infertile men. Selenium supplementation in these circumstances may improve sperm motility and enhance fertility. In a study of 64 infertile men living in an area of Scotland where low plasma levels of selenium are common, selenium supplementation over a two-year period significantly enhanced sperm motility compared with placebo. Five of the selenium-supplemented men fathered children; none of the men in the placebo group fathered children. There were 64 men in the study, including controls. Selenium appears to both protect sperm from oxidative damage and to help maintain the structural integrity of mature sperm. Follow-up is needed.

There is one report that selenium, in doses five times the recommended daily allowance (RDA) of this mineral, promoted modest weight gain among healthy men, aged 20 to 45. Supplementation continued for four months. The men all consumed the same diet, except for variations in selenium content. The diets were designed to maintain baseline body weight. The five men consuming the diet with high selenium content gained about 1.5 pounds. The six subjects consuming the diet low in selenium (providing about one fifth of the RDA) lost about 1 pound each. More research may be warranted.

CONTRAINDICATIONS, PRECAUTIONS, ADVERSE REACTIONS

CONTRAINDICATIONS

Selenium is contraindicated in those who are hypersensitive to any component of a selenium-containing preparation.

PRECAUTIONS

Pregnant women and nursing mothers should avoid selenium intakes greater than RDA amounts (60 and 70 micrograms daily, respectively).

ADVERSE REACTIONS.

Intakes of selenium less than 900 micrograms daily (for adults) are unlikely to cause adverse reactions. Prolonged intakes of selenium of doses of 1,000 micrograms (or one milligram) or greater daily may cause adverse reactions.

The most frequently reported adverse reactions of selenosis or chronic selenium toxicity are hair and nail brittleness and loss. Other symptoms include skin rash, garlic-like breath odor, fatigue, irritability and nausea and vomiting. Perhaps the most famous example of selenium toxicity was reported in 1984. About 11 days after starting to take supplemental selenium, a 57-year-old female who was otherwise in good health noted marked hair loss which progressed over a two-month period to almost total alopecia. She also noted white horizontal streaking on one fingernail, as well as tenderness and swelling on the fingertips and purulent discharge from the fingernail beds. All of her fingernails eventually became involved and she lost the entire fingernail of the first digit affected. She also experienced episodes of nausea, vomiting, a sour-milk breath odor, and increase in fatigue. She learned a little over three months later that the selenium tablets she had taken were recalled by the distributor because they, in error, contained over 27 milligrams of selenium per tablet, 182 times higher than labeled. Others who took the same preparation suffered similar symptoms. Hair loss and fingernail changes (horizontal streaking, blackening, loss) were the most common symptoms.

Daily intake of 3.20 to 6.69 milligrams of selenium (average of 4 mg) by Chinese subjects in China produced loss of hair and nails, skin rash, garlic breath, fatigue, irritability and hyperreflexia. The same report described a 62 year old man who took supplemental selenium in the form of sodium selenite; after two years he developed thickened, fragile nails and a garlic-like skin odor.

INTERACTIONS

DRUGS

There are no known interactions with drugs in clinical practice.

NUTRITIONAL SUPPLEMENTS

Iodine: Intake of selenium and iodide may have synergistic activity in the treatment of Kashin-Beck disease.

Vitamin C: Concomitant intake of selenium and the selenite form of selenium may decrease the absorption of selenium.

Vitamin E: Intake of vitamin E and selenium may produce synergistic beneficial effects.

OVERDOSAGE

Selenium overdosage has been reported in the literature. (See Adverse reactions).

DOSAGE AND ADMINISTRATION

Available forms of selenium supplements include high-selenium yeast, L-selenomethionine, sodium selenate and sodium selenite. Typical dosage ranges from 50 to 200 micrograms (as elemental selenium) daily. Se-methylseleno-cysteine is a predominant form of selenium found in garlic.

The average daily intake of selenium in the United States is about 100 micrograms.

The Food and Nutrition Board of the Institute of Medicine of the National Academy of Sciences has recommended the following Adequate Intake (AI) and Recommended Dietary Allowance (RDA) for selenium:

Infants	(AI)
0-6 months	15 micrograms/day
	(2.1 microgams/kg)
7-12 months	20 micrograms/day
	(2.2 micrograms/kg)
Children	(RDA)
1-3 years	20 micrograms/day
4-8 years	30 micrograms/day
Boys	
9-13	40 micrograms/day
14-18 years	55 micrograms/day
Girls	
9-13 years	40 micrograms/day
14-18 years	55 micrograms/day
Men	
19-30 years	55 micrograms/day
31-50 years	55 micrograms/day
51-70 years	55 micrograms/day
Greater than 70 years	55 micrograms/day
Women	
19-30 years	55 micrograms/day
31-50 years	55 micrograms/day
51-70 years	55 micrograms/day
Greater than 70 years	55 micrograms/day
Pregnancy	
14-18 years	60 micrograms/day
19-30 years	60 micrograms/day

31-50 years	60 micrograms/day
Lactation	
14-18 years	70 micrograms/day
19-30 years	70 micrograms/day
31-50 years	70 micrograms/day

The Food and Nutrition Board has recommended the following Tolerable Upper Intake Levels (UL) for selenium:

Infants	(UL)
0-6 months	45 micrograms/day
7-12 months	60 micrograms/day
Children	
1-3 years	90 micrograms/day
4-8 years	150 micrograms/day
9-13 years	280 micrograms/day
Adolescents	
14-18 years	400 micrograms/day
Adults	
19 years and older	400 micrograms/day
Pregnancy	
14-18 years	400 micrograms/day
19 years and older	400 micrograms/day
Lactation	
14-18 years	400 micrograms/day
19 years and older	400 micrograms/day

The Lowest-Observed-Adverse-Effects-Level (LOAEL) for adults is about 900 micrograms daily.

HOW SUPPLIED
Capsules — 50 mcg, 100 mcg, 200 mcg
Extended Release Tablets — 200 mcg
Tablets — 50 mcg, 100 mcg, 126 mcg, 150 mcg, 200 mcg

LITERATURE

Alaejos MS, Romero FJD, Romero CD. Selenium and cancer: some nutritional aspects. *Nutrition.* 2000; 16:376-383.

Beck MA, Shi Q, Morris VC, Levander OA. Rapid genomic evolution of a non-virulent Coxsackievirus B3 in selenium-deficient mice results in selection of identical virulent strains. *Nature Med.* 1995; 5:433-436.

Berry MJ, Banu L, Larsen PR. Type I iodothyronine deiodinase is a selenocysteine-containing enzyme. *Nature.* 1991; 349:438-440.

Burk RF, ed. *Selenium in Biology and Human Health.* New York, NY: Springer-Verlag; 1994.

Burk RF, Levander OA. Selenium. In: Shils ME, Olson JA, Shike M, Ross AC, eds. *Modern Nutrition in Health and Disease.* Baltimore, MD: Williams and Wilkins; 1999:265-276.

Clark LC, Combs GF Jr, Turnbull BW, et al. Effects of selenium supplementation for cancer prevention in patients with carcinoma of the skin. *JAMA.* 1996; 276:1957-1963.

Colditz GA. Selenium and cancer prevention. Promising results indicate further trials required (editorial). *JAMA.* 1996; 276:1984-1985.

Dietary Reference Intakes for Vitamin C, Vitamin E, Selenium, and Carotenoids. Washington, DC: National Academy Press; 2000.

Dworkin BM. Selenium deficiency in HIV infection and the acquried immunodeficiency syndrome (AIDS). *Chem Biol Interact.* 1994; 91:181-186.

Fleet JC. Dietary selenium repletion may reduce cancer incidence in people at high risk who live in areas with low soil selenium. *Nutr Rev.* 1997; 55:277-279.

Hendler SS. Micronutrition: vitamins, minerals, and trace elements. In: Newcomer VD, Young EM, eds. *Geriatric Dermatology. Clinical Diagnosis and Practical Therapy.* New York and Tokyo: Igaku-Shoin; 1989:365-393.

Huttunen JK. Selenium and cardiovascular diseases — an update. *Biomed Environ Sci.* 1997; 10:220-226.

Ip C, Thompson HJ, Zhu HJ, Ganther HE. In vitro and in vivo studies of methylseleninic acid: evidence that a monomethylated selenium metabolite is critical for cancer chemoprevention. *Cancer Res.* 2000; 60:2882-2886.

Ip C, Zhu Z, Thompson HJ, et al. Chemoprevention of mammary cancer with Se-allylselenocysteine and other selenoaminoacids in the rat. *Anticancer Res.* 1999; 19(4B):2875-2880.

Ip C. Lessons from basic research in selenium and cancer prevention. *J Nutr.* 1998; 128:1845-1854.

Ip C. Interaction of vitamin C and selenium supplementation in the modification of mammary carcinogenesis in rats. *J Natl Cancer Inst.* 1986; 77:299-303.

Jiang C, Jiang W, Ip C, et al. Selenium-induced inhibition of angiogenesis in mammary cancer at chemopreventive levels of intake. *Mol Carcinog.* 1999; 26:213-225.

Kardinaal AF, Kok FJ, Kohlmeier L, et al. Association between toenail selenium and risk of acute myocardial infarction in European men. The EURAMIC Study. European Antioxidant Myocardial Infarction and Breast Cancer. *Am J Epidemiol.* 1997; 145:373-379.

Kohrle J. Thyroid hormone deiodinases — a selenoenzyme family acting as gate keepers to thyroid hormone action. *Acta Med Austriaca.* 1996; 23:17-30.

Low SC, Berry MJ. Knowing when not to stop: selenocysteine incorporation in eukaryotes. *Trends Biochem Sci.* 1996; 21:203-208.

Moreno-Reyes R, Suetens C, Mathieu F, et al. Kashin-Beck osteoarthropathy in rural Tibet in relation to selenium and iodine status. *N Eng J Med.* 1998; 339:1112-1120.

Mukhopadhyay-Sardar S, Rana MP, Chatterjee M. Antioxidant associated chemoprevention by selenomethionine in murine tumor model. *Mol Cellul Biochem.* 2000; 206:17-25.

Olmsted L, Schrauzer GN, Flores-Arce M, Dowd J. Selenium supplementation of symptomatic human immunodeficiency virus infected patients. *Biol Trace Elem Res.* 1989; 20:59-65.

Reilly C. Selenium: a new entrant into the functional food arena. *Trends Food Sci Technol.* 1998; 9:114-118.

Schrauzer GN. Selenomethionine: a review of its nutritional significance, metabolism and toxicity. *J Nutr.* 2000; 130:1653-1656.

Scott R, MacPherson A, Yates RWS, et al. The effect of oral selenium supplementation on human sperm motility. *J Urol.* 1998; 82:76-80.

Selenium Intoxication-New York. *Morbidity and Mortality Weekly.* 1984; Report 33, No.12:157-158.

Suadicani P, Hein HO, Gyntelberg F. Serum selenium concentration and risk of ischaemic heart disease in a prospective cohort study of 3,000 males. *Atherosclerosis.* 1992; 96:33-42.

Ursini F, Heim S, Kiess M, et al. Dual function of the selenoprotein PHGPx during sperm maturation. *Science.* 1999; 285:1393-1396.

Yang G, Wang S, Zhou R, Sun S. Endemic selenium intoxication of humans in China. *Am J Clin Nutr.* 1988; 37:872-881.

Yu MW, Horng IS, Hsu KH, et al. Plasma selenium levels and risk of hepatocellular carcinoma among men with chronic virus infection. *Am J Epidemiol.* 1999; 150:367-374.

Yu SY, Zhu YJ, Li WG. Protective role of selenium against hepatitis B virus and primary liver cancer in Qidong. *Biol Trace Elem Res.* 1997; 56:117-124.

Shark Cartilage

TRADE NAMES

Shark Cartilage is available from numerous manufacturers generically. Branded products include Cartilade (Solgar, BioTherapies, Source Naturals), Mega Shark Cartilage (Twinlab), Sharkilage (Futurebiotics) and BeneFin Shark Cartilage (Lane Labs).

DESCRIPTION

Shark cartilage became popular as a nutritional supplement a few years ago, based on the claim that sharks do not get cancer and that this substance must therefore be useful for the prevention and treatment of cancer. The fact is that sharks do get cancer.

Cartilage is a tissue that lacks blood vessels and rarely develops malignancies. Angiogenesis, the formation of new capillaries, is now known to be important in a number of pathological conditions, including solid tumors, proliferative retinopathy, neovascular glaucoma and rheumatoid arthritis. The process is also important in other physiological events as well, such as neovascularization following coronary artery occlusion.

In 1976, Judah Folkman and his colleagues reported on the isolation of a fraction from the scapular cartilage of calves, which inhibited the growth of new blood vessels supporting implanted tumors in rabbits. It also stopped the growth of the tumors. Subsequent reports demonstrated a fraction in shark cartilage that also inhibited tumor neovascularization and growth.

The study of angiogenesis inhibitors has become a new field in cancer research. Since the earliest anti-angiogenesis substances discovered were derived from cartilage, research continues looking at cartilage to try to identify and characterize novel anti-angiogenic agents. Because sharks are an abundant source of cartilage, shark cartilage is being used by several research groups.

Sharks have an endoskeleton comprised entirely of cartilage, and while cartilage comprises less than 0.6% of the body weight of calves, it comprises about 6% of the body weight of sharks. Shark cartilage, like other forms of cartilage, is mainly composed of collagen, which participates in giving cartilage its tensile strength, and proteoglycans, themselves composed of a core protein to which is attached polysaccharides known as glycosaminoglycans or mucopolysaccharides. Proteoglycans impart resilience to cartilage. The main glycosaminoglycans in shark cartilage are the chondroitin sulfates. In addition to collagen and chondroitin sulfate, shark cartilage contains about 5 to 10% water, a large percentage of calcium and phosphate, and other molecules, several of low molecular weight. These appear to possess anti-angiogenic activity, as well as other activities. These substances are being researched as possible therapeutic candidates.

ACTIONS AND PHARMACOLOGY

ACTIONS

Shark cartilage has putative antitumor, antioxidant, anti-inflammatory and anti-atherogenic actions, although these putative actions are so far poorly supported by credible clinical research.

MECHANISM OF ACTION

The mechanism of the possible actions of shark cartilage is unclear. It appears that any possible therapeutic benefit derives mainly from low-molecular-weight molecules that are currently being researched. Some of these molecules possess anti-angiogenic activity and inhibit metalloproteinases, activities that could help explain any possible antitumor activity. Small-molecular-weight substances from shark cartilage are also demonstrating antioxidant and anti-inflammatory activities. The antioxidant and anti-inflammatory activities may play roles in any putative anti-atherogenic action of shark cartilage.

PHARMACOKINETICS
There is little known about the pharmacokinetics of shark cartilage. The absorption, distribution, metabolism and excretion of collagen should be similar to that of dietary proteins. See Chondroitin Sulfate for the pharmacokinetics of that substance. The small-molecular-weight substances appear to be absorbed from the lumen of the small intestine, but not much more is known about the pharmacokinetics of these substances.

INDICATIONS AND USAGE
Widespread claims are made for shark cartilage, including anti-cancer, anti-inflammatory, anti-arthritic, anti-psoriasis and anti-atherosclerotic effects. At present there is no credible clinical data sufficient to support any of these claims.

RESEARCH SUMMARY
Shark cartilage has been heavily promoted as an anti-cancer agent. Some *in vitro* and animal studies show some anti-angiogenic properties. Inhibition of wound angiogenesis has recently been demonstrated in one study of human subjects given liquid shark cartilage extract, but there are no other human data related to shark cartilage's putative anti-angiogenic effects and certainly none that show this effect in cancer patients.

Recently, shark cartilage was tested directly in human subjects with advanced cancers of various types. In this phase I/II trial of the safety and efficacy of shark cartilage in cancer treatment, the substance was found to be inactive ''and had no salutary effect on quality of life.''

Some anti-inflammatory effects of shark cartilage have been demonstrated *in vitro* and in animal models, but no useful conclusion can yet be drawn from this very preliminary research. Because shark cartilage contains some chondroitin sulfate, it might have some favorable activity in osteoarthritis, but this has not yet been demonstrated.

CONTRAINDICATIONS, PRECAUTIONS, ADVERSE REACTIONS
CONTRAINDICATIONS
Shark cartilage is contraindicated in those who are hypersensitive to any component of a shark cartilage-containing product. It is also contraindicated in those with hypercalcemia (shark cartilage contains a high percentage of calcium).

PRECAUTIONS
Pregnant women and nursing mothers should avoid shark cartilage supplementation.

Those with renal failure or liver failure should exercise caution in the use of shark cartilage.

Those with cancer who wish to try shark cartilage must only do so under medical supervision.

ADVERSE REACTIONS
The major adverse reactions are gastrointestinal and include nausea and vomiting, bloating and constipation. Some find the taste of shark cartilage disagreeable. There is one report of hepatitis associated with the use of shark cartilage.

OVERDOSAGE
There are no reports of overdosage in the literature.

DOSAGE AND ADMINISTRATION
Shark cartilage supplements are available in powders, tablets and capsules. There are no typical doses.

HOW SUPPLIED
Capsules — 250 mg, 500 mg, 740 mg, 750 mg
Powder — 6 g/scoop
Tablets — 740 mg, 750 mg

LITERATURE
Ashar B, Vargo E. Shark cartilage-induced hepatitis. *Ann Int Med.*1996; 125: 780-781.

Berbari P, Thibodeau A, Germain L, et al. Antiangiogenic effects of the oral administration of liquid cartilage extract in humans. *J Surg Res.* 1999; 87:108-113.

Dupont E, Brazeau P, Juneau C, Maes DH, Marenus K. Methods of using extracts of shark cartilage. United States Patent Number 6,028,118. Feb. 22, 2000.

Dupont E, Lachance Y, Lessard D, Auger S. Low molecular weight components of shark cartilage, processes for their preparation and therapeutic uses thereof. World patent W0004910A2. Feb. 3, 2000.

Dupont E, Savard PE, Jourdain C, et al. Antiangiogenic properties of a novel shark cartilage extract: potential role in the treatment of psoriasis. *J Cutan Med Surg.* 1998; 2:146-152.

Felzenszwalb I, Pelielo de Mattos JC, Bernardo-Filho M, et al. Shark cartilage-containing preparation: protection against reactive oxygen species. *Food Chem Toxicol.* 1998; 36:1079-1084.

Fontenele JB, Araujo GB, de Alencar JW, Viana GS. The analgesic and anti-inflammatory effects of shark cartilage are due to a peptide molecule and are nitric oxide (NO) system dependent. *Biol Pharm Bull.* 1997; 20:1151-1154.

Lee A, Langer R. Shark cartilage contains inhibitors of tumor angiogenesis. *Science.* 1983; 221:1185-1187.

Miller DR, Anderson GT, Stark JJ, et al. Phase I/II trial of the safety and efficacy of shark cartilage in the treatment of advanced cancer. *J Clin Oncol.* 1998; 16:3649-3655.

Oikawa T, Ashino-Fuse H, Shimamura M, et al. A novel angiogenic inhibitor derved from Japanese shark cartilage (I).

Extraction and estimation of inhibitory activities toward tumor and embryonic angiogenesis. *Cancer Lett.* 1990; 15:181-186.

Silicon

DESCRIPTION
Silicon is a non-metallic element with atomic number 14 and symbol Si. In the periodic table, it is in the same group as carbon and is carbon's closest relative. Silicon is, next to oxygen, the most abundant element in the earth's crust and is found in plants, animals and in most living organisms.

Silicon is not currently considered an essential nutrient for humans. Silicon deficiency states have been reported in chicks and rats, and silicon is an essential nutrient for some plants. Chicks fed silicon-deficient diets are found to have abnormalities in their skulls and long bones. Abnormalities include poorly formed joints, defective endochondral growth and defective articular cartilage. Bone and cartilage abnormalities have also been found in rats fed silicon-deficient diets. In these animals, silicon appears to be involved in collagen and glycosaminoglycan formation. Silicon may play such a role in other animals, including humans, but this has not yet been established. Silicon has also been reported to inhibit experimental atheromas induced by an atheromatous diet in rabbits.

Daily dietary intake of silicon in the United States ranges from approximately 20 to 50 milligrams. The richest sources of silicon are cereal products and unrefined grains of high fiber content. Significant amounts of silicon in the diet occur in the form of silicon dioxide (silica), which is poorly absorbed. Animal foods are low in silicon.

Magnesium trisilicate is frequently used as an antacid, either alone or in combination products. In the stomach, magnesium trisilicate is converted to silicon dioxide and magnesium chloride.

ACTIONS AND PHARMACOLOGY
ACTIONS
The actions of supplemental silicon are not known.

PHARMACOKINETICS
Little is known about the pharmacokinetics of supplemental and dietary silicon in humans. There is great variability in the absorption of the various forms of silicon in the diet. Most forms of dietary silicon are poorly absorbed. Most of the silicon food additives are hardly absorbed at all. Silicon dioxide or silica is more poorly absorbed than orthosilic acid, which is formed by the hydration of silicon dioxide. The mechanisms of silicon absorption are unknown. Silicon is not bound in plasma, where it is believed to exist almost entirely as monomeric silicic acid. Most of the silicon in the body is found in connective tissues, such as in bone, tendons, the trachea, the aorta, skin, hair and nails. Absorbed silicon is mainly excreted in the urine.

INDICATIONS AND USAGE
There is, at present, insufficient evidence to support any indication for the use of supplemental silicon. A very preliminary animal study suggests that it might have some positive impact in atherosclerosis. There is no support for claims that supplemental silicon is helpful in osteoporosis.

RESEARCH SUMMARY
It has been hypothesized that lack of silicon may play a role in the etiology of atherosclerosis. Intravenous administration of silicon inhibited experimental atheromas in an animal model, making atheromatous plaques fewer in number and the lipid deposits more superficial. This research was conducted many years ago and needs followup.

Claims that supplemental silicon is of benefit in osteoporosis and joint disease are not confirmed.

CONTRAINDICATIONS, PRECAUTIONS, ADVERSE REACTIONS
CONTRAINDICATIONS
None known.

PRECAUTIONS
There are reports of high doses of silicon intake, usually in the form of the antacid magnesium trisilicate, causing siliceous renal calculi. Those who form renal calculi should be cautious about the use of supplemental silicon.

ADVERSE REACTIONS
High doses of silicon have been reported to form siliceous renal calculi.

INTERACTIONS
Silicon may inhibit aluminum absorption.

OVERDOSAGE
No reports of overdosage.

DOSAGE AND ADMINISTRATION
No recommended dosage. Silicon is available in multivitamin preparations, usually in the form of silicon dioxide or magnesium trisilicate, typically at doses of about 2 milligrams. Supplemental silicon is also available as orthosilicic acid. The stems of the herb horsetail (*Equisetum arvense*) are rich in silicon dioxide. *Equisetum* is also used as a homeopathic remedy. Silicon may be found in colloidal or liquid minerals.

LITERATURE
Calomme MR, Vandem Berghe DA. Supplementation of calves with stabilized orthosilicic acid. Effect on the Si, Ca, Mg, and P concentrations in serum and the collagen concentration in skin and cartilage. *Biol Trace Elem Res.* 1997; 56:153-165.

Carlisle EM. Silicon as a trace nutrient. *Sci Total Environ.* 1988; 73:95-106.

Carlisle EM. The nutritional essentiality of silicon. *Nutr Rev.* 1982; 40:193-198.

Loeper J, Goy-Loeper J, Rozensztajn L, Fragny M. The antiatheromatous action of silicon. *Atherosclerosis.* 1979; 33:397-408.

Nielsen FH. Ultratrace minerals. In: Shils ME, Olson JA, Shike M, Ross AC, eds. *Modern Nutrition in Health and Disease.* 9th ed. Baltimore, MD: Williams and Wilkins; 199:283-303.

Rico H, Gallego-Lago JL, Hernandez ER, at al. Effect of silicon supplement on osteopenia induced by ovariectomy in rats. *Calcif Tissue Int.* 2000; 66:53-55.

Schwarz K. A bound form of silicon in glycosaminoglycans and polyuronides. *Proc Nat Acad Sci.* 1973; 70:1608-1612.

Schwarz K. Silicon, fibre, and atherosclerosis. *Lancet.* 1977; 1:454-457.

Sodium Alginates and other Phyco-Polysaccharides

TRADE NAMES
Blue-green algae is available from numerous manufacturers; branded products include Klamath Shores Blue Green Algae (Klamath). Red seaweed products available on the market include Irish Moss Herb (Quantum Herbal) and Irish Moss Tea (Alvita Tea).

DESCRIPTION
The algal plants or seaweeds are classified into four principal groups: the green algae or *Chlorophyceae*, the blue-green algae or *Cyanophyceae*, the brown algae or *Phaeophyceae*, and the red algae or *Rodophyceae*. The study of algae is called phycology. The brown and red algae are important commercially because of their polysaccharide content. These phyco-polysaccharides have broad applications in foods, pharmaceuticals and cosmetics, and as nutritional supplements. Agar and carrageenan are extracted from various types of red seaweeds, and algin is derived from brown seaweeds.

Agar is comprised of two major polysaccharides, neutral agarose and charged agaropectin. Both of these polysaccharides are composed of linear chains of alternating beta-D-galactose and 3,6-anhydro-alpha-L-galactose residues. These polysaccharides are resistant to digestion by intestinal digestive enzymes. Agar is also known as agar-agar. Agar is marketed in flakes and powder form and is commonly used to replace gelatin in various recipes. Agar is sometimes used to promote bowel regularity.

Carrageenans are polysaccharides also derived from certain red seaweeds. They are polysulfated, straight-chain galactans comprised of residues of D-galactose and 3,6-anhydro-D-galactose. The principal carrageenans are called kappa-carrageenan, lambda-carrageenan and iota carrageenan. Carrageenans are also resistant to digestion by intestinal digestive enzymes. Carrageenans have been reported to lower cholesterol levels in animals and also to have anti-viral activity against some membrane-containing viruses in culture.

Algin is a polysaccharide derived from the brown seaweeds or *Phaeophyceae*. Algin is present in these organisms as a mixed salt (sodium, potassium, calcium, magnesium) of alginic acid. Alginic acid is a high molecular polymer comprised of two types of uronic acid residues, beta-D-mannuronic acid and its C_5 epimer alpha-L-guluronic acid. The uronic acids are simple monosaccharides in which the primary hydroxyl group at C_6 has been oxidized to the corresponding carboxylic acid. For example, D-mannuronic acid is derived from D-mannose.

Algin is principally extracted from the giant kelp *Macrocystis pyrifera*. Its derivatives have wide application in the food industry (gelling, water-holding, emulsifying and stabilizing properties), in the cosmetic industry, and in medicine and dentistry (dental impressions). Calcium alginate, the calcium salt of alginic acid, is used as a wound dressing for the treatment of exudative wounds. Sailors have been treating their wounds with seaweed for hundreds of years. Sodium alginate, the sodium salt of alginic acid, is present in some antacid products and is effective for the treatment of gastroesophageal reflux disease or GERD. Sodium alginate reacts with gastric acid to form a viscous gel called the alginate raft. The alginate raft floats on top of the gastric contents and acts as a barrier to acid and food reflux.

Sodium alginate binds tightly to such substances as strontium, calcium, barium, cadmium and radium. Cows have been fed sodium alginate, which binds to radioactive strontium 90, causing it to pass out of the body without any of it getting absorbed. Sodium alginate has also been used to treat ouch-ouch or Itai-Itai-Byo disease. This disease has been found in Japan and is believed to be due to poisoning by cadmium-containing water used to irrigate rice. Painful joints are the major symptom of ouch-ouch disease.

Sodium alginate may be considered a soluble fiber. And, similar to other soluble fibers like pectin and psyllium, sodium alginate may have hypocholesterolemic and glycemic-regulatory activities.

ACTIONS AND PHARMACOLOGY

ACTIONS

Sodium alginate may have hypocholesterolemic and glycemic-regulatory activities. It may also have detoxification activity.

MECHANISM OF ACTION

Sodium alginate has been found to lower cholesterol in animal studies. It is speculated that this may be due to alginate-stimulated increase of fecal bile acid excretion.

Sodium alginate has also been demonstrated to lower glucose levels in diabetic animals. The mechanism of this activity is unknown.

Sodium alginate binds tightly to such substances as strontium, cadmium, radium and barium. It also binds to lead, but not as well. Sodium alginate's binding to these substances reduces their absorption.

PHARMACOKINETICS

There is little on the pharmacokinetics of sodium alginate in humans. It appears to be resistant to digestion by the digestive enzymes and is probably fermented, in part, by colonic bacteria to the short-chain fatty acids acetate, propionate and butyrate.

INDICATIONS AND USAGE

Sodium alginate may have some usefulness as a lipid-lowering agent, but the evidence for this possible indication is preliminary. Similarly, there is preliminary evidence that it may be of benefit in diabetes. It has demonstrated detoxifying effects and may be helpful in some with gastroesophageal reflux disease. Seaweed, rich in iodine, is used in many parts of the world to prevent and treat goiter. Carrageenans found in some red seaweeds have demonstrated some antiviral activity. Agar is used by some for regulating bowels. Calcium alginate has been used for wound healing, and sodium alginate has been effective in treating ouch-ouch disease. Some other polysaccharide components of seaweed have exhibited immunomodulating and anticarcinogenic effects in the laboratory. Folk remedy uses of seaweed products have included fever, eczema, gallstone and liver disease, gout, menstrual problems, hypertension, kidney disease and scabies. There is no credible research to support these folk uses.

RESEARCH SUMMARY

There are some preliminary animal studies in which sodium alginate and agar have been shown to reduce cholesterol levels. In one of these studies, sodium alginate enhanced cholesterol excretion into feces. It also inhibited blood glucose and insulin levels from rising 30 minutes after glucose administration. In another animal study, both algin and agar had favorable cholesterol effects but did not affect triglycerides. There are also preliminary reports that carrageenans derived from red seaweeds have some experimental cholesterol-lowering properties.

In a small human trial, consumption of 175 mg/kg/day of sodium alginate for seven days followed by consumption of 200 mg/kg/day for an additional 16 days resulted in no significant effects on hematological indices, plasma biochemistry and urinalysis parameters, blood glucose and plasma insulin concentrations, and breath hydrogen concentrations. No allergic responses were noted. There were only five subjects in this study—all with normal health at the outset.

Alginates have been used for heartburn and acid reflux for decades. Numerous *in vitro* and *in vivo* studies have demonstrated that alginate-based rafts effectively provide physical barriers to acidic gastric contents and can thus significantly reduce reflux episodes. Alginates are present in some over-the-counter antacids.

Calcium alginate is often used as a dressing for exudative wounds. It is an effective absorbable hemostatic and is often used to pack sinuses, bleeding wounds of various types and burns. Sodium alginate is also used for this purpose. In one study, the use of calcium alginate hemostatic swabs was credited with significantly reducing blood loss in various surgeries and with significantly reducing duration of operations. Calcium alginate was shown to be four times as absorbent per unit weight as gauze.

The alginates have been shown to bind tightly to strontium, barium, cadmium and radium so that these toxins pass out of the body with little or no absorption. It also binds with lead, but not as completely. Ouch-ouch disease, characterized by painful joints and believed to be caused by oral cadmium exposure, has been successfully treated with alginates in Japan. Reduction in the absorption of strontium has been noted in children given an alginate derivative. Retention of radioactive barium has been reduced in rats fed sodium alginate derivatives. In one human trial, 10 grams of sodium alginate ameliorated acute radiation effects due to exposure to radiation doses of 50 to 3,000 rads.

Calcium alginate has shown anti-viral activity in some *in vitro* and animal studies. It is sufficiently effective that diagnostic laboratories caution against the use of calcium alginate swabs in some diagnostic sampling, owing to calcium alginate's toxicity to herpes viruses and chlamydia, among other infective agents.

The carrageenans, sulfated polysaccharides derived from red seaweeds like Irish moss, have inhibited both HSV1 and HSV2 *in vitro*. They also inhibit some other viruses, including HIV. The natural alginates, on the other hand, do not show anti-herpetic or anti-HIV activity.

In one animal study, preparations from various edible seaweeds significantly reduced the incidence of chemically induced cancers, compared with controls that were unsupplemented with these preparations. In another animal study, an extract of the brown alga hijiki recently showed immuno-enhancing activity. The polysaccharide fraction of the extract, more than the nonpolysaccharide fraction, had immuno-enhancing effects on the proliferative response of spleen cells. This response was associated with B-cell, but not T-cell, populations. More research is needed.

CONTRAINDICATIONS, PRECAUTIONS, ADVERSE REACTIONS

CONTRAINDICATIONS

Sodium alginate is contraindicated in those who are hypersensitive to any component of a sodium alginate-containing product.

PRECAUTIONS

Pregnant women and nursing mothers should avoid supplementation with sodium alginate unless it is recommended by their physicians.

ADVERSE REACTIONS

Gastrointestinal symptoms such as flatulence may occur with sodium alginate supplements.

INTERACTIONS

NUTRITIONAL SUPPLEMENTS

Sodium alginate may decrease the absorption of the carotenoids beta-carotene, lycopene and lutein if used concomitantly. It may also decrease the absorption of such minerals as calcium, zinc, manganese, chromium and magnesium if used concomitantly.

FOODS

Sodium alginate may reduce the absorption of food carotenoids, such as beta-carotene, lycopene and lutein and such minerals in foods as calcium, magnesium, zinc, manganese and chromium.

DOSAGE AND ADMINISTRATION

Sodium alginate supplements can be found in the marketplace, but there are no typical doses. Various algaes and seaweeds are available as supplements as well. Among algae or seaweeds often used as foods and supplements are hijiki, kombu, wakame and arame. These are all brown seaweeds or algae. The red seaweeds and some of their constituents are also widely used. These include nori, agar or agar-agar, dulse and Irish moss. There are no typical doses.

HOW SUPPLIED

Blue-green algae is supplied as follows:

Capsules — 500 mg, 750 mg

Powder — 1 g/teaspoon

Tablets — 375 mg, 500 mg

Irish moss is supplied as follows:

Liquid

Tea

LITERATURE

Anderson DM, Brydon WG, Eastwood MA, Sedgwick DM. Dietary effects of sodium alginate in humans. *Food Addit Contam.* 1991; 8:237-248.

Carr TE, Harrison GE, Humphreys ER, Sutton A. Reduction in the absorption and retention of dietary strontium in man by alginate. *Int J Radiat Biol Relat Stud Phys Chem Med.* 1968; 14:225-233.

Harmuth-Hoene AE, Schelenz R. Effect of dietary fiber on mineral absorption in growing rats. *J Nutr.* 1980; 110:1774-1784.

Hendler SS. *The Doctors' Vitamin And Mineral Encyclopedia.* New York, NY: Simon and Schuster; 1990.

Kimura Y, Watanabe K, Okuda H. Effects of soluble sodium alginate on cholesterol excretion and glucose tolerance in rats. *J Ethnopharmacol.* 1996; 54:47-54.

Mandel KG, Daggy BP, Brodie DA, Jacoby HI. Review article: alginate-raft formulations in the treatment of heartburn and acid reflux. *Aliment Pharmacol Ther.* 2000; 14:669-690.

Ohta A, Taguchi A, Takizawa T, et al. The alginate reduce the postprandial glycaemic response by forming a gel with dietary calcium in the stomach of the rat. *Int J Vitam Nutr Res.* 1997; 67:55-61.

Okai Y, Higashi-Okai K, Ishizaka S, et al. Possible immunomodulating activities in an extract of edible brown alga, *Hijikia fusiforme* (Hijiki). *J Sci Food Agric.* 1998; 76:56-62.

Riedl J, Linseisen J, Hoffmann J, Wolfram G. Some dietary fibers reduce the absorption of carotenoids in women. *J Nutr.* 1989; 129:2170-2176.

Sayag J, Meaume S, Bohbot S. Healing properties of calcium alginate dressings. *J Wound Care.* 1996; 5:357-362.

Silva AJ, Fleshman DG, Shore B. The effects of sodium alginate on the absorption and retention of several divalent cations. *Health Phys.* 1970; 19:245-251.

Sutton A, Harrison GE, Carr TE, Barltrop D. Reduction in the absorption of dietary strontium in children by an alginate derivative. *Int J Radiat Biol Relat Stud Phys Chem Med.* 1971; 19:79-85.

Sutton A, Humphreys ER, Shepherd H, Howells GR. Reduction in the retention of radioactive barium in rats following the addition of sodium alginate derivatives to the diet. *Int J Radiat Biol Relat Stud Phys Chem Med.* 1972; 22:297-300.

Wu J, Peng SS. Comparison of hypolipidemic effect of refined konjac meal with several common dietary fibers and their mechanisms of action. *Biomed Environ Sci.* 1997; 10:27-37.

Soy Isoflavones

TRADE NAMES

Soy Choice (Vitanica), Soy Protein Isoflavone Powder (MotherNature.com), EasySoy Gold Super Isoflavone Concentrate (Carlson Laboratories), MaxiLife Mega Soy (Twinlab), Soy Essentials (Health From the Sun) and Phyto-Est (BioTherapies), Healthy Woman Soy Menopause (Personal Products), Soy & Red Clover Isoflavones (Nature's Answer).

DESCRIPTION

Soy isoflavones are phytoestrogens found in soybeans. Phytoestrogens are plant-derived nonsteroidal compounds that possess estrogen-like biological activity. Soy isoflavones have both weak estrogenic and weak anti-estrogenic effects. They have been found to bind to estrogen receptors-alpha (ER-alpha) and beta (ER-beta). They appear to bind better to ER-beta than to ER-alpha.

Soy isoflavones comprise three main isoflavones and their glycosylated forms. The three main isoflavones are the aglycones genistein, daidzein and glycitein. They can be represented by the following structural formulas:

Soy isoflavones

	R_1	R2	R3	R4
Daidzen	H	H	OH	OH
Genistein	OH	H	OH	OH
Glycitein	H	OCH3	OH	OH

The glycosylated forms of genistein are genistin, 6'' -O-malonylgenistin and 6''-O-acetylgenistin; those of daidzein are daidzin, 6''-O-malonyldaidzin and 6''-O-acetyldaidzin, and those of glycitein are glycitin, 6''-O-malonylglycitin and 6'' -O-acetylglycitin. The malonyl glycosides of genistein are the major forms of the soy isoflavones that are found in soybeans. Fermented soy foods, such as tempeh and miso, are rich in the soy isoflavone aglycones. The most abundant of the soy isoflavones in soybeans are the genistein glycosides (about 50%), followed by the daidzein glycosides (about 40%). The least abundant of the soy isoflavones in soybeans are the glycitein glycosides (about 5 to 10%). Soy protein derived from soybeans contains about 2 mg of genistin and daidzin per gram of protein. In soy germ, the order is different. Glycitein glycosides comprise about 40% of soy germ, daidzein glycosides about 50% and genistein glycosides about 10%.

Soy isoflavones, when marketed as nutritional supplements, are mainly present as the isoflavone glycosides genistin, daidzin and glycitin.

ACTIONS AND PHARMACOLOGY

ACTIONS

Soy isoflavones have estrogenic activity. Soy isoflavones may have antioxidant activity. They may also have anticarcinogenic, anti-atherogenic, hypolipidemic and anti-osteoporotic activities.

MECHANISM OF ACTION

Soy isoflavones have weak estrogenic activity. The order of activity in *in vivo* assays is glycitein greater than genistein greater than daidzein. They bind to estrogen receptors-alpha and beta. They appear to bind better to estrogen receptor-beta than to estrogen receptor-alpha.

The most studied of the soy isoflavones is genistein. Genistein has been found to have a number of antioxidant activities. It is a scavenger of reactive oxygen species and inhibits lipid peroxidation. It also inhibits superoxide anion generation by the enzyme xanthine oxidase. In addition, genistein, in animal experiments, has been found to increase the activities of the antioxidant enzymes superoxide dismutase, glutathionine peroxidase, catalase and glutathione reductase. Daidzein and glycitein also appear to have reactive oxygen scavenging activity. However, these isoflavones have not been studied as much as genistein has.

Regarding possible anticarcinogenic activity, again genistein has been the most studied of the soy isoflavones. Several mechanisms have been proposed for genistein's possible anticarcinogenic activity. These include upregulation of apoptosis, inhibition of angiogenesis, inhibition of DNA topoisomerase II and inhibition of protein tyrosine kinases. Genistein's weak estrogenic activity may be involved in its putative activity against prostate cancer. Other possible anti-prostate cancer mechanisms include inhibition of NF (nuclear factor)-kappa B in prostate cancer cells, downregulation of TGF (transforming growth factor)-beta and inhibition of EGF (epidermal growth factor)- stimulated growth. Genistein's anti-estrogenic action may be another possible mechanism to explain its putative activity against breast cancer. Additional possible anti-breast cancer mechanisms include inhibition of aromatase activity and stimulation of sex hormone binding globulin, both of which might lower endogenous estrogen levels.

The possible anti-atherogenic activity of soy isoflavones may be accounted for, in part, by their possible antioxidant activity, particularly with regard to inhibition of lipid peroxidation and oxidation of LDL. Soy isoflavones may have some cholesterol-lowering activity, but the mechanism of this possible effect is unclear.

Soy isoflavone's weak estrogenic effect may help protect against osteoporosis by preventing bone resorption and promoting bone density. However, the mechanism of this possible effect is entirely speculative at this time.

PHARMACOKINETICS

See Genistein, Daidzein and Glycitein.

INDICATIONS AND USAGE

Soy isoflavones may be helpful in preventing and treating some forms of heart disease and cancer. They may ameliorate some menopausal symptoms and may be beneficial in preventing osteoporosis.

RESEARCH SUMMARY

Epidemiological data suggest that higher intakes of foods containing soy isoflavones are significantly correlated with reduced incidence of heart disease and some forms of cancer. Animal, *in vitro* and human studies have provided further support for the epidemiological findings. Soy proteins were shown to lower plasma levels of cholesterol in animal models of hypercholesterolemia, and, subsequently, a meta-analysis of human studies has more recently established that soy consumption is significantly associated with reduction in plasma cholesterol levels in humans, as well. These effects are largely attributed to the isoflavone components of soy.

Epidemiological data indicate that consumption of soy is particularly associated with reduced risk of breast, lung and prostate cancers, as well as leukemia. Here again, *in vitro* and animal research has further supported these observations.

Problems associated with menopause, including osteoporosis, also appear to be favorably affected by higher intakes of soy products and by soy isoflavones specifically. The "hot flashes" that some menopausal women experience are significantly reduced in some who consume soy products and/or soy isoflavone supplements. These benefits have been demonstrated in randomized, double-blind studies.

Soy isoflavones have also been shown to prevent bone resorption and to help increase bone density in some *in vitro* and animal studies. The synthetic isoflavone ipriflavone (see Ipriflavone), the major metabolite of which is the soy isoflavone daidzein, has demonstrated a significant ability to prevent osteoporosis in both animal models and in humans.

One negative finding related to soy intake was reported recently. The authors of an epidemiological study associated high intake of tofu by men during midlife with significantly poorer cognitive test performance, enlargement of ventricles and diminished brain weight. The study, however, was not able to control for many potentially important dietary and other variables that may have affected outcome. The results of the study, while provocative, are too preliminary to support any conclusions. More research may be warranted.

CONTRAINDICATIONS, PRECAUTIONS, ADVERSE REACTIONS

CONTRAINDICATIONS

Soy isoflavones are contraindicated in those who are hypersensitive to any component of a soy isoflavone-containing product.

PRECAUTIONS

Pregnant women and nursing mothers should avoid the use of soy isoflavone supplements pending long-term safety studies. Men with prostate cancer should discuss the advisability of the use of soy isoflavones with their physicians before deciding to use them.

Women with estrogen receptor-positive tumors should exercise caution in the use of soy isoflavones and should only use them if they are recommended and monitored by a physician.

Soy isoflavone intake has been associated with hypothyroidism in some.

DOSAGE AND ADMINISTRATION

Soy isoflavone supplements containing genistin, daidzin and glycitin are available with much smaller amounts of the aglycones genistein, daidzein and glycitein. The percentages of the soy isoflavones present in a standard soy isoflavone supplement reflect the percentages of these substances as found in soybeans and are: genistin, about 50%; daidzin, about 38%; and glycitin, about 12%. A 50-mg dose of soy isoflavones—a typical daily dose—delivers 25 mg of genistin, 19 mg of daidzin and about 6 mg of glycitin. Usually, 40% of the formula is comprised of soy isoflavones. Therefore, to get a dose of 50 milligrams of soy isoflavones, 125 mg daily of soy isoflavones are required. Various observational and epidemiological studies suggest 50 mg daily of soy isoflavones approximates the dose that may have health benefits.

Soy isoflavones are also available in some functional food products.

HOW SUPPLIED

Capsules — 12 mg, 18 mg, 40 mg, 56 mg, 80 mg
Powder
Tablets — 130 mg

LITERATURE

Barnes S. Evolution of the health benefits of soy isoflavones. *Proc Soc Exp Biol Med.* 1998; 217:386-392.

Constantinou AI, Mehta RG, Vaughan A. Inhibition of N-methyl-N-nitrosourea-induced mammary tumors in rats by the soybean isoflavones. *Anticancer Res.* 1996; 16:3293-3298.

Grodstein F, Mayeux R, Stampfer MJ. Tofu and cognitive function: food for thought (Editorial). *J Am Coll Nutr.* 2000; 19:207-209.

Klein KO. Isoflavones, soy-based infant formulas, and relevance to endocrine function. *Nutr Rev.* 1998; 56:193-204.

Kurzer MS, Xu X. Dietary phytoestrogens. *Annu Rev Nutr.* 1997; 17:353-381.

Merz-Demlov BE, Duncan AM, Wangen KE, et al. Soy isoflavones improve plasma lipids in normocholesterolemic premenopausal women. *Am J Clin Nutr.* 2000; 71:1462-1469.

Third International Symposium on the Role of Soy in Preventing and Treating Chronic Disease. *J Nutr.* 2000; 130:653S-711S.

Tikkanen MJ, Adlercreutz H. Dietary soy-derived isoflavone phytoestrogens. *Biochem Pharmacol.* 2000; 60:1-5.

White LR, Petrovitch H, Ross GW, et al. Brain aging and midlife tofu consumption. *J Am Coll Nutr.* 2000; 19:242-255.

Soy Protein

TRADE NAMES

Genisoy Protein Shake (MLO Products), Genista Soy Protein (Biotherapies), Soytein (Solaray), Vege Fuel (Twinlab), Premium Soy Protein Booster (Naturade).

DESCRIPTION

In October, 1999, the Food and Drug Administration (FDA) approved labeling claims for dietary soy protein stating that it may reduce the risk of heart disease. This is the 11th health claim allowed by the FDA. The health claim that can be used on labels of products containing soy protein states: "Diets low in saturated fat and cholesterol that include 25 grams of soy protein a day may reduce the risk of heart disease." In order to carry the health claim, one serving of a product must contain at least 6.25 grams of soy protein and must also be low in total and saturated fat, cholesterol and sodium.

This latest FDA health claim was based on animal studies, epidemiological studies and human studies demonstrating that diets high in soy protein and low in animal protein lead to decreased levels of total cholesterol, low-density lipoprotein (LDL) cholesterol and triglycerides. The mechanism of the lipid-lowering effect of soy protein remains unclear.

Soy protein isolates have become popular items in the nutritional supplement marketplace. Most of these supplements also contain the soy isoflavones genistin, daidzin and glycitin.

ACTIONS AND PHARMACOLOGY

ACTIONS

Soy protein may have lipid-lowering, antiatherogenic, antioxidant, anticarcinogenic and antiosteoporotic activities.

MECHANISM OF ACTION

Diets rich in soy protein have been found to reduce serum levels of total cholesterol, LDL-cholesterol, triglycerides and apolipoprotein B (apo B). The mechanism of the lipid-lowering activity of soy protein is unclear. There are a few possible explanations. Soy protein is much richer in L-arginine than is animal protein, which is richer in L-lysine. Some animal studies indicate that dietary increases in L-arginine are accompanied by decreases in cholesterol levels. Further, some studies have demonstrated that, under certain conditions, e.g., hypercholesterolemia, high intakes of L-arginine could enhance endothelial-dependent vasodilation and nitric oxide or NO production (see L-Arginine). This could contribute to the possible antiatherogenic activity of soy protein.

The soy isoflavones may also contribute to the lipid-lowering activity of soy protein as well as its antiatherogenic activity. Most soy protein products contain the isoflavones genistin, daidzin and glycitin, which have weak estrogenic effects and also may have antiestrogenic activity (see Soy Isoflavones). Oral estrogens have been shown to decrease total cholesterol and LDL-cholesterol. The soy isoflavones may have similar actions.

Interestingly, a few studies have shown that when the isoflavones are removed from the soy protein, the protein itself has little hypocholesterolemic activity. Soy isoflavones themselves do not have the same hypocholesterolemic activity as the combination of soy protein and soy isoflavones. There are probably synergistic effects of these substances that are not understood at this time.

There are also other substances associated with soy protein, including saponins, trypsin inhibitor and bioactive peptides, which may also contribute to the lipid-lowering activity of soy protein. The soy isoflavones are antioxidants, and their antioxidant activity may contribute to the possible antiatherogenic effect of soy protein.

The antioxidant, anticarcinogenic and antiosteoporotic activities of soy protein are probably due, in large part, to the soy isoflavones (see Soy Isoflavones). Soy protein has been found to reduce intestinal mucosa polyamine levels in rats, which may be another anticarcinogenic mechanism. Also, a bioactive peptide has recently been isolated from soybeans and has been found to have potent antimitotic activity.

PHARMACOKINETICS

The digestion, absorption, distribution and metabolism of soy protein occurs by normal physiological processes. See Soy Isoflavones, Genistin, Daidzin and Glycitin for the pharmacokinetics of these substances.

INDICATIONS AND USAGE

The FDA has allowed the following health claim for soy protein: "25 grams of soy protein a day, as part of a diet low in saturated fat and cholesterol, may reduce the risk of heart disease." The isoflavone constituents of soy protein may confer some additional benefits. See Soy Isoflavones.

RESEARCH SUMMARY

The FDA-approved health claim—see Indications above—that soy protein, in adequate amounts, may help protect against heart disease is based upon numerous *in vitro*, animal, epidemiological and human studies. Evidence has accumulated over many decades showing that soy protein, but not animal protein, has significant cholesterol-lowering properties in animal studies.

In a meta-analysis of clinical studies, most of them well-controlled, investigators concluded that soy protein significantly lowered serum concentrations of total cholesterol, LDL-cholesterol and triglycerides without significantly altering HDL-cholesterol concentrations.

Since the meta-analysis cited above was conducted, other clinical research has continued to confirm the lipid-lowering ability of soy protein. Recently it was demonstrated that administration for six weeks of as little as 20 grams of soy protein per day, in place of animal protein, achieved significant reductions of non-HDL-cholesterol and apolipoprotein (apo) B in moderately hypercholesterolemic men.

CONTRAINDICATIONS, PRECAUTIONS, ADVERSE REACTIONS

CONTRAINDICATIONS

Soy protein supplements are contraindicated in those who are hypersensitive to any component of a soy protein-containing product.

PRECAUTIONS

Pregnant women and nursing mothers should avoid the use of soy protein supplements pending long-term safety studies or unless these supplements are recommended by their physicians.

Women with estrogen receptor-positive tumors should exercise caution in the use of soy protein supplements and should only use them if they are recommended and monitored by their physicians.

INTERACTIONS

NUTRITIONAL SUPPLEMENTS AND FOODS

Soy contains phytic acid, which may bind with certain minerals, such as calcium, magnesium, manganese, zinc, copper and iron, reducing their availability.

OVERDOSAGE

There are no reports of overdosage.

DOSAGE AND ADMINISTRATION

There are several soy protein supplements available. Typically the soy protein supplements contain soy isoflavones. Dosage is variable.

A total intake of 25 to 50 grams of soy protein and 50 milligrams of soy isoflavones daily may have cardiovascular and other health benefits. This can come from nutritional intake, as well as supplemental intake.

HOW SUPPLIED

Bar

Liquid

Powder

LITERATURE

Anderson JW, Johnstone BM, Cook-Newell ME. Meta-analysis of the effects of soy protein intake on serum lipids. *N Engl J Med*. 1995; 333:276-282.

Aoyama T, Fukui K, Takamatsu K, et al. Soy protein isolate and its hydrolysate reduce body fat of dietary obese rats and genetically obese mice (yellow KK). *Nutrition*. 2000; 16:349-354.

Carroll KK. Review of clinical studies on cholesterol-lowering response to soy protein. *J Am Diet Assoc*. 1991; 91:820-827.

Carroll KK, Kurowska EM. Soy consumption and cholesterol reduction: review of animal and human studies. *J Nutr*. 1995; 125(3Suppl):594S-597S.

Crouse JR III, Morgan T, Terry JG, et al. A randomized trial comparing the effect of casein with that of soy protein containing varying amounts of isoflavones on plasma concentrations of lipids and lipoproteins. *Arch Intern Med*. 1999; 159:2070-2076.

Erdman JW Jr. Control of serum lipids with soy protein (Editorial). *N Eng J Med*. 1995; 333:313-315.

Gaddi A, Decovich GC, Noseda G, et al. Hypercholesterolemia treated by soybean protein diet. *Arch Dis Childhood*. 1987; 62:274-278.

Galvez AF, deLumen BO. A soybean cDNA encoding a chromatin-binding peptide inhibits mitosis of mammalian cells. *Nat Biotechol*. 1999; 17:495-500.

Greaves KA, Wilson MD, Rudel LL, et al. Consumption of soy protein reduces cholesterol absorption compared to casein protein alone or supplemented with an isoflavone extract or conjugated equine estrogen in ovariectomized cynomolgus monkeys. *J Nutr*. 2000; 130:820.

Teixeira SR, Potter SM, Weigel R, et al. Effects of feeding 4 levels of soy protein for 3 and 6 wk on blood lipids and apolipoproteins in moderately hypercholesterolemic men. *Am J Clin Nutr*. 2000; 71:1077-1084.

Wang W, Higuch CM. Dietary soy protein is associated with reduced intestinal mucosal polyamine concentration in male Wistar rats. *J Nutr*. 2000; 130:1815-1820.

Spirulina

TRADE NAMES

Fingerprinted Spirulina (GNC), Hawaiian Spirulina (Source Naturals, Rainbow Light), Chinese Spirulina (Nature's Way), Spirulina Pacific (Nutrex), Spirulina Green Superfood for Life (Earthrise), Spirulina Gold (Earthrise), Spirulina Sunrise Bar (Glenny's).

DESCRIPTION

Spirulina is a genus of the phylum *Cyanobacteria. Cyanobacteria* are classified as either blue-green algae or as blue-green bacteria. Spirulina is a popular food supplement in Japan and is marketed as a nutritional supplement in the United States. Spirulina, wheat grass, barley grass and chlorella are sometimes referred to as "green foods." There are several species of spirulina. The ones most commonly used in nutritional supplements are *Spirulina platensis* (also called *Arthrospira platensis*) and *Spirulina maxima.*

Spirulina used for the production of nutritional supplements is either grown in outdoor tanks or harvested from lakes in as Mexico, Central and South America, and Africa.

Spirulina is a rich source of protein. It also contains chlorophyll, carotenoids, minerals, gamma-linolenic acid (GLA) and some unique pigments. These pigments, called phycobilins, include phycocyanin and allophycocyanin. The pigments give spirulina their bluish tinge. Phycobilins are similar in structure to bile pigments such as bilirubin. In the spirulina cell, phycobilins are attached to proteins; the phycobilin-protein complex is called phycobiliprotein.

ACTIONS AND PHARMACOLOGY

ACTIONS

Spirulina has putative antiviral, hypocholesterolemic, antioxidant, hepatoprotective, antiallergic and immune-modulatory activities.

MECHANISM OF ACTION

A sulfated polysaccharide called calcium spirulan isolated from *Spirulina platensis (Arthrospira platensis)* was found to inhibit a number of membraned viruses. The viruses inhibited by the polysaccharide included herpes simplex virus 1 (HSV-1), cytomegalovirus, measles virus, mumps virus and HIV-1. Calcium spirulan appears to inhibit the penetration of these viruses into host cells. These studies were performed *in vitro.*

Spirulina has been shown to have hypocholesterolemic activity in experimental animals. The mechanism of this activity is unknown.

The spirulina pigment phycocyanin has demonstrated antioxidant activity. It scavenges peroxyl radicals.

Phycocyanin has been found to protect against hepatotoxins in rats. The mechanism may be via its antioxidant activity. An extract of *Spirulina maxima* also protected against carbon tetrachloride hepatotoxicity in rats. The phycocyanin contained in the extract, as well as other antioxidants, probably account for the hepatoprotective effect.

Mast-cell mediated immediate-type allergic reactions were found to be inhibited in rats by spirulina. It is speculated that there are substances in spirulina that may inhibit mast-cell degranulation, possibly by affecting the mast-cell membrane.

Spirulina platensis extracts have been demonstrated to enhance macrophage function in cats and to enhance humoral and cell-mediated immune functions in chickens. The mechanism of these effects is unknown.

PHARMACOKINETICS

The pharmacokinetics of spirulina in humans have not been studied. However, the proteins, lipids and carbohydrates in spirulina should be digested, absorbed and metabolized by normal physiological processes.

INDICATIONS AND USAGE

Spirulina has shown some indication of having antiviral effects in preliminary *in vitro* and animal studies. There is also evidence of a preliminary nature that it might favorably affect some immune functions and have some hepatoprotective capability. It has shown some promise of inhibiting some allergic reactions in recent experimental studies. Hypocholesterolemic effects have been reported in some animal studies.

RESEARCH SUMMARY

An extract of spirulina inhibited *in vitro* replication of HSV-1 simplex virus type 1. It also significantly prolonged survival time of HSV-1-infected hamsters. It seemed to act, not through direct virucidal effects, but rather through inhibition of viral penetration into cells. Subsequently, further experiments demonstrated that spirulina extract significantly inhibited *in vitro* replication of several enveloped viruses, including human cytomegalovirus, measles virus, mumps virus, influenza A virus and HIV-1. Again, the mechanism of action was said to be selective inhibition of viral penetration into host cells.

More recently still, other researchers have focused specifically on the ability of a spirulina extract to inhibit HIV-1 replication in human T-cell lines, peripheral blood mononuclear cells (PBMC) and Langerhans cells (LC). The researchers stated: "We conclude that aqueous *A platensis* extracts contain antiretroviral activity that may be of potential clinical interest."

Spirulina and some of its constituents have shown an ability to favorably affect various immune functions. In one animal experiment, it boosted phagocytic activity and increased natural killer (NK)-cell activity two-fold, compared with controls.

Spirulina has significantly inhibited chemically induced anaphylactic shock and serum histamine levels in rats, leading to the conclusion that spirulina may inhibit mast-cell degranulation. In another animal experiment, spirulina significantly inhibited local allergic reactions induced by anti-dinitrophenyl (DNP) IgE. It demonstrated, more specifically, a significant inhibitory effect on anti-DNP IgE-induced tumor necrosis factor-alpha production, leading the researchers to conclude that spirulina inhibits mast-cell mediated immediate-type allergic reactions both *in vitro* and *in vivo*.

Finally, a constituent of spirulina, administered intraperitoneally, significantly reduced the hepatotoxicity of a carbon tetrachloride challenge. A more recent study confirmed this finding.

CONTRAINDICATIONS, PRECAUTIONS, ADVERSE REACTIONS.

CONTRAINDICATIONS

Spirulina is contraindicated in those who are hypersensitive to any component of a spirulina-containing supplement.

PRECAUTIONS

Pregnant women and nursing mothers should avoid spirulina-containing supplements.

Spirulina can accumulate heavy metals, such as mercury, from contaminated waters. Those who use spirulina supplements should select reputable products that are free of any heavy metal contamination.

ADVERSE REACTIONS

Occasional gastrointestinal symptoms, such as nausea, have been reported. Also, there are a few reports of allergic reactions to spirulina-containing supplements.

DOSAGE AND ADMINISTRATION

There are various forms of spirulina supplements, including capsules, tablets, flakes and powders. Spirulina is also found in some functional foods and in combination ''green food'' products with barley grass, chlorella and wheat grass. Doses range from 250 mg to 5 grams daily.

HOW SUPPLIED

Bar — 1000 mg
Capsules — 350 mg, 380 mg, 400 mg, 429 mg, 500 mg
Powder
Tablets — 5250 mg, 00 mg, 750 mg

LITERATURE

Ayehunie S, Belay A, Baba TW, Ruprecht RM. Inhibition of HIV-1 replication by an aqueous extract of Spirulina platensis (Arthrospira platensis). *J Acquir Immune Defic Synd Hum Retrovirol.* 1998; 18:7-12.

Chamorro G, Salazar M, Favil L, Bourges H. [Pharmacology and toxicology of Spirulina alga.] [Article in Spanish.] *Rev Invest Clin.* 1996; 48:389-399.

Devi MA, Venkataraman LV. Hypocholesterolemic effect of blue-green algae Spirulina platensis in albino rats. *Ann Nutr Reports Int.* 1983; 28:519-530.

Hayashi T, Hayashi K. Calcium spirulan, an inhibitor of enveloped virus replication, from a blue-green alga *Spirulina platensis.* 1996; 59:83-87.

Hayashi K, Hayashi T, Morita N, Kajima I. An extract from Spirulina platensis is a selective inhibitor of herpes simplex virus type 1 penetration into HeLa cells. *Phytotherapy Res.* 1993; 7:76-80.

Johnson PE, Shubert LE. Accumulation of mercury and other elements by spirulina (cyanophyceae). *Nutr Rep Intl.* 1986; 34:1063-1071.

Kim HM, Lee EH, Cho HH, Moon YH. Inhibitory effect of mast cell-mediated immediate-type allergic reactions in rats by spirulina. *Biochem Pharmacol.* 1998; 55:1071-1076.

Lissi EA, Pizarro M, Aspee A, Romay C. Kinetics of phycocyanine bilin groups destruction by peroxyl radicals. *Free Rad Biol Med.* 2000; 28:1051-1055.

Miranda MS, Cintra RG, Barros SB, Mancini Filho J. Antioxidant activity of the microalga Spirulina maxima. *Braz J Med Biol Res.* 1998; 31:1075-1079.

Quereshi MA, Ali RA. Spirulina platensis exposure enhances macrophage phagocytic function in cats. *Immunopharmacol Immunotoxicol.* 1996; 18:457-463.

Quereshi MA, Garlich JD, Kidd MT. Dietary Spirulina platensis enhances humoral and cell-mediated functions in chickens. *Immunopharmacol Immunotoxicol.* 1996; 18:465-476.

Romay C, Armesto J, Ramirez D, et al. Antioxidant and anti-inflammatory properties of C-phycocyanin from blue-green algae. *Inflamm Res.* 1998; 47:36-41.

Torres-Durán PV, Miranda-Zamora R, Paredes-Carbajal MC, et al. Studies on the preventive effect of *Spirulina maxima* on fatty liver development induced by carbon tetrachloride. *J Ethnopharmacol.* 1999; 64:141-147.

Watanabe F, Katsura H, Takenaka S, et al. Pseudovitamin B_{12} is the predominant cobamide of an algal health food, spirulina tablets. *J Agric Food Chem.* 1999; 47:4736-4741.

Yang H-N, Lee E-H, Kim H-M. *Spirulina platensis* inhibits anaphylactic reaction. *Life Sciences.* 1997; 61:1237-1244.

Squalene

TRADE NAMES

Branded products include Squalene + (Biotherapies US).

DESCRIPTION

Squalene, a 30-carbon isoprenoid, is a lipid found in large quantities in shark liver oil and in smaller amounts (0.1 to 0.7 %) in olive oil, wheat germ oil, rice bran oil and yeast. It is a key intermediate in the biosynthesis of cholesterol. Squalene is an all-trans isoprenoid containing six isoprene units. Chemically, it is known as (all-E)-2, 6, 10, 15, 19, 23-Hexamethyl-2, 6, 10, 14, 18, 22-tetracosahexaene. It is represented structurally as:

Squalene

It is also known as spinacene and supraene. Squalene is also found in human sebum. Squalene has the ability to absorb oxygen. However, the amount of oxygen absorbed would be physiologically significant only for the shark.

ACTIONS AND PHARMACOLOGY

ACTIONS

Squalene has demonstrated proliferative activity in animal cancer studies; to date no human data are available. Squalene may have some radioprotective effects, but, again, there are no human data. Animal work suggests that squalene may also have a cholesterol-lowering effect, but this has not been tested in humans.

MECHANISM OF ACTION

Squalene is a key precursor in the biosynthesis of cholesterol. It inhibits 3-hydroxy-3-methylglutaryl coenzyme A reductase activity, thus reducing farnesyl pyrophosphate availability for prenylation of the ras oncogene, an activity that could account for its anti-proliferative effect in some animal cancer models. Apoptosis inhibition may also play a role in the anti-tumor effects of squalene in animals. The mechanism of the radioprotective effect of squalene is unknown.

PHARMACOKINETICS

Over 60% of ingested squalene is absorbed from the small intestine; from there it is carried in the lymph in the form of chylomicrons into the systemic circulation. In the blood, squalene is carried mainly in very-low-density lipoproteins and distributed to the various tissues of the body. A large percentage of squalene gets distributed to the skin. Squalene is metabolized to cholesterol.

INDICATIONS AND USAGE

Animal work suggests that indications could one day emerge for squalene in the prevention and treatment of some cancers, for immune enhancement and possibly for lowering cholesterol. It is not indicated for gastritis, joint pain and inflammation or to improve lung function.

RESEARCH SUMMARY

Squalene is being investigated as an adjunctive therapy in some cancers. In animal models, it has proved effective in inhibiting lung tumors. It has also demonstrated chemopreventive effects against colon cancer in animal models. Supplementation of squalene in mice has produced enhanced immune function and, in other animal studies, it has reduced cholesterol levels, prompting one researcher to suggest that it might be used to potentiate cholesterol-lowering drugs.

A mouse study showed squalene to confer radioprotection against lethal whole-body radiation.

CONTRAINDICATIONS, PRECAUTIONS, ADVERSE REACTIONS

CONTRAINDICATIONS

None known.

PRECAUTIONS

Squalene supplementation should be avoided in infants, children, pregnant women and nursing mothers.

ADVERSE REACTIONS

Those taking squalene supplements may have mild gastrointestinal symptoms such as diarrhea.

INTERACTIONS

None known.

OVERDOSAGE

There have been no reports of overdosage.

DOSAGE AND ADMINISTRATION

Squalene is a liquid that is available in capsules for oral use. Doses of 500 milligrams to 4 grams are used; the higher doses are used by some cancer sufferers. The source of squalene is usually from shark liver oil and sometimes from olive oil.

Squalene should not be confused with squalamine, which is an unusual steroid found in the dogfish shark and which has antibiotic properties.

HOW SUPPLIED

Capsules — 450 mg, 500 mg, 1000 mg

LITERATURE

Kelly GS. Squalene and its potential clinical uses. *Altern Med Rev.* 1999; 4:29-36.

Newmark HL, Squalene, olive oil, and cancer risk: a review and hypothesis. *Cancer Epidemiol Biomarkers Prev.* 1997; 6:1101-1103.

Rao CV, Newmark HL, Reddy BS. Chemopreventive effect of squalene on colon cancer. *Carcinogenesis.* 1998; 19:287-290.

Smith TJ, Yank GY, Seril DN, et al. Inhibition of 4-(methylnitrosamino)-1-(3-pyridyl)-1-butanone-induced lung tumorogenesis by dietary olive oil and squalene. *Carcinogenesis.* 1998; 19:703-706.

Storm HM, Oh SY, Kimler BF, Norton S. Radioprotection of mice by dietary squalene. *Lipids.* 1993; 28:555-559.

Sulforaphane

DESCRIPTION

Sulforaphane is the aglycone breakdown product of the glucosinolate glucoraphanin, also known as sulforaphane glucosinolate (SGS). Glucosinolates are beta-thioglucoside-N-hydroxysulfates and are primarily found in cruciferous vegetables (cabbage, broccoli, broccoli sprouts, brussels sprouts, cauliflower, cauliflower sprouts, bok choy, kale, collards, arugula, kohlrabi, mustard, turnip, red radish and watercress). Young broccoli sprouts and young cauliflower sprouts are especially rich in glucoraphanin.

Sulforaphane may have cancer chemopreventive activity. However, glucosinolates themselves typically have low anticancer activity. Sulforaphane is produced from sulforaphane glucosinolate via the action of the enzyme myrosinase (thioglucoside glucohydrolase), an enzyme present in cruciferous vegetables that is activated upon maceration of the vegetables.

Sulforaphane is also classified as an isothiocyanate. Its molecular formula is $C_6H_{11}NOS_2$, and its molecular weight is 177.29 daltons. It is also known as 4-methylsulfinylbutyl isothiocyanate and (-)-1-isothiocyanato-4(R)-(methylsulfinyl) butane. Sulforaphane glucosinolate (glucoraphanin) is also known as 4-methylsufinylbutyl glucosinolate. The structural formula is:

Sulforaphane

ACTIONS AND PHARMACOLOGY

ACTIONS

Sulforaphane may have anticarcinogenic activity.

MECHANISM OF ACTION

Sulforaphane's possible anticarcinogenic activity is accounted for by its ability to induce phase II detoxication enzymes, such as glutathione S-transferase and quinone reductase [NAD(P)H: (quinone-acceptor) oxidoreductase]. These enzymes may afford protection against certain carcinogens and other toxic electrophiles, including reactive oxygen species.

PHARMACOKINETICS

Little is presently known about the pharmacokinetics of sulforaphane in humans. Some preliminary studies indicate that sulforaphane is absorbed and that it is metabolized by first undergoing conjugation with reduced glutathione to form a dithiocarbamate. The dithiocarbamate is then converted sequentially to conjugates with cysteinylglycine, cysteine and N-acetylcysteine.

INDICATIONS AND USAGE

Experimental data suggest that sulforaphane may have anticarcinogenic effects.

RESEARCH SUMMARY

Sulforaphane has significantly reduced the incidence, multiplicity and rate of development of chemically induced mammary tumors in rats. It has demonstrated an ability to detoxify a number of carcinogens and thus might have the ability to protect against a variety of cancers. It has been shown that dietary supplementation with sulforaphane enhances glutathione S-transferase (GST) enzyme activity, which is known to detoxify many carcinogens.

One group of researchers has reported that three-day-old sprouts of certain broccoli and cauliflower cultivars contain 10 to 100 times higher levels of glucoraphanin, the glucosinolate of sulforaphane, than do mature broccoli and cauliflower sprouts. Thus they have concluded that "small quantities of crucifer sprouts may protect against the risk of cancer as effectively as much larger quantities of mature vegetables of the same variety." Additionally they have noted that the indole glucosinates that are prevalent in mature broccoli, for example, are present in only small quantities in the sprouts. One report suggested that the degradation products (e.g., indole-3-carbinol) of these glucosinates might themselves promote tumorigenesis, but several other investigators have not confirmed this.

CONTRAINDICATIONS, PRECAUTIONS, ADVERSE REACTIONS

CONTRAINDICATIONS

Sulforaphane is contraindicated in those who are hypersensitive to any component of a sulforaphane-containing product.

PRECAUTIONS

Pregnant women and nursing mothers should avoid sulforaphane supplementation pending long-term safety data.

ADVERSE REACTIONS

No adverse reactions reported.

DOSAGE AND ADMINISTRATION

Sulforaphane is available in a few different formulations, usually in combination with other dietary phytochemicals. There are no typical doses.

Sulforaphane, in the form of its glucosinolate glucoraphanin, is abundant in three-day old broccoli sprouts, which are available in the marketplace. The levels of glucoraphanin in three-day old broccoli sprouts are from 10 to 100 times greater than in mature broccoli.

LITERATURE

Fahey JW, Talalay P. Antioxidant functions of sulforaphane: a potent inducer of Phase II detoxification enzymes. *Food Chem Toxicol.* 1999; 37:973-979.

Fahey JW, Zhang Y, Talalay P. Broccoli sprouts: an exceptionally rich source of inducers of enzymes that protect against chemical carcinogens. *Proc Natl Acad Sci USA.* 1997; 94:10367-10372.

Faulkner K, Mithen R, Williamson G. Selective increase of the potential anticarcinogen 4-methylsulphinylbutyl glucosinolate in broccoli. *Carcinogenesis.* 1998; 19:605-609.

Singletary K, MacDonald C. Inhibition of benzo[a]pyrene- and 1, 6-dinitropyrene-DNA adduct formation in human mammary epithelial cells by dibenzoylmethane and sulforaphane. *Cancer Letters.* 2000; 155:47-54.

Zeligs MA. Diet and estrogen status: the cruciferous connection. *J Med Food.* 1998; 1:67-82.

Zhang Y. Role of glutathione in the accumulation of anticarcinogenic isothiocyanates and their glutathione conjugates by murine hepatoma cells. *Carcinogenesis.* 2000; 21:1175-1182.

Zhang Y. Talalay P, Cho CG, Posner GH. A major inducer of anticarcinogenic protective enzymes from broccoli: isolation and elucidation of structure. *Proc Natl Acad Sci USA.* 1992; 89:2399-2403.

Supplemental Enzymes

TRADE NAMES

Lactaid (McNeil Consumer)

DESCRIPTION

Enzymes are biological catalysts. Until recently, it was thought that all enzymes were protein in nature. It is now known that ribonucleic acids and other non-protein substances can have enzymatic activity, as well. Enzymes have important roles in medicine. They are used for the rapid lysis of blood clots (streptokinase, tissue plasminogen activator or TPA, urokinase) and for the treatment of Gaucher's disease (glucocerebrosidase), among other things. Enzymes are also used in the treatment of pancreatic insufficiency secondary to such disorders as cystic fibrosis and chronic alcoholic pancreatitis. Enzymes, in addition to being used therapeutically, are marketed as nutritional supplements. They are principally used as digestants. Some enzymes, in particular proteolytic enzymes, have putative anti-inflammatory and anticarcinogenic activities. The enzymes marketed for supplemental use are derived from animal, plant and fungal sources. The following describes the enzymes that are available in the nutritional supplement market place.

ALPHA-GALACTOSIDASE

Alpha-galactosidase is an enzyme that is derived from selected strains of the fungus *Aspergillus niger*. Alpha-galactosidase catalyzes the hydrolysis of the alpha-1→6 linkages in such carbohydrates as the disaccharide melibiose, the trisaccharide raffinose, the tetrasaccharide stachyose and the nonsaccharide verbascose. These oligosaccharides are widely found in legumes and cruciferous vegetables, including beans, peas, broccoli, brussels sprouts and cabbage. These carbohdyrates are gas productive in some. Hydrolysis of melibiose yields D-galactose and D-glucose; hydrolysis of raffinose yields D-galactose and sucrose; hydrolysis of stachyose yields D-galactose and sucrose; and verbascose yields D-galactose, D-glucose and D-fructose. The activity of alpha galactosidases is expressed in galactose units or GalU. A tablet of alpha-galactosidase typically contains 150 GalU.

AMYLASE

Amylases are enzymes that catalyze the hydrolysis of alpha-1, 4-glycosidic linkages of polysaccharides to yield dextrins, oligosaccharides, maltose and D-glucose. Amylases are derived from animal, fungal and plant sources. Pancreatin and pancrelipase contain amylase derived from the pancreas of animals, usually porcine pancreas. Amylase is also derived from barley malt and the fungus *Aspergillus oryzae*. There are a few different amylases. These enzymes are classified according to the manner in which the glysosidic bond is attacked. Alpha-amylases hydrolyze alpha-1, 4-glycosidic linkages, randomly yielding dextrins, oligosaccharides and monosaccharides. Alpha-amylases are endo-amylases. Exoamylases hydrolyze the alpha-1, 4-glycosidic linkage only from the non-reducing outer polysaccharide chain ends. Exoamylases include beta-amylases and glucoamylases (gamma-amylases, amyloglucosidases). Beta-amylases yield beta-limit dextrins and maltose. Gamma-amylases yield glucose. Amylases are used as digestants. Amylase activity is expressed as Dextrinizing Units or DU.

BROMELAIN

Bromelain refers to proteolytic enzymes which are derived from the ripe and unripe fruit, as well as the stem and leaves, of the pineapple plant, *Ananas comosus (Ananas sativus)*.

Bromelain is comprised of several proteolytic enzymes which differ in their specificities. These enzymes hydrolyze proteins to form oligopeptides and amino acids. Bromelain is used as a digestive aid. It also has putative anti-inflammatory activity. The activity of bromelain may be expressed in bromelain units or BU. The assay is based on a 60-minute proteolytic hydrolysis of casein at pH 6.0 and 40°C. One BU is defined as that quantity of enzyme that liberates the equivalent of one microgram of L-tyrosine per hour. The bromelain proteolytic enzymes are cysteine proteinases. There are at least four distinct bromelain cysteine proteinases. The activity of bromelain may also be expressed in gelatin dissolving units (GDU) or milk clotting units (MCU). One GDU is equivalent to about 1.5 MCU.

CELLULASE
Cellulase is an enzyme derived from the fungi *Aspergillus niger* and *Trichoderma longbrachiatum* or other sources. Cellulose is an indigestible plant polysaccharide. It is the principal constituent of the cell wall of plants. Cellulase has cellulolytic activity, meaning that it hydrolyzes cellulose. Cellulase hydrolyzes the beta-D-1, 4-glycosidic bonds of cellulose. Cellulase derived from *Trichoderma longbrachiatum* is comprised of an enzyme complex consisting of cellulase, a glucosidase, cellobiohydrolase and a glucanase. This complex converts cellulose to beta-dextrins and ultimately to D-glucose. Cellulase is used as a digestive aid, particularly in animals, and for the management of flatulence. The activity of cellulase is expressed in cellulose units or CU.

CHYMOTRYPSIN
Chymotrypsin is a proteolytic enzyme that is principally derived from ox pancreas. Chymotrypsin is a serine proteinase, referring to the fact that serine and histidine residues at the active site are involved in catalysis. Trypsin, also a serine proteinase, and chymotrypsin have similar tertiary structures although very different substrate specificities. Trypsin hydrolyzes peptides at Lys/Arg residues while chymotrypsin recognizes large hydrophobic residues. Chymotrypsin is found in pancreatic preparations, such as pancreatin and pancrelipase. It is used in ophthalmology for the dissection of the zonule of the lens. It is also used as a digestant and it has putative anti-inflammatory activity.

LACTASE
Lactase or beta-galactosidase is an enzyme that is derived from the fungus *Kluyveromyces lactis* (formerly known as *Saccharomyces lactis*) or from the fungus *Aspergillus oryzae*. Lactase hydrolyzes the lactose beta-D-galactoside linkage, yielding D-galactose and D-glucose. Lactase may be helpful to those with lactose or milk sugar intolerance. The activity of lactase supplements is expressed in acid lactase units or ALU. A regular strength lactase caplet typically contains 4,500 ALU. Lactase derived from *Kluyveromyces lactis* is used to pretreat milk for use by those with lactose intolerance. The activity of lactase in milk is expressed in neutral lactase units or NLU. The maximum recommended dose of lactase in milk is 3,000 NLU per liter.

PANCREATIN
Pancreatin is a pancreatic enzyme preparation derived from hog pancreas. Pancreatin is comprised of the pancreatic enzymes trypsin, amylase and lipase. Pancreatin and pancrelipase are similar except that pancrelipase has relatively more lipase activity than does pancreatin. Trypsin hydrolyzes proteins to oligopeptides, amylase hydrolyzes starch to oligosaccharides and the disaccharide maltose, and lipase hydrolyzes triglycerides to fatty acids and glycerol. Pancreatin is a digestant that is used in the treatment of pancreatic insufficiency as pancreatic enzyme replacement. A typical 500-milligram tablet of pancreatin contains 12,500 USP units of trypsin, 12,500 USP units of amylase and 1,000 USP units of lipase.

PANCRELIPASE
Pancrelipase is a standardized preparation of porcine pancreas that principally contains the pancreatic enzymes lipase, trypsin and amylase. Pancrelipase is similar to pancreatin except that it has relatively more lipase activity than pancreatin. Lipase hydrolyzes triglycerides to fatty acids and glycerol. Amylase hydrolyzes starch to oligosaccharides and the disaccharide maltose, and trypsin hydrolyzes proteins to oligopeptides. Pancrelipase is a digestant. It is used in the treatment of steatorrhea secondary to pancreatic insufficiency such as occurs in cystic fibrosis or in chronic alcoholic pancreatitis. A typical capsule of pancrelipase contains 4,500 USP (United States Pharmacopoeia) units of lipase, 25,000 USP units of trypsin and 20,000 USP units of amylase.

PAPAIN
Papain is a mixture of proteolytic enzymes derived from the juice of the unripe fruit of the tropical plant *Caroica papaya*, commonly known as papaya. Papain hydrolyzes proteins to form oligopeptides and amino acids. Papain also contains the proteolytic enzyme chymopapain which differs from papain in electrophoretic mobility, solubility and substrate specificity. The molecular weight of chymopapain is approximately 27,000 daltons. Papain is used as a digestive aid. It is also used as a meat tenderizer. Papain has putative anti-inflammatory activity. The activity of papain is expressed in papain units or PU. The assay of papain activity is based on the hydrolysis of casein.

PEPSIN
Pepsin is a proteolytic enzyme which is secreted by the stomach where it hydrolyzes proteins to polypeptides and oligopeptides. Pepsin that is derived from animal tissue is

sometimes used in combination with dilute hydrochloric acid or betaine hydrochloride as an adjunct in the management of gastric hypochlorhydria.

TRYPSIN

Trypsin is a proteolytic enzyme which is principally derived from porcine pancreas. It is a serine proteinase, referring to the fact that serine and histidine residues at the active site are involved in catalytic activity. Chymotrypsin, also a serine proteinase, and trypsin have similar tertiary structures, although very different substrate specificities. Trypsin hydrolyzes peptides at Lys/Arg residues, while chymotrypsin recognizes large hydrophobic residues. Trypsin is found in pancreatic preparations, such as pancreatin and pancrelipase; it has been used for the debridement of wounds. It is used as a digestant and it has putative anti-inflammatory activity.

SUPEROXIDE DISMUTASE

Superoxide dismutases are enzymes that play major roles in the protection of cells against oxidative damage. The two major forms of superoxide dismutase (SOD) in humans are the mitochondrial manganese SOD and the cytosolic copper/zinc SOD. A copper/zinc SOD, isolated from beef liver, has been used intra-articularly for degenerative joint disorders as an anti-inflammatory agent. SOD is also marketed as a nutritional supplement. Oral SOD has putative anti-inflammatory activity.

WOBE-MUGOS/WOBENZYME

Wobe-Mugos and Wobenzyme are proprietary enzyme preparations that have putative anti-inflammatory and anticarcinogenic activities. Wobe-Mugos contains the proteolytic enzymes papain, trypsin and chymotrypsin. The papain is derived from the fruit of the papaya plant. Trypsin and chymotrypsin are derived from bovine pancreas. Wobenzyme contains pancreatin, papain, bromelain, trypsin and chymotrypsin. Pancreatin, which contains amylase, trypsin and lipase, is derived from porcine pancreas. Bromelain is derived from the pineapple plant. The activity of the proteolytic enzymes in Wobe-Mugos and Wobenzyme is expressed in FIP units. The FIP unit is the measurement of enzyme activity according to the test methods of the Federation Internationale Pharmaceutique. Wobe-Mugos (papain, trypsin and chymotrypsin) is an orphan drug for the treatment of multiple myeloma.

ACTIONS AND PHARMACOLOGY
ACTIONS

Alpha-galactosidase, amylase, bromelain, cellulase, chymotrypsin, lactase, pancreatin, pancrelipase, papain and pepsin have digestant activities. Bromelain, chymotrypsin, papain, and trypsin have putative anti-inflammatory activity. Superoxide dismutase has putative anti-inflammatory activity.

Wobe-Mugos and Wobenzyme have putative anti-inflammatory and anticarcinogenic activities.

MECHANISM OF ACTION

Alpha-galactosidase hydrolyzes melibiose to D-galactose, and D-glucose; raffinose to D-galactose and sucrose; stachyose to D-galactose; and sucrose and verbascose to D-galactose, D-glucose and D-fructose. Amylase hydrolyzes starch to oligosaccharides and maltose. Bromelain hydrolyzes proteins to oligopeptides and amino acids. Cellulase hydrolyzes cellulose to D-glucose. Chymotrypsin hydrolyzes proteins to oligopeptides. Lactase hydrolyzes lactose to D-galactose and D-glucose. Pancreatin and pancrelipase hydrolyze triglycerides to fatty acids and glycerol, proteins to oligopeptides and starch to oligosaccharides and maltose. Papain hydrolyzes proteins to oligopeptides and amino acids. Pepsin hydrolyzes proteins to polypeptides and oligopeptides. Trypsin hydrolyzes proteins to oligopeptides.

The mechanism of the putative anti-inflammatory activity of the proteolytic enzymes bromelain, chymotrypsin, papain and trypsin are not well understood. It is believed that a fraction of these proteolytic enzymes is absorbed probably via the enteropancreatic circulation. It is speculated that the putative anti-inflammatory activity of these enzymes may be accounted for, in part, by their activation of plasmin production from plasminogen and by their reduction of kinin via inhibition of the conversion of kininogen to kinin. Degradation of circulating immune complexes may be another possible mechanism.

The putative anti-inflammatory and anticarcinogenic activities of Wobe-Mugos and Wobenzyme are also open to speculation. Possibilities include a decrease of circulating immune complexes, disruption of adhesion molecules on tumor and endothelial cells, degradation of cytokines and cytokine receptors and possible immunomodulatory effects. Bromelain is speculated to play a role in differentiation of malignant cells.

The mechanism of the putative anti-inflammatory activity of superoxide dismutase is unknown.

PHARMACOKINETICS

The fungal- and plant-derived enzymes appear more resistant to inactivation and denaturation by stomach acid than are the animal-derived enzymes. Pancreatin and pancrelipase require enteric coating to prevent denaturation and inactivation by stomach acid. In the small intestine, a fraction of the enzymes may be absorbed via the enteropancreatic circulation. Much is unknown regarding the pharmacokinetics of oral enzymes in humans.

INDICATIONS AND USAGE

Supplemental enzymes (alpha-galactosidase, chymotrypsin lactase, pancreatin, pancrelipase, papain and pepsin) are used as digestive aids in some circumstances. Some (bromelain, superoxide dismutase, chymotrypsin, papain and trypsin) are said to have some anti-inflammatory activity. There is some evidence that Wobe-Mugos and Wobenzyme may have some anti-inflammatory and anticarcinogenic activities.

RESEARCH SUMMARY

Supplemental enzymes have been used for some time as digestive aids with various degrees of efficacy. Those with digestive disorders, however, should not use digestive enzymes unless they are approved by their physicians. Pancreatin is used pharmaceutically in some with pancreatic insufficiency secondary to such disorders as cystic fibrosis and chronic alcoholic pancreatitis. It is used in this context as pancreatic enzyme replacement therapy. Pancrelipase is used in the treatment of steatorrhea secondary to pancreatic insufficiency related, again, to such disorders as cystic fibrosis and chronic alcoholic pancreatitis.

Pepsin, in combination with dilute hydrochloric acid has been used as an adjunctive treatment of gastric hypochlorhydria. Papain is used as a digestant. Lactase is effective in some with milk sugar (lactose) intolerance, and cellulase has reportedly been of benefit in some with flatulence. Amylases have been used as digestants, as has chymotrypsin and bromelain. Alpha-galactosidase is used to manage flatulence in those who develop ''gas'' from the consumption of certain foods, such as beans. Superoxide dismutase, used intra-articularly, has reportedly shown some anti-inflammatory effects in animals, but clinical studies are lacking.

More studies have been done on bromelain, Wobe-Mugos and Wobenzyme. Bromelain is a major constituent of Wobenzyme, which also includes pancreatin, papain, trypsin and chymotrypsin. Wobe-Mugos contains papain, trypsin and chymotrypsin. These enzyme preparations have demonstrated some anti-inflammatory and anticarcinogenic activity. Wobe-Mugos is an orphan drug for use in the treatment of multiple myeloma.

Wobe-Mugos and Wobenzyme have shown an ability to clear circulating immune complexes from the body, in both animal and human experiments. These antibody/antigen complexes have been implicated in some inflammatory processes, including those related to rheumatoid arthritis and some other autoimmune diseases. Antigen-induced experimental arthritis in rabbits was inhibited by these enzyme preparations in one experiment. Wobenzyme reportedly improved the condition of patients with chronic polyarthritis in another study. No side effects were noted. Recently, significant pain reduction was associated with use of these proteolytic enzyme preparations in subjects with osteoarthritis of the knee and periarthritis of the shoulder.

Long-term rectal administration of Wobe-Mugos has been reported to inhibit growth of solid tumors and development of experimental metastases in mice inoculated with B16 melanoma cells. In another recent study, Wobe-Mugos significantly increased survival time in mice with Lewis lung carcinoma. In a recent randomized trial, Wobe-Mugos was said to significantly reduce the acute sequelae of radiation in head and neck cancers.

There is a report in which Wobe-Mugos was tested in comparison with acyclovir in subjects with herpes zoster. The enzyme preparation was said to be as efficacious as acyclovir in alleviating pain. Effects on skin lesions were largely equal. More study is needed.

CONTRAINDICATIONS, PRECAUTIONS, ADVERSE REACTIONS

CONTRAINDICATIONS

Supplemental enzymes are contraindicated in those hypersensitive to any component of an enzyme-containing preparation.

PRECAUTIONS

The use of digestive enzymes for the treatment of pancreatic insufficiency requires medical supervision.

Those who wish to use supplemental enzymes for any indication should first discuss their use with their physicians.

Pregnant women and nursing mothers should avoid supplemental enzymes unless prescribed by their physicians.

Galactosemics should avoid the use of alpha-galactosidase. D-galactose is one of the substances formed via the action of alpha-galactosidase.

Those on anticoagulants or antithrombotic agents should be cautious in the use of bromelain. Bromelain may have blood-thinning activity in some.

ADVERSE REACTIONS

Alpha-galactosidase: Gastrointestinal symptoms such as cramping and diarrhea have been reported. Allergic-type reactions, including rash and pruritis, have also been reported.

Amylase: Allergic-type reactions, including rash and pruritis, have been reported.

Bromelain: Gastrointestinal symptoms such as nausea and vomiting, diarrhea and cramping, have been reported. Metrorrhagia and menorrhagia have been occasionally reported. Hypersensitivity reactions have been reported, including rashes and exacerbation of asthma.

Pancreatin: The most frequently reported adverse reactions are gastrointestinal and include diarrhea, abdominal pain, nausea and vomiting. Hyperuricemia has been reported with the use of pancreatin products.

Pancrelipase. The most frequently reported adverse reactions are gastrointestinal and include diarrhea, abdominal pain, nausea and vomiting, constipation, melena and perianal irritation. Hyperuricemia and hyperuricosuria have been reported with the use of pancrelipase products, primarily with non-enteric coated formulations. Cases of fibrosing colonopathy have been reported primarily in cystic fibrosis patients.

Wobe-Mugos/Wobenzyme: The most frequently reported adverse reactions are gastrointestinal and include diarrhea, abdominal pain, nausea and vomiting. There is a report of an anaphylactic reaction in a woman receiving intramuscular injections of Wobe-Mugos. There is a report of circulatory shock in a woman receiving injections and suppositories of Wobe-Mugos, as well as Wobenzyme tablets.

INTERACTIONS

DRUGS

Acarbose: Concomitant intake of enzyme preparations (containing amylase, pancreatin, pancrelipase) and acarbose may decrease the efficacy of acarbose.

Anticoagulants (e.g., warfarin): Bromelain may enhance the anticoagulant activity of such drugs as warfarin.

Antithrombotic agents (e.g., aspirin): Bromelain may enhance the antithrombotic activity of such drugs as aspirin.

NUTRITIONAL SUPPLEMENTS

Folic acid: Pancreatic enzymes (pancreatin, pancrelipase) have been reported to decrease the absorption of folic acid if taken concomitantly. However, this has not been substantiated.

Soy oligosaccharides: Concomitant intake of alpha-galactosidase and soy oligosaccharide prebiotics, may inactivate the prebiotic activity of the soy oligosaccharides.

DOSAGE AND ADMINISTRATION

Supplemental enzymes are available in the nutritional supplement marketplace; pancreatin and pancrelipase are available as pharmaceutical agents for the treatment of pancreatic insufficiency. Supplemental enzymes that are available include alpha-galactosidase, alpha-amylase, amyloglucosidase, bromelain, cellulase, chymotrypsin, hemicellulase, lactase, lipase, pepsin, protease, superoxide dismutase, trypsin and Wobenzyme. A plant-derived analogue of pancreatin is also available. Those who wish to use supplementary enzymes should first discuss their use, as well as dosage, with their physicians.

LITERATURE

Anthony H, Collins CE, Davidson G, et al. Pancreatic enzyme replacement therapy in cystic fibrosis: Australian guidelines. *J Pediatr—Child Health.* 1999; 35:125-129.

Billigmann P. [Enzyme therapy—an alternative in treatment of herpes zoster. A controlled study of 192 patients]. [Article in German]. *Fortschr Med.* 1995; 113:43-48.

Bock U, Kolac C, Borchard G, et al. Transport of proteolytic enzymes across Caco-2 cell monolayers. *Pharm Res.* 1998; 15:1393-1400.

Coenen TMM, Bertens AMC, De Hoog SCM, Verspeek-Rip CM. Safety evaluation of a lactase enzyme preparation derived from *Kluyveromyces lactis. Food Chem Toxicol.* 2000; 38:671-677.

de Smet PA, Pegt GW, Meyboom RH. [Acute circulatory shock following administration of the non-regular enzyme preparation Wobe-Mugos]. [Article in Dutch]. Ned Tijdschr *Geneeskd.* 1991; 135:2341-2344.

Dominguez-Munoz JE, Birckelbach U, Glassbrenner B, et al. Effect of oral pancreatic enzyme administration on digestive function in healthy subjects: comparison between two enzyme preparations. *Aliment Pharmacol Ther.* 1997; 11:403-408.

Eckert K, Grabowska E, Stange R, et al. Effects of oral bromelain administration on the impaired immunocytotoxicity of mononuclear cells from mammary tumor patients. *Oncol Rep.* 1999; 6:1191-1199.

Farkas G, Takacs T, Baradnay G, Szasz Z. [Effect of pancreatin replacement on pancreatic function in the postoperative period after pancreatic surgery]. [Article in Hungarian]. *Orv Hetil.* 1999; 140:2751-2754.

Greenberger NJ. Enzymatic therapy in patients with chronic pancreatitis. *Gastrenterol Clin North Am.* 1999; 28:687-693.

Kaul R, Mishra BK, Sutrador P, et al. The role of Wobe-Mugos in reducing acute sequelae of radiation in head and neck cancers—a clinical phase-III randomized trial. *Indian J Cancer.* 1999; 36:141-148.

Kiessling WR. [Anaphylactic reaction in enzyme therapy of multiple sclerosis]. [Article in German]. *Fortschr Neurol Psychiatr.* 1987; 55:385-386.

Klein G, Kullich W. [Reducing pain by oral enzyme therapy in rheumatic diseases]. [Article in German]. *Wien Med Wochenschr.* 1999; 149:577-580.

Rowan AD, Buttle DJ, Barrett AJ. The cysteine proteinases of the pineapple plant. *Biochem J.* 1990; 266:869-875.

Stauder G, Ransberger K, Streichhan P, et al. The use of hydrolytic enzymes as adjuvant therapy in AIDS/ARC/LAS patients. *Biomed Pharmacother.* 1988; 42:31-34.

Steffen C, Menzel J. [Enzyme breakdown of immune complexes]. [Article in German]. *Z Rheumatol.* 1983; 42:249-255.

Steffen C, Smolen J, Miehlke K, et al. [Enzyme therapy in comparison with immune complex determinations in chronic polyarthritis]. [Article in German]. *Z Rheumatol.* 1985; 44:51-56.

Wald M, Olejár T, Pouková P, Zadinova M. Proteinases reduce metastatic dissemination and increase survival time in C57B16 mice with the Lewis lung carcinoma. *Life Sciences.* 1998; 63:PL237-243.

Wald M, Závadová E, Pouková P, et al. Polyenzyme preparation Wobe-Mugos inhibits growth of solid tumors and development of experimental metastases in mice. *Life Sciences.* 1998; 62:PL43-48.

Wolf M, Ransberger K. [Effect of proteolytic enzymes on the reciprocal growth modification of normal and tumor tissues]. [Article in German]. *Arch Geschwultstforsch.* 1968; 31:317-331.

Synbiotics

DESCRIPTION

Synbiotics refer to combination nutritional supplements comprised of probiotics and prebiotics. Probiotics (see Probiotics) are live microbial food supplements that beneficially affect the host by improving its intestinal microflora balance. Prebiotics (see Prebiotics) are nondigestible dietary substances, typically oligosaccharides and disaccharides, that beneficially affect the host by selectively stimulating the growth and/or activity of a limited number of bacterial species already resident in the large intestine.

Synbiotics could improve the survival of the probiotic organism by providing the specific substrate to the probiotic organism for its fermentation.

Synbiotic supplements that are currently available, include combinations of bifidobacteria and fructo-oligosaccharides (FOS), *Lactobacillus* GG and inulins and bifidobacteria and lactobacilli and FOS or inulins.

ACTIONS AND PHARMACOLOGY

ACTIONS

Synbiotics may have antimicrobial, anticarcinogenic, immunomodulatory, antidiarrheal, antiallergenic, hypolipidemic and hypoglycemic activities. They may also have activity in improving mineral absorption and balance and may have anti-osteoporotic activity.

MECHANISM OF ACTION

The antimicrobial activity of the synbiotics can be accounted for by the probiotic component of these substances. The bacteria can reinforce the barrier function of the intestinal mucosa, helping in the prevention of the attachment of pathogenic bacteria to the intestinal wall, essentially by crowding them out. These bacteria may also produce antimicrobial substances and stimulate antigen specific and nonspecific immune responses.

The possible anticarcinogenic activity of synbiotics is not well understood. The prebiotic oligosaccharides are fermented by the probiotic bacteria, as well as other bacteria that reside in the colon, to butyrate and other short-chain fatty acids. Butyrate may induce growth arrest and cell differentiation and may also upregulate apoptosis, three activities which could be significant for the possible anticarcinogenic activity of butyrate. The prebiotic oligosaccharides may also aid in increasing the concentrations of calcium and magnesium in the colon. Elevated concentrations of these cations in the colon may help to control the rate of cell turnover. Elevated concentrations of calcium in the colon may also help to control the formation of insoluble bile or salts of fatty acids. This might reduce the potential damaging effects of bile or fatty acids on colonocytes. The probiotic bacteria may bind to and inactivate some carcinogens and may directly inhibit the growth of some tumors as well as some bacteria that may convert precarcinogens into carcinogens.

The probiotic bacteria may increase levels of circulating immunoglobulin A (IgA) and enhance nonspecific immune mechanisms, such as increasing phagocytic activity.

Probiotics that colonize the colon may be helpful in the management of some with food allergies, helping to reinforce the barrier function of the intestinal mucosa, thus possibly preventing aberrant absorption of intraluminal antigens.

The prebiotics may lower triglyceride levels in some. The mechanism of this possible effect is unclear. Decreased hepatocyte *de novo* synthesis of triglycerides is one hypothetical possibility. The prebiotics may also lower total cholesterol and LDL-cholesterol levels in some. Again, the mechanism of this possible effect is unclear. Propionate, a product of prebiotic oligosaccharide fermentation in the colon, may inhibit HMG-CoA reductase.

The mechanism of the possible effect of the prebiotic oligosaccharides on modulating serum levels glucose is not well understood, but could be accounted for in a few ways. The oligosaccharides may delay gastric emptying and/or shorten small-intestinal tract transit time. This may be via the short-chain fatty acids produced from the oligosaccharides in the colon. Short-chain fatty acids may also stimulate contractions of the ileum and shorten ileal emptying. In addition, propionate may inhibit gluconeogenesis, reduce serum levels of free fatty acids and enhance glycolysis.

The oligosaccharides may bind/sequester such minerals as calcium and magnesium in the small intestine. The short-chain fatty acids formed from the bacterial fermentation of the oligosaccharides may facilitate the colonic absorption of calcium and, possibly, also magnesium ions. This could be beneficial in the prevention of osteoporosis.

PHARMACOKINETICS

The effectiveness of probiotics is related to their ability to survive in the acid stomach environment and the alkaline conditions in the duodenum as well as to their ability to adhere to the intestinal mucosa of the large intestine and to colonize the colon. After passage through the stomach and the small intestine, those probiotics that do survive become established transiently in the colon.

Following ingestion, the prebiotic oligosaccharides reach the colon with little of them being digested in the upper gastrointestinal tract. The oligosaccharides are fermented by bifidobacteria, lactobacilli and some other bacteria in the colon to produce the short-chain fatty acids acetate, propionate and butyrate; the gases hydrogen, hydrogen sulfide, carbon dioxide and methane; and lactate, pyruvate, succinate and formate. Acetate, propionate and butyrate that are not metabolized in colonocytes are absorbed from the colon and transported via the portal circulation to the liver. These short-chain fatty acids are extensively metabolized in hepatocytes. Acetate, propionate and butyrate that are not metabolized in hepatocytes are transported by the circulation to various tissues where they undergo further metabolism. Butyrate is an important respiratory fuel for colonocytes.

INDICATIONS AND USAGE

Synbiotics are useful for the same indications as prebiotics and probiotics. Some may protect against intestinal pathogens and ameliorate the severity of some inflammatory bowel diseases. Some may be helpful in antibiotic associated diarrhea, as well as some infectious and viral diarrheas. They may have some immune-enhancing, anticarcinogenic, anti-osteoporotic, glucose-modulating and lipid-modulating effects.

RESEARCH SUMMARY

See Probiotics and Prebiotics.

CONTRAINDICATIONS, PRECAUTIONS, ADVERSE REACTIONS

CONTRAINDICATIONS

Synbiotics are contraindicated in those who are hypersensitive to any component of a synbiotic-containing supplement.

PRECAUTIONS

Pregnant women and nursing mothers should only use synbiotic supplementation if prescribed by their physicians.

ADVERSE REACTIONS

The most common adverse reaction to synbiotics is flatulence.

INTERACTIONS

NUTRITIONAL SUPPLEMENTS

Minerals (calcium, magnesium): Concomitant intake of calcium or magnesium supplements and synbiotics may enhance the colonic absorption of these minerals.

FOODS

Synbiotics, via their prebiotic oligosaccharides, may enhance the colonic absorption of calcium and magnesium in foods.

DOSAGE AND ADMINISTRATION

Synbiotic supplements that are currently available include combinations of bifidobacteria and fructo-oligosaccharides (FOS), Lactobacillus GG and inulins and bifidobacteria and lactobacilli and FOS or inulins. New combinations are currently being developed.

Probiotic intake typically ranges from one to ten billion colony-forming units a few times a week. Doses of prebiotics, in the form of synbiotics, are variable.

LITERATURE

Collins MD, Gibson GR. Probiotics, prebiotics, and synbiotics: approaches for modulating the microbial ecology of the gut. *Am J Clin Nutr.* 1999; 69(suppl):1052S-1057S.

Macfarlane GT, Cummings JH. Probiotics and prebiotics: can regulating the activities of intestinal bacteria benefit health? *West J Med.* 1999; 17:187-191.

Roberfroid MB. Prebiotics and synbiotics: concepts and nutritional properties. *Br J Nutr.* 1998; 80:S197-S202.

For additional Literature, see Prebiotics and Probiotics.

Taurine

TRADE NAMES

Mega Taurine (Twinlab)

DESCRIPTION

Taurine is a nonprotein amino acid. It is an end product of L-cysteine metabolism and the principal free intracellular amino acid in many tissues of humans and other animal species. Taurine is present in high amounts in the brain, retina, myocardium, skeletal and smooth muscle, platelets and neutrophils. It is classified as a conditionally essential amino acid because it is necessary to be supplied in the diet of infants for normal retinal and brain development.

Research of taurine was greatly stimulated by the finding that it is an essential nutrient for cats. Taurine deficiency in cats can result in a variety of clinical abnormalities, including central retinal degeneration, dilated cardiomyopathy and platelet function abnormalities. Shortly after the discovery that dietary taurine deficiency leads to retinal degeneration in cats, it was observed that infants who were fed formulas lacking taurine had lower plasma levels of this amino acid than did infants fed human milk. Further, it was discovered that children receiving total parenteral nutrition not containing taurine had abnormal electroretinograms, as well as low plasma taurine levels. Taurine has been added to most human infant formulas since the mid-1980s.

Taurine is produced in the body from L-cysteine. The first reaction in the pathway is the formation of cysteine sulfinic acid. Cysteine sulfinic acid (CSA) is converted to hypotaurine via the enzyme CSA-decarboxylase, and taurine is formed from hypotaurine. Cats have low activity of CSA-decarboxylase. Dietary taurine mainly comes from animal food. Taurine is present in very low levels in plant foods. Taurine is found in seaweeds.

The most understood role of taurine in humans is its involvement in the formation of taurine bile acid conjugates in the liver, which are essential for micelle formation and fat absorption. Taurine is involved in the pre-and post-natal development of the central nervous system and visual system, although the details of its involvement in these processes are unclear. Taurine also has antioxidant and membrane-stabilizing activities. Much remains to be learned about the role of taurine in human physiology.

Taurine is different from most biological amino acids in a few particulars. It is a sulfonic acid rather than a carboxylic acid; it is a beta-amino acid rather than an alpha-amino acid and it does not have a chiral center. Taurine is also known as 2-aminoethane sulfonic acid. Its molecular formula is $C_2H_7NO_3 S$, and its molecular weight is 215.15 daltons.

ACTIONS AND PHARMACOLOGY
ACTIONS
Taurine has antioxidant activity. It has putative hypocholesterolemic, hypotensive, antiatherogenic and detoxifying activities. It may also have steatorrhea-reducing activity in those with cystic fibrosis and has putative antidiabetic, inotropic and antiseizure activities.

The major antioxidant activity of taurine derives from its ability to scavenge the reactive oxygen species hypochlorite, which is generated in neutrophils during respiratory-burst activity of these cells. Taurine reacts with excess hypochlorite produced in the process of phagocytosis to form the relatively harmless N-chlorotaurine. N-chlorotaurine is then reduced to taurine and chloride. This activity may protect against collateral tissue damage that can occur from the respiratory burst of neutrophils. Taurine may also suppress peroxidation of membrane lipoproteins by other reactive oxygen species. It is thought that this effect is not due to taurine's scavenging of these reactive oxygen species, but rather to taurine's membrane-stabilizing activity, which confers greater resistance to the membrane lipoproteins against lipid peroxidation.

Taurine has been demonstrated to reduce cholesterol levels in animals, but results in humans have been contradictory. The hypocholesterolemic effect of taurine in animals is thought to be due, in large part, to the stimulation of bile acid synthesis and enhancement of cholesterol 7 alpha-hydroxylase activity. Taurine has been found to have antiatherogenic activity in animals, but there is less evidence that it does in humans. The antiatherogenic activity of taurine in animals is thought to be due, in large part, to its hypocholesterolemic activity.

Taurine has been found to normalize blood pressure in spontaneous hypertensive rats, and there is some evidence from human studies that it also has hypotensive activity in hypertensive, but not normotensive, individuals. It is speculated that the hypotensive effect of taurine may result from the normalization of increased sympathetic activity in hypertensive individuals.

Taurine has been found to ameliorate bleomycin-induced lung fibrosis in hamsters and also to ameliorate the side effects of some nitrogen mustards. It is thought that the possible antioxidant and membrane-stabilizing activities of taurine may account for these detoxifying actions.

Some studies have shown decreased steatorrhea in cystic fibrosis patients receiving taurine. It is though that the mechanism of this effect is taurine's stimulation of bile acid formation resulting in increased fat absorption in these individuals.

Again in animals, but not in humans, taurine has been found to have antidiabetic activity. The mechanism of this effect is unclear. It is thought that taurine may decrease insulin resistance.

Cats who are deficient in taurine develop dilated cardiomyopathy and congestive heart failure. Taurine has an inotropic effect when given to these animals. Some studies suggest that taurine has an inotropic effect in humans with congestive heart failure. The mechanism of this possible effect is unclear. It is thought that taurine may modulate the calcium current.

The mechanism of taurine's putative antiseizure activity is unknown.

PHARMACOKINETICS
Following ingestion, taurine is absorbed from the small intestine via the beta-amino acid or taurine transport system, a sodium- and chloride-dependent carrier system that serves gamma-aminobutyric acid and beta-alanine, as well as taurine. This carrier system is located in the apical membrane of intestinal mucosa cells. Taurine is transported to the liver via the portal circulation, where much of it forms conjugates with bile acids. Taurocholate, the bile salt conjugate of taurine and cholic acid, is the principal conjugate formed via the action of the enzyme choloyl-CoA N-acyltransferase. The taurine conjugates are excreted via the biliary route. Taurine that is not conjugated in the liver is distributed via the systemic circulation to various tissues in

the body. Taurine is not usually completely reabsorbed from the kidneys, and some fraction of an ingested dose of taurine is excreted in the urine.

INDICATIONS AND USAGE

Taurine may be helpful in some with congestive heart failure and hypertension. It has demonstrated some antiatherogenic effects in both animal and human studies. There is the suggestion, mostly from animal data, that taurine might improve glucose tolerance and protect against some toxins. Some older studies suggest if might have some antiseizure activity. There is preliminary evidence that it might be helpful in some with cystic fibrosis.

RESEARCH SUMMARY

In a study of 24 subjects with congestive heart failure, administration of 2 grams of taurine, twice a day, resulted in clinical improvement in 19 patients. Roentgenographic data helped confirm the improvement. These positive results were subsequently confirmed in a double-blind, randomized, crossover, placebo-controlled study in which taurine was added to conventional treatment for a four-week period. Compared with placebo, taurine produced significant improvement as evaluated by a number of measures, including chest films. In still another study, supplemental taurine, but not coenzyme Q10, was said to have significant benefit in patients with congestive heart failure secondary to ischemic or idiopathic dilated cardiomyopathy. This was a double-blind study using 3 grams of taurine daily.

Taurine has demonstrated hypotensive effects in some animal studies. In humans, it has lowered blood pressure in borderline hypertensive patients using 6 grams of taurine daily for seven days. Lipid-lowering effects have been seen in animals, but human data are few and contradictory. There is some preliminary evidence from one small study that 0.4 to 1.6 grams of taurine daily for eight days inhibited platelet aggregation in a dose-dependent manner. Supplementation with 1.5 grams of taurine daily decreased platelet aggregation in subjects with type 1 diabetes. Insulin sensitivity was significantly improved by taurine supplementation in a rat model of spontaneous type 2 diabetes. Serum cholesterol and triacylglycerol were decreased in the supplemented animals. Taurine was also effective in another animal model of insulin resistance.

Taurine has exerted some detoxifying effects in animal experiments. It helped prevent bleomycin-induced lung injury and fibrosis in mice. It also appeared to have protective effects, as measured by changes in memory and lipid peroxidation levels in the brain, in rats exposed to ozone. Additionally, it has inhibited ethanol-induced elevation of plasma acetaldehyde in other animal studies. In one

of these, it prevented the development of ethanol-induced hypertension in rats.

In some older studies, taurine demonstrated some preliminary ability to suppress some epileptic seizures. Follow-up is needed.

Finally, taurine was shown to be of benefit in a study of 22 Canadian children with cystic fibrosis and documented steatorrhea. They were given taurine (30 mg/kg/day) and placebo during separate six-month periods. Severity of fat malabsorption was significantly reduced in most of the subjects, especially in those with the most severe steatorrhea. A more recent study, however, failed to note these benefits, but significant differences in the two study groups may account for this discrepancy. A second study by the Canadian group showed positive effects of taurine on fat absorption in cystic fibrosis patients. Again, those with the greatest malabsorption at baseline seemed to benefit the most.

CONTRAINDICATIONS, PRECAUTIONS, ADVERSE REACTIONS
CONTRAINDICATIONS

Taurine is contraindicated in those hypersensitive to any component of a taurine-containing nutritional supplement.

PRECAUTIONS

Pregnant women and nursing mothers should avoid taurine supplements unless recommended by their physicians. Those with congestive heart failure should only use taurine under medical supervision.

ADVERSE REACTIONS

No reports of adverse reactions.

INTERACTIONS
DRUGS

In animal studies, taurine was found to ameliorate the pulmonary side effects (pulmonary fibrosis) of bleomycin.

DOSAGE AND ADMINISTRATION

Doses are variable and range from 500 mg to 3 grams daily.

HOW SUPPLIED

Capsules — 500 mg, 1000 mg
Powder
Tablets — 500 mg, 1000 mg

LITERATURE

Azuma J, Sawamura A, Awata N, et al. Therapeutic effect of taurine in congestive heart failure: a double-blind, crossover trial. *Clin Cardiol.* 1985; 8:267-282.

Azuma J, Sawamura Z, Awata N. Usefulness of taurine in congestive heart failure and its prospective application. *Jpn Circ J.* 1992; 56:95-99.

Barbeau A, Donaldson J. Taurine in epilepsy. *Lancet.* 1973; 2(7825):387.

Chesney RW. Taurine: its biological role and clinical implications. Advances in Pediatrics. 1985:22:1-42.

Chesney RW. Taurine: is it required for infant nutrition? *J Nutr.* 1988; 118:6-10.

Darling PB, Lepage G, Leroy C, et al. Effect of taurine supplements on fat absorption in cystic fibrosis. *Pediatr Res.* 1985; 19:578-582.

Geggel HS, Ament ME, Heckenlively JR, et al. Nutritional requirement for taurine in patients receiving long-term parenteral supplementation. *N Eng J Med.* 1985; 312:142-146.

Gurujeyalakshmi G, Wang Y, Giri SN. Taurine and niacin block lung injury and fibrosis by down-regulating bleomycin-induced activation of transcription nuclear factor-kappa B in mice. *J Pharmacol Exp Ther.* 2000; 293:82-90.

Hayes KC, Carey RE. Retinal degeneration associated with taurine deficiency in the cat. *Science.* 1975; 188:949-951.

Hayes KC, Sturman JA. Taurine in metabolism. *Ann Rev Nutr.* 1981; 1:401-425.

McCarty MF. The reported clinical utility of taurine in ischemic disorders may reflect a down-regulation of neutrophil activation and adhesion. *Med Hypothesis.* 1999; 53:290-299.

Murakami S, Kondo Y, Tomisawa K, Nagate T. Prevention of atherosclerotic lesion development in mice by taurine. *Drugs Exp Clin Res.* 1999; 25:227-234.

Nakamura T, Ogasawara M, Koyama I, et al. The protective effect of taurine on the biomembrane against damage produced by oxygen radicals. *Biol Pharm Bull.* 1993; 16:970-972.

Niitynen L, Nurminen M-L, Korpela R, et al. Role of arginine, taurine and homocysteine in cardiovascular diseases. *Ann Med.* 1999; 31:318-326.

Pierson HF, Fisher JM, Rabinovitz M. Modulation by taurine of the toxicity of taumustine, a compound with antitumor activity. *J Natl Canc Inst.* 1985; 75:905-909.

Pion PD, Kittleson MD, Rogers QR, Morris JG. Myocardial failure in cats associated with low plasma taurine: a reversible cardiomyopathy. *Science.* 1987; 237: 764-767.

Rivas-Arancibia S, Dorado-Martínez C, Borgonio-Pérez G, et al. Effects of taurine on ozone-induced memory deficits and lipid peroxidation in brains of young, mature, and old rats. *Environ Res.* 2000; 82:7-17.

Stipanuk MH. Homocysteine, Cysteine, and Taurine. In: Shils ME, Olson JA, Shike M, Ross AC, eds. *Modern Nutrition in Health and Disease*, 9th ed. Baltimore, MD: Williams and Wilkins; 1999:543-558.

Wang Q, Giri SN, Hyde DM, Nakashima JM. Effects of taurine on bleomycin-induced lung fibrosis in hamsters. *Proc Soc Exp Biol Med.* 1989; 190:330-338.

Thiamin (Vitamin B1)

TRADE NAMES

Thiamilate (Tyson Neutraceuticals), Bethamine (Ampharco Inc.).

DESCRIPTION

In 1911, the chemist Casimir Funk isolated a substance from rice bran extracts which he thought was the anti-beriberi factor. Because the substance was an amine and because he thought the substance had a vital dietary function, he named it vitamine. As it turned out, Funk's vitamine was not the anti-beriberi factor which was subsequently isolated and called thiamin or vitamin B1. Nevertheless, Funk did coin the term vitamin and the concept that vitamins are essential dietary factors.

Thiamin is a water-soluble vitamin. Structurally it consists of a substituted pyrimidine ring joined by a methylene bridge to a substituted thiazole ring. The free vitamin is a base. The thiazolium salts of thiamin, thiamin hydrochloride and thiamin mononitrate, are the forms of thiamin which are typically used in nutritional supplements and for food fortification. In addition to being known as vitamin B1, thiamin is known as thiamine, aneurin and 3-[(4-amino-2-methyl-5-pyrimidinyl) methyl]-5-(2-hydroxyethyl)-4-methyl-thiazonium. The structural formula of thiamin follows:

Thiamin

The classic deficiency state of thiamin is beriberi. An analogous disorder in fowl is called polyneuritis. The term beriberi is derived from the Sinhalese word meaning extreme weakness. Beriberi was very common during the early part of the last century in those whose diets consisted principally of highly polished rice. Interestingly, those who ate parboiled rice—partially boiled rice—did not develop beriberi. Milling removes the husk, which contains most of the thiamin, while parboiling the rice before husking disperses thiamin throughout the grain. Beriberi still occurs in those whose diet mainly consists of polished rice. Thiamin deficiency is also associated with alcoholism and occurs in some cases of malnutrition, those receiving total parenteral nutrition without thiamin, malabsorption syndromes, increased carbohydrate intake, major catabolic and physiologic stress states, acute infection, folate deficiency, thyrotoxicosis and those on long-term loop diuretics (furosemide, ethacrynic acid, bumetanide). Subclinical thiamin deficiency may not be uncommon.

There are three types of beriberi: dry beriberi, wet beriberi and cerebral beriberi or Wernicke-Korsakoff syndrome. Dry or neurologic beriberi occurs when thiamin deficiency affects the peripheral nervous system resulting in peripheral neuropathy. The peripheral neuropathy is characterized by a bilateral, symmetric impairment of sensory, motor and reflex functions involving predominantly the lower extremities. Symptoms and signs of dry beriberi, include paresthesias of the toes, burning of the feet, calf muscle tenderness and cramps, difficulty in rising from a squatting position, a decrease in the vibratory sensation in the toes, loss of ankle and knee jerks and footdrop and toedrop. Wet or cardiovascular beriberi involves the heart and circulatory system. Cardiovascular manifestations of thiamin deficiency are characterized by peripheral vasodilatation with increased cardiac output, sodium and water retention and myocardial failure. The most extreme form of wet beriberi is shoshin beriberi. Shoshin is Japanese for damage to the heart and is characterized by global heart failure with lactic acidosis in the context of blood tests showing thiamin deficiency. Shoshin beriberi, if not promptly treated, is rapidly fatal. Alcoholics who present with unexplained lactic acidosis, a hyperdynamic state and high output failure, or cardiogenic shock without evidence of a myocardial infarction, are unlikely to have anything but Shoshin beriberi.

Alcoholism is the major cause of thiamin deficiency in Wernicke-Korsakoff syndrome or cerebral beriberi. Wernicke-Korsakoff syndrome is characterized by abnormal ocular motor signs, ataxia and derangement of mental functions. The ocular motor signs include paresis of abduction which is accompanied by horizontal diplopia, strabismus and nystagmus. Derangement of mental functions include a global-confusional apathetic state and amnesia. Wernicke-Korsakoff syndome represents the full-blown clinical state of cerebral beriberi. Wernicke's disease itself is characterized by abnormal ocular motor signs and ataxia without an evident amnesic state. Korsakoff's psychosis itself is characterized by the mental derangements mentioned above.

Thiamin occurs in cells principally in its active coenzyme form called thiamin pyrophosphate (TPP, cocarboxylase). Thiamin, in the form of thiamin pyrophosphate, plays an essential role as a cofactor in key reactions in carbohydrate metabolism. It is also involved in the metabolism of branched-chain amino acids and may have non-coenzyme (non-cofactor) roles in excitable cells. TPP is a coenzyme in the oxidative decarboxylation of pyruvate to acetyl-coenzyme A (acetyl-CoA), of alpha-ketoglutarate to succinyl-CoA, and of the oxidative decarboxylation of the branched-chain alpha-keto acids, which are metabolites of the

branched-chain amino acids L-leucine, L-isoleucine and L-valine. TPP is also a cofactor in the reversible transketolase reactions in the phosphogluconate pathway, also know as the pentose phosphate pathway and the hexose monophosphate shunt. The two transketolase reactions are the reversible conversions of D-xylulose 5-phosphate and D-ribose 5-phosphate to D-sedoheptulose 7-phosphate and D-glyceraldehyde 3-phosphate, and D-xylulose-5-phosphate and D-erythrose-4-phosphate to D-fructose 6-phosphate and D-glyceraldehyde 3-phosphate. The first of these two reactions represents the pathway for the non-oxidative production of ribose.

The total metabolic pool of thiamin in the body is approximately 30 milligrams. The predominant form of thiamin in the body is thiamin pyrophosphate (TPP, also known as thiamin diphosphate or TDP and cocarboxylase). Approximately 80% of thiamin in blood is present in erythrocytes as TPP. About 50% of total body thiamin is present in skeletal muscles. Thiamin is also found in heart, liver kidneys and brain. Other forms of thiamin present in the body include, thiamin triphosphate (TTP, about 10%), thiamin monophosphate (TMP) and free thiamin. TMP and free thiamin comprise about 10% of total body thiamin. The most reliable method of evaluating thiamin status is the measurement of erythrocyte transketolase activity and the percentage enhancement of the transketolase activity resulting from added thiamin pyrophosphate.

All plant and animal foods contain thiamin. Good dietary sources of the vitamin, include whole-grain products, brown rice, meat products, vegetables, fruits, legumes and seafood.

ACTIONS AND PHARMACOLOGY

ACTIONS

Thiamin may have antioxidant, erythropoietic, cognition-and mood-modulatory, antiatherosclerotic and detoxification activities. It has putative ergogenic activity.

MECHANISM OF ACTION

Thiamin has been found to protect against lead-induced lipid peroxidation in rat liver and kidney. Thiamin deficiency results in selective neuronal death in animal models. The neuronal death is associated with increased free radical production, suggesting that oxidative stress may play an important early role in brain damage associated with thiamin deficiency. The mechanism of the possible antioxidant activity of thiamin is unknown.

Even though anemia is not one of the consequences of thiamin deficiency, there is a type of anemia, called thiamin-responsive megaloblastic anemia, that responds well to large doses of thiamin. It is thought that those with thiamin-responsive megaloblastic anemia may actually be thiamin-deficient secondary to reduced thiamin transport and absorption, and to impaired intracellular thiamin pyrophosphorylation.

Thiamin deficiency is associated with cognitive and emotional changes. For example, Korsakoff's psychosis is characterized by the inability to form new memories, the poorly organized retrieval of remote memories, apathy and emotional blandness. The treatment of Korsakoff's patients with thiamin often results in significant improvement in these symptoms. Marginal thiamin deficiency may also result in cognitive and emotional changes. There are a few studies suggesting that high-dose thiamin supplementation may have a positive effect on mood and cognition in those with marginal deficiency, and even adequate status, of the vitamin. In one study with female subjects, improved thiamin status was associated with improved mood, and a decline in thiamin status was associated with poorer mood. In another study, again with female subjects, those taking 50 milligrams of thiamin daily for 20 months were found to have improvement in thiamin status associated with reports of being more clearheaded, composed and energetic. Reaction times were also faster. The study was placebo-controlled and performed in subjects whose thiamin status was adequate. The mechanism of the neurophysiological actions of thiamin are not well understood. Thiamin may play a role in neurophysiology independent of its coenzyme function. Thiamin is located in nerve cell membranes and phosphorylated forms of thiamin are associated with sodium channel proteins. It is thought that phosphorylated forms of thiamin may play roles in the control of sodium conductance at axonal membranes and in other neurological processes.

Migration and proliferation of arterial smooth muscle cells are thought to play an important role in the development of atherosclerosis. Glucose and insulin have been found to have an additive effect on the proliferation of infragenicular arterial smooth muscle cells *in vitro*. Thiamin has been found to inhibit human infragenicular arterial muscle cell proliferation induced by high glucose and insulin, in cell culture. Thiamin plays a key role in intracellular glucose metabolism and it is thought that thiamin inhibits the effect of glucose and insulin on arterial smooth muscle cell proliferation. However, the mechanism of this *in vitro* effect is not well understood. Inhibition of endothelial cell proliferation may also promote atherosclerosis. Endothelial cells in culture have been found to have a decreased proliferative rate and delayed migration in response to hyperglycemic conditions. Thiamin has been shown to inhibit this effect of glucose on endothelial cells. It is thought that the mechanism of action of thiamin on endothelial cells is related to a reduction in intracellular protein glycation by redirecting the glycolytic flux. Atherosclerosis and peripheral artery disease are significant problems in those with type 2 diabetes mellitus.

Further study of the possible anti-atherosclerotic activity of thiamin, particularly in those with type 2 diabetes, is warranted.

Some animal studies have found that high doses of thiamin block some of the toxic symptoms from orally administered lead. Thiamin may protect against lead toxicity by inhibiting lead-induced lipid peroxidation.

There are few studies investigating the effect of large doses of thiamin as an aid to exercise performance. In one such study, carbohydrate-loaded mice administered very high doses of thiamin demonstrated an improvement in swim time to exhaustion. In another study, experienced cyclists administered 900 milligram daily of thiamin for three days were found to have lower exercise heart rates, blood glucose and blood lactate concentrations. In still another study, thiamin supplementation at 100 milligram/day was found to decrease exercise-induced fatigue in male athletes. A recent study, however, using a thiamin derivative, thiamin tetrahydrofurfuryl disulfide, which is better absorbed than thiamin, showed no effect on high-intensity exercise performance. There is insufficient evidence to suggest that thiamin may have exercise performance-enhancing activity. The possible mechanism of this putative effect is unknown.

PHARMACOKINETICS

Thiamin is absorbed from the lumen of the small intestine—mainly the jejunum—by active transport and passive diffusion mechanisms. At lower amounts, absorption from the small intestine is by an active, carrier-mediated process that is energy-dependent as well as sodium-dependent. Passive diffusion occurs with higher amounts of thiamin. Absorption of thiamin appears to be limited by a saturable rate-limiting transport mechanism. Only a small percentage of a high dose of thiamin is absorbed. Certain lipid-soluble thiamin derivatives known as allithiamins, do not appear to be subject to the rate-limiting transport mechanism. Thiamin is transported by the portal circulation to the liver and by the systemic circulation to various tissues in the body. Thiamin is metabolized to thiamin monophosphate (TP, TMP), thiamin pyrophosphate (TPP, cocarboxylase, thiamin diphosphate, TDP) and thiamin triphosphate (TTP). Thiamin is phosphorylated directly to thiamin pyrophosphate by thiamin diphosphokinase and thiamin pyrophosphate is dephosphorylated to thiamin monophosphate via thiamin diphosphatase. Approximately 80% of thiamin in blood is present in erythrocytes as TPP. The transport of thiamin into erythrocytes appears to occur by facilitated diffusion; it enters other cells by an active process. Total thiamin content in the adult body is about 30 milligrams. Thiamin and its metabolites are mainly excreted by the kidneys.

INDICATIONS AND USAGE

Frank and marginal thiamin deficiency may not be uncommon and may be a particular problem among alcoholics, the elderly and the chronically ill. Thiamin supplementation may be useful in these subgroups, among others. There is evidence that supplemental thiamin can help protect against some of the metabolic imbalances caused by heavy alcohol consumption. It may help protect against Wernicke's encephalopathy and some other forms of brain damage seen in some alcoholics, some with HIV-disease, some with anorexia nervosa and others. It may be helpful in alcohol withdrawal. It is needed in those who receive total parenteral nutrition, particularly to prevent lactic acidosis due to thiamin deficiency. It may increase glucose tolerance and may help prevent atherosclerosis, particularly in diabetics. It has been used in congestive heart failure with benefit under certain circumstances and may be helpful in some other forms of heart disease. There is preliminary evidence that it can improve mood and cognition in some. Data are in short supply and results mixed with respect to claims that thiamin can enhance exercise performance and increase energy. Thiamin's use in cancer might be ill-advised, as there is evidence that it may promote tumor-cell proliferation.

RESEARCH SUMMARY

Alcoholics are at particularly high risk of thiamin deficiency. Alcohol interferes with the absorption of thiamin and its storage in tissue. It also inhibits conversion of thiamin to its active form. In addition, alcoholics generally have unbalanced diets low in thiamin. Some alcoholics suffer from frank beriberi, which, among other things, can lead to congestive heart failure. More frequently, alcoholics suffer from such beriberi symptoms as mental confusion, visual disturbances and staggering gait. Beriberi can be prevented and, in some cases, successfully treated with high doses of thiamin (up to 100 milligrams daily).

Thiamin can also help prevent some cases of Wernicke's encephalopathy, a potentially fatal disorder that occurs in some who consume very large amounts of alcohol. Symptoms include double vision, mental confusion, muscle weakness and disturbed gait. Untreated, this disorder can result in permanent brain damage and memory impairment. In extreme cases it leads to coma and death. It is often reversible with prompt thiamin treatment. Some use thiamin as part of alcohol-withdrawal therapy.

Others at higher than average risk of Wernicke's encephalopathy include those suffering from anorexia nervosa, typically young women. Older people are also at higher risk. So are people with HIV disease. Thiamin deficiency was found in 23% of HIV patients in one study, and brain lesions characteristic of those found in sufferers of Wernicke's encephalopathy have been seen in some with HIV-disease.

Some researchers have recommended dietary thiamin supplementation in all newly diagnosed cases of HIV-disease.

It is now recognized that thiamin deficiency may occur with total parenteral nutrition (TPN). Several cases of lactic acidosis have been reported in TPN patients not receiving thiamin. Administration of thiamin has resolved the acidosis with attendant clinical improvement. Researchers stress that thiamin deficiency should always be included in the differential diagnosis of lactic acidosis. A recent shortage of multivitamin preparations for TPN is said to have resulted in a number of cases of lactic acidosis due to thiamin deficiency. A previous shortage led to several TPN-related deaths.

Thiamin deficiency is associated with abnormal glucose tolerance, and there is some evidence that supplemental thiamin may, in some cases, help correct the abnormality. In a recent in vitro study, thiamin inhibited accelerated proliferation of arterial smooth muscle cells. This proliferation contributes to atherosclerosis and preferentially affects the infragenicular vasculature in patients with diabetes mellitus. High insulin and glucose levels demonstrate additive effects in this process in vitro. This research gives some preliminary indication that thiamin may help prevent or delay atherosclerotic complications in some diabetics.

Thiamin supplementation has improved left ventricular function in patients with congestive heart failure being administered long-term furosemide therapy and, as noted above, supplemental thiamin can help prevent and treat heart disease related to beriberi. In addition, intravenous injection of thiamin proved helpful in an animal model of myocardial infarction, increasing strength of contractions and decreasing oxygen demand. Russian researchers have reported similar results in humans. Thiamin pyrophosphate (cocarboxylase) was used in these heart attack experiments. Research is needed to see whether thiamin itself might be beneficial.

Thiamin was found to have positive effects on mood and cognitive functioning in a recent study of 120 young females. In a previous study, females receiving a multivitamin supplement for three months were said to have improved mood compared with controls who received placebo. Using biochemical indices, an association was made between thiamin status and improved mood. These same measures did not support an association between any of eight other vitamins and elevated mood.

In this recent study, focus was on thiamin alone among the vitamins. All but one of the 120 women had normal thiamin levels at baseline. They were randomized to receive 50 milligrams of thiamin daily or placebo. After two months, the thiamin group significantly improved (more than doubled) their scores on the clear-headedness and mood subsets of the bipolar profile of mood states psychological test. There was no change in these measures in the placebo group. The thiamin group also showed nonsignificant improvement in feelings of confidence, composure and elation. The researchers considered their findings remarkable given that they were obtained in a group which, as measured by transketolase activation, had normal thiamin nutrition. More research is warranted.

Thiamin and a thiamin derivative have not shown any effect on exercise performance in two studies. High-dose thiamin (100 milligrams daily) was found to be helpful in preventing or accelerating recovery from exercise-induced fatigue in a third study. This trial tested thiamin in 16 male volunteer athletes using bicycle ergometer exercises. Followup is needed.

Finally, a group of researchers have recently called thiamin supplementation "a double-edged sword" in cancer patients. Like other seriously ill patients, cancer sufferers may benefit from improved thiamin status in terms of general nutrition, but, as these researchers observed, there is some evidence that thiamin may also, in effect, nourish some cancers. There is some indication that high-dose thiamin supplementation may promote tumor cell proliferation. More research is needed to help clarify this issue.

CONTRAINDICATIONS, PRECAUTIONS, ADVERSE REACTIONS

CONTRAINDICATIONS

Thiamin contraindicated in those hypersensitive to any component of a thiamin-containing product.

PRECAUTIONS

The use of thiamin for the treatment of a thiamin-deficiency state, lactic acidosis secondary to thiamin-deficiency, Wernicke-Korsakoff syndrome, Wernicke's encephalopathy, Korsakoff's psychosis or any medical condition must only be undertaken under medical supervision.

A typical dose of thiamin used in pre- and postnatal multivitamin/multimineral supplements is three milligrams daily. Pregnant women and nursing mothers should avoid intakes of thiamin greater than this amount unless higher doses are prescribed by their physicians.

Those who are treated with parenteral thiamin for thiamin deficiency, should be given the thiamin prior to receiving parenteral glucose. Administration of intravenous glucose prior to receiving thiamin could result in severe lactic acidosis.

ADVERSE REACTIONS

Oral thiamin is well tolerated even at doses up to 200 milligrams daily or higher. There have been occasional reports of serious and even fatal responses to parenteral thiamin. These have probably been anaphylactic reactions.

There are also reports of less serious allergic reactions to parenteral thiamin.

There is some animal evidence that high doses of parenteral thiamin may promote tumor growth.

INTERACTIONS

DRUGS

Loop diuretics (furosemide, ethacrynic acid, bumetanide): Chronic use of loop diuretics may result in thiamin deficiency. Chronic use of furosemide for the treatment of congestive heart failure has been reported to result in thiamin deficiency. Thiamin repletion in such patients can improve left ventricular function.

FOODS

Substances in food that inactivate thiamin are called anti-thiamin factors.

Sulfites: Concomitant intake of thiamin and foods and beverages containing sulfites may inactivate thiamin.

Tea, coffee and decaffeinated coffee: Concomitant intake of these beverages and thiamin may inactivate thiamin. Tannic acid is most likely the substance in tea that inactivates thiamin by forming a tannin-thiamin adduct.

OVERDOSAGE

Overdosage of thiamin has not been reported in the literature.

DOSAGE AND ADMINISTRATION

Thiamin is available in nutritional supplements in the form of thiamin hydrochloride and thiamin nitrate. These are also the forms used for food fortification. Thiamin pyrophosphate or cocarboxylase may also be available in some products. Supplemental doses of thiamin are variable and range from the U.S. RDA amount of 1.5 milligrams/day to 10 milligrams/day or higher. There is a rapid decline in absorption that occurs at oral doses above five milligrams. Thiamin is typically found in the form of multivitamin, multivitamin/ multimineral or B-complex preparations. Single ingredient thiamin supplements are also available. Pre- and postnatal supplements typically deliver a thiamin dose of 3 milligrams daily.

Lipid-soluble thiamin derivatives called allithiamins are also available. These forms are better absorbed at higher intakes than is thiamin.

The Food and Nutrition Board of the Institute of Medicine of the National Academy of Sciences recommends the following dietary reference intakes (DRIs) for thiamin:

Infants		Adequate Intakes (AI)
0-6 months	0.2 mg/day	0.03 mg/kg
7-12 months	0.3 mg/day	0.03 mg/kg

Recommended Dietary
Allowances (RDA)

Children
1-3 years   0.5 mg/day
4-8 years   0.6 mg/day

Boys
9-13 years   0.9 mg/day
14-18 years   1.2 mg/day

Girls
9-13 years   0.9 mg/day
14-18 years   1.0 mg/day

Men
19 years and older   1.2 mg/day

Women
19 years and older   1.1 mg/day

Pregnancy
14-50 years   1.4 mg/day

Lactation
14-50 years   1.4 mg/day

The U.S. RDA for thiamin, which is used for determining percentage of daily values on nutritional supplement and food labels, is 1.5 milligrams.

HOW SUPPLIED
Vitamin B1 is available in the following forms and strengths for Rx use:

Injection — 100 mg/mL

Vitamin B1 is available in the following forms and strengths for OTC use:

Capsules — 100 mg, 500 mg

Enteric Coated Tablets — 20 mg

Tablets — 25 mg, 50 mg, 100 mg, 250 mg, 500 mg

LITERATURE

Avena R, Arora S, Carmody BJ, et al. Thiamin (vitamin B1) protects against glucose- and insulin-mediated proliferation of human infragenicular arterial smooth muscle cells. *Ann Vasc Surg.* 2000; 14:37-43.

Bakker SJL, Hoogeveen EK, Nijpels G, et al. The association of dietary fibres with glucose tolerance is partly explained by concomitant intake of thiamin: The Hoorn Study. *Diabetologia.* 1998; 41:1168-1175.

Benton D, Griffiths R, Haller J. Thiamin supplementation mood and cognitive functioning. *Psychopharmacol.* 1997; 129:66-71.

Bettendorff L. A non-cofactor role of thiamin derivatives in excitable cells? *Arch Physiol Biochem.* 1996; 104:745-751.

Blanc P, Boussuges A. [Cardiac beriberi]. [Article in French]. *Arch Mal Coeur Vaiss.* 2000; 93:371-379.

Boros LG. Population thiamine status and varying cancer rates between western, Asian and African countries. *Anticancer Res.* 2000; 20(3B):2245-2248.

Boros LG, Brandes JL, Lee WN, et al. Thiamine supplementation to cancer patients: a double edge sword. *Anticancer Res.* 1998; 18(1B):595-602.

Boros LG, Comin B, Boren J, et al. Over-expression of transketolase: a mechanism by which thiamine supplementation promotes cancer growth. *Am Assoc Cancer Res.* 2000; 41:66(Ab #4234).

Butterworth RF, Gaudreau C, Vincelette J, et al. Thiamin deficiency and Wernicke's encephalopathy in AIDS. *Metab Brain Dis.* 1991; 6:207-212.

Dietary Reference intakes for Thiamin, Riboflavin, Niacin, Vitamin B6, Folate, Vitamin B12, Pantothenic Acid, Biotin, and Choline. Washington, DC: National Academy Press; 1998.

Frank T, Bitsch R, Maiwald J, Stein G. High thiamine diphosphate concentrations in erythrocytes can be achieved in dialysis patients by oral administration of benfotiamine. *Eur J Clin Pharmacol.* 2000; 56:251-257.

Härdig L, Daae C, Dellborg M, et al. Reduced thiamine phosphate, but not thiamine diphosphate, in erythrocytes in elderly patients with congestive heart failure treated with furosemide. *J Int Med.* 2000; 247:597-600.

La Selva M, Beltramo E, Pagnozzi F, et al. Thiamine corrects delayed replication and decreases production of lactate and advanced glycation end-products in bovine retinal and human umbilical vein endothelial cells cultured under high glucose conditions. *Diabetologia.* 1996; 39:1263-1268.

Muri RM, Von Overbeck J, Furrer J, Ballmer PE. Thiamin deficiency in HIV-positive patients: evaluations by erythrocyte transketolase activity and thiamin pyrophosphate effect. *Clin Nutr.* 1999; 18:375-378.

Pekovich SR, Martin PR, Singleton CK. Thiamine deficiency decreases steady-state transketolase and pyruvate dehydrogenase but not alpha-ketoglutarate dehydrogenase mRNA levels in three human cell types. *J Nutr.* 1998; 128:683-687.

Romanski SA, McMahon MM. Metabolic acidosis and thiamine deficiency. *Mayo Clin Proc.* 1999; 74:259-263.

Sato Y, Nakagawa M, Higuchi I, et al. Mitochondrial myopathy and familial thiamine deficiency. *Muscle Nerve.* 2000; 23:1069-1075.

Senapati SK, Dey S, Dwivedi SK, et al. Effect of thiamine hydrochloride on lead induced lipid peroxidation in rat liver and kidney. *Vet Hum Toxicol.* 2000; 42:236-237.

Shimon I, Almog S, Vered Z, et al. Improved left ventricular function after thiamine supplementation in patients with congestive heart failure receiving long-term furosemide therapy. *Am J Med.* 1995; 98:485-490.

Suter PM, Haller J, Hany A. Diuretic use: a risk for subclinical thiamine deficiency in elderly patients. *J Nutr Health Aging.* 2000; 4:69-71.

Suzuki M, Itokawa Y. Effects of thiamine supplementation on exercise-induced fatigue. *Metab Brain Dis.* 1996; 11:95-106.

Tanphaichitr V. Thiamin. In: Shils ME, Olson JA, Shike M, Ross AC, eds. *Modern Nutrition in Health and Disease.* 9th ed. Baltimore, MD: Williams and Wilkins; 1999:381-389.

Todd K, Butterworth RF. Mechanisms of selective neuronal cell death due to thiamine deficiency. *Ann NY Acad Sci.* 1999; 893:404-411.

Webster MJ. Physiological and performance responses to supplementation with thiamin and pantothenic acid derivatives. *Eur J Appl Physiol Occup Physiol.* 1998; 77:486-491.

Webster MJ, Scheett TP, Doyle MR, Branz M. The effect of a thiamin derivative on exercise performance. *Eur J Appl Physiol.* 1997; 75:520-524.

Tin

DESCRIPTION

Tin is a metallic element with atomic number 50 and symbol Sn. It is a heavy metal. Tin is not considered an essential nutrient for humans. A tin-deficiency state has been reported in rats.

Rats fed a diet low in tin showed poor growth, alopecia and lowered response to sound compared with rats fed a tin-rich diet. Abnormalities in mineral status were also noted in the tin-deficient rat group. At least for rats tin, may serve as an essential nutrient.

The typical daily dietary intake of tin ranges from about 1 to 40 milligrams. Tin intake is essentially dependent on food stored in tin cans. Higher intakes of tin are obtained from foods preserved in unlacquered tin cans than from foods preserved in lacquered tin cans.

Regarding potential drug applications of tin, an organotin compound, tin protoporphyrin or Sn-P, a potent inhibitor of heme oxygenase and bilirubin formation, is being studied as a treatment for controlling severe hyperbilirubinemia in full-term breast-fed newborns with high bilirubin levels after birth. It is also being studied as a treatment for neuropathic and incisional pain.

ACTIONS AND PHARMACOLOGY

ACTIONS

The actions and pharmacology of dietary tin are not known.

INDICATIONS AND USAGE

There is no evidence that supplemental tin has immune-enhancing activity in humans; nor is there any evidence that it has anticarcinogenic activity in humans.

RESEARCH SUMMARY

It has been hypothesized that the thymus gland secretes tin-containing substances that possess immune-enhancing properties. There are some animal studies suggesting that tin may have immune-modulating activity and may also have anti-proliferative activity. There is no evidence that tin has these activities in humans. Such studies are needed, especially if the animal studies have any validity.

CONTRAINDICATIONS, PRECAUTIONS, ADVERSE REACTIONS

CONTRAINDICATIONS

None known.

PRECAUTIONS

Given our present state of knowledge regarding tin, supplemental tin is not recommended for anyone.

DOSAGE AND ADMINISTRATION

No recommended dosage. Tin may be found in colloidal or liquid mineral preparations. It is also found in some multivitamin preparations, typically at a dose of about 10 micrograms.

LITERATURE

Arakawa Y. [Biological activity of tin and immunity.] [Article in Japanese.] *Sangyo Eiseigaku Zasshi.* 1997; 39:1-20

Biego GH, Joyeux M, Hartemann P, Debry G. Determination of tin intake in an adult French citizen. *Arch Environ Contam Toxicol.* 1999; 36:227-232.

Cardarelli N. Tin and the thymus gland: a review. *Thymus.* 1990; 15:223-231.

Martinez JC, Garcia HO, Otheguy LE, et al. Control of severe hyperbilirubinemia in full-term newborns with the inhibitor of bilirubin production Sn-mesoporphyrin. *Pediatrics.* 1999; 103:1-5.

Nielsen FH. Ultratrace minerals. In: Shils ME, Olson JA, Shike M, Ross AC, eds. *Modern Nutrition in Health and Disease.* 9th ed. Baltimore, MD: Williams and Wilkins; 1999; 283-303.

Pekelharing HL, Lemmens AG, Beynan AC. Iron, copper and zinc status in rats fed on diets containing various concentrations of tin. *Br J Nutr.* 1994; 71:103-109.

Yokoi K, Kimura M, Itokawa Y. Effect of dietary tin deficiency on growth and mineral status in rats. *Biol Trace Elem Res.* 1990; 223-231.

Tiratricol (TRIAC)

DESCRIPTION

Tiratricol is an orphan drug for use in combination with levothyroxine to suppress thyroid stimulating hormone in patients with well-differentiated thyroid cancer who are intolerant to adequate doses of levothyroxine alone. Tiratricol is a metabolite of the thyroid hormone triiodothyronine (T_3) and has thyroid hormone activity.

Tiratricol is also marketed as a dietary supplement for weight-loss purposes. In November, 1999, the Food and Drug Administration (FDA) warned against consuming products containing tiratricol. This was based on reports of individuals using tiratricol developing side effects, such as fatigue, lethargy, profound weight loss and severe diarrhea. They were also found to have abnormal thyroid function tests. Further action by the FDA is being considered.

Tiratricol is also known as triiodothyroacetic acid, TRIAC, 3,5,3' -triiodothyroacetic acid and [4-(4-hydroxy-3-iodophenoxy)-3,5-di-iodophenyl]acetic acid. Its molecular formula is $C_{14}H_9I_3O_4$, and its molecular weight is 621.9 daltons.

ACTIONS AND PHARMACOLOGY

ACTIONS
Tiratricol has thyroid hormone activity, including various metabolic effects. It also inhibits the secretion of thyroid-stimulating hormone (TSH) by the pituitary gland.

MECHANISM OF ACTION
The mechanism by which thyroid hormones exert their various actions has not been completely elucidated. Tiratricol is known to act as a feedback inhibitor of TSH secretion by the pituitary gland.

PHARMACOKINETICS
Much is unknown about the pharmacokinetics of tiratricol in humans. The pharmacokinetics of tiratricol appear to be similar to those of thyroxine and triiodothyronine. Tiratricol is absorbed from the small intestine following ingestion. Distribution of tiratricol in the body has not been fully elucidated. Most of this substance appears to be bound to serum proteins, including thyroxine-binding protein and albumin. It appears to be less firmly bound to serum proteins than are T_4 and T_3. The liver appears to be the major site of degradation of tiratricol. Tiratricol appears to be conjugated with glucuronic acid and sulfuric acid and excreted in the bile. Mainly because it is less tightly bound to serum proteins, tiratricol has a shorter half-life than T_4 or T_3.

INDICATIONS AND USAGE
The FDA has warned consumers not to purchase tiratricol-containing products due to risk of serious health consequences, including heart attacks and strokes. Tiratricol should be used only under a physician's supervision. Tiratricol is currently used by some as a supplement to burn fat. The doses required to achieve this effect pose significant health risks.

RESEARCH SUMMARY
Tiratricol is an orphan drug. The FDA has determined that it should not be used as a nutritional supplement due to serious potential health risks including heart attack and stroke.

CONTRAINDICATIONS, PRECAUTIONS, ADVERSE REACTIONS

CONTRAINDICATIONS
Tiratricol is contraindicated in those with untreated thyrotoxicosis of any etiology and in those with uncorrected adrenal insufficiency. Thyroid hormones increase tissue demands for adrenocortical hormones and may thereby precipitate acute adrenal crisis. Tiratricol is also contraindicated in those who are hypersensitive to any component of a tiratricol-containing product.

PRECAUTIONS
Tiratricol should only be used for specific approved indications and only under strict medical supervision. Tiratricol should not be used as a treatment for obesity. Tiratricol should be used with extreme caution in those with cardiovascular disorders (including angina, coronary artery disease and hypertension) and in the elderly who have a greater likelihood of occult cardiac disease. Concomitant use of tiratricol and sympathomimetic agents in those with coronary artery disease may increase the risk of coronary insufficiency.

Use of tiratricol in those with concomitant diabetes mellitus, diabetes insipidus or adrenal cortical insufficiency may aggravate the intensity of their symptoms.

ADVERSE REACTIONS
Reported adverse reactions include fatigue, lethargy, profound weight loss and severe diarrhea. Tiratricol has also been reported to cause abnormal thyroid function tests.

INTERACTIONS

DRUGS
Anticoagulants (oral). The hypoprothrombinemic effect of anticoagulants, such as warfarin, may be potentiated.

Sympathomimetic agents. There is a possible increased risk of coronary insufficiency in those with coronary artery disease.

Thyroid drugs (levothyroxine, triiodothyronine, thyroid). Concomitant use of tiratricol with these thyroid drugs is likely to produce additive effects.

LABORATORY TESTS
Tiratricol is likely to alter thyroid function tests, including TSH, T_4 and T_3.

OVERDOSAGE
There have been no reports of overdosage with tiratricol. Excessive doses of tiratricol theoretically may result in a hypermetabolic state indistinguishable from thyrotoxicosis.

DOSAGE AND ADMINISTRATION

Tiratricol is not recommended for use as a dietary supplement.

LITERATURE

Anon. FDA warns against consuming dietary supplements containing tiratricol. *FDA Talk Paper.* Nov 21, 2000.

Bracco D, Morin O, Schutz Y, et al. Comparison of the metabolic effects of 3,5,3'-triiodothyroacetic acid and thyroxine. *J Clin Endocrin Met.* 1993; 77:221-228.

Radetti G, Persani L, Molinaro G, et al. Clinical and hormonal outcome after two years of triiodothyroacetic acid treatment in a child with thyroid hormone resistance. *Thyroid.* 1997; 7:775-778.

Takeda T, Suzuki S, Liu RT, DeGroot LJ. Triiodothyroacetic acid has unique potential for therapy of resistance to thyroid hormone. *J Clin Endocrinol Metab.* 1995; 80:2033-2040.

Tocotrienols

DESCRIPTION

Tocotrienols comprise one of the two groups of molecules belonging to the vitamin E family, the other group being the tocopherols. Tocotrienols and tocopherols are sometimes collectively called tocols. Just as there are four natural tocopherols, alpha-, beta-, gamma- and delta-tocopherol, there are also four natural tocotrienols, alpha-, beta-, gamma- and delta-tocotrienol. The tocotrienols differ from the tocopherols in the chemical nature of the side chain or tail. Tocopherols have a saturated phytyl side chain, whereas tocotrienols have an unsaturated isoprenoid or farnesyl side chain possessing three double bonds.

The major source of tocotrienols are plant oils, and the richest sources are palm oil, rice bran oil, palm kernel oil and coconut oil. Tocotrienols are also found in such cereal grains as oat, barley and rye. Vegetable oils, such as those from canola, cottonseed, olive, peanut, safflower, soybean and sunflower, contain little to no tocotrienols. However, those oils do contain tocopherols. Corn oil has small amounts of tocotrienols.

All of the natural tocotrienols are fat-soluble, water-insoluble oils. The tocotrienols, as well as the tocopherols, possess chain-breaking, peroxyl radical scavenging activities. In contrast to tocopherols, tocotrienols inhibit the rate-limiting enzyme of the cholesterol biosynthetic pathway beta-hydroxy-beta-methylglutaryl-coenzyme A (HMG-CoA) reductase.

The four natural tocotrienols are characterized by the number of methyl groups and their position in the chromanol ring. Alpha-tocotrienol has three methyl groups located on positions 5, 7 and 8 of the chromanol ring; beta-tocotrienol has two methyl groups located on positions 5 and 8 of the ring; gamma-tocotrienol has two methyl groups located on positions 7 and 8 of the ring and delta-tocotrienol has one methyl group located on position 8 of the ring.

While tocopherols have three chiral centers, tocotrienols have only one chiral center. Therefore, each tocotrienol has two stereoisomeric possibilities in comparison with eight such possibilities for each of the tocopherols. The natural tocotrienols exist as d-stereoisomers: d-alpha-tocotrienol, d-beta-tocotrienol, d-gamma-tocotrienol and d-delta-tocotrienol. The chiral center in the tocotrienol structure is at the point where the isoprenoid side chain bonds to the chromanol ring, the 2 position of the ring. The natural tocotrienols are E, E in reference to the geometric configuration of the double bonds of the side chain.

D-Alpha-tocotrienol is also known as 2R, 3'E, 7'E-alpha tocotrienol and is abbreviated alpha-T_3; d-beta-tocotrienol is known as 2R, 3'E, 7'E-beta-tocotrienol and abbreviated beta-T_3; d-gamma-tocotrienol is known as 2R, 3'E, 7'E-gamma-tocotrienol and abbreviated gamma-T3; delta-tocotrienol is known as 2R, 3'E, 7'E-delta-tocotrienol and abbreviated delta-T_3. Tocotrienols are presently available in nutritional supplement form as mixed tocotrienols. Typically, the gamma form is the most abundant one in the mixture.

Occasionally tocotrienol is used in the singular but refers to the entire group of natural tocotrienols.

ACTIONS AND PHARMACOLOGY

ACTIONS

Tocotrienols have antioxidant activity. They may also have hypocholesterolemic, anti-atherogenic, antithrombotic, anti-carcinogenic and immunomodulatory actions.

MECHANISM OF ACTION

All the tocotrienols are lipid soluble, chain-breaking, peroxyl radical scavengers. As such, they can protect polyunsaturated fatty acids (PUFAs) within membrane phospholipids as well as PUFAs within plasma lipoproteins, such as low density lipoproteins, from lipid peroxidation. Which of the tocols have the highest antioxidant activity is still open to debate. For many years, alpha-tocopherol was thought to be the most potent antioxidant in the vitamin E family. Some studies have shown tocotrienols to be more effective inhibitors of both lipid peroxidation and protein oxidation than alpha-tocopherol. In these same studies, the order of antioxidant potency was gamma-tocotrienol followed by the alpha and delta tocotrienol homologues. Gamma-tocopherol is a peroxynitrite scavenger, and gamma-tocotrienol may be, as well. The possible greater antioxidant activity of the tocotrienols, compared with alpha-tocopherol, may be accounted for by a more efficient interaction of the chromanol ring with reactive oxygen species, a higher recycling efficiency of the chromanoxyl radicals of the tocotrienols and a more uniform distribution of the tocotrienols in cellular membranes. In any case, alpha-tocopherol is the dominant tocol in human plasma and tissue, and, therefore, would be expected to be the dominant antioxidant form, as well.

Tocotrienols inhibit the rate-limiting enzyme of the cholesterol biosynthetic pathway, beta-hydroxy-beta-methlyglutaryl-coenzyme A (HMG-CoA) reductase. Tocopherols do not have this activity. This hypocholesterolemic effect of tocotrienols is accounted for by the tocotrienol isoprenoid sidechain's ability to increase the concentration of cellular farnesol. Farnesol is derived from mevalonate, the product of the HMG-CoA reductase reaction. Farnesol, post-transcriptionally, suppresses HMG-CoA reductase synthesis and enhances the proteolytic catabolism of this enzyme. This mechanism is different from that of the statin hypocholesterolemic drugs (atorvastatin, cerivastatin, fluvastatin, lovastatin and pravastatin) which are competitive inhibitors of the enzyme. Gamma-tocotrienol and delta-tocotrienol are significantly more active than alpha-tocotrienol in suppressing HMG-CoA reductase activity.

The possible anti-atherogenic activity of tocotrienols can be accounted for by a few mechanisms. These include inhibition of LDL oxidation, suppression of HMG-CoA reductase activity and inhibition of platelet aggregation. Additional possible mechanisms include tocotrienol-mediated reduction of plasma apolipoprotein B-100 (apoB) levels, reduction of lipoprotein (a) [Lp (a)] plasma levels and inhibition of adhesion molecule (e.g., ICAM-1 and VCAM-1) expression and monocyte cell adherence. High plasma levels of apoB as well as Lp (a) are considered risk factors for coronary artery disease.

Tocotrienols' possible antithrombotic effect may be due to tocotrienols' (especially gamma-tocotrienol's) inhibition of thromboxane B_2 synthesis, as well as their suppression of plasma levels of platelet factor 4.

Tocotrienols have been found to inhibit the growth of several tumor cell lines in culture, including both estrogen receptor-negative and estrogen receptor-positive human breast cancer cells. The mechanism of this effect is unclear, but there is some speculation about it. Tocotrienols may upregulate apoptosis in these lines. Another possible mechanism may relate to tocotrienols' post-transcriptional suppression of HMG-CoA reductase. The suppression of mevalonate synthesis depletes tumor tissues of farnesyl pyrophosphate and geranylgeranylpyrophosphate. These intermediates in the cholesterol biosynthetic pathway play important roles in growth control-associated proteins. Suppressing the production intermediates could result in suppression of prenylation of the oncogene ras protein. Post-translational farnesylation of Ras is required for the cytoplasmic localization of the active Ras p21 to the cell membrane, enabling this oncogene to stimulate growth and induce malignant transformation.

PHARMACOKINETICS

The efficiency of absorption of tocotrienol is low and variable. Absorption from the lumen of the small intestine is lower on an empty stomach than with meals. Prior to their absorption, tocotrienols are emulsified with the aid of bile salts and form micelles with dietary fats and products of lipid hydrolysis. Tocotrienols, after absorption into the enterocytes, are secreted by these cells into the lymphatics in the form of chylomicrons. The chylomicrons are transported by the lymphatics to the circulation where they are metabolized to chylomicron remnants. Some tocotrienols are transferred to various tissues, including adipose tissue, muscle and possibly the brain. Chylomicrons transfer tocotrienols to HDL, which, in turn, transfers them to LDL and VLDL. These remnants can also acquire apolipoprotein E, which directs them and the tocotrienols they contain to the liver for further metabolism.

Chylomicron remnants are taken up by the liver. Tocotrienols do not bind very well to the hepatic alpha-tocopherol transfer protein. It is this protein that is involved in the secretion from the liver of alpha-tocopherol in VLDLs. Very little tocotrienol is secreted by the liver to the circulation in VLDLs.

Some tocotrienol is metabolized, and the metabolites are excreted in the urine. Fecal excretion is the main route of exertion of oral tocotrienols. Fecal excretion products include non-absorbed tocotrienols and tocotrienols that may be excreted by the biliary route.

INDICATIONS AND USAGE

Indications and uses of the tocotrienols are, generally, the same as those of vitamin E. (See Vitamin E.) The tocotrienols may, in some conditions, be more potent and, in others, less potent than vitamin E, but research related to this issue is preliminary. There are some data suggesting that tocotrienols may have greater hypolipidemic effects than the tocopherols. The tocotrienols show some promise in inhibiting breast cancer and some other malignancies, though this work, too, is preliminary. Tocotrienols were reported, in one recent animal study, to promote healing of ethanol-induced gastric lesions.

RESEARCH SUMMARY

There is evidence, in animal models, that tocotrienols decrease serum cholesterol levels. Both total and LDL-cholesterol levels have been significantly reduced in swine, 44% and 60% respectively. Serum cholesterol levels were lowered 29% in hypercholesterolemic chickens fed a tocotrienol-enriched diet. In some animal studies, it has also inhibited platelet aggregation.

In some small, case-controlled human trials, tocotrienol preparations showed an ability to reduce cholesterol, principally LDL-cholesterol, while leaving HDL-cholesterol essentially unchanged. Despite good results in these studies and in animal and *in vitro* studies, coupled with epidemiological data suggesting that high tocotrienol status confers protection against cardiovascular disease, some recent, small studies have not been quite as promising.

In one randomized, placebo-controlled trial of 50 subjects with cerebrovascular disease (including carotid stenosis), a daily supplement containing 64 milligrams of alpha-tocopherol and 160 milligrams of gamma-tocotrienol failed to produce any positive lipid effects. The lack of effect persisted even when the dose was boosted to 96 milligrams of alpha-tocopherol and 240 milligrams of gamma-tocotrienol.

But, even though there was no lipid-lowering effect, the treated group showed improvement, compared with controls receiving placebo in terms of ultrasonigraphically measured rate of progression and, in some cases, regression of carotid stenosis. It was hypothesized that the treatment might have inhibited protein kinase C stimulation and may thus have prevented proliferation of smooth muscle cells among other possible mechanisms of action.

More recently, another randomized, double-blind, placebo-controlled study found no lipid effects from a supplement containing 35 milligrams of tocotrienols and 20 milligrams of alpha-tocopherol in 20 men with slightly elevated lipid concentrations. Larger studies, perhaps using higher doses of tocotrienols in subjects with more pronounced hyperlipidemia, are needed.

In one small, double-blind, crossover study of hypercholesterolemic subjects, 200 milligrams of a tocotrienol-enriched fraction of palm oil daily for four weeks significantly lowered total cholesterol, LDL-cholesterol, Apo B, thromboxane, platelet factor 4 and glucose. The crossover confirmed these findings.

Subsequently, both gamma-tocotrienol and the same tocotrienol-enriched fraction of palm oil described above were tested in more hypercholesterolemic subjects. Both supplements produced significant cholesterol reduction in these subjects. Gamma tocotrienol (200 milligrams daily) was more effective than the palm oil preparation (which contained 40 milligrams of alpha-tocotrienol and 60 milligrams of delta-tocotrienol).

Gamma and delta-tocotrienols, but not alpha- and gamma-tocopherols, have shown significant tumor-inhibition activity in several *in vitro* studies. In one of these, a tocotrienol-rich fraction of palm oil significantly inhibited the growth of a human breast cancer cell line, whereas alpha-tocopherol did not. Additional *in vitro* studies have demonstrated that tocotrienols inhibit the growth of human breast cancer cells in culture irrespective of the estrogen receptor status of the cells. It has been suggested by some researchers that tocotrienols might productively be combined with tamoxifen as a breast cancer treatment. The efficacy and safety of such a combination have not been tested, but the potential for such a treatment might be considerable, particularly with respect to treating hormone-responsive breast cancer that has become resistant to tamoxifen and other antiestrogens.

Tocotrienols have shown experimental activity against a number of other cancers. Research continues.

Recently, a tocotrienol-enriched fraction of palm oil was found to enhance the healing of ethanol-induced gastric mucosal lesions in rats. It was not, however, able to prevent such injuries. It was hypothesized that tocotrienols may abet healing through inhibition of lipid peroxidation. Further study is needed.

CONTRAINDICATIONS, PRECAUTIONS, ADVERSE REACTIONS
CONTRAINDICATIONS
Tocotrienols are contraindicated in those with known hypersensitivity to these substances.

PRECAUTIONS
Those on warfarin should be cautious in using doses of tocotrienols greater than 100 milligrams daily and, if they do so, they should have their INRs carefully monitored and their warfarin dose appropriately adjusted if indicated. Likewise, those with vitamin K deficiencies, such as those with liver failure, should be cautious in using doses of tocotrienols greater than 100 milligrams daily. Tocotrienols should also be used with caution in those with lesions with a propensity to bleed (e.g., bleeding peptic ulcers), those with a history of hemorrhagic stroke and those with inherited bleeding disorders (e.g., hemophilia).

High dose tocotrienol supplementation (greater than 100 milligrams daily) should be stopped about one month before surgical procedures and may be resumed following recovery from the procedure.

Those taking iron supplements should not take tocotrienols and iron at the same time.

ADVERSE REACTIONS
Tocotrienol supplements have only recently been introduced in the nutritional supplement marketplace. No adverse reactions have been reported.

INTERACTIONS

DRUGS

Antiplatelet drugs, such as aspirin, dipyridamole, eptifibatide, clopidogrel, ticlopidine, tirofiban and abciximab: Tocotrienol supplementation may potentiate the effects of these antiplatelet drugs.

Cholestyramine: may decrease tocotrienol absorption.

Colestipol: may decrease tocotrienol absorption.

Isoniazid: may decrease tocotrienol absorption.

Mineral oil: may decrease tocotrienol absorption.

Neomycin: may impair utilization of tocotrienols.

Orlistat: is likely to inhibit tocotrienol absorption.

Statins: atorvastatin, cerivastatin, fluvastatin, lovastatin, pravastatin: The possible cholesterol-lowering action of tocotrienols may be additive to that of the statins.

Sucralfate: may interfere with tocotrienol absorption.

Warfarin: Tocotrienol doses greater than 100 milligrams daily may enhance the anticoagulant response of warfarin. Monitor INRs and appropriately adjust warfarin dose if necessary.

NUTRITIONAL SUPPLEMENTS

Desiccated ox bile: may increase the absorption of tocotrienols.

Iron: Most iron supplements contain the ferrous form of iron. This form can oxidize tocotrienols, marketed in their unesterified forms, to their pro-oxidant forms if taken concomitantly.

Medium-chain triglycerides: may enhance absorption of tocotrienols if taken concomitantly.

Phytosterols and phytostanols, including beta-sitosterol and beta-sitostanol: may lower plasma tocotrienol levels.

FOOD

Olestra: is likely to inhibit the absorption of tocotrienols. Alpha-tocopherol is the only member of the vitamin E family that is added to olestra.

HERBS

Some herbs, including ginkgo and garlic, possess antithrombotic activity, and tocotrienols, if taken concomitantly with these herbs, may enhance their antithrombotic activity.

OVERDOSAGE

Tocotrienol overdosage has not been reported in the literature.

DOSAGE AND ADMINISTRATION

Presently marketed forms of tocotrienols contain mixed tocotrienols in their unesterified forms. These products typically contain d-alpha-tocotrienol, d-gamma-tocotrienol and d-delta-tocotrienol. Gamma-tocotrienol is usually the major tocotrienol in these preparations, which are marketed in the form of softgel capsules (tocotrienol is an oil).

Doses of 200 to 300 milligrams daily, with food, have been used in clinical trials studying possible cholesterol-lowering activity of tocotrienol.

The unesterified forms of tocotrienols, as well as tocopherols, are susceptible to oxidation and should therefore be stored in tightly closed, opaque containers in a cool, dry place. Tocotrienols should not be taken concomitantly with iron supplements.

LITERATURE

Elson CE. Suppression of mevalonate pathway activities by dietary isoprenoids: protective roles in cancer and cardiovascular disease. *J Nutr.* 1995; 125(6 Suppl):1666S-1672S.

Guthrie N, Gapor A, Chambers AF, Carroll KK. Inhibition of proliferation of estrogen receptor-negative MDA-MB-435 and— positive MCF-7 human breast cancer cells by palm oil tocotrienols and tamoxifen, alone and in combination. *J Nutr.* 1997; 127:544S-548S.

Kamat JP, Devasagayam TP. Tocotrienols from palm oil as inhibitors of lipid peroxidation and protein oxidation in rat brain mitochondria. *Neurosci Lett.* 1995; 195:179-182.

Kamat JP. Sarma HD, Devasagayam TPA, et al. Tocotrienols from palm oil as effective inhibitors of protein oxidation and lipid peroxidation in rat liver microsomes. *Mol Cell Biochem.* 1997; 170:131-137.

Mc Intyre BS, Briski KP, Tirmenstein MA, et al. Antiproliferative and apoptotic effects of tocopherols and tocotrienols on normal mouse mammary epithelial cells. *Lipids.* 2000; 35:171-180.

Mensink RP, van Houwelingen AC, Kromhout D, Hornstra G. A vitamin E concentrate rich in tocotrienols had no effect on serum lipids, lipoproteins, or platelet function in men with mildly elevated serum lipid concentrations. *Am J Clin Nutr.* 1999; 69:213-219.

Nesaretnam K, Guthrie N, Chambers AF, Carroll KK. Effects of tocotrienols on the growth of a human breast cancer cell line in culture. *Lipids.* 1995; 30:1139-1143.

Nesaretnam K, Stephen R, Dils R, Dabre P. Tocotrienols inhibit the growth of human breast cancer cells irrespective of estrogen receptor status. *Lipids.* 1998; 33:461-469.

Parker RA, Pearce BC, Clark RW, et al. Tocotrienols regulate cholesterol production in mammalian cells by post-transcriptional suppression of 3-hdroxy-3-methylglutaryl-coenzyme A reductase. *J Biol Chem.* 1993; 268:11230-11238.

Pearce BC, Parker RA, Deason ME, et al. Inhibitors of cholesterol biosynthesis. 2. Hypocholesterolemic and antioxidant activities of benzopyran and tertrahydronaphthalene analogues of the tocotrienols. *J Med Chem.* 1994; 37:526-541.

Quereshi AA, Bradlow BA, Manganello J, et al. Response of hypercholesterolemic subjects to administration of tocotrienols. *Lipids.* 1995; 30:1171-1177.

Qureshi AA, Pearce BC, Nor RM, et al. Dietary alpha-tocopherol on hepatic 3-hydroxy-3-methlyglutaryl coenzyme A reductase activity in chickens. *J Nutr.* 1996; 126:389-394.

Qureshi AA, Qureshi N, Hasler-Rapacz JO, et al. Dietary tocotrienols reduce concentrations of plasma cholesterol, apolipoprotein B, thromboxane B2 and platelet factor 4 in pigs with inherited hyperlipidemica. *Am J Clin Nutr.* 1991; 53(Suppl):1042S-1046S.

Serbinova E, Khwaja S, Catudioc J, et al. Palm oil vitamin E protects against ischemia reperfusion injury in the isolated perfused Langendorff heart. *Nutr Res.* 1992; 12(Suppl 1):S203-S215.

Theriault A, Chao J-T, Wang Q, et al. Tocotrienol: a review of its therapeutic potential. *Clinic Biochem.* 1999; 32:309-319.

Theriault A, Wang Q, Gapor A, Adeli K. Effects of gamma-tocotrienol on ApoB synthesis, degradation, and secretion in Hep G2 cells. *Arterioscler Thromb Vasc Biol.* 1999; 19:704-712.

Tomeo AC, Geller M, Watkins TR, et al. Antioxidant effects of tocotrienols in patients with hyperlipidemia and carotid stenosis. *Lipids.* 1995; 30:1179-1183.

Wang Q, Theriault A, Gapor A, Adeli K. Effects of tocotrienol on the intracellular translocation and degradation of apolipoprotein B: possible involvement of a proteasome independent pathway. *Biochem Biophys Res Commun.* 1998; 246:640-643.

Watkins T, Lenz P, Gapor A, et al. Gamma-tocopherol as a hypocholesterolemic and antioxidant agent in rats fed atherogenic diets. *Lipids.* 1993; 28:1113-1118.

Transgalacto-Oligosaccharides

DESCRIPTION

Transgalacto-oligosaccharides (TOS), also known as galactooligosaccharides (GOS), are a mixture of oligosaccharides consisting of D-glucose and D-galactose. Transgalacto-digosaccharides are produced from D-lactose via the action of the enzyme beta-galactosidase obtained from *Aspergillus oryzae*.

TOS are not normally digested in the small intestine. They are, however, fermented by a limited number of colonic bacteria. This could lead to changes in the colonic ecosystem in favor of some bacteria, such as bifidobacteria, which may have health benefits, including protection against certain cancers and lowering of cholesterol levels. TOS and other non-digestible oligosaccharides are sometimes referred to as bifidogenic factors.

Substances such as TOS that promote the growth of beneficial bacteria in the colon are called prebiotics. Prebiotics are typically non-digestible oligosaccharides.

ACTIONS AND PHARMACOLOGY

ACTIONS

Transgalacto-oligosaccharides may have antitumor, antimicrobial, hypolipidemic and hypoglycemic actions. They may also help improve mineral absorption and balance.

MECHANISM OF ACTION

The possible antitumor activity of TOS might be accounted for by the possible antitumor action of butyrate, one of the substances produced from TOS in the colon. Butyrate, the anion of the naturally occurring short-chain fatty acid butyric acid, is produced by bacterial fermentation of TOS in the colon. Studies suggest that butyrate induces growth arrest and cell differentiation and may upregulate apoptosis, three activities that could be significant for antitumor activity. Interestingly, butyrate also appears to inhibit vascular smooth muscle cell proliferation, at least in the rat, an activity that could have relevance with regard to a possible antiatherogenic role. TOS may promote the growth of favorable bacterial populations, such as bifidobacteria, in the colon. Bifidobacteria may inhibit the growth of pathogenic bacteria, such as *Clostritium perfringens* and diarrheogenic strains of *Escherichia coli*.

There is evidence, again from rat studies, that butyrate may suppress cholesterol synthesis in the liver and intestine. Propionate, another short-chain fatty acid produced from the bacterial fermentation of TOS in the colon, may reduce plasma free fatty acids. This might be good for blood glucose and insulin sensitivity in the long term, since high levels of plasma free fatty acids lower tissue glucose utilization and induce insulin resistance. Propionate may also aid in lowering cholesterol levels in some by possibly inhibiting HMG-CoA reductase.

TOS, similar to dietary fiber, may bind/sequester such minerals as calcium and magnesium in the small intestine. The short-chain fatty acids (acetate, propionate, butyrate) formed from the bacterial fermentation of TOS may facilitate the colonic absorption of calcium and magnesium ions. This could have both bone- and cardiovascular-health benefits.

PHARMACOKINETICS

Under normal conditions, following ingestion of TOS, no digestion of these oligosaccharides takes place in the small intestine. A small amount of TOS may undergo some acid hydrolysis in the stomach. TOS are fermented in the colon by bifidobacteria and some other bacteria to produce the short-chain fatty acids acetate, propionate and butyrate. Lactate is also produced. Acetate, propionate and butyrate that are not metabolized in colonocytes are absorbed from the colon and transported via the portal circulation to the liver. These short-chain fatty acids are extensively metabolized in hepatocytes. Acetate, propionate and butyrate that are not metabolized in hepatocytes are transported by the circulation to various tissues, where they undergo further metabolism. Butyrate is an important respiratory fuel for the colonocytes and is metabolized in them to CO_2 and H_2O. Energy is produced (ATP) from the catabolism of butyrate. Those with ileostomies may have a microbial population colonizing their ileums. In those cases, TOS could be fermented by some of the bacteria to short-chain fatty acids and lactic acid.

INDICATIONS AND USAGE

Transgalacto-oligosaccharides are being investigated for possible protective effects against colorectal cancer and infectious bowel diseases, for modulation of lipids and prevention of bone loss. Animal research suggests a role for TOS in those situations, but there is still little substantial clinical research.

RESEARCH SUMMARY

TOS, through their stimulation of bifidobacteria, have shown some protective effects against colorectal cancer and infectious bowel diseases in animal and *in vitro* experiments. TOS inhibit putrefactive bacteria (*Clostridium perfringens*) and pathogenic bacteria, such as *Escherichia coli, salmonella, listeria* and *shigella*.

A recent human study showed that supplemental TOS (in doses of 7.5 and 10 grams daily) are completely fermented in the human colon but that they did not, in this study, beneficially change the composition of the intestinal microflora. Another study, however, did show some alteration in the fermentative activity of colonic flora in humans given 10 grams of TOS per day for 21 days.

TOS have demonstrated some preliminary positive effects on calcium absorption and lipid metabolism in animal studies. Reduced serum triglyceride levels have been noted. A significant TOS hypocholesterolemic effect was observed in ovariectomized rats that had elevated total cholesterol at baseline. This same study also demonstrated a significant positive TOS effect on calcium absorption and prevention of bone loss in these animals. The stimulatory effect of TOS on calcium absorption has been observed in additional studies. Research continues.

CONTRAINDICATIONS, PRECAUTIONS, ADVERSE REACTIONS

CONTRAINDICATIONS

Transgalacto-oligosaccharides are contraindicated in those who are hypersensitive to any component of a TOS-containing product.

PRECAUTIONS

Because of absence of long-term safety studies, pregnant women and nursing mothers should exercise caution in the use of TOS supplements.

Those with lactose intolerance should be cautious in the use of TOS supplements.

ADVERSE REACTIONS

Doses of 10 grams daily are well tolerated. Higher doses may cause some gastrointestinal symptoms, such as flatulence, bloating and diarrhea.

INTERACTIONS

NUTRITIONAL SUPPLEMENTS

TOS may enhance the colonic absorption of calcium and magnesium supplements if used concomitantly with them.

Probiotics. The possible beneficial effects of TOS may be enhanced if used in combination with probiotics.

FOODS

TOS may enhance the colonic absorption of calcium and magnesium in foods.

DOSAGE AND ADMINISTRATION

Transgalacto-oligosaccharides are available in Japan and Europe as nutritional supplements and as functional foods. They are also expected to enter the U.S. marketplace. Typical dosage is about 10 grams daily, usually taken in divided doses.

LITERATURE

Bouhnik Y, Flourié B, D'Agay-Abensour L, et al. Administration of transgalacto-oligosaccharides increases fecal bifidobacteria and modifies colonic fermentation metabolism in healthy humans. *J Nutr*. 1997; 127:444-448.

Chonan O, Matsumoto K, Watanuki M. Effect of galactooligosaccharides on calcium absorption and preventing bone loss in ovariectomized rats. *Biosci Biotechnol Biochem*. 1995; 59:236-239.

Chonan O, Watanuki M. Effect of galactooligosaccharides on calcium absorption in rats. *J Nutr Sci Vitaminol (Tokyo)*. 1995; 11:95-104.

Ito M, Deguchi Y, Matsumoto K, et al. Influence of galactooligosaccharides on the human fecal microflora. *J Nutr Sci Vitaminol (Tokyo)*. 1993; 39:635-640.

Vanadium

DESCRIPTION

Vanadium is a metallic element with atomic number 23 and atomic symbol V. Vanadium is a transition element that exists in several oxidation states, including +2, +3, +4 and +5. Vanadium compounds are striking for their varied colors. For this reason, vanadium was first named panchromium. The element chromium, another colorful element, is vanadium's next-door neighbor to the left in the periodic table. Vanadium is widely found in nature in the form of minerals, as well as in living matter, such as the human body. In living matter, vanadium is found mainly as the tetravalent vanadyl cation and the pentavalent vanadate form.

Nutritional essentiality for humans has not been established for vanadium. Vanadium-deficiency states have been reported in some animals. Goats fed diets deficient in vanadium had an elevated spontaneous abortion rate and depressed milk production, and approximately 40% of kids from these goats died between days 7 and 91 of life, with some deaths preceded by convulsions. Only 8% of kids from vanadium-supplemented goats died during the same period. Rats fed vanadium-deficient diets were found to have decreased growth.

Vanadyl and vanadate compounds act as insulin-mimetics and are being studied as potentially orally active replacements for insulin. However, these substances are poorly absorbed from the gastrointestinal tract, and the amounts needed for an effective oral dose are likely to be toxic. Vanadium-containing compounds are being developed for the treatment of diabetes with higher therapeutic-to-toxicity ratios. Such compounds include peroxovanadiums, bis(picolinato) oxovanadium and the vanadium ligand L-glutamic acid gamma-monohydroxamate.

Typical diets supply less than 30 micrograms of vanadium daily. The average daily dietary intake of vanadium is approximately 15 micrograms. Foods rich in vanadium include black pepper, mushrooms, shellfish, parsley, dill seed and some prepared foods. Foods low in vanadium include fresh fruits and vegetables, oils and beverages.

Tetravalent vanadium compounds are sometimes designated as vanadium (IV) and pentavalent vanadium compounds are designated as vanadium (V).

ACTIONS AND PHARMACOLOGY

ACTIONS

Vanadium salts have insulin-mimetic activity, and vanadium compounds are being studied as potentially orally active replacements for insulin. The doses of supplemental vanadium that may affect blood glucose levels are potentially toxic, and supplemental vanadium is not recommended for the management of diabetes, hyperglycemia, hypoglycemia or insulin resistance.

MECHANISM OF ACTION

Vanadium salts mimic most of the effects of insulin *in vitro* and also induce normoglycemia and improve glucose homeostasis in insulin-deficient and insulin-resistant diabetic rodents *in vivo*. Vanadium salts appear to have these effects via alternative pathways not involving insulin receptor tyrosine kinase activation or phosphorylation of insulin receptor substrate. Vanadium's mechanisms of action appear to involve inhibition of protein-phosphotyrosine phosphatase and activation of nonreceptor protein-tyrosine kinases.

PHARMACOKINETICS

The absorption of dietary vanadium and supplemental vanadium (usually vanadyl sulfate) is poor, and most ingested vanadium is excreted in the feces. It is estimated that less than 5% of dietary vanadium is absorbed. Most ingested vanadium appears to be converted to tetravalent vanadyl in the stomach. Any absorbed vanadate is converted to cationic vanadyl in the blood. The vanadyl cation complexes with transferrin and ferritin in plasma and other body fluids. Vanadium is removed from the plasma and is found in highest amounts in the kidney, liver, testes, bone and spleen. Absorbed vanadium is mainly excreted in the urine in both high- and low-molecular weight complexes. Some absorbed vanadium may be excreted via the bile.

INDICATIONS

The use of supplemental vanadium is not indicated for any purpose at this time. Vanadium is showing promise in the treatment of both type 1 and type 2 diabetes, but this work is still preliminary and utilizes pharmacological doses of vanadium with unknown long-term safety consequences. Claims that vanadium increases muscle mass have no research support.

RESEARCH SUMMARY

Both experimental and clinical trials indicate that vanadium has significant insulin-mimetic properties in pharmacological doses. *In vitro*, vanadium salts have most of the major effects of insulin itself on insulin-sensitive tissues. Favorable results are seen, as well, in animal models of insulin deficiency, where vanadium significantly reduces blood glucose levels, and in insulin-resistant diabetic animals, where vanadium improves glucose homeostasis.

In *in vivo* animal studies examining the relationship between hyperinsulinemia, insulin resistance and hypertension, vanadium compounds produce significant, sustained decreases in both plasma insulin concentration and blood pressure. Restoring plasma insulin levels reversed the blood-pressure effect.

Clinical trials with vanadium compounds have produced benefits in both type 1 and type 2 diabetic patients. Results have been better, however, in type 2 patients. Six type 2 diabetic subjects treated with 100 milligrams of vanadyl sulfate daily for four weeks had significant reductions in fasting plasma glucose; beneficial effects on insulin sensitivity persisted for up to four weeks after vanadium treatment ended.

Recently, new vanadium compounds have been developed that are reportedly less toxic and more effective. Animal studies are underway, and clinical trials are planned.

Reports that vanadium promotes muscle-mass development are refuted by research.

CONTRAINDICATIONS, PRECAUTIONS, ADVERSE REACTIONS

CONTRAINDICATIONS
None known.

PRECAUTIONS
Those with diabetes or hyperglycemia are cautioned not to use supplemental vanadium to manage their diabetes or hyperglycemia. Those with hypoglycemia should avoid using vanadium supplements.

ADVERSE REACTIONS
The amount of vanadium in typical diets (less than 30 micrograms daily) appears to have low toxicity. In one study, 12 subjects were given 13.5 milligrams of vanadium daily for two weeks, followed by 22.5 milligrams daily for five months, Five subjects experienced gastrointestinal symptoms — nausea, vomiting, diarrhea, cramps — and five subjects developed green tongues. In another study, six subjects receiving daily doses of 4.5 to 18 milligrams of vanadium for six to 10 weeks developed green tongues, diarrhea and cramps at the higher doses.

INTERACTIONS

Chromium, ferrous ion, chloride, aluminum hydroxide and EDTA may decrease absorption of vanadium.

OVERDOSAGE

Overdosage with supplemental vanadium in humans has not been reported.

DOSAGE AND ADMINISTRATION

No recommended dosage. Vanadium, usually as the tetravalent vanadyl sulfate, is available in some vitamin and mineral preparations. Doses range from 10 micrograms to about 10 milligrams (expressed as vanadium). Tetravalent bis (maltolato) oxovanadium (BMOV) is available in some nutritional supplements as is bis-glycinato oxovanaduim (BGOV). Colloidal or liquid vitamins also may contain vanadium.

HOW SUPPLIED

Vanadyl sulfate is available in the following forms and strengths:

Capsules — 500 mcg
Tablets — 10 mg

LITERATURE

Badmaev V, Prakash S, Majeed M. Vanadium: a review of its potential role in the fight against diabetes. *J Altern Complement Med.* 1999; 5:273-291.

Boden G, Chen X, Ruiz J, et al. Effects of vanadyl sulfate on carbohydrate and lipid metabolism in patients with non-insulin dependent diabetes mellitus. *Metabolism.* 1996; 45:1130-1135.

Clarkson PM, Rawson ES. Nutritional supplements to increase muscle mass. *Crit Rev Food Sci Nutr,* 1999; 39:317-328.

Goldwaser I, Li J, Gershonov E, et al. L-glutamic acid gamma-monohydroxamine. A potentiator of vanadium-evoked glucose metabolism *in vitro* and *in vivo. J Biol Chem* 1999; 274:26617-26624.

Meyerovitch J, Rothenberg P, Schechter Y, et al. Vanadate normalizes hyperglycemia in two mouse models of non-insulin-dependent diabetes mellitus. *J Clin Invest.* 199; 87:1286-1294.

Nielsen FH. Ultratrace minerals. In: Shils ME, Olson JA, Shike M, Ross AC, eds. *Modern Nutrition in Health and Disease.* 9th ed. Baltimore, MD: Williams and Wilkins; 1999:283-303.

Pepato MT, Magnani MR, Kettelhut IC, Bruneti IL. Effect of oral vanadyl sulfate treatment on serum enzymes and lipids of streptzotocin-diabetic young rats. *Mol Cell Biochem.* 1999; 198:157-161.

Thompson KH. Vanadium and diabetes. *Biofactors.* 1999; 10:43-51.

Verma S, Cam MC, Mac Neill JH. Nutritional factors that can favorably influence the glucose/insulin system: vanadium. *J Amer Col Nutr.* 1998; 17:11-18.

Vinpocetine

TRADE NAMES
Intelectol (Covex)

DESCRIPTION
Vinpocetine is a semi-synthetic derivative of vincamine. Vincamine is an alkaloid derived from the plant *Vinca minor* L., a member of the periwinkle family. Vinpocetine, as well as vincamine, are used in Europe, Japan and Mexico as pharmaceutical agents for the treatment of cerebrovascular and cognitive disorders. In the United States, vinpocetine is marketed as a dietary supplement. It is sometimes called a nootropic, meaning cognition enhancer, from the Greek *noos* for mind.

Vinpocetine is also known as ethyl apovincaminate; ethyl apovincaminoate; eburnamenine-14-carboxylic acid ethyl ester; 3 alpha, 16 alpha-apovincaminic acid ethyl ester; ethyl apovincamin-22-oate; and cavinton, which is sometimes used generically for a branded product with that name. Another vinca alkaloid called vinconate is also being researched as a possible cognition enhancer. The structural formula of vinpocetine is:

Vinpocetine

ACTIONS AND PHARMACOLOGY

ACTIONS

Vinpocetine has several possible actions, including increasing cerebral blood flow and metabolism, anticonvulsant, cognition enhancement, neuroprotection and antioxidant. Vincamine, the parent compound of vinpocetine, is believed to be a cerebral vasodilator.

MECHANISM OF ACTION

Several mechanisms have been proposed for the possible actions of vinpocetine. Vinpocetine has been reported to have calcium-channel blocking activity, as well as voltage-gated sodium channel blocking activity. It has also been reported to inhibit the acetylcholine release evoked by excitatory amino acids and to protect neurons against excitotoxicity. In addition, vinpocetine has been shown to inhibit a cyclic GMP phosphodiesterase, and it is speculated that this inhibition enhances cyclic GMP levels in the vascular smooth muscle, leading to reduced resistance of cerebral vessels and increase of cerebral flow. In some studies, vinpocetine has demonstrated antioxidant activity equivalent to that of vitamin E.

PHARMACOKINETICS

Vinpocetine is absorbed from the small intestine, from whence it is transported to the liver via the portal circulation. From the liver via the systemic circulation, it is distributed to various tissues in the body, including the brain. Absorption of vinpocetine is significantly higher when given with food and can be up to about 60% of an ingested dose. On an empty stomach, absorption of an ingested dose can be as low as 7%. Peak plasma levels are obtained one to one and a half hours after ingestion. Extensive metabolism to the inactive

apovincaminic acid occurs in the liver. Only small amounts of unmetabolized vinpocetine are excreted in the urine, the major route of excretion of apovincaminic acid. Most of a dose is excreted within 24 hours as this metabolite. The elimination half-life of vinpocetine following ingestion is one to two hours.

INDICATIONS AND USAGE

The primary claim made for vinpocetine is that it decreases fatality and dependency in ischemic stroke. Research results are mixed. Vinpocetine has not been helpful in Alzheimer's disease, but there is some suggestion that it might help some with other dementias and cerebral dysfunction. Very preliminary research additionally suggests that vinpocetine may help protect the eye and ear from injuries caused by trauma (and, in the case of the eye, from infection) and that it might be gastroprotective, ameliorate symptoms of motion sickness and help prevent atherosclerosis.

RESEARCH SUMMARY

Several small studies, in both animals and humans, have reported significant vinpocetine-associated protective effects in ischemic stroke. A review of these studies, however, found only one positive study of a truly randomized, unconfounded clinical trials that compared the effect of vinpocetine to either placebo or another reference treatment for acute stroke where treatment started no later than 14 days after stroke onset. There is currently not enough evidence to determine whether vinpocetine does or does not reduce fatalities and dependence in ischemic stroke. Further research is needed.

There is some evidence vinpocetine may be useful in some other cerebral maladies. In one multi-center, double-blind, placebo-controlled study lasting 16 weeks, 203 patients described as having mild to moderate psychosyndromes, including primary dementia, were treated with varying doses of vinpocetine or placebo. Significant improvement was achieved in the vinpocetine-treated group as measured by "global improvement" and cognitive performance scales. Three 10-milligram doses daily were as effective or more effective than three 20-milligram doses daily. Similarly good results were found in another double-blind clinical trial testing vinpocetine versus placebo in elderly patients with cerebrovascular and central nervous system degenerative disorders. Studies of Alzheimer's disease, however, have shown no vinpocetine benefit.

Some preliminary research suggests that vinpocetine may have some protective effects in both sight and hearing. One study of patients with mild burn trauma in the eyes showed that vinpocetine enhanced healing, most likely as a result of increased blood flow to the damaged tissue. Vinpocetine has also been associated with improvements seen in retinas damaged by hepatitis B virus. Damage from acoustic trauma has similarly been reduced by vinpocetine treatment.

Vinpocetine gastroprotective effects have been reported in animal models challenged with noxious agents. There are anecdotal reports that vinpocetine is protective against some of the gastric and neurological toxicity of excessive alcohol consumption.

There are some reports that vinpocetine may be an effective motion sickness preventative and some early findings in animals that it may exert some anti-atherosclerotic effects through a reported ability to decalcify cholesterol-induced atherosclerotic lesions.

CONTRAINDICATIONS, PRECAUTIONS, ADVERSE REACTIONS

CONTRAINDICATIONS
None known.

PRECAUTIONS
Pregnant women and nursing mothers should avoid vinpocetine supplements. Those with a history of allergic reactions or hypersensitivity reactions during treatment with other vinca alkaloids, such as vinblastine and vincristine, should avoid vinpocetine. Those on warfarin are advised to have their INRs (international normalized ratios) regularly monitored when using vinpocetine supplements (see Interactions). Those with hypotension or orthostatic hypotension should be cautioned that prolonged use of vinpocetine may lead to slight reductions in systolic and diastolic blood pressure.

ADVERSE REACTIONS
Reported adverse reactions include nausea, dizziness, insomnia, drowsiness, dry mouth, transient hypotension, transient tachycardia, pressure-type headache and facial flushing. Slight reductions in both systolic and diastolic blood pressure with prolonged use of vinpocetine have been reported, as well as slight reductions in blood glucose.

INTERACTIONS
Warfarin—Slight changes in prothrombin time have been noted in those adding vinpocetine to warfarin dosing. The changes appear minimal. However, regular monitoring of INR is advised in those using warfarin and vinpocetine concomitantly. There are no other known drug or nutritional supplement, herb or food interactions.

OVERDOSAGE
There are no reports of vinpocetine overdosage.

DOSAGE AND ADMINISTRATION
Vinpocetine is available as an individual supplement and in combination products. Typical doses for supplement use are 5 to 10 milligrams daily with food. Some take up to 20 milligrams daily. Higher doses are not advised.

LITERATURE

Bereczki D, Fekete I. A systematic review of vinpocetine therapy in acute ischaemic stroke. *Eur J Clin Pharmacol.* 1999; 55:349-352.

Bukanova YV, Solntseva EI. Nootropic agent vinpocetine blocks delayed rectified potassium currents more strongly than high-threshold calcium currents. *Neurosci Behav Physiol* 1998; 28:116-120.

Cholnoky E, Domok LI. Summary of safety tests of ethyl apovincaminate. *Arzneimittelforschung.* 1976; 26(10a):1938-1944.

Gulyas B, Halldin C, Karlsson P, et al. Brain uptake and plasma metabolism of [11C] vinpocetine: a preliminary PET study in a cynomolgus monkey. *J Neuroimaging.* 1999; 9:217-222.

Hindmarch I, Fuchs HH, Erzigkeith H. Efficacy and tolerance of vinpocetine in ambulant patients suffering from mild to moderate organic psychosyndromes. *Int Clin Psychopharmacol.* 1991; 6:31-43.

Kiss B, Karpati E. [Mechanism of action of vinpocetine.] [Article in Hungarian.] *Acta Pharm Hung.* 1996; 66:213-224.

Lakics V, Sebestyén MG, Erdö SL. vinpocetine is a highly potent neuroprotectant against veratridine-induced cell death in primary cultures of rat cerebral cortex. *Neurosci Lett.* 1995; 185:127-130.

Miskolczi P, Vereczkey L, Szalay L, Gondoc C. Effect of age on the pharmacokinetics of vinpocetine (Cavinton) and apovincaminic acid. *Eur J Clin Pharmacol.* 1987; 33:185-189.

Nosalova V, Machova J, Babulova A. Protective action of vinpocetine against experimentally induced gastric damage in rats. *Arzneimittelforschung.* 1993; 43:981-985.

Pudleiner P, Vereczkey L. Study of the absorption of vinpocetine and apovincamic acid. *Eur J Drug Metab Pharmacokinet.* 1993; 18:317-321.

Subhan Z, Hindmarch I. Psychopharmacological effects of vinpocetine in normal healthy volunteers. *Eur J Clin Pharmacol.* 1985; 28:567-571.

Szakall S, Boros I, Balkay L, et al. Cerebral effects of a single dose of intravenous vinpocetine in chronic stroke patients: a PET study. *J Neuroimaging.* 1998; 8:197-204.

Thal LJ, Salmon DP, Lasker B, et al. The safety and lack of efficacy of vinpocetine in Alzheimer's disease. *J Am Geriatr Soc.* 1989; 37:515-520.

Vereczkey L, Czira G, Tamas J, et al. Pharmacokinetics of vinpocetine in humans. *Arzneimittelforschung.* 1979; 29:957-960.

Vitamin A

TRADE NAMES
Ultra Carotenoids (Westlake Labs), A-25 (Bio-Tech Pharmacal), Palmitate-A (Akorn Inc.) Mycel Vitamin A (Ethical Nutrients), Dry A (Solaray).

DESCRIPTION

Vitamin A refers to a group of fat-soluble substances that are structurally related to and possess the biological activity of the parent substance of the group called all-*trans* retinol or retinol. Vitamin A plays vital roles in vision, epithelial differentiation, growth, reproduction, pattern formation during embryogenesis, bone development, hematopoiesis and brain development. It is also important for the maintenance of the proper functioning of the immune system. Certain carotenoids, such as beta-carotene alpha-carotene and beta-cryptoxanthin, are dietary precursors of vitamin A. Collectively, these substances are called provitamin A. (See Beta-Carotene). The term retinoids refers to retinol and its metabolites, such as retinoic acid, as well as to synthetic analogues that are structurally similar to retinol but may not have the same biological activities as retinol.

Vitamin A deficiency can result in night blindness (defective vision at low illumination), xerosis of the conjunctiva and cornea (destruction of the cornea secondary to vitamin A deficiency or xerophthalmia is a major cause of blindness in children), keratinization of the lung, gastrointestinal tract and urinary tract epithelia, growth retardation, follicular hyperkeratosis of the skin, increased susceptibility to infections and death. Children are particularly susceptible to the effects of vitamin A deficiency. Deficiency of the vitamin is a serious public health issue in developing countries.

Vitamin A deficiency was probably the first nutritional deficiency to be recognized. The ancient Egyptians and Greeks apparently treated the corneal changes due to deficiency of the vitamin and night blindness by the topical application and the feeding of liver, a rich source of vitamin A. In addition to liver, other rich sources of vitamin A are fish liver oils (e.g., cod liver oil), egg yolks, butter and cream. Vitamin A occurs naturally in the form of fatty acid esters, such as vitamin A palmitate (retinyl palmitate).

Vitamin A deficiency occurs under certain conditions. These include inadequate dietary intake of vitamin A or provitamin A, malabsorption syndromes (cystic fibrosis, Whipple's disease, Crohn's disease, ulcerative colitis, short bowel syndrome), pancreatic disease and chronic liver disease (e.g., cirrhosis).

The effects of vitamin A are mediated by two different mechanisms. The eye illustrates both of these mechanisms. Vitamin A (all-*trans* retinol) is converted in the retina to the 11-*cis*-isomer of retinaldehyde or 11-*cis*-retinal. 11-*cis*-retinal functions in the retina in the transduction of light into the neural signals necessary for vision. 11-*cis*-retinal, while attached to opsin in rhodopsin is isomerized to all-*trans*-retinal by light. This is the event that triggers the nerve impulse to the brain which allows for the perception of light.

All-*trans*-retinal is then released from opsin and reduced to all-*trans*-retinol. All-*trans*-retinol is isomerized to 11-*cis*-retinol in the dark, and then oxidized to 11-*cis*-retinal. 11-*cis*-retinal recombines with opsin to re-form rhodopsin. Night blindness or defective vision at low illumination results from a failure to resynthesize 11-*cis* retinal rapidly. This is a consequence of vitamin A deficiency. Vitamin A deficiency results in the depletion of the vitamin A storage pool (retinyl ester) in the retinal pigment epithelial cells.

The normal differentiation of the cells of the cornea and conjunctiva is dependent on another metabolite of vitamin A, retinoic acid. Retinoic acid acts as a hormone and is involved in signal transduction. Retinoic acid signaling and signaling by other retinoids are mediated by two classes of nuclear receptors, retinoic acid receptors (RAR-alpha, -beta and -gamma) and retinoid X receptors (RXR-alpha, -beta and -gamma). The RARs and RXRs belong to the superfamily of nuclear hormone receptors. Members of this family, which, in addition to retinoic acid, include receptors for small hydrophobic hormones, such as steroids, the biologically active form of vitamin D, thyroid hormones and metabolites of long-chain fatty acids, associate with DNA response elements in the promoter region of target genes and act either to activate or repress transcription. The response elements to which retinoic acid and other retinoids bind to are called retinoid response elements. The role of vitamin A in epithelial differentiation, as well as in other physiological processes, is thought to be mediated via retinoic acid's hormonal activity.

High-dose vitamin A has been used in the management of various skin disorders, including acne; Darier's disease or keratosis follicularis, an autosomal dominant disorder of keratinization; pityriasis rubra pilaris, an abnormality of follicular keratinization; Kyrle's disease, a focal derangement of orientation of keratinization and xerosis. None of the above uses are FDA approved. FDA-approved retinoids, include tretinoin (all-trans-retinoic acid), which is used topically for acne vulgaris; isotretinoin (13-*cis*-retinoic acid), for cystic acne; etretinate, a synthetic analog of retinoic acid ethyl ester, for psoriasis; and acitretin, a metabolite of etretinate, also for psoriasis. FDA-approved retinoids used for the treatment of malignancies, include alitretinoin (9-*cis*-retinoic acid), a topical treatment for Kaposi's sarcoma; all-*trans*-retinoic acid, for acute promyelocytic leukemia; and bexarotene, for refractory cutaneous T-cell lymphoma.

The parent compound of the vitamin A family is all-*trans*-retinol. It is also the most abundant dietary form of vitamin A. All-*trans*-retinol occurs naturally in the form of fatty acid esters, such as vitamin A palmitate (retinyl palmitate). Vitamin A palmitate and vitamin A acetate (retinyl acetate) are the principal forms used as nutritional supplements.

All-*trans*-retinol, as is the case of all forms of vitamin A, is a derivative of beta-ionone. All-*trans*-retinol is also known as retinol, vitamin A$_1$, anti-infective vitamin, vitamin A alcohol and (all-*E*)-3, 7-dimethyl-9- (2, 6, 6-trimethyl-1-cyclohexen-1-y1)-2, 4, 6, 8-nonatetraen-1-o1. Its molecular formula is C$_{20}$H$_{30}$O and its molecular weight is 286.46 daltons. Its structural formula is:

Vitamin A

Other naturally occurring forms of vitamin A, include retinal (retinaldehyde, retinene, vitamin A$_1$ aldehyhde), retinoic acid (vitamin A$_1$ acid), retinoyl-beta-glucuronide (vitamin A$_1$ beta-glucuronide), retinyl phosphate (vitamin A$_1$ phosphate), 3-dehydroretinol (vitamin A$_2$), 11-*cis*-retinal (11-*cis*-retinaldehyde, 11-*cis* or neo b vitamin A$_1$ aldehyde), 5, 6-epoxyretinol (5, 6-epoxy vitamin A$_1$ alcohol), anhydroretinol (anhydro vitamin A$_1$) and 4-ketoretinol (4-keto-vitamin A$_1$ alcohol). Except for all-*trans*-retinol, retinyl palmitate and retinyl acetate, all the other above-mentioned forms are minor dietary components.

Amounts of vitamin A are expressed in four ways: international units (IU), United States Pharmacopia (USP) units, micrograms and retinol equivalents. One IU is equal to one USP unit. One IU of vitamin A activity is defined as either equal to 0.30 micrograms of all-*trans* retinol or to 0.60 micrograms of the provitamin A, all-*trans*-beta-carotene. One retinol equivalent (RE) is defined as one microgram of all-*trans* retinol, six micrograms of all-*trans*-beta-carotene or 12 micrograms of other provitamin A carotenoids.

ACTIONS AND PHARMACOLOGY

ACTIONS

Vitamin A may prevent loss of vision or restore lost vision. Vitamin A may have anticarcinogenic, immunomodulatory and antioxidant activities.

MECHANISM OF ACTION

Vitamin A deficiency can result in night blindness and blindness due to the destruction of the cornea (xerophthalmia). The ability of vitamin A to prevent these two visual problems and its mechanism of action in doing so is well known (see Description). There are a couple of recent reports that suggest vitamin A may affect some visual problems in those who are not vitamin A-deficient. Sorsby's fundus dystrophy (SFD) is an autosomal dominant retinal degeneration disorder which, among other things, can result in night blindness. SFD, both clinically and histopathologically,

shares similarities with age-related macular degeneration, the most common cause of loss of vision in the elderly. In an SFD family, it was found that vitamin A at 50,000 IU daily resolved night blindness within a week in those members of the family who were at early stages of the disease. The mechanism of this effect is not clear. The researchers hypothesized that the abnormally thickened Bruch's membrane, with its lipid deposits, acts as a barrier to the diffusion of vitamin A presented from the choroidal vasculature, essentially causing vitamin A deficiency in the retina. According to this hypothesis, large doses of vitamin A override the reduced transport efficiency of retinol across the defective Bruch's extracellular matrix. Direct or indirect effects of retinol on retinal pigment epithelial (RPE) cells are other possibilities. Vitamin A is known to modulate RPE cellular function and behavior. In another study, an oral retinoid was found to restore visual pigment and function in a mouse model of childhood blindness. Leber's congenital amaurosis (LCA) is an autosomal recessive mitochondrial disease which results in retinal degeneration. It is a rare variant of the more common disease, retinitis pigmentosum. Researchers found that administration of the vitamin A form 9-*cis*-retinal to the mice led to signs of visual improvement. The researchers hypothesized that 9-*cis*-retinal bypassed the biochemical block in the retina caused by the disease. Human studies are needed. It must be noted, however, that high doses of vitamin A have the potential for serious side effects.

Vitamin A and retinoids have been found to inhibit tumor development, especially those of epithelial origin, in a variety of *in vitro* studies. All-*trans*-retinol has been demonstrated to suppress the malignant behavior of cultured cells transformed by radiation, chemicals or viruses, to delay the development of transplanted tumors and to prevent malignancy in animals exposed to various potent carcinogens. It is thought that the anticarcinogenic effect of preformed vitamin A (all-*trans*-retinol) in these cases are mediated by its conversion to retinoic acid. Retinoic acid, via its binding to nuclear receptors (retinoic acid receptors, retinoid X receptors), may induce cell differentiation, inhibit proliferation and/or induce apoptosis. Many of these results were obtained using doses of all-*trans*-retinol that were very high and that would be too toxic for general, preventive use. Further, it is unclear whether sufficient conversion of all-*trans*-retinol to retinoic acid occurs to make a significant anticarcinogenic impact. A recent two-year study (EUROSCAN) of high-dose retinyl palmitate showed no benefit—in terms of survival, event-free survival, or secondary primary tumors—for patients with head and neck cancer or with lung cancer, most of whom were previous or current smokers.

Some retinoids, however, have shown anticancer effects in certain situations. All-*trans*-retinoic acid is an approved drug for the treatment of acute promyelocytic leukemia (APL). The mechanism of action of all-*trans*-retinoic acid in the treatment of APL is not fully understood. Those with APL possess an abnormal gene for retinoic acid receptor-alpha (RAR-alpha). Treatment with all-*trans*-retinoic acid induces expression of the remaining normal RAR-alpha allele, which may rebalance the receptor system toward normal differentiation. Bexarotene is a synthetic retinoid analogue which is approved for the treatment of cutaneous T-cell lymphoma. The mechanism of action of bexarotene is unknown. It is known to activate retinoid X receptors (RXR), which pair with other cellular receptors to control the expression of genes involved in cellular differentiation and growth. The use of retinoids in the treatment of cancer is known as differentiation therapy.

Vitamin A deficiency results in decreased resistance to infection. Vitamin A deficiency affects both cell-mediated and antibody-mediated immune responses. Nonspecific immune responses involving neutrophils, macrophages and natural killer cells, are also affected by vitamin A deficiency. It is thought that vitamin A's participation in the immune response is via signal transduction pathways which are necessary for the normal functioning of the immune system. Retinol may also stimulate the immune response in animals and humans who are not vitamin A deficient. High doses of retinyl palmitate have been found to stimulate the nonspecific immune system in animals. Retinol and retinoic acid have also been found to enhance the antibody response to specific antigens, again, in animals. In surgery patients treated with high doses of vitamin A for seven days after surgery, lymphocyte proliferation did not differ from the control group after one day, but was significantly greater after seven days. The mechanism of action of the possible immunomodulatory effect of vitamin A is not well understood. Further, the studies of immunomodulation in animals that were not vitamin A-deficient, used vitamin A doses that would be toxic in humans.

Vitamin A deficiency has been found to cause oxidative damage to liver mitochondria in rats. In these animals, a deficit of Vitamin A produced an increase in oxidized glutathione, malondialdehyde, 8-oxo-deoxyguanosine, a drop in the mitochondrial membrane potential and an 80% decrease in the reduced glutathione to oxidized glutathione ratio. Vitamin A has also been found to protect against lipid peroxidation induced by doxorubicin in heart and brain membrane lipids and to inhibit chemiluminescence and lipid peroxidation in isolated rat liver microsomes and mitochondria. The antioxidant mechanism of vitamin A is thought to be due, in part, to the hydrophobic chain of polyene units, which can quench singlet oxygen, neutralize thiyl radicals and stabilize and combine with peoroxyl radicals.

PHARMACOKINETICS

Preformed vitamin A is present in food in the form of retinyl esters. The principal nutritional supplement forms of preformed vitamin A are retinyl palmitate and retinyl acetate. Retinyl palmitate is also used in food fortification. Preformed vitamin A is efficiently absorbed from the small intestine. The efficiency of absorption ranges from 60%-90%. Vitamin A absorption requires bile salts, pancreatic enzymes and dietary fat. Vitamin A is delivered to the enterocytes in the form of micelles. Prior to its absorption, the retinyl esters are hydrolyzed by a pancreatic hydrolase. Long-chain retinyl esters, such as retinyl palmitate, appear to be hydrolyzed by a hydrolyase which is a component of the brush border. Within the enterocytes, all-*trans*-retinol is re-esterified to retinyl esters and the retinyl esters are secreted by the enterocytes into the lymphatics in the form of chylomicrons.

The chylomicrons enter the circulation via the thoracic duct. Chylomicrons undergo metabolism in the circulation via lipoprotein lipase to form chylomicron remnants. Most of the retinyl esters in chylomicron remnants are rapidly taken up into liver parenchymal cells. Within the liver parenchymal cells, retinyl esters are again hydrolyzed to all-*trans*-retinol and fatty acids. All-*trans*-retinol may be stored in the liver as retinyl esters or may be transported in the circulation bound to serum retinol binding protein (RBP). RBP delivers retinol to the various tissues. Approximately 50%-85% of the total body vitamin A content is stored in the liver. Greater than 95% of serum retinol is present in its unesterified form.

Serum retinol binding (RBP) protein is the principal carrier of all-*trans*-retinol, which comprises over 90% of serum vitamin A. RBP is found in serum in association with a cotransport protein called transthyretin or prealbumin. The mechanism of the transport of retinol into target cells is not known. Within cells, retinol and its metabolites are bound to retinoid-binding proteins in the cytosol and nucleus. The cytosolic retinoid-binding proteins are: cellular retinol-binding protein I (CRBP-I), cellular retinol-binding protein II (CRBP-II), cellular retinoic acid-binding protein I (CRABP-I) and cellular retinoic acid-binding protein II (CRABP-II). The nuclear retinoid-binding proteins are: retinoic acid receptor-alpha (RAR-alpha), retinoic acid receptor-beta (RAR-beta), retinoic acid receptor-gamma (RAR-gamma), retinoid X receptor-alpha (RXR-alpha), retinoid X receptor-beta (RXR-beta) and retinoid X receptor-gamma (RXR-gamma). The cytosolic retinoid-binding proteins limit the amounts of unbound or free retinoids and channel them to specific enzymes responsible for their metabolism. The nuclear retinoid-binding proteins bind retinoids and regulate the activities of retinoid-responsive genes.

All-trans retinol is oxidized to retinal via retinol dehydrogenase: retinal is metabolized to retinoic acid via retinal dehydrogenase. All-trans-retinol is delivered to the cornea via the tears and by diffusion through eye tissue. Retinol and retinoic acid form a number of oxidized metabolites. The metabolites of retinol and retinoic acid undergo glucuronidation, glucosylation and amino acylation and are excreted mainly via the biliary route. Some excretion of retinol and its metabolites occurs via the kidneys.

INDICATIONS AND USAGE

A major role has emerged for vitamin A in the treatment of malnourished children, principally in developing countries. It is credited with significantly reducing mortality and the incidence of blindness, diarrhea, measles and some other infections in these populations. Vitamin A appears to have many positive effects in the immune system and may have some anti-cancer effects. It can help with some skin conditions and may be useful in some with Sorsby's fundus dystrophy. There is emerging evidence that vitamin A plays crucial roles in embryonic development, and some believe it will eventually be used to prevent teratogenesis under some circumstances. Pregnant women, however, should not use doses of vitamin A greater than the U.S. RDA (5,000 IU/day) without a physician's recommendation and supervision.

RESEARCH SUMMARY

Several large, well-controlled, double-blind intervention trials have shown that intermittent high-dose vitamin A supplementation in malnourished children can significantly reduce mortality and the incidence of blindness, diarrhea, measles and some other infections. In one of these trials, there was a significant 27% relative reduction in mortality from all causes in children who received vitamin A supplementation. In another study, this one involving 11,200 children in Indonesia, there was a 30% lower mortality in supplemented children. Six of eight such intervention studies have shown significant reductions in mortality.

Other studies have shown significant reduction in morbidity in similar populations supplemented with vitamin A. Significant reductions in xerophthalmia, blindness, measles, diarrhea and some parasitic infections have been reported. Less dramatic effects have been seen in respiratory infections. The World Health Organization estimates that there are 250 million preschool-age children worldwide whose health may be compromised by vitamin A deficiency. For some years, WHO and some other health organizations have recommended administering large doses of vitamin A to at-risk children at the time they are vaccinated for measles. This practice caused concern when one study suggested that the vitamin A

dose was interfering with seroconversion to live measles vaccine in infants with maternal antibodies. A more recent study, however, has refuted this finding to the satisfaction of many. The researchers concluded that "there is no indication that simultaneous administration of measles vaccine and vitamin A supplements has a negative effect on measles immunity."

Vitamin A's effects on immunity generally appear to be broad. It was demonstrated some years ago that high-dose vitamin A can significantly protect against some of the immune-depressing effects of radiation and cancer chemotherapy. Animal and *in vitro* work, as well as some human work, has shown that vitamin A can protect immune function by helping to maintain the integrity of epithelial barriers to infection and by activating phagocytes and cytotoxic T-cells, among other activities.

There is some evidence that vitamin A can stimulate and otherwise favorably affect the immune system even in the absence of frank or marginal vitamin A deficiency. Such effects have been demonstrated in a number of animal models.

An *in vitro* experiment showed that a form of vitamin A found in breast milk inhibits herpes simplex virus-1. And vitamin A, administered to surgical patients in large daily doses (90 to 135 milligrams) for seven days, significantly increased lymphocyte proliferation. Research on the immune-modulating effects of vitamin A continues. Many *in vitro* and some animal studies have shown that vitamin A can inhibit malignant activity in various types of cells adversely affected by radiation, chemicals and viruses. The vitamin variously delayed or prevented malignancy in animals exposed to several different carcinogens. Drug derivatives of vitamin A have demonstrated efficacy against some cancers and pre-cancerous lesions, including oral leukoplakia, myelodisplastic syndrome, cutaneous T-cell lymphoma and cervical cancer. Retinoids have been shown to help regulate the expression of some proto-oncogenes and protein growth factors. And retinoic acid has demonstrated an ability to inhibit proliferation of some tumor cells and to promote differentiation of some other cancer cells *in vitro*.

On the other hand, vitamin A, in combination with beta-carotene, showed no anti-cancer efficacy in an aborted intervention study of smokers, former smokers and workers exposed to asbestos. There was a statistically non-significant increase in incidence of lung cancer and mortality in the treated group. (See Beta-carotene.)

Vitamin A and its drug derivatives have been used with significant success in the treatment of several skin disorders, including cystic acne, acne vulgaris, psoriasis and photoaged skin. High-dose vitamin A and theses drugs require careful medical supervision and must not be used during pregnancy, owing to risk of birth defects.

One study has shown that high-dose vitamin A (50,000 IU per day) significantly reversed night blindness in some with Sorsby's fundus dystrophy, a rare autosomal retinal degeneration disorder that is clinically similar to age-related macular degeneration. Lower doses (5,000 IU daily) had no effect, but it was suggested that lower doses begun early in disease progression might be helpful. Testing with intermediate doses was also proposed.

Recently, research has suggested that vitamin A might be helpful in preventing some birth defects—surprising to some, since high-dose vitamin A supplementation is itself associated with risk of birth defects. But so is vitamin A deficiency. Current research shows that retinoic acid signaling is crucial for proper development of the early embryonic mesoderm. There are further suggestions that impaired retinoid signaling could have negative effects not only on the embryo but later in life, as well, in terms of neurologic and behavioral development and function. Even schizophrenia, some researchers believe, may be promoted by retinoid defects. Obviously, much more research will be required before any possible strategies for safely and effectively utilizing vitamin A for the prevention of birth defects emerge.

CONTRAINDICATIONS, PRECAUTIONS, ADVERSE REACTIONS
CONTRAINDICATIONS
Doses of vitamin A above 5,000 IU are contraindicated in pregnant women.

Vitamin A is contraindicated in those hypersensitive to any component of a vitamin A-containing product.

Vitamin A is contraindicated in those with hypervitaminosis A.

PRECAUTIONS
The use of vitamin A for the treatment of vitamin A deficiency requires medical supervision.

The use of vitamin A or any retinoid for the treatment of any medical condition must be prescribed and supervised by a physician.

Nursing mothers should avoid doses of vitamin A great than the U.S. RDA (5,000 IU daily), unless prescribed by a physician.

Supplemental vitamin A may add to the toxicity of retinoids or retinoid analogues which are used pharmaceutically. These include acitretin, all-*trans*-retinoic acid, bexarotene, etretinate and isotretinoin. Those taking any of these drugs should avoid the use of supplemental vitamin A.

ADVERSE REACTIONS
High intakes of vitamin A may cause acute or chronic toxicity. (see overdosage for acute toxicity). Symptoms and signs of chronic toxicity, include dry rough skin, cracked lips, sparse coarse hair and alopecia of the eyebrows. These are early signs. Late symptoms and signs, include irritability, headache, pseudotumor cerebri (benign intracranial hypertension), elevated serum liver enzymes, reversible noncirrhotic portal hypertension, hepatic fibrosis and cirrhosis. There are a few reports of death secondary to liver failure.

Supplemental doses of 10,000 IU of vitamin A daily or greater have been reported to increase the risk of birth defects when used by pregnant women.

Subjects in the EUROSCAN study were given 300,000 IU/day of vitamin A for one year followed by 150,000 IU/day for the second year. Typical side effects were mucocutaneous ones (dryness, desquamation, itching, bleeding and hair loss).

Hepatotoxicity has been reported in one patient who took 25,000 IU/day of vitamin A over a six-year period.

INTERACTIONS
DRUGS
Cholestyramine: Concomitant intake of cholestyramine and vitamin A may reduce the absorption of vitamin A.

Colestipol: Concomitant intake of colestipol and vitamin A may reduce the absorption of vitamin A.

Mineral Oil: Concomitant intake of mineral oil and vitamin A may reduce the absorption of vitamin A.

Oral Contraceptives: Oral contraceptives may increase serum retinol.

Orlistat: Orlistat may decrease the absorption of vitamin A.

Retinoid Drugs (acitretin, all-trans-retinoic acid, bexarotene, etretinate and isotretinoin): Supplemental vitamin A may add to the toxicity of these drugs (see Precautions).

NUTRITIONAL SUPPLEMENTS
Vitamin K: Intake of large doses of vitamin A may decrease the absorption of vitamin K.

FOODS
Olestra: The fat substitute olestra inhibits the absorption of vitamin A as well as the other fat-soluble vitamins D, E and K. These vitamins are added to olestra to compensate for this. Olestra contains 170 IU of vitamin A per gram (51 retinol equivalents per gram).

OVERDOSAGE
Acute toxicity in infants or children can occur with a single dose of 25,000 IU per kilogram of body weight. Vomiting, increased intracranial pressure and death may occur. A dose

of 2,000,000 IU or greater in adults, can cause a similar clinical picture. Some Arctic explorers have ingested several million units of vitamin A from eating polar bear or seal liver, two of the richest sources of vitamin A. The Arctic explorers developed irritability, drowsiness, headache and vomiting. There are few reports of fatalities with such high doses of vitamin A.

DOSAGE AND ADMINISTRATION

The two principal forms of vitamin A supplements are retinyl acetate and retinyl palmitate. Multivitamin preparations contain vitamin A in one of these forms, a combination of vitamin A and beta-carotene (provitamin A) or beta-carotene alone. Rarely are doses higher than 5,000 IU of vitamin A exceeded in these formulas. Supplemental doses of vitamin A greater than 10,000 IU daily are not recommended. Many take beta-carotene for vitamin A supplementation (see Beta-Carotene). Vitamin A is also available in the form of cod liver oil.

The current recommended dietary allowances (RDA) for vitamin A by the Food and Nutrition Board of the U.S. National Academy of Sciences are:

Category	Age (years) or conditions	RDS (micrograms RE) day	IU/day
Infants	0.0-1.0	375	1,250
Children	1 through 3	400	1,333
	4 through 6	500	1,667
	7 through 10	700	2,333
Males	11 years and older	1,000	3,333
Females	11 years and older	1,000	3,333
Pregnant/Lactating	1st 6 months	1,300	4,333
	2nd 6 months	1,200	4,000

One IU or one USP unit equals 0.30 micrograms of all-*trans* retinol, 0.344 micrograms of retinyl acetate or 0.55 micrograms of retinyl palmitate.

The U.S. RDA is different than the RDAs. The U.S. RDA, which is used on nutritional supplement labels and food labels, is usually the highest RDA value. In the case of vitamin A, the U.S. RDA is 5,000 IU which is slightly higher than the highest RDA value (4,333) for the vitamin.

HOW SUPPLIED

Vitamin A is available in the following forms and strengths for Rx use:

Capsules — 50,000 IU

Vitamin A is available in the following forms and strengths for OTC use:

Capsules — 8000 IU, 10,000 IU, 15,000 IU, 25,000 IU

Liquid — 3000 IU/drop

Tablets — 5000 IU, 10,000 IU, 15,000 IU, 25,000 IU

LITERATURE

Acott TS, Weleber RG. Vitamin A megatherapy for retinal abnormalities. *Nature Med.* 1995; 1:884-885.

Barber T, Borrás E, Torres L, et al. Vitamin A deficiency causes oxidative damage to liver mitochondria in rats. *Free Rad Biol Med.* 2000; 29:1-7.

Barreto ML, Santos LMP, Assis AMO, et al. Effect of vitamin A supplementation on diarrhoea and acute lower-respiratory-tract infections in young children in Brazil. *Lancet.* 1994; 344:228-231.

Bates CJ. Vitamin A. *Lancet.* 1995; 345:31-35.

Benn CS, Aaby P, Balé C, et al. Randomized trial of effect of vitamin A supplementation on antibody response to measles vaccine in Guinea-Bissau, West Africa. *Lancet.* 1997; 350:101-105.

Collins MD, Mao GE. Teratology of retinoids. *Annu Rev Pharmacol Toxicol.* 1999; 39:399-430.

Chiang M-Y, Misner D, Kempermann G, et al. An essential role for retinoid receptors RARbeta and RXRgamma in long-term potentiation and depression. *Neuron.* 1998; 21:1353-1361.

Futoryan T, Gilchrest BA. Retinoids and the skin. *Nutr Rev.* 1994; 52:299-310.

Gilchrest B. Anti-sunshine vitamin A. *Nature Med.* 1999; 5:376-377.

Hadi H, Stoltzfus RJ, Dibley MJ, et al. Vitamin A supplementation selectively improves the linear growth of Indonesian preschool children: results from a randomized controlled trial. *Am J Clin Nutr.* 2000; 71:507-513.

Humphrey JH, Rice AL. Vitamin A supplementation of young infants. *Lancet.* 2000; 356:422-424.

Jacobson SG, Cideciyan AV, Regunath G, et al. Night blindness in Sorsby's fundus dystrophy reversed by vitamin A. *Nature Gen.* 1995; 11:27-32.

Kowalski TE, Falestiny M, Furth E, Malet PF. Vitamin A hepatotoxicity: a cautionary note regarding 25,000 IU supplements. *Am J Med.* 1994; 97:523-528.

Lee M-O, Han S-Y, Jiang S, et al. Differential effects of retinoic acid on growth and apoptosis in human colon cancer cell lines associated with the induction of retinoic acid receptor beta. *Biochem Pharmacol.* 2000; 59:485-496.

Ross AC. Vitamin A and retinoids. In: Shils ME, Olson JA, Shike M, Ross AC, eds. *Modern Nutrition in Health and Disease.* 9th ed. Baltimore, MD: Williams and Wilkins; 1999:305-327.

Ross AC, Stephensen CB. Vitamin A and retinoids in antiviral responses. *FASEB J.* 1996; 10:979-985.

Rothman KJ, Moore LL, Singer MR, et al. Teratogenicity of high vitamin A intake. *N Engl J Med.* 1995; 333:1369-1373.

Russell RM. The vitamin A spectrum: from deficiency to toxicity. *Am J Clin Nutr.* 2000; 71:878-884.

Sohlenius-Sternbeck A-K, Appelkvist E-L, De Pierre JW. Effects of vitamin A deficiency on selected xenobiotic-metabolizing enzymes and defenses against oxidative stress in mouse liver. *Biochem Pharmacol.* 2000; 59:377-383.

Underwood BA, Arthur P. The contribution of vitamin A to public health. *FASEB J.* 1996; 10:1040-1048.

Van Hooser JP, Aleman TS, He Y-G, et al. Rapid restoration of visual pigment and function with oral retinoid in a mouse model of childhood blindness. *Proc Natl Acad Sci USA.* 2000; 97:8623-8628.

Varani J, Warner RL, Gharaee-Kermani M, et al. Vitamin A antagonizes decreased cell growth and elevated collagen-degrading matrix metalloproteinases and stimulates collagen accumulation in naturally aged human skin. *J Invest Dermatol.* 2000; 114:480-486.

Wang Z, Boudjelal M, Kang S, et al. Ultraviolet irradiation of human skin causes functional vitamin A deficiency, preventable by all-*trans* retinoic acid pre-treatment. *Nature Med.* 1999; 5:418-422.

West KP Jr, Pokhrel RP, Katz J, et al. Efficacy of vitamin A in reducing preschool child mortality in Nepal. *Lancet.* 1991; 338:67-71.

Wolf G. A regulatory pathway of thermogenesis in brown fat through retinoic acid. *Nutr Rev.* 1995; 53:230-231.

Wolf G. A history of vitamin A and retinoids. *FASEB J.* 1996; 10:1102-1107.

Wolf G. Vitamin A functions in the regulation of the dopaminergic system in the brain and pituitary gland. *Nutr Rev.* 1998; 56:354-358.

Vitamin B6

TRADE NAMES

Releaf PMS (Lake Consumer Products), Bedoxine 100 (Ampharco Inc.), VitaBee 6 (Consolidated Midland Corp.), Pyri-500 (Miller Pharmacal), Rodex (Legere Pharmaceuticals), Aminoxin (Tyson Neutraceuticals), Vitelle Nestrex (Fielding Pharmaceutical), Ginkai (Lichtwer Pharm).

DESCRIPTION

Vitamin B_6 is the collective term for a group of three related compounds, pyridoxine (PN), pyridoxal (PL) and pyridoxamine (PM), and their phosphorylated derivatives, pyridoxine 5'-phosphate (PNP), pyridoxal 5'-phosphate (PLP) and pyridoxamine 5'-phosphate (PMP). Although all six of these vitamers should technically be referred to as vitamin B_6, the term vitamin B_6 is commonly used interchangeably with just one of the vitamers, pyridoxine. Vitamin B_6, principally in the form of the coenzyme pyridoxal 5'-phosphate, is involved in a wide range of biochemical reactions, including the metabolism of amino acids and glycogen, the synthesis of nucleic acids, hemoglobin, sphingomyelin and other sphingolipids, and the synthesis of the neurotransmitters serotonin, dopamine, norepinephrine and gamma-aminobutyric acid (GABA).

Food sources of vitamin B_6, include meat, poultry, fish, eggs, white potatoes and other starchy vegetables, noncitrus fruits, fortified ready-to-eat cereals and fortified soy-based meat substitutes. The principal forms of vitamin B_6 in animal products are pyridoxal 5'-phosphate and pyridoxamine 5'-phosphate. In plant-derived foods, the major forms of vitamin B_6 are pyridoxine, pyridoxine 5'-phosphate and pyridoxine glucosides. Glycosylated forms of pyridoxine range from approximately 5% to 75% of the total vitamin B_6 content in fruits, vegetables and grains, with little to none in animal products. Pyridoxine appears to be the only glycosylated form of vitamin B_6. The major glycosylated form of pyridoxine in most plant-derived foods is pyridoxine 5'-beta-D-glucoside. Pyridoxine hydrochloride is the form of vitamin B_6 most commonly used for fortification of foods and in nutritional supplements.

The classical symptoms and signs of vitamin B_6 deficiency are a microcytic, hypochromic anemia, seizure activity, seborrheic dermatitis, confusion and depression. Vitamin B_6-deficiency states in infants and children primarily result in electroencephalogram abnormalities and seizure activity, while in adults, vitamin B_6 deficiency primarily results in cheilosis (chapping and fissuring of the lips), glossitis (inflammation of the tongue), stomatitis (inflammation of the oral mucosa), anemia, irritability, confusion and depression. Many of these signs are not specific for vitamin B_6 deficiency and may be due to deficiencies of other vitamins or result from other causes. Vitamin B_6 deficiency may result from the use of certain drugs, including isoniazid (isonicotinic acid hydrazide or INH), penicillamine, cycloserine, ethionamide, hydralazine and theophylline. Subclinical vitamin B_6 deficiency frequently occurs in those with malabsorption syndromes, uremia, cancer, heart failure and cirrhosis, and in alcoholics, the elderly and adolescent females and during pregnancy. In the elderly and in those with malabsorption syndromes, clinical deficiency of the vitamin may occur.

In addition to vitamin B_6 deficiency conditions, vitamin B_6-dependency conditions exist. Certain inborn errors of metabolism exist in which a vitamin B_6-dependent enzyme is defective in the coenzyme (pyridoxal 5'-phosphate) binding site, and the enzyme only has significant activity when the tissue concentration of pyridoxine 5'-phosphate, the biologically active form of vitamin B_6, is much higher than normal. These vitamin B_6-dependent conditions, which may be responsive to treatment with large doses of the vitamin, include convulsions of the newborn secondary to glutamate decarboxylase (GAD) deficiency, cystathionuria secondary to cystathionase deficiency, gyrate atrophy with ornithinuria secondary to ornithinine-delta-aminotransferase deficiency, homocystinuria secondary to cystathionine beta-synthase deficiency, primary hyperoxaluria type 1 secondary to peroxisomal alanine-glyoxylate transaminase deficiency, sideroblastic anemia secondary to delta-aminolevulinate synthase deficiency and xanthurenic aciduria secondary to kynureninase deficiency. These genetic disorders are all rare.

Vitamin B6 in the form of pyridoxal 5'-phosphate is a coenzyme for over 100 enzymes. Most of these enzymes are involved in amino acid metabolism and include aminotransferases (transaminases), decarboxylases. Pyridoxal 5'-phosphate is sometimes referred to as codecarboxylase, dehydratases and racemases. The basic chemistry accounting for the broad range of reactions of B6 is Schiff's base formation. Schiff's bases are reaction products of aldehyde and amino groups. In the resting state of the above enzymes, the aldehyde group of pyridoxal 5'-phosphate is covalently linked to the epsilon-amino group of a lysine residue at the active site of the enzyme. Upon binding of the amino acid substrate, the lysine is exchanged for the alpha-amino group of the substrate, forming a Schiff's base with the aldehyde group of pyridoxal 5'-phosphate. A quinonoid intermediate follows the formation of the Schiff's base, which in turn is followed by the formation of the reaction products. Schiff's base chemistry is the mechanism of almost all of the reactions in which pyridoxal 5'-phosphate participates. One exception is the glycogen phosphorylase reaction. Glycogen phosphorylase catalyzes the breakdown of the storage polysaccharide glycogen to yield glucose 1-phosphate. Much of the total pyridoxal 5'-phosphate in the body is found in muscle bound to glycogen phosphorylase. In glycogen phosphorylase, the phosphate group of pyridoxal 5'-phosphate, rather than its aldehye group, participates in the catalytic role of the enzyme.

Vitamin B6 is involved in several key biological processes. Pyridoxal 5'-phosphate is the coenzyme for delta-aminolevulinate synthase, the first step in the synthesis of porphyrins. Heme is derived from protoporphyrin IX. Heme is the iron-containing prosthetic group that is an essential component of such proteins as hemoglobin, myoglobin and the cytochromes. Homocysteine is an intermediate in methionine metabolism and may undergo one of two metabolic fates, remethylation to L-methionine or further metabolism, leading to the synthesis of L-cysteine. The pathway leading to the synthesis of cysteine is known as the transsulfuration pathway. This pathway has two pyridoxal 5'-phosphate-dependent enzymes: cystathionine beta-synthase and cystathionase. The conversion of tryptophan to niacin also requires pyridoxal-5'-phosphate, this time as a cofactor for the pyridoxal 5'-phosphate-dependent enzyme kynureninase. And, via its role in transamination, pyridoxal 5'-phosphate is involved in the production of energy.

Decarboxylation of amino acids yields amines, including gamma-aminobutyrate, dopamine, norepinephrine, epinephrine and serotonin, which play important roles as neurotransmitters or hormones. The amino acid decarboxylases are also pyridoxal 5'-phosphate-dependent enzymes. Pyridoxal 5'-phosphate plays a role in the regulation of steroid hormone activity: Physiological levels of pyridoxal 5'-phosphate interact with glucocorticoid receptors to downregulate their activity. Pyridoxal 5'-phosphate has also been shown to negatively modulate steroid-dependent gene expression induced by progesterone, androgen and estrogen hormones. Finally, serine hydroxymethyltransferase is a pyridoxal 5'-phosphate-dependent enzyme which catalyzes the interconversion of serine and glycine, both of which are major sources of one-carbon units necessary for the *de novo* synthesis of purine nucleotides and thymidylate. Purine nucleotides are precursors of DNA and RNA, and thymidylate is a precursor of DNA.

The vitamers comprising the vitamin B6 family are pyridine derivatives. Specifically, they are derivatives of 3-hydroxy-5-hydroxymethyl-2-methyl pyridine. The vitamers differ by the nature of the chemical group occupying the 4 position of the parent compound. In the case of pyridoxine, the 4 position is occupied by an hydroxymethyl group. Pyridoxine is also known as 5-hydroxy-6-methyl-3, 4-pyridinedimethanol, 2-methyl-3-hydroxy-4,5-bis(hydroxymethyl)pyridine and pyridoxol. Its molecular formula is $C_8H_{11}NO_3$ and its molecular weight is 169.17 daltons. Pyridoxine hydrochloride is the principal form of vitamin B6 used in nutritional supplements and for food fortification.

Pyridoxal is also known as 3-hydroxy-5-(hydroxymethyl)-2-methyl-4-pyridinecarboxaldehyde and 2-methyl-3-hydroxy-4-formyl-5-hydroxymethylpyridine. In the case of pyridoxal, the 4 position of the parent compound is occupied by a formyl group. The molecular formula of pyridoxal is $C_8H_9NO_3$ and its molecular weight is 167.16 daltons. Pyridoxamine has an aminomethyl group occupying the 4 position of the parent structure. Pyridoxamine is also known as 4-(aminomethyl)-5-hydroxy-6-methyl-3-pyridinemethanol and 2-methyl-3-hydroxy-4-aminomethyl-5-hydroxymethylpyridine. Its molecular formula is $C_8H_{12}N_2O_2$ and its molecular weight is 168.18.

ACTIONS AND PHARMACOLOGY

ACTIONS

Vitamin B6 has antineurotoxic activity and may have activity in a number of inborn errors of metabolism, including pyridoxine-dependent seizures in infants, sideroblastic anemia, primary hyperoxaluria, homocystinuria and cystathioninuria. Vitamin B6 has putative antiatherogenic, immunomodulatory, anticarcinogenic and mood-modulatory activities.

MECHANISM OF ACTIONS
Vitamin B6 is used in the prophylaxis and treatment of vitamin B6 deficiency and peripheral neuropathy in those receiving isoniazid (isonicotinic acid hydrazide, INH). The antituberculosis drug isoniazid reacts non-enzymatically with pyridoxal 5'-phosphate to form a metabolically inactive hydrazone. This can result in vitamin B6 deficiency and peripheral neuropathy. It may also result in pellagra. The formation of niacin from tryptophan is catalyzed by, among other enzymes, kynureninase. Kynureninase is a vitamin B6-dependent enzyme. Therefore, vitamin B6 deficiency resulting from isoniazid, particularly in the context of marginal or clinical niacin deficiency, may lead to the niacin deficiency disorder pellagra. The peripheral neuropathy resulting from isoniazid does not appear to be due to vitamin B6 deficiency, but to isoniazid itself. The antineurotoxic effect of vitamin B6 in the case of isoniazid appears to be accounted for by the reaction of the vitamin with the drug, thus lowering its tissue level and its neurotoxicity.

High theophylline levels may cause seizures. It is thought that this is due to reaction of theophylline with pyridoxal 5'-phosphate, leading to lowered plasma levels of the vitamin. Pyridoxal 5'-phosphate is involved in the metabolism of gamma-aminobutyric acid (GABA). GABA is a major inhibitory neurotransmitter in the central nervous system. When the concentration of GABA in the brain decreases to below a threshold level, seizures and other neurological disorders, may occur. The concentration of GABA in the brain is controlled by two pyridoxal 5'-phosphate-dependent enzymes, glutamate decarboxylase (GAD) and GABA transaminase (GABA-T). A decrease in the levels of GABA in the brain secondary to decreased levels of pyridoxal 5'-phosphate can lead to seizures. It has been found that the administration of vitamin B6 to mice treated with theophylline reduced the number of seizures, and the vitamin administered to rabbits reversed electroencephalogram changes caused by high doses of theophylline.

Seven inborn errors of metabolism are known in which a vitamin B6-dependent enzyme has a defect in the coenzyme (pyridoxal 5'-phosphate) binding site, and the enzyme only has significant activity when the tissue concentration of pyridoxine 5'-phosphate is much higher than normal. The disorders and their enzyme defects are pyridoxine-dependent seizures in infants (glutamate decarboxylase deficiency resulting in decreased CNS levels of GABA), pyridoxine-responsive sideroblastic anemia (delta-aminolevulinate syn-

thase deficiency resulting in decreased synthesis of hemoglobin), primary hyperoxaluria type 1 (peroxisomal alanine-glyoxylate transaminase deficiency), homocystinuria (cystathionine beta-synthase deficiency), cystathioninuria (gamma-cystathionase deficiency), xanthurenic aciduria (kynureninase deficiency) and gyrate atrophy of the choroid and retina (ornithine-delta-aminotransferase deficiency). These disorders may be responsive to high doses of vitamin B6, which increase tissue levels of pyridoxal 5'-phosphate.

The putative antiatherogenic activity of vitamin B6 may be accounted for by a few different mechanisms. Hyperhomocysteinemia is an independent risk factor for atherosclerosis and coronary heart disease. Homocysteine is an intermediate in the metabolism of L-methionine and is either remethylated to L-methionine or, via the transsulfuration pathway, is converted to L-cysteine. Two pyridoxal 5'-phosphate-dependent enzymes are involved in the conversion of homocysteine to cysteine: cystathionine beta-synthase and gamma-cystathionase. Studies to date, indicate that folic acid (see Folate) is more important than vitamin B6 in lowering homocysteine levels in those with moderate hyperhomocysteinemia (folic acid is involved in the remethylation of homocysteine), but it has not been ruled out that supplementary vitamin B6 may also aid in lowering homocysteine levels in some with hyperhomocysteinemia. Those who are deficient in vitamin B6 would be expected to have their homocysteine levels lowered with administration of the vitamin.

Vitamin B6, in the form of pyridoxine hydrochloride, has been found to lower systolic and diastolic blood pressure in a small group of subjects with essential hypertension. Hypertension is another risk factor for atherosclerosis and coronary heart disease. The mechanism of action of the antihypertensive effect of vitamin B6 is unknown. Another study showed pyridoxine hydrochloride to inhibit ADP- or epinephrine-induced platelet aggregation and to lower total cholesterol levels and increase HDL-cholesterol levels, again in a small group of subjects. The mechanisms of action of the possible platelet and lipid effects of vitamin B6 are unknown. Vitamin B6, in the form of pyridoxal 5'-phosphate, was found to protect vascular endothelial cells in culture from injury by activated platelets. Endothelial injury and dysfunction are critical initiating events in the pathogenesis of atherosclerosis. The mechanism of the possible endothelial-protective effect of vitamin B6 is unclear. It is thought that vitamin B6 plays a role in the maintenance of endothelial integrity. Finally, vitamin B6 has been shown to have singlet oxygen quenching activity *in vitro*. Single oxygen is a reactive oxygen species and oxidative stress is thought to play a major role in the pathogenesis of atherosclerosis.

Both animal and human studies have demonstrated that vitamin B₆ deficiency affects cellular and humoral responses of the immune system. Vitamin B₆ deficiency results in altered lymphocyte differentiation and maturation, reduced delayed-type hypersensitivity (DTH) responses, impaired antibody production, decreased lymphocyte proliferation and decreased interleukin (IL)-2 production, among other immunologic activities. Those at risk for vitamin B₆ deficiency and associated immunological dysfunction are the elderly, those with uremia and those with HIV (human immunodeficiency virus) disease. Repletion of vitamin B₆ in those with vitamin B₆ deficiency can correct immunological dysfunctions. Supplementation of the vitamin in those who are vitamin B₆ sufficient, has not to date shown immune-enhancing or immunomodulatory effects. The mechanism through which vitamin B₆ deficiency alters immune responses is not well understood. Vitamin B₆ deficiency appears to impair nucleic acid synthesis. The impaired nucleic acid synthesis is associated with altered one-carbon metabolism, particularly the activity of serine hydroxymethyltransferase. Serine hydroxymethyltransferase is a pyridoxal 5'-phosphate-dependent enzyme which catalyzes the interconversion of serine and glycine, both of which are major sources of one-carbon units necessary for the synthesis of purine nucleotides and thymidylate. Impairment of purine nucleotide and thymidylate synthesis would impair the synthesis of nucleic acids. Serine hydroxymethyltransferase activity appears to be low in resting lymphocytes. Antigenic or mitogenic stimulation of immune cells triggers their proliferation. Serine hydroxymethyltransferase activity increases in immune cells under the influence of antigenic or mitogenic stimulation, thus supplying the increased demand for nucleic acid synthesis during an immune response. Since vitamin B₆ is involved in the synthesis of nucleic acids, via serine hydromethyltransferase, deficiency of the vitamin would result in decreased DNA replication, with consequent decreases in RNA and protein synthesis and immune cell proliferation.

Pyridoxal has been found to inhibit the growth of human malignant melanoma cells *in vitro*. It has also been found to inhibit the growth of melanoma cells injected into mice. There is one report of topical vitamin B₆ inducing lesion regression in two patients with melanoma. The mechanism of the putative anticarcinogenic activity of vitamin B₆ is unknown.

Vitamin B₆ may be useful in managing the depressive symptoms in some women with premenstrual dysphoric disorder (PMDD), also known as premenstrual syndrome (PMS). However, the evidence for this comes mainly from poor-quality trials. The mechanism of this putative effect may be accounted for, in part, by the participation of pyridoxal 5'-phosphate as a coenzyme in the synthesis of the neurotransmitters serotonin and dopamine. Modulation of steroid-dependent gene expression, by the vitamin, may also play some role in this putative effect.

PHARMACOKINETICS

The major forms of vitamin B₆ from animal products are pryridoxal 5'-phosphate and pyridoxamine 5'-phosphate. The major forms of vitamin B₆ from plant-derived foods are pyridoxine, pyridoxine 5'-phosphate and pyridoxine glucosides. Pyridoxine hydrochloride is the principal form of vitamin B₆ used for food fortification and in nutritional supplements. Pyridoxal 5'-phosphate is also available as a nutritional supplement.

The phosphylated forms of vitamin B₆ undergo hydrolysis in the small intestine via alkaline phosphatase, and the non-phosphorylated forms of the vitamin are absorbed by a nonsaturable passive diffusion process, mainly in the jejunum. The efficacy of absorption of vitamin B₆ is high and even extremely high doses of vitamin B₆ are well absorbed. The pyridoxine glucosides are less efficiently absorbed than the other vitamin B₆ forms. The pyridoxine glucosides are deconjugated by a mucosal glucosidase. A fraction of the pyridoxine glucosides is absorbed intact and hydrolyzed in various tissues.

Some vitamin B₆ is converted to pyridoxal 5'-phosphate in the enterocytes where it is used in various metabolic reactions. Most of the absorbed vitamin B₆ is transported via the portal circulation to the liver. In the liver, pyridoxine, pyridoxal and pyridoxamine are metabolized to pyridoxine 5'-phosphate, pyridoxal 5'-phosphate and pyridoxamine 5'-phosphate, by pyridoxal 5'-phosphate kinase. Pyridoxal 5'-phosphate is secreted by the liver and transported by the systemic circulation to the various tissues of the body. Pyridoxal 5'-phosphate is the primary form of vitamin B₆ in the circulation and is bound to serum albumin.

The major body pool of vitamin B₆ is in muscle, where most of the vitamin is present as pyridoxal 5'-phosphate bound to glycogen phosphorylase. The principal catabolite of vitamin B₆ is 4-pyridoxic acid which is the primary form of the vitamin excreted in the urine. 4-Pyridoxic acid, which is principally formed in the liver, accounts for approximately 50% of the vitamin B₆ compounds in the urine. At very high doses of vitamin B₆, which is mainly in the form of pyridoxine, much of the dose is excreted unchanged in the urine.

INDICATIONS AND USAGE

Vitamin B₆ is used for the treatment of vitamin B₆ deficiency and for the prophylaxis of isoniazid-induced peripheral neuropathy. It may also be helpful in treatment of convulsions of the newborn secondary to glutamate decarboxylase deficiency, sideroblastic anemia secondary to delta-aminole-vulinate synthase deficiency, primary hyperoxaluria type 1 secondary to peroxisomal alanine-glyoxylate transaminase deficiency, homocystinuria secondary to cystathionine beta-synthase deficiency, cystathioninuria secondary to gamma-cystathionase deficiency, xanthurenic aciduria secondary to kynureninase deficiency and gyrate atrophy of choroid and retina secondary to ornithinine-delta-aminotransferase deficiency.

Vitamin B_6 may be helpful in some women with premenstru-al dysphoric disorder (PMDD), also known as premenstrual syndrome (PMS), and may be useful in some cases of gestational diabetes and for protection against metabolic imbalances associated with the use of some oral contracep-tives. Results are mixed and largely negative with the respect to claims that vitamin B_6 is an effective treatment of carpal tunnel syndrome. There is very preliminary evidence that vitamin B_6 may help protect against atherosclerosis, that it might show some activity against melanoma and that it might be helpful in some neurologic conditions. It has some immune stimulating properties. It is an anti-emetic in some circumstances. There is little evidence to support claims that vitamin B_6 is an effective treatment for depression (other than, possibly, the depression associated with premenstrual syndrome), autism, schizophrenia, atopic dermatitis, alcohol-ism, diabetic peripheral neuropathy, Down's syndrome, dental caries, Huntington's chorea or steroid-dependent asthma.

RESEARCH SUMMARY
A recent review of randomized, double-blind, placebo-con-trolled trials of vitamin B_6 in the treatment of premenstrual syndrome (PMS) concluded that the treatment significantly relieves overall premenstrual and premenstrual-associated depressive symptoms. Doses ranged between 50 milligrams and 600 milligrams of vitamin B_6 daily. Only one of 940 subjects included in these studies reported symptoms sugges-tive of sensory neuropathy, the principal adverse reaction of high dose vitamin B_6. Premenstrual symptoms were signifi-cantly relieved by 100 milligrams of vitamin B_6 daily (typically in divided 50 milligrams doses). There was less evidence of efficacy at a 50 milligram daily dose. Though the review authors found methodological flaws in many of the studies, they have stated that the available evidence warrants a large scale multicenter clinical trial. Vitamin B_6's apparent efficacy in PMS has been speculatively attributed, in part, to its role as a cofactor in the synthesis of serotonin and dopamine, deficits in the availability and function of which may play a part in the pathogenesis of PMS.

There are reports that vitamin B_6 supplementation can help normalize disturbances in the metabolism of tryptophan associated with the use of some oral contraceptives. Studies suggest that 5 to 50 milligrams daily are adequate for this purpose. Improved glucose tolerance has been reported in some of these studies. Some other studies, however, have shown no vitamin B_6 effect on the nausea, vomiting, dizziness and irritability sometimes associated with the use of oral contraceptives. Evidence is conflicting and inconclu-sive with respect to vitamin B_6's impact on depression linked to the use of oral contraceptives.

Claims that vitamin B_6 is useful in improving glucose tolerance in diabetics in general is poorly supported except in gestational diabetes where the evidence is somewhat better, though still far from conclusive. More research is needed.

Studies on the use of vitamin B_6 in the treatment of carpal tunnel syndrome have produced mixed results which, on balance, suggest little benefit. Some open trials have found that vitamin B_6 is helpful, but most double-blind, placebo-controlled trials have reported no benefit. Until larger, better-designed studies are conducted, no useful conclusion can be reached with respect to vitamin B_6's role, if any, in treating carpal tunnel syndrome.

It has been suggested that vitamin B_6 might have cardiopro-tective effects. Reduced levels of vitamin B_6 have been associated with elevated levels of homocysteine, a risk factor for atherosclerosis. Results have been mixed on the ability of supplemental vitamin B_6 to lower homocysteine levels. There is one uncontrolled report associating supplemental vitamin B_6 use with reduced incidence of acute cardiac chest pain and myocardial infarction. And there is a recent study showing a significant protective effect of vitamin B_6 on function and integrity of vascular endothelium subjected to experimental injury by activated platelets. There are also preliminary reports that supplemental vitamin B_6 can reduce hypertension in some. This work needs confirmation.

There was a report in 1985 that a topical application of pyridoxal produced significant regression in the metastatic melanoma of two patients. Greater than 50% regression of lesions was noted after two weeks of treatment. Untreated lesions did not regress. This preliminary report needs followup.

Vitamin B_6 is an effective treatment for seizures in infants caused by a specific inborn metabolic disorder. Deficiencies in vitamin B_6 have been associated with a number of neurologic and behavioral disorders, but interventive data are largely lacking. There is a study of Egyptian mothers and their infants significantly relating the vitamin B_6 nutritional status of the mother to infant behavior. Some studies have indicated that, even in the United States, a significant percentage of women of child-bearing age, as well as pregnant and lactating women, may have vitamin B_6 intakes below the recommended dietary allowance.

Studies are needed to determine the effects of low maternal vitamin B6 intake on neurologic and behavioral development in offspring: Experiments with vitamin B6-deficient maternal rats have demonstrated effects that might impair developmental processes related to learning and memory in offspring.

Vitamin B6 plays an active role in the immune system. Even marginal deficiency, such as is found in many of the elderly, may result in some immune deficits. Chronically ill patients, notably those with HIV-disease, also often exhibit marginal or frank vitamin B6 deficiency. Both humoral and cell-mediated immune responses have been shown to be impaired in those with vitamin B6 deficiencies. Supplementation to normal levels generally restores immune function due to deficiency. Higher doses have not been reported to further stimulate or modulate the immune system.

In one study, approximately one-third of a healthy elderly population had marginal vitamin B6 deficiency. Supplementation with the vitamin in elderly subjects has produced significant improvement in immune function as determined by a number of laboratory measures, including lymphocyte proliferative responses to both T- and B-cell mitogens. Percentages of CD3+ and CD4+ (but not CD8+) cells increased significantly in elderly subjects receiving 50 milligrams of vitamin B6 daily.

Vitamin B6 has been used with some success as an anti-emetic in a dose range of 50-200 milligrams daily. It has been effective in treating nausea subsequent to radiotherapy and nausea associated with pregnancy (''morning sickness''). In one double-blind trial, vitamin B6 alleviated the severe nausea and significantly reduced the vomiting of those who received the vitamin in 25 milligram doses every eight hours for three days.

CONTRAINDICATIONS, PRECAUTIONS, ADVERSE REACTIONS

CONTRAINDICATIONS

Vitamin B6 is contraindicated in those hypersensitive to any component of a vitamin B6-containing product.

PRECAUTIONS

Pre- and postnatal vitamin/mineral supplements typically deliver vitamin B6 (as pyridoxine) at a dose of between 2 to 20 milligrams daily. Pregnant women and nursing mothers should avoid doses of vitamin B6 greater than these doses, unless higher doses are prescribed by their physicians.

Those who are being treated with levodopa without concurrently taking carbidopa should avoid doses of vitamin B6 of 5 milligrams or greater daily.

The use of vitamin B6 for the treatment of vitamin B6 deficiency, for the prophylaxis of isoniazid-induced peripheral neuropathy, for the treatment of vitamin B6-dependency disorders (see Indications) or for the treatment of any other medical condition requires medical supervision.

ADVERSE REACTIONS

Doses of vitamin B6, typically in the form of pyridoxine, of up to 200 milligrams daily are generally well tolerated. One report showed severe sensory neuropathy in seven adults after pyridoxine intakes that started at 50 to 100 milligrams/day and were steadily increased to 2 to 6 grams/day over 2 to 40 months. None of the subjects in the report showed sensory neuropathy at doses of pyridoxine of less than 2 grams/day. There is one report of a woman who had been taking 200 milligrams/day of pyridoxine for 2 years without showing sensory neuropathy who developed sensory neuropathy after she increased her pyridoxine dose to 500 milligrams/day. There are rare reports of sensory neuropathy occurring at pyridoxine doses in the range of 100 to 200 milligrams/day. The Food and Nutrition Board of the Institute of Medicine of the U.S. National Academy of Sciences has concluded that reports and studies showing sensory neuropathy at doses of pyridoxine less than 200 milligrams/day are weak and inconsistent, with the weight of evidence indicating that sensory neuropathy is unlikely to occur in adults taking pyridoxine at doses less than 500 milligrams/day.

Other adverse reactions reported with high doses of pyridoxine, include nausea, vomiting, abdominal pain, loss of appetite and breast soreness. Rare cases of pyridoxine-induced photosensitivity have been reported.

INTERACTIONS

DRUGS

Amiodarone: Concomitant use of vitamin B6 and amiodarone may enhance amiodarone-induced photosensitivity reactions. Doses of vitamin B6 greater than 5-10 milligrams/day should be avoided by those taking amiodarone.

Carbamazepine: Chronic use of carbamazepine may result in a significant decrease in plasma pyridoxal 5'-phosphate levels.

Cycloserine: Cycloserine may react with pyridoxal 5'-phosphate to form a metabolically inactive oxime, which may result in a functional vitamin B6 deficiency.

Ethionamide: The use of ethionamide may increase vitamin B6 requirements.

Fosphenytoin: High doses of vitamin B6 may lower plasma levels of phenytoin. Fosphenytoin is a prodrug of phenytoin.

Hydralazine: The use of hydralazine may increase vitamin B6 requirements.

Isoniazid: (isonicotinic acid, INH). Isoniazid reacts with pyridoxal 5'-phosphate to form a metabolically inactive hydrazone, which may result in functional vitamin B_6 deficiency.

Levodopa: Concomitant use of levodopa and vitamin B_6 in doses of 5 milligrams or more daily may reverse the therapeutic effects of levodopa. Vitamin B_6 does not reverse the therapeutic effects of levodopa if levodopa is taken concurrently with the levodopa decarboxylase inhibitor carbidopa. Levodopa is typically administered as a combination product with carbidopa.

Oral contraceptives: The use of oral contraceptives may increase vitamin B_6 requirements. This was more the case with the older oral contraceptive agents with high-dose estrogen/progestin. It appears to be less the case with the newer low-dose estrogen/progestin products.

Penicillamine: Penicillamine may react with pyridoxal 5'-phosphate to form a metabolically inactive thiazolidine, which may result in a functional vitamin B_6 deficiency.

Phenelzine: Phenelzine may react with pyridoxal 5'-phosphate to yield a metabolically inactive hydrazone compound.

Phenobarbital: High doses of vitamin B_6 may lower plasma levels of phenobarbital.

Phenytoin: High doses of vitamin B_6 may lower plasma levels of phenytoin.

Theophylline: Theophylline may react with pyridoxal 5'-phosphate leading to low plasma levels of the coenzyme. This may increase the risk of theophylline-induced seizures.

Valproic acid: Chronic use of valproic acid may result in a significant decrease in plasma pyridoxal 5'-phosphate levels.

FOODS
Alcoholic beverages: Alcohol may increase the catabolism of pyridoxal 5'-phosphate. Chronic and excessive use of alcoholic beverages can result in vitamin B_6 deficiency.

OVERDOSAGE
No reports.

DOSAGE AND ADMINISTRATION
Vitamin B_6 is available in nutritional supplements principally in the form of pyridoxine hydrochloride. Pyridoxal 5'-phosphate is also available as a nutritional supplement. Pyridoxine hydrochloride is available in multivitamin and multivitamin/multimineral products as well as products that, in addition to vitamins and minerals, contain other nutritional substances. Single ingredient pyridoxine products are also available. Some products are available which contain mixtures of pyridoxine hydrochloride and pyridoxal 5'-phosphate. Typical doses of pyridoxine used for nutritional supplementation range from 2 to 20 milligrams/day.

Those who use pyridoxine for the management of premenstrual syndrome, typically use doses ranging from 50 to 100 milligrams/day. Those who use pyridoxine for the management of carpal tunnel syndrome, typically use doses ranging from 100 to 200 milligrams/day.

The Food and Nutrition Board of the Institute of Medicine of the National Academy of Sciences has recommended the following Dietary Reference Intakes (DRI) for vitamin B_6:

Infants	Adequate Intakes (AI)
0 through 6 months	0.1mg/day $\approx$ 0.014 mg/Kg
7 through 12 months	0.3 mg/day $\approx$ 0.033 mg/Kg

	Recommended Dietary Allowances (RDA)
Children	
1 through 3 years	0.5 mg/day
4 through 8 years	0.6 mg/day
Boys	
9 through 13 years	1.0 mg/day
14 through 18 years	1.3 mg/day
Girls	
9 through 13 years	1.0 mg/day
14 through 18 years	1.2 mg/day
Men	
19 through 50 years	1.3 mg/day
51 through 70 years	1.7 mg/day
70 years and older	1.7 mg/day
Women	
19 through 50 years	1.3 mg/day
51 through 70 years	1.5 mg/day
70 years and older	1.5 mg/day
Pregnancy	
14 through 50 years	1.9 mg/day
Lactation	
14 through 50 years	2.0 mg/day

The U.S. RDA for vitamin B_6, which is used for determining percentage of nutrient daily values on nutritional supplement and food labels, is 2.0 mg/day.

The Food and Nutrition Board has identified a Lowest-Observed-Adverse-Effect Level (LOAEL) for vitamin B_6 of 500 milligrams/day (See Adverse Reactions) and a No-Observed-Adverse-Effect Level (NOAEL) of 200 milligrams/day. Based on the NOAEL and an uncertainty factor of 2, the Food and Nutrition Board has recommended the following Tolerable Upper Intake Levels (UL) for vitamin B_6:

Infants	UL
0 through 12 months	Not possible to establish

Children
1 through 3 years .... 30 mg/day
4 through 8 years .... 40 mg/day
9 through 13 years .... 60 mg/day

Adolescents .... 80 mg/day

Pregnancy
14 through 18 years .... 80 mg/day
19 years and older .... 100 mg/day

Lactation
14 through 18 years .... 80 mg/day
19 years and older .... 100 mg/day

Adults
19 years and older .... 100 mg/day

HOW SUPPLIED
Vitamin B6 is available in the following forms and strengths for OTC use:

Capsules — 150 mg, 500 mg
Enteric Coated Tablets — 20 mg
Tablets — 10 mg, 25 mg, 32.5 mg, 50 mg, 100 mg, 250 mg, 500 mg
Tablets Extended Release — 200 mg

Vitamin B6 is available in the following forms and strengths for Rx use:

Injection — 100 mg/mL

LITERATURE

Anon. Vitamin B6 for melanoma. *Medical World News.* February 11, 1985.

Aybak M, Sermet A, Ayylidiz MO, Karakilcik AZ. Effect of oral pyridoxine hydrochloride supplementation on arterial blood pressure in patients with essential hypertension. *Arzneimittelforschung.* 1995; 45:1271-1273.

Bender DA. Non-nutritional uses of vitamin B6. *Br J Nutrition.* 1999; 81:7-20.

Bendich A, Cohen M. Vitamin B6 safety issues. *Ann NY Acad Sci.* 1990; 585:321-330.

Bernstein AL. Vitamin B6 in clinical neurology. *Ann NY Acad Sci.* 1990; 585:250-260.

Bernstein AL, Dinesen JS. Brief communication: effect of pharmacologic doses of vitamin B6 on carpal tunnel syndrome, electroencephalographic results, and pain. *J Am Coll Nutr.* 1993; 12:73-76.

Bilski P, Li MY, Ehrenshaft M, et al. Vitamin B6 (pyridoxine) and its derivatives are efficient singlet oxygen quenchers and potential fungal antioxidants. *Photochem Photobiol.* 2000; 71:129-134.

Chang S-J. Vitamin B6 protects vascular endothelial injury by activated platelets. *Nutr Res.* 1999; 19:1613-1624.

Dakshinamurti, K, ed. *Vitamin B6.* New York, NY: The New York Academy of Sciences; 1990.

Dietary Reference Intakes for Thiamin, Riboflavin, Niacin, Vitamin B6, Folate, Vitamin B12, Pantothenic Acid, Biotin, and Choline. Washington, DC: National Academy Press; 1998; 150-195.

DiSorbo DM, Wagner R Jr, Nathanson L. In vivo and in vitro inhibition of B16 melanoma growth by vitamin B6. *Nutr Cancer.* 1985; 7:43-52.

Ellis J, Folkers K, Watanabe T, et al. Clinical results of a cross-over treatment with pyridoxine and placebo of the carpal tunnel syndrome. *Am J Clin Nutr.* 1979; 32:2040-2046.

Ellis JM, McCully KS. Prevention of myocardial infarction by vitamin B6. *Res Commun Mol Pathol Pharmacol.* 1995; 89:208-220.

Franzblau A, Rock CL, Werner RA, et al. The relationship of vitamin B6 status to median nerve function and carpal tunnel syndrome among active industrial workers. *J Occup Environ Med.* 1996; 38:485-491.

Gregory JF III. Nutritional properties and significance of vitamin glycosides. *Annu Rev Nutr.* 1998; 18:277-296.

Gridley DS, Schultz TD, Stickney DR, Slater JM. In vivo and in vitro stimulation of cell-mediated immunity by vitamin B6. *Nutr Res.* 1988; 8:201-207.

Guilarte TR. Vitamin B6 and cognitive development: recent research findings from human and animal studies. *Nutr Rev.* 1993; 51:193-198.

Khatami M. Role of pyridoxal phosphate/pyridoxine in diabetes. Inhibition of nonenzymatic glycosylation. *Ann NY Acad Sci.* 1990; 585:502-504.

Laso Guzman FJ, Gonzalez-Buitrago JM, de Arriba F, et al. Carpal tunnel syndrome and vitamin B6. *Klin Wochenschr.* 1989; 67:38-41.

Leklem JE. Vitamin B6. In: Shils ME, Olson JA, Shike M, Ross AC, eds. *Modern Nutrition in Health and Disease.* 9th ed. Baltimore, MD: Williams and Wilkins; 1999; 413-421.

Maksymowych AB, Robertson NM, Litwack G. Efficacy of pyridoxal treatment in controlling the growth of melanomas in cell culture and an animal pilot study. *Anticancer Research.* 1993; 13:1925-1937.

Okada H, Moriwaki K, Kanno Y, et al. Vitamin B6 supplementation can improve peripheral polyneuropathy in patients with chronic renal failure on high-flux haemodialysis and human recombinant erythropoietin. *Nephrol Dial Transplant.* 2000; 15:1410-1413.

Rall LC, Meydani SN. Vitamin B6 and immune competence. *Nutr Rev.* 1993; 51:217-225.

Rimland B, Calloway E, Dreyfus P. The effects of high doses of vitamin B6 on autistic children: a double-blind crossover study. *Am J Psychiatry.* 1978; 135:472-475.

Schaumburg H, Kaplan J, Windebank A, et al. Sensory neuropathy from pyridoxine abuse. *N Engl J Med.* 1983; 309:445-448.

Schneider G, Käck H, Lindquist Y. The manifold of vitamin B6 dependent enzymes. *Structure.* 2000; 8:R1-R6.

Sermet A, Aybak M, Ulak G, et al. Effect of oral pyridoxine hydrochloride supplementation on *in vitro* platelet sensitivity to different agonists. *Arzneimittelforschung.* 1995; 45:19-21.

Seto T, Inada H, Kobayashi N, et al. [Depression of serum pyridoxal levels in theophylline-related seizures]. [Article in Japanese]. *No To Hattatsu.* 2000; 32:295-300.

Shimizu T, Maeda S, Arakawa H, et al. Relation between theophylline and circulating vitamin levels in children with asthma. *Pharmacology.* 1996; 53:384-389.

Shimizu T, Maeda S, Mochizuki H, et al. Theophylline attenuates circulating vitamin B6 levels in children with asthma. *Pharmacology.* 1994; 49:392-397.

Spooner GR, Desai HB, Angel JF, et al. Using pyridoxine to treat carpal tunnel syndrome. Randomized control trial. *Can Fam Physician.* 1993; 39:2122-2127.

Stern F, Berner YN, Polyak Z, et al. [Nutritional status and vitamin B6 supplementation in the institutionalized elderly]. [Article in Hebrew]. *Harefuah.* 2000; 139:97-102,167,166.

Stransky M, Rubin A, Lava NS, Lazaro RP. Treatment of carpal tunnel syndrome with vitamin B6: a double-blind study. *South Med J.* 1989; 82:841-842.

Ubbink JB, Hayward Vermaak WJ, Delport R, Serfontein WJ. The relationship between vitamin B6 metabolism, asthma, and theophylline therapy. *Ann NY Acad Sci.* 1990; 585:285-294.

Wyatt KM, Dimmock PW, Jones PW, Shaughn O'Brien PM. Efficacy of vitamin B6 in the treatment of premenstrual syndrome: systemic review. *Br Med J.* 1999; 318:1375-1381.

Vitamin B12

TRADE NAMES

Vitamin B12 is available generically from numerous manufacturers. Branded products include: Twelve Resin-K (The Key Company), B12 Dots (Twinlab), Vitamin B12 Nuggets (Solgar)

DESCRIPTION

The term vitamin B_{12} (cobalamin) is used in two different ways. Vitamin B_{12}, a member of the B-vitamin family, is a collective term for a group of cobalt-containing compounds known as corrinoids. The principal cobalamins are cyanocobalamin, hydroxocobalamin and the two coenzyme forms of vitamin B_{12}, methylcobalamin and 5-deoxyadenosylcobalamin (adenosylcobalamin). The term vitamin B_{12} is more commonly used to refer to only one of these forms, cyanocobalamin. Cyanocobalamin is the principal form of the vitamin used for fortification of foods and in nutritional supplements. In this monograph, vitamin B_{12} will be used in both ways. The meaning will be clear from its context. The cobalamins are comprised of a nucleotide (base, ribose and phosphate) attached to a corrin ring. The corrin ring is made up of four pyrrole groups and an atom of cobalt in its center. The cobalt atom attaches to a methyl group, a deoxyadenosyl group, an hydroxyl group or a cyano group, to yield the four cobalamin forms mentioned above.

Vitamin B_{12} is the most chemically complex of all the vitamins. It is also one of the most biologically interesting ones. Because of the striking dark red color of its crystals, vitamin B_{12} has been called ''nature's most beautiful cofactor.'' Its close relatives hemoglobin, chlorophyll and the cytochromes are also brightly colored complex organometallic substances, which, along with vitamin B_{12} and some others derived from the parent molecule called uroporphyrinogen III, have led to their being known as the pigments of life. Vitamin B_{12} works in close partnership with folate in the synthesis of the building blocks for DNA and RNA synthesis as well as the synthesis of molecules important for the maintenance of the integrity of the genome. It is also essential for the maintenance of the integrity of the nervous system and for the synthesis of molecules which are involved in fatty acid biosynthesis and the production of energy. The human body does all of this with just two to three milligrams of the vitamin, which is much less than the weight of a tenth of a drop of water. It is even speculated that B_{12} was mainly responsible for the origin of the DNA world from the RNA world.

Deficiency of vitamin B_{12} results in hematological, neurological and gastrointestinal effects. The hematological effects of the deficiency are identical to that of folate deficiency and are caused by interference with DNA synthesis. The hematologic symptoms and signs of B_{12} deficiency, include hypersegmentation of polymorphonuclear leukocytes, macrocytic, hyperchromic erythrocytes, elevated mean corpuscular volume (MCV), elevated mean corpuscular hemoglobin concentration (MCH, MCHC), a decreased red blood cell count, pallor of the skin, decreased energy and easy fatigability, shortness of breath and palpitations. The resulting anemia of B_{12} deficiency, as is the case of the anemia of folate deficiency, is a megaloblastic macrocytic anemia. However, in the context of a simultaneous iron deficiency anemia, which is a microcytic one, anemia secondary to B_{12} deficiency may not result in macrocytic erythrocytes.

The neurological effects of the vitamin deficiency may occur even in the absence of anemia. This is particularly true in those who are over 60 years old. Vitamin B_{12} deficiency principally affects the peripheral nerves, and in later stages, the spinal cord. The symptoms and signs of the neurological effects of B12 deficiency, include tingling and numbness in the extremities (particularly the lower extremities), loss of vibratory and position sensation, abnormalities of gait, spasticity, Babinski's responses, irritability, depression and cognitive changes (loss of concentration, memory loss, dementia). Visual disturbances, impaired bladder and bowel control, insomnia and impotence may also occur. Gastrointestinal effects of B12 deficiency, include intermittent diarrhea and constipation, abdominal pain, flatulence and burning of the tongue (glossitis). Anorexia and weight loss are general symptoms of B12 deficiency. Recently, age-related hearing loss has been associated with poor vitamin B12 and folate status. Poor B12 status has also been associated with Alzheimer's disease.

Pernicious anemia is the most common cause of clinical B12 deficiency in temperate regions. Pernicious anemia is the result of an autoimmune process in which parietal cell autoantibodies against the gastric H^+/K^+-adenosine triphosphatase (the gastric proton pump) cause loss of gastric parietal cells. The loss of parietal cells results in diminished production of the intrinsic factor. The intrinsic factor is necessary for B12 absorption (see Pharmacokinetics). Deficiency of intrinsic factor results in B12 deficiency. Inadequate B12 intake is another cause of B12 deficiency. Breastfed infants of vegan mothers are particularly at risk for B12 deficiency. Total gastrectomy results in B12 deficiency secondary to lack of intrinsic factor. Pancreatic insufficiency and atrophic gastritis result in B12 deficiency secondary to inability to digest dietary protein-bound B12. Small bowel disorders, including ileal resection or bypass, Crohn's disease, malignancy, tropical sprue, celiac sprue (gluten-induced enteropathy) and amyloidosis result in B12 deficiency secondary to decreased absorption of the vitamin. Bacterial overgrowth of the small intestine results in B12 deficiency secondary to bacterial competition for uptake of the vitamin. Certain drugs, including proton pump inhibitors can interfere with absorption of the vitamin (see Interactions). Nitrous oxide anesthesia can cause a functional B12 deficiency via degradation of B12 coenzymes (see Interactions). Rare congenital disorders such as transcobalamin II deficiency and defective intrinsic factor production result in B12 deficiency. Finally, infestation with the tapeworm *Diphyllobothrium latum* can cause B12 deficiency secondary to competition for uptake of B12 by the parasite. In this regard, in the early 1900s, B12 deficiency was common in Jewish women in the United States who prepared their own gefilte fish. They used fresh-water fish, including pike, pickeral and carp, which hosted the wormlike larvae of the parasite. The women would sample the fish, by tasting it, from the time it was quite raw until it was well cooked. Although their children totally enjoyed the prepared gefilte fish, the Jewish mothers wound up with forty-foot parasites in their digestive tracts and B12 deficiencies.

The two coenzyme forms of vitamin B12 are methylcobalamin and 5'-deoxyadenosylcobalamin (adenosylcobalamin). Methylcobalamin is a cofactor for the enzyme methionine synthase, while adenosycobalamin is a cofactor for the enzyme L-methylmalonyl coenzyme A (methylmalonyl-CoA) mutase. Methionine synthase is one of the key enzymes in intermediary metabolism. It catalyzes the conversion of homocysteine to methionine. Its folate partner in the reaction is 5-methyltetrahydrofolate (intracellular folates are present in their polyglutamate forms). This is the only reaction in the body in which folate and B12 are coparticipants. In addition to forming methionine, 5-methyltetrahydrofolate is converted to tetrahydrofolate. The reactions occur in the following manner: methylcobalamin transfers its methyl group to homocysteine yielding methionine and 5-methyltetrahydrate transfers its methyl group to cobalamin reconverting it to methylcobalamin. Methionine is converted to S-adenosylmethionine (SAMe), the major donor of methyl groups in transmethylation reactions, including reactions that are involved in the synthesis of basic myelin basic protein.

Tetrahydrofolate is converted to 5,10-methylenetetrahydrofolate via the action of the enzyme serine hydroxymethyltransferase. 5,10-Methylenetetrahydrofolate is presented with three metabolic opportunities. It can be converted to 5-methyltetrahydrofolate—the folate cofactor of the methionine synthase reaction—via the enzyme 5,10-methylenetetrahydrofolate reductase; it can transfer its one-carbon residue to deoxyuridylic acid to form thymidylic acid or it can be converted to 5-formyltetrahydrofolate, which is a one-carbon donor in the *de novo* synthesis of purine nucleotides.

The hematological effects of B12 deficiency are accounted for as follows: B12 deficiency leads to reduced synthesis of tetrahydrofolate as well as methionine. Decreased tetrahydrofolate results in decreased 5,10-methylenetetrahydrofolate which in turn, results in decreased conversion of deoxyuridylate to thymidylate and decreased *de novo* synthesis of purine nucleotides. In addition, because of decreased synthesis of methionine and S-adenosylmethionine, the enzyme 5,10-methylenetetrahydrofolate reductase converts most of the 5,10-methylenetetrahydrofolate to 5-methyltetrahydrofolate, the so-called methyl trap. To summarize, decreased B12 results in a decrease in the nucleotide precursor pool for DNA synthesis (thymidylic acid, purine nucleotides) which results in decreased DNA replication and cell division and finally to a megaloblastic anemia. Since the megaloblastic anemia induced by B12 deficiency is caused by a functional cellular folate deficiency, it is not surprising that it can be corrected with administration of folate. On the other hand, the neurological deficits of vitamin B12 deficiency can not be corrected with folate administration. Further, high doses of folate administered to those with an undiagnosed B12 deficiency can cause progression of neurological symptoms.

The neurological effects of B12 deficiency are accounted for as follows: Consequences of B12 deficiency, in addition to those mentioned above, include increased serum levels of homocysteine, decreased levels of methionine and S-adenosylmethionine and a decreased ratio of S-adenosylmethionine to S-adenosylhomocysteine, the product of S-adenosylmethionine methyltransferase reactions. Decreased S-adenosylmethionine in the central nervous system results in decreased methylation reactions and an overall state of hypomethylation. Transmethylation reactions are important in the synthesis of a number of substances in the central nervous system, including myelin basic protein which is involved in the process of myelination. Much research is needed to better elucidate the mechanism of the neurological effects of B12 deficiency.

In addition to methionine synthase, B12 is a cofactor in the methylmalonyl-CoA mutase reaction. In this reaction, the coenzyme form of B12 is adenosylcobalamin. A number of substances, including the branched-chain amino acids isoleucine and valine, as well as methionine, threonine, thymine and odd-chain fatty acids are metabolized via methylmalonyl semialdehyde or propionyl-CoA to methylmalonyl-CoA. Methylmalonyl-CoA mutase converts methylmalonyl-CoA to succinyl-CoA. This occurs in the mitochondria. Succinyl-CoA can be metabolized in the tricarboxylic acid cycle to produce energy and it is also involved in the synthesis of fatty acids. Methylmalonic acid is elevated in the serum and urine in those with B12 deficiency.

Animal products are the principal food sources of vitamin B12. B12 cannot be made by plants or by animals. It is thought that only bacteria (eubacteria, archaebacteria) manufacture the vitamin. The B12 in animal products is derived from bacterial B12 sources. The richest dietary sources of cobalamin are the liver, brain and kidney. Other sources, include egg yolk, clams, oysters, crabs, sardines, salmon and heart. Lower amounts of cobalamin are found in fish, beef, lamb, pork, chicken, cheese and milk. Plant foods are generally devoid of B12. Some fermented plant products, e.g., tempeh, may have some vitamin B12. Pseudovitamin B12 refers to B12-like substances which are found in certain organisms, such as *Spirulina* spp. (blue-green algae, cyanobacteria). However, these substances do not have B12 biological activity for humans. Food-form B12 is comprised of protein-bound methylcobalamin and adenosylcobalamin.

Vitamin B12, B12 and cobalamin are terms that are used interchangeably. Vitamin B12 most commonly refers to one of the cobalamin forms, cyanocobalamin. Cyanocobalamin is also known as 5,6-dimethylbenzimidazolyl cyanocobamide.

Its molecular formula is $C_{63}H_{88}CoN_{14}O_{14}P$ and its molecular weight is 1355.38 daltons. The structural formula is:

Vitamin B12

ACTIONS AND PHARMACOLOGY

ACTIONS

Vitamin B12 is used in the treatment of B12 deficiency states, including megaloblastic anemia. It may have antiatherogenic, neuroprotective, anticarcinogenic and detoxifying activities. B12 has putative anti-allergic and mood-modulatory activities.

MECHANISM OF ACTION

Vitamin B12, in the form of methylcobalamin, is a cofactor in the methionine synthase reaction. The enzyme converts homocysteine to methionine. Folate, in the form of 5-methyltetrahydrofolate (as the pentaglutamate) is the other cofactor in the reaction. In addition to methionine, tetrahydrofolate (again, as the pentaglutame) is also formed. Tetrahydrofolate is converted to 5,10-methylenetetrahydrofolate which is a cofactor in the formation of thymidylic acid from deoxyuridylic acid and which is also converted to 5-formyltetrahydrofolate, a one-carbon donor in the *de novo* synthesis of purine nucleotides. B12 deficiency results in decreased formation of thymidylic acid and purine nucleotides, precursors of DNA synthesis and which are necessary for normal cell division. Megaloblastic anemia is the consequence of this and administration of B12, which yields the B12 cofactor for methionine synthase, corrects this problem. Methionine is a precursor of S-adenosylmethionine

(SAMe). SAMe is the principal transmethylating agent and is involved in, among many other things, the synthesis of myelin basic protein. Abnormal myelin basic protein resulting in defective myelination, is thought to be responsible for many of the neurological effects of B_{12} deficiency. The neurological effects may or may not be corrected with administration of B_{12} in those with B_{12} deficiency. Whether the neurological effects are reversible after treatment depends on their duration.

Hyperhomocysteinemia is thought to be an independent risk factor for coronary heart disease and other vascular disorders. B_{12} works in concert with folate in the methionine synthase reaction, which metabolizes homocysteine to methionine. This is a key reaction in the maintenance of low serum homocysteine levels. The mechanism by which elevated homocysteine levels might increase the risk of developing vascular disease is unclear. It has been shown that homocysteine increases platelet adhesiveness, promotes the growth of smooth muscle cells and causes endothelial dysfunction. Homocysteine may also promote oxidative stress resulting in, among other things, the oxidation of low-density lipoproteins (LDL) to oxidized-LDL. All of these possible activities of homocysteine can play roles in atherogenesis.

B_{12} deficiency can result in a number of neurological effects, including peripheral neuropathy and cognitive changes, including memory loss and dementia. Administration of B_{12} successfully reverses mild memory impairment and peripheral neuropathy, if not advanced neurological deficits, in most elderly subjects deficient in the vitamin. The mechanism by which B_{12} deficiency causes neurological effects and by which B_{12} administration may reverse them is not well understood. B_{12} and folate are cofactors in the conversion of homocysteine to methionine and methionine is the precursor of the transmethylating agent S-adenosylmethionine (SAMe). SAMe is involved in the synthesis of myelin basic protein which can become defective in the context of B_{12} deficiency. Defective myelin basic protein and resultant defective myelination can account, in large part, for the peripheral neuropathy of B_{12} deficiency. Hyperhomocysteinemia, another consequence of B_{12} deficiency, may also contribute to the neurological effects of deficiency of the vitamin. Elevated homocysteine levels may cause cerebrovascular effects which could lead to cognitive changes. Decreased brain levels of SAMe may result in disturbances in certain neurotransmitters. SAMe is involved in key methylation reactions in catecholamine synthesis and metabolism in the brain. These neurotransmitters are known to be important in maintaining the affective state. In the elderly, depression often presents as cognitive changes, including dementia.

Vitamin B_{12} deficiency has been associated with Alzheimer's disease, at least in some with this neurodegenerative disorder.

It is hypothesized that the altered B_{12} status that may occur in those with the disorder is due, in part, to a defect in the protein megalin. Megalin is a member of the low-density lipoprotein receptor family, and mediates the ileal uptake of the cubulin-bound B_{12}-intrinsic factor complex (see Pharmacokinetics). The low-density lipoprotein receptors, include receptors that bind apolipoprotein E, amyloid precursor protein and alpha$_2$-macroglobulin, substances that have been linked to Alzheimer's disease. Impaired transport of B_{12} to the central nervous system may, in part, account for the pathogenesis of the disorder.

There is some evidence, mainly epidemiological, that B_{12} may protect against certain types of cancer. A couple of clinical studies have shown that a combination of B_{12} and folic acid significantly reduces the number of abnormal bronchial cells thought to be cancer cell precursors. The mechanism of the possible anticarcinogenic effect of B_{12} is unclear. B_{12} deficiency results in decreased levels of SAMe and thymidylic acid, as discussed above. SAMe, among other things, is involved in DNA methylation which results in regulation of its genetic expression via a process known as gene silencing. Abnormal DNA methylation patterns are characteristic of neoplastic cells. Decreased SAMe and thymidylic acid levels may also lead to increased errors in DNA replication, increased DNA strand breaks and defective DNA repair.

Hydroxocobalamin is used in conditions which are associated with cyanide toxicity, such as may occur with sodium nitroprusside therapy and Leber's optic atrophy. Hydroxocobalamin is used parenterally in these cases; it combines with cyanide to form cyanocobalamin. Clearly, cyanocobalamin is not the right form of B_{12} for use in these conditions. B_{12} can also combine with sulfite and has been found to be effective in the management of sulfite-induced hypersensitivity conditions in some preliminary studies. The studies used cyanocobalamin. Perhaps better results could have been obtained with hydroxocobalamin. There is no evidence that B_{12} has any effect in the management of other hypersensitive or allergic conditions.

Vitamin B_{12} may have mood-modulatory activity in some, e.g., the elderly, who are B_{12} deficient. There is no evidence that B_{12} has mood-modulatory activity in those who are not deficient in the vitamin. As discussed above, SAMe is involved in key methylation reactions in catecholamine synthesis in the brain and these neurotransmitters are known to be important in maintaining the affective state.

PHARMACOKINETICS

Vitamin B_{12} is found naturally in food sources (principally animal products) in protein-bound forms. Cyanocobalamin is the principal form of vitamin B_{12} used in nutritional supplements and for fortification of foods. Methylcobalamin is also available for nutritional supplementation and hydroxocobalamin is available for parenteral administration.

Naturally found B_{12} is dissociated from proteins in the stomach via the action of acid and the enzyme pepsin. The forms of B_{12} released by this process are methylcobalamin and adenosylcobalamin. All forms of B_{12} bind to proteins called haptocorrins or R proteins, which are secreted by the salivary glands and the gastric mucosa. This binding occurs in the stomach. Pancreatic proteases partially degrade the B_{12}-haptocorrin complexes in the small intestine where the B_{12} that is released then binds to intrinsic factor (IF). Intrinsic factor is a glycoprotein which is secreted by gastric parietal cells. The B_{12}-intrinsic factor complex is absorbed from the terminal ileum into the ileal enterocytes via a process that first requires the complex to bind to a receptor called cubilin. Within the enterocytes, B_{12} is released from the B_{12}-IF complex and then binds to another protein called transcobalamin II which delivers it to the portal circulation. The portal circulation transports B_{12} to the liver which takes up about 50% of the vitamin; the reminder is transported to the other tissues of the body via the systemic circulation.

Vitamin B_{12} in the circulation is bound to the plasma proteins transcobalamin I (TCI), transcobalamin II (TCII) and transcobalamin III (TCIII). Approximately 80% of plasma B_{12} is bound to TCI. TCII is the principal B_{12} binding protein for the delivery of B_{12} to cells, via specific receptors for TCII. This B_{12} binding protein (TCII) is identical to the one that delivers B_{12} from the enterocytes to the portal circulation (see above).

Total absorption increases with increased intake of the vitamin. However, the absorption efficacy of the vitamin decreases with increased dosage. Studies with cyanocobalamin found that 50% of the vitamin was absorbed at a dose of one microgram, 20% at a dose of 5 micrograms and about 5% at a dose of 25 micrograms. Significantly, very large doses of B_{12} are absorbed with an absorption efficiency of about one percent. This occurs via passive diffusion even in the absence of intrinsic factor. Thus, large oral doses may be given for the treatment of B_{12} deficiency instead of using the parenteral route (usually, intramuscularly). There are now several studies confirming this. The absorption efficiency of B_{12} from foods is approximately 50%.

The vitamin B_{12}-transcobalamin II complex is degraded intracellularly via lysosomal proteases to yield cobalamin (cyanocobalamin, methylcobalamin, adenosylcobalamin, hydroxocobalamin). Cobalamin is metabolized to methylcobalamin in the cytosol and to adenosylcobalamin in the mitochondria. Methylcobalamin is the principal circulating form of cobalamin. Adenosylcobalamin comprises more than 70% of cobalamin in the liver, erythrocytes, kidney and

brain. The total body content of cobalamin ranges from two to three milligrams, with approximately 50% of it residing in the liver.

Vitamin B_{12} is secreted in the bile and reabsorbed via the enterohepatic circulation. Some of the B_{12} secreted in the bile is excreted in the feces. Also, oral B_{12} that is not absorbed is excreted in the feces. Reabsorption of B_{12} via the enterohepatic circulation requires the intrinsic factor. If the circulating level of B_{12} exceeds the B_{12} binding capacity of the blood, a situation that usually occurs following parenteral administration of the vitamin, the excess is excreted in the urine.

INDICATIONS AND USAGE

Vitamin B_{12} is indicated in those with vitamin B_{12} deficiency. It is especially important for the elderly and for those who have had gastric surgery. Both groups are at high risk for vitamin B_{12} deficiency. There is evidence that it may be beneficial in some others with low vitamin B_{12} status and in some with malabsorption of B_{12}, including some who are chronically ill, as well as some vegetarians, among others. There is some preliminary indication that vitamin B_{12} may be helpful in inhibiting a pre-cancerous condition in the lungs of smokers, that it might help ameliorate the symptoms of some neuropsychiatric disorders and that it might be useful in some with chronic fatigue and HIV disease. It has been suggested that vitamin B_{12} might help prevent some vascular diseases and breast cancer, based upon epidemiological and theoretical considerations. Claims that it is a general ''energizer'' are anecdotal. There is some evidence that vitamin B_{12} can protect against hypersensitivity to sulfites. Earlier open trials suggested that methylcobalamin was effective in the management of sleep-wake rhythm disorders. However, a recent double-blind controlled trial with this form of B_{12} failed to confirm this.

RESEARCH SUMMARY

Clinically, overt vitamin B_{12} deficiency manifests as megaloblastic anemia and neurologic dysfunction. There are more clinically silent and subtle forms of cobalamin deficiency which are also reversible with vitamin B_{12} therapy. In addition, mild deficiency may be present in a number of populations, including, most significantly, the elderly. It is estimated that 10-15% of those over 60 have vitamin B_{12} deficiency, due, principally, to decreased absorption of naturally occurring vitamin B_{12} caused by an age-related atrophic gastritis that diminishes the acid-pepsin secretions that normally release free vitamin B_{12} from food proteins.

Neurologic symptoms of vitamin B_{12} deficiency can occur, contrary to what was previously believed, in the absence of predecessor hematologic abnormalities. Among neurologic abnormalities noted are those involving the spinal cord, peripheral nerves, optic nerves and cerebrum. Sensory disturbances, such as paresthesias in the extremities, are considerably more common than motor disturbances. Neuropathies and myelopathies can occur alone or in combination. Cognitive impairment and mood changes are more common than dementia, psychosis, paranoia and violent behavior. There are rare instances of visual impairment. Age-related hearing loss has been associated with B12 and folate deficiency in the elderly. Researchers stress the need for prompt treatment. These conditions, if left untreated, often become irreversible.

Those with mild deficiency usually suffer only from neuropathy and modest memory impairment. Some immunologic deficits are also sometimes noted, but it is not known if these are caused by the deficiency. Supplemental vitamin B12 successfully reverses mild memory impairment and neuropathy in most elderly subjects deficient in this vitamin.

The Food and Nutrition Board has recommended that elderly people obtain 2.4 micrograms of vitamin B12 daily—from verifiable sources, e.g., either from eating fortified foods, such as cereals, that clearly identify the amount of vitamin B12 per serving and/or from vitamin B12 supplements. And some researchers, again noting the danger of irreversibility of neurologic symptoms that go untreated, have recently recommended regular periodic screening of the elderly for detection of vitamin B12 deficiency at an early stage.

A high prevalence of vitamin B12 deficiency has also been reported in those who have had gastric surgery. A recent study detected this deficiency in 31% of those who had undergone this type of surgery, compared with 2% of controls of similar age and race. Previous studies had noted an incidence of vitamin B12 deficiency of 1%-20% in gastric surgery patients, but the most recent study used more metabolic variables to detect the deficiency and tested an older patient sample. It also looked for the deficiency over a longer period of time. Median age of subjects in this study was 67 years.

These researchers found that vitamin B12 deficiency is often undetected in post-gastric surgery patients whose subsequent neurologic symptoms are often misdiagnosed. Most had not been advised, after surgery, to be monitored for vitamin B12 deficiency. These researchers stress the need for regular vitamin B12 screening in all gastric surgery patients, no matter how many years elapsed since the surgery. They point out that vitamin B12 deficiency may develop many years after surgery.

Vitamin B12 deficiencies have been reported in some chronically ill populations. Vitamin B12 has been found to be malabsorbed in some with HIV disease. There have also been reports of vitamin B12 deficiency in individuals with chronic fatigue of various etiologies. There are anecdotal reports that supplemental vitamin B12 is helpful in these disorders. Controlled trials are lacking.

Two placebo-controlled trials have shown that a combination of vitamin B12 and folic acid inhibited a precursor of bronchial squamous cell cancer of the lung in humans. In one of these studies, supplementation with 10 milligrams of folic acid daily, combined with 500 micrograms of vitamin B12 daily, for four months, produced a significant reduction in the number of subjects, all heavy smokers, who exhibited the abnormal bronchial cells said to be cancer precursors.

Many researchers have noted that diminished vitamin B12 status is strongly associated with hyperhomocysteinemia, a significant risk factor for cardiovascular disease. Two researchers have noted that, "although folate deficiency is a far more common cause of elevated homocysteine levels than are vitamin B12 and vitamin B6 deficiencies, an elevated homocysteine value in an older person should not be considered due to folate deficiency alone. Because elderly people may have elevated homocysteine levels due to vitamin B12 deficiency, lowering serum total homocysteine levels to reduce the high incidence of vascular disease among the elderly by supplying adequate amounts of all three vitamins may become an important public health issue."

Recently, diminished vitamin B12 status has been identified as an additional nutritional risk factor for breast cancer among post-menopausal women. This preliminary finding needs followup before its significance, if any, can be assessed.

Claims that vitamin B12 can enhance exercise performance and that it is an "energizer" have not been tested and are based upon anecdotal accounts.

There is evidence that some who are on strict vegetarian or macrobiotic diets may need supplemental vitamin B12. Children and the elderly who are on these diets may, in particular, have need of this supplementation. Some have claimed that miso, tamari, tempeh and other soy products can provide adequate B12 in the absence of meats and dairy products. This has not been demonstrated. Nor has the claim that adequate B12 can be obtained from spirulina, sea weeds and other sea vegetables. Even unpasteurized miso, claimed to be an excellent source of B12, appears to have very little to none of the vitamin. Nor can vegetarians get adequate B12 from brewer's yeast, grains, cereals or mushrooms. Some sea vegetables are said to contain significant amounts of vitamin B12, but accumulating evidence suggests that, instead, these foods contain vitamin B12 analogues (pseudovitamin B12) that do not confer the functions and protection of vitamin B12 itself.

Again, vitamin B_{12} supplementation is highly advised for vegetarians, especially children who are vegetarians. Vegetarians whose diets allow for the regular use of eggs and dairy products can generally obtain enough vitamin B_{12} from their diets. Vegetarians consume certain foods (garlic, onions) that contain certain substances (e.g., inulins) which stimulate the growth of certain bacteria (e.g., *lactobacillus*) in the colon. These bacteria produce B_{12} and may supply some of the vitamin to the body. However, this needs to be proven.

Finally, there is evidence that vitamin B_{12} can protect some from allergy to the sulfites that are added to some foods and wines. In one study, 2,000 micrograms of sublingual vitamin B_{12} significantly prevented reactions to sulfites in 17 of 18 sulfite-sensitive subjects challenged with sulfites. Subsequent placebo-controlled trials confirmed this protective effect.

CONTRAINDICATIONS, PRECAUTIONS, ADVERSE REACTIONS
CONTRAINDICATIONS
Vitamin B_{12} (cyanocobalamin, hydroxocobalamin, methylcobalamin) is contraindicated in those hypersensitive to any component of a vitamin B_{12}-containing product.

PRECAUTIONS
The use of vitamin B_{12} to treat vitamin B_{12} deficiency or to treat any medical condition requires medical supervision.

Cyanocobalamin should not be used in those with Leber's optic atrophy. This is a congenital disorder associated with chronic cyanide intoxication (e.g., from tobacco smoke). Decreased levels of B_{12} have been associated with reduced ability to detoxify the cyanide in exposed individuals and cyanocobalamin may increase the risk of irreversible neurological damage from optic atrophy in those affected with the disorder. Hydroxocobalamin can aid in the detoxification of cyanide. This form of B_{12} is an acceptable form for B_{12} supplementation in those with this disorder.

A typical dose of B_{12} (cyanocobalamin) in nutritional supplements used by pregnant women and nursing mothers is 12 micrograms daily. Pregnant women and nursing mothers should only use doses higher than this if recommended by their physicians.

Administration of doses of vitamin B_{12} greater than 10 micrograms daily may produce a hematological response in those with anemia secondary to folate deficiency.

ADVERSE REACTIONS
Oral vitamin B_{12} is well tolerated even at high doses. There are occasional reports of hypersensitivity reactions (urticaria, rash, pruritis) in those receiving parenteral B_{12}. Those who have experienced hypersensitivity reactions from use of parenteral B_{12} may experience similar reactions from oral B_{12}, although there are very few reports of this occurring.

INTERACTIONS
DRUGS
Antibiotics: The use of antibiotics may alter the intestinal microflora and may decrease the possible contribution of B_{12} by certain inhabitants of the microflora (e.g., *Lactobacillus* species) to the body's requirement for the vitamin. This may particularly be a problem for vegetarians. Garlic, onions, leeks, bananas, asparagus and artichokes, among other vegetables and fruits, contain inulins which promote the growth of certain colonic bacteria, including *Lactobacillus* species (see Inulins).

Cholestyramine: Cholestyramine may decrease the enterohepatic reabsorption of B_{12}.

Colchicine: Colchicine may cause decreased absorption of B_{12}.

Colestipol: Colestipol may decrease the enterohepatic reabsorption of B_{12}.

H₂ blockers (cimetidine, famotidine, nizatidine, ranitidine): Chronic use of H_2 blockers may result in decreased absorption of vitamin B_{12} naturally found in food sources. They are unlikely to affect the absorption of supplemental B_{12}.

Metformin: Metformin may decrease the absorption of vitamin B_{12}. This possible effect may be reversed with oral calcium supplementation.

Nitrous oxide: Inhalation of the anesthetic agent nitrous oxide (not to be confused with nitric oxide) can produce a functional vitamin B_{12} deficiency. Nitrous oxide forms a complex with cobalt in methylcobalamin, the cofactor for methionine synthase, resulting in inactivation of the enzyme.

Para-aminosalicylic acid: Chronic use of the anti-tuberculosis drug may decrease the absorption of B_{12}.

Potassium chloride: It has been reported that potassium chloride may decrease the absorption of dietary B_{12} in some.

Proton pump inhibitors (lansoprazole, omeprazole, pantoprazole, rabeprazole): Chronic use of proton pump inhibitors may result in decreased absorption of vitamin B_{12} naturally found in food sources. They are unlikely to affect the absorption of supplemental B_{12}.

NUTRITIONAL SUPPLEMENTS
Calcium: Calcium supplementation may reverse the possible metformin-induced decrease of B_{12} absorption.

Folate: Folic acid may work synergistically with vitamin B_{12} in lowering homocysteine levels.

Vitamin B6: Vitamin B6 may work synergistically with vitamin B12 and folate in lowering homocysteine levels.

Vitamin C: Low serum B12 levels reported in those receiving large doses of vitamin C were artifacts of the effect of ascorbate on the radioisotope assay for B12. There are no known interactions between vitamin C and vitamin B12.

OVERDOSAGE

There are no reports of vitamin B12 overdosage in the literature.

DOSAGE AND ADMINISTRATION

The principal form of B12 used in nutritional supplements is cyanocobalamin. Methylcobalamin is also available for nutritional supplementation. Hydroxocobalamin is presently only available for parenteral use.

Cyanocobalamin is available as a single ingredient product and in multivitamin, multivitamin/multimineral and B complex products. Lozenges of cyanocobalamin and methylcobalamin are also available. Prenatal and postnatal vitamin/mineral formulas typically deliver a dose of 12 micrograms of B12 daily. A general range of B12 dosage is 3 to 30 micrograms daily. Some use much higher doses. Absorption of naturally occurring B12 decreases with age. Because of this, the Food and Nutrition Board advises that those older than 50 years should consume foods fortified with B12 or take a vitamin B12-containing nutritional supplement in order to meet the RDA (2.4 micrograms daily).

Those with B12 deficiency may be managed with high doses of oral B12. However, this requires prescription and management by a physician.

The Food and Nutrition Board of the Institute of Medicine of the National Academy of Sciences has recommended the following Dietary Reference Intakes (RDI) for vitamin B12:

Infants	Adequate Intakes (AI)
0 through 6 months	0.4 micrograms/day ≈ 0.05 micrograms/Kg
7 through 12 months	0.5 micrograms/day ≈ 0.05 micrograms/Kg
	Recommended Dietary Allowance (RDA)
Children	
1 through 3 years	0.9 micrograms/day
4 through 8 years	1.2 micrograms/day
Boys	
9 through 13 years	1.8 micrograms/day
14 through 18 years	2.4 micrograms/day
Girls	
9 through 13 years	1.8 micrograms/day
14 through 18 years	2.4 micrograms/day
Men	
19 years and older	2.4 micrograms/day
Women	
19 years and older	2.4 micrograms/day
Pregnancy	
14 through 50 years	2.6 micrograms/day
Lactation	
14 through 50 years	2.8 micrograms/day

The U.S. RDA, for vitamin B12, the value used for nutritional supplement and food labeling purposes, is 6 micrograms daily.

HOW SUPPLIED

Vitamin B12 is available by prescription in the following forms and strengths:

Injection — 100 mcg/mL, 1000 mcg/mL

Nasal Gel — 500 mcg/0.1 mL

Vitamin B12 is available in the following forms and routes for OTC use:

Lozenges — 100 mcg, 250 mcg, 500 mcg

Sublingual Tablets — 500 mcg, 1000 mcg, 2000 mcg, 2500 mcg, 5000 mcg

Tablets — 50 mcg, 100 mcg, 250 mcg, 500 mcg, 1000 mcg

LITERATURE

Adachi S, Kawamoto T, Otsuka M, et al. Enteral vitamin B12 supplements reverse postgastrectomy B12 deficiency. *Ann Surg.* 2000; 232:199-201.

Baik HW, Russell RM. Vitamin B12 deficiency in the elderly. *Annu Rev Nutr.* 1999; 19:357-377.

Battersby AR. How nature builds the pigments of life: The conquest of vitamin B12. *Science.* 1994; 264:1551-1557.

Bauman WA, Shaw S, Jayatilleke E, Spungen AM, Herbert V. Increased intake of calcium reverses vitamin B12 malabsorption induced by metformin. *Diabetes Care.* 2000; 23:1227-1231.

Bottiglieri T. Folate, vitamin B12, and neuropsychiatric disorders. *Nutr Rev.* 1996; 54:382-390.

Butzkueven H, King JO. Nitrous oxide myelopathy in an abuser of whipped cream bulbs. *J Clin Neurosci.* 2000; 7:73-75.

Carmel R. Subtle cobalamin deficiency. *Ann Intern Med.* 1996; 124:338-339.

Carmel R, Gott PS, Waters CH, et al. The frequency of low cobalamin levels in dementia usually signify treatable metabolic, neurologic and electrophysiologic abnormalities. *Eur J Haematol.* 1995; 54:245-253.

Choi S-W. Vitamin B12 deficiency: A new risk factor for breast cancer? *Nutr Rev.* 1999; 57:250-253.

Clarke R, Smith AD, Jobst KA, Refsum H, Sutton L, Ueland PM. Folate, vitamin B$_{12}$, and serum total homocysteine levels in confirmed Alzheimer's disease. *Arch Neurol.* 1998; 55:1449-1455.

Dagnelie PC, van Staveren WA, van den Berg H. Vitamin B$_{12}$ from algae appears not to be bioavailable. *Am J Clin Nutr.* 1991; 53:695-697.

Delpre G, Stark P, Niv Y. Sublingual therapy for cobalamin deficiency as an alternative to oral and parenteral cobalamin supplementation. *Lancet.* 1999; 354:740-741.

Dietary Reference Intakes for Thiamin, Riboflavin, Niacin, Vitamin B$_6$, Folate, Vitamin B$_{12}$, Pantothenic Acid, Biotin, and Choline. Washington, DC: National Academy Press; 1998:306-356.

Drennan CL, Huang S, Drummond JT, et al. How a protein binds B$_{12}$: A 3.0 A X-ray structure of B$_{12}$-binding domains of methionine synthase. *Science.* 1994; 266:1669-1674.

Elia M. Oral or parenteral therapy for B$_{12}$ deficiency (commentary). *Lancet.* 1998; 352:1721-1722.

Ellenbogen L. Vitamin B$_{12}$. In: Machlin LJ, ed. *Handbook of Vitamins.* New York, NY: Marcel Dekker, Inc; 1984:497-547.

Farquharson J, Adams JF. Conversion of hydroxo(aquo)cobalamin to sulfitocobalamin in the absence of light: a reaction of importance in the identification of the forms of vitamin B$_{12}$, with possible clinical significance. *Am J Clin Nutr.* 1977; 30:1617-1622.

Fata FT, Herzlich BC, Schiffman G, Ast AL. Impaired antibody responses to pneumococcal polysaccharide in elderly patients with low serum vitamin B$_{12}$ levels. *Ann Intern Med.* 1996; 124:299-304.

Funada U, Wada M, Kawata T, et al. Changes in CD4+CD8+/CD4-CD8+ ratio and humoral immune functions in vitamin B$_{12}$-deficient rats. *Int J Vitam Nutr Res.* 2000; 70:167-171.

Harriman GR, Smith PD, Horne MK, et al. Vitamin B$_{12}$ malabsorption in patients with acquired immunodeficiency syndrome. *Arch Intern Med.* 1989; 149:2039-2041.

Heimburger DC, Alexander CB, Birch R, et al. Improvement in bronchial squamous metaplasia in smokers treated with folate and vitamin B$_{12}$. Report of a preliminary randomized, double-blind intervention trial. *JAMA.* 1988; 259:1525-1530.

Higginbottom MC, Sweetman L, Nyhan WL. A syndrome of methylmalonic aciduria, homocystinuria, megaloblastic anemia and neurological abnormalities in a vitamin B$_{12}$-deficient breast-fed infant of a strict vegetarian. *N Eng J Med.* 1978; 299:317-323.

Houeto P, Hoffman JR, Imbert M, et al. Relation of blood cyanide to plasma cyanocobalamin concentration after a fixed dose of hydroxycobalamin in cyanide poisoning. *Lancet.* 1995; 346:605-608.

Houston DK, Johnson MA, Nozza RJ, et al. Age-related hearing loss, vitamin B$_{12}$, and folate in elderly women. *Am J Clin Nutr.* 1999; 69:564-571.

Jacobsen DW, Simon RA, Singh M. Sulfite oxidase deficiency and cobalamin protection in sulfite sensitive asthmatics. *J Allergy Clin Immunol.* 1984; 73(Suppl):135.

Kaptan K, Beyan C, Ural AU, et al. Helicobacter pylori—is it a novel causative agent in Vitamin B$_{12}$ deficiency? *Arch Int Med.* 2000; 160:1349-1353.

Kozyraki R, Fyfe J, Kristiansen M, et al. The intrinsic factor-vitamin B$_{12}$ receptor, cabilin, is a high-affinity apolipoprotein A-1 receptor facilitating endocytosis of high-density lipoprotein. *Nat Med.* 1999; 5:656-661.

Kristiansen M, Kozyraki R, Jacobsen C, et al. Molecular dissection of the intrinsic factor-vitamin B$_{12}$ receptor, cubilin, discloses regions important for membrane association and ligand binding. *J Biol Chem.* 1999; 274:20540-20544.

Kuzuminski AM, Del Giacco EJ, Allen RH, Stabler SP, Lindenbaum J. Effective treatment of cobalamin deficiency with oral cobalamin. *Blood.* 1998; 92:1191-1198.

Laine L, Ahnen D, McClain C, et al. Review article: potential gastrointestinal effects of long-term acid suppression with proton pump inhibitors. *Aliment Pharmacol Ther.* 2000; 14:651-668.

Langdon FW. Nervous and mental manifestations of pre-pernicious anemia. *JAMA.* 1905; 45:1635-1638.

Lindenbaum J, Healton EB, Savage DG, et al. Neuropsychiatric disorders caused by cobalamin deficiency in the absence of anemia or macrocytosis. *N Engl J Med.* 1988; 318:1720-1728.

Lindstedt G. [Nitrous oxide can cause cobalamin deficiency. Vitamin B$_{12}$ is a simple and cheap remedy]. [Article in Swedish]. *Lakartidningen.* 1999; 96:4801-4805.

McCaddon A, Kelly CL. Familial Alzheimer's disease and vitamin B$_{12}$ deficiency. *Age Ageing.* 1994; 23:334-337.

Nilsson-Ehle H. Age-related changes in cobalamin (vitamin B$_{12}$) handling. Implications for therapy. *Drugs Aging.* 1998; 12:277-292.

Okawa M, Takahashi K, Egashira K, et al. Vitamin B$_{12}$ treatment for delayed sleep phase syndrome. *Psychiatry Clin Neurosci.* 1997; 51:275-279.

Ostreicher DS. Vitamin B$_{12}$ supplements as protection against nitrous oxide inhalation. *NY State Dent J.* 1994; 60:47-49.

Rosener M, Dichgans J. Severe combined degeneration of the spinal cord after nitrous oxide anaesthesia in a vegetarian. *J Neurol Neurosurg Psychiatry.* 1996; 60:354.

Salom IL, Silvis SE, Doscherholmen A. Effect of cimetidine on the absorption of vitamin B$_{12}$. *Scan J Gastroenterol.* 1982; 17:129-131.

Scalabrino G, Tredici G, Buccellato FR, Manfridi A. Further evidence for the involvement of epidermal growth factor in the signaling pathway of vitamin B$_{12}$ (cobalamin) in the rat central nervous system. *J Neuropathol Exp Neurol.* 2000; 59:808-814.

Stubbe J. Binding site of nature's most beautiful cofactor. *Science.* 1994; 266:1663-1664.

Sumner AE, Chin MM, Abrahm JL, et al. Elevated methylmalonic acid and total homocysteine levels show high prevalence of vitamin B12 deficiency after gastric surgery. *Ann Int Med.* 1996; 124:469-476.

van Asselt DZ, Blom HJ, Zuiderent R, et al. Clinical significance of low cobalamin levels in older hospital patients. *Neth J Med.* 2000; 57:41-49.

Watanabe F, Katsura H, Takenaka S, et al. Pseudovitamin B12 is the predominant cobamide of an algal health food, spirulina tablets. *J Agric Food Chem.* 1999; 47:4736-4741.

Weir DG, Scott JM. Brain function in the elderly: role of vitamin B12 and folate. *Br Med Bull.* 1999; 55:669-682.

Weir DG, Scott JM. Vitamin B12 "Cobalamin." In: Shils ME, Olson JA, Shike M, Ross AC, eds. *Modern Nutrition in Health and Disease.* 9th ed. Baltimore, MD; Williams and Wilkins; 1999:447-458.

Vitamin C

TRADE NAMES

Asco-Caps-1000 (The Key Company), Asco-Caps-500 (The Key Company), Ester-C (Swanson Health Products), C-Time (Time-Cap Labs), C-Tym (Economed Pharmaceuticals), Fruit C (Freeda Vitamins), Sunkist Vitamin C (Novartis Consumer Health), Cecon (Abbott Pharmaceutical), Vicks Vitamin C (Procter & Gamble), Dull-C (Freeda Vitamins), Mega-C (Merit Pharmaceuticals), C-Max (Bio-Tech Pharmacal), Cemill (Miller Pharmacal), Cevi-Bid (Lee Pharmaceuticals), Honey C Chews (Nature's Life), Halls Defense (Warner Lambert).

DESCRIPTION

VITAMIN C

The term vitamin C applies to substances that possess antiscorbutic activity and includes two compounds and their salts: L-ascorbic acid, commonly called ascorbic acid, and L-dehydroascorbic acid. Ascorbic acid is the major dietary form of vitamin C. The terms vitamin C, ascorbic acid and ascorbate are commonly used interchangeably.

Vitamin C is a hexose derivative, similar in structure to the six-carbon sugar glucose. It is an essential nutrient for humans, and, as pointed out by Linus Pauling in 1970, "differs from other nutrients in that it is required in the diet by only a few species of animals—man, other primates, the guinea pig, an Indian fruit-eating bat, and the red-vented barbul and some related species of Passeriform birds." It is also an essential nutrient for Coho salmon, rainbow trout, carp and some insects. Most other animals, all higher plant species and probably all algal classes can synthesize vitamin C from glucose or other sugars. Molecules similar to ascorbic acid are made by some fungi but not by bacteria.

All vitamin C requiring animals lack the enzyme L-gulano-gamma-lactone oxidase, the final step in the synthesis of ascorbic acid from glucose.

The major deficiency syndrome of vitamin C is scurvy. Symptoms of scurvy include inflamed and bleeding gums, petechiae, ecchymosis, follicular hyperkeratosis, coiled hairs, perifollicular hemorrhages, impaired wound healing, dry eyes and mouth (Sjögren's syndrome), arthralgia, joint effusions, muscle weakness, myalgia, fatigue, depression, frequent infections, anemia, anorexia, diarrhea, and pulmonary and kidney problems that can lead to coma and death. All systems of the body are affected by scurvy.

The antiscorbutic factor was isolated from the ox adrenal cortex in 1928 by the Hungarian biochemist Albert Szent-Györgyi and his colleagues. In 1932, the American biochemist Glen King and his colleagues isolated this factor from lemon juice. Structural studies revealed this factor to be a sugar acid and, before it was named ascorbic acid, it was called hexuronic acid and godnose.

Many of the symptoms of scurvy, particularly those having to do with connective tissue, can be explained by the known biochemical roles of vitamin C, particularly its role as a cofactor for prolyl and lysyl hydroxylase, enzymes important in the formation of collagen. Collagen synthesized in the absence of ascorbic acid—as occurs in scurvy—cannot properly form fibers, resulting in blood-vessel fragility, among other defects. In the prolyl and lysyl hydroxylase reactions, as well as in most of the biochemical reactions ascorbic acid participates in, it acts as a reducing agent. In these reactions, the vitamin reduces ferric and cupric ions to their ferrous and cuprous states, forms which are required for the reactions to proceed.

Ascorbic acid is also involved in the biosynthesis of other connective-tissue components, including elastin, fibronectin, proteoglycans, bone matrix and elastin-associated fibrillin. It also appears to play a role in collagen gene expression and cellular procollagen secretion.

The fatigue and weakness of scurvy may be due to L-carnitine deficiency. Ascorbic acid is a cofactor for crucial reactions in the carnitine biosynthetic pathway.

Ascorbic acid is involved in modulating iron absorption, transport and storage. It aids in the intestinal absorption of iron by reducing ferric iron to ferrous iron and may stimulate ferritin synthesis to promote iron storage in cells. It is involved in the biosynthesis of corticosteroids, aldosterone, the conversion of cholesterol to bile acids and functions as a reducing agent for mixed-function oxidases.

For all of this, ascorbic acid is best known for its antioxidant properties and its possible role in the prevention of certain chronic degenerative disorders, such as coronary heart disease and cancer. In fact, ascorbic acid may be the most important water-soluble antioxidant in the body.

The daily dietary intake of vitamin C necessary to prevent scurvy is about 5 to 10 milligrams. Scurvy is rare in developed countries, since most people living in these countries typically consume much more than this amount.

About 90% of vitamin C in the average diet comes from fruits and vegetables. Peppers—sweet green and red peppers and hot red and green chili peppers—are especially rich in vitamin C. Other good sources include citrus fruits and juices, brussels sprouts, cauliflower, cabbage, kale, collards, mustard greens, broccoli, spinach and strawberries. Nuts and grains contain very little vitamin C. Cooking destroys vitamin C activity.

About 5% to 10% of the total vitamin C content of fresh fruits and vegetables is comprised of dehydroascorbic acid. In the case of processed foods, dehydroascorbic acid makes up about 30% of the vitamin C content. D-ascorbic acid (erythorbic acid or isoascorbic acid), the epimer of L-ascorbic acid, is frequently added to food as an antioxidant preservative. Erythorbic acid has very low vitamin C activity.

In addition to being known as ascorbic acid and L-ascorbic acid, vitamin C is also known as 2, 3-didehydro-L-*threo*-hexano-1, 4-lactone, 3-oxo-L-gulofuranolactone, L-*threo*-hex-2-enonic acid gamma-lactone, L-3-keto-*threo*-hexuronic acid lactone, L-*xylo*-ascorbic acid and antiscorbutic vitamin. It is abbreviated AA. Ascorbic acid is a crystalline, water-soluble substance with a pleasant (to some), sharp acidic taste. Its molecular weight is 176.13 daltons, and its molecular formula is $C_6H_8O_6$. The structural formula of vitamin C is represented as follows:

Vitamin C

The other form of vitamin C is the oxidation product of L-ascorbic acid, L-dehydroascorbic acid or DHA.

VITAMIN C WITH BIOFLAVONOIDS
Vitamin C with bioflavonoids are mixtures of vitamin C, either as ascorbic acid or as an ascorbate, with flavonoids. Typically, the flavonoids are citrus flavonoids and are derived from lemons, oranges and grapefruits. It is believed that flavonoids work synergistically with vitamin C. This

belief originates from the work and writings of the Hungarian biochemist Albert Szent-Györgyi, the co-discoverer of ascorbic acid. Szent-Györgyi also isolated substances from citrus fruits and Hungarian paprika which he called vitamin P. Vitamin P is now referred to as bioflavonoids or flavonoids. Flavonoids are not vitamins.

Szent-Györgyi believed that bioflavonoids and vitamin C worked synergistically to maintain blood capillary health and prevent capillary fragility. There is some *in vitro* evidence that flavonoids and vitamin C do work synergistically. One study showed that ascorbic acid acts synergistically with the flavonoid quercetin to protect cutaneous tissue cells in culture against oxidative damage induced by glutathione deficiency. However, there is, as yet, no good evidence that vitamin C and flavonoids work synergistically *in vivo*. A recent study, in cell culture, suggested that flavonoids may even inhibit the uptake of vitamin C into cells.

Flavonoids have biological effects independent of any interaction with vitamin C. (See various monographs on flavonoids.) Flavonoids from grapefruit include quercetin, naringenin and kaempferol. Lemon flavonoids include hesperidin (hesperitin 7-0-beta-rutinoside) and eriocitrin (eriodictyol 7-0-beta-rutinoside). These flavonoids, along with rutin and others, may be found in vitamin C/bioflavonoid supplements. Some formulations use flavonoids from the sour orange *Citrus aurantium*.

EFFERVESCENT VITAMIN C
Effervescent vitamin C is comprised of L-ascorbic acid, citric acid and sodium bicarbonate. It is similar to Alka Seltzer with ascorbic acid added. When the tablet is placed in water, the citric acid reacts with sodium bicarbonate to form sodium citrate and carbon dioxide. Also, some sodium bicarbonate reacts with ascorbic acid to form some sodium ascorbate. Some find effervescent C a more tolerable supplement than ascorbic acid.

ACEROLA VITAMIN C
Acerola vitamin C is vitamin C derived from acerola fruit. Acerola is the fruit of the small tree or shrub known as *Malphighia glabra* L. *Malphighia glabra* is native to the Antilles and northern South America. Acerola is also known as Barbados cherry, Antilles cherry, West Indies cherry, Puerto Rican cherry, cereso, cereja-das-antilhas and cereja-do-para. In 1945, the Barbados cherry was analyzed by researchers at the School of Medicine, University of Puerto Rico, and was found to be very rich in vitamin C. Interestingly, the analysis was inspired by the use of the fruit for colds by the local people.

Acerola is one of the richest sources of vitamin C in the world. The vitamin C content of the fruit depends on ripeness, seasons, climates and localities. Content is highest when the fruit is still green and lowest when ripe. The vitamin C content of unripe fruits can range up to 4.7 grams per 100 grams of fruit or 4.7% and is about 2 grams per 100 grams or 2% in very ripe fruit. For comparison, the vitamin C content of a peeled orange is 0.05% or 50 milligrams per 100 grams. Acerola also contains flavonoids, other vitamins, such as thiamin, riboflavin, niacin, pantothenic acid and beta carotene, and minerals, such as magnesium and potassium.

Malphighia glabra has also shown active anti-fungal properties. Folk medicine uses of acerola include treatment of liver ailments, diarrhea, dysentery, coughs, colds and sore throats.

ROSE HIP VITAMIN C

Rose hips are the fruit of roses. The rose hip is the swollen ovary of the flower which produces seed after the petals of a blossom wither and fall. Once the petals have fallen off a rose all that remains attached to the stem is the rose hip. Rose hips are rich sources of Vitamin C. In fact, one species, *Rosa rugosa* Thunb, contains the highest amount of vitamin C of any organism in the world. *Rosa rugosa* Thunb rose hips can contain up to 7 grams of vitamin C per 100 grams of rose hips or 7%. Acerola, the next richest source of natural vitamin C produces up to 4.7% vitamin C, and, for comparison, the peeled orange contains 0.05% vitamin C.

During World War II, England, Norway and Sweden were faced with a scurvy crisis. Since the war had restricted normal shipping, the British could not obtain enough citrus fruit for vitamin C. Children began showing the symptoms of early scurvy. The British discovered rose hips to be an excellent source of vitamin C and made the fruit of the rose into teas, soups and syrups. The children received these supplements daily, and this prevented any problem with scurvy.

Rose hips are the major source of natural vitamin C. A few species are used to obtain the vitamin, including *Rosa canina*, *Rosa mosqueta* and *Rosa rugosa* Thunb. In addition to vitamin C, rose hips contain such carotenoids as beta-carotene, lycopene, zeaxanthin, rubixanthin, gazaniaxanthin, beta cryptoxanthin, gamma-carotene, lutein, violaxanthin, and antheraxanthin. They also contain flavonoids, catechins, polyphenols, procyanidins and pectins.

Rose hips have other applications. The oil extracted from its seeds is included in many cosmetic preparations for its high content of alpha-linolenic acid (45%-50%) and linoleic acid (40%). The fruit has been used as food, mainly for preparing jams, teas and alcoholic beverages.

REDUCED-ACIDITY VITAMIN C

Reduced-acidity vitamin C consists of a mixture of 50% ascorbic acid and 50% sodium ascorbate. Some find this form of vitamin C a more tolerable supplement than ascorbic

acid. Since the first pKa of ascorbic acid is 4.2, the pH of the mixture dissolved in water would be 4.2. Reduced-acidity vitamin C is also known as buffered vitamin C.

NON-ACID VITAMIN C

Non-acid vitamin C consists of an ascorbate salt of sodium or calcium which has a neutral pH when dissolved in water. The calcium salt consists of two molecules of ascorbate and one atom of calcium. The molecular formula is $C_{12}H_{14}CaO_{12}$. Calcium ascorbate is freely soluble in water. The sodium salt consists of one molecule of ascorbate and one atom of sodium. The molecular formula is $C_6H_7NaO_6$. Some find sodium ascorbate and calcium ascorbate more acceptable forms for vitamin C supplementation.

ASCORBATE AND VITAMIN C METABOLITES

Ascorbate and vitamin C metabolites refer to marketed vitamin C supplements containing vitamin C in a salt form, typically as calcium ascorbate, and vitamin C metabolites. Vitamin C metabolites can include the aldonic acids L-threonic acid, L-xylonic acid and L-lyxonic acid. Typically, the vitamin C metabolite present in these products is L-threonic acid, also known as 2, 3, 4-trihydroxy- [threo] butanoic acid. L-threonic acid is usually also present as the calcium salt or calcium L-threonate, and the percentage of calcium L-threonate in the product is usually 1% of the amount of ascorbate. That is, a tablet supplying 500 milligrams of ascorbate would supply 5 milligrams of L-threonate.

Ascorbate and vitamin C metabolites are sometimes referred to as metabolite-supplemented ascorbate. Some *in vitro* studies have shown that the addition of L-threonate to ascorbate enhances the transfer efficiency of ascorbate into cells. Animal studies have reported increased absorption and higher retention of vitamin C when the animals were supplemented with ascorbate plus threonate than when supplemented with ascorbate alone. One cell-culture study showed that the addition of threonate to ascorbate enhanced the production of collagenous protein and mineralized tissue when compared with ascorbate alone. The authors concluded that this finding could have relevance with respect to wound healing and bone regeneration.

Although the *in vitro* and animal studies appear interesting, what is wanting are well-designed and well-executed clinical trials in humans to determine if vitamin C metabolites, such as L-threonate, positively affect vitamin C status.

ACTIONS AND PHARMACOLOGY

ACTIONS

Vitamin C has antioxidant activity. It may also have anti-atherogenic, anticarcinogenic, antihypertensive, antiviral, antihistaminic, immunomodulatory, opthalmoprotective and airway-protective actions. Vitamin C may aid in the detoxification of some heavy metals, such as lead and other toxic chemicals.

MECHANISM OF ACTION

Vitamin C is arguably the most important water-soluble biological antioxidant. It can scavenge both reactive oxygen species and reactive nitrogen species. Ascorbic acid or, more specifically, ascorbate is an excellent reducing agent, and it acts as a cofactor in various biochemical reactions to reduce the transition metals, iron and copper.

Ascorbate can be oxidized by most reactive oxygen and nitrogen species thought to play roles in tissue injury associated with various diseases. These species include superoxide, hydroxyl, peroxyl and nitroxide radicals, as well as such non-radical reactive species as singlet oxygen, peroxynitrite and hypochlorite. By virtue of this scavenging activity, ascorbate inhibits lipid peroxidation, oxidative DNA damage and oxidative protein damage.

Ascorbate is oxidized by reactive oxygen and nitrogen species to the semidehydroascorbate radical that is either reconverted to ascorbate via the enzyme NADH semidehydroascorbate reductase or is converted to dehydroascorbate

Dehydroascorbate in turn can be converted back to ascorbate via glutathione-dependent enzymes or catabolized.

Ascorbate can act as a secondary antioxidant. At least *in vitro*, ascorbate regenerates the major lipid antioxidant alpha-tocopherol from the alpha-tocopheroxyl radical form. Ascorbate may also participate in regenerating and sparing alpha-tocopherol *in vivo*, though this has not been clearly demonstrated. Vitamin C does preserve intracellular reduced glutathione concentrations.

The possible anti-atherogenic activity of vitamin C may be explained in a few ways. Oxidation of low-density lipoprotein (LDL) is thought to be a key early step in atherogenesis. Vitamin C protects against LDL peroxidation by scavenging peroxyl radicals in the aqueous phase. Vitamin C may enhance endothelial function by promoting the synthesis of nitric oxide (also known as NO and EDRF for endothelium-derived relaxing factor) or by preventing its inactivation by scavenging superoxide radicals. Superoxide reacts with nitric oxide to form peroxynitrite. High concentrations of vitamin C are required to prevent the interaction of superoxide with nitric oxide, extracellularly. Although such high plasma concentrations are feasible if vitamin C is given parenterally, they are likely not to occur with oral administration of vitamin C.

As noted above, vitamin C helps preserve intracellular reduced glutathione concentrations. This activity likely helps maintain nitric oxide levels and potentiates its vasoactive effects. Oral vitamin C can reach high enough concentrations

intracellularly to scavenge superoxide radicals. Thus, intracellular sources of superoxide that impair nitric oxide may be scavenged by oral vitamin C. Recently, it has been found that ascorbic acid enhances nitric oxide synthase activity by increasing intracellular tetrahydrobiopterin.

Vitamin C may modulate prostaglandin synthesis to favor the production of eicosanoids with antithrombotic and vasodilatory activity. The possible sparing and regeneration of alpha-tocopherol by vitamin C could be yet another factor in the vitamin's possible anti-atherogenic action.

Vitamin C's possible anticarcinogenic effects may be accounted for, in part, by its ability to detoxify carcinogens, as well as its ability to block carcinogenic processes through its antioxidant activity. Vitamin C can prevent the formation of such carcinogens as nitrosamines in foods and in the gastrointestinal tract and can detoxify such chemical mutagens and carcinogens as anthracene, benzo[a]pyrene, organochlorine pesticides and heavy metals. High concentratins of ascorbic acid in gastric juice may reduce the risk of gastric cancer by inhibiting, as noted, the formation of carcinogenic N-nitroso compounds. Additionally, increased oxidative stress to the gastric mucosa has been reported in *Helicobacter pylori*-associated gastritis, a condition that predisposes to gastric cancer. There is preliminary evidence that vitamin C can inhibit growth of *Helicobacter pylori*.

Evidence appears to suggest that vitamin C may have cancer-preventive activity, at least for certain types of cancer. However, the role of vitamin C, if any, in the treatment of cancer remains very unclear. A recent cell-culture study of human breast carcinoma lines showed vitamin C to improve the antineoplastic activity of doxorubicin, cisplatin and paclitaxel. The mechanism of the effect may be pro-oxidant, not antioxidant, activity of the vitamin in potentiating the effects of these chemotherapeutic agents. Another study suggests that the pro-oxidant form of vitamin C may upregulate some of the enzymes involved in DNA repair. This possible activity may play some anticarcinogenic role.

Vitamin C may have anti-hypertensive activity in some. The mechanism of this possible effect is a matter of speculation. Some *in vitro* studies show that vitamin C increases the synthesis of the vasodilatory prostaglandin PGE_1. However, this may not have relevance in the regulation of vascular tone in humans. As observed above, vitamin C may help maintain nitric oxide levels and potentiate its vasoactive effects. There is an indication that vitamin C may improve endothelial-dependent vasodilation in those with essential hypertension, as well as in those with hypercholesterolemia, and may help restore nitric oxide-mediated flow-dependent vasodilation in those with congestive heart failure.

There is some evidence that vitamin C inhibits the replication of human immunodeficiency virus 1 (HIV-1) *in vitro*. One study showed upregulation of the expression of glucose transporter 1 (Glut1) in HIV-infected cells Glut1 is one of the transport proteins for ascorbic acid. Increased cellular concentrations of ascorbate may be toxic to HIV-infected cells due to degradation of the viral nucleic acid by the action of the pro-oxidant form of vitamin C. The mechanism of the anti-HIV effect of the vitamin *in vitro*, however, is unclear, as is the relevance of this finding to HIV-positive individuals.

There is no evidence that vitamin C affects the replication of the viruses that cause the common cold *in vivo*. There is some evidence that vitamin C supplementation decreases the incidence, severity and duration of common cold symptoms in some. It is thought that this is due, at least in part, to antihistaminic activity of vitamin C.

The possible immunomodulatory activity of vitamin C may also be due, in part, to an antihistaminic effect of the vitamin. Vitamin C may enhance neutrophilic chemotaxis indirectly by reducing immunosuppressive effects of histamine. Some studies have shown that vitamin C, *in vitro*, enhances mitogen-stimulated lymphocyte proliferation, delayed-type hypersensitivity (DTH) response to skin antigens, natural killer cell activity and neutrophil chemotaxis. However, other studies have shown no effect of the vitamin on these and other indices of immune function.

Some studies suggest a protective effect of vitamin C supplementation against cataracts. Age-related lens opacities are thought to be due to oxidative stress. Ocular tissue concentrates vitamin C, and the antioxidant action of the vitamin could account for its possible effect in protection against cataracts.

Vitamin C may protect against asthma and other obstructive pulmonary diseases, as well as protect the airways against the effects of allergens, viral infections and irritants in some. Allergens, viruses and irritants, including ozone, nitrogen oxides and sulfur oxides, subject the airways to increased oxidative stress which can lead to bronchoconstriction. The possible protective action of vitamin C appears clearly due to its antioxidant properties.

The antioxidant properties of vitamin C can also account for its role in protecting against the tissue-damaging effect of some toxic chemicals and heavy metals. High serum levels of ascorbic acid have been reported to be associated with a decreased prevalence of elevated blood lead levels. The mechanism of the possible lead-lowering action of vitamin C is unclear. One study compared the chelating properties of ascorbic acid and the known lead-chelating agent EDTA and found them to have equivalent activity with respect to lead.

PHARMACOKINETICS

Absorption of vitamin C from the lumen of the small intestine depends on the amount of dietary intake. At a dietary intake of 30 milligrams daily, the vitamin is nearly completely absorbed from the lumen of the small intestine into the enterocytes. At an intake of 30 to 180 milligrams daily, about 70% to 90% is absorbed. About 50% of a single dose of 1 to 1.5 grams is absorbed. The percentage of a single dose absorbed decreases with increasing amounts. For example, only 16% of a single dose of 12 grams is absorbed. Maximum vitamin C absorption of large doses is attained by ingestion of several spaced doses throughout the day rather than by a single large dose. Further, sustained-release forms of large doses will give a higher efficiency of absorption than an equivalent dose that is not sustain-released. The type of food consumed does not appear to affect the absorption of supplemental vitamin C or vitamin C found in food.

The intestinal absorption of vitamin C from foods and from supplements, up to about 500 milligrams, occurs via a sodium-dependent active transport process. At doses higher than 500 milligrams, diffusion processes come into play. The major intestinal vitamin C transporter is SVCT1 (sodium-dependent vitamin C transporter 1). Some ascorbic acid may be oxidized to dehydroascorbic acid and transported into enterocytes via glucose transporters. Dietary dehydroascorbic acid is absorbed from the lumen of the small intestine into the enterocytes in such a manner. All dehydroascorbic acid within the enterocytes is reduced to ascorbic acid via reduced glutathione, and ascorbic acid leaves the enterocytes to enter, first, the portal and, subsequently, the systemic circulation. Ascorbic acid is distributed to the various tissues of the body.

Higher levels of ascorbic acid are found in the pituitary gland, the adrenal glands, the various white blood cells and the brain. Ascorbic acid itself cannot cross the blood-brain barrier. In order to enter the brain, ascorbic acid is first oxidized to dehydroascorbic acid or DHA. DHA is then transported across the blood-brain barrier by facilitative diffusion via glucose transporter 1 (GLUT1). DHA is next transported through GLUT1 at the surface of the blood-brain barrier endothelial cells. DHA is transported out of the endothelial cells through GLUT1. DHA in the brain is reduced to ascorbic acid. Ascorbic acid, once formed, is essentially trapped in the brain since it cannot be transported through GLUT1.

Ascorbic acid appears to be transported into intestinal cells, liver cells and kidney cells by a sodium-dependent active transport process via SVCT1 (sodium-dependent vitamin C transporter 1). The transporter SVCT2 (sodium-dependent vitamin C transporter 2) appears to aid in the transport of vitamin C into the aqueous humor of the eyes. Uptake of ascorbic acid into neutrophils appears to be by facilitative diffusion via GLUT1.

Regarding the metabolism of ascorbic acid, it is oxidized to dehydroascorbic acid which can either be reduced back to ascorbic acid or hydrolyzed to diketogulonate. Other metabolites include oxalic acid, threonic acid, L-xylose and ascorbate-2-sulfate. The principal route of excretion of ascorbic acid and its metabolites is via the kidney. In order to maintain ascorbic acid homeostasis, very little unmetabolized ascorbate is excreted with dietary intakes up to about 80 milligrams daily. Renal excretion of ascorbate increases proportionately with higher doses. As mentioned earlier, as the dose of supplemental ascorbic acid increases, the percentage of its absorption proportionately decreases. Consequently, there is significant fecal excretion of ascorbic acid with high supplemental intakes of the vitamin.

INDICATIONS AND USAGE

Vitamin C may be helpful in chronic diseases characterized by oxidative damage to biological molecules. Though vitamin C also has a pro-oxidant potential under some circumstances, fears raised in that regard in recent years appear overblown. There is currently no credible evidence for vitamin C pro-oxidant damage in humans except, possibly, in rare circumstances involving iron overload.

Vitamin C's antioxidant activity, on the other hand, is well established, and that activity may be helpful in the prevention of some cancers and cardiovascular disease. Vitamin C may also be helpful in protecting against some of the lipid oxidation caused by smoking. Vitamin C's demonstrated ability to reduce some forms of oxidative DNA damage and indications that it may also reduce protein oxidation under some circumstances further suggest that it may be of benefit in smokers and some with chronic stress and disease, in general.

Vitamin C may also be useful as an immune stimulator and modulator in some circumstances. Claims that it is a "cure" for common colds are unsubstantiated, although several studies have shown that vitamin C can significantly reduce the duration and severity of colds in some and reduce incidence in others. There is also preliminary evidence that vitamin C can be useful in ameliorating some other respiratory infections.

Vitamin C may help prevent cataracts.

Recently it was demonstrated that vitamin C can inhibit growth of *Helicobacter pylori* and may thus be protective against some ulcers and gastric carcinomas. There is also the suggestion in a recent report that low serum levels of ascorbic acid may be associated with a higher incidence of gall bladder disease in women. In another recent report,

vitamin C supplementation was associated with reduced risk of reflex sympathetic dystrophy after wrist fracture. It may be of benefit in some burn victims and may be helpful, generally, in promoting wound healing and gum health. It has also shown benefit in some with asthma.

RESEARCH SUMMARY

Vitamin C's antioxidant effects are well established. It has been reported to protect plasma lipids from oxidative damage. It also significantly protects DNA and protein from various oxidative processes, as demonstrated in numerous studies.

There is still controversy around claims that vitamin C can be a dangerous pro-oxidant in humans. These claims are now generally discounted, and the research that led to these fears has been widely challenged as being flawed in a number of respects. One researcher recently reviewed this controversy and concluded: "there is nothing in current data to worry members of the public who take ascorbate supplements."

Other researchers have also recently reviewed this controversy, noting that *in vitro* observations of DNA damage arising in the presence of vitamin C and redox-active transition metal ions are unlikely to have relevance *in vivo*. The damaging effect demonstrated *in vitro*, these researchers point out, "requires the availability of free, redox-active metal ions and a low ratio of vitamin C to metal ion, conditions unlikely to occur *in vivo* under normal circumstances. Furthermore, it was shown recently that in biological fluids such as plasma, vitamin C acts as an antioxidant toward lipids even in the presence of free, redox-active iron ... there is no convincing evidence for a pro-oxidant effect of vitamin C in humans."

On the other hand, vitamin C's antioxidant activity is marked and appears to play an important role in its possible cardioprotective activity. Several studies have shown that vitamin C, either alone, or in combination with other nutrients significantly inhibits LDL-cholesterol oxidation. This effect is most consistent when vitamin C is combined with vitamin E and/or beta-carotene, but it has also been observed when vitamin C is used alone. In the latter case, some hypothesize that it works by sparing or recycling vitamin E, an activity that has been observed *in vitro*. Results have been mixed in smokers in whom lipid oxidation is a serious problem. One of the better designed studies, utilizing a particularly sensitive measure of lipid oxidation, found that heavy smokers benefited from 2,000 milligrams of vitamin C administered for only five days, as measured by a significant reduction in a specific lipid oxidation marker, the F2 isoprostane 8-*epi*-PGF$_2$-alpha.

Where there have been discrepancies in results from lipid (and other) biomarkers studies, some researchers attribute these, in part, to the failure of some investigators to differentiate between subjects whose tissues are already saturated with vitamin C at baseline and those whose tissues are not thus saturated. Even dietary, non-supplemental, vitamin C intake, they argue, can readily result in saturation sufficient to rule out further reductions in oxidative damage, no matter what supplemental dose is administered.

Vitamin C supplementation has also been shown, in some studies, to significantly reduce total serum cholesterol. Some others have not shown this benefit. And there have been several observational reports associating high plasma vitamin C concentrations with higher levels of HDL-cholesterol.

Platelet aggregation has been reduced in two studies utilizing 2,000-3,000 milligrams of vitamin C daily for one to six weeks. No effect was noted on platelets in another study using 250 milligrams of vitamin C daily for eight weeks. Leukocyte adhesion to endothelium, an activity implicated in atherogenesis, was significantly inhibited in smokers receiving 2,000 milligrams of vitamin C daily for ten days.

Several studies have shown that vitamin C has positive effects on hypertension. Here, too, there have been some conflicting results, but the preponderance of evidence suggests a positive effect. Epidemiological studies also consistently show that lower vitamin C intake is associated with hypertension. In one recent randomized, double-blind, placebo-controlled study, hypertensive patients received placebo or 500 milligrams of vitamin C daily for 30 days. Vitamin C resulted in a 13 mm Hg reduction in systolic blood pressure. Placebo had no effects.

Several other studies have shown that both oral administration (1,000-2,000 milligrams) and intra-arterial infusion with vitamin C can exert significant, positive effects on vasodilation in coronary artery disease patients. Similar benefits have been found in several other test groups, including smokers and those with both type 1 and type 2 diabetes.

Vitamin C's potential impact on incidence of heart attack, stroke and death related to cardiovascular disease may be quite significant according to the findings of several epidemiological studies. In an analysis of findings from the First National Health and Nutrition Examination Survey, researchers found that "the relation of the standardized mortality ratio (SMR) for all causes of death to increasing vitamin C intake is strongly inverse for males and weakly inverse for females." Among males with the highest vitamin C intake, SMRs were 0.65 for all causes, 0.78 for all cancers and 0.58 for all cardiovascular disease. Among females with the highest vitamin C intake, SMRs were 0.90 for all causes, 0.86 for all cancers and 0.75 for all cardiovascular disease. Comparisons were made relative to the U.S. white population, for which the SMR was defined as 1.00.

In a 20-year followup study of a cohort of randomly selected elderly people in Britain, Scotland and Wales, mortality from stroke was highest in those with the lowest vitamin C status, as measured by dietary intake and plasma ascorbic acid concentration. Adjustments were made for age, sex and established cardiovascular risk factors. The association noted was independent of social class and other dietary variables. No association was found in this study between vitamin C status and risk of death from coronary artery disease, but the researchers noted this may have been due to the age of their observed population. "Factors that may predict premature death from coronary heart disease may become less important when measured in a population of elderly survivors," they noted. The subjects in this cohort were 65-74 years of age.

Recently, a five-year prospective population study of 1,605 Finnish men aged 42-60, who were free of atherosclerotic heart disease at baseline, concluded with these results: risk of myocardial infarction was considerably higher among those with the lowest baseline plasma vitamin C concentrations than among those with higher levels; 13.2% of those with the lowest levels suffered MIs versus 3.8% of those with higher levels.

What made this study particularly significant was its finding that increased risk of MI, in relation to plasma vitamin C concentrations, was confined to that group of subjects who were frankly deficient in vitamin C. In men with normal to high concentrations, there was no increased risk. This may have significance for some other studies that found no benefit from vitamin C in reducing cardiovascular disease risk.

It has been established by prior research that the Finnish population suffers high mortality from coronary heart disease and that many Finnish men have low plasma ascorbate concentrations. A reviewer of the Finnish study thus concluded that the finding in this study "that only individuals who are vitamin C-deficient are at increased risk may explain to some extent why no significant relationship was observed in many studies of relatively well-nourished populations."

This observation might apply, some believe, to the Nurses' Health Study and the Health Professionals' Study, both followup investigations that showed a relationship between increased vitamin E intake and reduced coronary heart disease risk but no similar relationship with respect to vitamin C.

As the reviewer further observed: "Both of these studies involved generally health-conscious study subjects. The vast majority of antioxidant-disease studies, even controlled intervention studies, involve generally healthy, well-nourished populations, primarily because these populations are much easier to study. The Finnish study results, therefore, provide a special perspective that may help us to understand the mixed results from past studies and better plan future studies.''

Vitamin C has, experimentally, demonstrated an ability to protect against various cancers, most likely through its ability to inhibit DNA oxidation, through reactive nitrogen species scavenging and other antioxidant actions, as well as through its possible effects on the immune system, among other activities. There are numerous epidemiological and case-control studies showing a consistent relationship between higher dietary intakes of vitamin C and lower incidence of cancer, particularly colo-rectal, stomach, lung, breast, esophageal, oral cavity and larynx-pharynx cancers. In one review of 75 epidemiologic studies, 54 found significant evidence of reduced cancer risk in those with higher dietary vitamin C intake.

Several *in vitro* and animal studies have demonstrated benefits. Results of some animal studies suggested that vitamin C therapy could reduce the toxicity and/or increase the effectiveness of some standard cancer therapies. Currently some researchers have expressed fear that vitamin C might reduce the effectiveness of some radiation and cancer chemotherapies by reducing their toxicity in cancer cells, as well as in normal ells. This idea has neither been confirmed nor refuted in animal or human studies and requires further investigation. Meanwhile, other researchers have expressed doubts about this hypothesis. They point out, as noted above, that several experimental studies indicate that high doses of vitamin C not only protect normal cells from toxic cancer therapies but may simultaneously fight the cancer cells, as well.

Many population studies have found evidence of a vitamin C protective effect against some cancers. Some other studies, however, have been negative. One group of researchers reported a significant 29% reduction in risk of all cancer in males consuming 113 milligrams or more of vitamin C daily, compared with males consuming less than 82 milligrams daily. Another found that consumption of 300 milligrams of vitamin C daily, derived from diet and from supplementation, was associated with a 21% reduction in risk from all cancers in men compared with daily consumption of less than 49 milligrams daily.

In a review of many of the epidemiological studies, the authors noted: ''Interestingly, virtually all of the studies in which vitamin C intakes were greater than 87 milligrams a day in the lowest intake group (quantile) found no or nonsignificant effects on cancer risk reduction with higher

intakes of vitamin C .... More studies investigating cancer risk in persons with lower vitamin C intakes are warranted.''

Studies of those using higher dose vitamin C supplements have generally not shown protective effects against cancer, ''possibly,'' these reviewers observed, ''because the dietary intake of vitamin C was already sufficient for tissue saturation.'' Intervention trials with high dose vitamin C have also been mostly negative.

At present, it appears that vitamin C helps protect against a number of cancers, and the amounts of vitamin C needed for this protection can generally be obtained from a diet that includes several servings of fruits and vegetables daily—or from low-dose vitamin C supplementation. More research will be needed before vitamin C's role, if any, in treating, as opposed to preventing cancer is established.

Vitamin C has shown a variety of activities in the immune system. It has been shown, in animal and *in vitro* studies, to favorably modulate lymphocytes and phagocytes. It can regulate natural killer cells under some circumstances and affect production of cytokines, antibodies and complement components.

Because supplemental vitamin C was not shown, in several studies, to reduce the incidence of the common cold, many concluded that it was of no use whatever in colds. That is still the impression of some physicians, but it is probably an erroneous one. First, a few studies have, in fact, shown a reduction in incidence of colds. Most studies have been done in normally nourished subjects in western countries; these have, typically, shown no effect on incidence. But in three trials of subjects under acute physical stress, vitamin C supplementation resulted in a 50% reduction in common cold incidence. And in four British trials, there was an average 30% reduction in incidence among those receiving vitamin C. Dietary vitamin C intake is known to be low in the UK.

Placebo-controlled trials have consistently found that supplemental vitamin C, in doses of 1 gram or greater daily, alleviated the duration and severity of cold symptoms. In several of these studies, the alleviation has been significant. For unexplained reason, there seems to be a greater effect in children than in adults and possibly, a greater effect in males than in females. The best results have been obtained with 2-gram (or greater) daily doses. There was a 6% median reduction in cold duration in five studies in which adults were administered 1 gram of vitamin C daily. There was a median decrease of 26% in two studies of children given 2 grams of vitamin C daily.

Vitamin C has also been found to be of benefit in patients with pneumonia and bronchitis. Incidence of pneumonia was significantly reduced in three controlled vitamin C studies, and substantial vitamin C treatment benefit was noted in elderly UK patients hospitalized with pneumonia or bronchitis.

There is evidence that supplemental vitamin C can inhibit the growth of *Helicobacter pylori* in both *in vitro* and animal studies. Thus it might have the potential to reduce the incidence of *H. pylori*-induced ulcers and subsequent gastric carcinoma. *In vitro*, high concentrations of vitamin C inhibited up to 90% of *H. pylori* growth. There was also significant inhibition of growth in animal experiments using oral administration of vitamin C.

High intake of vitamin C is strongly associated with reduced incidence of cataracts, according to the findings of case-control studies. In one study, intake of 300 milligrams or more per day was associated with a 70% reduction in risk. Another study found a 75% reduction in risk with daily intake of 490 milligrams or more per day, compared with intakes less than 125 milligrams per day. An intervention study using 120 milligrams of vitamin C daily produced a nonsignificant reduction in cataract risk of 22%, but a significant 36% reduction was observed in the same trial in subjects who consumed a multivitamin/mineral supplement.

Laboratory work has shown that vitamin C can slow chemical reactions that lead to cataracts by causing various lens proteins to aggregate. This has been demonstrated in animal work and in the human eye.

In a study of women who took vitamin C for at least ten years, incidence of cataract was significantly reduced compared with controls who did not take vitamin C. The vitamin C-supplemented women were only 23% as likely to develop cataracts compared with the women who did not take supplements. In women not taking supplements, mean daily dietary intake of vitamin C was 130 milligrams per day, about twice the recommended intake but still less than one-third the average of women taking supplements.

Recently, serum ascorbic acid levels were found to be inversely related to prevalence of gall bladder disease among women but not among men. Previously, it was shown that vitamin C-deficient guinea pigs have a high incidence of gallstones. Further clinical investigation is warranted.

In another recent study, this one a double-blind, placebo-controlled trial of vitamin C in patients with conservatively treated wrist fractures, treatment with 500 milligrams of vitamin C daily for 50 days significantly reduced the incidence of reflex sympathetic dystrophy (RSD). Followup continued for one year. The researchers proposed that "this simple and cheap means of prevention could also be useful in the prophylaxis of RSD after other injuries, such as trauma of the foot or ankle, talar and calcaneal fractures, or crural fractures."

It was the use of vitamin C as an antioxidant therapy in dermal burns that led the researchers to believe that an antioxidant therapy might also be of benefit in preventing post-traumatic dystrophy (after wrist fracture). Researchers have found that vitamin C helps protect endothelial cells and reduces capillary permeability by reducing lipid peroxidation after burns. Some of these same mechanisms apparently account for reported beneficial effects of vitamin C in a variety of wounds, in addition to burns. There is some evidence that supplemental vitamin C may decrease permeability of gum surface tissue and may, by that and other mechanisms, help protect against periodontal gum disease.

Evidence that vitamin C can sometimes counteract the symptoms of asthma comes, in part, from a study showing that vitamin C (taken in a 500 milligram dose 90 minutes before exercise) reduces bronchial spasms in some asthma sufferers and from another study in which 1 gram of vitamin C daily reduced airway reactivity to various harmful inhalants in asthmatics.

CONTRAINDICATIONS, PRECAUTIONS, ADVERSE REACTIONS
CONTRAINDICATIONS
Vitamin C is contraindicated in those with known hypersensitivity to the substance or to any ingredient in a vitamin C-containing product.

Rose hip vitamin C
Rose hip vitamin C is contraindicated in those with known hypersensitivity to rose hips. There are reports of allergic reactions in those working with rose hips.

PRECAUTIONS
Although oxalic acid is formed when ascorbic acid is metabolized, this is highly unlikely to cause renal problems in healthy individuals without preexisting renal problems or who are not predisposed to increased crystal aggregation. Those with preexisting kidney stone disease or a history of renal insufficiency, defined as serum creatine greater than 2 and/or creatinine clearance less than 30, should exercise caution in the use of higher than RDA amounts of vitamin C (see Dosage and Administration).

Ascorbic acid is involved in modulating iron absorption and transport. It is highly unlikely that healthy individuals who take supplemental vitamin C will have any problem with iron overload. On the other hand, those with hemochromatosis, thalassemia, sideroblastic anemia, sickle cell anemia and erythrocyte G6PD deficiency might have such a problem if they use large amounts of vitamin C.

Pregnant women and nursing mothers should avoid using supplemental doses of vitamin C higher than RDA amounts.

ADVERSE REACTIONS

In healthy adults, oral doses up to 3 grams daily of vitamin C are unlikely to cause adverse reactions. The most common adverse reaction in those who take oral doses greater than 3 grams daily are gastrointestinal and include nausea, abdominal cramps, diarrhea and flatulent distention. These reactions are attributed to the osmotic effect of unabsorbed vitamin C passing through the intestine. Some advocates of megadose vitamin C use recommend titrating the daily dose of vitamin C to what they refer to as "bowel tolerance", i.e., the point at which the user begins experiencing diarrhea. This is not recommended.

Rare adverse reactions have been reported in healthy individuals taking high oral doses of vitamin C. These include elevation of serum glucose in an adult male taking 4.5 grams daily, a gastrointestinal obstruction in a 66-year-old woman taking 4.5 grams daily of ascorbic acid and esophagitis in one person taking a single 500 milligram dose.

INTERACTIONS

DRUGS

Aluminum-containing antacids: The intake of large doses of vitamin C used at the same time as aluminum-containing antacids has been reported to increase urinary aluminum excretion, suggesting increased aluminum absorption from these antacids. However, this is not well documented.

Aspirin: Chronic use of high dose aspirin may lead to impaired vitamin C status.

Chemotherapeutic agents: Vitamin C may potentiate the antineoplastic activity of cisplatin, doxorubicin and paclitaxel. It may also help ameliorate the cardiotoxic effect of doxorubicin and the nephrotoxic effect of cisplatin. This is based on *in vitro* and animal studies. There is a concern by some researchers that supplemental doses of vitamin C may diminish the efficacy of some chemotherapeutic agents.

Estrogen: Ascorbic acid may enhance 17 beta-estradiol inhibition of oxidized LDL formation.

Vitamin C/Bioflavonoid combinations and drugs that inhibit cytochrome P-450 3A4: Preparations containing grapefruit flavonoids may interact with some drugs. Some drugs have up to a three-fold greater bioavailability when coadministered with grapefruit juice. It is thought that the grapefruit flavonoid naringenin plays some role in this effect. Naringenin and/or other substances found in grapefruit juice inhibit cytochrome P-450 3A4 (CYP 3A4). Drugs affected include the calcium channel blocker felodipine, as well as carbamazepine, cyclosporine, lovastatin, simvastatin, saquinavir and nisoldipine. Those taking these drugs need to exercise some caution in the use of any grapefruit products.

NUTRITIONAL SUPPLEMENTS

Copper: One study showed that high doses of vitamin C negatively affected copper status in men. Other studies have not shown such effects.

Flavonoids: Vitamin C may act synergistically with various flavonoids. This is the basis of combining flavonoids with vitamin C in some supplements. However, it is not known if any synergism occurs to any extent in humans. There is a report that the vitamin acts synergistically with the flavonoid quercetin to protect cutaneous cells against oxidative damage. The study was performed with cells in culture. There are other reports, again from cell culture studies, that certain flavonoids such as quercetin and hesperetin may inhibit the uptake of vitamin C into cells.

Glutathione: Ascorbic acid may help maintain reduced glutathione levels in cells.

Iron: Vitamin C used concomitantly with nonheme iron supplements may increase the uptake of iron. This may cause problems in those with high iron stores or with propensity for iron overload, such as those with hemochromatosis, sideroblastic anemia, sickle cell anemia, thalassemia and erythrocyte G6PD deficiency.

Selenium: One animal study reported that the protective effect of selenite in tumorogenesis was nullified by vitamin C. The chemopreventive action of selenomethionine, a form of selenium derived from foods, was not affected by the vitamin. Selenite may be reduced by vitamin C to a form that is not available for uptake by tissue.

Vitamin E: Vitamin C may regenerate or spare d-alpha-tocopherol. However, this is based on *in vitro* and animal studies. It is not yet known if this occurs in humans and, if it does, to what extent.

LABORATORY TESTS

Bilirubin assay: High intakes of vitamin C may cause falsely elevated bilirubin values.

Creatine assay: Large intakes of vitamin C may cause falsely elevated urine and serum creatinine levels. However, this is not well documented.

Glucose assay: Large intakes of vitamin C may cause false positive glucose readings measured by copper reduction methods (e.g., Clinitest) and false negative glucose results as measured by the oxidase methods (e.g., Clinistix and Tes-Tape).

Guaiac assay for occult blood: Intakes of vitamin C greater than 1 gram daily may cause a false negative guaiac test.

OVERDOSAGE

There are no reports of vitamin C overdosage in the literature.

DOSAGE AND ADMINISTRATION

A dose of 200 milligrams daily is almost enough to maximize plasma and lymphocyte levels. Doses of vitamin C vary from those equivalent to the RDAs up to 5 to 10 grams daily and, in some, even higher. Typical doses used range from 500 milligrams to 2 grams daily. Some increase their dose to 4 to 5 grams daily when coming down with a cold. Such doses may have antihistaminic action. A dose of vitamin C of 5 grams daily for 4 weeks was found to significantly inhibit *Helicobacter pylori* in one report. Although a dose of 200 milligrams daily is almost enough to maximize plasma and lymphocyte levels, high doses may aid in detoxifying some carcinogens in the stomach prior to absorption of the vitamin.

Absorption of supplemental vitamin C is most efficient if spaced throughout the day or if taken in time-release form.

In the United States, the average intake of vitamin C is about 95 milligrams for women and 107 milligrams for men. Children between the ages of one to five consume about 83 milligrams daily.

The most recent (2000) dietary reference intakes (DRI) for vitamin C are as follows:

Infants	Adequate Intake (AI)
0 — 6 months	40 milligrams daily or 6mg/kg
7 — 12 months	50 milligrams daily or 6mg/kg

	Recommended Dietary Allowances
Children	(RDA)
1 — 3 years	15 mg daily
4 — 8 years	25 mg daily
Boys	
9 — 13 years	45 mg daily
14 — 18 years	75 mg daily
Girls	
9 — 13 years	45 mg daily
14 — 18 years	65 mg daily
Men	
19 — 30 years	90 mg daily
31 — 50 years	90 mg daily
51 — 70 years	90 mg daily
70 years and older	90 mg daily
Women	
19 — 30 years	75 mg daily
31 — 50 years	75 mg daily
51 — 70 years	75 mg daily
70 years and older	75 mg daily
Pregnancy	
14 — 18 years	80 mg daily
19 — 30 years	85 mg daily
31 — 50 years	85 mg daily
Lactation	
14 — 18 years	115 mg daily
19 — 30 years	120 mg daily
31 — 50 years	120 mg daily
Smokers	
Men	125 mg daily
Women	110 mg daily

A LOAEL (Lowest-Observed-Adverse-Effect Level) of 3 grams daily has been established for vitamin C for adults. Based on this LOAEL, a Tolerable Upper Level Intake (UL) for the vitamin has been set at 2 grams daily for men and women 19 years and older.

Ascorbate and vitamin C metabolites are available in a few forms. The basic form contains calcium ascorbate and calcium L-threonate (present at 1% of the ascorbate dose). Some formulations contain such substances as flavonoids, in addition. Intravenous forms of vitamin C are also available.

HOW SUPPLIED

Vitamin C is available in the following forms and strengths for Rx use:

Injection: 222 mg/mL, 250 mg/mL, 500 mg/mL

Vitamin C is available in the following forms and strengths for OTC use:

Capsules: 100 mg, 250 mg, 500 mg, 1000 mg
Capsules, Extended Release: 500 mg, 1000 mg
Cream: 10%
Chewable Tablets: 60 mg, 100 mg, 200 mg, 250 mg, 500 mg, 1000 mg
Granules
Liquid: 100 mg/mL, 500 mg/5 mL
Lozenges: 25 mg
Powder
Syrup: 500 mg/5 mL
Tablets: 100 mg, 250 mg, 500 mg, 1000 mg
Tablets, Extended Release: 500 mg, 1000 mg, 1500 mg, 2000 mg

LITERATURE

Agus DB, Gambhir SS, Pardridge WM, et al. Vitamin C crosses the blood-brain barrier in the oxidized form through the glucose transporters. *J Clin Invest.* 1997; 100:2842-2848.

Antunes LMG, Darin JDC, Bianchi MDLP. Protective effects of vitamin C against cisplatin-induced nephrotoxicity and lipid peroxidation in adult rats: a dose-dependent study. *Pharmacol Res.* 2000; 41:405-411.

Bors W, Michel C, Schikora S. Interaction of flavonoids with ascorbate and determination of their univalent redox potentials: a pulse radiolysis study. *Free Rad Biol Med*. 1995; 19:45-52.

Bush MJ, Verlangieri AJ. An acute study on the relative gastro-intestinal absorption of a novel form of calcium ascorbate. *Res Commun Chem Pathol Pharmacol*. 1987; 57:137-140.

Carr A, Frei B. Does vitamin C act as a pro-oxidant under physiological conditions? *FASEBJ*. 1999; 13:1007-1024.

Carr AC, Tijerina T, Frei B. Vitamin C protects against and reverses specific hypochlorous acid- and chloramine-dependent modifications of low-density lipoprotein. *Biochem J*. 2000; 346 Pt 2:491-496.

Cooke MS, Evans MD, Podmore ID, et al. Novel repair action of vitamin C upon in vivo oxidative DNA damage. *FEBS Lett*. 1998; 439:363-367.

Dietary Reference Intakes for Vitamin C, Vitamin E, Selenium, and Carotenoids. Washington, D.C.: National Academy Press; 2000.

Duffy SJ, Gokce N, Holbrook M, et al. Treatment of hypertension with ascorbic acid. *Lancet*. 1999; 354:2048-2049.

Enstrom JE, Kanim LE, Klein MA. Vitamin C intake and mortality among a sample of the United States population. *Epidemiology*. 1992; 3:194-202.

Fay MJ, Bush MJ, Verlangieri AJ. Effect of aldonic acids on the uptake of ascorbic acid by 3T3 mouse fibroblasts and human T lymphoma cells. *Gen Pharmacol*. 1994; 25:1465-1469.

Fay MJ, Verlangieri AJ. Stimulatory action of calcium L-threonate on ascorbic acid uptake by a human T-lymphoma cell line. *Life Sci*. 1991; 49:1377-1381.

Friedman PA, Zeidel ML. Victory at C. *Nature Med*. 1999; 5:620-621.

Gamble J, Grewal PS, Gartside IB. Vitamin C modifies the cardiovascular and microvascular responses to cigarette smoke inhalation in man. *Clin Science*. 2000; 98:455-460.

Halliwell B. Vitamin C: poison, prophylactic or panacea? *Trends Biochem Sci*. 1999; 24:255-259.

Harakeh S, Jariwalla RJ, Pauling L. Suppression of human immunodeficiency virus replication by ascorbate in chronically and acutely infected cells. *Proc Natl Acad SciUSA*. 1990; 87:7245-7249.

Harding JJ, Hassett PC, Rixon KC, et al. Sugars including erythronic and threonic acids in the human aqueous humor. *Curr Eye Res*. 1999; 19:131-136.

Hemila H, Douglas RM. Vitamin C and acute respiratory infections. *Int J Tuberc Lung Dis*. 1999; 3:756-761.

Hodison T, Socaciu C, Ropan I, Neamtu G. Carotenoid composition of *Rosa canina* fruits determined by thin-layer chromatography and high performance liquid chromatography. J *Pharmaceut Biomed Anal*. 1997; 16:521-528.

Hornero-Méndez D, Minguez-Mosquera MI. Carotenoid pigments in *Rosa mosqueta* hips, an alternative carotenoid source for foods. *J Agric Food Chem*. 2000; 48:825-828.

Hwang J, Peterson H, Hodis HN, et al. Ascorbic acid enhances 17 beta-estradiol-mediated inhibition of oxidized low density lipoprotein formation. *Atherosclerosis*. 2000; 150:275-284.

Ip C. Interaction of vitamin C and selenium supplementation in the modification of mammary carcinogenesis in rats. *J Nat Cancer Inst*. 1986; 77:299-303.

Jacob RA. Vitamin C In: Shils ME, Olson JA, Shike M, Ross AC, eds. *Modern Nutrition in Health and Disease*. 9th ed. Baltimore, MD: William and Wilkins; 1999:467-483.

Jarosz M, Dzieniszewski J, Dabrowska-Ufniarz E, et al. Effects of high dose vitamin C treatment on Helicobacter pylori ingestion and total vitamin C concentration in gastric juice. *Eur J Cancer Prev*. 1998; 7:449-454.

Kurbacher CM, Wagner U, Kolster B, et al. Ascorbic acid (vitamin C) improves the antineoplastic activity of doxorubicin, cisplatin, and paclitaxel in human breast carcinoma cells in vitro. *Cancer Letters*. 1996; 103:183-189.

Kwaselow A, Rowe M, Sears-Ewald D, Ownby D. Rose hips: a new occupational allergen. *J Allergy Clin Immunol*. 1990; 85:704-708.

Lykkesfeldt J, Christen S, Wallock LM, et al. Ascorbate is depleted by smoking and repleted by moderate supplementation: a study in male smokers and nonsmokers with matched dietary intakes. *Am J Clin Nutr*. 2000; 71:530-536.

Markham RG. Compositions and methods for administering vitamin C. United States Patent Number 4, 822, 816. April 18, 1989.

Moertel CG, Fleming TR, Creagan ET, et al. High-dose vitamin C versus placebo in the treatment of patients with advanced cancer who had no prior chemotherapy. A randomized double-blind comparison. *N Engl J Med*. 1985; 312:137-141.

Mowat C, Carswell A, Wirz A, McColl KEL. Omeprazole and dietary nitrate independently affect levels of vitamin C and nitrite in gastric juice. *Gastroenterology*. 1999; 116:813-822.

Ness AR, Chee D, Elliot P. Vitamin C and blood pressure—an overview. *J Hum Hypertens*. 1997; 11:343-350.

Panda K, Chattopadhyay R, Ghosh MK, et al. Vitamin C prevents cigarette smoke induced oxidative damage of proteins and increased proteolysis. *Free Rad Biol Med*. 1999; 27:1064-1079.

Park JB, Levine M. Intracellular accumulation of ascorbic acid is inhibited by flavonoids via blocking of dehydroascorbic acid and ascorbic acid uptakes in HL-60, U937 and Jurkat cells. *J Nutr*. 2000; 130:1297-1302.

Pauling L. Evolution and the need for ascorbic acid. *Proc Natl Acad SciUSA*. 1970; 67:1643-1648.

Pauling L. The significance of the evidence about ascorbic acid and the common cold. *Proc Natl Acad SciUSA*. 1971; 68:2678-2681.

Podmore ID, Griffiths HR, Herbert KE, et al. Vitamin C exhibits pro-oxidant effects. *Nature.* 1998; 392:559.

Raitakari OT, Adams MR, McCredie RJ, et al. Oral vitamin C and endothelial function in smokers: short-term improvement, but no sustained beneficial effect. *J Amer Coll Cardiol.* 2000; 35:1616-1621.

Rehman A, Collis CS, Yang M, et al. The effects of iron and vitamin C co-supplementation on oxidative damage to DNA in healthy volunteers. *Biochem Biophys Res Commun.* 1998; 246:293-298.

Rivas CI, Vera JC, Guaiquil VH, et al. Increased uptake and accumulation of Vitamin C in human immunodeficiency virus 1-infected hematopoietic cell lines. *J Biol Chem.* 1997; 272:5814-5820.

Rowe DJ, Ko S, Tom XM, et al. Enhanced production of mineralized nodules and collagenous proteins in vitro by calcium ascorbate supplemented with vitamin C metabolites. *J Periodontol.* 1999; 70:992-929.

Sakagami H, Satoh K, Hakeda Y, Kumegawa M. Apoptosis-inducing activity of vitamin C and vitamin K. *Cell Mol Biol.* 2000; 46:129-143.

Simon JA, Hudes ES. Relationship of ascorbic acid to blood lead levels. *J Amer Med Assoc.* 1999; 281:2298-2293.

Simon JA, Hudes ES. Serum ascorbic acid and gallbladder disease prevalence among US adults. The Third National Health and Nutrition Examination Survey (NHANES III). *Arch Intern Med.* 2000; 160:931-936.

Skaper SD, Fabris M, Ferrari V, et al. quercetin protects cutaneous tissue-associated cell types including sensory neurons from oxidative stress induced by glutathione depletion: cooperative effects of ascorbic acid. *Free Rad Biol Med.* 1997; 22:669-678.

Taddei S, Virdis A, Ghiadoni L, et al. Vitamin C improves endothelium-dependent vasodilation by restoring nitric oxide activity in essential hypertension. *Circulation.* 1998; 97:2222-2229.

Tsukaguchi H, Tokui T, Mackenzie B, et al. A family of mammalian Na+-dependent L-ascorbic acid transporters. *Nature.* 1999; 399:70-75.

Valkonen MM, Kuusi T. Vitamin C prevents the acute atherogenic effects of passive smoking. *Free Rad Biol Med.* 2000; 28:428-436.

Verlangieri AJ, Fay MJ, Bannon AW. Comparison of L-ascorbic acid and Ester C in the non-ascorbate synthesizing Osteogenic Disorder Shionogi (ODS) rat. *Life Sci.* 1991; 48:2275-2281.

WangY, Mackenzie B, Tsukaguchi H, et al. Human vitamin C (L-ascorbic acid) transporter SVCT1. *Biochem Biophys Res Commun.* 2000; 267:488-494.

Zhang HM, Wakisaka N, Maeda O, Yamamoto T. Vitamin C inhibits the growth of a bacterial risk factor for gastric carcinoma: Helicobacter pylori. *Cancer.* 1997; 80:1897-1903.

Zollinger PE, Tuinebreijer WE, Kreis RW, Breederveld RS. Effect of vitamin C on frequency of reflex sympathetic dystrophy in wrist fractures: a randomized trial. *Lancet.* 1999; 354:2025-2028.

Vitamin D

TRADE NAMES

Vitamin D is available from numerous manufacturers generically. Branded products include: Allergy D Caps (Twinlab).

DESCRIPTION

The term vitamin D refers to the secosterols ergocalciferol or vitamin D_2 and cholecalciferol or vitamin D_3 as well as to the metabolites and analogues of these substances. All forms of vitamin D possess antirachitic activity. Vitamin D is different from all of the other vitamins in human nutrition because it is the only vitamin that is a conditional one. Vitamin D_3 is synthesized in the skin from 7-dehydrocholesterol via photochemical reactions using ultraviolet B (UV-B) radiation from sunlight. However, there are conditions where the synthesis of vitamin D_3 in the skin is not sufficient to meet physiological requirements. Humans who are not exposed to sufficient sunlight due to reason of geography, shelter or clothing, require dietary intake of vitamin D. Under these conditions, vitamin D is an essential nutrient. Vitamin D without a subscript refers to either vitamin D_2 or vitamin D_3.

Vitamin D is the principal regulator of calcium homeostasis in the body. It is particularly important in skeletal development and bone mineralization. Vitamin D is a prohormone. That is, it has no hormone activity itself, but is converted to a molecule which does.

The active form of vitamin D is 1alpha, 25-dihydroxyvitamin D or $1,25(OH_2)D$ (again, when D is used without a subscript it refers to either D_2 or D_3). The vitamin D hormone $1,25(OH_2)D$ mediates its actions via binding to vitamin D receptors (VDRs) which are principally located in the nuclei of target cells. $1,25(OH_2)D$ enhances the efficiency of calcium absorption, and, to a much lesser extent, phosphorus absorption, from the small intestine. Vitamin D deficiency is characterized by inadequate mineralization or demineralization of the skeleton. Inadequate mineralization of the skeleton is the cause of rickets in children (vitamin D is also known as the antirachitic factor), while demineralization of the skeleton results in osteomalcia in adults. Further, vitamin D deficiency in adults can lead to osteoporosis. This results from a compensatory increase in the production of parathyroid hormone resulting in resorption of bone.

Very few foods are natural sources of vitamin D. Foods that do contain vitamin D include fatty fish, fish liver oils (e.g., cod liver oil) and eggs from hens that have been fed vitamin D. Nearly all the vitamin D intake from foods comes from fortified milk products and other foods, such as breakfast cereals, that have been fortified with vitamin D. Vitamin D is a fat-soluble vitamin and therefore its absorption is adversely affected in those with malabsorption disorders. Those with chronic liver disease, cystic fibrosis, Crohn's disease, Whipple's disease and sprue are prone to vitamin D deficiency. Others at risk for vitamin D deficiency, include those that do not drink milk and who do not receive much sunlight, those who live in regions where they receive little natural light and alcoholics. The elderly are at risk for vitamin D deficiency for several reasons, including inadequate exposure to sunlight, consumption of low amounts of vitamin D-containing foods and the use of certain drugs which interfere with the absorption and/or metabolism of vitamin D (see Interactions). The use of sunscreens may be another factor that may negatively affect vitamin D status.

The two forms of vitamin D used for nutritional supplementation are the secosterols ergocalciferol (vitamin D₂) and cholecalciferol (vitamin D₃). Secosterols or secosteroids are derived from the cyclopentanoperhydrophenanthrene ring structure, the basic structure of all steroids. The cyclopentanoperhydrophenanthrene structure is comprised of four rings (A, B, C and D). Secosterols or secosteroids are steroids in which one of the rings has been broken. In the case of vitamin D, the bond between carbons 9 and 10 of ring B is broken, and this is indicated by the inclusion of "9, 10-seco" in the chemical name of the molecule. Seco is from the Greek word for split.

Vitamin D₂ is derived from fungal and plant sources. Vitamin D₂ is also known as ergocalciferol. Its chemical names are 9, 10-seco (5Z, 7E)-5, 7, 10(19), 22-ergostatetraene-3beta-ol and (3 beta, 5Z, 7E, 22E)-9, 10-secoergosta-5, 7, 10(19), 22-tetraen-3-ol. Its molecular formula is $C_{28}H_{44}O$ and its molecular weight is 396.66 daltons. The configuration of the double bonds are notated *E* for entgegen (from the German, meaning to stand opposite to) or *trans*, and *Z* for zusammen (from the German, meaning together) or *cis*. Vitamin D₂ is represented by the following structural formula:

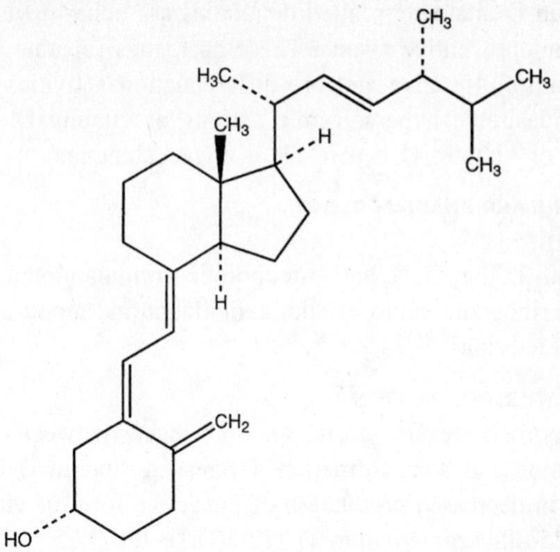

Vitamin D₂

Vitamin D₃ is derived from animal sources. Vitamin D₃ is also known as cholecalciferol and calciol. Its chemical names are 9, 10-seco (5Z, 7E)-5, 7, 10(19) cholestatriene-3beta-ol and (3beta, 5Z, 7E)-9, 10-secocholesta-5, 7, 10(19)-trien-3-ol. Its molecular formula is $C_{27}H_{44}O$, and its molecular weight is 384.65 daltons. The only structural difference between vitamin D₂ and vitamin D₃ is in their side chains. The side chain of vitamin D₂ contains a double bond between carbons 22 and 23 and a methyl group on carbon 24. The structural formula of vitamin D₃ can be represented as follows:

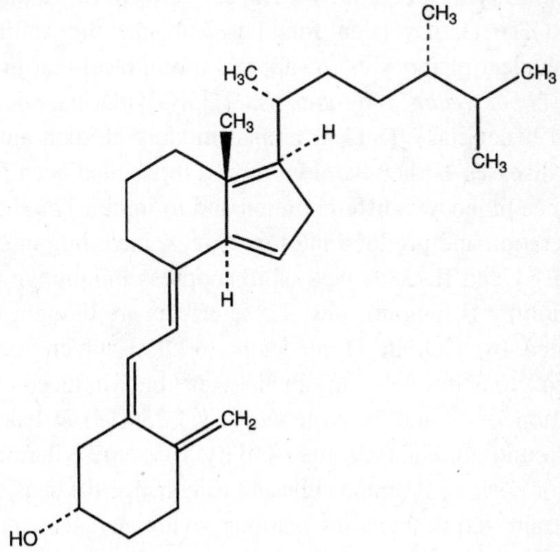

Vitamin D₃

Pharmaceutical forms of vitamin D include calcitriol (1alpha, 25-dihydroxycholecalciferol), doxercalciferol and calcipotriene. Calcitriol and doxercalciferol are used to treat certain metabolic disorders; calcipotriene is used topically for the treatment of psoriasis.

Vitamin D analogues called deltanoids are being developed as chemopreventive agents. These analogues separate desirable antiproliferative and pro-differentiation activities from the undesirable hypercalcemic activity of vitamin D. High doses of vitamin D can result in hypercalcemia.

ACTIONS AND PHARMACOLOGY

ACTIONS

Vitamin D may have anti-osteoporotic, immunomodulatory, anticarcinogenic, antipsoriatic, antioxidant and mood-modulatory activities.

MECHANISM OF ACTION

Osteoporosis results from an imbalance between bone resorption and bone formation. Decreased vitamin D levels result in decreased production of the active form of vitamin D, 1,25-dihydroxyvitamin D (1,25(OH)$_2$ D). 1,25 (OH)$_2$ D enhances the efficiency of calcium absorption. Chronic vitamin D deficiency results in decreased calcium absorption and secondary hyperparathyroidism. Increased bone resorption may be a consequence of vitamin D deficiency, resulting from secondary hyperparathyroidism. Therefore, vitamin D supplementation might be expected to protect against osteoporosis and fractures in those with occult vitamin D deficiency. Vitamin D may also be effective in the treatment of corticosteroid-induced osteoporosis by virtue of its stimulation of calcium absorption from the small intestine and its inhibition of the secretion and production of parathyroid hormone.

Vitamin D deficiency has long been suspected to increase the susceptibility to tuberculosis. The active form of vitamin D, 1,25 (OH)$_2$ D, has been found to enhance the ability of mononuclear phagocytes to suppress the intracellular growth of *Mycobacterium tuberculosis*. 1,25(OH)$_2$D has demonstrated beneficial effects in animal models of such autoimmune diseases as rheumatoid arthritis. It has also been found to induce monocyte differentiation and to inhibit lymphocyte proliferation and production of cytokines, including interleukin (IL)-1 and IL-2, as well as to suppress immunoglobulin secretion by B lymphocytes. These effects are thought to be mediated by vitamin D receptors (VDRs) which are expressed constitutively in monocytes but induced upon activation of T and B lymphocytes. 1,25(OH)$_2$D has also been found to enhance the activity of some vitamin D-receptor positive immune cells and to enhance the sensitivity of certain target cells to various cytokines secreted by immune cells. Vitamin D appears to demonstrate both immune-enhancing and immunosuppressive effects.

1, 25-dihydroxyvitamin D has been found to induce differentiation and/or inhibit cell proliferation in a number of malignant cell lines including human prostate cancer cells. 1, 25-dihydroxyvitamin D suppresses the *in vivo* growth of human cancer (colon cancer, malignant melanoma) solid tumor xenografts. It has been demonstrated in various cancer cell lines that 1, 25-dihydroxyvitamin D causes a dose-dependent inhibition of cell proliferation and switches cellular activity from proliferation to differentiation. 1, 25-dihydroxyvitamin D has also been demonstrated to inhibit the growth of renal cell carcinoma cells in culture, to inhibit the growth of retinoblastoma in mice and to be antiproliferative and pro-differentiating for leukemia cells. The anticarcinogenic activity of the active form of vitamin D appears to be correlated with cellular vitamin D receptor (VDR) levels. Vitamin D receptors belong to the superfamily of steroid-hormone zinc-finger receptors. VDRs selectively bind 1, 25-dihydroxyvitamin D and retinoic acid X receptor (RXR) to form a heterodimeric complex that interacts with specific DNA sequences known as vitamin D-responsive elements. VDRs are ligand-activated transcription factors. The receptors activate or repress the transcription of target genes upon binding their respective ligands. For example, the binding of 1, 25-dihydroxyvitamin D to the VDR in intestinal cells activates the transcription of the calcium-binding protein which enhances the absorption of calcium. It is thought that the anticarcinogenic effect of vitamin D is mediated via VDRs in cancer cells.

The mechanism of action of the anticarcinogenic activity of vitamin D, however, is not fully understood. 1, 25-dihydroxyvitamin D has been found to induce apoptosis of cancer cells *in vitro* and *in vivo*. It downregulates the antiapoptotic bcl-2 protein and upregulates p53 expression, resulting in active cell death. It also upregulates clusterin and cathepsin B. 1, 25-dihydroxyvitamin D has also been shown to have antiangiogenesis activity. *In vitro*, it was found to inhibit vascular endothelial growth factor (VEGF)-induced endothelial sprouting and elongation and to have a significant inhibitory effect on VEGF-induced endothelial cell proliferation. *In vivo*, it was found to produce tumors that were less vascularized than tumors formed in mice treated with vehicle alone.

1, 25-dihydroxyvitamin D and its analogues have been found to be effective in the treatment of psoriasis when applied topically. Psoriasis is a cutaneous disorder involving abnormal cellular proliferation and differentiation. The mechanism of action of 1, 25-dihydroxyvitamin D and its analogues in the treatment of psoriasis is accounted for by their antiproliferative activity for keratinocytes and their stimulation of epidermal cell differentiation.

Vitamin D$_3$ has been found to inhibit lipid peroxidation in rat hepatocytes *in vivo*, to inhibit iron-dependent lipid peroxidation in liposomes and to modulate cellular antioxidant defense in lymphoma-bearing mice. The mechanism of the antioxidant effect of vitamin D is unknown.

Vitamin D$_3$, in two human studies, was found to significantly enhance positive affect and possibly reduce negative affect. The mechanism of this possible mood-modulating effect is unclear. It is speculated that vitamin D may affect brain serotonin levels.

PHARMACOKINETICS

Vitamin D is principally absorbed in the small intestine. It is absorbed from the lumen of the small intestine into the enterocytes by passive diffusion. Vitamin D is delivered to the enterocytes in micelles formed from bile acids and other substances. The efficiency of absorption of vitamin D is high. Approximately 50% to 80% of ingested vitamin D is absorbed. Vitamin D is secreted by the enterocytes into the lymphatics in the form of chylomicrons. It enters the circulation via the thoracic duct. Vitamin D is transported in the blood bound to an alpha-globulin vitamin D binding protein. This protein is also known as the vitamin D-binding protein (DBP) and the group-specific component (Gc) protein. A large faction of circulating vitamin D is extracted by the hepatocytes. It is metabolized to 25-hydroxyvitamin D (25(OH)D) or calcidiol via the enzyme vitamin D 25-hydroxylase in the hepatocytes. 25(OH)D is the major circulating form of vitamin D. This metabolite of vitamin D, however, is not biologically active under physiological conditions. The biologically active hormone form of vitamin D, 1, 25-dihydroxyvitamin D (1, 25(OH)$_2$ D) or calcitriol, is produced in the kidney via the enzyme 25-hydroxyvitamin D-1-alpha hydroxylase.

25-hydroxyvitamin D-1-alpha hydroxylase 25(OH) D and 1, 25(OH)$_2$ D may undergo hydroxylation to form 24, 25-dihydroxyvitamin D (24, 25(OH)$_2$ D) and 1, 24, 25-trihydroxyvitamin D (1, 24, 25(OH)$_3$ O), respectively. Other metabolites of 1, 25 (OH)$_2$ D include calcitroic acid and the lactone 1alpha, 25R (OH)$_2$-26,23S-lactone cholecalciferol. Vitamin D and its metabolites are excreted primarily via the biliary route. The final degradation product of 1, 25 (OH)$_2$ D$_3$ is calcitroic acid, which is excreted by the kidney.

INDICATIONS AND USAGE

Vitamin D's usefulness in reducing bone loss and fracture incidence in the elderly remains somewhat unclear, but the preponderance of evidence suggests that this use is merited. There is evidence that it may also be helpful in preventing or limiting some perinatal growth retardation and that it is of benefit in some cases of psoriasis. Current research suggests that a broad range of additional indications may eventually emerge, including uses in cancer, immunomodulation, diabetes (and some other endocrinopathies) and infertility. There is also the suggestion, in preliminary research, that vitamin D and its analogues might be helpful in diminishing depression associated with seasonality, that it might increase resistance to some seizures and that it might help with bilateral cochlear deafness, sick sinus syndrome and multiple sclerosis.

RESEARCH SUMMARY

Various studies have found an association between low serum levels of vitamin D and incidence of osteoarthritis and bone fracture. Moreover, low dietary intake of vitamin D has itself been associated with progression of osteoarthritis of the knee in participants in the Framingham study. Progression was confirmed by knee radiography at various intervals over a ten-year period. Risk for progression increased threefold in those subjects in the middle and lower tertiles for both vitamin D intake and serum levels of vitamin D. Loss of cartilage was also predicted by low serum levels of vitamin D.

More recently, a high incidence of occult vitamin D deficiency was found in a group of postmenopausal women who had suffered hip fractures. The researchers suggested that "repletion of vitamin D and suppression of parathyroid hormone at the time of fracture may reduce future fracture risk and facilitate hip fracture repair." They added that "supplements of about 800 IU of vitamin D per day and calcium may be necessary to attenuate bone loss in the winter and to reduce fractures."

Some have doubted that supplemental vitamin D would have much direct impact on osteoporosis and bone fracture. Vitamin D deficiency has not been shown to be a direct cause of osteoporosis. It produces osteomalacia, a defect in bone mineralization, rather than the reduction in bone mass that characterizes osteoporosis. Nonetheless, osteomalacia itself may predispose to bone fracture. Others have observed that vitamin D deficiency, now known to be considerably more prevalent in elderly populations than previously suspected, can also result in muscle weakness, another possible contributor to falls and fractures. And recently at least one function of vitamin D in osteoblasts associated with the development of clinical osteoporosis has been found.

Some studies have, in fact, failed to find any benefit from supplemental vitamin D in the prevention and treatment of osteoporosis. The majority of studies, however, have reported significant benefits, evidenced by a review of 23 studies. Positive outcomes, measured primarily by increase in bone density, were associated, in this review, with higher doses, longer duration of use and more sensitive methods of measuring bone mass.

Some of the best results have been obtained in studies using considerably higher than the typical 400 IU doses daily and administering calcium simultaneously. Response also appears sensitive to the subject population. More geriatric and infirm populations that are indoors more tend to have lower vitamin D levels and greater suppression of serum parathyroid hormone levels, and these populations seem to show greater response to vitamin D therapy.

In a three-year study, supplemental vitamin D was given at a dose of 800 IUs daily in combination with a calcium supplement. The population group included nursing home residents who were indoors most of the time. The vitamin D-calcium combination was found to significantly protect against hip fracture in this randomized, double-blind, placebo-controlled study.

In another recent three-year double-blind, placebo-controlled study, a combination of vitamin D (700 IUs daily) and calcium (500 milligrams daily) was tested for its effects on nonvertebral fracture incidence and bone mass maintenance in 389 men and women older than 65. The researchers concluded that this combination "led to a positive change in biochemical markers related to bone turnover, slowed the rate of bone loss and significantly decreased fracture incidence."

There is evidence from *in vitro*, animal and clinical research that supplemental vitamin D, administered during pregnancy in appropriate circumstances and under a physician's supervision, can be of benefit to the neonate, helping to ensure healthy osteogenesis and to prevent low-birth weight. There is also evidence that supplemental vitamin D enhances lactational performance in some. Again, supplemental vitamin D in greater than U.S. RDA amounts should be used during pregnancy and breast feeding only with the recommendation and monitoring of a physician.

Because vitamin D and its analogues are potent antiproliferative agents for keratinocytes and stimulators of epidermal cell differentiation, they have been investigated as possible therapies for psoriasis. Calcipotriol, a synthetic vitamin D analogue with relatively low toxicity, has been demonstrated to significantly improve psoriatic lesions in a number of double-blind, placebo-controlled trials.

In a recent review of 37 trials involving 6,038 subjects with plaque psoriasis, topical calcipotriol was found to be as effective as topical corticosteroids in treating this condition. The researcher concluded that "although calcipotriol caused more skin irritation than tropical corticosteroids this has to be balanced against the potential long-term effects of corticosteroids."

Vitamin D's antiproliferative activity has also suggested a possible role for it in the treatment or prevention of some cancers. It has demonstrated a dose-dependent inhibition of cell proliferation in a number of cancer cell lines. It also has a pro-differentiation effect on these cells, resulting in potent anti-cancer activity in some preliminary work. It and its analogues show significant experimental activity against colorectal, renal cell, breast and prostate cancers, among others. They are also active against leukemic cells and retinoblastoma. With respect to the latter, these substances seem to inhibit angiogenesis.

Vitamin D's observed immunomodulatory abilities may also play a role in its anti-cancer activity. Vitamin D has been shown to enhance the activity of immune cells that have vitamin D receptors. There is some evidence that vitamin D increases the potency of cytokines and enhances the phagocyte activity and antibody-dependent cytotoxicity of macrophages and that it boosts natural killer cell activity and helps regulate T cells, among other things. Vitamin D-deficient subjects given supplemental vitamin D have reportedly had significantly fewer infections.

One researcher has observed that vitamin D is a "flexible," bi-directional immunomodulator that, in some circumstances, can also dampen immune activity in favorable ways. It has been reported, for example, to improve joint symptoms caused by autoimmune psoriatic arthritis. Animal experiments suggest efficacy in some other disorders with autoimmune components, such as multiple sclerosis and rheumatoid arthritis. It has also shown some preliminary ability to control graft rejection and thus may prove helpful in transplantation. Some have suggested that vitamin D and its analogues may be superior to cyclosporine in suppressing transplant rejection and without the serious side effects of cyclosporine.

Finally, with respect to immunity, attention is again focusing on vitamin D as a tuberculosis preventive. In the 1800s sunlight and vitamin D-rich cod-liver oil were the treatments of choice for tuberculosis. With the development of antimycobacterial drugs, these earlier treatments, which had proved quite effective in many cases, were set aside and largely forgotten. *In vitro* studies have shown that vitamin D can enhance the macrophage activity that inhibits intracellular growth of *Mycobacterium tuberculosis*. With the incidence of tuberculosis again rising, some researchers have recently suggested that consideration be given to administering vitamin D to those in high-risk groups as preventive therapy.

Very preliminary work suggests that vitamin D may be able to improve glucose tolerance in some diabetics, that it may have some favorable effects on spermatogenesis, that it may increase seizure threshold in some circumstances, that it might be helpful in some cases of bilateral cochlear deafness and some cases of seasonal-related depression. There is a case study in which it seemed to obliterate the symptoms of sick sinus syndrome, a disorder of sinus node function that is generally treated with antiarrhythmia drugs. Followup research is needed.

Finally, researchers have found evidence for a correspondence between frequency of multiple sclerosis (MS) lesions and season. These investigators postulate that vitamin D levels, whether enhanced by diets or sunlight, contribute to the lessening of MS lesion activity. They conclude: "The impressive correlation also supports the need for proper clinical trials to test whether vitamin D nutrition can reduce formation of CNS lesions and slow the progression of MS.''

CONTRAINDICATIONS, PRECAUTIONS, ADVERSE REACTIONS.

CONTRAINDICATIONS

Vitamin D is contraindicated in those with hypercalcemia and in those with evidence of vitamin D toxicity. Vitamin D is contraindicated in those with hypersensitivity to any component of a vitamin D-containing product.

PRECAUTIONS

Pregnant women and nursing mothers should avoid vitamin D supplemental intakes greater than U.S. RDA amounts of the vitamin unless higher amounts are prescribed by their physicians. The U.S. RDA for vitamin D is 400 IU or 10 micrograms daily.

Pharmaceutical use of vitamin D must only be undertaken under medical supervision.

Supplemental vitamin D should be used cautiously in those on digoxin or any cardiac glycoside. Hypercalcemia in those on digoxin may precipitate cardiac arrhythmias. Supplemental doses of vitamin D greater that upper limit intake levels (UL) should only be used if medically prescribed and should be avoided by those on digoxin or other cardiac glycoside. The UL for adults is 2,000 IU or 50 micrograms daily.

Concomitant use of thiazides and pharmacologic doses of vitamin D may cause hypercalcemia in some.

ADVERSE REACTIONS

Dosage of vitamin D up to 60 micrograms (2,400 IU)/day in healthy individuals rarely causes adverse reactions. Chronic dosage of 95 micrograms (3,800 IU)/day or greater in healthy individuals may cause hypercalcemia. Early symptoms of hypercalcemia, include nausea and vomiting, weakness, headache, somnolence, dry mouth, constipation, metallic taste, muscle pain and bone pain. Late symptoms and signs of hypercalcemia, include polyuria, polydipsia, anorexia, weight loss, nocturia, conjunctivitis, pancreatitis, photophobia, rhinorrhea, pruritis, hyperthermia, decreased libido, elevated BUN, albuminuria, hypercholesterolemia, elevated ALT (SGPT) and AST (SGOT), ectopic calcification, nephrocalcinosis, hypertension and cardiac arrhythmias.

INTERACTIONS

DRUGS

Cholestyramine: Concomitant intake of cholestyramine and vitamin D may reduce the absorption of vitamin D.

Colestipol: Concomitant intake of colestipol and vitamin D may reduce the absorption of vitamin D.

Ketoconazole: Ketoconazole may inhibit the biosynthesis and catabolism of 1, 25-dihydroxyvitamin D. Reductions in serum 1, 25-dihydroxyvitamin D concentrations have been observed following the administration of 300 to 1,200 milligrams daily of ketoconazole to healthy men for seven days.

Mineral Oil: Concomitant use of mineral oil and vitamin D may reduce the absorption of vitamin D.

Orlistat: Orlistat may decrease the absorption of vitamin D.

Phenobarbital and Phenytoin: Phenobarbital and phenytoin may reduce plasma levels of 25-hydroxyvitamin D by inhibiting vitamin D 25-hydrolyase activity in the liver.

NUTRITIONAL SUPPLEMENTS

Calcium: Concomitant intake of calcium and vitamin D may be more effective than no therapy or calcium alone in corticosteroid-induced osteoporosis.

FOODS

Olestra: The fat substitute olestra inhibits the absorption of vitamin D as well as the other fat-soluble vitamins A, E and K. Vitamins A, D, E (alpha-tocopherol) and K are added to olestra to compensate for this. Olestra contains 12 IU (0.3 micrograms) of vitamin D per gram.

OVERDOSAGE

Hypercalcemia can result either from excess intakes of prescribed forms of vitamin D or from consumption of high amounts of vitamin D_2 or vitamin D_3. The hypercalcemia associated with hypervitaminosis D may cause multiple debilitating effects. Anorexia, nausea and vomiting have been observed in hypercalcemic individuals treated with 1,250 to 5,000 micrograms (50,000 to 200,000 IU)/day of vitamin D. Hypercalcemia can result in a loss of the urinary concentrating mechanism of the kidney tubule, resulting in polyuria and polydipsia. The prolonged ingestion of excessive amounts of vitamin D and the accompanying hypercalcemia can result in metastatic calcification of soft tissues, including the kidney, blood vessels, heart and lungs. Typically, chronic ingestion of 50,000 to 100,000 IU/day of vitamin D is required to produce hypercalcemia. Since vitamin D stores in fat may be substantial, vitamin D intoxication may persist for weeks after vitamin D ingestion is terminated. The elimination half-life of vitamin D is about 20 to 29 days.

DOSAGE AND ADMINISTRATION

Supplemental vitamin D is available as vitamin D_2 (ergocalciferol) or vitamin D_3 (cholecalciferol). Usually, vitamin D is present in a multi-vitamin, multi-mineral preparation. Typical dosage is 200 to 400 IU (5 to 10 micrograms) daily. Pre- and postnatal multi-vitamin, multi-mineral supplements typically deliver a dose of 400 IU daily.

Pharmaceutical preparations containing 50,000 IU (1,250 micrograms) of vitamin D_2 are used in the treatment of vitamin D deficiency in the elderly and in those with malabsorption syndromes, nephrotic syndrome and hepatic failure. Dosage used is 50,000 IU once weekly for eight weeks. This must be done under medical supervision.

The Food and Nutrition Board of the Institute of Medicine of the U.S. National Academy of Sciences has recommended the following adequate intakes (AI) for vitamin D (the biological activity of one microgram of vitamin D_2 or vitamin D_3 is 40 IU [international units]):

Infants	(AI)
0 through 12 months	5.0 micrograms (200 IU)/day

Children	
1 through 8 years	5.0 micrograms (200 IU)/day

Boys	
9 through 18 years	5.0 micrograms (200 IU)/day

Girls	
9 through 18	5.0 micrograms (200 IU)/day

Men	
19 through 50 years	5.0 micrograms (200 IU)/day
51 through 70 years	10.0 micrograms (400 IU)/day
Greater than 70 years	15.0 micrograms (600 IU)/day

Women	
19 through 50 years	5.0 micrograms (200 IU)/day
51 through 70 years	10.0 micrograms (400 IU)/day
Greater than 70 years	15.0 micrograms (600 IU)/day

Pregnancy	
14 through 50 years	5.0 micrograms (200 IU)/day

Lactation	
14 through 50 years	5.0 micrograms (200 IU)/day

The LOAEL (lowest-observed-adverse-effect level) for vitamin D is set at 95 micrograms (3,800 IU)/day. The adverse effect referenced is hypercalcemia which is defined as a serum calcium level above 2.75 mmoles per liter or 11 milligrams per deciliter. The NOAEL (no observed-adverse-effect level) for vitamin D is set at 60 micrograms (2,400 IU)/day.

The Food and Nutrition Board of the Institute of Medicine has recommended the following tolerable upper limit intake levels (UL) for vitamin D:

Infants	(UL)
0 through 12 months	25 micrograms (1,000 IU)/day

Children	
1 through 18 years	50 micrograms (2,000 IU)/day

Adults	
Greater than 18 years	50 micrograms (2,000 IU)/day

Pregnancy	
14 through 50 years	50 micrograms (2,000 IU)/day

Lactation	
14 through 50 years	50 micrograms (2,000 IU)/day

The U.S. RDA for vitamin D is 400 IU. This is the value used on nutritional supplement and food labels.

HOW SUPPLIED

Capsules — 400 IU, 1000 IU

Tablets — 400 IU

LITERATURE

Amin S, La Valley MP, Simms RW, Felson DT. The role of vitamin D in corticosteroid-induced osteoporosis. A meta-analytic approach. *Arthritis Rheum.* 1999; 42:1740-1751.

Ashcroft DM, Po ALW, Williams HC, Griffiths CEM. Systemic review of comparative efficacy and tolerability of calcipotriol in treating chronic plaque psoriasis. *Br Med J.* 2000; 320:963-967.

Barger-Lux MJ, Heaney RP, Dowell S, et al. Vitamin D and its major metabolites: serum levels after graded oral dosing in healthy men. *Osteoporosis Int.* 1998; 8:222-230.

Basha B, Rao DS, Han Z-H, Parfitt AM. Osteomalacia due to vitamin D depletion: a neglected consequence of intestinal malabsorption. *Am J Med.* 2000; 108:296-300.

Bishop N. Rickets today—children still need milk and sunshine (editorial). *N Engl J Med.* 1999; 341:602-603.

Blutt SE, Weigel NL. Vitamin D and prostate cancer. *Proc Soc Exp Biol Med.* 1999; 221:89-98.

Chapuy MC, Arlot ME, Duboeuf F, et al. Vitamin D_3 and calcium to prevent hip fractures. *N Engl J Med.* 1992; 327:1637-1642.

De Luca HF, Zierold C. Mechanisms and functions of vitamin D. *Nutr Rev.* 1998; 56:S4-S10.

Dietary Reference Intakes for Calcium, Phosphorus, Magnesium, Vitamin D, and Fluoride. Washington, DC: National Academy Press; 1997.

Embry AF, Snowden LR, Vieth R. Vitamin D and seasonal fluctuations of gadolinium-enhancing magnetic resonance imaging lesions in multiple sclerosis. *Ann Neurol.* 2000; 48:271-272.

Fraser DR. Vitamin D. *Lancet.* 1995; 345:104-107.

Fleet JC. Vitamin D receptors: not just in the nucleus anymore (review). *Nutr Rev.* 1999; 57:60-62.

Fujita T. Vitamin D in the treatment of osteoporosis. *Proc Soc Exp Biol Med.* 1992; 199:394-399.

Glorieux FH, Feldman D, eds. *Vitamin D.* San Diego, CA: Academic Press; 1997.

Gloth FM III, Gundberg CM, Hollis BW, et al. Vitamin D deficiency in homebound elderly persons. *JAMA*. 1995; 274:1683-1686.

Holick MF. Vitamin D In: Shils ME, Olson JA, Shike M, Ross AC, eds. *Modern Nutrition in Health and Disease*. 9th ed Baltimore, MD: Williams and Wilkins; 1999:329-345.

Kato S. The function of vitamin D receptor in vitamin D action. *J Biochem*. 2000; 127:717-722.

Kensler TW, Dolan PM, Grange SJ, et al. Conceptually new deltanoids (vitamin D analogues) inhibit multistage skin tumorigenesis. *Carcinogenesis*. 2000; 21:1341-1345.

Kreiter SR, Schwartz RP, Kirkman HN Jr., et al. Nutritional rickets in African American breast-fed infants. *J Pediatr*. 2000; 137:153-157.

Lal H, Pandey R, Aggarwal SK. Vitamin D: non-skeletal actions and effects on growth. *Nutr Res*. 1999; 19:1683-1718.

Landsdowne ATG, Provost SC. Vitamin D3 enhances mood in healthy subjects during winter. *Psychopharmacol*. 1998; 135:319-323.

Lane NE, Gore L, Cummings SR, et al. Serum vitamin D levels and incident changes of radiographic osteoarthritis. *Arthritis Rheum*. 1999; 42:854-860.

LeBoff MS, Kohlmeier L, Hurwitz S, et al. Occult vitamin D deficiency in postmenopausal US women with acute hip fracture. *JAMA*. 1999; 281:1505-1511.

Lips P, Graafmans WC, Ooms ME, et al. Vitamin D supplementation and fracture incidence in elderly persons. A randomized, placebo-controlled clinical trial. *Ann Intern Med*. 1996; 124:400-406.

Lowe KE, Norman AW. Vitamin D and psoriasis. *Nutr Rev* 1992; 50:138-142.

Malloy PJ, Feldman D. Vitamin D resistance. *Am J Med*. 1999; 106:355-370.

Malloy PJ, Pike JW, Feldman D. The vitamin D receptor and the syndrome of hereditary 1, 25-dihydroxyvitamin D-resistant rickets. *Endocrine Reviews*. 1999; 20:156-188.

Manolagas SC, Provvedini DM, Tsoukas CD. Interactions of 1, 25-dihydroxyvitamin D3 and the immune system. *Mol. Cell Endocrinol*. 1985; 43:113-122.

Mantell DJ, Owens PE, Bundred NJ, et al. 1alpha, 25-Dihydroxyvitamin D3 inhibits angiogenesis in vitro and in vivo. *Circ Res*. 2000; 87:214-220.

McAlindon TE, Felson DT, Zhang Y, et al. Relation of dietary intake and serum levels of vitamin D to progression of osteoarthritis of the knee among participants in the Framingham study. *Ann Int Med*. 1996; 125:353-359.

Mukhopadhyay S, Singh M, Chatterjee M. Vitamin D3 as a modulator of cellular antioxidant defense in murine lymphoma. *Nutr Res*. 2000; 20:91-102.

O'Brien KO. Combined calcium and vitamin D supplementation reduces bone loss and fracture incidence in older men and women. *Nutr Rev*. 1998; 56(5 Pt 1):148-150.

Prabhala A, Garg R, Dandona P. Severe myopathy associated with vitamin D deficiency in Western New York. *Arch Intern Med*. 2000; 160:1199-1203.

Sardar S, Chakraborty A, Chatterjee M. Comparative effectiveness of vitamin D3 and dietary vitamin E on peroxidation of lipids and enzymes of the hepatic antioxidant system in Sprague-Dawley rats. *Int J Vitam Nutr Res*. 1996; 66:39-45.

Sato Y, Asoh T, Oizumi K. High prevalence of vitamin D deficiency and reduced bone mass in elderly women with Alzheimer's disease. *Bone*. 1998; 23:555-557.

Tsoukas CD, Watry D, Escobar SS, et al. Inhibition of interleukin-1 production by 1, 25-dihydroxyvitamin D3. *J Clin Endocrinol Metabolism*. 1989; 69:127-133.

Vieth R. Vitamin D supplementation, 25-dihydroxyvitamin D concentrations and safety. *Am J Clin Nutr*. 1999; 69:842-856.

Wilkinson RJ, Llewelyn M, Toossi Z, et al. Influence of vitamin D deficiency and vitamin D receptor polymorphisms on tuberculosis among Gujarati Asians in west London: a case-control study. *Lancet*. 2000; 355:618-621.

Vitamin E

TRADE NAMES

Alph-E (The Key Company), Vitamin E-d-Alpha (Mason Vitamins), Vitamin E-dl Alpha (Health Products Corp., Mason Vitamins), E Mixed (Rexall Consumer), Vitamin E Dry (Swanson Health Products), Total E (Westlake Labs), Vitamin E MTC (National Vitamin), Nutr-E-Sol (Advanced Nutritional), Aquasol E (Astra Zeneca), Aquavit-E (Cypress Pharmaceutical), Liquid E (Freeda Vitamins), E-Pherol (Vitaline Corp.), Dry E (Nature's Life).

DESCRIPTION

Vitamin E is the collective term for a family of chemical substances that are structurally and, in some cases, biologically related to the best known member of this family, alpha-tocopherol. Vitamin E is a fat-soluble vitamin and an essential nutrient for humans. However, in contrast with the other vitamins present in human nutrition, its exact biochemical role remains unknown.

Vitamin E does not appear to play roles in reproduction and lactation in humans as it does in such animals as rats, and overt deficiency states of this vitamin are rare. Deficiency states of vitamin E, however, do exist in humans, and suboptimal nutriture of the vitamin may increase the risk of certain degenerative disorders, such as coronary heart disease, Alzheimer's disease and cancer.

Vitamin E deficiency occurs as a result of rare genetic abnormalities affecting the alpha-tocopherol transfer protein (alpha-TTP), as a result of various malabsorption syndromes and as a result of protein-energy malnutrition. Alpha-TTP is a protein found in the liver, heart, cerebellum and retina. Alpha-TTP selectively recognizes alpha-tocopherol and is believed to mediate the secretion of alpha-tocopherol taken up by the liver cells into the circulation. It may also function in delivering alpha-tocopherol to the cerebellum and retina.

Genetic defects in alpha-TTP are associated with a characteristic syndrome, ataxia with vitamin E deficiency or AVED, previously called familial isolated vitamin E (FIVE) deficiency. AVED patients suffer from neurologic symptoms that are characterized by progressive peripheral neuropathy.

Vitamin E deficiency can also be caused by genetic defects in lipoprotein synthesis. Lipoproteins containing apolipoprotein (apo-B) are necessary for absorption and transport of vitamin E. Those with homozygous hypobetalipoproteinemia have a defect in the apo-B gene and those with abetalipoproteinemia have genetic defects in the microsomal triglyceride-transfer protein. Homozygous hypobetalipoproteinemics and abetalipoproteinemics become vitamin E-deficient and develop the progressive peripheral neuropathy characteristic of vitamin E deficiency.

Fat malabsorption syndromes can result in vitamin E deficiency. Since vitamin E requires biliary and pancreatic secretions, as well as an intact and healthy intestine for its absorption, a wide range of hepatobiliary, pancreatic and intestinal disorders can lead to deficiency of the vitamin. These disorders include cholestatic hepatobiliary disease in children, cystic fibrosis, primary biliary cirrhosis, chronic pancreatitis, short bowel syndromes, Crohn's disease, celiac disease, mesenteric vascular thrombosis, blind loop syndrome, intestinal pseudo-obstruction, intestinal lymphangiectasia, Whipple's syndrome and sclerodermal bowel disease. In adults with these disorders, the development of the neurological symptoms of vitamin E deficiency takes many years. In children, the deficiency symptoms of vitamin E deficiency can be reversed by supplementation with vitamin E but only if it is provided before irreversible neurological injury occurs.

The primary syndrome of vitamin E deficiency, whether genetic or secondary to fat malabsorption syndromes or protein-calorie malnutrition, is peripheral neuropathy. This neuropathy is characterized by the degeneration of the large-caliber axons in the sensory neurons. The cardinal neuropathological changes consist of marked dying back-type degeneration of the posterior columns of the spinal cord. In addition, spinocerebellar ataxia, skeletal myopathy and pigmented retinopathy have been observed in vitamin E deficiency in humans. Vitamin E-deficiency anemia may also occur in premature infants as a result of peroxidation damage to red blood-cell membranes.

The vitamin E family of molecules can be divided into two groups, the tocopherols and the tocotrienols. Vitamin E occurs naturally in eight different forms: four tocopherols, alpha-, beta-, gamma- and delta-tocopherol and four tocotrienols, alpha- beta gamma- and delta-tocotrienol. All of these forms consist of a substituted hydroxylated ring system (the chromanol ring or head group) with a long phytyl side chain or tail. The phytyl tail is bonded to the chromanol ring at the 2 position of the ring. It is the hydroxyl group of the chromanol ring that confers antioxidant activity to vitamin E.

Tocopherols differ from tocotrienols in that tocopherols have three chiral centers, (at positions 2, 4' and 8') while the tocotrienols have only one chiral center (at position 2) and three double bonds in the tail. That is, tocotrienols possess polyunsaturated phytyl side chains. The chiral center of the tocotrienols is located at the point where the phytyl side chain bonds to the chromanol ring (the 2 position of the ring).

The various natural tocopherols and tocotrienols are characterized by the number of methyl groups and the pattern of methylation in the chromanol ring. Alpha-tocopherol and tocotrienol have three methyl groups, beta- and gamma-tocopherol and tocotrienol have two methyl groups and delta-tocopherol and tocotrienol have one methyl group.

Of the eight naturally occurring forms of vitamin E, it appears that only alpha-tocopherol is maintained in human plasma. This is most likely due to the fact that alpha-tocopherol transfer protein (alpha-TTP) selectively recognizes alpha-tocopherol and is believed to mediate the secretion of alpha-tocopherol taken up by the liver cells into the circulation. This does not rule out possible important roles for the other natural forms of vitamin E. It does, however, indicate that alpha-tocopherol is probably the most important member of the vitamin E family in human physiology.

Alpha-tocopherol is commonly known as d-alpha-tocopherol. Chemically, this implies that alpha-tocopherol has only one chiral center. In fact, alpha-tocopherol has three chiral centers. Its correct name is RRR-alpha-tocopherol or 2, 5, 7, 8-tetramethyl-2R- (4'R, 8'R, 12' trimethyltridecyl)-6-chromanol. Since alpha-tocopherol has 3 chiral centers, it can have 2^3 or eight stereoisomeric forms. d-alpha-tocopherol is represented by the following chemical structure:

d-Alpha-Tocopherol

Synthetic vitamin E, which is produced by coupling trimethylhydroquinone with racemic isophytol, does contain all eight stereoisomers of alpha-tocopherol in equal amounts Synthetic alpha-tocopherol is commonly known as dl-alpha-tocopherol. This would be correct if alpha-tocopherol had only one chiral center, but since it has three, this nomenclature is incorrect. Synthetic alpha-tocopherol is correctly called *all racemic*-or *all rac*-alpha-tocopherol. It is also known as 2, 5, 7, 8-tetramethyl —2RS-(4⁹RS, 8⁹RS, 12⁹ trimethyltridecyl)-6-chromanol. *All rac*-alpha-tocopherol consists of four 2R-stereoisomers: RRR-alpha-tocopherol, RSR-alpha-tocopherol, RRS-alpha-tocopherol and RSS-alpha-tocopherol and four 2S-stereoisomers: SRR-alpha-tocopherol, SSR-alpha-tocopherol, SRS-alpha-tocopherol and SSS-alpha-tocopherol. 2R and 2S refer to the configuration of the phytyl tail at the point it meets the chromanol ring or the 2 position of the ring.

The only forms of alpha-tocopherol that are maintained in human plasma are the 2R-stereoisomers. The 2S-stereoisomers of alpha-tocopherol are not maintained in human plasma or tissue. Therefore, the only forms of alpha-tocopherol maintained in human plasma are the natural RRR-alpha-tocopherol and the four 2R synthetic stereoisomers.

Vitamin E is found in plants, animals and in some green, brown and blue/green algae. The richest sources of the vitamin are found in unrefined edible vegetable oil, including wheat germ, safflower, sunflower, cottonseed, canola and olive oils. In these oils, approximately 50% of the tocopherol content is in the form of alpha-tocopherol. Soybean and corn oils contain about ten times as much gamma-tocopherol as they do alpha-tocopherol. Palm, ricebran and coconut oils are rich sources of tocotrienols. Alpha-tocopherol is the major form of vitamin E in animal products and is found mainly in the fatty portion of the meat. Other foods containing vitamin E include unrefined cereal grains, fruits, nuts and vegetables.

Most of the marketed supplemental RRR-alpha-tocopherol (d-alpha-tocopherol) is derived from unrefined soy oil. Since soy oil contains mainly gamma-tocopherol, a synthetic process is necessary to convert the gamma-tocopherol to the alpha-tocopherol. Therefore, alpha-tocopherol derived from soy oil is a semi-synthetic product for which reason it is called natural-source alpha-tocopherol, rather than natural alpha-tocopherol.

D-ALPHA-TOCOPHERYL ACETATE

d-Alpha-tocopheryl acetate is the acetate ester of natural-source d-alpha-tocopherol. Its molecular weight is 472.75 daltons. It is obtained by the vacuum steam distillation and acetylation of edible vegetable oil products. It is found in nutritional supplement products either as a light brownish yellow, nearly odorless, clear viscous oil or as a water-dispersible solid substance with a melting point of 25° centigrade. The water-dispersible solid form of d-alpha-tocopheryl acetate is about 96 to 100% d-alpha-tocopheryl acetate, while the typical oil supplement is comprised of about 40-50% d-alpha-tocopheryl acetate.

d-Alpha-tocopheryl acetate is also known as RRR-alpha-tocopheryl acetate and 2R, 4', 8'R-d-alpha-tocopheryl acetate.

d-Alpha-tocopheryl acetate, in addition to being available as a nutritional supplement, is used in topical skin care products. It appears that it can diffuse into skin cells where it is converted to d-alpha-tocopherol. The acetate itself does not have antioxidant activity. d-alpha-tocopherol may protect skin against ultraviolet damage and is also a skin moisturizer. Some are hypersensitive to topical d-alpha-tocopherol and may develop dermatitis from its use.

DL-ALPHA-TOCOPHERYL ACETATE

dl-alpha-tocopheryl acetate is an all-synthetic form of alpha-tocopherol. It is produced by coupling racemic isophytol with trimethylhydroquinone to form dl-tocopherol. This product is then acetylated to produce dl-alpha-tocopheryl acetate. Since alpha-tocopherol has three chiral centers, eight stereoisomers are formed in the coupling reaction in equal amounts, four 2R-stereoisomers and four 2S-stereoisomers. 2R and 2S refer to the configuration of the phytyl tail at the point it bonds to the chromanol ring, the 2 position of the ring. The four 2R-stereoisomers are RRR-alpha tocopherol, RRS-alpha-tocopherol, RSS-alpha-tocopherol and RSR-alpha tocopherol. The four 2S-stereoisomers are SRR-alpha-tocopherol, SSR-alpha-tocopherol, SRS-alpha-tocopherol and SSS-alpha-tocopherol.

The 2R-stereoisomers are the only forms of alpha-tocopherol that are maintained in human plasma and tissue. The activity of natural or natural-source alpha-tocopherol (RRR alpha-tocopherol), on an equal weight basis, is at least twice as high as synthetic alpha-tocopherol. This is mainly because half of the stereoisomers of synthetic alpha-tocopherol are not maintained in human plasma and are, therefore, not bioavailable.

Although synthetic alpha-tocopheryl acetate is commonly referred to as dl-alpha-tocopheryl acetate, this is not chemically correct. Chemically correct names are *all-racemic-* or *all-rac*-alpha-tocopheryl acetate and 2, 5, 7, 8-tetramethyl-2RS-(4'RS, 8'RS, 12' trimethyldecyl)- 6-chromanol hydrogen acetate.

D-ALPHA-TOCOPHEROL SUCCINATE

d-Alpha-tocopherol succinate is the succinate ester of natural-source d-alpha-tocopherol. It is a white to off-white crystalline powder with a molecular weight of 530.79 daltons. d-Alpha-tocopherol succinate is obtained by the vacuum steam distillation and succinylation of edible vegetable oil. It is insoluble in water, but is water-dispersible.

d-Alpha-tocopheryl succinate is also known as RRR-alpha-tocopheryl succinate and 2R, 4', 8'R-alpha-tocopheryl succinate. It is sometimes called ''dry'' vitamin E, referring to its solid nature.

Some cell culture studies show that d-alpha-tocopheryl succinate can enter into cells as the intact ester and is then hydrolyzed intracellularly to d-alpha-tocopherol. Most ingested d-alpha-tocopheryl succinate is hydrolyzed to d-alpha-tocopherol prior to absorption from the lumen of the small intestine into enterocytes. A small percentage of ingested d-alpha-tocopheryl succinate may enter enterocytes as the ester and is subsequently hydrolyzed to d-alpha-tocopherol within the enterocytes. d-Alpha-tocopheryl succinate itself has no antioxidant activity.

DL-ALPHA-TOCOPHERYL SUCCINATE

dl-Alpha-tocopheryl succinate is an all-synthetic form of alpha-tocopherol. It is produced by coupling racemic isophytol with trimethylhydroquinone to form dl-tocopherol. The dl-tocopherol product is then succinylated to dl-alpha-tocopheryl succinate. Since alpha-tocopherol has three chiral centers, eight stereoisomers are formed in the coupling reaction in equal amounts, four 2R-stereoisomers and four 2S-stereoisomers. 2R and 2S refer to the configuration of the phytyl tail at the point it bonds to the chromanol ring, the 2 position of the ring. The four 2R- stereoisomers are RRR-alpha-tocopherol, RRS-alpha-tocopherol, RSS-alpha-tocopherol and RSR-alpha-tocopherol. The four 2S-stereoisomers: SRR-alpha-tocopherol, SSR-alpha-tocopherol, SRS-alpha-tocopherol and SSS-alpha-tocopherol.

The 2R-stereoisomers are the only forms of alpha-tocopherol that are maintained in human plasma and tissue. The activity of natural or natural-source alpha-tocopherol (RRR-alpha-tocopherol), on an equal weight basis, is at least twice as high as synthetic alpha-tocopherol. This is due to the fact that 50% of the stereoisomers of synthetic alpha-tocopherol are not maintained in human plasma.

Although synthetic alpha-tocopheryl succinate is commonly referred to as dl-alpha-tocopheryl succinate, this is not chemically correct. Chemically correct names for this substance are *all-racemic-* or *all-rac*-alpha-tocopheryl succinate and 2, 5, 7, 8-tetramethyl-2RS- (4' RS, 8'RS, 12'trimethyldecyl)-6-chromanol hydrogen succinate.

MIXED TOCOPHEROLS

Mixed tocopherols consist of mixtures of the natural tocopherol homologues: d-alpha-tocopherol, d-beta-tocopherol, d-gamma-tocopherol and d-delta-tocopherol. These tocopherols are present in their unesterified forms. Mixed tocopherols are obtained by the vacuum steam distillation of edible vegetable oil products.

There are two types of mixed tocopherol products available for nutritional supplementation: high-alpha-mixed-tocopherols and low-alpha-mixed-tocopherols. High-alpha-mixed-tocopherols contain mainly d-alpha-tocopherol with much smaller amounts of beta-, gamma- and delta-tocopherol. Low-alpha-mixed-tocopherols typically contain gamma-tocopherol as the major tocopherol homologue. High-alpha-mixed-tocopherols are labeled to indicate the milligrams of d-alpha-tocopherol present, as well as the milligrams of total tocopherols present. Low-alpha-mixed-tocopherols are usually labeled to indicate the total amount of tocopherols and sometimes tocotrienols-present, as well as the amounts of gamma-, beta- and delta-tocopherols. Mixed tocopherols occur as brownish-red to red, clear viscous oils.

ACTIONS AND PHARMACOLOGY

ACTIONS

Vitamin E has antioxidant activity. It may also have anti-atherogenic, antithrombotic, anticoagulant, neuroprotective, antiproliferative, immunomodulatory, cell membrane-stabilizing and antiviral actions.

MECHANISM OF ACTION

All forms of vitamin E possess antioxidant activity. However, the only forms maintained in human plasma and tissue are the 2R-alpha forms, including the natural RRR-alpha-tocopherol, commonly known as d-alpha-tocopherol. Vitamin E is the principal antioxidant of the lipid domains of the body, such as cellular membranes. It is a chain-breaking antioxidant that prevents the propagation of free radical activities. It is a peroxyl radical scavenger and especially protects the polyunsaturated fatty acids (PUFAs) within membrane phospholipids and in plasma lipoproteins (LDL) against oxidation. The hydroxyl group of the chromanol ring reacts with an organic peroxyl radical to form the corresponding organic hydroperoxide and the tocopheroxyl radical. The tocopheroxyl radical is the pro-oxidant form of vitamin E and is thought to be regenerated to the antioxidant form by a network of other antioxidants, including vitamin C and glutathione.

The relative antioxidant activity of the tocopherols with regard to peroxyl radical scavenging is alpha > beta > gamma > delta. The order is similar among the tocotrienols. Interestingly, this order also parallels the relative order of their biological activities as determined by the classical rat fetal gestation-resorption assay.

This is the case, though, only for the natural tocopherols. All eight stereoisomers of the synthetic *all rac*-alpha-tocopherol, commonly known as dl-alpha-tocopherol, have equivalent peroxyl radical scavenging activity but different activities in the rat fetal resorption assay. And, alpha-tocotrienol has about one-third the activity of alpha-tocopherol in this assay but is a better peroxyl radical scavenger than alpha-tocopherol.

It can be concluded that antioxidant activity of vitamin E is not sufficient to explain the vitamin's biological activity. Recently, it has been demonstrated that vitamin E has activity against reactive nitrogen species (peroxyl radicals are reactive oxygen species). In this regard, gamma-tocopherol inhibits peroxynitrite-induced lipid peroxidation more effectively than alpha-tocopherol (see Gamma-Tocopherol).

Several mechanisms have been proposed to account for vitamin E's possible anti-atherogenic activity. Oxidation of LDL is believed to be a key early step in atherogenesis. It is thought that oxidation of LDL triggers a number of events which lead to the formation of atherosclerotic plaque. These events include uptake of oxidized (ox) LDL by monocytes leading to foam cell formation, promotion of apoptosis by oxLDL, induction of endothelial-cell damage and stimulation of cytokine and growth factor release from cells in the artery wall. LDL contains alpha-tocopherol and smaller amounts of gamma-tocopherol. Alpha-tocopherol inhibits the oxidation of LDL and the accumulation of oxLDL in the arterial wall. It, as well as gamma-tocopherol, also appears to reduce oxLDL-induced apoptosis in human endothelial cells.

A non-antioxidative mechanism of vitamin E is its inhibition of protein kinase C (PKC) activity. PKC is involved in smooth muscle cell proliferation, and, consequently, inhibition of PKC results in inhibition of smooth muscle cell proliferation. Smooth muscle cell proliferation is involved in atherogenesis. PKC inhibition by alpha-tocopherol is, in part, attributable to its attenuating effect on the generation of membrane-derived diacylglycerol, a lipid that facilitates PKC translocation thus increasing its activity. Mitogen-activated protein kinase (MAPK) is also involved in smooth muscle proliferation, and both alpha-tocopherol and gamma-tocopherol inhibit this activity.

Vitamin E enrichment of endothelial cells in culture downregulates the expression of intracellular cell adhesion molecule(ICAM)-1 and vascular cell adhesion molecule(VCAM)-1, both induced by exposure to oxLDL, thereby decreasing the adhesion of blood-cell components to the endothelium. Vitamin E also upregulates the expression of cytosolic phospholipase A_2 and cyclooxygenase (COX)-1. The enhanced expression of these two rate-limiting enzymes in the arachidonic acid cascade appears to explain the observation that vitamin E, in a dose-dependent fashion, enhances the release of prostacyclin, a vasodilating factor and inhibitor of platelet aggregation in humans.

Vitamin E appears to inhibit platelet adhesion, aggregation and platelet release reactions. Enhancing the release of prostacyclin may play a role in these effects. Also, it is known that platelet aggregation is mediated by a common mechanism that involves the binding of fibrinogen to the glycoprotein IIb/IIIa (GPIIb/ IIIa) complex of platelets. GPIIb/IIIa is the major membrane receptor protein that is central to the role of the platelet aggregation response. Glycoprotein IIb (GPIIb) is the alpha-subunit of this platelet membrane protein. It has been shown in tissue culture that alpha-tocopherol downregulates, in a dose-dependent manner, GPIIb promoter activity. This could result in reduction of GPIIb protein expression and decreased platelet aggregation.

Vitamin E has also been found in culture to decrease plasma production of thrombin, a protein which binds to platelets and induces aggregation. A metabolite of vitamin E called vitamin E quinone or alpha-tocopheryl quinone (TQ) is a potent anticoagulant. This metabolite inhibits vitamin K-dependent carboxylase, which is a major enzyme in the coagulation cascade.

A number of mechanisms are proposed to account for the possible neuroprotective effects of high doses of vitamin E. Oxidative stress is thought to be a factor in the pathogenesis of many disorders of the nervous system. Since the nervous system is rich in lipids and since vitamin E is the principal lipid antioxidant, the vitamin has become attractive as a possible preventive, as well as therapeutic agent, for nervous system disorders. Also, the primary syndrome of overt deficiency of this vitamin is peripheral neuropathy.

Vitamin E may play a special role in the cerebellum because concentrations of the vitamin are the lowest in this part of the brain, and the vitamin is more quickly depleted in the cerebellum than in other parts of the brain during vitamin E deficiency. Electrophysiologic investigations in vitamin E-deficient humans show signs of a distal ''dying-back'' axonal neuropathy, especially in the posterior columns and the gracile and cuneate nuclei.

Vitamin E may also be involved in signal-transduction. Vitamin E may play a number of roles associated with neuronal cell membranes and other lipids in the nervous system. However, a specific and unique mechanism of action of the vitamin in the nervous system has not been elucidated.

Several animal and human studies have shown that vitamin E can improve the immune response in aged animals and humans. *In vitro*, alpha-tocopherol increases mitogenic response of T lymphocytes from aged mice. The mechanism of this response by vitamin E is not well understood. It has been suggested that vitamin E itself may have mitogenic activity independent of its antioxidant activity. All four homologues of tocopherol, alpha-, beta-, gamma- and delta-tocopherol, were found to enhance both spontaneous and mitogen-stimulated lymphocyte proliferation in mouse splenocytes in culture.

Alpha-tocopherol was reported to have potent activity against human immunodeficiency virus (HIV)-1. Oxidative stress is thought to contribute to HIV-1 pathogenesis, as well as to the pathogenesis of other viral infections. The anti-HIV-1 activity may be due, in part, to alpha-tocopherol's antioxidant activity. Vitamin E also affects membrane integrity and fluidity. HIV-1 is a membraned virus. Altering membrane fluidity of HIV-1 may interfere with its ability to bind to cell-receptor sites, thus decreasing its infectivity. It is unclear, however, how much vitamin E would bind to HIV-1 if administered *in vivo*, since vitamin E can bind to several different sites including alpha-tocopherol transfer protein (alpha-TTP) and LDL.

In conclusion, oxidative stress appears to play a major role in the pathogenesis of many chronic degenerative disorders, and, as the principal lipophilic antioxidant in the body, vitamin E may play a significant role in the prevention, as well as treatment of these disorders. Vitamin E may also have roles independent of its antioxidant action. The action and mechanisms of action of this vitamin are a work in progress.

PHARMACOKINETICS
The precise rate of vitamin E absorption is not known with certainty. The absorption of this vitamin is typically low and variable. The absorption of one form of vitamin E, d-alpha-tocopheryl polyethylene glycol 1000 succinate or vitamin E TPGS, is different (see d-Alpha-Tocopheryl Polyethylene Glycol 1000 Succinate).

Reported rates of absorption of vitamin E following intake with food have varied from as high as 51% to 86% to as low as 21% to 29%. It is likely the higher values are an overestimation and that the lower numbers represent a truer picture. Absorption is significantly lower on an empty stomach and may be somewhat higher with the esterified acetate and succinate delivery forms of vitamin E. However, some studies show that the free and esterified tocopherols have similar absorption efficiency. All forms of vitamin E, including all of the tocopherol and tocotrienol homologues, are absorbed in a similar manner.

Vitamin E is absorbed from the lumen of the small intestine into the enterocytes by passive diffusion. Prior to its absorption, vitamin E is emulsified together with dietary lipids. Bile acids and salts secreted by the liver aid in the emulsification process. Lipolysis and emulsification of the formed lipid droplets lead to the spontaneous formation of mixed micelles. Esterified forms of vitamin E, alpha-tocopheryl acetate and succinate, undergo hydrolysis via esterases secreted by the pancreas. The micelles containing vitamin E are absorbed at the brush border of the intestinal mucosa in the enterocytes. Vitamin E is secreted by the enterocytes into the lymphatics in the form of chylomicrons. The chylomicrons contain the various forms of vitamin E, including alpha-, beta-, gamma-, and delta-tocopherol, alpha-, beta-, gamma- and delta-tocotrienol and, if consumed either in supplement form or in fortified foods, all eight stereoisomers of *all rac*-alpha-tocopherol (dl-alpha-tocopherol).

Chylomicrons undergo metabolism in the circulation via lipoprotein lipase to form chylomicron remnants. During this process, some vitamin E, including all the above-cited forms, is transferred to various tissues, such as adipose tissue, muscle and possibly the brain. Lipoprotein lipase appears to be required for the transfer of vitamin E to these tissues. Chylomicron remnants can transfer tocopherols to high density lipoproteins (HDL), which, in turn, can transfer tocopherols to LDL and very low density lipoproteins (VLDL). Chylomicron remnants can also acquire apolipoprotein E (apoE), which directs them to the liver for metabolism. The remnants are taken up by the liver, which, in turn, secretes vitamin E in VLDLs.

The secretion by the liver of vitamin E in VLDLs is, arguably, the most important singular event in the biochemistry of vitamin E. The only forms of the vitamin secreted by the liver are the natural RRR-alpha-tocopherol and the four 2R forms of synthetic tocopherol. The four 2S synthetic forms of *all rac*-alpha-tocopherol are not secreted by the liver in VLDLs, and only very small amounts of the other tocopherol and tocotrienol homologues are secreted. It is this step that discriminates between all the various forms of vitamin E; the reason for this is that hepatic alpha-tocopheryl transfer protein (alpha-TTP) is selective for the binding of RRR-alpha-tocopherol and the 2R forms of alpha-tocopherol. The secretion of RRR-alpha-tocopherol in VLDLs by the liver is also the mechanism that maintains the plasma concentration of vitamin E. Following secretion of VLDL in the circulation, lipoprotein lipase and triglyceride lipase convert VLDL to LDL. Alpha-tocopherol is transported in the plasma mainly in LDL and also in HDL. Alpha-tocopherol is distributed to the central nervous system (CNS) via LDL. Newly absorbed vitamin E slowly accumulates in the CNS. Sebaceous gland secretion is a major route of vitamin E delivery to the skin.

Alpha-tocopherol can be oxided to the tocopheroxyl radical, which is the pro-oxidant form of this molecule. Reduction back to the antioxidant form is thought to take place with the help of such reducing agents as vitamin C and glutathione. Alpha-tocopherol, vitamin C, glutathione and alpha-lipoic acid are major components of the so-called antioxidant network. Metabolites of alpha-tocopherol include alpha-tocopheryl quinone, alpha-tocopheryl hydroquinone and 2, 5, 7, 8-tetramethyl-2- (2^9-carboxyethyl)-6-hydroxychroman (alpha-CEHC). A gamma-tocopherol metabolite is 2, 7, 8-trimethyl-2- (2^9-carboxyethyl)-6-hydroxychroman (gamma-CEHC).

Fecal excretion is the major route of excretion of oral vitamin E. Fecal excretion of the vitamin includes non-absorbed vitamin E, as well as vitamin E forms not utilized. For example, the forms not secreted by the liver, such as the 2S alpha-tocopherol forms and the beta-, gamma- and delta-tocopherol homologues, are excreted via the biliary route.

Vitamin E metabolites, such as alpha-CEHC and gamma-CEHC, are excreted via the urinary route. About three times as much *all rac*-alpha-tocopherol, compared with RRR-alpha-tocopherol, is excreted as alpha-CEHC. Alpha-CEHC is the major urinary metabolite of alpha-tocopherol.

INDICATIONS AND USAGE

Vitamin E, widely recognized for its antioxidant activities, appears to be protective against cardiovascular disease and some forms of cancer in some individuals. It has demonstrated immune-enhancing effects. It may be of limited benefit in some with asthma and rheumatoid arthritis. It may be effective in protecting against air pollution and some other toxins and may be helpful in some neurological diseases (including Alzheimer's disease) and in some eye disorders (particularly cataracts) and to some individuals with diabetes and premenstrual syndrome. It may also help protect skin from ultraviolet irradiation. Claims that it reverses skin aging, enhances male fertility and exercise performance are poorly supported. There is no credible evidence that it increases sexual prowess. It may help relieve some muscle cramps.

RESEARCH SUMMARY

The results of a very large number of studies, including *in vitro* and animal studies, epidemiological and intervention trials, support a role for vitamin E in the prevention of cardiovascular disease. Recently, however, some large intervention trials have raised some doubts about that role; concurrently, controversy has erupted over the design of these trials. The situation, in some ways, parallels that of the conflicting evidence related to beta-carotene's possible role in preventing lung cancer. (See Beta-Carotene.) Vitamin E has been shown to inhibit the oxidation of LDL-cholesterol in various *in vitro*, animal and human experiments. Other *in vitro*, animal and some human studies demonstrate that

vitamin E also acts on coagulation, platelet aggregation and endothelial relaxation, among other factors, in ways that may reduce cardiovascular risk.

In one study of hyperlipidemic rabbits, supplemental vitamin E significantly reduced oxidation of LDL-cholesterol and surface area of atherosclerotic lesions. In male monkeys, 108 IUs of vitamin E daily decreased progression (and produced some regression) of atherosclerosis over a three-year study period. Rabbits on high cholesterol diets given supplemental vitamin E or beta-carotene exhibited aortas with normal endothelial function, compared with controls receiving only the high-cholesterol diet. A number of animal studies have consistently shown that supplemental vitamin E can reduce formation of atheromas by 25% to 50%.

In humans supplemented with vitamin E, their LDL-cholesterol was subsequently shown to contain elevated amounts of the vitamin. Concurrently, increased oxidation resistance was measured in these LDL samples.

Many epidemiological studies have associated low-vitamin E status with significantly increased risk of cardiovascular disease. Angina sufferers, in some case-control studies, were found to have lower vitamin E levels than controls. In a much larger case-control study, results were obtained suggesting that higher concentrations of vitamin E in adipose tissue indirectly helped protect against myocardial infarction through vitamin E's favorable effects on beta-carotene.

Among prospective cohort studies examining the possible role of vitamin E in cardiovascular disease, The Nurses' Health Study has yielded some significant findings. In a cohort of 87,000 of these nurses, all free of cardiovascular disease at baseline, there was a 34% reduction in coronary heart disease risk among those women in the highest versus the lowest quintile of vitamin E intake after adjustment for age, smoking and other relevant variables. Dietary intake alone did not show this significant inverse relationship, but total intake (diet plus supplementation) did. The nurses were followed for eight years. In nurses in the highest quintile of vitamin E intake from supplementation extending for at least two years, risk reduction was even greater: 46%. Similar risk reduction was seen in a large cohort of men free of heart disease at baseline (the Health Professionals Follow-Up Study). Almost all of the benefit was restricted to those men who took daily supplements of vitamin E in doses of 100 IUs or greater for at least two years.

Several other smaller cohort studies have similarly reported significant evidence of vitamin E's protective role in cardiovascular disease. High dietary intake alone (without supplementation) has also been associated with significantly reduced risk in some of these studies.

A number of other studies have correlated blood levels of vitamin E with risk of cardiovascular disease. In many, but not all, of these, high levels of the vitamin have correlated with reduced risk. Additionally, there are angiography and ultrasound studies that provide some further evidence that vitamin E helps protect the arteries.

Some small clinical intervention trials have found supplemental vitamin E to be beneficial in some with intermittent claudication and angina. More recently, however, the large Alpha-Tocopherol Beta-Carotene Cancer Prevention (ATBC) study of 29,000 Finnish male smokers failed to find any overall significant cardiovascular benefit from low dose (50 milligrams daily) vitamin E (synthetic). However, a subsequent analysis showed some slight benefit from vitamin E among those smokers who had no history of myocardial infarction. After a median follow-up of 6.1 years, there was an observed 4% reduction in primary major coronary events in this subset. Vitamin E decreased the incidence of fatal coronary heart disease by 8%. These findings were statistically non-significant. There was also a significant increase in fatal hemorrhagic stroke in the vitamin E group, although use of the vitamin was associated with a reduction in ischemic stroke, and, overall, there was no statistically significant difference in stroke between those taking the vitamin and those not taking it.

This study has been criticized for using doses of vitamin E significantly lower than those generally shown to have positive preventive effects. Additionally this study involved subjects who had been smoking, in many cases, for decades and thus, some argued, posed a far greater challenge for antioxidant therapy.

Much was made, by some, of the small but statistically significant increase in hemorrhagic stroke associated with vitamin E supplementation in this study. Others, however, have pointed out that some other long-term studies, using considerably higher doses of vitamin E, found no increased risk. There was a statistically non-significant reduction in risk of ischemic stroke in the vitamin E-supplemented subjects in the Nurses' Health Study. There was also a statistically non-significant reduction in cerebrovascular mortality in the vitamin E-supplemented group in the large interventive Linxian China study. And there was a statistically non-significant reduction in total stroke incidence among those receiving vitamin E in the recently concluded GISSI-Prevenzione trial.

In the Cambridge Heart Antioxidant Study (CHAOS), 2002 subjects with cardiovascular disease confirmed by angiography were given 400-800 IUs of natural source vitamin E daily or placebo. A significant 77% reduction in risk of nonfatal myocardial infarction was reported after 510 days of vitamin E administration. There was, however, no effect on cardiovascular death or total mortality.

There was, in fact, a small statistically non-significant increase in cardiovascular death in the vitamin E group. This was a group with serious cardiovascular disease at baseline, and there were considerably more deaths in the early stages of the study, at a point when vitamin E had been used for a relatively short period of time, than at later stages. Thus, there was little concern that the vitamin itself was contributing to an increase in death. Additionally, a recent further analysis has shown that most of these deaths occurred in subjects who were non-compliant with the vitamin E regimen.

The study's reliability has been questioned by some due to purported design flaws, small size and short duration. Defenders of the study, however, say that its results are all the more dramatic, given that the subjects who benefited were already beset with advanced cardiovascular disease. Moreover, the benefit came in relatively short order. This suggested, they said, that the vitamin might be affecting more than just lipid oxidation in these subjects.

One reviewer, commenting on this possibility, has noted that in subgroup analyses of the Cholesterol Lowering Atherosclerosis Study (CLAS), vitamin E supplementation, in doses greater than 100 IUs daily, was shown to reduce the rate of angiographic progression of mild-to-moderate lesions over a two-year period. On the other hand, some critics of the CHAOS trial said the reported results were improbable in so short a study period, and they concluded that the results occurred by chance alone rather than owing to any real vitamin E effect.

In the Linxian China study, supplemental beta-carotene (15 milligrams daily), synthetic vitamin E (30 IUs daily) and selenium (50 micrograms daily) significantly protected against total mortality and total cancer (which was the primary focus of the study) and non-significantly protected against cerebrovascular disease. The vitamin E dose used in this study was even smaller than that used in the ATBC study. In both cases, synthetic alpha-tocopherol was used.

In the GISSI-Prevenzione trial, 11,324 Italian survivors of myocardial infarction were given 300 milligrams of synthetic vitamin E daily or a mixture of n-3 polyunsaturated fatty acids (PUFA) in a combination of docosahexaenoate (DHA) and eicosapentaenoate (EPA), or both the vitamin E and the n-3 PUFA combination, or neither. The primary end points were nonfatal myocardial infarction, stroke and death. Comparing each treatment against no treatment, the n-3 PUFA combination achieved a statistically significant 15% reduction in primary endpoint risk, while vitamin E achieved a statistically non-significant 11% reduction in the same risks. Vitamin E produced a non-significant reduction in risk of stroke, while the n-3 PUFA combination non-significantly increased risk of stroke.

The GISSI researchers noted that "a possible beneficial effect of vitamin E" was suggested "in the secondary analyses of the individual components of cardiovascular death of the combined endpoints, for which the increasing benefit (from 20% for all cardiovascular deaths to 35% for sudden death) is similar to the picture for n-3 PUFA. The absence of a difference in the rate of non-fatal cardiovascular events between vitamin E and the control group is also similar to the findings related to n-3 PUFA." They added: "The significant decrease of cardiovascular deaths ... cannot be easily dismissed."

The multi-center GISSI study has been criticized by some for not being placebo-controlled and for dispensing with independent monitors at each participating center. One reviewer noted that synthetic vitamin E was used in this study, reducing the potency of the 300 milligram daily doses, he said, to the equivalent of 150 milligrams of natural-source vitamin E. The greater potency of natural-source vitamin E is widely recognized, and some studies have indicated that natural-source alpha-tocopherol is at least twice as bioavailable as synthetic vitamin E.

Some other researchers said the GISSI trial made too little of the reduction in deaths apparently attributable to vitamin E. Two researchers stated that "cardiovascular mortality was significantly reduced by vitamin E in GISSI, and the effect on overall survival showed a very favorable trend." Others argued that a longer follow-up period was needed. The GISSI trial lasted for 3.5 years.

One of the CHAOS researchers commented on the GISSI trial: "Whether patients who have an MI despite a lifetime of Mediterranean diet and are subsequently treated with a statin would be expected to benefit from vitamin E is not clear, especially since many of the complications of MI depend more on the state of the myocardium than of the coronary arteries." Since the Mediterranean diet is generally higher in vitamin E than the English diet consumed in the CHAOS study, this researcher suggested that the English subjects might be more responsive to vitamin E supplementation.

In this same commentary, the CHAOS researcher observed that investigators in that trial have reported that the English patients had a 3.5-fold increased frequency for a polymorphism in the gene for endothelial nitric oxide synthase (eNOS). Vascular endothelial function is reduced in such individuals, and he speculated that vitamin E may thus have worked in these subjects through an avenue other than the inhibition of LDL-cholesterol oxidation. Conceivably this might help explain the more rapid activity of vitamin E seen in the CHAOS study and might explain why some other populations (with possibly lower frequency of the eNOS gene) are less responsive. More research is needed to clarify these issues.

Recently, results of the Heart Outcomes Prevention Evaluation (HOPE) study were released. This study of 2,545 women and 6,996 men 55 years and older with cardiovascular disease or diabetes tested 400 IUs of natural-source vitamin E against placebo (it also tested the angiotension-converting-enzyme inhibitor ramipril against placebo) and found no significant protective effect for vitamin E with respect to either primary or secondary endpoints: myocardial infarction, stroke and death from cardiovascular causes, unstable angina, congestive heart failure, revascularization or amputation, death from any cause, complications of diabetes and cancer. Neither did it find any adverse vitamin E effects. Subjects were supplemented for a mean of 4.5 years.

If there was an inconsistency in this study it was that, in contrast with the previous large intervention trials, it appeared to consistently show virtually no vitamin E activity, positive or negative.

The HOPE researchers hypothesized that this lack of activity could be due, in part, to the moderate duration of the trial, to the characteristics of the population studied and/or to the fact that vitamin E was used by itself without some of the co-factors found in some other studies to potentiate its effects. They noted that some trials in which vitamin E is used with some other antioxidants are now in progress. Clearly, these and other studies may be needed before vitamin E's role in various populations with various forms and stages of cardiovascular disease can be adequately evaluated. Some do not expect antioxidants to have notable effects in established disease and say their real strength is in preventing disease in healthy populations.

Though it has long been assumed that vitamin E's starring role would be in heart disease, it may turn out to have as big a part to play in preventing and treating some cancers. The same study that dealt a blow to claims that beta-carotene supplementation prevents lung cancer raised hopes that vitamin E might effectively help prevent prostate cancer. In the ATBC study of Finnish smokers, low-dose synthetic vitamin E (50 milligrams daily) reduced the incidence of prostate cancer by a significant 32% and prostate cancer deaths by a significant 41%. This unexpected result was sufficiently impressive that the National Cancer Institute is considering a follow-up study.

Reduction in prostate cancer incidence became evident in the ATBC study within two years of beginning supplementation. Some believe there is the suggestion in this and other research that vitamin E blocks the progression of latent prostate cancer, particularly important, if verified, because latent prostate cancer cannot be detected clinically, and many deaths occur because of this. There is often little or no warning of the transition from latent to aggressive disease. A lesser reduction in colon cancer associated with vitamin E supplementation was also seen in this study.

In the Linxian China study, another randomized long-term intervention study, administration of synthetic vitamin E, in combination with selenium and beta-carotene, resulted in a significant reduction in total mortality and total cancer incidence. Only this combination of nutrients, among four regimens tested, was effective with respect to these endpoints. The combination was particularly protective against esophageal and stomach cancers. This was the only regimen tested that included vitamin E. Dosage was low—30 IUs daily.

In a recent further analysis of data from the ATBC study, researchers found that "higher serum alpha-tocopherol status is associated with reduced lung cancer risk; this relationship appears stronger among younger persons and among those with less cumulative smoke exposure. These findings suggest that high levels of alpha-tocopherol, if present during the early critical stages of tumorigenesis, may inhibit lung cancer development." Those in the highest versus the lowest quintile of serum vitamin E concentrations had a 19% reduction in incidence of lung cancer in this study. The researchers further noted that "There was a stronger inverse association among younger men .... And possibly among men receiving supplementation."

Did vitamin E supplementation, then, help protect against lung cancer? The conclusion in the original study report was that it did not. Secondary analyses of the ATBC trial, however, suggested that study subjects who supplemented with vitamin E for the longest periods of time experienced a 10-15% reduction in lung cancer risk in this cohort of smokers. Supplementation was low-dose (50 milligrams daily of synthetic alpha-tocopherol).

In the serum vitamin E analysis, the researchers further concluded that there was "synergism between usual intake and the controlled intervention." Those who had higher pre-trial serum levels of vitamin E did better than those with lower pre-trial serum levels, and still better results were seen in those with higher pre-trial serum levels who also received vitamin E supplements during the trial. Thus there is the suggestion that epidemiology may coincide here with intervention.

The researchers concluded that "while it is tempting, based on the present data, to speculate that the administration of greater quantities of alpha-tocopherol might have produced a substantial reduction in lung cancer incidence in the ATBC study, only future studies, and controlled trials in particular, can shed light on this question."

Numerous epidemiological studies have associated higher vitamin E status with reduced cancer, including lung, colorectal, prostate, colon, stomach, reproductive organs, upper gastrointestinal tract, bladder, breast, cervix, mouth, pharynx and thyroid cancer. Reduced serum vitamin E levels are also associated with a higher incidence of lymphoma and leukemia in some populations. Not all epidemiological studies have shown an inverse relationship between vitamin E status and cancer risk, but the majority have.

Vitamin E has shown significant activity against various cancers *in vitro* and in experimental animal models of carcinogenesis. In a review of animal work, results overall strongly indicated that vitamin E significantly reduced the incidence of a variety of cancers. Vitamin E has shown significant anti-cancer activity in these experiments when used alone and when used in combination with vitamin C and/or selenium, among other antioxidant companions. Mammary tumors have been significantly inhibited in rat experiments using vitamin E and selenium. Chemically induced skin cancers in mice were inhibited with vitamin E and beta-carotene.

In one intervention trial, neither beta-carotene, vitamin C, nor vitamin E reduced the incidence of colorectal adenoma recurrence in subjects who had undergone removal of colorectal adenoma prior to entering this study. Supplementation continued for four years. Critics of the study said far longer supplementation would be required to have any impact on this problem.

Vitamin E (400 IUs twice daily for 24 weeks) achieved clinical improvement (disappearance of at least 50% of lesions) in 20 of 43 patients with oral leukoplakia. In a randomized, double blind, placebo-controlled study, a topical preparation of vitamin E completely resolved the oral lesions of subjects with chemotherapy-induced mucositis.

High plasma vitamin E levels have been associated with greater resistance to infection in some, but not all, epidemiological studies. Some of these have shown a stronger protective effect in the elderly. *In vitro* and animal studies have demonstrated that vitamin E can enhance some immune functions. In animals, there is evidence that supplemental vitamin E increased resistance to a number of pathogens including *Escherichia coli* and *Pneumoccocus pneumonia* type I. Influenza viral lung titers were significantly reduced in elderly mice supplemented with vitamin E, compared with unsupplemented controls who were also infected and who consumed normal amounts of vitamin E in their diets. A number of immunologic studies have tested vitamin E alone and in combination with other nutrients in humans. The number of CD4 and CD8 T cells were high and lymphocyte proliferative response to mitogen was significantly enhanced in elderly subjects given supplemental vitamins A, E and C for four weeks, compared with those given placebo. In some other human studies, supplementation with vitamin E alone or in combination with vitamin C, beta-carotene and some other nutrients has favorably affected T-cell counts, lymphocyte response, levels of interleukin-2 and natural killer cell activity.

One reviewer of the vitamin E literature concluded: "Evidence from animal and human studies indicates that vitamin E plays an important role in the maintenance of the immune system. Even a marginal vitamin E deficiency impairs the immune response, while supplementation with higher than recommended dietary levels of vitamin E enhances humoral and cell-mediated immunity."

In one double-blind, placebo-controlled study, 88 healthy elderly subjects were randomized to receive 60, 200 or 800 milligrams of synthetic vitamin E daily or placebo for 235 days. The objective was to determine the effects, if any, of these varying doses of vitamin E on various measures of cell-mediated immunity. Some older healthy people have been shown to have an impaired ability to produce an effective delayed-type hypersensitivity skin response (DTH), which, in turn, has been associated with greater mortality. Decreased DTH appears to be indicative of diminished capacity to deal with infectitious and neoplastic challenges and prolonged illness.

Subjects receiving 200 milligrams of vitamin E daily in this study had a significant 65% increase in DTH and a six-fold increase in antibody titer to hepatitis B, compared with subjects receiving placebo. Subjects receiving the 200 milligram dose also had significant increases in antibody titer to tetanus vaccine, compared with controls. Supplementation did not affect antibody titer to diphtheria, immunoglobulin levels or levels of T and B cells. Nor was there any observed effect on antibody levels.

The 60 milligram dose did not produce statistically significant results in some of the parameters measured. The 200 milligram dose generally produced better results than the 800 milligram dose. Thus the researchers concluded that there may be a threshold level for vitamin E's observed immunostimulatory effects and that the 200 milligram dose, pending possible different findings in future research, appears to be the optimal dose for healthy elderly individuals seeking to preserve immune function. Very high doses of vitamin E have been associated with adverse effects on immunity in some studies. Subjects given 1,600 milligrams of vitamin E daily for one week, for example, were shown to have diminished polymorphonuclear leukocyte bactericidal activity.

Finally, with respect to immunity, there have been some reports that vitamin E may be helpful in some with HIV-disease. In a study of 311 HIV-infected individuals followed over a period of nine years, those with the highest blood levels of vitamin E were 34% less likely than those with low levels to progress to fully-developed AIDS. The higher vitamin E status was also associated in this study with higher T helper lymphocyte counts.

In another study, there was the suggestion that low vitamin E status might be associated with elevated immunoglobulin E (IgE) levels and consequent increased inflammation in HIV-infected individuals. This inflammation is postulated to increase HIV replication.

And in an animal model of AIDS, vitamin E supplementation reportedly helped restore some T cell functions and reduced production of inflammation-promoting interleukin-6 and tumor necrosis factor.

Results of an additional study showed that vitamin E, in combination with erythropoietin and interleukin-3, increased survival and weight of fetuses in pregnant rats administered AZT. Thus it has been suggested that vitamin E might help protect against some of the toxic effects of AZT and similar drugs. Research continues.

As for autoimmune disorders, here too there is epidemiological evidence linking low vitamin E status with a higher incidence of rheumatoid arthritis. In one small interventive trial, 1,200 IUs of vitamin E daily reportedly reduced pain in rheumatoid arthritis patients but not inflammation, compared with subjects receiving placebo. Other studies have also reported significant pain reduction.

Vitamin E has been used with benefit in some with asthma. Lung function measures were significantly improved in one double-blind, placebo-controlled study of asthmatic volunteers exposed to ozone and sulfur dioxide who received 400 IUs of vitamin E and 500 milligrams of vitamin C daily for five weeks.

Various animal and human experiments have demonstrated that supplemental vitamin E can protect against some of the toxic effects of cigarette smoke and smog. In a recent study of Dutch bicyclists, 100 milligrams of vitamin E and 500 milligrams of vitamin C daily for 15 weeks significantly protected measures of lung function against effects of ozone, compared with controls receiving placebo.

Vitamin E (50 milligrams daily) did not have any effect on the recurrence or incidence of chronic obstructive bronchopulmonary diseases in the ATBC study of Finnish smokers.

Higher dietary intake of vitamin E, however, was associated in this study with lower incidence of chronic bronchitis and dyspnea.

Supplemental vitamin E has shown some positive activity in neurological disorders. In a well-designed double-blind, multicenter, placebo-controlled study, 2,000 IUs of synthetic vitamin E daily, alone or in combination with the drug selegiline (10 milligrams daily), were administered to subjects with moderate Alzheimer's disease over a two-year period. Primary endpoints were death, severe dementia, loss of ability to perform everyday tasks and need of institutionalization. Those receiving vitamin E alone had a 53% reduction in risk of reaching any of these endpoints, while those on selegiline had a 43% reduction in risk, and those taking both vitamin E and selegiline had a 31% reduction. There was an increase of 230 days in the time it took on vitamin E to reach a primary endpoint, compared to those on placebo. There were 341 subjects in this study which warrants follow-up.

Partly because of this study, the American Psychiatric Association updated its treatment guidelines for Alzheimer's disease. Those guidelines include the use of vitamin E in newly diagnosed, mildly impaired and moderately impaired victims of this disease and some other diseases that also cause dementia.

In another trial, selegiline but not vitamin E was shown to significantly delay the need for levodopa in patients with Parkinson's disease (a benefit that was not sustained during follow-up).

Results have been mixed with respect to vitamin E's effects on tardive dyskinesia. In one study, the vitamin significantly out-scored placebo at 400-800 IUs daily. In a more recent randomized, multicenter, placebo-controlled study, vitamin E (1,600 IUs daily) showed no effect in the treatment of tardive dyskinesia over a two-year supplementation period.

In a study of 3,385 elderly men, age 71 to 93 years, use of either vitamin E or vitamin C supplements, ascertained by questionnaire, was significantly associated with better cognitive test performance and protection against vascular dementia.

Pre-treatment and post-treatment with vitamin E enhanced neurologic recovery after experimental spinal cord compression injury in cats. Four weeks post-injury, treated cats recovered 72% of pre-injury function, compared with 20% recovery in untreated controls.

Epidemiological associations have been made between high blood levels of vitamin E and reduced incidence of cataract. In a study of 764 elderly subjects, those taking vitamin E supplements had a 50% reduced risk that their cataracts would progress over a 4-5 year period. Multivitamin use was associated with a 33% reduction in the same risk. Vitamin E supplementation has prevented cataract development and significantly inhibited its progression in several animal models.

Results of a population-based study of 2,584 French subjects recently showed that high plasma vitamin E levels are associated with decreased risk of late age-related macular degeneration (AMD). The risk of late AMD was reduced by 82% in those individuals in the highest vitamin E quintile compared with the lowest quintile. There was also a lesser but still significant reduction in risk of early signs of AMD associated with high vitamin E status. The study adjusted for smoking and factors related to cardiovascular disease including diabetes, all of which are associated with increased AMD risk. No association was found between reduced risk of AMD and plasma retinol, ascorbic acid levels or with red blood cell glutathione values.

The controlled, clinical intervention trial that could demonstrate supplemental vitamin E's possible benefit in the treatment of AMD has yet to be conducted, but, as several researchers have noted, such a study is clearly warranted.

Through its cardiovascular-protective effects, vitamin E is hypothesized by some to be beneficial in some cases of diabetes. Additionally, in animal studies, vitamin E has exerted various effects in the kidneys, eyes and nerves that may be helpful in combating some of the damage of diabetes. Vitamin E did not show any benefit with respect to incidence of complications of diabetes in the HOPE study previously discussed. Some said the follow-up was of insufficient duration to show and any effect.

A recent report indicated serum vitamin E concentrations at baseline, in a case-control study nested within a 21-year follow-up study, were inversely associated with insulin-dependent diabetes mellitus incidence 4-14 years later. Risk was diminished 85% among those with the highest vitamin E status versus those with the lowest. This reduced risk persisted after adjustment for serum cholesterol levels.

Recently, researchers reported that supplemental oral vitamin E normalized retinal hemodynamic abnormalities and improved renal function in type 1 diabetic patients of short disease duration. This was a randomized, double-blind, placebo-controlled crossover trial of eight-months duration. Vitamin E dose was 1,800 IUs daily.

In another recent double-blind, placebo-controlled study 1,600 IUs of vitamin E daily did not improve postulated receptor-specific vascular endothelial dysfunction in subjects with type 2 diabetes mellitus. Vitamin E has, however, been shown to prevent and reverse some of the vascular complications of diabetes in *in vitro*, animal and human studies. Vitamin E has demonstrated an ability to inhibit hyperglycemia-induced activation of protein kinase C (PKC) and to also inhibit diacylglycerol (DAG) levels. Both PKC and DAG have been implicated in diabetic complications, and inhibition of PKC has reversed some of the vascular dysfunctions in retina, kidney and cardiovascular systems caused by hyperglycemia or diabetes.

Preliminary research has indicated that supplemental vitamin E might be helpful in some with premenstrual syndrome (PMS). In a double-blind, placebo-controlled trial, vitamin E (in doses of 150, 300 or 600 IUs daily administered for two months) significantly outperformed placebo. It reportedly significantly improved three of four classes of PMS symptoms. A subsequent double-blind, placebo-controlled study found significant improvement in some affective and physical symptoms of PMS in subjects treated with 400 IUs of vitamin E daily for three menstrual cycles. The same research group conducted both of these studies in the 1980s. They need follow-up.

There is evidence from *in vitro* and animal studies that both oral and topically applied vitamin E can help protect against UV light-induced skin changes and protect against skin cancer. In animals and humans, studies have shown that UV irradiation diminishes both skin and plasma levels of various nutrients, including vitamin E.

In one experiment, the UVB irradiation that is considered to be the most carcinogenic suppressed immune functions in the skin of mice. This suppression was blocked with vitamin E. *In vitro*, vitamin E has also blocked some of the immune-suppressing effects UVA radiation has on human cells. Topically applied vitamin E prevented UVB-induced skin tumors in an animal model.

Some studies in humans have demonstrated that topical vitamin E can protect skin against photo-damage and subsequent wrinkling. In one placebo-controlled study, topically applied vitamin E, more than placebo, reportedly reduced eyelid wrinkling over a four-week period. And, in another human study, a patented cream containing, among other things, vitamin E and C, reportedly produced significant improvement in wrinkling. An oral preparation of vitamin E and C had no effect. Placebos were used. Treatment continued for 18 months. More rigorous follow-up studies are required before vitamin E's ability, if any, to reverse photo-damage is established.

In a recent double-blind study, vitamin E ointment did not improve the cosmetic appearance of surgical scars. Application of topical vitamin E was associated with contact dermatitis in 33% of the subjects.

It has been claimed that supplemental vitamin E increases male sexual performance and enhances male fertility. There is no evidence that supplemental vitamin E has any effect on sexual performance in either males of females. An Israeli research group has reported that 200 milligrams of oral vitamin E daily for one month apparently helped two men overcome their long-term infertility. Both had very high levels of lipid peroxidation as measured by elevated levels of malondialdehyde prior to beginning vitamin E supplementation. Within one month of starting vitamin E supplementation, the malondialdehyde levels dropped significantly. Both men were able to impregnate their wives.

A combination of vitamin E and selenium seemed to improve sperm motility and morphology in one group of men. Similar results were obtained in a second study, this one using 600 IUs of vitamin E daily. It is possible that these changes might enhance male fertility, but that endpoint was not investigated in these studies.

More recently, a more rigorous randomized placebo-controlled, double-blind study found no improvement in semen parameters in infertile men supplemented with 1,000 milligrams of vitamin C and 800 milligrams of vitamin E for 56 days. Semen parameters studied included semen volume, sperm concentration and motility, sperm count and viability.

Also poorly supported are claims that vitamin E can enhance exercise/athletic performance. There is some evidence that supplemental vitamin E can reduce some measures of oxidative stress in some exercisers but no evidence that it enhances performance.

Notable relief from persistent nocturnal cramps of legs and feet was seen in 82% of 125 subjects taking 300 IUs or less of vitamin E daily.

CONTRAINDICATIONS, PRECAUTIONS, ADVERSE REACTIONS
CONTRAINDICATIONS
Vitamin E is contraindicated in those with known hypersensitivity to any component of a vitamin E-containing product.

PRECAUTIONS
Those on warfarin should be cautious in using high doses of vitamin E (i.e., doses greater than 100 milligrams daily of d-alpha-tocopherol or 200 milligrams daily of dl-alpha-tocopherol), and if they do use such doses, they should have their INRs monitored and their warfarin dose appropriately adjusted if indicated. Likewise, those with vitamin K deficiencies, such as those with liver failure, should be cautious in using high doses of vitamin E. Vitamin E should be used with extreme caution in those with any lesions that have a propensity to bleed (e.g., bleeding peptic ulcers), those with a history of hemorrhagic stroke and those with inherited bleeding disorders (e.g., hemophilia). Supplemental

doses of vitamin E higher than RDA amounts should be avoided by pregnant women and nursing mothers.

High dose vitamin E supplementation should be stopped about one month before surgical procedures and may be resumed following recovery from the procedure. Use of supplemental vitamin E in low birth weight premature infants must be undertaken with extreme caution and only by trained medical personnel.

ADVERSE REACTIONS

The risk of adverse reactions to vitamin E supplementation (in doses up to one gram daily of alpha-tocopherol) generally appears to be very low. A large randomized trial, the Alpha-Tocopherol Beta Carotene (ATBC) Cancer Prevention Study, the subjects of which were Finnish male smokers, reported that subjects consuming 50 milligrams daily of dl-alpha-tocopherol for 6 years had a 50% increase in mortality from hemorrhagic stroke. The numbers were 66 versus 44 strokes in the supplemented versus the control groups. This result was statistically significant. Interestingly, an increase in hemorrhagic stroke has not been observed in other large, long-term studies using much higher doses of the vitamin. The overall stroke rate between the two groups was not statistically significant in the ATBC study. In their most recent report (April, 2000) on vitamin E, the National Research Council comments "The unexpected finding in the ATBC study was considered preliminary and provocative, but not convincing until it can be corroborated or refuted in further large-scale clinical trials."

Adverse reactions reported for vitamin E supplementation include fatigue, breast soreness, emotional disturbances, thrombophlebitis, retinuria, gastrointestinal disturbances, altered serum lipid levels and thyroid problems. These adverse reactions were rare and none of these has been reported in controlled studies. An increased incidence of necrotizing enterocolitis has been reported in premature, very-low birth weight infants receiving 200 milligrams daily of alpha-tocopheryl acetate.

INTERACTIONS

DRUGS

Amiodarone: Alpha-tocopherol may ameliorate some of the adverse side effects of this drug. This is based on the results of cell culture studies.

Anticonvulsants such as phenobarbitol, phenytoin and carbamazepine: Anticonvulsants may lower plasma vitamin E levels.

Antiplatelet drugs such as aspirin, dipyridamole, eptifibatide, clopidogrel, ticlopidine HCl tirofiban and abciximab: High doses of vitamin E may potentiate the effects of these antiplatelet drugs.

Cholestyramine: may decrease vitamin E absorption.

Colestipol: may decrease vitamin E absorption.

Cyclosporine: Based on cell culture studies, alpha-tocopherol may help to ameliorate the renal side effects of cyclosporin.

Isoniazid: may decrease vitamin E absorption.

Mineral oil: may decrease vitamin E absorption.

Multidrug-resistance (MDR) modifying agents: Based on cell culture studies, alpha-tocopherol is reported to antagonize the multidrug-resistance (MDR)-modifying activity of the chemosensitizing agents cyclosporin A, verapamil, clofazimine, GF120918 and B669 to both doxorubicin and vinblastine.

Neomycin: may impair utilization of vitamin E.

Orlistat: inhibits vitamin E absorption. Absorption of a vitamin E acetate supplement was inhibited by approximately 60% by orlistat.

Sucralfate: interferes with vitamin E absorption.

Warfarin: Vitamin E may enhance anticoagulant response. Monitor INRs and appropriately adjust dose of warfarin if necessary.

Zidovudine: Vitamin E may ameliorate myelosuppressive side effects of zidovudine.

NUTRITIONAL SUPPLEMENTS

Beta-carotene: Some studies have suggested that oral supplements of beta carotene may cause a decrease in serum levels of alpha-tocopherol. However, more recent and much larger and longer studies have demonstrated that supplementation with beta carotene does not alter serum concentrations of vitamin E.

Desiccated ox bile: Desiccated ox bile may increase the absorption of vitamin E.

Dietary fiber: Dietary fiber supplementation may decrease the antioxidative effect of a supplement containing alpha-tocopherol and carotenoids.

Iron: Most iron supplements contain the ferrous form of iron. This cation can oxidize unesterified vitamin E to its pro-oxidant form if taken concomitantly. This does not occur with esterified vitamin E (alpha-tocopheryl acetate and succinate).

Medium—chain triglycerides: Medium-chain triglycerides, if taken concomitantly with vitamin E, may enhance its absorption.

Phytosterols and phytostanols, including beta-sitosterol and beta-sitostanol: Phytosterols and phytostanols may lower plasma vitamin E levels.

Plant phenolic compounds and flavonoids: These substances may participate in redox cycling reactions and help maintain levels of reduced vitamin E.

Polyunsaturated fatty acids (PUFAs): Supplementary PUFAs, including alpha-linolenic acid (in flaxseed oil and perilla oil), gamma-linolenic acid (in borage oil, blackcurrant oil, evening primrose oil), docahexaenoic acid, eicosapentaenoic acid and conjugated linoleic acid may increase vitamin E requirements. In most cases this can be satisfied by supplemental use of either at least 15 milligrams daily of d-alpha-tocopherol or 30 milligrams daily of dl-alpha-tocopherol.

Selenium: Selenium may function synergistically with vitamin E.

Vitamin C: Vitamin C may spare vitamin E. It, along with other antioxidants, such as glutathione, alpha-lipoic acid and coenzyme Q_{10}, are thought to be involved in a so-called antioxidant network which helps to regenerate reduced alpha-tocopherol from the tocopheroxyl radical.

FOOD

Dietary polyunsaturated fat: High polyunsaturated fatty acid intakes should be accompanied by increased vitamin E intakes to prevent their oxidation.

Olestra: The fat substitute olestra inhibits the absorption of vitamin E, as well as the other fat-soluble vitamins A, D and K, carotenoids and flavonoids. Vitamins A, D, E (alpha-tocopherol) and K are added to olestra to partly compensate for this.

HERBS

Some herbs, including garlic and ginkgo, possess antithrombotic activity. High doses of vitamin E used at the same time as these herbs may enhance their antithrombotic activity.

OVERDOSAGE

There are no reports of overdosage with vitamin E in any form.

DOSAGE AND ADMINISTRATION

There are several forms of vitamin E available commercially. These are available as nutritional supplements or in functional and fortified foods. The following table lists these forms and their common names.

Vitamin E Forms

Correct Name	Common Name
RRR-alpha-tocopherol	d-alpha-tocopherol
RRR-alpha-tocopheryl acetate	d-alpha-tocopheryl acetate
RRR-alpha-tocopheryl succinate	d-alpha-tocopheryl succinate
all rac-alpha-tocopherol	dl-alpha-tocopherol
all rac-alpha-tocopheryl acetate	dl-alpha-tocopheryl acetate
all rac-alpha-tocopheryl succinate	d1-alpha-tocopheryl succinate
gamma-tocopherol	gamma-tocopherol
mixed tocopherols	mixed tocopherols
RRR-alpha-tocopheryl polyethylene glycol 1000 succinate	TPGS
all *rac*-alpha-tocopheryl nicotinate	d1-alpha-tocopheryl nicotinate
mixed tocotrienols	mixed tocotrienols

For the purpose of defining dietary reference intakes (RDI) for vitamin E, the National Research Council, in its most recent report, restricted vitamin E activity to only one of the homologues of the tocopherol family, alpha-tocopherol. And the term alpha-tocopherol includes only the naturally occurring form, RRR-alpha-tocopherol, commonly called d-tocopherol, and four out of the eight forms of synthetic alpha-tocopherol called *all rac*-alpha-tocopherol, commonly known as d1-alpha-tocopherol. The four included forms are 2R structures: RRR-, RSR-, RRS- and RSS-alpha-tocopherol. RRR-alpha-tocopherol, natural alpha-tocopherol (called natural-source alpha-tocopherol when sold commercially), has approximately twice the availability of the all-synthetic d1-alpha-tocopherol and is probably the better form for supplementation.

The new RDA for alpha-tocopherol for both men and women is 15 milligrams/day. This is for natural or natural-source alpha-tocopherol. Since only 4 out of the 8 stereoisomers of the *all rac*-alpha-tocopherol have vitamin E activity, 30 milligrams daily of *all rac*-alpha-tocopherol daily are needed to supply the RDA for the vitamin.

To determine the number of milligrams of alpha-tocopherol in a supplement labeled in internationals units, one of two conversion factors is used. If the forms are d-alpha-tocopherol, d-alpha-tocopheryl acetate or d-alpha-tocopheryl succinate, multiply IU times 0.67. If the forms are d1-alpha-tocopherol, dl-alpha tocopheryl acetate or dl-tocopheryl succinate, multiply IU times 0.45.

Regarding doses, vitamin E-deficiency conditions need to be managed by medical personnel.

Recommended doses for supplementation range from 100 to 400 milligrams daily with a cap of 1000 milligrams/day for d-alpha-tocopherol in the form of d-alpha-tocopheryl acetate or succinate or 200 to 800 milligrams/day with a cap of 1000 milligrams/day for dl-alpha-tocopherol in the form of dl-alpha-tocopheryl acetate or succinate.

The average intake of alpha-tocopherol derived from various dietary surveys ranges from about 7.5 to 10.3 milligrams daily for men and 5.4 to 7.3 milligrams daily for women. It is believed that these intake estimates may be low due to underreporting of fat and caloric intake and uncertainties about the particular fats or oils consumed. It is thought that an average daily intake of about 15 milligrams may be closer to reality, but this is not clear. The principal vitamin E form in the American diet is gamma-tocopherol.

The Food and Nutrition Board of the National Academy of Sciences has recently issued its report on dietary reference intakes (RDI) for vitamin E, as well as for some other antioxidant nutrients. In establishing the Recommended Dietary Allowance (RDA) for vitamin E, only alpha-tocopherol was taken into account. Other naturally occurring forms of vitamin E (beta-, gamma-, and delta-tocopherol and tocotrienols) were not considered to meet the vitamin E requirement since they are not converted to alpha-tocopherol in humans and have significantly lower binding affinities to the alpha-tocopherol transfer protein. For establishing RDAs of vitamin E, alpha-tocopherol is defined as the natural RRR-alpha-tocopherol and the 2R-stereoisomers of synthetic vitamin E (found in supplements and fortified foods), RRR-, RSR-, RRS-, and RSS-alpha-tocopherols. The 2S-stereoisomers are excluded by this definition. All forms of supplemental vitamin E are included in calculating the Tolerable Upper Intake Level (UL).

The new RDA for vitamin E (again, defined as only alpha-tocopherol) for both men and women is 15 milligrams daily, To convert from milligrams to International Units (UI), the conversion factor is 1.49. Therefore, 15 milligrams of alpha-tocopherol is equal to 22.4 IU. The UL for vitamin E is 1,000 milligrams or 1,490 IU/day expressed as alpha-tocopherol.

The following summarizes the DRIs for various age groups and conditions:

Infants	Adequate Intake (AI)	
0-6 months	4mg/day	0.6mg/kg
7-12 months	5 mg/day	0.6mg/kg

	Recommended Daily Allowance (RDA)
Children	
1-3 years	6mg/day
4-8 years	7mg/day
Boys	
9-13 years	11mg/day
14-18 years	15mg/day

Girls	
9-13 years	11mg/day
14-18 years	15mg/day
Men	
19-30 years	15mg/day
31-50 years	15mg/day
51-70 years	15mg/day
70 years or older	15mg/day
Women	
19-30 years	15mg/day
31-50 years	15mg/day
51-70 years	15mg/day
70 years or older	15mg/day
Pregnancy	
14-18 years	15mg/day
19-30 years	15mg/day
31-50 years	15mg/day
Lactation	
14-18 years	19mg/day
19-30 years	19mg/day
31-50 years	19mg/day

The following summarizes the Tolerable Upper Intake Level (UL) for various age groups and conditions:

Children	(UL)
1-3 years	200mg/day
4-8 years	300mg/day
9-13 years	600mg/day
Adolescents	
14-18 years	800mg/day
Adults	
19 years and older	1,000mg/day
Pregnancy	
14-18 years	800mg/day
19 years and older	1,000mg/day
Lactation	
14-18 years	800mg/day
19 years and older	1,000mg/day

D-ALPHA-TOCOPHEROL

d-alpha-tocopherol is available as a stand-alone supplement and in the form of mixed tocopherols. d-alpha-tocopherol is unesterified and thus much more susceptible to oxidation. It should be stored in a tightly closed, opaque bottle and in a cool, dry place. Typical doses for supplementation range from 100 to 400 milligrams daily. d-alpha-tocopherol is also available for cosmetic application as an antioxidant and moisturizer. Some are hypersensitive to topical d-alpha-tocopherol and may develop dermatitis from its use. To convert from International Units (IU) of d-alpha-tocopherol to milligrams, multiply by 0.67. To convert from milligrams of d-alpha-tocopherol to IU, multiply by 1.49.

D-ALPHA-TOCOPHERYL ACETATE

d-Alpha-tocopheryl acetate is available as a stand-alone supplement and in multivitamin preparations. Since the acetate group protects the hydroxyl group of the chromanol ring against oxidation, it is a more stable form than d-alpha-tocopherol, the free or unesterified form.

Typical doses for supplementation range from 100 to 400 milligrams daily (as d-alpha-tocopherol). To convert from International Units (IU) of d-alpha-tocopheryl acetate to milligrams of d-alpha-tocopherol, multiply byy 0.67. To convert milligrams of d-alpha-tocopheryl acetate to d-alpha-tocopherol, multiply by 0.91.

DL-ALPHA-TOCOPHERYL ACETATE

dl-alpha-tocopheryl acetate is available as a stand-alone supplement and in combination products. Typical doses for supplementation range from 200 to 800 milligrams daily (as alpha-tocopherol). To convert from International Units (IU) of dl-alpha-tocopheryl acetate to milligrams of d-alpha-tocopherol, multiply by 0.45.

D-ALPHA-TOCOPHERYL SUCCINATE

d-Alpha-tocopheryl succinate is available as a stand-alone supplement and in combination vitamin preparations. Since the succinate group protects the hydroxyl group of the chromanol ring against oxidation, it is a more stable form than d-alpha-tocopherol, the free or unesterified form.

Typical doses for supplementation range from 100 to 400 milligrams daily (as d-alpha-tocopherol). To convert from International Units (IU) of d-alpha-tocopheryl succinate to milligrams of d-alpha-tocopherol, multiply by 0.67. To convert milligrams of d-alpha-tocopheryl succinate to d-alpha-tocopherol, multiply by 0.81.

Dl-ALPHA-TOCOPHERYL SUCCINATE

dl-Alpha-tocopheryl succinate is available as a stand-alone supplement and in combination vitamin products. Typical doses for supplementation range from 200 to 800 milligrams daily (as alpha-tocopherol). To convert from International Units (IU) of dl-alpha-tocopheryl succinate to milligrams of d-alpha-tocopherol, multiply by 0.45.

MIXED TOCOPHEROLS

Typical doses for supplementation of high-alpha-mixed-tocopherols range from 100 to 400 milligrams daily, determined as d-alpha-tocopherol. Typical doses for supplementation of low-alpha-mixed-tocopherols are around 200 milligrams daily, determined as d-gamma-tocopherol.

Since the tocopherols are present in their unesterified forms, forms which are much more susceptible to oxidation than esterified forms, mixed tocopherols should be stored in a tightly closed, opaque bottle and in a cool, dry place.

HOW SUPPLIED

Capsules: 100 IU, 200 IU, 400 IU, 600 IU, 800 IU, 1000 IU

Cream

Liquid: 15 IU/0.3 mL, 200 IU/mL, 400 IU/15 mL

Lotion

Ointment

Powder

Tablets: 100 IU, 200 IU, 400 IU, 500 IU, 800 IU

LITERATURE

Adler LA, Rotrosen J, Edson R, et al. Vitamin E treatment for tardive dyskinesia. Arc*h Gen Psychiatry.* 1999; 56:836-841.

Anderson DK, Waters TR, Means ED. Pretreatment with alpha-tocopherol enhances neurologic recovery after experimental spinal cord compression injury. *J Neurotrauma.* 1998; 5:61-67.

Baumann LS, Spencer J. The effects of topical vitamin E on the cosmetic appearance of scars. *Dermatol Surg.* 1999; 25:311-315.

Bozbuga M, Izgi N, Canbolat A. The effects of chronic alpha-tocopherol administration on lipid peroxidation in an experimental model of acute spinal cord injury. *Neurosurg Rev.* 1998; 21:36-42.

Brigelius-Flohe R, Traber MG. Vitamin E: function and metabolism. *FASEB J.* 1999; 13:1145-1155.

Bursell S-E, King GL. Can protein kinase C inhibition and vitamin E prevent the development of diabetic vascular complications? *Diabetes Res Clin Pract.* 1999; 45:169-182.

Burton GW, Traber MG, Acuff RV, et al. Human plasma and tissue alpha-tocopherol concentrations in response to supplementation with deuterated natural and synthetic vitamin E. *Am J Clin Nutr.* 1998; 67:669-684.

Delcourt C, Cristol J-P, Tessier F, et al. Age-related macular degeneration and antioxidant status in the POLA study. *Arch Opthalmol.* 1999; 117:1384-1390.

Dietary Reference Intakes for Vitamin C, Vitamin E, Selenium and Carotenoids. Washington, D.C.: National Academy Press; 2000.

Dowd P, Zheng ZB. On the mechanism of the anticlotting action of vitamin E quinone. *Proc Natl Acad Sci USA.* 1995; 92:8171-8175.

GISSI-Prevenzione Investigators. Dietary supplementation with n-3 polyunsaturated fatty acids and vitamin E after myocardial infarction: results of the GISSI-Prevenzioni trial. *Lancet.* 1999; 354:447-455.

Gogu SR, Lertora JJL, George WJ, et al. Protection of zidovudine-induced toxicity against murine erythroid progenitor cells by vitamin E. *Exp Hematol.* 1999; 19:649-652.

Grundman M. Vitamin E and Alzheimer's disease: the basis for additional clinical trials. *Am J Clin Nutr.* 2000; 71:630S-636S.

Heinonen OP, Albanes D, Virtamo J, et al. Prostate cancer and supplementation with alpha-tocopherol and beta-carotene: incidence and mortality in a controlled trial. *J Natl Cancer Inst.* 1998; 90:440-446.

Hendler SS, Sanchez R. Tocopherol-based antiviral agents and method of using same. United States Patent Number 5, 114, 957. 1992.

Kayden HJ, Traber M. Absorption, lipoprotein transport and regulation of plasma concentrations of vitamin E in humans. *J Lipid Res.* 1993; 34:343-358.

Knekt P, Reunanen A, Marniemi J, et al. Low vitamin E status is a potential risk factor for insulin-dependent diabetes mellitus. *J Intern Med.* 1999; 245:99-102.

Lee I-K, Koya D, Ishi H, et al. Alpha-tocopherol prevents the hyperglycemia induced activation of diacylglycerol (DAG)-protein kinase C (PKC) pathway in vascular smooth muscle cell by an increase of DAG kinase activity. *Diabetes Res Clin Pract.* 1999; 45:189-190.

Meydani SN, Meydani M, Blumberg JB, et al. Vitamin E supplementation and in vivo immune response in healthy elderly subjects. *JAMA.* 1997; 277:1380-1386.

Paolisso G, Gambardella A, Giugliano D, et al. Chronic intake of pharmacological doses of vitamin E might be useful in the therapy of elderly patients with coronary heart disease. *Am J Clin Nutr.* 1995; 61:848-852.

Pryor WA. Vitamin E and heart disease: basic science to clinical intervention trials. Free *Rad Biol Med.* 2000; 28:141-164.

Rapola JM, Virtamo J, Ripatti S, et al. Effects of alpha-tocopherol and beta-carotene supplements on symptoms, progression, and prognosis of angina pectoris. *Heart.* 1998; 79:454-458.

Rimm EB, Stampfer MJ, Ascherio A, et al. Vitamin E consumption and the risk of coronary heart disease in men. *N Engl J Med.* 1993; 328:1450-1456.

Sano M, Ernesto C, Thomas RG, et al. A controlled trial of selegiline, alpha-tocopherol, or both as treatment for Alzheimer's disease. *N Engl J Med.* 1997; 336:1216-1222.

Shoulson I. DATATOP: a decade of neuroprotective inquiry. Parkinson Study Group. Deprenyl and tocopherol antioxidative therapy of Parkinsonism. *Ann Neurol.* 1998; 44(3 Suppl 1): S160-S166.

Stahl W, Heinrich U, Jungmann H, et al. Carotenoids and carotenoids plus vitamin E protect against ultraviolet light-induced erythrema in humans. *Am J Clin Nutr.* 2000; 71:795-798.

Stampfer MJ, Hennekens CH, Manson JE, et al. Vitamin E consumption and the risk of coronary disease in women. *N Engl J Med.* 1993; 328:1444-1449.

Steinberg D, Parthsarathy S, Carew TE, et al. Beyond cholesterol: modifications of low-density lipoprotein that increases its atherogenicity. *N Engl J Med.* 1989; 320:915-924.

Steiner M. Vitamin E, a modifier of platelet function: rationale and use in cardiovascular disease. *Nutr Rev.* 1999; 57:306-309.

Stephens NG, Parsons A, Schofield PM, et al. Randomized controlled trial of vitamin E in patients with coronary disease: Cambridge Heart Antioxidant Study (CHAOS). *Lancet.* 1996; 347:781-786.

Stone WL, Pappas AM. Tocopherols and the etiology of colon cancer. *J Natl Cancer Inst.* 1997; 89:1006-1014.

Takanami Y, Iwane H, Kawai Y, Shimomitsu T. Vitamin E supplementation and endurance exercise: are there benefits? *Sports Med.* 2000; 29:73-83.

The Alpha-Tocopherol Beta-Carotene Cancer Prevention Study Group. The effect of vitamin E and beta-carotene on the incidence of lung cancer and other cancers in male smokers. *N Engl J Med.* 1994; 330:1029-1035.

The Heart Outcomes Prevention Evaluation Study Investigators. Vitamin E supplementation and cardiovascular events in high-risk patients. *N Engl J Med.* 2000; 342:154-160.

Traber MG, Arai H. Molecular mechanisms of vitamin E transport. *Annu Rev Nutr.* 1999; 19:343-355.

Traber MG. Vitamin E. In: Shils ME, Olson JA, Shike M, Ross AC, eds. *Modern Nutrition in Health and Disease.* 9th ed. Baltimore, MD: Williams and Wilkins; 1999: 347-362.

Trevithick JR, Xiong H, Lee S, et al. Topical tocopheryl acetate reduces post-UVB, sunburn-associated erythema, edema, and skin sensitivity in hairless mice. *Arch Biochem Biophys.* 1992; 296:575-582.

Vatassery GT, Bauer T, Dysken M. High doses of vitamin E in the treatment of the central nervous system in the aged. *Amer J Clin Nutr.* 1999; 70:793-801.

Wadleigh RG, Redman RS, Graham ML, et al. Vitamin E in the treatment of chemotherapy-induced mucositis. *Ann J Med.* 1992; 92:481-484.

Woodson K, Tangrea JA, Barrett MJ, et al. Serum alpha-tocopherol and subsequent risk of lung cancer among male smokers. *J Natl Cancer Inst.* 1999:91; 1738-1743.

Wu D, Meydani M, Beharka AA, et al. In vitro supplementation with different tocopherol homologues can affect the function of immune cells in old mice. *Free Rad Biol Med.* 2000; 28:643-651.

Yokota T, Uchihara T, Shiojiri T, et al. Postmortem study of ataxia with retinitis pigmentosa by mutation of the alpha-tocopherol transfer protein gene. *J Neurol Neurosurg Psychiatry.* 2000; 68:521-525.

Vitamin K

TRADE NAMES

Vitamin K is available from numerous manufacturers generically.

DESCRIPTION

Vitamin K is a generic term for a group of substances which contain the 2-methyl-1, 4-naphthoquinone ring structure and which possess hemostatic activity. Substances with vitamin K activity were originally identified in green leafy vegetables, hemp seeds, liver and fish meal. These substances were found to have antihemorrhagic activity and their collective name was derived from koagulation, the German word for clotting. In addition to its essential role in hemostasis, vitamin K is involved in bone metabolism, among other processes.

Vitamin K_1 or phylloquinone is the principal dietary source of vitamin K and its predominant circulating form. Green leafy vegetables are rich in vitamin K_1 and contribute 40%-50% of total dietary intake of the vitamin. The next largest contributors to dietary vitamin K intake are the vegetable oils olive oil, canola oil, soybean oil and cottonseed oil. These vegetable oils also contain vitamin K_1. Vitamin K_1 is a fat-soluble substance. Vitamin K_2, which is also fat soluble, is the collective term for a number of substances known as menaquinones. Vitamin K_2 is found in chicken egg yolk, butter, cow liver, certain cheeses and fermented soybean products such as natto. This form of vitamin K is also produced by certain bacteria, including some of the bacteria that comprise the microflora of the intestine. The dietary contribution of vitamin K_2 is much less than that of vitamin K_1. The amount of vitamin K contributed to the body by the intestinal microflora remains unclear. Vitamin K_3 or menadione is a fat-soluble synthetic compound which is used in animal feed and dog and cat food. It is metabolized to vitamin K_2.

Vitamin K is involved as a cofactor in the posttranslational gamma-carboxylation of glutamic acid residues of certain proteins in the body. These proteins include the vitamin K-dependent coagulation factors II (prothrombin), VII (proconvertin), IX (Christmas factor), X (Stuart factor), protein C, protein S, protein Zv and a growth-arrest-specific factor (Gas6). In contrast to the other vitamin K-dependent proteins in the blood coagulation cascade, protein C and protein X serve anticoagulant roles. The two vitamin K-dependent proteins found in bone are osteocalcin, also known as bone Gla (gamma-carboxyglutamate) protein or BGP, and the matrix Gla protein or MGP. Gamma-carboxylation is catalyzed by the vitamin K-dependent gamma-carboxylases. The reduced form of vitamin K, vitamin K hydroquinone, is the actual cofactor for the gamma-carboxylases. Proteins containing gamma-carboxyglutamate are called Gla proteins.

Vitamin K deficiency can occur under certain conditions. These include, inadequate dietary intake, malabsorption syndromes (cystic fibrosis, Crohn's disease, ulcerative colitis, Whipple's disease, celiac sprue, short bowel syndrome) and loss of storage sites due to hepatocellular disease. Vitamin K deficiency frequently occurs in those with chronic liver disease, such as primary biliary cirrhosis. Coumarin anticoagulants, such as warfarin, induce a state analogous to vitamin K deficiency by inhibiting the reduction and recycling of vitamin K, and certain cephalosporin antibiotics (see Interactions) may also induce a vitamin K deficiency state by inhibiting the reduction and recycling of the vitamin. Recently, it has been found that space flight may impair vitamin K metabolism and also induce a state of vitamin K deficiency. Symptoms of vitamin K deficiency include easy bruisability, epistaxis, gastrointestinal bleeding, menorrhagia and hematuria. Chronic vitamin K deficiency may also result in osteoporosis and increased risk of fractures. There is some evidence that chronic warfarin use may also cause osteoporosis.

Vitamin K_1, in addition to being known as phylloquinone, is also known as phytonadione and 2-methyl-3-phytyl-1, 4-naphthoquinone. The lipophilic side chain is located at position 3 of the naphthoquinone ring. Its molecular formula is $C_{31}H_{46}O_2$ and its molecular weight is 450.71 daltons. The structural formula is:

Vitamin K_1

Vitamin K_2 is the collective term for a group of vitamin K compounds called menaquinones. The menaquinone homolgues are characterized by the number of isoprene residues comprising the side chain. The side chain is located at position 3 of the naphthoquinone ring. The group chemical name of the menaquinones is 2-methyl-3-all-*trans*-polyprenyl-1, 4-naphthoquinones. Menaquinones with side chains of up to 15 isoprene units have been described. Menaquinones of from two to 13 isoprene units have been found in human and animal tissues. Menaquinones are designated by the name menaquinone followed by a number. The number refers to the number of isoprene residues in the structure. Thus, menaquinone-4, abbreviated MK-4, possesses four isoprene residues in the side chain. Menaquinone-7 possesses seven isoprene units in the side chain. The menaquinones may also be designated by the number of carbons in the side chain. An isoprene residue contains five carbons. Thus, menaquinone-4 is also called vitamin K_2 (20) and menaquinone-7 is also called vitamin K_2 (35). Menaquinone-4 is also known as menatetrenone. The fermented soybean product natto is rich in menaquinone-7. Menaquinone-4 is the predominant form of vitamin K in the rat brain.

Vitamin K_3 or menadione is a synthetic naphthoquinone derivative. It is also known as 2-methyl-1, 4-naphthoquinone. Its molecular formula is $C_{11}H_8O_2$ and its molecular weight is 172.18 daltons. Vitamin K_3 does not possess a lipophilic side chain.

The nutritional supplement forms of vitamin K are vitamin K_1 and vitamin K_2.

ACTIONS AND PHARMACOLOGY

ACTIONS
Vitamin K has hemostatic activity and may have anti-osteoporotic, antioxidant and anticarcinogenic activities.

MECHANISM OF ACTION
The hemostatic activity of vitamin K is well known. Vitamin K is used to treat anticoagulant-induced prothrombin deficiency caused by warfarin, hypoprothrombinemia secondary to antibiotic therapy and hypoprothrombinemia secondary to vitamin C deficiency from various causes, including malabsorption syndromes. The pharmacological action of vitamin K in the treatment of hypoprothrombinemia is related to the normal physiological function of the vitamin. Vitamin K is an essential cofactor for the gamma-carboxylase enzymes which catalyze the posttranslational gamma-carboxylation of glutamic acid residues in inactive hepatic precursors of coagulation factors II, VII, IX and X. Gamma-carboxylation converts these inactive precursors into active coagulation factors which are secreted by hepatocytes into the blood. Supplement vitamin K has no hemostatic activity in those who are not vitamin K-deficient.

The mechanism of the possible anti-osteoporotic activity of vitamin K is not completely understood. Two vitamin K-dependent proteins are found in bone: osteocalcin or bone Gla protein (BGP) and the matrix Gla protein or MGP. Osteocalcin appears to be the most abundant non-collagenous protein in the bone. Most of the osteocalcin synthesized by the osteoblasts during bone matrix formation is incorporated into bone. This is due to the high specificity of the gamma-carboxyglutamyl residues for the calcium ions of hydroxyapatite. A small amount of osteocalcin is released into the circulation. Osteocalcin appears to act as a regulator of bone mineralization. High levels of circulating undercarboxylated (under-gamma-carboxylated) osteocalcin have been associated with low bone mineral density and increased risk of hip fractures. The serum level of undercarboxylated

osteocalcin may be a more sensitive marker of vitamin K status than blood coagulation tests. High levels of undercarboxylated osteocalcin are frequently found in the context of normal blood coagulation tests.

In vivo and *in vitro* studies have shown that vitamin K may directly act on bone metabolism. *In vitro* studies have demonstrated that vitamin K_2 inhibits bone resorption by, in part, inhibiting the production of bone resorbing substances such as prostaglandin E_2 and interleukin-6. Vitamin K_2 has been reported to enhance human osteoblast-induced mineralization *in vitro* and to inhibit bone loss in steroid-treated rats and ovariecomized rats.

The reduced form of vitamin K, vitamin K-hydroquinone, is the active cofactor for the gamma-carboxylase enzymes. Vitamin K hydroquinone is produced in the vitamin K cycle. In the vitamin K cycle, vitamin K-hydroquinone is continuously regenerated. Vitamin K-hydroquinone is a potent reactive oxygen species scavenger. Vitamin K-hydroquinone has been found to inhibit lipid peroxidation.

Certain naphthoquinones, in particular the synthetic vitamin K menadione, have been found to have antitumor activity *in vitro* and *in vivo*. Vitamin K_2 has been found to induce the in vitro differentiation of myeloid leukemic cell lines. The mechanism of the possible anticarcinogenic activity of vitamin K is not well understood. Menadione is an oxidative stress inducer and its possible anticarcinogenic activity may, in part, be explained by induction of apoptotic cell death. One study suggested that the induction of apoptosis by menadione is mediated by the Fas/Fas ligand system. Another study reported that menadione induces cell cycle arrest and cell death by inhibiting Cda 25 phosphatase.

PHARMACOKINETICS
Vitamin K, mainly in the form of vitamin K_1, is principally absorbed from the jejunum and ileum. The efficiency of absorption is variable and ranges from 10% to 80%. Vitamin K is delivered to the enterocytes in micelles formed from bile salts and other substances. Vitamin K is secreted by enterocytes into the lymphatics in the form of chylomicrons. It enters the circulation via the thoracic duct and is carried in the circulation to various tissues including hepatic, bone and spleen, in the form of chylomicron remnants. In the liver, some vitamin K is stored, some is oxidized to inactive end products and some secreted with VLDL (very low-density lipoprotein). Approximately 50% of vitamin K is carried in the plasma in the form of VLDL, about 25% in LDL (low-density lipoprotein) and about 25% in HDL (high-density lipoprotein). Vitamin K undergoes some oxidative metabolism. Excretion of vitamin K and its metabolites is mainly via the feces. Some urinary excretion of vitamin K also occurs.

INDICATIONS AND USAGE

Vitamin K is indicated in those with vitamin K deficiency, in some cases of hemorrhagic disease of the newborn, in some malabsorption syndromes and in some on long-term total parenteral nutrition. There is emerging evidence that adequate vitamin K intake may help protect against osteoporosis generally. There is the suggestion in early research that vitamin K may also have some anti-atherosclerotic effects. Claims that vitamin K is an anti-cancer agent derive from very preliminary work utilizing, primarily, vitamin K$_3$ or menadione. There is little or no reliable data yet available to support further claims that vitamin K inhibits platelet aggregation, that it has favorable effects on insulin and glucose, that it is helpful in Alzheimer's disease and that it favorably modulates immunity and has anti-inflammatory effects.

RESEARCH SUMMARY

Though primary vitamin K deficiency is uncommon, deficiencies secondary to disease or drug therapy arise more often. The most significant instance of acquired vitamin K deficiency manifests as hemorrhagic disease of the newborn (HDN). Causes of HDN are varied and include exclusive breast feeding (vitamin K is in short supply in breast milk) and liver dysfunction. Vitamin K prophylaxis, via oral and intramuscular administration at birth, has been widely used for decades with apparent efficacy. Intramuscular administration is considerably more effective but has been less used in recent years following publication of an epidemiological study suggesting an association between this treatment and a reported doubling of cancer risk in later life. Whether this association is genuinely causal has yet to be confirmed. No such association is seen with oral administration.

A number of drug therapies, including vitamin A and E in pharmacologic doses, some broad-spectrum antibiotics, the 4-hydroxycoumarins and salicylates, antagonize the action of vitamin K and, in some instances, result in deficiencies requiring additional vitamin K intake under a physician's supervision. TPN is frequently another indication for supplemental vitamin K, as are some malabsorption syndromes and gastrointestinal disorders. Those with parenchymal liver disease often have vitamin K deficiency. Recently vitamin K deficiency was found to be significant in many with cystic fibrosis.

Over the past decade, some very important vitamin K roles in bone metabolism have begun to be elucidated. Vitamin K has been demonstrated to promote the gamma-carboxylation of glutamyl residues on many bone proteins. This carboxylation is associated with increased bone mineral density, while undercarboxylation results in diminished bone mineral density and increased risk of bone fracture.

In a prospective analysis, the diets of 72,327 women 38-63 years of age were assessed and the incidence of hip fractures monitored over a ten-year period. A significant association was found between low dietary vitamin K intake and increased risk of hip fracture. This study looked at several specific dietary components and found a significant protective effect from lettuce, a source rich in vitamin K. Women who consumed lettuce (iceberg and romaine) one or more times daily had a significant 45% lower risk of hip fracture than did women who ate lettuce once a week or less.

In another study, gammacarboxyglutamate (Gla) proteins, the formation of which, as noted above, are promoted by vitamin K activity, were observed to play regulatory roles in calcification processes in both bone tissue and atherosclerotic vessel wall. This research suggested that reduced vitamin K status increases vessel wall calcification and reduces bone calcification and that increased vitamin K status might do the opposite. Thus, it is suggested that vitamin K might simultaneously protect against some atherosclerosis and osteoporosis. More research is needed to confirm or refute supplemental vitamin K's possible role in atherosclerosis.

CONTRAINDICATIONS, PRECAUTIONS, ADVERSE REACTIONS.

CONTRAINDICATIONS

Vitamin K is contraindicated in those hypersensitive to any component of a vitamin K-containing product.

PRECAUTIONS.

Those taking warfarin should avoid supplementation with vitamin K unless specifically prescribed by their physicians.

Pregnant women and nursing mothers should avoid supplemental intakes of vitamin K greater than RDA amounts (65 micrograms daily) unless higher amounts are prescribed by their physicians.

Use of vitamin K for the treatment of vitamin K deficiency must be done under medical supervision.

ADVERSE REACTIONS.

The supplemental forms of vitamin K, vitamin K$_1$ and vitamin K$_2$ are well tolerated. In one study, doses of 90 milligrams daily of vitamin K$_2$ were given for 24 weeks. Few adverse effects were noted. Reversible elevations of some liver tests were noted in a few subjects in the study. Menadione (vitamin K$_3$), which is not used as a nutritional supplemental form of vitamin K for humans, has been reported to cause adverse reactions, including hemolytic anemia.

INTERACTIONS

DRUGS

Broad-Spectrum Antibiotics: Broad-spectrum antibiotics may sterilize the bowel and decrease the vitamin K contribution to the body by the intestinal microflora.

Cephalosporins: Cephalosporins containing side chains of N-methylthiotetrazole (cefmenoxime, cefoperazone, cefotetan, cefamandole, latamoxef) or methylthiadiazole (cefazolin) can cause vitamin K deficiency and hypoprothrombinemia. These cephalosporins are inhibitors of hepatic vitamin K epoxide reductase.

Cholestyramine: Concomitant intake of cholestyramine and vitamin K may reduce the absorption of vitamin K.

Colestipol: Concomitant intake of colestipol and vitamin K may reduce the absorption of vitamin K.

Mineral Oil: Concomitant intake of mineral oil and vitamin K may reduce the absorption of vitamin K.

Orlistat: Orlistat may decrease the absorption of vitamin K.

Salicylates: Salicylates in large doses may inhibit vitamin K epoxide reductase resulting in vitamin K deficiency.

Warfarin: Vitamin K can antagonize the effect of warfarin.

NUTRITIONAL SUPPLEMENTS
Medium Chain Triglycerides: Concomitant intake of medium-chain triglycerides and vitamin K may enhance the absorption of vitamin K.

Squalene: Concomitant intake of squalene and vitamin K may decrease the absorption of vitamin K.

Vitamin A: Intake of high doses of vitamin A may decrease the absorption of vitamin K.

Vitamin E: Intake of very large doses of vitamin E may result in vitamin K deficiency. A vitamin E metabolite, vitamin E quinone, can inhibit vitamin K-dependent gamma-glutamyl carboxylase activity.

FOODS
Olestra: The fat substitute olestra inhibits the absorption of vitamin K as well as the other fat-soluble vitamins A, D and E. These vitamins are added to olestra. Olestra contains 8 micrograms of vitamin K per gram.

DOSAGE AND ADMINISTRATION
There is no typical dosage for vitamin K. Some multivitamin preparations contain vitamin K as vitamin K_1 (phylloquinone or phytonadione) or vitamin K_2 (menaquinones) at doses of 25 to 100 micrograms. The amount of vitamin K in these products is stated as the percentage of the daily value (DV) for vitamin K. The DV is the highest RDA for the vitamin, or 80 micrograms. Vitamin K_1 is also available in 10 milligram doses. In Japan, vitamin K, usually in the form of vitamin K_2, is used for the management of osteoporosis. The fermented soybean product natto is rich in menaquinone-7 or vitamin K_2 (35). The bacteria that is used in the preparation of natto, *Bacillus natto*, is also used in Japan as a dietary supplement source of vitamin K_2.

The Food and Nutrition Board of the U.S. National Academy of Sciences has indicated the following recommended dietary allowances (RDA) for vitamin K:

Category	Age (Years)	RDA (micrograms/day)
Infants	0.0 to 0.5	5
	0.5 to 1.0	10
Children	1 through 3	15
	4 through 6	20
	7 through 10	30
Males	11 through 14	45
	15 through 18	65
	19 through 24	70
	25 through 50	80
	51 years and older	80
Females	11 through 14	45
	15 through 18	55
	19 through 24	60
	25 through 50	65
	51 years and older	65
Pregnant		65
Lactating		65

HOW SUPPLIED
Vitamin K is available in the following forms and strengths for OTC use:

Tablets — 100 mcg

Vitamin K is available in the following forms and strengths for Rx use:

Injection — 10 mg/mL

Tablets — 5 mg

LITERATURE
Blackwell GJ, Radkomski M, Moncada S. Inhibition of human platelet aggregation by vitamin K. *Throm Res.* 1985; 37:103-114.

Booth SL, Mayer J. Warfarin and fracture risk. *Nutr Rev.* 2000; 58:20-22.

Booth SL, O'Brien-Morse ME. Dallal GE, et al. Response of vitamin K status to different intakes and sources of phylloquinone-rich food: comparison of younger and older adults. *Am J Clin Nutr.* 1999; 70:368-377.

Booth SL, Tucker KL, Chen H, et al. Dietary vitamin K intakes are associated with hip fracture but not with bone mineral density in elderly men and women. *Am J Clin Nutr.* 2000; 71:1201-1208.

Booth SL Suttie JW. Dietary intake and adequacy of vitamin K. *J Nutr.* 1998; 128:785-788.

Caillot-Augusseau A, Vico L, Herr M, et al. Space flight is associated with rapid decreases of under carboxylated osteocalcin and increases of markers of bone resorption without changes in their circadian variation: observations in two cosmonauts. *Clin Chem.* 2000; 46:1136-1143.

Caricchio R, Kovalenko D, Kaufmann WK, Cohen PL. Apoptosis provoked by the oxidative stress inducer menadione (vitamin K_3) is mediated by the Fas/Fas ligand system. *Clin Immunol.* 1999; 93:65-74.

Chlebowski RT, Akman SA, Block JB. Vitamin K in the treatment of cancer. *Cancer Treatment Rev.* 1985; 12:49-63.

Craciun AM, Wolf J, Knapen MH, et al. Improved bone metabolism in female elite athletes after vitamin K supplementation. *Int J Sports Med.* 1998; 19:479-484.

Feskanich D, Weber P, Willett WC, et al. Vitamin K intake and hip fractures in women: a prospective study. *Am J Clin Nutr.* 1999; 69:74-79.

Jamal SA, Browner WS, Bauer D, Cummings SR. Warfarin use and risk for osteoporosis in elderly women. Study of Osteoporotic Fractures Research Group. *Ann Intern Med.* 1998; 128:829-832.

Jie K-SG, Bots ML, Vermeer C, et al. Vitamin K status and bone mass in women with and without aortic atherosclerosis: a population-based study. *Calcif Tissue Int.* 1996; 59:352-356.

Kawashima H, Nakajima Y, Matubara Y, et al. Effects of vitamin K_2 (menatetrenone) on atherosclerosis and blood coagulation in hypercholesterolemic rabbits. *Jpn J Pharmacol.* 1997; 75:135-143.

Lipsky JJ. Nutritional sources of vitamin K. *Mayo Clin Proc.* 1994; 69:462-466.

Olson RE. Osteoporosis and vitamin K intake (editorial). *Am J Clin Nutr.* 2000; 71:1031-1032.

Olson RE. Vitamin K. In: Shils ME, Olson JA, Shike M, Ross AC, eds. *Modern Nutrition in Health and Disease.* 9th ed. Baltimore, MD: Williams and Wilkins; 1999:363-380.

Philip WJ, Martin JC, Richardson JM, et al. Decreased axial and peripheral bone density in patients taking long-term warfarin. *QJM.* 1995; 88:635-640.

Rashid M, Durie P, Andrew M, et al. Prevalence of vitamin K deficiency in cystic fibrosis. *Am J Clin Nutr.* 1999; 70:378-382.

Sakamoto N, Wakabayashi I, Sakamoto K. Low vitamin K intake effects on glucose tolerance in rats. *Int J Vitam Nutr Res.* 1999; 69:27-31.

Sakagami H, Satoh K, Hakeda Y, Kumegawa M. Apoptosis-inducing activity of vitamin C and vitamin K. *Cell Mol Biol (Noisy-le-grand).* 2000; 46:129-143.

Sano M, Fujita H, Morita I, et al. Vitamin K_2 (menatetrenone) induces iNOS in bovine vascular smooth muscle cells: no relationship between nitric oxide production and gamma-carboxylation. *J Nutr Sci Vitaminol.* (Tokyo). 1999; 45:711-723.

Shearer MJ. Vitamin K. *Lancet.* 1995; 345:229-234.

Takami A, Nakao S, Ontachi Y, et al. Successful therapy of myelodysplastic syndrome with menatetrenone, a vitamin K_2 analog. *Int J Hematol.* 1999; 69:24-26.

Tsaioun KI. Vitamin K-dependent proteins in the developing and aging nervous system. *Nutr Rev.* 1999; 57:231-240.

Vermeer C, Jie KS, Knapen MH. Role of vitamin K in bone metabolism. *Annu Rev Nutr.* 1995; 15:1-22.

Vervoort LM, Ronden FE, Thijssen HH. The potent antioxidant activity of the vitamin K cycle in microsomal lipid peroxidation. *Biochem Pharmacol.* 1997; 54:871-876.

Wu FY, Sun TP. Vitamin K_3 induces cell cycle arrest and cell death by inhibiting Cdc25 phosphatase. *Eur J Cancer.* 1999; 35:1388-1393.

Wheat Grass/Barley Grass

TRADE NAMES

Trade names for barley grass include Pure Energy Greens (Montana Big Sky) and Green Magma (Green Foods). Trade names for wheat grass include Green Energy Wheat Grass (Pines Wheat Grass).

DESCRIPTION

Cereal grass is the young green plant that grows to produce the cereal grain. Grasses belong to the *Gramineae* family that provides all the world's cereals and most of the world's sugar. Wheat grass and barley grass are popular nutritional supplements. These cereal grasses, along with spirulina (see Spirulina), chlorella (see Chlorella), oat grass and alfalfa are sometimes referred to as "green foods." Wheat grass and barley grass are rich sources of chlorophyll (see Chlorophyll/Chlorophyllin), which is believed to have some health-promoting activities.

ACTIONS AND PHARMACOLOGY

ACTIONS

Wheat grass and barley grass have putative anticarcinogenic activity.

MECHANISM OF ACTION

Wheat sprout extracts have demonstrated antimutagenic activity *in vitro*. The mechanism of the antimutagenic effect is unclear. Wheat sprouts and wheat grass are rich in chlorophyll, and the antimutagenic activity of wheat sprouts may be accounted for by the presence of this substance, which is known to have antimutagenic and anticarcinogenic activities (see Chlorophyll/Chlorophyllin). Other substances, including flavonoids, may also play a role in these possible activities. Barley grass extracts have been found to protect human fibroblasts against carcinogenic agents. Again, chlorophyll may, in part, account for this effect. Barley grass contains several substances other than chlorophyll that have antioxidant activity and that may contribute to its possible antimutagenic and anticarcinogenic activities.

PHARMACOKINETICS
The proteins, lipids and carbohydrates in wheat grass and barley grass are digested, absorbed and metabolized by normal physiological processes.

INDICATIONS AND USAGE
Wheat grass/barley grass supplements are promoted for multiple uses. Claims have been made that they help prevent and fight cancer, lower cholesterol, detoxify many pollutants, protect against solar and other forms of radiation, boost energy and immunity, enhance wound healing, help with digestion, fight tooth decay and bad breath, promote healthy skin, reverse graying of hair and lower blood pressure, among other things. There is no credible evidence to support any of these claims at this time.

RESEARCH SUMMARY
Research is lacking on the possible effects of wheat grass and barley grass. Given that they contain chlorophyll, it is possible that they might have some of the activities exhibited by that substance, including antimutagenic and anticarcinogenic activities. See Chlorophyll/Chlorophyllin.

CONTRAINDICATIONS, PRECAUTIONS, ADVERSE REACTIONS
CONTRAINDICATIONS
Wheat grass and barley grass are contraindicated in those who are hypersensitive to any component of a wheat grass- or barley grass-containing supplement.

PRECAUTIONS
Pregnant women and nursing mothers should avoid wheat grass- or barley grass-containing supplements.

Wheat grass supplements may contain high amounts of vitamin K. Those on warfarin should exercise caution in the use of wheat grass supplements.

ADVERSE REACTIONS
No reports of adverse reactions.

INTERACTIONS
Some wheat grass supplements may be rich in vitamin K and may affect the INR of those on warfarin.

DOSAGE AND ADMINISTRATION
There are various forms of wheat grass and barley grass supplements. Both are available as a powder, in tablets and as a juice. It is also available as a juice. Wheat grass and barley grass are also found in combination ''green food'' products with spirulina, chlorella, oat grass and alfalfa. Those who use wheat grass typically take 3.5 grams daily. The typical dose of barley grass is also about 3.5 grams daily.

HOW SUPPLIED
Barley grass is supplied as follows:

Capsules — 470 mg, 475 mg, 500 mg
Powder
Tablets — 350 mg, 500 mg

Wheat grass is supplied as follows:

Capsules — 500 mg
Powder
Tablets — 500 mg

LITERATURE
Lai C-N. Chlorophyll: the active factor in wheat sprout extract inhibiting the metabolic activation of carcinogens in vitro. *Nutr Cancer.* 1979; 1:19-21.

Lai C-N, Dabney BJ, Shaw CR. Inhibition of in vitro metabolic activation of carcinogens by wheat sprout extracts. *Nutr Cancer.* 1978; 1:27-30.

Peryt B, Miloszewska J, Tudek B, et al. Antimutagenic effects of several subfractions of extract from wheat sprout toward benzo[a]pyrene-induced mutagenicity in strain TA98 of *Salmonella typhimurium. Mutat Res.* 1988; 206:221-225.

Peryt B, Szymczyk T, Lesca P. Mechanism of antimutagenicity of wheat sprout extracts. *Mutat Res.* 1992; 269:201-215.

Tudek B, Peryt B, Miloszewska J, et al. The effect of wheat sprout extract on benzo(a)pyrene and 7,2-dimethylbenz(a)anthracene activity. *Neoplasma.* 1998; 35:515-523.

Whey Proteins

TRADE NAMES
Whey Ahead (Pinnacle), Isopure (Nature's Best), 100% Ion Exchange Whey Amino Acids (Healthy 'N Fit), N-Large 2 (Prolab Nutrition), Whey Protein Stack (Champion Nutrition), Just Whey Powder (SportPharma), Designer Protein (Next Nutrition).

DESCRIPTION
Whey proteins comprise one of the two major protein groups of bovine milk, the other group being the caseins. Caseins account for about 80% of the total protein in bovine milk, while whey proteins account for the remaining approximately 20%. Whey is derived as a natural byproduct of the cheese-making process. In addition to proteins, the raw form contains fat, lactose and other substances. The raw form is processed to produce protein-rich whey protein concentrates (WPC) and whey protein isolates (WPI), among other things.

Whey proteins are comprised of high-biological-value proteins and proteins that have different functions. The main whey proteins are beta-lactoglobulin and alpha-lactoglobulin, two small globular proteins that account for about 70 to 80% of total whey protein. Proteins present in lesser amounts include the immunoglobulins IgG, IgA and IgM, but especially IgG, glycomacropeptides, bovine serum albumin, lactoferrin, lactoperoxidase and lysozyme. Whey proteins also contain smaller peptides derived from various proteins which are called biopeptides.

A few different types of whey proteins are marketed. Whey protein concentrates are rich in whey proteins and also contain fat and lactose. Some whey protein concentrates contain higher amounts of immunoglobulins than others. Whey protein isolates are low in fat and lactose.

There are various processes for preparing whey protein isolates. Ion-exchange whey protein isolates are high in protein but low in glycomacropeptides, lactoferrin, lactoperoxidase and some bioactive peptides. Microfiltration/ultrafiltration whey protein isolates have higher amounts of glycomacropeptides, lactoferrin, lactoperoxidase and the bioactive peptides, but are lower in bovine serum albumin. Interestingly, bovine serum albumin, along with beta-lactoglobulin and IgG1, are proteins with abundant glutamylcysteine sequences. Glutamylcysteine is the precursor to glutathione. Cross-flow microfiltration gives a whey protein isolate which is greater than 90% in protein that is undenatured and that retains all important sub-fractions in natural ratios, with no fat or lactose.

ACTIONS AND PHARMACOLOGY
ACTIONS
Whey proteins may have antimicrobial and immunomodulatory actions. They may also have antioxidant activity.

MECHANISM OF ACTION
The mechanism of the possible antimicrobial actions of whey proteins may be accounted for by examining the activities of some of the whey proteins. Lactoferrin binds iron very tightly. Iron is a nutrient essential to support microbial growth, especially the growth of pathogenic bacteria. Lactoferrin may also inhibit the adsorption and/or penetration of bacteria and viruses in the intestinal wall. Lactoperoxidase may inactivate or kill microorganisms via an enzymatic activity producing reactive oxygen species. The immunoglobulins may also play a passive immunity role.

The possible immunomodulatory activity of whey proteins may also be due, in part, to the immunoglobulins playing a role in passive immunity. Whey proteins are rich in L-cysteine and L-glutamate, two amino acids that are precursors to the tripeptide glutathione. Some are also abundant in the dipeptide sequence of glutamylcysteine. This dipeptide is also a precursor to glutathione. There is some indication that intake of whey proteins enhance monocyte glutathione

levels. Enhanced glutathione levels may also contribute to a possible immunomodulatory role of whey proteins, as well as to the possible antioxidant activity of these proteins. In addition, lactoferrin may modulate immune function.

PHARMACOKINETICS
The pharmacokinetics of whey proteins should be similar to those for dietary proteins. There is indication that lactoferrin and some of the immunoglobulins in whey proteins may be more resistant to proteolytic degradation than are other types of proteins. Some proteins may be digested to peptides that may be absorbed and may have various activities (bioactive peptides). Some (e.g., bovine serum albumin, beta-lactoglobulin) may yield glutamylcysteine during their digestion, which may be absorbed and serve as a precursor to glutathione in some tissues.

INDICATIONS AND USAGE
Whey proteins may be useful in the nutrition of some infants and others, and there is some very preliminary evidence that they may have some immune-modulating and anticancer effects. There is no credible evidence that they build muscle faster than other protein sources.

RESEARCH SUMMARY
Whey proteins have been used as the sole proteins in some infant formulas, and this has reportedly resulted in fewer allergies in these infants. In one study, the use of a whey protein formula in the first six months of life significantly reduced atopic disease up to one year of age. In another study, infants receiving a whey protein-hydrolysate formula during the first six months of life had a lower incidence of cow's milk protein sensitivity at age six months, less eczema during the first year of life and less diarrhea of non-infectitious origin during the first half-year of life.

There are several animal studies in which whey and whey factors are said to exert some positive effects on immunity and cancer. Observed immuno-enhancing properties are believed by some researchers to be related only partially to whey's nutritional effects. Enhancement of host humoral immune response has been associated, in some of these studies, with whey's role in increasing glutathione levels in the body.

In animal studies, whey proteins were found to be protective against colon cancer, relative to red meat and some other protein sources. A whey protein diet significantly decreased tumor burden and extended life in mice with colon cancer, compared to mice with colon cancer fed-standard diet.

Whey protein concentrate was administered to five patients with metastatic cancers (30 grams daily for six months). Two of these patients exhibited some evidence of tumor regression, normalization of hemoglobin and peripheral lymphocyte counts. In two other patients, there was stabilization of tumor growth and increased hemoglobin levels. More research is needed.

CONTRAINDICATIONS, PRECAUTIONS, ADVERSE REACTIONS

CONTRAINDICATIONS
Whey proteins are contraindicated in those who are hypersensitive to milk proteins.

PRECAUTIONS
See Contraindications.

ADVERSE REACTIONS
No reports. However, those who are hypersensitive to milk products are expected to experience allergy symptoms, including possible serious ones, if they use whey protein products.

INTERACTIONS
No known interactions with drugs, nutritional supplements, food or herbs.

DOSAGE AND ADMINISTRATION
There are several types of whey protein supplements available, including whey protein concentrates, ion exchange whey protein isolates, microfiltration/ultrafiltration whey protein isolates and whey protein hydrolysates. Some preparations contain mixtures of these various forms, and some are enriched with other substances, including branched-chain amino acids and L-glutamine. Dosages are variable. Some (athletes, for example) use whey proteins as a protein supplement and take 10 to 25 grams daily and, in some cases, higher doses.

HOW SUPPLIED
Packets
Powder

LITERATURE
Barth CA, Behnke U. [Nutritional physiology of whey and whey components.] [Article in German.] *Nahrung.* 1997; 41:2-12.

Bell S J. Whey protein concentrates with and without immunoglobulins: a review. *J med Food.* 2000; 3:1-13.

Bounous G, Batist G, Gold P. Immunoenhancing property of a dietary whey protein in mice: role of glutathione. *Clin Invest Med.* 1989; 12:154-161.

Bounous G, Batist G, Gold P. Whey proteins in cancer prevention. *Cancer Left.* 1991; 57:91-94.

Bounous G, Gervais F, Amer V, et al. The influence of dietary whey protein on tissue glutathione and the diseases of aging. *Clin Invest Med.* 1989; 12:343-349.

Kennedy RS, Konok GP, Bounous G, et al. The use of a whey protein concentrate in the treatment of patients with metastatic carcinoma: a phase I-II clinical study. *Anticancer Res.* 1995; 15(6B):2643-2649.

Kinsella JE, Whitehead DM. Proteins in whey: chemical, physical, and functional properties. *Adv Food Nutr Res.* 1989; 33:343-438.

Papenburg R, Bounous G, Fleiszner D, Gold P. Dietary milk proteins inhibit the development of dimethylhydrazine-induced malignancy. *Tumor Biol.* 1990; 11:129-136.

Tong LM, Sasaki S, McClements DJ, Decker EA. Mechanisms of the antioxidant activity of a high molecular weight fraction of whey. *J Agric Food Chem.* 2000; 48:1473-1478.

Vandenplas Y, Hauser B, Van den Borre C, et al. Effect of a whey hydrolysate prophylaxis of atopic disease. *Ann Allergy.* 1992; 68:419-424.

Wong CW, Watson DL. Immunomodulatory effects of dietary whey proteins in mice. *J Dairy Res.* 1995; 62:359-368.

Yeast Beta-D-Glucan

TRADE NAMES
Immunition Beta Glucan Extra Strength (Nutritional Supply Corp.), Beta Glucan Support Healthy Macrophage Activity (Solaray), NSC-100 Immune Enhancer (Nutritional Supply Corp.), NSC-24 Immune Enhancer (Nutritional Supply Corp.).

DESCRIPTION
Beta-D-glucans are nondigestible polysaccharides widely found in nature in such sources as cereal grains, including oats and barley, as well as in yeast, bacteria, algae and mushrooms. Beta-D-glucans are primarily located in the cell walls. Yeast beta-D-glucan is marketed as a nutritional supplement. The yeast beta-D-glucan in the supplement is a polyglucose polysaccharide derived from the cell walls of baker's yeast or *Saccharomyces cerevisiae.*

Yeast beta-D-glucan, usually referred to as yeast beta-glucan, consists of straight-chain and branched polymers. The straight-chain structures are (1/3)-beta-D-linked glucose polymers and (1/6)-beta-D-linked glucose polymers. The branched polymers consist of a (1/3)-beta-D-linked backbone containing varying degrees of (1-6)-beta branches. Yeast beta-glucan is sometimes designated as beta 1, 3/1, 6 glucan.

Yeast beta-glucan appears to have immunomodulatory properties. It can bind to various cells of the non-specific immune system, such as macrophages and neutrophils. PGG-glucan or poly- [1, 6]-beta-D-glucopyranosyl- [1,3]-beta-D-glucopyranose is a genetically modified *Saccharomyces cerevisiae* beta-glucan. It is being evaluated in clinical studies as an immunomodulatory agent and a biological response modifier.

Zymosan is the name of a cell wall preparation derived from *Saccharomyces cerevisiae*, which contains beta (1/3)-glucan, beta (1/6)-glucan and other components of the cell wall, such as chitin and mannoprotein. Zymosan's immunological effects are mainly attributed to the beta-glucans.

ACTIONS AND PHARMACOLOGY

ACTIONS

Yeast beta-glucan may have immunomodulatory and lipid-lowering activity.

MECHANISM OF ACTION

Most of the studies done with yeast beta-glucan have been performed in tissue culture, in animals and with PGG-glucan, which is administered parenterally. Yeast beta-glucan can bind to a beta-glucan receptor in macrophages and stimulate the production of such cytokines as TNF (tumor necrosis factor)-alpha and IL (interleukin)-I beta. Binding to the beta-glucan receptor may also induce the release of such reactive oxygen species as superoxide anions and hydrogen peroxide. Yeast beta-glucan may also stimulate such cells as neutrophils NK (natural killer cells) and LAK (lymphokine-activated killer) cells. All of the above stimulation effects may result in antimicrobial and tumoricidal activities.

Research on PGG-glucan indicates that it interacts with receptors on monocytes and neutrophils. It is thought that this interaction primes these cells for production of cytokines and other immune-modulating substances when they are needed. In this sense, yeast beta-glucan may be considered an immune system primer.

The possible immunomodulatory effects of oral yeast beta-glucan remain unclear. Yeast beta-glucan is an indigestible polysaccharide and very little hydrolysis of it takes place in the stomach or small intestine. There is some digestion of yeast beta-glucan that does take place in the large intestine via bacterial beta-glucosidases, and some remnants of this digestion, oligosaccharides with molecular weights of up to 20,000 daltons, have been detected in the serum of animals, as well as of humans, following ingestion of yeast beta-glucan. However, it is not known if these absorbed oligosaccharides have any immunological or other biological activity. Oral yeast beta-glucan may have immunological activity by virtue of its interaction with gut-associated lymphoid tissue (GALT). Immune cells associated with GALT may be activated via their contact with yeast beta-glucan in the gut and migrate to other tissues where they may exert immunomodulatory effects.

Yeast beta-glucan has been found to lower total cholesterol levels as well as to increase levels of HDL-cholesterol. The mechanism of the HDL-elevation activity is unknown. Also, it is not well understood how beta-glucans, including oat beta-glucans, lower total cholesterol levels. It is thought that the cholesterol-lowering effect of oat beta-glucan may be accounted for, in large part, by its promotion of the excretion of bile acids. Yeast beta-glucan may also promote the excretion of bile acids.

PHARMACOKINETICS

Following ingestion, there is virtually no digestion of yeast beta-glucan in the small intestine. The glycosidic linkages of yeast beta-glucan are of the beta type, and there are no beta-glucosidases among the digestive enzymes. Some digestion of yeast beta-glucan does take place in the large intestine via the action of bacterial beta-glucosidases. Some oligosaccharides up to molecular weight of 20,000 daltons that are produced via the bacterial beta-glucosidases may get absorbed. A large percentage of the ingested yeast beta-glucan is excreted in the feces.

INDICATIONS AND USAGE

Yeast beta-glucan appears to be a non-specific immune enhancer via its ability, among other possible mechanisms, to activate macrophages. It may have some anticarcinogenic, antiatherosclerotic and anti-inflammatory effects, may enhance wound healing and promote skin health in some circumstances.

RESEARCH SUMMARY

Yeast beta-glucan has been demonstrated to have non-specific immune-enhancing effects in *in vitro* and some animal and human studies. This substance binds to an activating receptor site on macrophages in humans, as well as in many animal species. In some of these experiments, yeast beta-glucan has exhibited antibacterial, antifungal and antiviral effects.

A genetically modified yeast beta-glucan enhanced the ability of monocytes and neutrophils to kill microbes in healthy volunteers. Subsequently, high-risk surgical patients were given placebo or this yeast beta-glucan in a double-blind, randomized trial. Those receiving the beta-glucan had significantly fewer postoperative infections than did controls. They also had decreased antibiotic requirement and shorter length of stay in intensive care.

Macrophage activation may be one of the mechanisms that also accounts for some of the anti-inflammatory and anticarcinogenic activities associated with yeast beta-glucan in preliminary experimental work. This substance has shown some activity against human melanoma and basal cell carcinoma *in vitro*. Tumor growth inhibition and increased survival times have been observed in animals with transplanted melanoma, adenocarcinoma, mammary carcinoma and lymphocytic leukemia.

Used in combination with some antimicrobial and anticancer drugs, yeast beta-glucan appears to have beneficial synergistic effects in some circumstances. Synergy has been reported with respect to ampicillin, gentamicin, amphotericin B and 5-fluorouracil, among others, in certain situations.

Yeast beta-glucan has been shown to be radioprotective in some circumstances when administered either pre- or post-radiation. This largely *in vitro* and animal work needs clinical followup.

Given that the oat beta-glucan (see Oat Beta-Glucan) has established hypocholesterolemic effects, research has been conducted to see if yeast beta-glucan also has this activity. Recently, obese hypercholesterolemic men given 15 grams of yeast beta-glucan fiber daily for eight weeks had significantly reduced plasma total cholesterol. They had a non-significant decline in LDL-cholesterol. A significant increase in HDL-cholesterol levels was noted four weeks after cessation of fiber administration.

Lipid effects of yeast beta-glucan were said to be similar to those seen with the use of oat beta-glucan with respect to total cholesterol and superior with respect to HDL-cholesterol. This superiority, however, might be due to the use in this study of significantly higher doses of fiber than were used in the oat studies.

The ability of yeast beta-glucan to activate the macrophagic activity of the Langerhans cells of the skin may account for some of the reported significant wound healing properties of this substance. Yeast beta-glucan has also been reported to improve skin dryness and elasticity, and has thus been promoted for cosmetic uses.

There is one study that suggests this substance can have some revitalizing effects on aging skin. Among 150 female volunteers, aged 35 to 60, those given a cosmetic preparation containing yeast beta-glucan were said to have significantly reduced number, depth and length of wrinkles, compared with controls. Dryness and elasticity of skin were also improved. Further research is needed to confirm or refute these findings.

CONTRAINDICATIONS, PRECAUTIONS, ADVERSE REACTIONS
CONTRAINDICATIONS
Yeast beta-glucan is contraindicated in those who are hypersensitive to any component of a yeast beta-glucan containing product.

PRECAUTIONS
Pregnant women and nursing mothers should avoid yeast beta-glucan supplementation.

INTERACTIONS
DRUGS
Antibiotics, antifungal agents, cancer chemotherapeutic agents: Animal studies have shown some synergistic effects when these substances were used concomitantly with yeast beta-glucan.

OVERDOSAGE
There are no reports of overdosage.

DOSAGE AND ADMINISTRATION
The introduction of yeast beta-glucan supplements has been recent. There are no typical doses.

HOW SUPPLIED
Capsules — 2.5 mg, 3 mg, 7.5 mg, 10 mg, 20 mg

LITERATURE
Babineau TJ, Hackford A, Kenler A, et al. A phase II multicenter, double-blind, randomized, placebo-controlled study of three dosages of an immunomodulator (PGG-glucan) in high-risk surgical patients. *Arch Surg.* 1994; 129:1204-1210.

Babineau TJ, Marcello P, Swails W, et al. Randomized phase I/II trial of a macrophage-specific immunomodulator (PGG-glucan) in high risk surgical patients. *Ann Surg.* 1994; 220:601-609.

Bell S, Goldman VM, Bistrian BR, et al. Effect of beta-glucan from oats and yeast on serum lipids. *Crit Rev Food Sci Nutr.* 1999; 39:189-202.

Nicolosi R, Bell SJ, Bistrian BR, et al. Plasma lipid changes after supplementation with beta-glucan fiber from yeast. *Am J Clin Nutr.* 1999; 70:208-212.

Williams DL, Mueller A, Browder W. Glucan-based macrophage stimulators: a review of their anti-infective potential. *Clin Immunother.* 1996; 5:392-399.

Yogurt

DESCRIPTION
Yogurt is a coagulated milk product that results from the fermentation of milk by the bacteria *Lactobacillus bulgaricus* and *Streptococcus thermophilus*. In addition to *L. bulgaricus* and *S. thermophilus*, other members of the *Lactobacillus* genus, such as *L. acidophilus* and other lactic acid-bacteria, can be used in the process of producing yogurt. Collectively, the bacteria used to make yogurt are called lactic acid bacteria (LAB). All of the LAB produce lactic acid. The acid fermentation curdles the milk and preserves it from putrefaction and spoilage. For centuries, many have believed that fermented milk products such as yogurt are beneficial for health. Elie Metchnikoff, the father of modern immunology, wrote in his book, *The Prolongation of Life: Optimistic Studies*, that yogurt was beneficial for gastrointestinal health, as well as for the promotion of longevity. Some recent research on yogurt suggests that it may have immunostimulatory effects, as well as other benefits.

ACTIONS AND PHARMACOLOGY

ACTIONS

Yogurt may have immunostimulatory and other immunomodulatory activities. It may also have hypocholesterolemic activity.

MECHANISM OF ACTION

The possible immunostimulatory activity of yogurt is probably due to the presence of lactic acid bacteria, as well as nonbacterial components of yogurt. The cell wall of lactic acid bacteria is composed of peptidoglycans, teichoic acid and polysaccharides. The peptidoglycans may induce adjuvant activity at the mucosal surface. Muramyl dipeptide, a lower-molecular-weight breakdown product of the peptidoglycans, may stimulate cytokine production by macrophages, monocytes and lymphocytes. Teichoic acid may also stimulate the production of certain cytokines by monocytes. The lactic acid bacteria may increase secretory IgA activity in the gastrointestinal tract, as well.

Nonbacterial components of yogurt may also contribute to the possible immunostimulatory activity of yogurt. Oligopeptides produced via the fermentation process may enhance phagocytic activity. Some bioactive peptides resulting from the fermentation process may stimulate the proliferation and maturation of T lymphocytes and natural killer (NK) cells for defense against pathogenic enteric bacteria.

Yogurt may have a higher concentration of conjugated linoleic acid (CLA) than nonfermented milk. CLA may have immunomodulatory and anticarcinogenic activity, among other possible health benefits (see Conjugated Linoleic Acid). Whey proteins found in yogurt may be another nonbacterial contributor to yogurt's possible immunostimulatory and other beneficial activities. Whey proteins (see Whey Proteins) are especially high in L-cysteine, a key precursor in the biosynthesis of the tripeptide glutathione. Glutathione has antioxidant activity and is involved in the detoxification of many xenobiotics, including some carcinogens. Whey proteins, in addition to their involvement in the synthesis of glutathione, may have immunomodulatory activities.

The mechanism of the possible anti-allergic activity of yogurt is unclear. It is speculated that yogurt may stimulate interferon-gamma production, which in turn may modulate T cell function by downregulating the Th-2 response.

Some studies have suggested a possible hypocholesterolemic activity of yogurt. Again, the mechanism of this possible effect is unclear. It has been speculated that hydroxymethylglutarate in yogurt may inhibit hydroxymethylglutarate coenzyme A (HMG CoA) reductase activity.

PHARMACOKINETICS

The proteins, peptides and amino acids in yogurt are digested, absorbed and metabolized by normal physiological processes. The same is true for the carbohydrates and lipids in yogurt. Most of the lactic acid bacteria in yogurt adhere only temporarily to the mucosa of the colon. Some, *Lactobacillus acidophilus* for example, persist longer. Most of the lactic acid bacteria do not survive stomach acid. Again, some, such as *L. acidophilus*, are more resistant to stomach acid.

INDICATIONS AND USAGE

Yogurt may have a variety of positive immunologic effects and may help fight certain infections. Yogurt may be anticarcinogenic and antiatherogenic in some circumstances. It may also be useful in some gastrointestinal disorders and in some with allergies and asthma. See also Prebiotics, Probiotics and Symbiotics.

RESEARCH SUMMARY

In vitro, animal and a few human studies indicate that yogurt has a number of favorable immunologic effects. These studies have shown that yogurt consumption increases antibody production, cytokine production, phagocyte activity, natural killer cell activity and T cell function. Both bacterial and non-bacterial components in yogurt have been hypothesized to play roles in these effects on immune function.

In a recent study of long-term yogurt consumption among two different age groups (young adults 20 to 40 years of age and seniors 55 to 70), intake of live-culture yogurt, more than pasteurized yogurt, was associated with decreased allergic symptoms in both age groups. Seniors consuming 200 grams of yogurt daily for one year had consistently lower levels of total immunoglobulin than did control seniors who did not consume yogurt.

Some other studies have also shown that yogurt may be effective in reducing IgE-mediated disorders such as asthma. Results, however, have been mixed, and further research is needed.

Some years ago, a small study suggested that a cup of yogurt daily could significantly reduce the incidence of recurrent vaginitis. The study involved women who had at least five occurrences of vaginitis due to candidal infections annually. The yogurt used in the study was confirmed to contain *Lactobacillus acidophilus*. A three-fold reduction in vaginitis was reported in the women who received yogurt daily for six months.

Various yogurt preparations have been shown to inhibit the growth of several cancers in animal studies. Several of the bacterial components of yogurt have been shown to inhibit tumorigenesis, possibly by reducing nitrite concentrations, through immune-modulation and other mechanisms.

Epidemiological data are somewhat conflicting with respect to yogurt intake and cancer incidence. A significantly lower consumption of fermented milk products (primarily yogurt and buttermilk) was seen among breast-cancer patients in one case-control study. But, in another study, greater yogurt consumption was associated with a higher incidence of ovarian cancer. Further research is needed.

There is some evidence that the bacterial components of yogurt can protect against some gastrointestinal tract infections. Some studies have shown that yogurt products can enhance recovery from some forms of diarrhea. Yogurt has also been used with some success to help restore intestinal microflora diminished by antibiotic treatment. Yogurt is also helpful in some with lactose intolerance.

Several studies spanning many years have concluded that yogurt has hypocholesterolemic effects. In one study, animals were fed high-cholesterol diets. Some were supplemented with yogurt and some were not. The supplemented animals had reduced serum cholesterol and reduced low-density lipoproteins. No effects were noted on serum triglycerides.

Recently, a fermented milk product produced a small but statistically significant reduction in total cholesterol and LDL-cholesterol levels in a double-blind, placebo-controlled, crossover study.

For more information, see Prebiotics, Probiotics and Symbiotics.

CONTRAINDICATIONS, PRECAUTIONS, ADVERSE REACTIONS
CONTRAINDICATIONS
Yogurt is contraindicated in those who are hypersensitive to any component of a yogurt-containing preparation.

PRECAUTIONS
Although yogurt contains much less lactose than nonfermented milk, some with lactase-deficiency may still not be able to tolerate yogurt. Generally, however, it is much better tolerated by those with lactase-deficiency than nonfermented milk.

ADVERSE REACTIONS
There are some reports of flatulence and diarrhea in some with lactase-deficiency.

OVERDOSAGE
None known.

DOSAGE AND ADMINISTRATION
Yogurt is available in many different preparations. Yogurt may be considered a functional food. In some yogurt

preparations, the lactic acid bacteria have been killed during the processing of the product via pasteurization. Yogurt preparations in which the lactic acid bacteria have been killed may still confer some, but probably not all, of the possible health benefits.

Intake of yogurt is variable. One study showing a possible anti-allergy effect of yogurt used 200 grams daily for one year. Unpasteurized yogurt was found to be more effective than pasteurized yogurt in this study.

LITERATURE
Bertolami MC, Faludi AA, Batlouni M. Evaluation of the effects of a new fermented milk product (G910) on primary hypercholesterolemia. *Eur J Clin Nutr*. 1999; 53:97-101.

Danielson AD, Peo ER Jr, Shahani KM, et al. Anticholesterolemic property of Lactobacillus acidophilus yogurt fed to mature boars. *J Anim Sci*. 1989; 67:966-974.

Hepner G, Fried R, St Jeor S, et al. Hypocholesterolemic effect of yogurt and milk. *Am J Clin Nutr*. 1979; 32:19-24.

Hitchins AD, McDonough FE. Prophylactic and therapeutic aspects of fermented milk. *Am J Clin Nutr*. 1989; 49:675-684.

Kolars JC, Levitt MD, Aouji M, Savaiano DA. Yogurt—an autodigesting source of lactose. *N Eng J Med*. 1984; 310:1-3.

Mann GV. A factor in yogurt which lowers cholesterolemia in man. *Atherosclerosis*. 1977; 28:335-340.

Metchnikoff E. *The Prolongation of Life: Optimistic Studies*. The English translation. Mitchell PC, ed. 1908; GP Putnam's Sons: New York.

Meydani SN, Ha W-K. Immunologic effects of yogurt. *Am Clin Nutr*. 2000; 71:861-872.

Van de Water J, Keen CL, Gershwin ME. The influence of chronic yogurt consumption on immunity. *J Nutr*. 1999; 129:1492S-1495S.

Zinc

TRADE NAMES
Cold-eeze (Quigley Corp.), Zinc-15 (The Key Company), Zn-50 (Bio-Tech Pharmacal), Ken-Zinc (Kenyon Drug Co.), Zinimin (The Key Company), Zinc-ease (Republic Drug Co.), Zinc Preferred (Reese Pharmaceutical), M2 Zinc 50 (Miller Pharmacal).

DESCRIPTION
Zinc is an essential element in human and animal nutrition with a wide range of biological roles. Zinc plays catalytic, structural or regulatory roles in the more than 200 zinc metalloenzymes that have been identified in biological systems. These enzymes are involved in nucleic acid and protein metabolism and the production of energy, among other things. Zinc plays a structural role in the formation of

the so-called zinc fingers. Zinc fingers are exploited by transcription factors for interacting with DNA and regulating the activity of genes. Another structural role of zinc is in the maintenance of the integrity of biological membranes resulting in their protection against oxidative injury, among other things.

Zinc is a metallic element with atomic number 30 and an atomic weight of 65.37 daltons. Its atomic symbol is Zn. Zinc exists under physiological conditions in the divalent state. The adult body contains about 1.5 to 2.5 grams of zinc. It is present in all organs, tissues, fluids and secretions. Approximately 90% of total body zinc is found in skeletal muscle and bone. Over 95% of total body zinc is bound to proteins within cells and cell membranes. Plasma contains only 0.1% of total body zinc. Most of the zinc (75% to 88%) in blood is found in the red blood cell zinc metalloenzyme carbonic anhydrase. In the plasma, approximately 18% of zinc is bound to alpha-2-macroglobulin, 80% to albumin and 2% to such proteins as transferrin and ceruloplasmin.

Physiologically, zinc is vital for growth and development, sexual maturation and reproduction, dark vision adaptation, olfactory and gustatory activity, insulin storage and release and for a variety of host immune defenses, among other things. Zinc deficiency can result in growth retardation, immune dysfunction, increased incidence of infections, hypogonadism, oligospermia, anorexia, diarrhea, weight loss, delayed wound healing, neural tube defects of the fetus, increased risk for abortion, alopecia, mental lethargy and skin changes.

Moderate to severe zinc deficiency is rare in industrialized countries. However, it is highly prevalent in developing countries. Many, however, are at risk for mild zinc deficiency in industrialized countries. Several diseases and situations predispose to zinc deficiency, including the autosomal recessive disease acrodermatitis enteropathica, alcoholism, malabsorption, thermal burns, total parenteral nutrition (TPN) without zinc supplementation and certain drugs, such as diuretics, penicillamine, sodium valproate and ethambutol. Zinc intake in many of the elderly may be suboptimal and, if compounded with certain drugs and diseases, can lead to mild or even moderate zinc deficiency.

Zinc acetate is an FDA-approved orphan drug for the treatment of the copper-overload disorder Wilson's disease.

ACTIONS AND PHARMACOLOGY
ACTIONS
Zinc may have immunomodulatory activity. It may also have antioxidant activity. Zinc has putative antiviral, fertility-enhancing and retinoprotective activities.

MECHANISM OF ACTION
Zinc is required for a number of immune functions, including T-lymphocyte activity. Zinc deficiency results in thymic involution, depressed delayed hypersensitivity, decreased peripheral T-lymphocyte count, decreased proliferative T-lymphocyte response to phytohemagglutinin (PHA), decreased cytotoxic T-lymphocyte activity, depressed T helper lymphocyte function, depressed natural killer cell activity, depressed macrophage function (phagocytosis), depressed neutrophil functions (respiratory burst, chemotaxis) and depressed antibody production. Zinc supplementation can restore impaired immune function in those with zinc deficiency, as found in malabsorption syndromes and acrodermatitis enteropathica.

There is little evidence that zinc supplementation will enhance immune responses in those who are not zinc deficient. High doses of zinc may even be immunosuppressive. Zinc supplementation may improve immune function in healthy elderly individuals who are marginally zinc deficient.

The mechanism underlying the immune effects of zinc is not fully understood. Some of these effects may be accounted for by zinc's membrane-stabilization effect. This could affect signaling processes involved in cell-mediated immunity. Zinc is known to be involved in such signaling processes. Zinc may also influence gene expression by structural stabilization of different immunological transcription factors. Zinc ions can induce blast formation of human peripheral blood monocytes (PBMCs). In PBMCs, zinc induces cytokines, including interleukin (IL)-1, IL-6 and tumor necrosis factor (TNF)-alpha. Cytokine induction by zinc is caused by a direct interaction of zinc with monocytes. The stimulation by zinc of T-lymphocytes appears to occur via monocyte released IL-1 and cell-cell contact. High zinc concentrations inhibit T-lymphocyte proliferation by blocking the IL-1 type 1 receptor-associated kinase. T-lymphocyte activation appears to be delicately regulated by zinc concentrations.

Zinc may have secondary antioxidant activity. Zinc does not have redox activity under physiological conditions. Zinc may influence membrane structure by its ability to stabilize thiol groups and phospholipids. It may also occupy sites that might otherwise contain redox active metals such as iron. These effects may protect membranes against oxidative damage. Zinc also comprises the structure of copper/zinc-superoxide dismutase (Cu/Zn-SOD). Zinc plays a structural role in Cu/Zn-SOD. Zinc may also have antioxidant activity via its association with the copper-binding protein metallothionein.

The role of zinc gluconate in the management of the common cold remains controversial (see Research Summary). The mechanisms proposed for zinc's effects on the duration of colds are inhibition by zinc of the replication of rhinoviruses and/or inhibition of virus entry into cells. Zinc ions, however, have only modest nonselective inhibitory effects for rhinoviruses *in vitro*.

Zinc is involved in sperm formation and testosterone metabolism. Zinc deficiency results in oligospermia. There is little evidence that zinc supplementation affects sperm production in those who are not zinc deficient.

The mechanism of the putative effect of zinc in age-related macular degeneration (ARMD) is unknown.

PHARMACOKINETICS

The efficiency of absorption (fractional absorption) of a zinc salt on an empty stomach ranges from 40% to 90%. The fractional absorption of zinc with food appears to be lower. Zinc-histidine, zinc-methionine and zinc-cysteine complexes appear to be more efficiently absorbed than other zinc supplementary forms. Zinc is absorbed all along the small intestine. Most ingested zinc appears to be absorbed from the jejunum. Zinc uptake across the brush border appears to occur by both a saturable barrier-mediated mechanism and a nonsaturable nonmediated mechanism. The exact mechanism of zinc transport into the enterocytes remains unclear. Zinc transporters have been identified in animal models. Once zinc is within the enterocyte, it can be used for zinc-dependent processes, become bound to metallothionein and held within the enterocyte or pass through the cell. Transport of zinc across the serosal membrane is carrier mediated and energy dependent.

Zinc is transported to the liver via the portal circulation. A fraction of zinc is extracted by the hepatocytes, and the remaining zinc is transported to the various cells of the body via the systemic circulation. Zinc is transported in the plasma bound to albumin (about 80%), alpha-2-macroglobulin (about 18%) and to such proteins as transferrin and ceruloplasmin (about 2%). The major route of zinc excretion is via the gastrointestinal tract. Fecal zinc excretion is comprised of unabsorbed zinc and zinc derived from biliary, pancreatic, and gastrointestinal secretions and zinc from sloughing of mucosal cells.

Much of the pharmacokinetics of zinc in humans is unknown. Research is ongoing.

INDICATIONS AND USAGE

Even borderline zinc deficiency or disturbances in zinc metabolism can have profound adverse health effects. Those at greatest risk of such deficiencies and disturbances include infants, children, the elderly and pregnant women. Due to conditions that can limit the bioavailability of zinc, even

when there is adequate zinc intake, zinc deficiency may affect still larger populations.

Among diseases and conditions associated with zinc deficiency are alcoholism, malabsorption syndromes, acrodermatitis enteropathica, anorexia nervosa, thermal burns and total parenteral nutrition (TPN) without zinc supplementation. Supplemental zinc may be helpful in some of the foregoing, in some conditions of immune impairment, in some complications of pregnancy, in the prevention of some cases of fetal neural tube defects, diarrhea, oligospermia, delayed wound healing and some cognitive disorders. It may also help protect against some inflammatory conditions.

Widely publicized claims that zinc is efficacious in preventing and ameliorating symptoms of the common cold are supported by some studies but not by others. There is the suggestion in some experimental research that zinc might have some anticarcinogenic effects. There is little evidence that zinc is helpful in diabetes. Topical zinc is useful in treating some skin conditions. Claims that it can prevent or reverse baldness are unsubstantiated except in some cases of severe zinc deficiency. It has no effect on typical male pattern baldness. It may be useful in dysguesia (taste disorder) in those who are zinc deficient. There is preliminary research suggesting that it might help some with macular degeneration.

RESEARCH SUMMARY

Zinc deficiency has been shown to impair immunity in many ways. It decreases T- and B-lymphocyte function and diminishes proliferative responses to mitogens. It also reduces the biological activity of many cytokines. Zinc deficiency has been shown to impair placental transport of antibodies from mother to fetus. Even mild zinc deficiency has been shown to produce an imbalance between cell-mediated and humoral immunity. Zinc supplementation has reversed many of these and other immune deficits in several *in vitro*, animal and human studies.

Supplementation with zinc reduced the incidence of childhood pneumonia by 41% and incidence of diarrhea in children by 25%, according to the findings of a review of ten randomized, controlled studies in the developing world. Zinc was found, in this review analysis, to be more effective than any other treatment for childhood pneumonia and was said to equal most other effective interventives for diarrhea in these populations. The diarrheas studied were related to diminished immune competence and high rates of exposure to infectious diseases. The significance of these findings is underscored by the fact that respiratory infections, and pneumonia in particular, are the cause of approximately one-third of all deaths among children in developing countries.

Many healthy elderly individuals and even more unhealthy elderly have marginal zinc deficiencies. There is both clinical and experimental evidence of impaired T-lymphocyte function, with associated increases in morbidity and mortality due to infectious diseases, among the elderly. Zinc deficiency has been shown to play a key role in this situation. Zinc supplementation in the elderly has produced mixed results with respect to immune restoration. Many researchers agree, however, that some of the negative results are probably due to the heterogeneity of elderly populations with respect to immune response, and most call for better-designed studies to bring hitherto ambiguous data into sharper focus.

Disturbances in metabolism, as well as zinc deficiency, have been associated with some inflammatory conditions, including some inflammatory bowel diseases and rheumatoid arthritis. The use of supplemental zinc in gastrointestinal inflammation, however, is highly experimental and is not without peril since inappropriate or uncontrolled administration can exacerbate, rather than ameliorate, some of these conditions. In some circumstances, however, supplemental zinc has enhanced the mucosal capacity of the small bowel to absorb water and electrolytes, thus easing inflammation. There is also some experimental evidence that zinc can stimulate tissue repair in some ulcer conditions.

There is some preliminary clinical evidence that supplemental zinc can produce benefit in some with rheumatoid arthritis. Diminished plasma zinc has been reported in some with this disease. Zinc has demonstrated an ability to inhibit mixed lymphocyte reaction in some of these subjects. Some researchers have suggested that further research is warranted to see if zinc might be a useful new therapy in T-cell-mediated auto-immune and graft-versus-host diseases.

Diminished zinc status has been associated with HIV disease and higher incidence of opportunistic infections. Zinc supplementation has produced higher CD4+ lymphocyte cell counts and reduced incidence of bacterial infections among patients with HIV disease in one study.

In a double-blind study, subjects were randomized to receive zinc lozenges containing 13.3 milligrams of zinc every two hours while awake for as long as they had symptoms of the common cold. Subjects were enrolled within 24 hours of first reporting cold symptoms. Median time to complete resolution of cold symptoms was 4.4 days in those supplemented with zinc, compared with 7.6 days in those receiving placebo. Patients dissolved the lozenges in their mouths, rather than immediately swallowing them.

A recent review of studies found findings similar to those reported above in three additional studies. Four other studies, however, found no benefit from zinc in shortening duration of cold symptoms. In one of the other positive studies, zinc supplementation reduced duration of symptoms by 42%, compared with placebo, when initiated on the first day of symptoms. When withheld until the second day, zinc reduced cold duration by 26%, compared with placebo.

Some have challenged the validity of the four studies that found no zinc effect ''on the basis of poor bioavailability of the zinc lozenge preparations, either due to a proposed failure of the lozenge formulations to provide adequate amounts of free zinc ions to the saliva and oral tissues or due to doses of zinc in the lozenge that were below a possible therapeutic threshold.''

On the other hand, some have also argued that there were significant methodological flaws in some of the positive studies. The only conclusion that can be reached at this time is that studies to date, when examined all together, are inconclusive.

Zinc supplementation has reversed some of the signs of anorexia nervosa, including weight loss, in some women. Weight has increased in some zinc-supplemented women with this condition, and menstruation has been restored in some supplemented with zinc.

Zinc supplementation has overcome some forms of both female and male infertility in those who are zinc deficient. Zinc is essential for proper formation and maturation of spermatozoa.

Zinc plays many roles in pregnancy, and disturbances in zinc metabolism, as well as zinc deficiency, can have serious adverse effects on the course of pregnancy and upon the growth of the fetus and newborn. Zinc deficiency can be teratogenic, producing neural tube defects. Zinc is also very important to the newborn when breast milk may be its only source of zinc (during the first few months of life). Premature infants may be at even greater risk of zinc deficiency. Impaired disease resistance and diminished vaccine efficacy in infants may result from zinc deficiency at this stage. Some studies have shown that giving 15 milligrams of zinc daily to breast-feeding mothers produced more weight gain in their babies than in the babies of unsupplemented mothers. Zinc supplementation in infants not breast fed have also shown benefits. Zinc supplementation has also shown benefit in regulating and promoting proper growth in some groups of young children with non-organic failure to thrive.

There is some evidence that zinc can promote and accelerate wound healing in some circumstances. There is very preliminary experimental evidence that it may have some protective effects against prostate cancer and some equally preliminary data suggesting that it might enhance neuropsychological performance in children, most likely those with zinc deficiencies.

There was an early report that 100 milligrams of zinc twice a day with meals significantly reduced visual loss in subjects with macular degeneration. This placebo-controlled, double-blind study warrants followup.

CONTRAINDICATIONS, PRECAUTIONS, ADVERSE REACTIONS
CONTRAINDICATIONS
Zinc is contraindicated in those who are hypersensitive to any component of a zinc-containing supplement.

PRECAUTIONS
Pregnant women and nursing mothers should avoid zinc doses higher than RDA amounts (15 milligrams/day for pregnant women, 19 mg/day for lactating women during the first six months and 16 mg/day for lactating women during the second six months).

ADVERSE REACTIONS
Doses of zinc up to 30 milligrams daily are generally well tolerated. Higher doses may cause adverse reactions. The most common adverse reactions are gastrointestinal and include nausea, vomiting and gastrointestinal discomfort. Other adverse reactions include a metallic taste, headache and drowsiness. There are some reports of decreased HDL-cholesterol in those taking high doses of zinc. Chronic intake of high doses of zinc can lead to copper deficiency and hypochromic, microcytic anemia secondary to zinc-induced copper deficiency.

High doses of zinc may be immunosuppressive.

INTERACTIONS
DRUGS
Bisphosphonates (alendronate, etidronate, risedronate): Concomitant intake of a bisphosphonate and zinc may decrease the absorption of both the bisphosphonate and zinc.

Quinolones (ciprofloxacin, gatifloxacin, levofloxacin, lomefloxacin, moxifloxacin, norfloxacin, ofloxacin, sparfloxacin, trovafloxacin): Concomitant intake of a quinolone and zinc may decrease the absorption of both the quinolone and zinc.

Penicillamine: Concomitant intake of penicillamine and zinc may depress absorption of zinc.

Tetracyclines (doxycycline, monocycline, tetracycline): Concomitant intake of a tetracycline and zinc may decrease the absorption of both the tetracycline and zinc.

NUTRITIONAL SUPPLEMENTS
Calcium: Concomitant intake of calcium and zinc may depress zinc absorption in postmenopausal women.

Copper: Concomitant intake of copper and zinc may depress the absorption of copper. Intake of large doses of zinc can negatively affect the copper status of the body. This is the basis for the use of high doses of zinc for the treatment of Wilson's disease. It is thought that high intakes of zinc induce synthesis of the copper-binding protein metallothionine in the gastrointestinal mucosal cells. Metallothionine can sequester copper. This makes copper unavailable for copper absorption.

L-cysteine: Concomitant intake of L-cysteine and zinc may enhance the absorption of zinc.

L-histidine: Concomitant intake of L-histidine and zinc may enhance the absorption of zinc.

Inositol Hexaphosphate: Concomitant intake of inositol hexaphosphate and zinc may depress the absorption of zinc.

Iron: Concomitant intake of iron and zinc may depress the absorption of both iron and zinc.

L-methionine: Concomitant intake of L-methionine and zinc may enhance the absorption of zinc.

N-acetyl-L-cysteine (NAC): Concomitant intake of NAC and zinc may enhance the absorption of zinc.

Phosphate Salts: Concomitant administration of zinc and phosphate salts may decrease the absorption of zinc.

FOODS
Caffeine: Concomitant intake of coffee, caffeinated beverages or caffeine and zinc may depress the absorption of zinc.

Cysteine-containing Proteins: Foods rich in cysteine-containing proteins (e.g., animal muscle tissue) may increase the absorption of zinc if ingested concomitantly.

Oxalic Acid: Concomitant intake of zinc with foods rich in oxalic acid (spinach, sweet potatoes, rhubarb and beans) may depress the absorption of zinc.

Phytic Acid Concomitant intake of zinc with foods rich in phytic acid (unleavened bread, raw beans, seeds, nuts and grains and soy isolates) may depress the absorption of zinc.

Tea: Concomitant intake of tea (tannins) and zinc may cause decreased absorption of zinc.

OVERDOSAGE
There are no reports of overdosage from use of zinc supplements.

DOSAGE AND ADMINISTRATION
There are several zinc supplementary forms. These include zinc gluconate, zinc oxide, zinc aspartate, zinc picolinate, zinc citrate, zinc monomethionine and zinc histidine. Zinc supplements are available in stand-alone or in combination products. A typical dose of zinc is about 15 milligrams (as elemental zinc) daily.

The Food and Nutrition Board of the National Academy of Sciences has recommended the following Recommended Dietary Allowances (RDA) for zinc:

Age (years) or Status	RDA (milligrams/day)
0-1	5
1-10	10
Males 11-51+	15
Females 11-51+	12
Pregnant	15
Lactating	
First 6 months	19
Second 6 months	16

HOW SUPPLIED

All strengths are expressed as total zinc content.

Zinc is available as a chelate in the following forms and strengths:

Tablets — 15 mg, 22.5 mg, 25 mg, 30 mg, 50 mg

Zinc gluconate is available in the following forms and strengths:

Liquid — 15 mg/mL

Lozenges — 10 mg, 13.3 mg, 23 mg

Tablets — 15 mg, 20 mg, 22 mg, 30 mg, 40 mg, 50 mg, 60 mg, 100 mg

Zinc picolinate is available in the following forms and strengths:

Capsules — 25 mg, 30 mg, 50 mg

Tablets — 50 mg

LITERATURE

Anon. Zinc lozenges reduce cold symptoms. *Nutr Rev.* 1997; 55:82-88.

Berg JM, Shi Y. The galvanization of biology: a growing appreciation for the roles of zinc. *Science.* 1996; 271:1081-1085.

Bhutta ZA, Black RE, Brown KH, et al. Prevention of diarrhea and pneumonia by zinc supplementation in children in developing countries: Pooled analysis of randomized controlled trials. *J Pediatr.* 1999; 135:689-697.

Chandra RK. Excessive intake of zinc impairs immune response. *JAMA.* 1984; 252:1443-1446.

Cuajungco MP, Lees GJ. Zinc metabolism in the brain; relevance to human neurodegenerative disorders. *Neurobiol Dis.* 1997; 4:137-169.

Duchateau J, Delepesse G, Vrijens R, et al. Beneficial effects of oral zinc duration on the immune response of old people. *Am J Med.* 1981; 70:1001-1004.

Fabris N, Mocchegiani E. Zinc, human diseases and aging. *Aging Clin Exp Res.* 1995; 7:77-93.

Grü ngreiff K, Grü ngreiff S, Reinhold D. Zinc deficiency and hepatic encephalopathy: results of a long-term follow-up on zinc supplementation. *J Trace Elem Exp Med.* 2000; 13:21-31.

Hambridge M. Human zinc deficiency. *J Nutr.* 2000; 130:1344S-1349S.

Jackson JL, Peterson C, Lesho E. A meta-analysis of zinc salts, lozenges and the common cold. *Arch Intern Med.* 1997; 157:2373-2376.

King JC, Keen CL. Zinc. In: Shils ME, Olson JA, Shike M, Ross AC, eds. Modern *Nutrition in Health and Disease.* Baltimore, MD: Williams and Wilkins; 1999:223-239.

Klug A, Rhodes D. "Zinc fingers": a novel protein motif for nucleic acid recognition. *Trends Biochem Sci.* 1987; 5:464-469.

Lonnerdal B. Dietary factors influencing zinc absorption. *J Nutr.* 2000; 130(5S Suppl): 1378S-1383S.

Macknin ML. Zinc lozenges for the common cold. *Cleveland Clin J Med.* 1999; 66:27-31.

Macknin ML. Piedmonte M, Calendine C, et al. Zinc gluconate lozenges for treating the common cold in children. A randomized controlled trial. *JAMA.* 1998; 279:1962-1967.

Mares-Perlman JA, Klein R, Klein BE, et al. Association of zinc and antioxidant nutrients with age-related maculopathy. *Arch Opthalmol.* 1996; 114:991-997.

Mc Mahon RJ, Cousins RJ. Mammalian zinc transporters. *J Nutr.* 1998; 128:667-670.

McMahon RJ, Cousins RJ. Regulation of the zinc transporter ZnT-1 by dietary zinc. *Proc Natl Acad Sci USA.* 1998; 95:4841-4846.

Mossad SB, Macknin ML, Medendorp SV, Mason PM. Zinc gluconate lozenges for treating the common cold. Ann Intern Med. 1996; 125:81-88.

Newsome DA, Swartz M, Leone NC. Oral zinc in macular degeneration. *Arch Opthalmol.* 1988; 106:192-198.

Noseworthy MD, Bray TM. Zinc deficiency exacerbates loss of blood-brain barrier integrity induced by hyperoxia measured by dynamic MRI. *Proc Soc Exp Biol Med.* 2000; 223:175-182.

O'Dell BL. Role of zinc in plasma membrane function. *J Nutr.* 2000; 130:1432S-1436S.

Olsen RJ, Olsen P. Zinc as a treatment for age related macular degeneration (review). *J Trace Elem Exp Med.* 1998; 11:137-145.

Prasad AS. Zinc deficiency in women, infants and children. *J Am Coll Nutr.* 1996; 15:113-120.

Prasad AS. Zinc: the biology and therapeutics of an ion. *Ann Intern Med.* 1996; 125:142-144.

Prasad AS. Discovery of human zinc deficiency and studies in an experimental human model. *Am J Clin Nutr.* 1991; 53:403-412.

Salgueiro MJ, Zubillaga M, Lysionek AK, et al. Zinc an essential micronutrient: a review. *Nutr Rev.* 2000; 20:737-755.

Sandstead HH, Frederickson CJ, Penland JG. History of zinc as related to brain function. *J Nutr*. 2000; 130:496S-502S.

Sazawal S, Black RE, Bhan MK, et al. Zinc supplementation in young children with acute diarrhea in India. *N Engl J Med*. 1995; 333:839-844.

Solomons NW. Mild human zinc deficiency produces an imbalance between cell-mediated and humoral immunity. *Nutr Rev*. 1998; 56:27-28.

Sturniolo GC, Di Leo V, Barollo M, et al. The many functions of zinc in inflammatory conditions of the gastrointestinal tract. *J Trace Elem Exp Med*. 2000; 13:33-39.

Umeta M, West CE, Haidar J, et al. Zinc supplementation and stunted infants in Ethiopia: a randomized controlled trial. *Lancet*. 2000; 355:2021-2026.

Combination Product Tables

On the following pages you'll find a series of tables designed to provide you with an at-a-glance comparison of related multi-ingredient products. Both prescription and over-the-counter supplements are included. The tables cover five product types:

■ Calcium Combination Products
■ Iron Combination Products
■ Multivitamin Products
■ Multivitamin and Mineral Products
■ Vitamin B Complex Products

Entries in each table have been organized roughly in order of the potency of the primary ingredients.

Products that contain equal amounts of the same ingredients are grouped together.

Secondary ingredients—nutrients found only in selected products—are covered in the "Other" column at the right of each table. In the table of Multivitamin and Mineral Products, many of which include a substantial number of trace elements and other nutrients, this column merely indicates whether or not other ingredients appear in the formulation. For a complete list of the extra ingredients found in each product, check the alphabetical product listings immediately following the table.

Calcium Combination Products

PRODUCT/FORM (MANUFACTURER)	CALCIUM (MG)	VITAMIN D (IU)	CALCIUM FORM	OTHER
Vita-Calcium Wafers (Vitaline Corporation)	1000	400	Calcium carbonate	
Cal-600 W/D Tablets (PDK Labs Inc.)	600	200	Calcium carbonate	
Calcarb 600 W/Vitamin D Tablets (Zenith Goldline Pharmaceuticals)				
Calcium 600/Vitamin D Tablets (Cardinal Health, Inc.)				
Calcium 600 + Vitamin D Tablets (Perrigo)				
Calcium-600 W/D Tablets (American Pharmacal, Inc.)				
Calcium/Vitamin D Tablets (Mckesson Drug Company)				
Caltrate 600 + D Tablets (Lederle Consumer Health)				
Liqua-Cal Capsules (The Key Company)				
Liquid Calcium Plus Vitamin D Capsules (Mason Vitamins, Inc.)				
Super Calcium W/Vitamin D Tablets (Mason Vitamins, Inc.)				
Calcium 600-D Tablets (Rugby Laboratories, Inc.)	600	125	Calcium carbonate	
Calcium 600/Vitamin D Tablets (Basic Vitamins)				
Calcium 600/Vitamin D Tablets (Bergen Brunswig Drug Company)				
Calcium 600 Plus Vitamin D Tablets (Nature's Bounty, Inc.)				
Calcium Carbonate/Vitamin D Tablets (Major Pharmaceuticals)				

PRODUCT/FORM (MANUFACTURER)	CALCIUM (MG)	VITAMIN D (IU)	CALCIUM FORM	OTHER
Calcium Carbonate/Vitamin D Tablets (National Vitamin Company, Inc.)	600	125	Calcium carbonate	
Calcium Carbonate/Vitamin D Tablets (PD-Rx Pharmaceuticals Inc.)				
Daily Calcium + Vitamin D Tablets (Nature's Bounty, Inc.)				
Oyster Shell Calcium/Vitamin D Tablets (Reese Pharmaceutical Company)				
Super Calcium W/Vitamin D Tablets (Mason Vitamins, Inc.)				
Calcium 1200 W/Vitamin D Capsules (Rexall Consumer Products)	600	100	Calcium carbonate	
Marblen Tablets (Fleming & Company)	520		Calcium carbonate	Magnesium carbonate 400 mg
Marblen Suspension (Fleming & Company)	520 mg/5 mL		Calcium carbonate	Magnesium carbonate 400 mg/5 mL
Calcium/Vitamin D Tablets (PD-Rx Pharmaceuticals Inc.)	500	200	Calcium carbonate	
Os-Cal 500 + D Tablets (Smithkline Beecham Consumer Healthcare)				
Oyster Shell Calcium/Vitamin D Tablets (American Pharmacal, Inc.)				
Oyster Shell Calcium/Vitamin D Tablets (Bergen Brunswig Drug Company)				
Oyster Shell Calcium/Vitamin D Tablets (Mckesson Drug Company)				
Oyster Shell Calcium/Vitamin D Tablets (Perrigo)				
Oyster Shell Calcium Natural/Vit D Tablets (Cardinal Health, Inc.)				
Calcium 500 W/Vitamin D Tablets (Basic Vitamins)	500	125	Calcium carbonate	

PRODUCT/FORM (MANUFACTURER)	CALCIUM (MG)	VITAMIN D (IU)	CALCIUM FORM	OTHER
Calcium 900 W/Vitamin D Capsules (Rexall Consumer Products)	300	100	Calcium carbonate	
Calcium Carbonate/Vitamin D Tablets (Heartland Healthcare Services)	250	125	Calcium carbonate	
Calcium Carbonate/Vitamin D Tablets (Sky Pharmaceuticals Packaging, Inc.)				
Os-Cal 250 + D Tablets (Smithkline Beecham Consumer Healthcare)				
Oysco D Tablets (Rugby Laboratories, Inc.)				
Oyst-Cal-D Tablets (Zenith Goldline Pharmaceuticals)				
Oyster Shell Calcium/Vitamin D Tablets (American Pharmacal, Inc.)				
Oyster Shell Calcium/Vitamin D Tablets (Basic Vitamins)				
Oyster Shell Calcium/Vitamin D Tablets (Bergen Brunswig Drug Company)				
Oyster Shell Calcium/Vitamin D Tablets (Dixon-Shane Drug Company)				
Oyster Shell Calcium/Vitamin D Tablets (Major Pharmaceuticals)				
Oyster Shell Calcium/Vitamin D Tablets (Mason Vitamins, Inc.)				
Oyster Shell Calcium/Vitamin D Tablets (Mckesson Drug Company)				
Oyster Shell Calcium/Vitamin D Tablets (National Vitamin Company, Inc.)				
Oyster Shell Calcium/Vitamin D Tablets (Rexall Consumer Products)				
Oyster Shell Calcium/Vitamin D Tablets (Vangard Labs, Inc.)				
Oystercal-D 250 Tablets (Nature's Bounty, Inc.)				

PRODUCT/FORM (MANUFACTURER)	CALCIUM (MG)	VITAMIN D (IU)	CALCIUM FORM	OTHER
Calcium 500 W/Vitamin D Tablets (Mason Vitamins, Inc.)	500	125	Calcium carbonate	
Calcium 500 W/Vitamin D Tablets (Rexall Consumer Products)				
Calcium Carbonate/Vitamin D Tablets (Compumed Pharmaceuticals, Inc.)				
Calcium Carbonate/Vitamin D Tablets (Heartland Healthcare Services)				
Calcium Carbonate/Vitamin D Tablets (Sky Pharmaceuticals Packaging, Inc.)				
Oysco 500 + D Tablets (Rugby Laboratories, Inc.)				
Oyst-Cal-D 500 Tablets (Zenith Goldline Pharmaceuticals)				
Oyster Shell Calcium 500 W/D Tablets (The Medicine Shoppe)				
Oyster Shell Calcium/Vitamin D Tablets (Major Pharmaceuticals)				
Oyster Shell Calcium/Vitamin D Tablets (Mason Vitamins, Inc.)				
Oyster Shell Calcium/Vitamin D Tablets (National Vitamin Company, Inc.)				
Oyster Shell Calcium/Vitamin D Tablets (Vangard Labs, Inc.)				
Oystercal-D 500 Tablets (Nature's Bounty, Inc.)				
Oyster Shell Calcium 1000/Vitamin D Tablets (Mason Vitamins, Inc.)	380	250	Calcium carbonate	
Oyster Shell Calcium 1000/Vitamin D Tablets (Rexall Consumer Products)				
Florical Capsules (Mericon Industries, Inc.)	364		Calcium carbonate	Sodium fluoride 8.3 mg
Florical Tablets (Mericon Industries, Inc.)				

PRODUCT/FORM (MANUFACTURER)	CALCIUM (MG)	VITAMIN D (IU)	CALCIUM FORM	OTHER
One-A-Day Bone Strength Tablets (Bayer Corp., Consumer Care Division)	500	100		Soybean 28 mg
Viactiv Chewable Tablets (Mead Johnson & Company)	500	100		Vitamin K 0.04 mg
AdvaCal Capsules (Lane Labs)	450			Minerals and Amino Acids
Calcium/Magnesium/Zinc Tablets (Cardinal Health, Inc.)	333			Magnesium 133 mg, Zinc 5 mg
Parva-Cal 250 Tablets (Freeda Vitamins, Inc.)	250	100		
Magnebind 400 Rx Tablets (Nephro-Tech, Inc.)	200			Folic Acid 1 mg, Magnesium carbonate 400 mg
Cal/Mag Chewable Tablets (Freeda Vitamins, Inc.)	200			Magnesium 100 mg
Calcium & Magnesium Chelate Capsules (The Key Company)	180			Magnesium 90 mg
Magnebind 200 Tablets (Nephro-Tech, Inc.)	160			Magnesium 57 mg
Calcet Tablets (Mission Pharmacal Co.)	150	100		
Ferosul Tablets (Major Pharmaceuticals)	112			Iron 50 mg
Cal/Mag Chelated Tablets (Freeda Vitamins, Inc.)	100			Magnesium 50 mg

PRODUCT/FORM (MANUFACTURER)	CALCIUM (MG)	VITAMIN D (IU)	CALCIUM FORM	OTHER
Magnebind 300 Tablets (Nephro-Tech, Inc.)	250		Calcium carbonate	Magnesium carbonate 300 mg
Monocal Tablets (Mericon Industries, Inc.)	250		Calcium carbonate	Sodium monofluorophosphate 3 mg
Liquid Calcium Capsules (Major Pharmaceuticals)	200	200	Calcium carbonate	Vitamin A 725 IU
Cal-Co3Y Capsules (Bio-Tech Pharmacal, Inc.)	200	100	Calcium carbonate	
Calcium Citrate W/Vitamin D Tablets (Mason Vitamins, Inc.)	1500	200	Calcium citrate	
Citracal + D Tablets (Mission Pharmacal Co.)		200		
Calcium Citrate + D Tablets (Cardinal Health, Inc.)	315	200	Calcium citrate	
Calcium Citrate/Vitamin D Tablets (Bergen Brunswig Drug Company)				
Citrus Calcium + D Tablets (Rugby Laboratories, Inc.)				
Calcium/Magnesium/Zinc Tablets (Rexall Consumer Products)	1000			Magnesium 500 mg, Zinc 50 mg
Healthy Woman Bone Health Supplement Tablets (Personal Products Company)	600	280		
One-A-Day Calcium Plus Chewable Tablets (Bayer Consumer)	500	100		Magnesium 50 mg

Iron Combination Products

PRODUCT/FORM (MANUFACTURER)	DEA	IRON SULFATE (MG)	IRON FUMARATE (MG)	IRON CARBONYL (MG)	IRON (MG)	POLYSACCHARIDE IRON COMPLEX (MG)	A (IU)	D (IU)	E (IU)	C (MG)	B1 (MG)	B2 (MG)	NIACIN/NIACINAMIDE B3 (MG)	CALCIUM PANTOTHENATE B5 (MG)	B6 (MG)	B12 (MG)	FOLIC ACID (MG)	OTHER
Fero-Folic 500 Extended Release Tablets (Abbott Pharmaceutical)	Rx	525								500							0.8	
Iberet-Folic-500 Extended Release Tablets (Abbott Pharmaceutical)	Rx	105								500	6	6	30	10	5	0.025	0.8	
Multi-Ferrous Folic Extended Release Tablets (United Research Laboratories, Inc.)																		
Multiret Folic-500 Extended Release Tablets (Amide Pharmaceuticals, Inc.)																		
Fero-Grad-500 Extended Release Tablets (Abbott Pharmaceutical)	OTC	105								500								
Vitelle Irospan Extended Release Tablets and Extended Release Capsules (Fielding Pharmaceutical Company)	OTC	60								150								
Slow FE W/Folic Acid Extended Release Tablets (Novartis Consumer Health, Inc.)	OTC	50															0.4	
Iron Advanced Tablets (Rexall Consumer)	OTC			25														Calcium 58.5 mg
Tolfrinic Tablets (Ascher, B.F. & Co., Inc.)	Rx		600							100						0.025		
Chromagen Forte Capsules (Savage Laboratories)	Rx		460							60						0.01	1	
Ed Cyte F Tablets (Edwards Pharmaceuticals, Inc.)	Rx		324														1	
Equi-Cyte F Tablets (Equipharm Corp.)																		
Hematin-F Tablets (Cypress Pharmaceutical Inc.)																		
Hemocyte-F Tablets (U.S. Pharmaceutical Corp.)																		

PRODUCT/FORM (MANUFACTURER)	DEA	IRON SULFATE (MG)	IRON FUMARATE (MG)	IRON CARBONYL (MG)	IRON (MG)	POLYSACCHARIDE IRON COMPLEX (MG)	A (IU)	D (IU)	E (IU)	C (MG)	B1 (MG)	B2 (MG)	NIACIN/NIACINAMIDE B3 (MG)	CALCIUM PANTOTHENATE B5 (MG)	B6 (MG)	B12 (MG)	FOLIC ACID (MG)	OTHER
Nephro-Fer Rx Tablets (R & D Laboratories, Inc.)	Rx		324														1	
Ircon-FA Tablets (Kenwood Therapeutics)	OTC		250														0.8	
Anemagen Capsules (Ethex Corporation)	Rx		200							250						0.01	1	
Chromagen FA Tablets (Savage Laboratories)																		
Anemagen FA Capsules (Ethex Corporation)	Rx		200							250						0.01	1	Stomach, Desiccated 100 mg
Fetrin Extended Release Capsules (Lunsco, Inc.)	Rx		200							60						0.005		
Fumatinic Extended Release Capsules (Laser, Inc.)																		
DSS W/Iron Extended Release Capsules (American Pharmacal, Inc.)	OTC		150															Docusate Sodium 100 mg
Ferro-DSS Extended Release Tablets (Time-Cap Labs)																		
Ferro-Sequels Extended Release Tablets (Inverness Medical, Inc.)																		
Ferrous Fumarate DS Extended Release Capsules (Vita-Rx Corp)																		
Iron W/Docusate Sodium Extended Release Tablets (Nature's Bounty, Inc.)																		
Vitron-C Plus Tablets (Novartis Consumer Health, Inc.)	OTC		132							250								
Promar Capsules (Marlop Pharmaceuticals, Inc.)	Rx		115							150						0.015	1	Intrinsic Factor 75 mg
Conison Capsules (Ethex Corporation)	Rx		110							75						0.015	0.5	Intrinsic Factor 240 mg
Contrin Capsules (Geneva Pharmaceuticals, Inc.)																		
Ferocon Capsules (Breckenridge Pharmaceutical Inc.)																		

PRODUCT/FORM (MANUFACTURER)	DEA	IRON SULFATE (MG)	IRON FUMARATE (MG)	IRON CARBONYL (MG)	IRON (MG)	POLYSACCHARIDE IRON COMPLEX (MG)	A (IU)	D (IU)	E (IU)	C (MG)	B1 (MG)	B2 (MG)	B3 (MG) NIACIN/NIACINAMIDE	B5 (MG) CALCIUM PANTOTHENATE	B6 (MG)	B12 (MG)	FOLIC ACID (MG)	OTHER
Ferotrinsic Capsules (Contract Pharmacal Corporation)	Rx	110								75						0.015	0.5	Intrinsic Factor 240 mg
Foltrin Capsules (Eon Labs Manufacturing, Inc.)																		
Martinic Capsules (Marlop Pharmaceuticals, Inc.)																		
Trinsicon Capsules (Marlex Pharmaceuticals, Inc.)																		
Vitron-C Tablets (Novartis Consumer Health, Inc.)	OTC		66							125								
Icar-C Plus Tablets (Hawthorn Pharmaceuticals)	Rx			100						250						0.025	1	
Multivitamins W/Iron Children's Chewable Tablets (Cardinal Health, Inc.)	OTC				15		2500	400	15	60	1.05	1.2	13.5		1.05	0.0045	0.3	
Irofol Tablets (Dayton Laboratories, Inc.)	Rx					150											1	
Ferrex 150 Forte Capsules (Breckenridge Pharmaceutical, Inc.)	Rx					150										0.025	1	
Fe-Tinic 150 Forte Capsules (Ethex Corporation)																		
Myferon 150 Forte Capsules (Me Pharmaceuticals)																		
Niferex-150 Forte Capsules (Schwarz Pharma)																		
Nu-Iron Plus Elixir (Merz Pharmaceuticals)	Rx					100*										0.025*	1*	
Icar-C Tablets (Hawthorn Pharmaceuticals)	OTC			100						250								
Infed Injection (Schein Pharmaceutical, Inc.)	Rx																	Iron Dextran 50 mg/mL

* per 5 mL

PRODUCT/FORM (MANUFACTURER)	DEA	IRON SULFATE (MG)	IRON FUMARATE (MG)	IRON CARBONYL (MG)	IRON (MG)	POLYSACCHARIDE IRON COMPLEX (MG)	A (IU)	D (IU)	E (IU)	C (MG)	B1 (MG)	B2 (MG)	NIACIN/NIACINAMIDE B3 (MG)	CALCIUM PANTOTHENATE B5 (MG)	B6 (MG)	B12 (MG)	FOLIC ACID (MG)	OTHER
Multi-Vitamin W/Iron Children's Liquid (Tri-Med Laboratories, Inc.)	OTC				10*		1500*	400*	5*	35*	0.5*	0.6*	8*		0.4*			
Chromagen Capsules (Savage Laboratories)	Rx				66					250						0.01		Stomach, Desiccated 100 mg
Ferragen Capsules (Pecos Pharmaceutical)																		
Iron-Folic 500 Tablets (Major Pharmaceuticals)	OTC				105					500	6	6	30	10	5	0.025	0.8	
Daily Multiple Vitamins/Iron Tablets (Vangard Labs, Inc.)	OTC				18		5000	400	30	60	1.5	1.7	20	10	2	0.006	0.4	
One Tablet Daily W/Iron Tablets (Zenith Goldline Pharmaceuticals)																		
Nutrinate Chewable Tablets (Ethex Corporation)	Rx				29		1000	400	11	120	2	3	20		10	0.012	1	
Prenafort Tablets (Cypress Pharmaceutical Inc.)	Rx				60		1000	400	11	120	2	3	20		10	0.012	1	
Thera Hematinic Tablets (Dixon-Shane Drug Company)	Rx				66.7		0.42†	0.0035†	5†	100	3.3	3.3	33.3	3.9		0.05	0.33	Calcium 11.7 mg, Copper 0.67 mg, Magnesium 41.7 mg
Theragran Hematinic Tablets (Apothecon Products)																		
Stress Formula + Iron Tablets (Cardinal Health, Inc.)	OTC				18					500	10	10	100	20	5	0.012	0.4	Biotin 0.045 mg
Vitamins W/Iron Children's Chewable Tablets (Marlex Pharmaceuticals, Inc.)	OTC				15		2500	400	15	60	1.05	1.2	13.5		1.05	0.0045	0.3	
Nephron FA Tablets (Nephro-Tech, Inc.)	Rx				66.6					300	1.5	1.7	20	10	10	0.006	1	Biotin 0.3 mg, Docusate Sodium 75 mg
Nephro-Vite + FE Tablets (R & D Laboratories, Inc.)	Rx				100					60	1.5	1.7	20	10	10	0.006	1	Biotin 0.3 mg

* per mL
† per mg

Multivitamin Products

PRODUCT/FORM (MANUFACTURER)	DEA	A (IU)	B1 (MG)	B2 (MG)	NIACIN, B3 (MG)	NIACINAMIDE B3 (MG)	CALCIUM PANTOTHENATE B5 (MG)	B6 (MG)	B12 (MG)	C (MG)	D (IU)	E (IU)	K (MG)	BIOTIN (MG)	FOLIC ACID (MG)	OTHER
Therapeutic Multivitamin Tablets (Bergen Brunswig Drug Company)	OTC	5000	3	3.4	20		0.01	3	0.009	90	400	30		0.03	0.4	Calcium 66 mg
Multivitamin Capsules (Numark Laboratories, Inc.)	OTC	5000	2.5	2.5		20	5	0.5	0.002	60	400	10				
Daily Multiple Vitamins Tablets (Marlex Pharmaceuticals, Inc.)	OTC	5000	2	2.5	20		1	1	0.001	50	800					
Once Daily Tablets (Prime Marketing)	OTC	5000	2	2.5		20	1	1	0.001	50	400					
Daily Multiple Vitamins W/Iron Tablets (Rexall Consumer Products)	OTC	5000	1.5	1.7		20	0.1	1	0.001	60	400				0.4	Iron 18 mg
Daily Multiple Vitamins Tablets (Rexall Consumer Products)	OTC	5000	1.5	1.7		20	1	1	0.001	60	400				0.4	
Daily Multivitamins Tablets (SKY Pharmaceuticals Packaging, Inc.)	OTC	5000	1.5	1.7		20	10	2	0.006	60	400	30			0.4	
One-A-Day Essential Tablets (Bayer Consumer)																
Multi-Vitamins Tablets (Rugby Laboratories, Inc.)	OTC	5000	1.5	2	20		1	0.1		37.5	400					
M.V.I.-12 Injection (AstraZeneca)	Rx	3300*	3*	3.6*		40*		4*	0.005*	100*	200*	10*		0.06*	0.4*	Dexpanthenol 15 mg/10 mL
Ultra Tabs Tablets (Major Pharmaceuticals)	Rx	2700	3	3.4		50		20	0.012	120	400	30			0.15	Calcium 200 mg, Copper 2 mg, Docusate Sodium 1 mg, Iodine 90 mg, Iron 20 mg, Zinc 25 mg
Bugs Bunny Plus Extra C Chewable Tablets (Bayer Consumer)	OTC	2500	1.05	1.2		13.5		1.05	0.0045	250	400	15			0.3	

* per 10 mL

PRODUCT/FORM (MANUFACTURER)	DEA	A (IU)	B1 (MG)	B2 (MG)	NIACIN, B3 (MG)	NIACINAMIDE, B3 (MG)	CALCIUM PANTOTHENATE, B5 (MG)	B6 (MG)	B12 (MG)	C (MG)	D (IU)	E (IU)	K (MG)	BIOTIN (MG)	FOLIC ACID (MG)	OTHER
Flintstones Plus Extra C Chewable Tablets (Bayer Consumer)	OTC	2500	1.05	1.2		13.5		1.05	0.0045	250	400	15			0.3	
Poly Vitamin Chewable Tablets (Rugby Laboratories, Inc.)	OTC	2500	1.05	1.2	13.5			1.05	0.0045	60	400	15			0.3	
Vitamins Children's Chewable Tablets (Prime Marketing)																
Circus Chews Children's Chewable Tablets (Rexall Consumer Products)	OTC	2500	1.05	1.2		13.5		1.05	0.0045	60	400	15			0.3	
Bugs Bunny Plus Iron Chewable Tablets (Bayer Consumer)	OTC	2500	1.05	1.2		13.5		1.05	0.0045	60	400	15			0.3	Iron 15 mg
Flintstones Original Children's Chewable Tablets (Bayer Consumer)																
Flintstones Plus Iron Chewable Tablets (Bayer Consumer)																
Flintstones Plus Calcium Chewable Tablets (Bayer Consumer)	OTC	2500	1.05	1.2		13.5		1.05	0.0045	60	400	15			0.3	Calcium 200 mg
M.V.I. Pediatric Powder for Injection (AstraZeneca)	Rx	2300	1.2	1.4		17		1	0.001	80	400	7	0.2	0.02	0.14	Dexpanthenol 5 mg
Key-Plex Injection (Hyrex Pharmaceuticals)	Rx		50*	5*		125*		5*	1*	50*						Dexpanthenol 6 mg/mL
BEC W/Zinc Tablets (Bergen Brunswig Drug Company)	OTC		15	10.2	100		25	10	0.006	600		45				Zinc 225 mg
Cefol Tablets (Abbott Pharmaceutical)	Rx		15	10	100		20	5	0.006	750		30			0.5	
Stress Formula Plus Zinc Tablets (Rexall Consumer Products)	OTC		10	10		100	20	5	0.012	500		30		0.045	0.4	Copper 3 mg, Zinc 24 mg

* per mL

PRODUCT/FORM (MANUFACTURER)	DEA	A (IU)	B1 (MG)	B2 (MG)	NIACIN, B3 (MG)	NIACINAMIDE, B3 (MG)	CALCIUM PANTOTHENATE, B5 (MG)	B6 (MG)	B12 (MG)	C (MG)	D (IU)	E (IU)	K (MG)	BIOTIN (MG)	FOLIC ACID (MG)	OTHER
Stress Formula Tablets (Rexall Consumer Products)	OTC		10	10		100	20	5	0.012	500		30		0.045	0.4	
Stress Formula Tablets (Cardinal Health, Inc.)	OTC		10	10	100		20	5	0.012	500		30		0.045	0.4	
Cardiotek Tablets (Stewart-Jackson Pharmacal, Inc.)	OTC							50	0.5	100		200			0.8	Arginine 75 mg

Multivitamin and Mineral Products

PRODUCT/FORM (MANUFACTURER)	DEA	A (IU)	D (IU)	E (IU)	B1 (MG)	B2 (MG)	B6 (MG)	B12 (MG)	C (MG)	FOLIC ACID (MG)	ZINC (MG)	SELENIUM (MG)	COPPER (MG)	CALCIUM (MG)	BIOTIN (MG)	CHROMIUM (MG)	MANGANESE (MG)	CALCIUM PANTOTHENATE (MG)	PANTOTHENATE, B5 (MG)	NIACINAMIDE, B3 (MG)	NIACIN, B3 (MG)	OTHER
Vita-Min Rx Tablets (Bio-Tech Pharmacal, Inc.)	Rx	10500	375	30	3	3.9	6	0.012	300	0.15	15	0.5		150	0.15	1	0.15	0.05			40	Yes
Circavite T Tablets (Circle Pharmaceuticals, Inc.)	Rx	10000	400	225	0.3	10	4.1	0.005	200		1.5						1.3	18.4			100	Yes
Mega-Multi Capsules (Innovative Health Products, Inc.)	OTC	10000	200	100	10	12.5	4.5	0.006	250	0.2	3.75	0.05	0.5	20	0.15	0.2	0.5	45			7	Yes
Super Plenamins Extra Strength Tablets (Rexall Consumer Products)	OTC	10000	400	30	10	10	5	0.006	250	0.4	15		2	7.8			1.3	20		100		Yes
Super Plenamins Tablets (Rexall Consumer Products)	OTC	8000	400	1	2.5	2.5	1	0.003	75		1		0.75	75	0.02		1.25	3		20		Yes
V-C Forte Capsules (Breckenridge Pharmaceutical, Inc.)	Rx	8000		50	10	5	2	0.01	150		80							10			25	No
Vicap Forte Capsules (Major Pharmaceuticals)																						
Vicon Forte Capsules (UCB Pharma, Inc.)																						
Vitacon Forte Capsules (Amide Pharmaceuticals, Inc.)																						
Total Formula Original Tablets (Vitaline Corporation)	OTC	7500	400	30	15	15	25	0.025	100	0.4	30	0.025	2	100	0.3	0.5	6	25		25		Yes
Sunvite Platinum Tablets (Rexall Consumer Products)	OTC	6000	400	45	1.5	1.7	3	0.025	60	0.2	15	0.025	2	200	0.03	0.025	2.5	10		20		Yes
Bacmin Tablets (Marnel Pharmaceuticals, Inc.)	Rx	5000		30	20	20	25	0.05	500	1	22.5	0.05	3		0.15	0.1	5	25			100	Yes
B-C W/Folic Acid Plus Tablets (Geneva Pharmaceuticals, Inc.)	Rx	5000		30	20	20	25	0.05	500	0.8	22.5		3		0.15	0.1	5	25			100	Yes
B-Complex Plus Tablets (United Research Laboratories, Inc.)																						

PRODUCT/FORM (MANUFACTURER)	DEA	A (IU)	D (IU)	E (IU)	B1 (MG)	B2 (MG)	B6 (MG)	B12 (MG)	C (MG)	FOLIC ACID (MG)	ZINC (MG)	SELENIUM (MG)	COPPER (MG)	CALCIUM (MG)	BIOTIN (MG)	CHROMIUM (MG)	MANGANESE (MG)	CALCIUM PANTOTHENATE, B5 (MG)	NIACINAMIDE, B3 (MG)	NIACIN, B3 (MG)	OTHER
B-Complex Vitamins Plus Tablets (Teva Pharmaceuticals USA)	Rx	5000		30	20	20	25	0.05	500	0.8	22.5		3		0.15	0.1	5	25		100	Yes
Becomax Rx Tablets (Ampharco, Inc.)																					
Berocca Plus Tablets (Roche Laboratories)																					
B-Plex Plus Tablets (Zenith Goldline Pharmaceuticals)																					
Protect Plus Liquid (Gil Pharmaceutical Corporation)	Rx	5000*	400*	100*	50*	50*	50*	0.05*	500*	1*	7.5*	0.1*	1*		0.15*	0.03*	5*	50*	50*		Yes
Cerovite Senior Tablets (Rugby Laboratories, Inc.)	OTC	5000	400	45	1.5	1.7	3	0.025	60	0.4	15	0.02	2	200	0.03	0.13	2.5	10		20	Yes
Daily Multiple Vitamins/ Minerals Tablets (Vangard Labs, Inc.)	OTC	5000	400	30	1.5	1.7	2	0.006	60	0.4	15	0.01	2	130	0.03	0.01	2.5	10	20		Yes
Dr. Art Ulene's Vitamin Formula Packets (Feeling Fine Company)	OTC	5000	400	200	4	5	10	0.1	420	0.4	10	0.2	2	400	0.1	0.4	3	50		20	Yes
One-A-Day 50 Plus Tablets (Bayer Consumer)	OTC	5000	400	60	4.5	3.4	6	0.03	120	0.4	22.5	0.105	2	120	0.03	0.180	4	15		20	Yes
Alpha Betic Tablets (Abkit)	OTC	5000	400	60	1.5	1.7	2	0.006	120	0.4	15	0.05	2	120	0.15	0.2	5	10		20	Yes
Theragran-M Tablets (Bristol-Myers Products)	OTC	5000	400	30	3	3.4	6	0.012	90	0.4	15	0.07	2	40	0.03	0.05	2	10		20	Yes
Equi-Roca Plus Tablets (Equipharm Corp.)	Rx	5000			20	20	25	0.05	500	0.8	22.5		3		0.15	0.1	5	25		100	Yes
Formula B Plus Tablets (Major Pharmaceuticals)																					
Glutofac-ZX Capsules (Kenwood Therapeutics)	Rx	5000	50	50	10	5	2		300	1	40		2				1.3				Yes
O-Cal FA Tablets (Pharmics, Inc.)	Rx	5000	400	30	3	3	4	0.012	90	1	15		2	200						20	Yes

* per 15 mL

PRODUCT/FORM (MANUFACTURER)	DEA	A (IU)	D (IU)	E (IU)	B1 (MG)	B2 (MG)	B6 (MG)	B12 (MG)	C (MG)	FOLIC ACID (MG)	ZINC (MG)	SELENIUM (MG)	COPPER (MG)	CALCIUM (MG)	BIOTIN (MG)	CHROMIUM (MG)	MANGANESE (MG)	CALCIUM PANTOTHENATE, B5 (MG)	NIACINAMIDE, B3 (MG)	NIACIN, B3 (MG)	OTHER
Bugs Bunny Complete Children's Chewable Tablets (Bayer Consumer)	OTC	5000	400	30	1.5	1.7	2	0.006	60	0.4	15		2	100	0.04			10		20	Yes
Flintstones Complete Children's Chewable Tablets (Bayer Consumer)																					
Sunvite Tablets (Rexall Consumer Products)	OTC	5000	400	30	1.5	1.7	2	0.006	60	0.4	15	0.025	2	162	0.03	0.025	2.5	10		20	Yes
One-A-Day Men's Tablets (Bayer Consumer)	OTC	5000	400	45	2.25	2.55	3	0.009	90	0.4	15	0.0875	2			0.15	3.33	10		20	Yes
One-A-Day Maximum Tablets (Bayer Consumer)	OTC	5000	400	30	1.5	1.7	2	0.006	60	0.4	15	0.020	2	162	0.03	0.065	3.5	10		20	Yes
One-A-Day Kids Complete Chewable Tablets (Bayer Consumer)	OTC	5000	400	30	1.5	1.7	2	0.006	60	0.4	15		2	100	0.04			10		20	Yes
Support 500 Capsules (A. G. Marin Pharmaceutical)	OTC	5000	50	400	20	20	20	0.025	500	0.4	28	0.05					1.3	10		25	Yes
Thera Vite M Tablets (PDK Labs, Inc.)	OTC	5000	400	30	3	3.4	3	0.009	90	0.4	15	0.021	2	40	0.03	0.026	3.5	10		20	Yes
Thera-M W/Minerals Tablets (Prime Marketing)																					
One-A-Day Women's Tablets (Bayer Consumer)	OTC	5000	400	30	1.5	1.7	2	0.006	60	0.4	15			450				10		20	Yes
Therapeutic Plus Vitamin Tablets (Rugby Laboratories, Inc.)	Rx	5000			20	20	25	0.05	500	0.8	22.5		3		0.15	0.1	5	25		100	Yes
Therobec Plus Tablets (Qualitest Products, Inc.)																					
Vitaplex Plus Tablets (Amide Pharmaceuticals)																					
Vitelle Nesentials Tablets (Fielding Pharmaceutical Company)	OTC	5000	400	30	3	3	2	0.006	120		15			370					25		Yes
One-A-Day Antioxidant Capsules (Bayer Consumer)	OTC	5000		200					250		7.5	0.015	1				1.5				No

PRODUCT/FORM (MANUFACTURER)	DEA	A (IU)	D (IU)	E (IU)	B1 (MG)	B2 (MG)	B6 (MG)	B12 (MG)	C (MG)	FOLIC ACID (MG)	ZINC (MG)	SELENIUM (MG)	COPPER (MG)	CALCIUM (MG)	BIOTIN (MG)	CHROMIUM (MG)	MANGANESE (MG)	CALCIUM PANTOTHENATE (MG)	PANTOTHENATE B5 (MG)	NIACINAMIDE B3 (MG)	NIACIN B3 (MG)	OTHER
Ferrex PC Tablets (Breckenridge Pharmaceutical, Inc.)	Rx	4000	400		3	3	2	0.003	50	1	18			125					10	10		Yes
Niferex-PN Tablets (Schwarz Pharma, Inc.)																						
Iromin-G Tablets (Mission Pharmacal Co.)	OTC	4000	400		4.8	2	20	0.002	100	0.8				57				1			10	Yes
Strovite Forte Tablets (Everett Laboratories, Inc.)	Rx	4000		60	20	20	25	0.05	500	0.8	15	0.05	3		0.15	0.1		25		100		Yes
Poly Vitamin W/Iron Chewable Tablets (Rugby Laboratories, Inc.)	OTC	2500	400	15	1.05	1.2	1.05	0.0045	60	0.3	8		0.8								13.5	Yes
Clusinex Syrup (Pharmakon Labs, Inc)	OTC	2500*	400*		1*	1*	0.6*	0.002*	15*		5*						5*	3*		3*		Yes
Protect Plus Capsules (Gil Pharmaceutical Corporation)	Rx	2500	200	200	25	25	25	0.025	250	0.5	15	0.05	0.5	50	0.15	0.1	2.5	30		25		Yes
Support Liquid (A. G. Marin Pharmaceutical)	Rx	1500*	100*		8*	2*	2*	0.01*		0.8*	7*									30*		Yes
Manly Machovites Tablets (Neurovites)	OTC	1041	16.67	16.67	4.17	4.17	50	0.017	250	0.07	4.17	0.017	0.08	20.83	0.017	0.017	1.67	4.17			4.17	Yes
PMS Formula Tablets (Neurovites)																						
Hematin Plus Tablets (Cypress Pharmaceutical Inc.)	OTC				10	6	5	0.015	200	1	18.2		0.8				1.3	10		30		Yes

* per 5 mL

OTHER INGREDIENTS:

Alpha Betic Tablets
Alpha Lipoic Acid 60 mg, Magnesium 200 mg, Potassium 100 mg, Vanadium 100 mcg

B-C W/Folic Acid Plus Tablets
Iron 27 mg, Magnesium 50 mg

B-Complex Plus Tablets
Iron 27 mg, Magnesium 50 mg

B-Complex Vitamins Plus Tablets
Iron 27 mg, Magnesium 50 mg

B-Plex Plus Tablets
Iron 27 mg, Magnesium 50 mg

Bacmin Tablets
Bioflavonoids 50 mg, Iron 27 mg, Magnesium 50 mg

Becomax Rx Tablets
Iron 27 mg, Magnesium 50 mg

Berocca Plus Tablets
Iron 27 mg, Magnesium 50 mg

Bugs Bunny Complete Children's Chewable Tablets
Iodine 150 mcg, Iron 18 mg, Magnesium 20 mg, Phosphorus 100 mg

Cerovite Senior Tablets
Boron 0.15 mg, Chloride 72 mg, Iodine 0.15 mg, Iron 4 mg, Magnesium 100 mg, Molybdenum 0.16 mg, Nickel 0.005 mg,

Phosphorus 48 mg, Potassium 80 mg, Silica 2 mg, Vitamin K 0.01 mg

Circavite T Tablets
Iron 12 mg

Clusinex Syrup
Magnesium 0.5 mg/5 mL

Daily Multiple Vitamins/Minerals Tablets
Iodine 0.15 mg, Iron 18 mg, Magnesium 100 mg, Molybdenum 0.01 mg, Phosphorus 100 mg, Potassium 40 mg

Dr. Art Ulene's Vitamin Formula Packets
Acetylcysteine 10 mg, Betaine 100 mg, Bioflavonoids 55 mg, Boron 1.3 mg, Borage Oil 100 mg, Choline 50 mg, Fish Oil 200 mg, Green Tea Extract 20 mg, Inositol 50 mg, Iodine 0.1 mg, Iron 8 mg, Magnesium 300 mg, Molybdenum 0.05 mg, Potassium 99 mg, Vitamin K 0.12 mg

Equi-Roca Plus Tablets
Iron 27 mg, Magnesium 50 mg

Ferrex PC Tablets
Iron 60 mg

Flintstones Complete Children's Chewable Tablets
Iodine 150 mcg, Iron 18 mg, Magnesium 20 mg, Phosphorus 100 mg

Formula B Plus Tablets
Iron 27 mg, Magnesium 50 mg

Glutofac-ZX Capsules
Magnesium 9.7 mg

Hematin Plus Tablets
Iron 324 mg, Magnesium 6.9 mg

Iromin-G Tablets
Iron 29.5 mg

Manly Machovites Tablets
Betaine 16.67 mg, Bioflavonoids 41.67 mg, Choline 52.08 mg, Inositol 4.17 mg, Iodine 0.013 mg, Iron 2.5 mg, Magnesium 41.67 mg, PABA 4.17 mg, Pancreatin GX 16.67 mg, Potassium 7.92 mg, Rutin 4.17 mg

Mega-Multi Capsules
Iodine 0.038 mg, Iron 4.5 mg, Magnesium 30 mg, Phosphorus 15 mg, Potassium 100 mg

Niferex-PN Tablets
Iron 60 mg

O-Cal FA Tablets
Iodine 0.15 mg, Iron 66 mg, Magnesium 100 mg, Sodium Fluoride 1.1 mg

One-A-Day 50 Plus Tablets
Chloride 34 mg, Iodine 150 mcg, Magnesium 100 mg, Molybdenum 94 mcg, Potassium 37.5 mg

One-A-Day Kids Complete Chewable Tablets
Iodine 150 mcg, Iron 18 mg, Magnesium 20 mg, Phosphorus 100 mg

One-A-Day Maximum Tablets
Boron 150 mcg, Chloride 72 mg, Iodine 150 mcg, Iron 18 mg, Magnesium 100 mg, Molybdenum 160 mcg, Nickel 5 mcg, Phosphorus 109 mg, Potassium 80 mg, Silicon 2 mcg, Tin 10 mcg, Vanadium 10 mcg

One-A-Day Men's Tablets
Chloride 34 mg, Iodine 150 mcg, Magnesium 100 mg, Molybdenum 75 mcg, Potassium 37.5 mg

One-A-Day Women's Tablets
Iron 27 mg

PMS Formula Tablets
Betaine 16.67 mg, Bioflavonoids 41.67 mg, Choline 52.08 mg, Inositol 4.17 mg, Iodine 0.013 mg, Iron 2.5 mg, Magnesium 41.67 mg, PABA 4.17 mg, Pancreatin GX 16.67 mg, Potassium 7.92 mg, Rutin 4.17 mg

Poly Vitamin W/Iron Chewable Tablets
Iron 12 mg

Protect Plus Capsules
Beta Carotene 2500 IU, Choline 25 mg, Glutathione 15 mg, Grape Seed Extract 0.25 mg, Inositol 25 mg, Magnesium 100 mg, Molybdenum 0.025 mg, Superoxide Dismutase 0.25 mg

Protect Plus Liquid
Choline 50 mg/15 mL, Inositol 50 mg/15 mL, Iron 10 mg/15 mL, Lysine 800 mg/15 mL, Magnesium 200 mg/15 mL, Molybdenum 0.025 mg/15 mL

Strovite Forte Tablets
Iron 10 mg, Magnesium 50 mg, Molybdenum 25 mg

Sunvite Platinum Tablets
Chloride 72 mg, Iodine 0.15 mg, Iron 9 mg, Magnesium 100 mg, Molybdenum 0.025 mg, Nickel 0.005 mg, Phosphorus 48 mg, Potassium 80 mg, Silicon 0.01 mg, Vanadium 0.01 mg, Vitamin K 0.01 mg

Sunvite Tablets
Boron 0.15 mg, Chloride 36.3 mg, Iodine 0.15 mg, Magnesium 100 mg, Molybdenum 0.025 mg, Nickel 0.005 mg, Phosphorus 125 mg, Potassium 40 mg, Silicon 2 mg, Tin 0.01 mg, Urib 18 mg, Vanadium 0.01 mg, Vitamin K 0.025 mg

Super Plenamins Extra Strength Tablets
Iodine 0.15 mg, Iron 24 mg, Magnesium 100 mg, Phosphorus 4 mg

Super Plenamins Tablets
Iodine 0.15 mg, Iron 30 mg, Liver 10 mg, Magnesium 10 mg, Phosphorus 58 mg

Support 500 Capsules
Glutathione 30 mg, Magnesium 9.7 mg

Support Liquid
Lysine 275 mg/5 mL, Magnesium 0.5 mg/5 mL

Thera Vite M Tablets
Boron 0.15 mg, Chloride 7.5 mg, Iodine 0.15 mg, Iron 18 mg, Magnesium 100 mg, Molybdenum 0.032 mg, Nickel 0.005 mg, Phosphorus 31 mg, Potassium 7.5 mg, Silicon 2 0.005 mg, Tin 0.1 mg, Vanadium 0.01 mg, Vitamin K 0.028 mg

Theragran-M Tablets
Boron 150 mcg, Chloride 7.5 mg, Iodine 150 mcg, Iron 9 mg, Magnesium 100 mg, Molybdenum 75 mcg, Nickel 5 mcg, Phosphorus 31 mg, Potassium 7.5 mg, Silicon 2 mg, Tin 10 mcg, Vanadium 10 mcg, Vitamin K 28 mcg

Thera-M W/Minerals Tablets
Chloride 7.5 mg, Iodine 0.15 mg, Iron 18 mg, Magnesium 100 mg, Molybdenum 0.032 mg, Phosphorus 31 mg, Potassium 7.5 mg, Vitamin K 0.028 mg

Therapeutic Plus Vitamin Tablets
Iron 27 mg, Magnesium 50 mg

Therobec Plus Tablets
Iron 27 mg, Magnesium 50 mg

Total Formula Original Tablets
Bioflavonoids 10 mg, Choline 10 mg, Hesperidin 10 mg, Inositol 10 mg, Iodine 0.1 mg, Iron 20 mg, Magnesium 100 mg, Molybdenum 0.1 mg, PABA 8 mg, Phosphorus 52 mg, Potassium 25 mg, Rutin 10 mg, Silicon 2.4 mg, Vanadium 0.025 mg, Vitamin K 0.07 mg

Vita-Min Rx Tablets
Iodine 200 mg, Magnesium 10 mg, Molybdenum 20 mg, Potassium 150 mg

Vitaplex Plus Tablets
Iron 27 mg, Magnesium 50 mg

Vitelle Nesentials Tablets
Phosphorus 130 mg

Vitamin B Complex Products

PRODUCT/FORM (MANUFACTURER)	DEA	B1 (MG)	B2 (MG)	NIACIN B3 (MG)	NIACINAMIDE B3 (MG)	CALCIUM PANTOTHENATE B5 (MG)	B6 (MG)	B12 (MG)	BIOTIN (MG)	C (MG)	FOLIC ACID (MG)	OTHER
Dialyvite Tablets (Hillestad Pharmaceuticals, Inc.)	Rx	1.5	1.7	20		10	10	0.006	0.3	100	1	
Nephplex Rx Tablets (Nephro-Tech, Inc.)	Rx	1.5	1.7	20		10	10	0.006	0.3	60	1	
Nephro-Vite Rx Tablets (R&D Laboratories, Inc.)												
Nephrocaps Capsules (Fleming & Company)	Rx	1.5	1.7	20		5	10	0.006	0.15	100	1	
Vitamin B Complex Capsules (Rugby Laboratories, Inc.)	OTC	3	3	20		5	0.5	0.001				Brewers Yeast 60 mg, Liver Desiccated 60 mg
Stress B Complex with Vitamin C Tablets (Mission Pharmacal Company)	OTC	13.8	10				4.1			300		Zinc 15 mg
Berocca Tablets (Roche Laboratories)	Rx	15	15		100	18	4	0.005		500	0.5	
B-Plex Tablets (Contract Pharmacal Corporation)												
B-Plex Tablets (Zenith Goldline Pharmaceuticals)												
Formula B Tablets (Major Pharmaceuticals)												
Strovite Tablets (Everett Laboratories, Inc.)												
Therobec Tablets (Qualitest Products, Inc.)												
Vitaplex Tablets (Amide Pharmaceuticals)												
Vitaplex Tablets (Medirex, Inc.)												
Vita-Bee W/C Tablets (Rugby Laboratories, Inc.)	OTC	15	10.2		50	10	5			300		

PRODUCT/FORM (MANUFACTURER)	DEA	B1 (MG)	B2 (MG)	NIACIN, B3 (MG)	NIACINAMIDE, B3	CALCIUM PANTOTHENATE B5 (MG)	B6 (MG)	B12 (MG)	BIOTIN (MG)	C (MG)	FOLIC ACID (MG)	OTHER
Marlbee W/C Capsules (Marlex Pharmaceuticals, Inc.)	OTC	15	10		50	10	5			300		
Thex Forte Tablets (Lee Pharmaceuticals)	OTC	25	15		100	10	5			500		
B-50 Complex Tablets (Rexall Consumer Products)	OTC	50	50		50	50	50	0.05	0.5		0.4	
Primaplex Injection (Primedics Laboratories)	Rx	50*	5*	125*		6*	5*	1*		50*		
Vicam Injection (Keene Pharmaceuticals, Inc.)												
Vitamin B Complex 100 Injection (Hyrex Pharmaceuticals)												
Vitamin B Complex W/Vitamin C & B12 Injection (McGuff Co.)												
B-100 Complex Tablets (Rexall Consumer Products)	OTC	100	100		100	100	100	0.1	0.1	0.1	0.4	
Vitamin B-100 Natural Tablets (Cardinal Health, Inc.)	OTC	100	100	100	100	100	100		0.1	0.1	0.4	Biotin 0.1 mg
B-Ject-100 Injection (Hyrex Pharmaceuticals)	Rx	100*	2*		100*		2*					Dexpanthenol 2 mg/mL
Vitamin B Complex 100 Injection (The Torrance Company)												
Vitamin B Complex 100 Injection (McGuff Co.)	Rx	100*	2*		100*		2*	1*				Dexpanthenol 2 mg/mL
Vitamin B Complex 100 Injection (Truxton Co., Inc.)												

* per mL

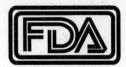

U.S. Food and Drug Administration

Professional and Consumer Information Numbers

Medical Product Reporting Programs

MedWatch (24-hour service) **800-332-1088**
*Reporting of problems with drugs, devices, biologics (except vaccines),
medical foods, dietary supplements.*

Vaccine Adverse Event Reporting System (24 hour service) **800-822-7967**
Reporting of vaccine-related problems.

Mandatory Medical Device Reporting...**301-827-0360**
*Reporting required from user-facilities (eg, hospitals, nursing homes)
regarding device-related deaths and serious injuries.*

Veterinary Adverse Drug Reaction Program **888-332-8387**
Reporting of adverse drug events in animals.

Medical Advertising Information **301-827-2828**
Inquiries from health professionals regarding product promotion.

USP Medication Errors **800-233-7767**
*Reporting of medication errors or near-errors to help avoid future problems through
improvement in product names and packaging.*

Information for Health Professionals

Center for Drugs Information Branch...**301-827-4573**
Information on human drugs including hormones.

Center for Biologics Office of Communications **301-827-2000**
Information on biological products including vaccines and blood.

Center for Devices and Radiological Health...**301-443-4190**
Automated request for information on medical devices and radiation-emitting products.

Emergency Operations **301-443-1240**
*Emergencies involving FDA-regulated products, tampering reports, and after-hours emergency
Investigational New Drug requests.*

Office of Orphan Products Development **301-827-3666**
Information on products for rare diseases.

General Information

General Consumer Inquiries..**888-463-6332**
Consumer information on regulated products/issues.

Freedom of Information **301-827-6500**
Requests for publicly available FDA documents.

Office of Public Affairs..**301-827-6250**
Interviews/press inquiries on FDA activities.

Center for Food Safety and Applied Nutrition **888-723-3366**
Information on food safety, seafood, dietary supplements, women's nutrition, and cosmetics.

Common Lab Test Values

Listed below are generally accepted normal values for a selection of common laboratory assays conducted on serum, plasma, and blood. Remember that norms may vary from laboratory to laboratory in accordance with the methodology and quality control measures employed by the facility. When in doubt, check with the laboratory that performed the analysis.

"SI range" refers to Système International d'Unités, a uniform system of reporting numerical values that permits interchangeability of information among nations and between disciplines.

Test	Range	Units	SI Range	Units
Acetone, serum	0.3-2.0	mg/dL	51.6-344.0	µmol/L
Acid phosphatase	0.1-5.0	U/L	2.7-10.7	IU/L
Alanine aminotransferase [ALT] (SGPT)	8-20	U/L	8-20	U/L
Albumin, serum	3.5-5.0	g/dL	35-50	g/L
Aldosterone	<16	ng/dL(fasting)	<0.45	nmol/L
	4-30	ng/dL(sitting)	0.11-0.84	nmol/L
Alkaline phosphatase	30-120	U/L	0.5-2	µkat/L
Ammonia [NH_4^+]	15-45	µg/dL	11-35	µmol/L
Amylase, serum	60-160	Somogyi U/dL	30-170	U/L
Antinuclear antibodies (ANA)	Negative at 1:20 dilution			
Aspartate aminotransferase [AST] (SGOT)	8-33	U/L	8-33	U/L
B_{12}	130-770	pg/mL		
Bilirubin, total (serum)	0.1-1	mg/dL	2-18	µmol/L
Bilirubin, conjugated (direct)	0.1-0.3	mg/dL	1.7-5.1	µmol/L
Blood urea nitrogen/ creatinine ratio	10:1-20:1		Average 15:1	
Calcium, serum	8.8-10-4	mg/dL	2.2-2.58	mmol/L
Calcium, ionized	4.4-5.0	mg/dL	1.1-1.24	mmol/L
Chloride, serum	95-105	mEq/L	95-105	mmol/L
Cholesterol				
Desirable level	<200	mg/dL	<5.20	mmol/L
Moderate risk	200-240	mg/dL	5.2-6.3	mmol/L
High risk	>240	mg/dL	>6.3	mmol/L
Copper	70-140	µg/dL	11-22	µmol/L
Cortisol, serum				
0800 hours	4-19	µg/L	110-520	nmol/L
1600 hours	2-15	µg/L	50-410	nmol/L
2400 hours	5	µg/L	140	nmol/L
Creatine kinase (CK)				
Isoenzymes	0-130	U/L	0-2.167	µkat/L
MB fraction	>5 in MI	%	>0.05	1
Creatine phosphokinase				
Male	5-35	µg/mL	55-170	U/L
Female	5-25	µg/mL	30-135	U/L
CPK-MB (heart)	0-6%			
Creatinine, serum	0.6-1.2	mg/dL	50-110	µmol/L
Creatinine clearance	75-125	mL/min	1.24-2.08	mL/sec
Digoxin				
Therapeutic	0.5-2.2	ng/mL	0.6 -2.8	nmol/L
	0.5-2.2	µg/L	0.6 -2.8	nmol/L
Toxic	> 2.5	ng/mL	>3.2	nmol/L
Erythrocyte count (RBC)				
Male	4.3-5.9	10^6/mm^3	4.3-5.9	10^{12}/L
Female	3.5-5	10^6/mm^3	3.5-5	10^{12}/L
Erythrocyte sedimentation rate (ESR)				
Male	0-20	mm/hr	0-20	mm/hr
Female	0-30	mm/hr	0-30	mm/hr
Ferritin				
Male	46-637	ng/mL		
Female	10-260	ng/mL		
Folate	1.5-20.6	pg/mL		
Follicle-stimulating hormone (FSH)				
Female	2-15	mIU/mL	2 -15	IU/L
Peak production	20-50	mIU/mL	20-50	IU/L
Male	1-10	mIU/mL	1-10	IU/L
Free thyroxine index (FTI)	1.1-4.7	µg/dL		
Gamma-glutamyl transferase (GGT)				
Male	4-23	IU/L	9-69	U/L
Female	3-13	IU/L	4-33	U/L
Gases, arterial blood				
pO_2	75-105	mm Hg	10-14	kPa
pCO_2	35-45	mm Hg	4.7-6	kPa
Glucose, plasma (fasting)	70-110	mg/dL	3.9-6.1	mmol/L
Glucose, postprandial (fasting)	<140	mg/dL/2 hr	<7.77	mmol/L

Test	Range	Units	SI Range	Units
Immunoglobulins (Ig)	900-2,200	mg/dL	9.0-22.0	g/L
Total				
IgG	600-1,900	mg/dL	6.0-19.0	g/L
IgA	60-330	mg/dL	0.6-3.3	g/L
IgM	45-145	mg/dL	0.45-1.45	g/L
IgD	0.5-3.0	mg/dL	0.005-0.03	g/L
IgE	10-506	U/mL	0.1-5.06	U/L
Iron, serum				
Male	80-180	µg/dL	14-32	µmol/L
Female	60-160	µg/dL	11-29	µmol/L
Iron binding capacity	250-460	µg/dL	45-82	µmol/L
Iron saturation	15-55	%		
Lactic acid				
Arterial	0.5-1.6	mEq/L	0.5-1.6	mmol/L
Venous	0.5-2.2	mEq/L	0.5-2.2	mmol/L
Lactic dehydrogenase (LDH)	70-250	U/L	70-250	U/L
Lead				
Normal	10-20	µg/dL	<0.9	µmol/L
Acceptable	20-40	µg/dL	<1.9	µmol/L
Leukocyte count (WBC)	4,500-10,000	mm^3	4.5-10	10^9/L
Lipase	14-280	mU/mL	14-280	U/L
	20-180	IU/L		
Lipoproteins				
Low density (LDL)	50-190	mg/dL	1.3-4.9	mmol/L
High density (HDL)				
Male	30-70	mg/dL	0.8-1.8	mmol/L
Female	30-85	mg/dL	0.8-2.2	mmol/L
Lithium ion — therapeutic	0.5 -1.5	mEq/L	0.5-1.5	mmol/L
		µg/dL		mmol/L
		mg/dL		mmol/L
Luteinizing hormone				
Male	3-25	mIU/mL	3-25	IU/L
Female	2-20	mIU/mL	2-20	IU/L
Peak production	30-140	mIU/mL	30-140	IU/L
Osmolality, plasma	280-300	mOsm/kg	280-300	mmol/kg
Phenytoin				
Therapeutic	10-20	mg/L	40-80	µmol/L
Toxic	>30	mg/L	>120	µmol/L
Phosphate, serum	2.5-5	mg/dL	0.8-1.6	mmol/L
Potassium, serum	3.5-5	mEq/L	3.5-5	mmol/L
Prolactin	<20	ng/mL	<20	µg/L
Prostate-specific antigen (PSA)				
Normal	0-4	ng/mL	Not available	Not available
BPH	4-19	ng/mL	Not available	Not available
Prostate CA	10-120	ng/mL	Not available	Not available
Protein				
Total	6-8	g/dL	60-80	g/L
Albumin	3.5-5.0	g/dL	35-50	g/L
Fibrinogen	0.2-0.4	g/dL	2-4	g/L
Globulin	1.5-3.0	g/dL	15-30	g/L
Reticulocyte count				
Male	0.5-1.5%		0.005-0.015 X 10^3	
Female	0.5-2.5%		0.005-0.025 X 10^3	
Rheumatoid factor	<1:20 titer			
Sodium, serum	135-147	mEq/L	135-147	mmol/L
Theophylline — therapeutic	10-20	mg/L	55-110	µmol/L
Thyroid binding globulin (TBG)	12-28	µg/dL	150-360	nmol/L
Thyroid stimulating hormone (TSH)	2-11	µU/mL	2-11	mU/L
Thyroxine (T$_4$)	5-12	µg/dL	51-142	nmol/L
Thyroxine, free serum	0.8-2.8	ng/dL	10-36	pmol/L
Transferrin	170-370	mg/dL	1.7-3.7	g/L
Triglycerides	<160	mg/dL	<1.8	mmol/L
Triiodothyronine (T$_3$)	0.075-0.2	mg/dL	1.2-3.4	nmol/L
T$_3$ uptake	25-35	%	0.25-0.35	1
T$_4$ uptake	0.8-1.1			
Urea nitrogen	5-20	mg/dL	1.8-7.1	mmol/L
Uric acid				
Male	3.5-7.0	mg/dL	202-416	µmol/L
Female	2.4-6.0	mg/dL	143-357	µmol/L
Warfarin — therapeutic	1-3	mg/L	3.3-9.8	µmol/L

Sources:

Chernecky, C.C., Krech, R.L., and Berger, B.J. (1993). Laboratory Tests and Diagnostic Procedures. Philadelphia, PA: W.B. Saunders.

Jacobs, D.S., Kaster, B.L., Demott, W.R., and Wolfson, W.L. (1988). Laboratory Test Handbook, 2nd ed. St. Louis, MO: Mosby/Lexi-Comp.

Kee, J.L. (1995). Laboratory and Diagnostic Tests with Nursing Implications, 4th ed., Norwalk, CT: Appleton & Lange.

Young, D.S. Implementation of SI Units for Clinical Laboratory Data. Annals of Internal Medicine 106:114-129, 1987. (Courtesy American College of Physicians.)

Poison Control Centers

Most of the centers listed below are certified by the American Association of Poison Control Centers. **Certified centers are marked by an asterisk after the name.** Each has to meet certain criteria. It must, for example, serve a large geographic area; it must be open 24 hours a day and provide direct-dial or toll-free access; it must be supervised by a medical director; and it must have registered pharmacists or nurses available to answer questions from the public.

The centers have a wide variety of toxicology resources, including a computerized database of some 750,000 substances maintained by MICROMEDEX, INC., an affiliate of *Physicians' Desk Reference.* Staff members are trained to resolve toxic situations in the home of the caller, though hospital referrals are given in some instances. The centers also offer a range of educational services to both the public and healthcare professionals. In some states, these larger centers exist side by side with smaller centers offering a more limited range of services.

Within each state, centers are listed alphabetically by city. Telephone numbers designated "TTY" are teletype lines for the hearing-impaired. "TDD" numbers reach a telecommunication device for the deaf.

ALABAMA

BIRMINGHAM

Regional Poison Control Center, The Children's Hospital of Alabama (*)

1600 7th Ave. South
Birmingham, AL 35233-1711
Business: 205-939-9720
Emergency: 205-933-4050
           205-939-9201
           800-292-6678 (AL)
Fax: 205-939-9245

TUSCALOOSA

Alabama Poison Center (*)

2503 Phoenix Dr.
Tuscaloosa, AL 35405
Business: 205-345-0600
Emergency: 205-345-0600
           800-462-0800 (AL)
Fax: 205-343-7410

ALASKA

ANCHORAGE

Anchorage Poison Control Center, Providence Hospital

P.O. Box 196604
3200 Providence Dr.
Anchorage, AK 99519-6604
Business: 907-562-2211,
            ext. 3193
Emergency: 907-261-3193
           800-478-3193 (AK)
Fax: 907-261-3684

FAIRBANKS

Fairbanks Poison Control Center

1650 Cowles St.
Fairbanks, AK 99701
Business and
Emergency: 907-456-7182
Fax: 907-458-5553

ARIZONA

PHOENIX

Samaritan Regional Poison Center (*)
Good Samaritan Regional Medical Center

Ancillary-1
1111 East McDowell Rd.
Phoenix, AZ 85006
Business: 602-495-4884
Emergency: 602-253-3334
           800-362-0101 (AZ)
Fax: 602-256-7579

TUCSON

Arizona Poison and Drug Information Center (*)
Arizona Health Sciences Center

1501 North Campbell Ave.
Room. 1156
Tucson, AZ 85724
Emergency: 520-626-6016
           800-362-0101 (AZ)
Fax: 520-626-2720

ARKANSAS

LITTLE ROCK

Arkansas Poison College of Pharmacy - UAMS

4301 West Markham St.
Mail Slot 522/2
Little Rock, AR 72205-7122
Business: 501-686-6161
Emergency: 800-376-4766
TDD/TTY: 800-641-3805

CALIFORNIA

FRESNO

California Poison Control System-Fresno/Madera (*)
Valley Children's Hospital

9300 Valley Children's Place
Madera, CA 93638-8762
Business: 559-353-3000
Emergency: 800-876-4766 (CA)

SACRAMENTO

California Poison Control System-Sacramento (*)

UCDMC-HSF Room 1024
2315 Stockton Blvd.
Sacramento, CA 95817
Business: 916-227-1400
Emergency: 800-876-4766 (CA)
TDD/TTY: 800-972-3323
Fax: 916-227-1414

SAN DIEGO

California Poison Control System-San Diego (*)
UCSD Medical Center

200 West Arbor Dr.
San Diego, CA 92103-8925
Emergency: 800-876-4766 (CA)
TDD/TTY: 800-972-3323

SAN FRANCISCO (*)

California Poison Control System-San Francisco
San Francisco General Hospital

1001 Potrero Ave., Room 1E86
San Francisco, CA 94110
Emergency: 800-876-4766 (CA)
TDD/TTY: 800-876-4766

COLORADO

DENVER

Rocky Mountain Poison and Drug Center (*)

1010 Yosemite Circle,
Bldg 752, Suite B
Denver, CO 80230-6800
Business: 303-739-1100
Emergency: 303-739-1123
           800-332-3073 (CO)
TTY: 303-739-1127 (CO)
Fax: 303-739-1119

CONNECTICUT

FARMINGTON

Connecticut Regional Poison Control Center (*)
University of Connecticut Health Center

263 Farmington Ave.
Farmington, CT 06030-5365
Business: 860-679-3056
Emergency: 800-343-2722 (CT)
TDD/TTY: 860-679-4346
Fax: 860-679-1623

DELAWARE

PHILADELPHIA, PA

The Poison Control Center of Philadelphia (*)

3535 Market St.
Suite 985
Philadelphia, PA 19104-3309
Business: 215-590-2003
Emergency: 800-722-7112
           215-386-2100
Fax: 215-590-4419

DISTRICT OF COLUMBIA

WASHINGTON, DC

National Capital Poison Center (*)

3201 New Mexico Ave., NW
Suite 310
Washington, DC 20016
Business: 202-362-3867
Emergency: 202-625-3333
TTY: 202-362-8563
Fax: 202-362-8377

FLORIDA

JACKSONVILLE

Florida Poison Information Center-Jacksonville (*) SHANDS Jacksonville Medical Center

655 W. 8th St.
Jacksonville, FL 32209
Emergency: 904-244-4480
    800-282-3171 (FL)
TDD/TTY: 800-282-3171 (FL)
Fax: 904-244-4063

MIAMI

Florida Poison Information Center-Miami (*) University of Miami, School of Medicine Department of Pediatrics

P.O. Box 016960 (R-131)
Miami, FL 33101
Business: 305-585-5253
Emergency: 305-585-8417
    800-282-3171 (FL)
Fax: 305-545-9762

TAMPA

Florida Poison Information Center-Tampa (*) Tampa General Hospital

P.O. Box 1289
Tampa, FL 33601
Emergency: 813-253-4444
    800-282-3171 (FL)
Fax: 813-253-4443

GEORGIA

ATLANTA

Georgia Poison Center (*) Hughes Spalding Children's Hospital, Grady Health System

80 Butler St., SE
P.O. Box 26066
Atlanta, GA 30335-3801
Emergency: 404-616-9000
    800-282-5846 (GA)
TDD: 404-616-9287
Fax: 404-616-6657

HAWAII

HONOLULU

Hawaii Poison Center

1319 Punahou St.
Honolulu, HI 96826
Emergency: 808-941-4411
    800-362-3585
    (outer islands only)
Fax: 808-535-7922

IDAHO

(DENVER, CO)

Rocky Mountain Poison & Drug Center (*)

1010 Yosemite Circle,
Bldg 752, Suite B
Denver, CO 80230-6800
Emergency: 800-860-0620 (ID)
    208-334-4570
TTY: 303-739-1127 (ID)
Fax: 303-739-1119

ILLINOIS

CHICAGO

Illinois Poison Center (*)

222 South Riverside Plaza
Suite 1900
Chicago, IL 60606
Business: 312-906-6136
Emergency: 800-942-5969 (IL)
TDD/TTY: 312-906-6185
Fax: 312-803-5400

URBANA

ASPCA/National Animal Poison Control Center

1717 S. Philo Rd., Suite 36
Urbana, IL 61802
Business: 217-337-5030
Emergency: 888-426-4435
Fax: 217-337-0599

INDIANA

INDIANAPOLIS

Indiana Poison Center (*)

I-65 at 21st St.
P.O. Box 1367
Indianapolis, IN 46206-1367
Emergency: 317-929-2323
    800-382-9097 (IN)
TTY: 317-929-2336
Fax: 317-929-2337

IOWA

SIOUX CITY

Iowa Statewide Poison Control Center

2720 Stone Park Blvd.
Sioux City, IA 51104
Business: 712-279-3710
Emergency: 800-352-2222 (IA)
    712-277-2222
Fax: 712-234-8775

KANSAS

KANSAS CITY

Mid-America Poison Control Center, University of Kansas Medical Center

3901 Rainbow Blvd.
Room B-400
Kansas City, KS 66160-7231
Business: 913-588-6638
Emergency: 800-332-6633 (KS)
TDD/TTY: 913-588-6639
Fax: 913-588-2350

TOPEKA

Stormont-Vail Regional Medical Center Emergency Department

1500 S.W. 10th
Topeka, KS 66604-1353
Business: 785-354-6000
Emergency: 785-354-6100
Fax: 785-354-5004

KENTUCKY

LOUISVILLE

Kentucky Regional Poison Center (*)

Medical Towers South
Suite 572
234 E. Gray St.
Louisville, KY 40202
Business: 502-629-7264
Emergency: 502-589-8222
    800-722-5725
    (Louisville only)
Fax: 502-629-7277

LOUISIANA

MONROE

Louisiana Drug and Poison Information Center (*) University of Louisiana at Monroe College of Pharmacy

Sugar Hall
Monroe, LA 71209-6430
Business: 318-342-1710
Emergency: 800-256-9822 (LA)
Fax: 318-342-1744

MAINE

PORTLAND

Maine Poison Center Maine Medical Center

22 Bramhall St.
Portland, ME 04102
Emergency: 207-871-2950
    800-442-6305 (ME)
TDD/TTY: 207-871-2879
Fax: 207-871-6226

MARYLAND

BALTIMORE

Maryland Poison Center (*) University of Maryland at Baltimore School of Pharmacy

20 North Pine St., PH 230
Baltimore, MD 21201
Business: 410-706-7604
Emergency: 410-706-7701
    800-492-2414 (MD)
TDD: 410-706-1858
Fax: 410-706-7184

MASSACHUSETTS

BOSTON

Regional Center for Poison Control and Prevention (*)

300 Longwood Ave.
Boston, MA 02115
Emergency: 617-232-2120
    800-682-9211
    (MA, RI)
TDD/TTY: 888-244-5313
Fax: 617-738-0032

MICHIGAN

DETROIT

Regional Poison Control Center (*) Children's Hospital of Michigan

4160 John R. Harper Prof.
Office Bldg.
Suite 616
Detroit, MI 48201
Business: 313-745-5335
Emergency: 313-745-5711
    800-764-7661 (MI)
TDD/TTY: 800-356-3232
Fax: 313-745-5493

GRAND RAPIDS

Spectrum Health Regional Poison Center (*)

1840 Wealthy SE
Grand Rapids, MI 49506-2968
Business: 616-774-7851
Emergency: 800-764-7661 (MI)
TDD/TTY: 800-356-3232
Fax: 616-774-7204

MINNESOTA

MINNEAPOLIS

Hennepin Regional Poison Center (*) Hennepin County Medical Center

701 Park Ave.
Minneapolis, MN 55415
Business: 612-347-3144
Emergency: 800-764-7661
    (MN, SD)
    612-347-3141
TTY: 612-904-4691
Fax: 612-904-4289

ST. PAUL

**PROSAR International
Poison Center**

1295 Bandana Blvd.
Suite 335
St. Paul, MN 55108
Business: 651-917-6100
Emergency: 888-779-7921
Fax: 651-641-0341

MISSISSIPPI

HATTIESBURG

**Poison Center,
Forrest General Hospital**

P. O. Box 16389
400 South 28th Ave.
Hattiesburg, MS 39404
Emergency: 601-288-2100
                601-288-2197
                601-288-2199
Fax: 601-288-2125

JACKSON

**Mississippi Regional Poison
Control Center, University of
Mississippi Medical Center**

2500 North State St.
Jackson, MS 39216
Business: 601-984-1675
Emergency: 601-354-7660
Fax: 601-984-1676

MISSOURI

ST. LOUIS

**Cardinal Glennon
Children's Hospital
Regional Poison Center (*)**

1465 South Grand Blvd.
St. Louis, MO 63104
Emergency: 800-366-8888 (MO)
                314-772-5200
TTY: 314-577-5336
Fax: 314-577-5355

MONTANA

(DENVER, CO)

**Rocky Mountain Poison
and Drug Center (*)**

1010 Yosemite Circle,
Bldg 752, Suite B
Denver, CO 80230-6800
Emergency: 800-525-5042 (MT)
                303-739-1123
Fax: 303-739-1119

NEBRASKA

OMAHA

**The Poison Center (*)
Children's Hospital**

8301 Dodge St.
Omaha, NE 68114
Emergency: 402-354-5555
                (Omaha)
                800-955-9119
                (NE, WY)

NEVADA

(DENVER, CO)

**Rocky Mountain Poison
and Drug Center (*)**

1010 Yosemite Circle,
Bldg 752, Suite B
Denver, CO 80230-6800
Emergency: 800-446-6179 (NV)
                303-739-1123
Fax: 303-739-1119

(PORTLAND, OR)

**Oregon Poison Center (*)
Oregon Health Sciences
University**

3181 SW Sam Jackson Park Rd,
CB550
Portland, OR 97201
Emergency: 503-494-8968
Fax: 503-494-4980

NEW HAMPSHIRE

LEBANON

**New Hampshire Poison
Information Center,
Dartmouth-Hitchcock
Medical Center**

1 Medical Center Dr.
Lebanon, NH 03756
Emergency: 603-650-8000
                800-562-8236 (NH)
Fax: 603-650-8986

NEW JERSEY

NEWARK

**New Jersey Poison Information
and Education System (*)**

201 Lyons Ave.
Newark, NJ 07112
Business: 973-926-7443
Emergency: 800-764-7661 (NJ)
TDD/TTY: 973-926-8008
Fax: 973-926-0013

NEW MEXICO

ALBUQUERQUE

**New Mexico Poison and
Drug Information Center (*)
University of New Mexico**

Health Science Center Library,
Room 130
Albuquerque, NM 87131-1076
Emergency: 505-272-2222
                800-432-6866 (NM)
Fax: 505-272-5892

NEW YORK

BUFFALO

**Western New York Regional
Poison Control Center (*)
Children's Hospital of Buffalo**

219 Bryant St.
Buffalo, NY 14222
Business: 716-878-7657
Emergency: 716-878-7654
                800-888-7655
(NY Western Regions Only)

MINEOLA

**Long Island Regional Poison
and Drug Information Center (*)
Winthrop University Hospital**

259 First St.
Mineola, NY 11501
Emergency: 516-542-2323
                516-663-2650
TDD: 516-747-3323
                (Nassau)
                516-924-8811
                (Suffolk)
Fax: 516-739-2070

NEW YORK CITY

**New York City
Poison Control Center (*)
NYC Dept. of Health**

455 First Ave., Room 123
New York, NY 10016
Business: 212-447-8152
Emergency: 800-210-3985
(English)   212-340-4494
                212-POISONS
                (212-764-7667)
Emergency: 212-VENENOS
(Spanish)   (212-836-3667)
TDD: 212-689-9014
Fax: 212-447-8223

ROCHESTER

**Finger Lakes Regional Poison
and Drug Information Center (*)
University of Rochester
Medical Center**

601 Elmwood Ave.
Box 321
Rochester, NY 14642
Business: 716-273-4155
Emergency: 716-275-3232
                800-333-0542 (NY)
TTY: 716-273-3854
Fax: 716-244-1677

SLEEPY HOLLOW

**Hudson Valley Regional Poison
Center (*) Phelps Memorial
Hospital Center**

701 N. Broadway
Sleepy Hollow, NY 10591
Emergency: 914-366-3030
                800-336-6997 (NY)
Fax: 914-366-1400

SYRACUSE

**Central New York
Poison Center (*)
SUNY Health Science Center**

750 East Adams St.
Syracuse, NY 13210
Business: 315-464-7078
Emergency: 315-476-4766
                800-252-5655 (NY)
Fax: 315-464-7077

NORTH CAROLINA

CHARLOTTE

**Carolinas Poison Center (*)
Carolinas Medical Center**

5000 Airport Center Pkwy.
Suite B
P.O. Box 32861
Charlotte, NC 28232
Business: 704-395-3795
Emergency: 704-355-4000
                800-848-6946

NORTH DAKOTA

FARGO

**North Dakota Poison
Information Center,
Meritcare Medical Center**

720 4th St. North
Fargo, ND 58122
Business: 701-234-6062
Emergency: 701-234-5575
                800-732-2200
                (ND, MN, SD)
Fax: 701-234-5090

OHIO

CINCINNATI

**Cincinnati Drug & Poison
Information Center
and Regional Poison
Control System (*)**

3333 Burnet Ave.
Vernon Place, 3rd floor
Cincinnati, OH 45229
Emergency: 513-558-5111
                800-872-5111 (OH)
TDD/TTY: 800-253-7955
Fax: 513-636-5069

CLEVELAND

**Greater Cleveland
Poison Control Center**

11100 Euclid Ave.
Cleveland, OH 44106-6010
Emergency: 216-231-4455
888-231-4455 (OH)
Fax: 216-844-3242

COLUMBUS

**Central Ohio
Poison Center (*)**

700 Children's Dr.
Room L032
Columbus, OH 43205-2696
Business: 614-722-2635
Emergency: 614-228-1323
800-682-7625 (OH)
800-762-0727 (OH)
937-222-2227
(Dayton Region)
TTY: 614-222-2272
Fax: 614-221-2672

TOLEDO

**Poison Information Center
of NW Ohio,
Medical College of Ohio
Hospital**

3000 Arlington Ave.
Toledo, OH 43614
Emergency: 419-383-3897
800-589-3897 (OH)
Fax: 419-383-6066

OKLAHOMA

OKLAHOMA CITY

**Oklahoma Poison Control
Center,
University of Oklahoma**

940 Northeast 13th St.
Room 3512
Oklahoma City, OK 73104
Business: 405-271-5062
Emergency: 800-764-7661 (OK)
405-271-5454
TDD: 405-271-1122
Fax: 405-271-1816

OREGON

PORTLAND

**Oregon Poison Center, CB 550 (*)
Oregon Health
Sciences University**

3181 S.W. Sam Jackson Park Rd.
Portland, OR 97201
Emergency: 503-494-8968
800-452-7165 (OR)
Fax: 503-494-4980

PENNSYLVANIA

HERSHEY

**Central Pennsylvania
Poison Center (*)
Pennsylvania State University
Milton S. Hershey Medical Center**

MC H043, P.O. Box 850
500 University Dr.
Hershey, PA 17033-0850
Emergency: 800-521-6110
717-531-6111
TTY: 717-531-8335
Fax: 717-531-6932

PHILADELPHIA

The Poison Control Center (*)

3535 Market St., Suite 985
Philadelphia, PA 19104-3309
Business: 215-590-2003
Emergency: 215-386-2100
800-722-7112
Fax: 215-590-4419

PITTSBURGH

**Pittsburgh Poison Center (*)
Children's Hospital of Pittsburgh**

3705 Fifth Ave.
Pittsburgh, PA 15213
Business: 412-692-5600
Emergency: 412-681-6669
Fax: 412-692-7497

PUERTO RICO

SANTURCE

**San Jorge Children's Hospital
Poison Center**

258 San Jorge St.
Santurce, PR 00912
Emergency: 787-726-5674

RHODE ISLAND

(BOSTON, MA)

**Regional Center for Poison
Control and Prevention
Serving Massachusetts and
Rhode Island (*)**

300 Longwood Ave.
Boston, MA 02115
Emergency: 800-682-9211
(MA, RI)
617-232-2120
TDD/TTY: 888-244-5313

SOUTH CAROLINA

COLUMBIA

**Palmetto Poison Center,
College of Pharmacy,
University of South Carolina**

Columbia, SC 29208
Business: 803-777-7909
Emergency: 803-777-1117
800-922-1117 (SC)
Fax: 803-777-6127

SOUTH DAKOTA

(FARGO, ND)

**North Dakota Poison
Information Center
Meritcare Medical Center**

720 4th St. North
Fargo, ND 58122
Business: 701-234-6062
Emergency: 701-234-5575
800-732-2200
(SD, MN, ND)
Fax: 701-234-5090

(MINNEAPOLIS, MN)

**Hennepin Regional Poison
Center (*) Hennepin County
Medical Center**

701 Park Ave.
Minneapolis, MN 55415
Business: 612-347-3144
Emergency: 800-764-7661
(MN, SD)
612-904-4691
TTY: 612-904-4289

TENNESSEE

MEMPHIS

Southern Poison Center

875 Monroe Ave.
Suite 104
Memphis, TN 38163
Business: 901-448-6800
Emergency: 901-528-6048
800-288-9999 (TN)
Fax: 901-448-5419

NASHVILLE

**Middle Tennessee
Poison Center (*)**

1161 21st Ave. South
501 Oxford House
Nashville, TN 37232-4632
Business: 615-936-0760
Emergency: 615-936-2034
(Greater Nashville)
800-288-9999 (TN)
Fax: 615-936-0756

TEXAS

AMARILLO

**Texas Panhandle
Poison Center
Northwest Texas Hospital**

1501 S. Coulter Dr.
Amarillo, TX 79106
Emergency: 806-354-1100
800-764-7661 (TX)

DALLAS

**North Texas Poison Center (*)
Texas Poison Center Network
Parkland Health and Hospital
System**

5201 Harry Hines Blvd.
P.O. Box 35926
Dallas, TX 75235
Business: 214-589-0911
Emergency: 800-764-7661 (TX)
Fax: 214-590-5008

EL PASO

**West Texas Regional
Poison Center (*)**

4815 Alameda Ave.
El Paso, TX 79905
Business   915-534-3800
Emergency: 800-764-7661 (TX)

GALVESTON

**Southeast Texas
Poison Center (*)
The University of Texas
Medical Branch**

3112 Trauma Bldg.
301 University Ave.
Galveston, TX 77555-1175
Business: 409-766-4403
Emergency: 800-764-7661 (TX)
409-765-1420
Fax: 409-772-3917

SAN ANTONIO

**South Texas
Poison Center (*)
The University of Texas Health
Science Center–San Antonio**

7703 Floyd Curl Dr., MC 7849
San Antonio, TX 78229-3900
Emergency: 210-567-5762
800-764-7661 (TX)
TDD/TTY: 800-764-7661 (TX)
Fax: 210-567-5718

TEMPLE

**Central Texas
Poison Center (*)
Scott & White
Memorial Hospital**

2401 South 31st St.
Temple, TX 76508
Emergency: 800-764-7661 (TX)
254-724-7401
Fax: 254-724-1731

UTAH

SALT LAKE CITY

Utah Poison Control Center (*)

410 Chipeta Way
Suite 230
Salt Lake City, UT 84108
Emergency: 801-581-2151
800-456-7707 (UT)
Fax: 801-581-4199

VERMONT

BURLINGTON

**Vermont Poison Center,
Fletcher Allen Health Care**

111 Colchester Ave.
Burlington, VT 05401
Business: 802-847-2721
Emergency: 802-658-3456
          877-658-3456
          (toll-free)
Fax: 802-847-4802

VIRGINIA

CHARLOTTESVILLE

**Blue Ridge Poison Center (*)
University of Virginia Health
System**

PO Box 800774
Charlottesville, VA 22908-0774
Emergency: 804-924-5543
       800-451-1428 (VA)
Fax: 804-971-8657

RICHMOND

**Virginia Poison Center (*)
Virginia Commonwealth
University**

P.O. Box 980522
Richmond, VA 23298-0522
Emergency: 800-552-6337 (VA)
       804-828-9123
TDD/TTY: 800-828-1120
Fax: 804-828-5291

WASHINGTON

SEATTLE

**Washington Poison
Center (*)**

155 NE 100th St.
Suite 400
Seattle, WA 98125-8012
Business: 206-517-2351
Emergency: 206-526-2121
       800-732-6985 (WA)
TDD: 800-572-0638 (WA)
       206-517-2394
Fax: 206-526-8490

WEST VIRGINIA

CHARLESTON

**West Virginia
Poison Center (*)**

3110 MacCorkle Ave. SE
Charleston, WV 25304
Business: 304-347-1212
Emergency: 304-348-4211
       800-642-3625 (WV)
Fax: 304-348-9560

WISCONSIN

MADISON

**Poison Control Center,
University of Wisconsin
Hospital and Clinics**

600 Highland Ave.
F6-133
Madison, WI 53792
Business: 608-262-7537
Emergency: 800-815-8855 (WI)

MILWAUKEE

**Children's Hospital
of Wisconsin Poison Center**

9000 W. Wisconsin Ave.
P.O. Box 1997
Milwaukee, WI 53201
Business: 414-266-2000
Emergency: 414-266-2222
       800-815-8855 (WI)
Fax: 414-266-2820

WYOMING

(OMAHA, NE)

**The Poison Center (*)
Children's Hospital**

8301 Dodge St.
Omaha, NE 68114
Emergency: 800-955-9119
       (WY, NE)

Drug Information Centers

ALABAMA

BIRMINGHAM

Drug Information Service
University of Alabama Hospital
619 S. 20th St.
1720 Jefferson Tower
Birmingham, AL 35249-6860
Mon.-Fri. 8 AM-5 PM
  205-934-2162
Fax: 205-934-3501

Global Drug Information Center
Samford University
McWhorter School of Pharmacy
800 Lakeshore Dr.
Birmingham, AL 35229-7027
Mon.-Fri. 8 AM-4:30 PM
  205-870-2659
Fax: 205-726-4012
samford. edu.schools/
pharmacy/dic/index.html

HUNTSVILLE

Huntsville Hospital Drug
Information Center
101 Sivley Rd.
Huntsville, AL 35801
Mon.-Fri. 8 AM-5 PM
  256-517-8284
Fax: 256-517-6558

ARIZONA

TUCSON

Arizona Poison and Drug
Information Center
Arizona Health Sciences Center
University Medical Center
1501 N. Campbell Ave.
Room 1156
Tucson, AZ 85724
7 days/week, 24 hours
  520-626-6016
  800-362-0101 (AZ)
Fax: 520-626-2720

ARKANSAS

LITTLE ROCK

Arkansas Poison and Drug
Information Center
4301 W. Markham St., Slot 522-2
Little Rock, AK 72205
7 days/week, 7 AM-Midnight
501-686-5540
Fax: 501-686-7357

CALIFORNIA

LOS ANGELES

Los Angeles Regional
Drug Information Center
LAC & USC Medical Center
1200 N. State St.
Room 1107 A & B
Los Angeles, CA 90033
Mon.-Fri. 8 AM-4:30 PM
  323-226-7741
Fax: 323-226-4194

SAN DIEGO

Drug Information Center
U.S. Naval Hospital
34800 Bob Wilson Dr.
San Diego, CA 92134-5000
Mon.-Fri. 8 AM-4 PM
  619-532-8417
Fax: 619-352-5898

Drug Information Service
University of California
San Diego Medical Center
135 Dickinson St.
San Diego, CA 92103-8925
Mon.-Fri. 9 AM-5 PM
  900-288-8273
Fax: 858-715-6323

STANFORD

Drug Information Center
Stanford Hospital and Clinics
Department of Pharmacy
300 Pasteur Dr.
Room H-0301
Stanford, CA 94305
Mon.-Fri. 8 AM-4 PM
  650-723-6422
Fax: 650-725-5028

COLORADO

DENVER

Rocky Mountain Poison and
Drug Consultation Center
1010 Yosemite Circle
Denver, CO 80230
Mon.-Fri. 8 AM-4:30 PM
  303-893-3784
  (For Denver County
  residents only)
Fax: 303-739-1119

Drug Information Center
University of Colorado
Health Science Center
4200 E. 9th Ave., Box C239
Denver, CO 80262
Mon.-Fri. 8:30 AM-4:30 PM
  303-315-8489
Fax: 303-315-3353

CONNECTICUT

FARMINGTON

Drug Information Service
University of Connecticut
Health Center
263 Farmington Ave.
Farmington, CT 06030
Mon.-Fri. 7 AM-4 PM
  860-679-2783
Fax: 860-679-1231
wnelson@nso.uchc.edu

HARTFORD

Drug Information Center
Hartford Hospital
P.O. Box 5037
80 Seymour St.
Hartford, CT 06102
Mon.-Fri. 8:30 AM-5 PM
  860-545-2221
  860-545-2961
Fax: 860-545-4371

NEW HAVEN

Drug Information Center
Yale-New Haven Hospital
20 York St.
New Haven, CT 06504
Mon.-Fri. 12 PM-4:30 PM
  203-688-2248
Fax: 203-688-3691

DISTRICT OF COLUMBIA

Drug Information Service
Howard University Hospital
Room BB06
2041 Georgia Ave. NW
Washington, DC 20060
7 days/week, 24 hours
  202-865-1325
Fax: 202-865-7410

FLORIDA

GAINESVILLE

Drug Information &
Pharmacy Resource Center
SHANDS Hospital at
University of Florida
P.O. Box 100316
Gainesville, FL 32610-0316
Mon.-Fri. 9 AM-5 PM
  352-395-0408
  (for healthcare
  professionals only)
Fax: 352-338-9860

JACKSONVILLE

Drug Information Service
SHANDS Jacksonville
655 W. 8th St.
Jacksonville, FL 32209
Mon.-Fri. 8 AM-5 PM
  904-244-4185
Fax: 904-244-4272

MIAMI

Drug Information Center (119)
Miami VA Medical Center
1201 NW 16th St.
Pharmacy 119
Miami, FL 33125
Mon.-Fri. 7:00 AM-3:30 PM
  305-324-3237
  (for healthcare
  professionals only)
Fax: 305-324-3394

ORLANDO

Orlando Regional Drug
Information Service
Orlando Regional
Healthcare System
1414 Kuhl Ave., MP 192
Orlando, FL 32806
Mon.-Fri. 8 AM-5 PM
  407-841-5111, ext. 8717
Fax: 407-650-9052

TALLAHASSEE

Drug Information
Education Center
Florida Agricultural and
Mechanical University
College of Pharmacy
Honor House, Room 200
Tallahassee, FL 32307
Mon.-Fri. 9 AM-5 PM
  850-488-5239
  850-599-3064
  800-451-3181
Fax: 850-412-7020

GEORGIA

ATLANTA

Emory University Hospital
Dept. of Pharmaceutical
Services-Drug Information
1364 Clifton Rd. NE
Atlanta, GA 30322
Mon.-Fri. 8:30 AM-5 PM
  404-712-4640
Fax: 404-712-7577

Drug Information Service
Northside Hospital
1000 Johnson Ferry Rd. NE
Atlanta, GA 30342
Mon.-Fri. 9 AM-4 PM
  404-851-8676 (GA)
Fax: 404-851-8682

AUGUSTA
Drug Information Center
University of Georgia
Medical College of GA
Room BIW201
1120 15th St.
Augusta, GA 30912-5600
Mon.-Fri. 8:30 AM-5 PM
  706-721-2887
Fax: 706-721-3827

IDAHO

POCATELLO
Idaho Drug Information Service
Campus Box 8092
Pocatello, ID 83209
Mon.-Fri. 8 AM-5 PM
  208-282-4689
Fax: 208-282-3003

ILLINOIS

CHICAGO
Drug Information Center
Northwestern Memorial Hospital
251 E. Huron
Feinberg LC-700B
Chicago, IL 60611
Mon.-Fri. 8 AM-5 PM
  312-926-7573
Fax: 312-926-7956

Saint Joseph Hospital Pharmacy
2900 N. Lake Shore Dr.
Chicago, IL 60657
7 days/week, 24 hours
  773-665-3140
Fax: 773-665-3462

Drug Information Services
University of Chicago
5841 S. Maryland Ave.
MC 0010
Chicago, IL 60637
Mon.-Fri. 8 AM-5 PM
  773-702-1388
Fax: 773-702-6631

Drug Information Center
University of Illinois at Chicago
833 S. Wood St.
Chicago, IL 60612
Mon.-Fri. 8 AM-4 PM
  312-996-0209
Fax: 312-996-0448

HARVEY
Drug Information Center
Ingalls Memorial Hospital
1 Ingalls Dr.
Harvey, IL 60426
Mon.-Fri. 8 AM-4:30 PM
  708-915-6413
  800-543-6543 (IL)
Fax: 708-915-4609

HINES
Drug Information Service
Hines Veterans Administration
Hospital
Inpatient Pharmacy (119B)
P.O. Box 5000
Hines, IL 60141-5000
Mon.-Fri. 8 AM-4:30 PM
  708-202-8387
Fax: 708-202-2201

PARK RIDGE
Drug Information Center
Lutheran General Hospital
1775 Dempster St.
Park Ridge, IL 60068
Mon.-Fri. 7:30 AM-4 PM
  847-723-8128
Fax: 847-723-2326

INDIANA

INDIANAPOLIS
Drug Information Center
St. Vincent Hospital
and Health Services
2001 W. 86th St.
P.O. Box 40970
Indianapolis, IN 46240
Mon.-Fri. 8 AM-4 PM
  317-338-3200
  (for healthcare
  professionals only)
Fax: 317-338-3041

IOWA

DES MOINES
Regional Drug Information
Center
Mercy Medical Center-
Des Moines
1111 Sixth Ave.
Des Moines, IA 50314
Mon.-Fri. 8 AM-4:30 PM
  515-247-3286
  (answered 7days/week,
  24 hours)
Fax: 515-247-3966

IOWA CITY
Drug Information Center
University of Iowa
Hospitals and Clinics
200 Hawkins Dr.
Iowa City, IA 52242
Mon.-Fri. 8 AM-5 PM
  319-356-2600
  (for healthcare
  professionals only)
Fax: 319-384-8840

SIOUX CITY
Iowa Statewide
Poison Center
2720 Stone Park Blvd.
Sioux City, IA 51104
7 days/week, 24 hours
  712-277-2222
  800-352-2222 (IA)
Fax: 712-234-8775

KANSAS

KANSAS CITY
Drug Information Center
University of Kansas
Medical Center
3901 Rainbow Blvd.
Kansas City, KS 66160
Mon.-Fri. 8 AM-6 PM
  913-588-2328
  (for healthcare
  professionals only)
Fax: 913-588-2350

KENTUCKY

LEXINGTON
Drug Information Center
Chandler Medical Center
College of Pharmacy
University of Kentucky
800 Rose St., C-117
Lexington, KY 40536-0293
Mon.-Fri. 8 AM-5 PM
  606-323-5320
Fax: 606-323-2049

LOUISIANA

NEW ORLEANS
Xavier University Drug
Information Center
Tulane University
Hospital and Clinic
Box HC12
1415 Tulane Ave.
New Orleans, LA 70112
Mon.-Fri. 9 AM-5 PM
  504-588-5670
Fax: 504-588-5862
mharris@tulane.edu

MARYLAND

ANDREWS AFB
Drug Information Services
89 MDTS/SGQP
1050 W. Perimeter Rd.
Suite D1-119
Andrews AFB, MD 20762-6660
Mon.-Fri. 7:30 AM-6 PM
  240-857-4565
Fax: 240-857-8892

ANNAPOLIS
The Anne Arundel
Medical Center
Dept. of Pharmacy
P.O. Box 64
Franklin St.
Annapolis, MD 21401
7 days/week, 24 hours
  410-267-1126
  410-267-1000
  (switchboard)
Fax: 410-267-1628

BALTIMORE
Drug Information Service
Johns Hopkins Hospital
600 N. Wolfe St.,
Halsted 503
Baltimore, MD 21287-6180
Mon.-Fri. 8:30 AM-5 PM
  410-955-6348
Fax: 410-955-8283

Drug Information Service
University of Maryland at
Baltimore School of Pharmacy
506 W. Fayette, 3rd Floor
Baltimore, MD 21201
Mon.-Fri. 8:30 AM-5 PM
  410-706-7568
Fax: 410-706-0897

BETHESDA
Drug Information Center
National Institutes of Health
Building 10, Room 1S-259
10 Center Drive (MSC1196)
Bethesda, MD 20892-1196
Mon.-Fri. 8:30 AM-5 PM
  301-496-2407
Fax: 301-496-0210

EASTON
Drug Information
Pharmacy Dept.
Memorial Hospital
219 S. Washington St.
Easton, MD 21601
Mon.-Fri. 7 AM-Midnight
Sat.-Sun. 7 AM-5:30 PM
  410-822-1000
Fax: 410-820-9489

MASSACHUSETTS

BOSTON
Drug Information Services
Brigham and Women's Hospital
75 Frances St.
Boston, MA 02115
Mon.-Fri. 7 AM-3:30 PM
  617-732-7166
Fax: 617-732-7497

Drug Information Center
New England Medical
Center Pharmacy
750 Washington St., Box 420
Boston, MA 02111
Mon.-Fri. 9 AM-5 PM
  617-636-8985
Fax: 617-636-4567

WORCESTER
Drug Information Center
U.M.M.H.C. Hospital
55 Lake Ave. North
Worcester, MA 01655
Mon.-Fri. 8:30 AM-5 PM
  508-856-3456
  508-856-2775
Fax: 508-856-1850

MICHIGAN

ANN ARBOR

**Drug Information and
Pharmacy Services
University of Michigan
Medical Center**
1500 East Medical Center Dr.
UHB2 D301 Box 0008
Ann Arbor, MI 48109/0008
Mon.-Fri. 8 AM-5 PM
    734-936-8200
    734-936-8251
Fax: 734-936-7027

DETROIT

**Drug Information Services
Harper Hospital**
3990 John R. St.
Detroit, MI 48201
Mon.-Fri. 8 AM-5 PM
    313-745-4556
    313-745-2006
Fax: 313-745-1628

PONTIAC

**Drug Information Center
St. Joseph Mercy Hospital**
900 Woodward
Pontiac, MI 48341
Mon.-Fri. 8 AM-4:30 PM
    248-858-3055
Fax: 248-858-3010

ROYAL OAK

**Drug Information Services
William Beaumont Hospital**
3601 West 13 Mile Rd.
Royal Oak, MI 48073-6769
Mon.-Fri. 8 AM-4:30 PM
    248-551-4077
Fax: 248-551-3301

SOUTHFIELD

**Drug Information Service
Providence Hospital**
16001 West 9 Mile Rd.
Southfield, MI 48075
Mon.-Fri. 8 AM-4 PM
    248-424-3125
Fax: 248-424-5364

MISSISSIPPI

JACKSON

**Drug Information Center
University of Mississippi
Medical Center**
2500 N. State St.
Jackson, MS 39216
Mon.-Fri. 8 AM-4:30 PM
    601-984-2060
Fax: 601-984-2064

MISSOURI

KANSAS CITY

**University of Missouri-Kansas
City
Drug Information Center**
2411 Holmes St., MG-200
Kansas City, MO 64108-2792
Mon.-Fri. 8 AM-5 PM
    816-235-5490
Fax: 816-235-5491

SPRINGFIELD

**Drug Information
St. Johns Regional
Health Center**
1235 E. Cherokee
Springfield, MO 65804
Mon.-Fri. 7:30 AM-4:30 PM
    417-885-3488
Fax: 417-888-7788

ST. JOSEPH

**Drug Information Service
Heartland Hospital West**
801 Faraon St.
St. Joseph, MO 64501
Mon.-Fri. 9 AM-5:30 PM
    816-271-7582
Fax: 816-271-7590

MONTANA

MISSOULA

**Drug Information Service
University of Montana
School of Pharmacy
and Allied Health Sciences**
Missoula, MT 59812-1077
Mon.-Fri. 8 AM-5 PM
406-243-5254
Fax: 406-243-4353

NEBRASKA

OMAHA

**Drug Information Service
School of Pharmacy
Creighton University**
2500 California Plaza
Omaha, NE 68178
Mon.-Fri. 8:30 AM-5:00 PM
    402-280-5101
Fax: 402-280-5149

NEW JERSEY

NEW BRUNSWICK

**Drug Information Service
Robert Wood Johnson
University Hospital
Pharmacy Department**
1 Robert Wood Johnson Place
New Brunswick, NJ 08901
Mon.-Fri. 8:30 AM-4:30 PM
732-937-8842
Fax: 732-937-8584

NEWARK

**New Jersey Poison Information
and Education System**
201 Lyons Ave.
Newark, NJ 07112
7 days/week, 24 hours
973-926-7443
Fax: 973-926-0013

NEW MEXICO

ALBUQUERQUE

**New Mexico Poison &
Drug Information Center
University of New Mexico**
Albuquerque, NM 87131
7 days/week, 24 hours
    505-272-2222
    800-432-6866 (NM)
Fax: 505-272-5892

NEW YORK

BROOKLYN

**International Drug
Information Center
Long Island University
Arnold & Marie Schwartz
College of Pharmacy & Health
Sciences**
1 University Plaza
RM-HS509
75 Dekalb Ave.
Brooklyn, NY 11201
Mon.-Fri. 9 AM-5 PM
    718-488-1064
Fax: 718-780-4056

**Drug Information Center
Brookdale University Hospital
and Medical Center**
1 Brookdale Plaza
Brooklyn, NY 11212
Mon.-Fri. 8 AM-4:30 PM
    718-240-5983
Fax: 718-240-5987

COOPERSTOWN

**Drug Information Center
Bassett Healthcare**
1 Atwell Rd.
Cooperstown, NY 13326
Mon.-Fri. 8:30 AM-5 PM
    607-547-3686
Fax: 607-547-3629

JAMAICA

**Drug Information Center
St. John's University College
of Pharmacy and Allied Health
Professions**
8000 Utopia Pkwy.
Jamaica, NY 11439
Mon.-Fri. 8:30 AM-3:30 PM
    718-990-2149
Fax: 718-990-2151

NEW YORK CITY

**Drug Information Center
Bellevue Hospital Center**
462 1st Ave.
New York, NY 10016
7 days/week, 24 hours
    212-562-6501
Fax: 212-562-2949

**Drug Information Center
Memorial Sloan-Kettering
Cancer Center**
1275 York Ave.
RM S-712
New York, NY 10021
Mon.-Fri. 9 AM-5 PM
    212-639-7552
Fax: 212-639-2171

**Drug Information Center
Mount Sinai Medical Center**
1 Gustave Levy Pl.
New York, NY 10029
Mon.-Fri. 9 AM-5 PM
    212-241-6619
Fax: 212-348-7927

**Drug Information Service
New York Presbyterian Hospital**
Room K04
525 E. 68th St.
New York, NY 10021
Mon.-Fri. 9 AM-5 PM
    212-746-0741
Fax: 212-746-8506

ROCHESTER

**Poison and Drug
Information Center
University of Rochester**
601 Elmwood Ave.
Rochester, NY 14642
7 days/week, 24 hours
    716-275-3718
    716-275-3232
    (after 5 PM)
Fax: 716-244-1677

STONY BROOK

**Suffolk Drug Information Center
University Hospital**
S.U.N.Y. - Stony Brook
Stony Brook, NY 11794-7310
Mon.-Fri. 8 AM-3:00 PM
    631-444-2675
    631-444-2680
    (after hours)
Fax: 631-444-7935

NORTH CAROLINA

BUIES CREEK

**Drug Information Center
School of Pharmacy
Campbell University**
P.O. Box 1090
Buies Creek, NC 27506
Mon.-Fri. 8:30 AM-4:30 PM
    910-893-1478
    800-327-5467 (NC)
Fax: 910-893-1476

CHAPEL HILL

Drug Information Center
University of North
Carolina Hospitals
101 Manning Dr.
Chapel Hill, NC 27514
Mon.-Fri. 8 AM-4:30 PM
   919-966-2373
Fax: 919-966-1791

GREENVILLE

Eastern Carolina Drug
Information Center
Pitt County
Memorial Hospital
Dept. of Pharmacy Service
2100 Stantonsburg Rd.
Greenville, NC 27834
Mon.-Fri. 8 AM-5 PM
   252-816-4257
Fax: 252-816-7425

WINSTON-SALEM

Drug Information
Service Center
Wake-Forest University
Baptist Medical Center
Medical Center Blvd.
Winston-Salem, NC 27157
Mon.-Fri. 8 AM-5 PM
   336-716-2037
Fax: 336-716-2186

NORTH DAKOTA

FARGO

North Dakota Institute for
Pharmaceutical Care
North Dakota State University
College of Pharmacy
110 Sudro Hall
Fargo, ND 58105-5055
Mon.-Fri. 8:30 AM-4:30 PM
701-231-7939
Fax: 701-231-7606

OHIO

ADA

Drug Information Center
Raabe College of Pharmacy
Ohio Northern University
Ada, OH 45810
Mon.-Fri. 9 AM-5 PM
   419-772-2307
Fax: 419-772-2289

CLEVELAND

Drug Information Center
Cleveland Clinic Foundation
9500 Euclid Ave.
Cleveland, OH 44195
Mon.-Fri. 8:30 AM-4:30 PM
   216-444-6456
Fax: 216-444-6157

COLUMBUS

Drug Information Center
Ohio State University Hospital
Dept. of Pharmacy
Doan Hall 368
410 W. 10th Ave.
Columbus, OH 43210-1228
Mon.-Fri. 8 AM-4 PM
   614-293-8679
Fax: 614-293-3264

Drug Information Center
Riverside Methodist Hospital
3535 Olentangy River Rd.
Columbus, OH 43214
Mon.-Fri. 8 AM-5 PM
   614-566-5425
Fax: 614-566-5447

TOLEDO

Drug Information Services
St. Vincent Mercy Medical
Center
2213 Cherry St.
Toledo, Ohio 43608-2691
Mon.-Fri. 8 AM-4 PM
   419-251-4227
Fax: 419-251-3662

OKLAHOMA

OKLAHOMA CITY

Drug Information Service
Integris Health
3300 Northwest Expressway
Oklahoma City, OK 73112
Mon.-Fri. 8 AM-4:30 PM
   405-949-3660
Fax: 405-951-8274

Drug Information Center
Presbyterian Hospital
700 NE 13th St.
Oklahoma City, OK 73104
Mon.-Fri. 8 AM-4:30 PM
   405-271-6226
Fax: 405-271-6281

TULSA

Drug Information Service
St. Francis Hospital
6161 S. Yale Ave.
Tulsa, OK 74136
Mon.-Fri. 7 AM-4:30 PM
   918-494-6339
   (for healthcare
   professionals only)
Fax: 918-494-1893

PENNSYLVANIA

PHILADELPHIA

Drug Information Center
Temple University Hospital
Dept. of Pharmacy
3401 N. Broad St.
Philadelphia, PA 19140
Mon.-Fri. 8 AM-4:30 PM
   215-707-4644
Fax: 215-707-3463

Drug Information Service
Dept. of Pharmacy
Thomas Jefferson
University Hospital
111 S. 11th St.
Philadelphia, PA 19107-5098
Mon.-Fri. 8 AM-5 PM
   215-955-8877
Fax: 215-923-3316

PITTSBURGH

The Christopher and Nicole
Browett Pharmaceutical
Information Center
Mylan School of Pharmacy
Duquesne University
431 Mellon Hall
Pittsburgh, PA 15282
Mon.-Fri. 8 AM-4 PM
   412-396-4600
Fax: 412-396-4488

Drug Information and
Pharmacoepidemiology Center
University of Pittsburgh Medical
Center
137 Victoria Hall
Pittsburgh, PA 15261
Mon.-Fri. 8:30 AM-4:30 PM
   412-624-3784
Fax: 412-624-6350

UPLAND

Drug Information Center
Crozer-Chester Medical Center
Dept. of Pharmacy
1 Medical Center Blvd.
Upland, PA 19013
Mon.-Fri. 8 AM-4:30 PM
   610-447-2851
   610-447-2862
   (after hours)
   (both numbers are
   for healthcare
   professionals only)
Fax: 610-447-2820

WILKES-BARRE

Drug Information Center
Nesbitt School of Pharmacy
Wilkes University
150-180 S. River St.
Stark Learning Center,
Room 1060
Wilkes-Barre, PA 18766
Mon.-Fri. 9 AM- 3 PM
   570-408-3295
Fax: 570-408-7828
dicenter@wilkes.edu

WILLIAMSPORT

Drug Information
Pharmacy Dept.
Susquehanna Health System
Rural Avenue Campus
Williamsport, PA 17701
24 hours/7 days a week
   570-321-3083
Fax: 570-321-3230

PUERTO RICO

PONCE

Centro Informacion
Medicamentos
Escuela de Medicina de Ponce
P.O. Box 7004
Ponce, PR 00732
Mon.-Fri. 8 AM-4:30 PM
   787-259-7085
   (Spanish and English)
   787-840-2575
   (switchboard)
Fax: 787-259-7085

RHODE ISLAND

PROVIDENCE

Rhode Island
Poison Control Center
Rhode Island Hospital, Dept. of
Pharmacy
593 Eddy St.
Providence, RI 02903
7 days/week, 24 hours
   401-444-5547
Fax: 401-444-8062

SOUTH CAROLINA

CHARLESTON

Drug Information Service
Medical University of
South Carolina
150 Ashley Ave.
Rutledge Tower Annex,
Room 604
P.O. Box 25058
Charleston, SC 29425-0810
Mon.-Fri. 9 AM-5:30 PM
   843-792-3896
   800-922-5250
Fax: 843-792-5532

SPARTANBURG

Drug Information Center
Spartanburg Regional
Medical Center
101 E. Wood St.
Spartanburg, SC 29303
Mon.-Fri. 8 AM-5 PM
   864-560-6910
Fax: 864-560-7323

TENNESSEE

MEMPHIS

South East Regional Drug
Information Center
VA Medical Center
1030 Jefferson Ave.
Memphis, TN 38104
Mon.-Fri. 7:30 AM-4 PM
   901-523-8990, ext. 6720
Fax: 901-577-7306

Drug Information Center
University of Tennessee
875 Monroe Ave.
Suite 116
Memphis, TN 38163
Mon.-Fri. 8 AM-5 PM
    901-448-5555
Fax: 901-448-5419

TEXAS

GALVESTON

Drug Information Center
University of Texas
Medical Branch
301 University Blvd. - G01
Galveston, TX 77555-0701
Mon.-Fri. 8 AM-5 PM
    409-772-2734
Fax: 409-747-5222

HOUSTON

Drug Information Center
Ben Taub General Hospital
Texas Southern
University/HCHD
1504 Taub Loop
Houston, TX 77030
Mon.-Fri. 8 AM-5 PM
    713-793-2917
Fax: 713-793-2998

Drug Information Center
Methodist Hospital
6565 Fannin (MSDB109)
Houston, TX 77030
Mon.-Fri. 8 AM-5 PM
    713-790-4190
Fax: 713-793-1224

LACKLAND A.F.B.

Drug Information Center
Dept. of Pharmacy
Wilford Hall Medical Center
2200 Berquist Dr., Suite 1
Lackland A.F.B., TX 78236
7 days/week, 24 hours
    210-292-5418
Fax: 210-292-3722

LUBBOCK

Drug Information and
Consultation Service
Covenant Medical Center
3615 19th St.
Lubbock, TX 79410
Mon.-Fri. 8 AM-5 PM
    806-725-0419
Fax: 806-725-0305

TEMPLE

Drug Information Center
Scott and White
Memorial Hospital
2401 S. 31st St.
Temple, TX 76508
Mon.-Fri. 8 AM-6 PM
    254-724-4636
Fax: 254-724-1731

UTAH

SALT LAKE CITY

Drug Information Service
University of Utah Hospital
Dept. of Pharmacy Services
Room A-050
50 N. Medical Dr.
Salt Lake City, UT 84132
Mon.-Fri. 8:30 AM-4:30 PM
    801-581-2073
Fax: 801-585-6688

VIRGINIA

CHARLOTTESVILLE

Drug Information Service
University of Virginia Health
System
Dept. of Pharmacy Services
P.O. Box 10002
Charlottesville, VA 22906
Mon.-Fri. 8 AM-4:30 PM
    804-924-8034
Fax: 804-982-1682

RICHMOND

Drug Information Service
Medical College of Virginia
Hospitals
Dept. of Pharmacy
Virginia Commonwealth
University
401 N. 12th St., Room B306
Richmond, VA 23298
Mon.-Fri. 8 AM-5 PM
    804-828-4636
Fax: 804-225-3919

WASHINGTON

SPOKANE

Washington State University
College of Pharmacy
601 W. First Ave.
Spokane, WA 99201-3899
Mon.-Fri. 8 AM-4 PM
    509-358-7662
Fax: 509-358-7627

WEST VIRGINIA

MORGANTOWN

West Virginia Drug
Information Center
WV University-
Robert C. Byrd
Health Sciences Center
1124 HSN, P.O. Box 9550
Morgantown, WV 26506
Mon.-Fri. 8:30 AM-5 PM
    304-293-6640
    800-352-2501 (WV)
Fax: 304-293-7672

WISCONSIN

MADISON

University of Wisconsin Hospital
& Clinics
Poison Control Center
600 Highland Ave.
Madison, WI 53792
    800-815-8855 (WI)
drug.info@hosp.wisc.edu
(for healthcare
professionals only)

WYOMING

LARAMIE

Drug Information Center
University of Wyoming
P.O. Box 3375
Laramie, WY 82071
Mon.-Fri. 8 AM-5 PM
    307-766-6988
Fax: 307-766-2953